EDELMAN'S Health Promotion THROUGHOUT the LIFE SPAN

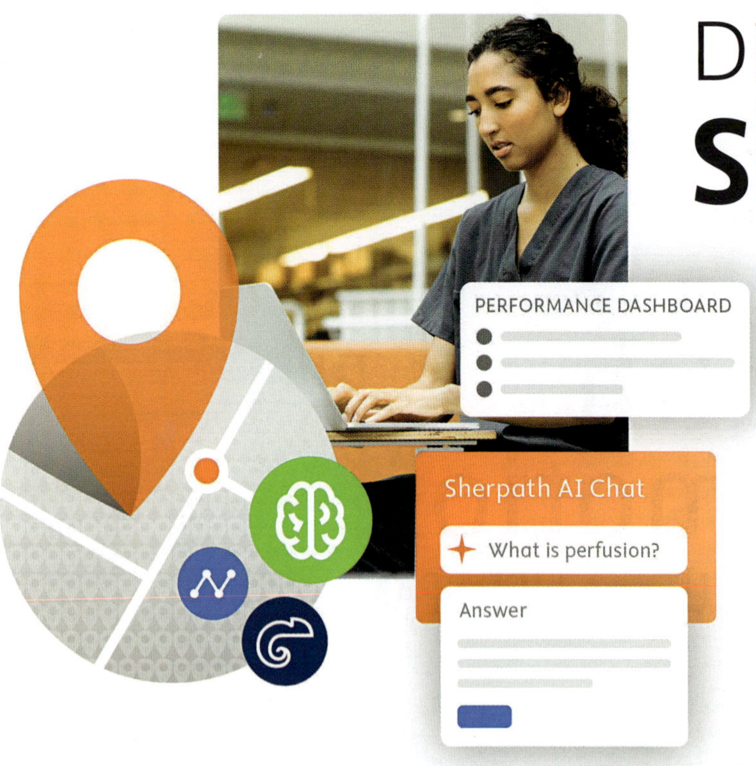

Discover Sherpath®

The digital teaching and learning technology **built specifically for healthcare education.**

Sherpath's all-in-one course delivery solution powers your textbook with innovative resources, including the following:

Digital lessons aligned with learning objectives create an interactive experience with multimedia, adaptive remediation, assignment assessments, and more.*

eBook and resources are seamlessly accessible within Sherpath for quick access to relevant course materials, activities, and reading recommendations.

Elsevier Adaptive Quizzing customizes quizzes based on performance and allows you to choose relevant quiz topics.

Performance dashboard offers a holistic view of course progress and areas of strength and weakness.

Sherpath AI is a conversational AI tool that generates personalized answers to questions, sourced solely from Elsevier's vast library of trusted, evidence-based content.

Osmosis® bite-sized, illustrated health education videos simplify complex concepts and promote active learning. A curated collection of Osmosis videos are seamlessly integrated into your Sherpath course.*

**Only available for select collections.*

And more!

STUDENTS — Ask your instructor about enhancing your course experience with Sherpath!

INSTRUCTORS — Scan code or visit **myevolve.us/spnu** to learn more!

24-0481 TM/AF

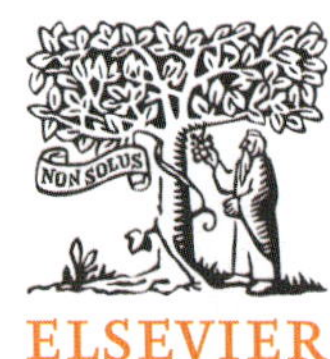

ELSEVIER

ELEVENTH EDITION

EDELMAN'S Health Promotion THROUGHOUT the LIFE SPAN

Elizabeth Connelly Kudzma, DNSc, MPH, RN, WHNP-BC
Professor Emerita
School of Nursing and Health Sciences
Curry College
Milton, Massachusetts

ASSOCIATE EDITORS

Susan A. LaRocco, PhD, MBA, RN, FNAP
Professor Emerita
School of Nursing and Health Sciences
Curry College
Milton, Massachusetts

Susan Natale, PhD, RN, CNE, NEA-BC
Associate Professor
School of Nursing and Health Sciences
Curry College
Milton, Massachusetts

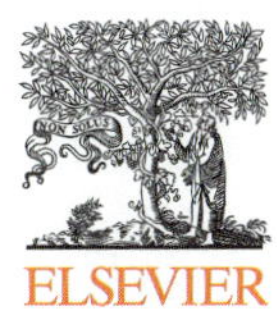
ELSEVIER

Elsevier
3251 Riverport Lane
St. Louis, Missouri 63043

EDELMAN'S HEALTH PROMOTION THROUGHOUT THE LIFE SPAN,
ELEVENTH EDITION

ISBN: 978-0-443-12176-0

Content Strategist: Grace Onderlinde
Content Development Manager: Laurie Gower
Content Development Specialist: Betsy McCormac
Publishing Services Manager: Deepthi Unni
Senior Project Manager: Kamatchi Madhavan
Book Designer: Margaret Reid

Printed in India

Last digit is the print number: 9 8 7 6 5 4 3 2 1

Dedication

First, to our families, friends, students, and colleagues—that they promote health in themselves and others.

Our students' and clinical preceptors' questions stretch our knowledge base and enlarge our thinking on community issues. Practicing nurse students enrich our understanding of various clinical workplaces and cultures. Colleagues teaching in the humanities and sciences show us ways to view clinical situations and application of theoretical bases from other disciplines. Our contributors continue to provide ideas and narratives that describe and enlarge their respective chapters.

This edition is dedicated to Carole Lium Edelman, who edited the book through ten editions. When the book was originally envisioned, she was teaching public health nursing and health promotion at Boston College; many of the original contributors were nursing faculty colleagues. Early manuscripts were handwritten/typewritten, with multiple drafts managed through the mail. When computerization became available, drafts were exchanged on floppy discs, and later via email attachments. Checking evidence/facts/sources in the later editions was easier with availability of online sources, but that posed its own problems of using digital software. Advances in safety science, application of evidence, biologic plausibility, and scientific breakthroughs over the timespan of the ten editions were enormous, as were upheaval and administrative changes in clinical nursing and other health disciplines. Many chapter contributors continued with the book through the various editions. Over forty years of theory and science transformations, Carole edited this book with determination to provide the most current information and best clinical practice. We are humbled to follow in her footsteps.

CONTRIBUTORS

Helen Bellenoit, MSN, RN
Associate Professor Nursing Practice
School of Nursing
Simmons University
Boston, Massachusetts
United States

Kevin K. Chui, PT, DPT, PhD, MBA, GCS, OCS, CEEAA, FAAOMPT
Endowed Chair and Professor
Department of Physical Therapy
Radford University
Roanoke, Virginia
United States

Courtney E. Coffey, DNP, CNM
Assistant Clinical Professor
Department of Nursing
University of New Hampshire
Durham, New Hampshire
United States

Michelle G. Criss, PhD, PT, DPT, Geriatric-Certified Specialist
Associate Professor
Physical Therapy Program, College of Health Sciences
Chatham University
Pittsburgh, Pennsylvania
United States

Donna M. Dello Iacono, PhD, NP, CNL
Senior Lecturer
School of Nursing and Health Sciences
Curry College
Milton, Massachusetts
United States;
Nurse Practitioner
Nursing/Anesthesia
Brigham and Women's Hospital
Boston, Massachusetts
United States

Stephanie Dribben, DNP, RN, AGACNP-BC
Assistant Professor
Department of Nursing
Webster University
St. Louis, Missouri
United States

Miriam Ford, PhD, FNP-BC
Assistant Professor
School of Nursing
Mercy University
Dobbs Ferry, New York
United States

June Andrews Horowitz, PhD, RN, PMHCNS-BC, FAAN
Associate Dean for Graduate Programs & Research & Professor
College of Nursing and Health Sciences
University of Massachusetts Dartmouth
Mattapoisett, Massachusetts
United States;
Professor Emeritus
William F. Connell School of Nursing
Boston College
Chestnut Hill, Massachusetts
United States

Kent E. Irwin, PT, DHS, MS, GCS
Professor
Physical Therapy Program
Midwestern University
Downers Grove, Illinois
United States

Susan Rowen James, PhD, RN
Professor Emerita
School of Nursing and Health Sciences
Curry College
Milton, Massachusetts
United States

Sallie Beth Johnson, PhD, MPH
Chair, Associate Professor
Public Health and Healthcare Leadership
Radford University
Roanoke, Virginia
United States;
Assistant Professor
Family and Community Medicine
Virginia Tech Carilion School of Medicine
Roanoke, Virginia
United States

Marni B. Kellogg, PhD, RN, CPN, CNE
Corporate Nurse Scientist
International Headquarters
Shriners Children's
Tampa, Florida
United States

Debora Elizabeth Kirsch, RN, MS, CNS
Clinical Assistant Professor Retired
College of Nursing
SUNY Upstate Medical University
Syracuse, New York
United States

Carolyn Cable Kleman, PhD, MHA, RN, CNE, BCPA
Associate Professor
School of Nursing
University of North Carolina Wilmington
Wilmington, North Carolina
United States

Elizabeth Connelly Kudzma, DNSc, MPH, RN, WHNP-BC
Professor Emerita
School of Nursing and Health Sciences
Curry College
Milton, Massachusetts
United States

Louise LaFramboise, PhD, RN
Emeritus Associate Professor and Assistant Dean
College of Nursing
University of Nebraska Medical Center
Omaha, Nebraska
United States

Susan A. LaRocco, PhD, MBA, RN, FNAP
Professor Emerita
School of Nursing and Health Sciences
Curry College
Milton, Massachusetts
United States

Carol Anne Martin, DNP, MS, CPNP-PC-Retired, RN
Associate Professor
Loretto Heights School of Nursing
Regis College
Weston, Massachusetts
United States

Maureen McDonald, MS, RN
Retired Department Chair
Nurse Education Department
Massasoit Community College
Brockton, Massachusetts
United States

Pari Mokhtari, RD, PhD
Manager, Health Sciences and Research Administration
Gastroenterology
Children's Hospital Orange County
Orange, California
United States

Susan Moscou, FNP, PMHNP, MPH, PhD
Professor
School of Nursing
Mercy University
Dobbs Ferry, New York
United States

Susan Natale, PhD, RN, CNE, NEA-BC
Associate Professor
School of Nursing and Health Sciences
Curry College
Milton, Massachusetts
United States

Daniele Piscitelli, PT, PhD
Assistant Professor
Department of Kinesiology, Doctor of Physical Therapy Program
University of Connecticut
Storrs, Connecticut
United States

Jessica N. Semin, DNP, MPH, RN
Assistant Professor
College of Nursing
University of Nebraska Medical Center
Omaha, Nebraska
United States

Valerie Seney, PhD, MA, LMHC, PMHNP-BC, FNAP
Assistant Professor
College of Nursing and Health Sciences
University of Massachusetts Dartmouth
Dartmouth, Massachusetts
United States;
Psychiatric Nurse Practitioner Board Certified
Foundations For Wellness, LLC
Fall River, Massachusetts
United States

Yvonne Marie Smith, PhD, APRN-CNS
Professor
Department of Nursing
Baldwin Wallace University
Berea, Ohio
United States;
Professor Emerita
College of Nursing
Kent State University
Kent, Ohio
United States

Jody Spiess, PhD, RN, GCPH
Associate Professor
Department of Nursing
Webster University
St. Louis, Missouri
United States

Lynnette Leeseberg Stamler, PhD, DLitt, RN, FAAN
Professor Emerita
College of Nursing
University of Nebraska Medical Center
Omaha, Nebraska
United States

Frank Tudini, PT, DScPT
Professor
Physical Therapy
University of Tennessee at Chattanooga
Chattanooga, Tennessee
United States

Renu A. Varughese, PhD, CNS, MBA
Associate Professor
School of Nursing
Mercy University
Dobbs Ferry, New York
United States

Julianne A. Walsh, PhD, RN
Associate Professor
School of Nursing and Health Sciences
Curry College
Milton, Massachusetts
United States

Diane Marie Welsh, DNP, APRN, CNE
Faculty
Young School of Nursing
Regis College
Weston, Massachusetts
United States;
Associate Professor of Nursing
Nursing Graduate Program
Regis College
Weston, Massachusetts
United States

Mariana Wingood, PT, DPT, PhD, MPH
Assistant Professor
Department of Implementation Science
Wake Forest University-School of Medicine
Winston-Salem, North Carolina
United States

Sheng-Che Yen, PT, PhD
Clinical Professor
Department of Physical Therapy, Movement and Rehabilitation Sciences
Northeastern University
Boston, Massachusetts
United States

REVIEWERS

Marie A. Bashaw, DNP, RN, NEA-BC
Professor and Director of Nursing
Wittenberg University Department of Nursing
Springfield, Ohio

Bethany Lynn McFann, MSN, RN
Assistant Professor of Nursing
Marshall University
Huntington, West Virginia

Donna Molyneaux PhD, MSN, BSN, RN, CNE
Professor
Gwynedd Mercy University
Gwynedd Valley, Pennsylvania

Emmanuel D. Paragas Jr., DNS, APRN, FNP-BC, CRRN
Associate Professor of Nursing
West Liberty University
West Liberty, West Virginia

Matthew Quilitzsch, MLIS
Curriculum & Instruction Librarian
Simmons University
Boston, Massachusetts

Lori M Rhudy, PhD, APRN, CNS, A-CNS BC, CNRN
Associate Professor and Chair, Department of Graduate Nursing
Winona State University
Rochester, Minnesota

Josie Veal, PhD, RN, APNP-BC
Public Health Officer
Milwaukee Area Technical College
Milwaukee, Wisconsin

PREFACE

PURPOSE OF THE BOOK

The case for promoting and protecting health, and preventing disease and injury, was established by accomplishments in the 20th and 21st centuries. Americans and global populations desire improved care; public concerns about physical fitness, good nutrition, and avoidance of health hazards such as environmental pollution have been adopted into the lifestyles of global citizens. Encouraging positive health changes has been a major effort of individuals; the local, state, and federal governments; health professionals; and society in general. In the United States, public and private attempts to improve the health status of individuals and groups traditionally focused on reducing communicable diseases and health hazards. These include delivery and best practices to improve access to and reduce costs of health services. As a result of the COVID-19 pandemic, Americans have greater awareness that the health of each person is influenced by the health of all individuals and environments worldwide.

Throughout the history of the United States, public health practice has assessed the health of Americans. In 1789 in New England, the Reverend Edward Wigglesworth developed the first American mortality tables. Population statistics gathered in England and America, including those of Florence Nightingale, proved that scientific data could change health outcomes. The *Report of a General Plan for the Promotion of Public and Personal Health* was completed by Lemuel Shattuck in Massachusetts in 1880 following British examples. *Healthy People, The Surgeon General's Report on Health Promotion and Disease Prevention,* was first published in 1979, and was followed by *Healthy People 2000, 2010, 2020* and now *2030*. The history of *Healthy People* investigations is described comprehensively in Chapter 1.

Professionals who undertake health-promotion strategies need to understand the basics of health protection and disease and injury prevention. Health protection is directed at population groups of all ages and involves adherence to standards, outcomes, infectious disease control, and governmental regulation and enforcement. These activities emphasize reducing exposure to various sources of hazards, including those related to air, water, foods, drugs, accidents, and other physical agents. Health care providers present individuals, families, and communities with disease- and injury-prevention services, which include immunizations, screenings, health education, and counselling. To implement prevention strategies effectively, it is essential to develop activities targeted to and tailored for all age groups in various settings including schools, industries, the home, the health care delivery system, the larger community, and the world.

Healthy People 2030 continued the tradition of earlier *Healthy People initiatives* but reduced the number of objectives to avoid overlap and better emphasize public health priorities. The vision statement for *Healthy People 2030* is "a society in which all people can achieve their full potential for health and well-being across the life span."

- The major goals of Healthy People for 2030 are:
  - Attain healthy, thriving lives and well-being free of preventable disease, disability, injury, and premature death.
  - Eliminate health disparities, achieve health equity, and attain health literacy to improve the health and well-being of all.
  - Create social, physical, and economic environments that promote attaining the full potential for health and well-being for all.
  - Promote healthy development, healthy behaviors, and well-being across all life stages.
  - Engage leadership, key constituents, and the public across multiple sectors to take action and design policies that improve the health and well-being of all.

Healthy People 2030 objectives are compared with data from earlier objectives of Healthy People so that objective data and investigations may be linked across decades. *Healthy People 2030* objectives are also arranged for easier search into five major topic areas:

- Health conditions
- Health behaviors
- Populations
- Settings and systems
- Social determinants of health

The databases within *Healthy People* continue to indicate targets and assessments of health status and risk for evaluations and future planning, not only for health policymakers and health care providers but also for individuals, families, and communities at the local, regional, national, and global levels.

APPROACH AND ORGANIZATION

This book focuses on primary prevention intervention; its three main components are (1) health promotion, (2) specific health protection, and (3) prevention of specific diseases. Primordial prevention is a subset of primary prevention, which addresses policy interventions to decrease risky lifestyle behaviors. Health promotion is an intervention designed to improve health, such as providing adequate nutrition, a healthy environment, and ongoing health education. Specific protection and prevention strategies, such as immunizations, periodic physical examinations, and safety plans in the workplace, are the interventions used to protect against illness.

In addition to primary prevention, this book discusses secondary prevention interventions, focusing specifically on screening and education. Such programs include blood pressure, cholesterol, and diabetes screening and referral. (The acute components of secondary prevention are generally not addressed in this book).

This text is presented in five parts, each portion forming the basis for the next.

Unit 1, *Foundations for Health Promotion,* describes the foundational concepts of promoting and protecting health and preventing diseases and injuries, including diagnostic, therapeutic, and ethical decision-making.

Unit 2, *Assessment for Health Promotion,* focuses on individuals, families, and communities and the factors affecting their health. The functional health pattern assessments developed by Gordon serve as the organizing framework for assessing the health of individuals, families, and communities. Next-Generation NCLEX® (NGN) Examination terminology is introduced.

Unit 3, *Interventions for Health Promotion,* discusses theories, methodologies, and case studies of nursing interventions, including screening, health-education counselling, stress management, and crisis intervention.

Unit 4, *Application of Health Promotion,* also uses Gordon's functional health patterns, emphasizing developmental, cultural, ethnic, and environmental variables in assessing the developing person. The intent is to address the health concerns of all Americans regardless of gender, race, age, or sexual orientation. The hope is to describe human development that more accurately reflects the complexity of human experiences throughout the life span.

Unit 5, *Emerging Global Health Issues,* in the final chapter discusses changing population groups and their health needs as well as related implications for research and practice in the 21st century. Throughout the text, boxes have been updated to highlight the science of nursing practice and demonstrate to the reader the relationship among evidence, practice, and outcomes. Bulleted text helps the reader remember important ideas and summarize concepts.

Throughout these units, the changing health care system, including future challenges for health care professionals and initiatives for health promotion, are described. Emphasis is placed on the current concerns of reducing health care costs while increasing life expectancy and improving the quality of life for all Americans.

Key Features

- Each chapter starts with a list of **objectives** to help focus the reader and emphasize the content the reader should acquire through reading the book.
- **Key Terms** including quality and safety terms are listed at the front to acquaint readers with the important terminology of the chapter.
- Each chapter's narrative begins with a **Think About It** section, the presentation of a clinical problem or scenario that relates to the topic of the chapter, followed by critical thinking questions. This promotes the reader's immediate interest in and thought about the chapter.
- Boxes throughout each chapter showcase important concepts and reinforce content areas.
- ***Healthy People 2030*** boxes present a list of selected objectives that are relevant to each chapter's topic.
- **Evidence-Based Practice** boxes provide brief synopses on current health-promotion research studies that demonstrate the links between research, theory, and practice.
- **Health and Social Determinants/Health Equity** boxes offer cultural perspectives on various aspects of health promotion.
- **Quality and Safety** boxes provide information regarding specific scenarios to improve health.
- **Genomics** boxes explore current genetic issues, controversies, and dilemmas with respect to health promotion, providing an opportunity for critical analysis of care issues.
- **Best Practice** boxes highlight inventive and resourceful projects, programs, and research studies that draw upon new ways of implementing health promotion.
- The **Case Study** highlights a realistic clinical situation relevant to the chapter topic.
- **Study Questions** are located on the book's website to offer additional review and self-study practice.

New Features

- Includes a greater emphasis on social determinants of health (SDOH)
- All chapters revised to current practice by field experts
- Content on increased health inequity in the US, the evolving global health outcomes as a result of COVID and increased involvement of at-risk communities.
- Evidence for health care decisions, and maintaining the health and well-being of professionals
- Updated photos, figures, and graphics freshen the view and feeling of the text
- Chapter language reflects the Clinical Judgment Model to align with the Next-Generation NCLEX®

An increased attention to genomics reflects increasing scientific evidence supporting the health benefits of using genetic information and family health history to guide public health interventions. Next-Generation NCLEX® (NGN) Examination–Style Case Studies for Health Promotion added to Evolve help guide instructors on the new question formats on the NCLEX®.

Evolve Resources

The expanded website for this book provides materials for both students and faculty and is accessible at http://evolve.elsevier.com/Edelman/.

For Students

Study Questions: Multiple choice NCLEX® examination format

For Instructors

- Next-Generation NCLEX® (NGN) Examination–Style Case Studies for Health Promotion
- **TEACH for Nurses** including Nursing Curriculum Standards, Teaching Activities, and Case Studies
- **Image Collection** with all images from the book
- **Lecture Slides** in PowerPoint
- **Test Bank:** 700 questions in NCLEX® examination format

It is crucial to attaining the highest level of wellness within community groups that health care professionals understand the many public health and environmental issues that individuals, families, national and world populations experience in social, work, and family settings. This includes biologic, inherited, cognitive, psychological, environmental, and sociocultural factors posing health risks. It is crucial to plan and advance interventions to promote health by understanding the diverse roles all factors play in the person's beliefs and health practices, particularly in the areas of disease and injury prevention, protection, and health promotion. Achieving such effectiveness requires collaboration with other health care providers and the integration of practice and policy while developing interventions and considering the ethical issues within individual, family, and both national and world communities' responsibilities for health.

Elizabeth Connelly Kudzma
Susan A. LaRocco
Susan Natale

ACKNOWLEDGMENTS

The authors received much assistance and support from many friends, relatives, and associates. Our contributors from many regions of the United States gave valuable advice and constructive suggestions, helped clarify concepts, and provided case examples. Many thanks to the Elsevier editorial and production team, especially Elizabeth McCormac and Heather Bays-Petrovic, along with all the Elsevier copyeditors, proofreaders, and print-production individuals. We appreciate and thank them for their ongoing help and support. It was a true pleasure working with them.

ABOUT THE AUTHORS

Elizabeth Connelly Kudzma is a Professor Emerita at the Curry College School of Nursing and Health Sciences.

Dr. Kudzma was on the Curry College nursing faculty, serving in various roles as undergraduate chairperson, and graduate nursing director. She is a certified Women's Health Nurse Practitioner (NCC) and a Clinical Nurse Leader-retired. Prior to her work at Curry, she taught nursing courses at Boston College, Laboure College, and in the nursing graduate program at Boston University. She has taught nursing courses at the undergraduate and graduate level in pathophysiology, research, maternal-child, leadership, ethics, and quality and safety. She was a short-term consultant for the World Health Association and continues to serve on committees and as an evaluator for the Commission on Collegiate Nursing Education. Dr. Kudzma graduated with bachelor's and master's degrees in nursing from the Connell School of Nursing at Boston College, and earned a Doctorate in Nursing Science (DNSc) from Boston University, and a Master of Public Health from the T. H. Chan School of Public Health at Harvard University.

Associate Editors

Susan A. LaRocco is a Professor Emerita at Curry College School of Nursing and Health Sciences.

Dr. LaRocco has been a nursing educator and administrator for more than 30 years and has held several interim or inaugural nursing dean positions. She spent an academic year as a Fulbright Scholar, teaching doctoral students at the University of Jordan in Amman. Dr. LaRocco has published extensively on clinical topics and on men in nursing and has served on the boards of several nursing organizations, including the American Association for the History of Nursing and the American Association for Men in Nursing. She has presented her research internationally, including in China, Russia, Australia, England, and Ireland. Dr. LaRocco is a Fellow in the National Academies of Practice. She received a bachelor's degree from Boston College, a master's degree in nursing administration from Boston University, an MBA from New York University, and a PhD in nursing from the University of Massachusetts Boston.

Susan Natale is an Associate Professor of Nursing at Curry College School of Nursing and Health Sciences. Prior to her work at Curry College, Dr. Natale was an Associate Chief Nursing Officer of Ambulatory Nursing at a nationally recognized safety-net healthcare system in the Boston area, dedicated to caring for at-risk populations. She teaches population health, health policy, and nursing administration courses to accelerated and graduate nursing students. Dr. Natale earned a bachelor's and master's degree from Northeastern University, and a PhD in nursing from the University of Massachusetts, Worcester, Graduate School of Nursing.

CONTENTS

UNIT 1 Foundations for Health Promotion

1

Health Defined: Health Promotion, Protection, and Prevention

Carolyn Cable Kleman and Yvonne M. Smith

http://evolve.elsevier.com/Edelman/

OBJECTIVES

After completing this chapter, the reader will be able to:

- Analyze concepts and models of *health* as used in this chapter.
- Evaluate the consistency of *Healthy People 2030* goals with various concepts of health.
- Analyze the progress made in this nation from the original *Healthy People* document to the foci in *Healthy People 2030.*
- Differentiate between health, illness, disease, disability, and premature death.
- Compare the four levels of prevention (primordial, primary, secondary, and tertiary) with the levels of service provision available across the life span.
- Critique the role of research and evidence as well as the nurse's role in health education and research for the promotion and protection of health for individuals and populations.

KEY TERMS

Adaptive model of health
Applied research
Asset planning
Clinical model of health
Community-based care
Cultural competence
Disease
Ecological model of health
Empathy
Endemic
Epidemic
Epidemiology
Ethnocentrism
Eudaimonistic
Eudaimonistic model of health
Evidence-based practice
Functional health
Health
Health disparities
Health in All Policies
Health promotion
Health-related quality of life (HRQoL)
High-level wellness
Illness
Interprofessional practice
Levels of prevention
Pandemic
Person-centered care
Population health
Public health
Qualitative studies
Quality of life
Quantitative studies
Role performance model of health
Salutogenesis
Social determinants of health
Social ecological model of health
Specific protection
Well-being
Wellness
Wellness-illness continuum

THINK ABOUT IT

Use of Complementary and Alternative Therapies

One of the biggest challenges to health care providers is the blending of Western medicine and health practices with the health practices of other cultures and ethnic groups. The federal government formed the National Center for Complementary and Integrative Health (NCCIH; https://nccih.nih.gov) to conduct and support basic and applied research and training and to disseminate information on complementary and alternative medicine to practitioners and the public. As demographics of the United States shift, more people use a combination of therapies in self-care and for the treatment of specific illnesses.

- What questions should you ask to obtain information from people about their use of complementary and alternative therapies?
- What information should you know about the benefits or limitations of using complementary therapies, such as acupuncture, spiritual healing, herbal remedies, or chiropractic?
- What resources should you trust for information on the efficacy and use of herbal remedies relative to prescription medications?
- Which ideas of health would be most compatible with the use of alternative therapies?
- How have alternative therapies been integrated into the *Healthy People 2030* objectives?

Health is a core concept in society. This concept is modified with qualifiers such as *excellent, good, fair,* or *poor* on the basis of a variety of factors. These factors may include age, sex, race or ethnic heritage, comparison group, current health or physical condition, past conditions, social or economic situation, geographical location, or the demands of various roles in society. In addition, there is evidence that larger societal and environmental concerns determine health outcomes. This chapter will discuss health as a concept and related concepts such as wellness, illness, disease, disability, and functioning. These concepts are frequently embedded in theories, such as theories of health behavior or health planning (Gehlert & Ward, 2019). Some motivating factors behind the move to disease prevention and health promotion in society will be examined with an introduction to *Healthy People*, the federal government's health objectives for the nation. The implementation of these concepts as nursing actions will also be addressed from ideal and pragmatic standpoints. Research and evidence supporting these concepts, and recommendations for further research, will be presented.

Nurses understand the pivotal role they play in promoting health and preventing disease, the important role of research in the knowledge of what is "healthy," and the central role of **epidemiology** (the study of health and disease in society) and public health theories in the everyday practice of nursing.

EXPLORING CONCEPTS OF HEALTH

Definitions of health in the nursing literature can be classified broadly within two major paradigms. The first paradigm is the **wellness-illness continuum**, a dichotomized portrayal of health and illness ranging from high-level wellness at the positive end to depletion of health at the negative end. **High-level wellness** is further conceptualized as a sense of **well-being**, life satisfaction, and **quality of life**. Movement toward the negative end of the continuum includes adaptation to disease and disability through various levels of functional ability (de Hond et al., 2019; Newman, 2003; Travis & Ryan, 2004). The wellness-illness conceptualization was the focus of early research and is consistent with some of the categories Smith (1983) identified in her philosophical analysis of health. Research based on this paradigm conforms primarily to scientific methods that seek to control contextual effects, provide the basis for causal explanations, and predict future outcomes (Hardin & Kaplow, 2017).

The second paradigm characterizes health as a perspective developmental phenomenon of unitary patterning of the person-environment. The developmental perspective of health has been present in the nursing literature since 1970, but it was not identified clearly with health until the late 1970s and early 1980s. It has been conceptualized as expanding consciousness, pattern or meaning recognition, personal transformation, and, tentatively, self-actualization. This shift toward a developmental perspective has had clear implications for the way in which health is conceptualized (Endo, 2017; Newman, 2003). Although not endorsing the developmental perspective to the extent of Rogers (1970) and Reed (1983), Murdaugh and colleagues (2019) and Allen and Warner (2002) state that health is an outcome of ongoing patterns of person and environment interactions throughout the life span. Research within this paradigm seeks to address the dynamic whole of the health experience through behavioral and social mechanisms over time. Health can be better understood if each person is seen as a part of a complex, interconnected biologic and social system. Research based on this paradigm conforms primarily to constructivist scientific methods that seek to describe and understand health experiences in more depth (Orchard & Mahler, 2018).

The **social ecological model of health** (Bronfenbrenner, 1977; Shelton, 2019) is a comprehensive developmental approach and is useful for promoting health at individual, family, community, and societal levels (Fig. 1.1). This model emphasizes the **social determinants of health**—those factors in society that influence health and the options available to people to improve or maintain their health, and how they affect people at all environmental levels, from the individual to the policy level. In this way, the **ecological model of health** is more compatible with Smith's (1983) descriptions of health as adaptation and eudemonia (self-actualization). The social determinants of health also form the basis for *Healthy People 2030* objectives. Each of these ideas will be examined in more detail throughout this chapter.

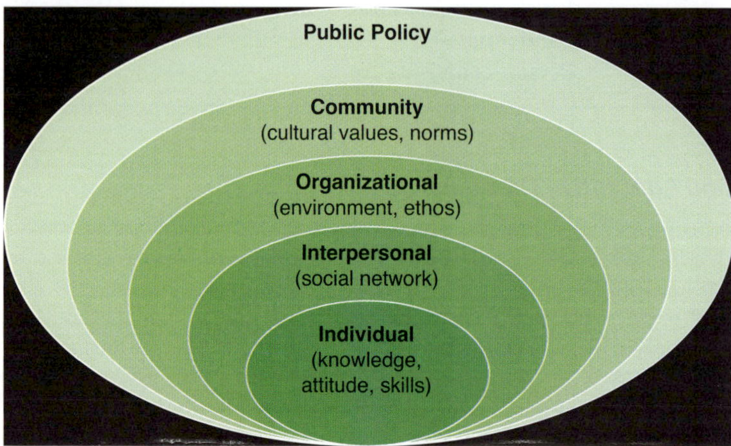

FIG. 1.1 Social Ecological Model. (Adapted from Bronfenbrenner, U. [1977]. Toward an experimental ecology of human development. *American Psychologist, 32*[7], 513–531.)

People involved in health promotion must consider the meaning of health for themselves and for others. Recognizing differences in the meaning of health can clarify outcomes and expectations in health promotion and enhance the quality of health care (Svalastog et al., 2017). Because health is used to describe a number of entities, including a philosophy of care, a health care delivery system, evidence-based health practices, personal health behaviors, health care costs, and health insurance, the confusion regarding the use of the term *health* becomes clear. People's use of the term *health* and its incorporation into these various entities have also changed over time.

Americans born before 1940 experienced the greatest changes in how health is defined. Because infectious diseases claimed the lives of many children and young adults at that time, health was viewed as the absence of disease. The physician in independent practice was the primary provider of health care services, with services provided in the private office. The federal government was only beginning to establish its role in working with states to address public health and welfare issues.

As the national economy expanded during and after World War II in the 1940s and 1950s, the idea of role performance became a focus in industrial research and entered the health care lexicon. Health became linked to a person's ability to fulfill a role in society. Increasingly, the physician was asked to complete physical examination forms for school, work, military, and insurance purposes, while physician practice became linked more directly to hospital-based services. The federal government expanded its role through funding for hospital expansion and establishment of the new Department of Health, Education, and Welfare, currently the Department of Health and Human Services (Barr et al., 2003). It was recognized that a person might recover from a disease and yet be unable to fulfill family or work roles because of residual changes from the illness episode. Concepts of disability and rehabilitation entered the health care arena. The work or school environment was viewed as a possible contributor to health, illness, disability, and death.

From the 1960s to the present, there have been incredible changes in the health care delivery system while health care costs have escalated and federal and state governments have attempted to control spending (Badash et al., 2017; Barr et al., 2003). Primary care providers, including advanced practice registered nurses (APRN), involve individuals and their families in the delivery of **person-centered care**, and teaching individuals about individual responsibilities and lifestyle choices has become an important part of their job. Health care has become an interdisciplinary endeavor even while managed care companies limit the health-promotion options available under insurance plans. During this time the idea of adaptation has had an important influence on the way Americans view health. Increasingly, health has become linked to individuals' reactions to the environment and their ability to adapt rather than being viewed as a fixed state. Adaptation fit well with the self-help movement during the 1970s and with the progressive increase in knowledge from research of disease prevention and health promotion at the individual level.

Emphasis is placed on the quality of a person's life as a component of health (USDHHS, Office of Disease Prevention and Health Promotion, 2022). Research on health and function from the patient's point of view (Gyasi & Phillips, 2018) indicates that multiple factors contribute to a person's perception of their health, sometimes referred to as **functional health** (Gordon, 2016) or **health-related quality of life (HRQoL)** (Andresen et al., 2003; Karimi & Brazier, 2016; USDHHS, Office of Disease Prevention and Health Promotion, 2022). Multiple tools are available for measuring quality of life, including the World Health Organization Quality of Life (WHOQOL)-BREF, a general measure established by the World Health Organization (WHO) (2004), and the Revised McGill Quality of Life Questionnaire (Cohen et al., 2017) for use at the end of life (Box 1.1: Quality and Safety Scenario). There is also an acknowledgment of the importance of resiliency as a factor that contributes to health. Resilience is one's ability to deal with stressful or traumatic life events. The Resilience Scale has been used to quantitatively measure resilience in many populations (The Resilience Center, 2024).

Models of Health

Throughout history, society has entertained a variety of conceptual models of health. Smith (1983) describes four distinct models in her classic work.

Clinical Model

In the **clinical model**, health is defined by the absence of signs and symptoms of disease, and illness is defined by the presence of signs and symptoms of disease. People who use this model may not seek preventive health services, or they may wait until they are very ill to seek care. The clinical model is the conventional model of the discipline of medicine.

Role Performance Model

The **role performance model of health** defines health in terms of an individual's ability to perform social roles. Role performance includes work, family, and social roles, with performance based on societal expectations. Illness would be the failure to perform roles at the level of others in society. This model is the basis for occupational health evaluations, school physical examinations, and physician-excused absences. The idea of the "sick role," which excuses people from performing their social functions, is a vital component of the role performance model. It is argued that the sick role is less relevant in health care nowadays (Burnham, 2012; Davis et al., 2011).

Adaptive Model

In the **adaptive model of health**, people's ability to adjust positively to social, mental, and physiologic change is the measure of their health. Illness occurs when the person fails to adapt or becomes maladaptive to these changes. As the concept of adaptation has entered other aspects of American culture, this model of health has become more accepted. For example, participating in goal-directed activities can be useful in adapting to a decreased level of functioning in older adults (Carpentieri et al., 2017).

BOX 1.1 QUALITY AND SAFETY SCENARIO

Fall Prevention in the Home

Falls in the home are a common yet preventable source of both fatal and nonfatal injuries. The age-adjusted fall death rate increased by 41% from 55.3 per 100,000 older adults in 2012 to 78.0 per 100,000 older adults in 2021 (https://www.cdc.gov/falls/data/index.html). In 2030 the number of estimated falls will be 49 million, with 12 million fall injuries. The Stopping Elderly Accidents, Deaths & Injuries (STEADI) initiative by the Centers for Disease Control and Prevention addresses coordination of fall prevention activities in primary care and implementation of fall prevention programs (https://www.cdc.gov/falls/index.html).

There are specific factors that contribute to fall risk, including changes to the person attributable to age, medication use, and environmental hazards. Nurses fulfill key roles in working with older adults to assess fall risks. The National Center for Injury Prevention and Control at the Centers for Disease Control and Prevention provides guidelines for fall prevention in older adults at https://www.cdc.gov/falls/index.html.

Risk factors attributable to the aging process include visual, hearing, and functional limitations. Although pets have proven to be a benefit for older adults by providing companionship and comfort, they can also scamper underfoot, or the older adult may trip over the pet because the pet is not seen or heard. Loss of night vision and depth perception can also contribute to falls when lighting is poor or when a person is moving from room to room. Older adults should be encouraged to always wear prescribed vision and hearing aids when moving about the house or apartment. Loss of upper- and lower-body strength can also contribute to fall risk. Lower-body strength is needed to lift the legs and feet high enough to navigate stairs and changes in texture of flooring. Upper-body strength allows for the use of supports when a person is moving about.

Medications can contribute to disequilibrium. A careful review of currently used medications, both prescribed and over the counter, can help identify medications that could contribute to fall risks. Environmental risks include clutter, too much furniture for the room, placement of items in walkways, lighting problems, necessary repairs to flooring and walls, and the need for supports such as grab bars and railings. Watching the person navigate the home is helpful in recognizing potential trip hazards and areas where additional supports are needed. Adequate hydration is another consideration, especially if the person is taking medications that contribute to dehydration without regular fluid replacement or if the temperature of the home and environment is too high.

Health outcomes for the person can be significant. Falls can cause minor injury and embarrassment, but they can also cause life-threatening injuries, such as fractures and head injuries. If a fall has occurred, it is helpful to do a root cause analysis to determine the factors that contributed to the fall. Ask permission before attempting to make any alteration to the home, because items and their placement may have sentimental importance. Address medication changes with the person, pharmacist, and/or primary care provider. Some medication habits may be hard for the person to change (Johnston et al., 2019).

The nursing implications of fall risk are many and varied. Assessment skills must be practiced in a variety of settings so that the nurse is vigilant for potential hazards and individual factors that might precipitate a fall. Older adults should be routinely observed performing their daily routines to identify visual, hearing, and functional decline. In addition, if a person reports a fall, that report should trigger a more extensive evaluation of that individual because falls may be indicative of future fall risk.

Questions

- Can you identify at least four items in your own environment that may contribute to your fall risk?
- How would you structure an interview with an older adult to determine the presence of fall risks in that person's home?
- What evidence and arguments would you use to encourage an older adult to modify the home environment to decrease the risk of a fall?

Eudaimonistic Model

In the **eudaimonistic model**, exuberant well-being indicates optimal health. This model emphasizes the interactions between physical, social, psychological, and spiritual aspects of life and the environment that contribute to goal attainment and create meaning. Illness is reflected by denervation or languishing, or a lack of involvement with life. Although these ideas may appear to be new when compared with the **clinical model of health**, aspects of the eudaimonistic model predate the clinical model of health. The eudaimonistic model is also more congruent with integrative modes of therapy (National Institutes of Health, NCCIH, n.d.), which are used increasingly by people of all ages in the United States and the rest of the world. In this eudaimonistic model, people dying of cancer may still consider themselves healthy if they are finding meaning in life.

These ideas of health provide a basis for how people view health and disease and how they view the roles of nurses, physicians, and other health care providers. For example, in the clinical model of health, a person may expect to see a health care provider only when there are obvious signs of illness. Personal responsibility for health may not be a motivating factor for this person because they may feel that the provider is responsible for dealing with their health problem and returning them to health. Therefore attempts to teach health-promoting activities may not be effective with this person. On the other hand, a person who adopts a **eudaimonistic model of health** may find that practitioners working under a clinical model do not address their more comprehensive health needs. They may instead seek out a practitioner of alternative medicine or the counsel of a priest, rabbi, or minister to complement the services of the more traditional health provider.

Wellness-Illness Continuum

The wellness-illness continuum is a dichotomous depiction of the relationship between the concepts of health and illness. In this paradigm, **wellness** is a positive state in which incremental increases in health can be made beyond the midpoint (Fig. 1.2). These increases involve improved physical and mental health states. The opposite end of the continuum is illness, with the possibility of incremental decreases in health beyond the midpoint. This depiction of the relationship between wellness and illness fits well with the conceptual and clinical model of health (McMahon & Fleury, 2012). This paradigm is useful when thinking about the transitions between wellness and illness (Polacsek et al., 2020).

High-Level Wellness

From a dichotomous representation of health and illness as opposites, Dunn (1961) developed a health-illness continuum that assessed a person not only in terms of their

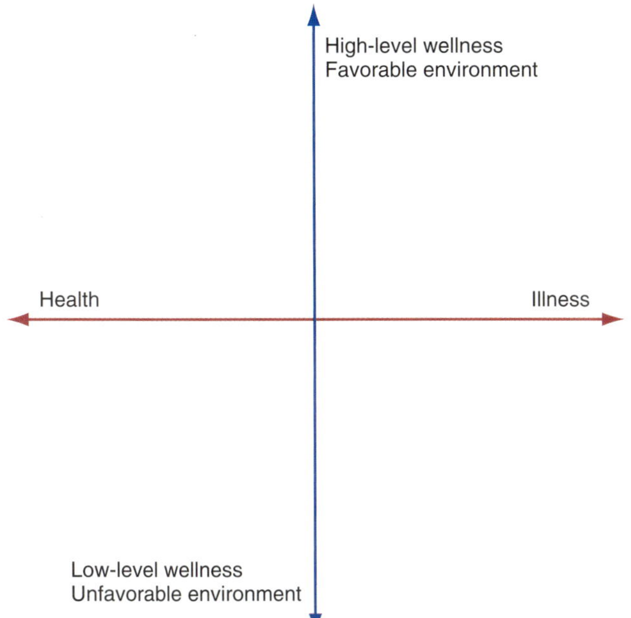

FIG. 1.2 Wellness-illness continuum with high-level wellness added. Moving from the center to the right demonstrates movement toward illness. Moving from the center to the left demonstrates movement toward health. Moving above the line demonstrates movement toward increasing wellness. Moving below the line demonstrates movement toward decreasing wellness. (Modified from US Department of Health and Human Services, Public Health Service [1982]; McMahon, S., & Fleury, J. [2012]. Wellness in older adults: A concept analysis. *Nursing Forum, 47*[1], 39–51. Becker, C. M., Glascoff, M. A., Felts, W. M., & Kent, C. [2015]. Adapting and using quality management methods to improve health promotion. *Explore, 11*[3], 222–228.)

relative health compared with that of others but also in terms of the favorability of the person's environment for health and wellness (see Fig. 1.2). Adding this second dimension to the health-illness continuum created a matrix in which a favorable environment allows high-level wellness to exist and an unfavorable environment allows low-level wellness to exist. Social and physical environmental factors can positively or negatively influence wellness.

With this addition, it became possible to combine the clinical model of health with models based on social and environmental parameters. The concept demonstrates that a person can have a terminal disease and be emotionally prepared for death while also acting as a support for other people and achieving high-level wellness. High-level wellness involves progression toward a higher level of functioning, an open-ended and ever-expanding future with its challenge of fuller potential and the integration of the whole being (Ardell, 2007). This definition of high-level wellness contains ideas similar to those in the eudaimonistic model of health. In addition, high-level wellness emphasizes the interrelationship between the environment and the ability to achieve health on both a personal and a societal level.

Health Ecology

An evolving view of health recognizes the interconnection between people and their physical and social environments. Newman (2003) expressed this interconnection within a developmental framework, and the work of Gordon (2016) applies this interconnection to functional health patterns as presented in subsequent chapters. Health from an ecological perspective is multidimensional, extending from the individual into the surrounding community, including the context within which the individual functions. It incorporates a systems approach in which the actions of one portion of the system affect the functioning of the system as a whole (National Academy of Medicine, 2013). This view of health expands on high-level wellness by recognizing that there are social and environmental factors that can enhance or limit health and healthy behaviors. For example, most people can benefit from physical activity such as walking, and people are more likely to walk in areas where there are sidewalks or walking paths and where they feel safe. Nurses can encourage people to walk but may also need to advocate safe areas for people to walk and work with others to plan for people-friendly community development.

Functioning

One of the defining characteristics of life is the ability to function. Functional health can be characterized as being present or absent, having high-level or low-level wellness, and being influenced by neighborhood and society. Functioning is integral to health. There are physical, mental, and social levels of function, and these are reflected in terms of performance and social expectations. Function can also be viewed from an ecological perspective, as in the example of walking used previously. Loss of function may be a sign or symptom of a disease. For example, sudden loss of the ability to move an arm or leg may indicate a stroke. The inability to leave the house may indicate overwhelming fear. In both cases the loss of function is a sign of disease, a state of ill health. Loss of function is a good indicator that the person may need nursing intervention. Research in older adults indicates that a decline in physical function is a sentinel event and may indicate the future loss of physical function and death (Gyasi & Phillips, 2018).

HEALTH, DISEASE, AND ILLNESS

Health

Health, as defined in this text, is a state of physical, mental, spiritual, and social functioning that realizes a person's potential and is experienced within a developmental context. Although health is, in part, an individual's responsibility, health also requires collective action to ensure a society and an environment in which people can act responsibly to support health. People's culture and beliefs can also influence health actions. This definition is consistent with the WHO's definition of health as the state of complete physical, mental, and social well-being and not merely the absence of disease and infirmity (WHO, 2023), but it moves beyond the WHO's definition to encompass spiritual, developmental, and environmental aspects over time. The physical aspect includes one's genetic makeup, which, when combined with the other aspects, influences one's longevity. This broader definition is applicable across the life span and in situations where illness may be a chronic state. For example, according to this broader definition of health, a person with diabetes may be considered healthy if they are able to adapt to their illness and live a meaningful, spiritually satisfying life. Health is considered to be part of the metaparadigm for nursing (Fawcett & Garity, 2009), which includes the four components of person, health, environment, and nursing. As can be seen in the discussion thus far, health can be viewed in a variety of ways.

Illness, Disease, and Health

It is easy to think of health or wellness as the lack of disease and to consider *illness* and *disease* as interchangeable terms. However, *health* and *disease* are not simply antonyms, and *disease* and *illness* are not synonyms. *Disease* literally means "without ease." **Disease** may be defined as the failure of a person's adaptive mechanisms to counteract stimuli and stresses adequately, resulting in functional or structural disturbances. This definition is an ecological concept of disease, which uses multiple factors to determine the cause of disease rather than describing a single cause. This multifactorial approach increases the chances of discovering multiple points of intervention to improve health.

Illness is composed of the subjective experience of the individual and the physical manifestation of disease (Hollingsworth & Didelot, 2010). Both are social constructs in which people are in an imbalanced, unsustainable relationship with their environment and are failing in their ability to survive and create a higher quality of life. Illness can be described as a response characterized by a mismatch between a person's needs and the resources available to meet those needs. In addition, illness signals to individuals and populations that the present balance is not working. Within this definition, illness has physical, psychological, spiritual, and social components. A person can have a disease without feeling ill (e.g., asymptomatic hypertension). A person can also feel ill without having a diagnosable disease (e.g., as a result of stress). Our understanding of disease and illness within society, overlaid with our understanding of the natural history of each disease, creates a basis for promoting health.

HEALTHY PEOPLE INITIATIVE

Planning for Health

Public health has always had the prevention of disease in society as its focus. However, during the latter half of the 20th century, the promotion of health and individual responsibility moved to the forefront within public health, becoming a driving force in health care reform.

A key milestone in promoting health was the advent of *Healthy People* (US Department of Health, Education, and Welfare, Public Health Service, 1979), the first Surgeon General's report on health promotion and disease prevention issued in the later years of President Carter's administration.

The document identified three causes of the major health issues in the United States as careless habits, environmental pollution, and harmful social conditions (e.g., hunger, poverty, and ignorance) to persist that destroy health, especially for infants and children.

Healthy People was a call to action and an attempt to set health goals for the United States for the next 10 years. Each decade overarching goals are identified for *Healthy People* (Table 1.1). Unfortunately, a change in political leadership, a lack of political and social priority, and the spiraling costs of

TABLE 1.1 Current and Historical Overarching Goals of *Healthy People*

	1990	2000	2010	2020	2030
1	Continue to improve infant health and reduce infant mortality.	Increase the span of healthy life.	Increase quality and years of healthy life.	Attain high-quality, longer lives free of preventable disease, disability, injury, and premature death.	Attain healthy, thriving lives and well-being, free of preventable disease, disability, injury, and premature death.
2	Improve child, adolescent, and young adult health and reduce deaths among these groups.	Reduce health disparities.	Eliminate health disparities.	Achieve health equity, eliminate disparities, and improve the health of all groups.	Eliminate health disparities, achieve health equity, and attain health literacy to improve the health and well-being of all.
3	Improve the health of adults and reduce deaths among this group.	Create access to preventive services for all.		Create social and physical environments that promote good health for all.	Create social, physical, and economic environments that promote attaining full potential for health and well-being for all.
4	Improve the health and quality of life of older adults and reduce the average annual number of days of restricted activity attributable to acute and chronic conditions.			Promote quality of life, healthy development, and healthy behaviors across all life stages.	Promote healthy development, healthy behaviors, and well-being across all life stages.
5					Engage leadership, key constituents, and the public across multiple sectors to take action and design policies that improve the health and well-being of all.

hospital-based health care intervened. The need to report progress toward these national objectives led to a larger, renewed effort in the form of *The 1990 Health Objectives for the Nation: A Midcourse Review* (USDHHS, Public Health Service, 1986). This midcourse review noted that although many goals were achievable, the unachieved goals were hindered by current health status, limited progress on risk reduction, difficulties in data collection, and a lack of public awareness.

Healthy People 2000 (USDHHS, Public Health Service, 1990) and *Healthy People 2000 Midcourse Review and 1995 Revisions* (USDHHS, Public Health Service, 1996) were landmark documents in that a consortium of people representing national organizations worked with US Public Health Service officials to create a more global approach to health. In addition, a management-by-objectives approach was used to address each problem area. These two documents became the blueprints for each state as funding for federal programs became linked to meeting these national health objectives. The core of these health objectives remained: prevention of illness and disease was the foundation for health.

Healthy People 2010 (US Department of Health and Human Services USDHHS, & Public Health Service, 2000) introduced two overarching goals (see Table 1.1). These goals addressed the issues of longevity and quality of life. Both longevity and quality of life address the concern that people are living longer but frequently with numerous chronic health problems that interfere with the quality of their lives. However, quality of life is also an issue for people who are unable to achieve a long life.

Eliminating **health disparities** addressed the continuing problems of access to care; differences in treatment based on race, sex, and ability to pay; and related issues such as urban versus rural health, insurance coverage, Medicare and Medicaid reimbursement for care, and satisfaction with service delivery.

Healthy People 2020 (USDHHS, Office of Disease Prevention and Health Promotion, 2022) topic areas included adolescent health; blood disorders and blood safety; dementias, including Alzheimer disease; early and middle childhood; genomics; global health; health care–associated infections; HRQoL and well-being; lesbian, gay, bisexual, and transgender health; older adults; preparedness; sleep health; and social determinants of health. These topic areas were an expansion on previous areas and incorporated recent evidence more directly in each area.

Healthy People 2030 Goals and Objectives

Healthy People 2030 has five health and well-being outcome goals for the overall program. The five goals relate to overall well-being and healthy life expectancy. Objectives were created to meet the program goals. There are three types of objectives in *Healthy People 2030*: developmental, research, and core. Developmental objectives relate to high-priority areas that may not have associated data but do have evidence-based interventions. An example developmental objective is to increase the proportion of children who are developmentally ready for school (EMC-DO1). Research objectives address areas that do not have evidence-based interventions. An example research objective is to increase the use of telehealth to improve access to health services (AHS-R02). The 359 core objectives are grouped into five categories: health conditions, health behaviors, populations, settings and systems, and social determinants of health. Twenty-three of the core objectives are considered leading health indicators (LHIs), which are a subset of high-priority objectives that cover the life span (USDHHS, Office of Disease Prevention and Health Promotion, n.d.). LHIs are core objectives focusing on risk factors and behaviors rather than disease outcomes. They address issues of national importance, social determinants of health, health disparities, and health equity that have a major effect on public health outcomes. The core objectives focus on behaviors that are modifiable in the short-term using evidence-based interventions and strategies to motivate action at the national, state, local, and community levels. Objective outcome data are collected and displayed on the *Healthy People* website (https://health.gov/healthypeople) (USDHHS, Office of Disease Prevention and Health Promotion, 2024). An example of an LHI is increasing the proportion of adults who do enough aerobic and muscle-strengthening activity (PA-05). A target measure is established for each objective, and data are collected periodically to document progress. Progress is described as baseline only, target met or exceeded, improving, little or no detectable change, or worsening. If an objective is documented as "baseline," that means that there are no data beyond the initial baseline data, so progress is unknown. One example core objective and its target measure is used here for illustration.

Objective NWS-03. Reduce the proportion of adults with obesity. This is an objective that is measured across populations (age groups, with or without activity limitations, country of birth, etc.). At this time the target is 36%, and the most recent data show that 41.8% have not achieved the target. This means that the objective progress is "getting worse." The *Healthy People* website (https://health.gov/healthypeople/objectives-and-data/browse-objectives/overweight-and-obesity/reduce-proportion-adults-obesity-nws-03) includes an objective overview, data, data methodology and measurement, and evidence-based resources for each objective. Some of the evidence-based resources for this objective are technology-supported multi-component coaching or counseling interventions, worksite programs, and physical activity interventions including activity monitors. Providing access to evidence-based interventions is a valuable addition to the *Healthy People* program.

Increasing physical activity in adults can help us reach the goal of reducing the proportion of adults with obesity (Box 1.2: Best Practice). There is a corresponding core objective of increasing the proportion of adults who do enough aerobic and muscle-strengthening activity (PA-05). Females, low-income populations, Black and Hispanic people, people with disabilities, and those older than 75 years exercise less than do White males with moderate-to-high incomes (USDHHS, National Institutes of Health, National Heart, Lung, and Blood Institute, 2020). The groups of people experiencing health disparities are more likely to develop high cholesterol levels, high blood pressure, and/or obesity, which increases their risk of heart disease and stroke. Although this objective addresses adults, other objectives address the need to begin exercise activities at an early age and to encourage young adults to actively engage in exercise. The target for this objective is

BOX 1.2 BEST PRACTICE

Process for Recognizing, Addressing, and Evaluating Overweight and Obesity in Adults

Overweight and obesity are major concerns in public health because they contribute to other health problems, such as high cholesterol, high blood pressure, diabetes mellitus, heart disease, functional limitations, and disability. As part of the National Heart, Lung, and Blood Institute's (2020) obesity education initiative, titled Aim for a Healthy Weight, nurses play an important role in health education related to obesity prevention and control. More complete information and guidelines can be obtained from https://www.nhlbi.nih.gov/health-topics/overweight-and-obesity.

Make the Most of the Individual's Visit and Set an Effective Tone for Communication: Nurses ask individuals about their weight history, weight-related health risks, and desire to lose weight. The approaches used must be respectful of a person's lifestyle, habits, and cultural influences. Discussions must be nonjudgmental and goal oriented.

Assess the Individual's Motivation/Readiness to Lose Weight: Nurses explain body mass index and why it is the preferred method of determining overweight and obesity in adults. Individuals must understand the methods of data collection and measurement of height and weight, as well as waist circumference, risk factors, and comorbidities. Nurses develop the skill of determining readiness and motivation to lose weight in their patients.

Build a Partnership With an Individual: Nurses work with individuals to determine what each person is willing to do to achieve a lower weight. This approach includes knowing the best practices in weight management and weight loss. Fad diets, dietary supplements, and weight-loss pills may be inappropriate for most people, and formal weight-loss programs may be too expensive for low- and moderate-income families. Use recommended diets that restrict caloric intake, set activity goals with your patients, encourage the person to keep a weekly food and activity diary, and provide information on diet and activity. Be sure to record individual goals and the treatment plan, including a health-education plan. Nurses are knowledgeable about current treatment options and their success. Holistic approaches are necessary because food behaviors are influenced by many factors. Listen to individuals' stories about food and its role in their lives. Therapies should fit the individual's goals and lead to lifestyle change.

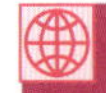

BOX 1.3 HEALTH AND SOCIAL DETERMINANTS/HEALTH EQUITY

Influence of Personal Cultural Values on Health Care Delivery

Culture influences every aspect of human life, including beliefs, values, and customs regarding lifestyle and health care. As health care providers, nurses must be aware of their own beliefs, values, and customs and how these ideas translate into behavior. It is easy to assume that an individual's own perspective is correct and shared by others. This is especially true when one is working with other health care providers who share the same culture. This concept is referred to as **ethnocentrism** and can lead to a devaluing of the beliefs, values, and customs of others. It can be associated with racism, leading to social inequities, discrimination, and prejudice. Although it is impossible for any person to ignore the cultural influences on their life, nurses and other health care providers have a special obligation to be aware of their own social and cultural biases. Our focus as nurses must be on the cultural influences in the daily lives of individuals through the development of **cultural competence** and cultural humility. The ability to view other people's situations from their perspective is known as **empathy**. Diversity awareness will continue to challenge providers to lifelong learning about the people for whom they provide care as the racial and ethnic mix in society changes (Červený, Kratochvílová, Hellerová, & Tóthová, 2022).

that 29.7% of adults engage in aerobic physical activity of at least moderate intensity for at least 150 minutes per week and muscle-strengthening activity at least 2 days per week.

Work sites and communities need to become partners in providing opportunities for people to lead healthy lives through flexible work schedules, work-site wellness programs, accessibility of safe parks, and availability of exercise facilities. Converting empty lots into community gardens provides beautification of the area, an opportunity for exercise in caring for the garden, and a source of fresh vegetables. The availability of bike paths encourages physical activity.

Faith communities can break economic, social, racial, and gender barriers, making them an excellent source for sharing information on health promotion and disease prevention. Parish nurses and Faith Community Nurses are becoming increasingly prevalent, and they incorporate *Healthy People* objectives into their activities (Westberg Institute, 2020).

Public health officials at all levels are necessary partners in meeting *Healthy People* objectives. As part of the core public health functions of assessment, policy development, and assurance, the US Public Health Service and all state, county, and local health departments need to collect data, make information available to the public, create policies that support *Healthy People* objectives, and ensure that needed services are available from a competent workforce.

Research in a variety of areas has clearly indicated that health disparities are directly and indirectly linked to longevity and quality-of-life issues (Clay et al., 2018; Xu et al., 2018). For example, Lillard and colleagues (2022) report that Black males die of prostate cancer more frequently than any other racial or ethnic group, with their death rate almost 2.2 times higher than that of White males (Box 1.3: Health and Social Determinants/Health Equity).

Healthy People can form the basis for planning, service delivery, evaluation, and research in every aspect of the health care system. The nurse needs to be familiar with this document and its intent. Nurses should compare their practices with the objectives of *Healthy People*. In addition, the nurse needs to be aware of the research and practice changes that occur as a result of the work toward these objectives.

LEVELS OF PREVENTION

Prevention, in a narrow sense, means averting the development of disease. In a broad sense, prevention consists of all measures that limit disease progression. Leavell and Clark (1965) defined three **levels of prevention**: primary, secondary, and tertiary (Fig. 1.3). Although the levels of prevention are related to the natural history of disease, they can be used to prevent disease and to provide nurses with starting points for making effective, positive changes in the health status of the persons for whom they provide care. Primordial prevention, the earliest form of prevention, has been added as a type of prevention that reflects policy-level intervention aimed at affecting health before at-risk lifestyle behaviors are

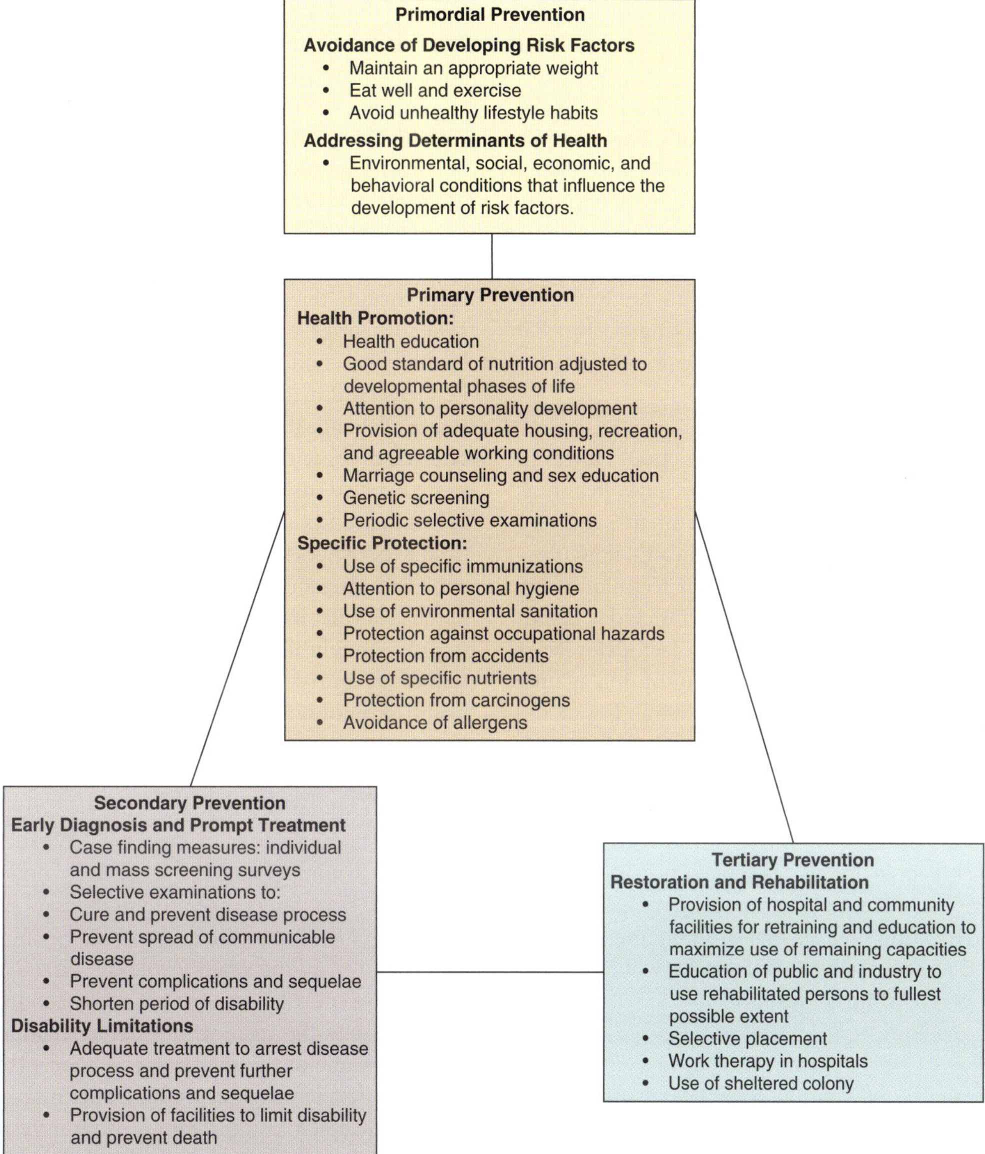

FIG. 1.3 The three levels of prevention developed by Leavell and Clark with primordial prevention added. (Modified from Leavell, H., & Clark, A. E. [1965]. *Preventive medicine for doctors in the community*. New York: McGraw Hill; Ali, A., & Katz, D. L. [2015]. Disease prevention and health promotion: How integrative medicine fits. *American Journal of Preventive Medicine, 49*[5], S230–S240; D'Ascenzi, F., Sciaccaluga, C., Cameli, M., Cecere, A., Ciccone, M. M., Di Francesco, S., Ganau, A., et al. [2019]. When should cardiovascular prevention begin? The importance of antenatal, perinatal and primordial prevention. *European Journal of Preventive Cardiology,* December 16, 2019, 1–12.)

chosen or become habit (Kisling & Das, 2023). Within the four levels of prevention are five steps. These steps include health promotion and specific protection (primordial and primary prevention); early diagnosis, prompt treatment, and disability limitation (secondary prevention); and restoration and rehabilitation (tertiary prevention). A fifth level of prevention has recently been introduced and is being discussed as the quaternary level of prevention; this level considers the potential for overmedicalization. Quaternary prevention is defined as steps taken to protect individuals from health-related interventions that are likely to cause more harm than good. Overdiagnosis and/or overprescription can result in overmedicalization (Martins et al., 2018).

Some confusion exists in the interpretation of these concepts; therefore, a consistent understanding of primordial, primary, secondary, tertiary, and quaternary prevention is essential. The levels of prevention operate on a continuum but may overlap in practice. The nurse must clearly understand the goals of each level to intervene effectively in keeping people healthy.

Primordial Prevention

Primordial refers to the time frame *before* a risk factor develops and *before* disease occurs. Primordial prevention can begin as early as childhood or even prenatally and is closely linked to the determinants of health and the environment in which one lives

(Kisling & Das, 2023). Determinants of health include income, education, literacy, employment, working conditions, social and physical environment, health practices, genetic makeup, health services, sex, and culture (Kindig & Stoddart, 2003). Primordial interventions are aimed at determinants of health. For example, if the social environment one grows up in discourages exercising or encourages eating high-fat food, that environment could be targeted for primordial prevention. Healthy eating and activity, school-based programs, reduction of sodium in the food supply, and creation of safe places to ride bikes and walk are examples of primordial prevention. Most health-promoting primordial prevention occurs at the national, state, and community levels.

Primary Prevention

Primary prevention precedes disease or dysfunction. However, primary prevention is therapeutic in that it includes health as beneficial to well-being; it uses therapeutic treatments; and, as a process or behavior geared toward enhancing health, it involves symptom identification when stress-reduction techniques are being taught. Primary prevention intervention includes health promotion, such as health education about risk factors for heart disease, and **specific protection**, such as immunization against hepatitis B. Its purpose is to decrease the vulnerability of the individual or population to disease or dysfunction. Interventions at this level encourage individuals and groups to become more aware of the means of improving health and the actions they can take at the primary preventive health level and the optimal health level. People are also taught to use appropriate primary preventive measures. However, primary prevention can also include advocating policies that promote the health of the community and electing public officials who will enact legislation that protects the health of the public.

Health Protection

Primordial and primary prevention activities focus on the reduction of threats and negative influences on health. Both types of prevention can occur at an individual level and at the community, state, national, and even global levels. Ensuring the availability of safe and adequate food, water, and medical therapies for all people and protecting them against workplace and environmental hazards are regional and global objectives. Ruger and colleagues (2015) suggest the formation of a global health fund that would unite efforts to ensure adequate protection of all the world's people concerning AIDS, tuberculosis, and malaria in recognition of the global responsibility for social protection.

Health Promotion

The definitions of **health promotion** differ. O'Donnell (1987) has defined *health promotion* as "the science and art of helping people change their lifestyle to move toward a state of optimal health." Devore and Kreuter (1980) proposed a more complex definition in an article commissioned by the US Public Health Service. They stated that health promotion is "the process of advocating health to enhance the probability that personal (individual, family, and community), private (professional and business), and public (federal, state, and local government) support of positive health practices will become a societal norm." *Healthy People* has adopted the definition of *health promotion* as "any planned combination of educational, political, regulatory, and organizational supports for actions and conditions of living conducive to the health of individuals, groups, or communities" (Health Education Curriculum Analysis Tool: Glossary, 2021).

The Theoretical Basis of Health Promotion. The theoretical underpinnings of health promotion have evolved since the early 1980s. Most of these theories are behaviorally based, derived from the social sciences, and extensively researched. These theories include the theory of reasoned action (Ajzen & Fishbein, 1980), theories of behavior (Bandura 1976, 1999, 2004), the health belief model by Rosenstock (Champion & Skinner, 2008), Pender's Health-Promotion Model (Murdaugh et al., 2019), and stages of change theory (Prochaska et al., 2015). Internet searches on each of these theories will provide numerous websites where more detailed information is available. The **salutogenesis** theory of health promotion, developed by Aaron Antonovsky, focuses on lived experiences that create a sense of coherence that one uses to cope with stressors (Mittlemark & Bauer, 2017). This sense of coherence is what influences action or inaction when attempting to improve one's health. The disease-related models of health promotion focus on risk factors and disease, whereas the salutogenesis health-promotion model directs attention to the assets that help patients make needed changes to health. This is an assets-based approach to health promotion as opposed to a disease-avoidance approach (Mittlemark & Bauer, 2017). The question Antonovsky developed a model to help answer is, "What can people do to be healthy?" In comparison, the prevention model of health promotion asks, "How can people prevent illness?" Essentially, these are two sides of the same coin and answering one might help answer the other. But asking what people can do to be healthy considers the positive contributions people and their environment provide, which regards the issue with a different, more growth-oriented mindset. Some of the salutogenesis concepts studied in current research include thriving, gratitude, learned optimism, quality of life, social capital, connectedness, humor, resilience, flourishing, well-being, and self-transcendence (Shorey, 2021).

The Social Nature of Health Promotion. Health promotion goes beyond providing information. It is also proactive decision-making at all levels of society, as reflected in the *Healthy People 2030* objectives. Health promotion holds the best promise for lower-cost methods of limiting the constant increase in health care costs and empowering people to be responsible for the aspects of their lives that can enhance well-being. Based on the need for health-promotion activities within the health care system, efforts must be made to identify the multiple determinants of health, determine relevant health-promotion strategies, and delineate issues relevant to social justice and access to care. Individuals, families, and communities must be active participants in this process so that the actions taken are socially relevant, economically feasible, and supportive of changes at the individual level.

The Active and Passive Nature of Health Promotion. Health-promotion efforts, unlike those efforts directed at specific protection from certain diseases, focus on maintaining or improving the general health of individuals, families, and communities. These activities are conducted at the public level (e.g., government programs promoting adequate housing or reducing pollutants in the air), at the community level (e.g., Habitat for Humanity or community health centers), and at the personal level (e.g., voting to offer low-income housing or to elect public officials who recognize the need for public oversight). Nursing interventions are actions directed toward developing people's resources to maintain or enhance their well-being—a form of assets-based planning.

Strategies of health promotion that involve the individual may be either passive or active. Passive strategies involve the individual as an inactive participant or recipient. Examples of passive strategies include public health efforts to maintain clean water and sanitary sewage systems to decrease infectious diseases and improve health, and efforts to introduce vitamin D in all milk to ensure that children will not be at high risk of rickets when living in areas where sunlight is scarce. These passive strategies must be used to promote the health of the public when individual participation might be low but the benefit to society is high. Policy plays a major role in passive health promotion. Nurses advocate for health-promoting policies at the local, state, federal, and global levels.

Active strategies depend on the individual becoming personally involved in adopting a proposed program of health promotion. Two examples of lifestyle change are performing daily exercise as part of a physical fitness plan and adopting a stress-management program as part of daily living. A combination of active and passive strategies is best for making an individual or society healthier. This text is concerned almost entirely with active strategies and the nurse's role in these strategies. Some passive strategies are presented, but they are presented with the implicit belief that each individual must take responsibility for improving their health. It is undeniable that passive strategies also have a valuable role, but they must be used within the context of encouraging and teaching individuals to assume more responsibility for their health.

An Application of Theory to the Practice of Health Promotion. The transtheoretical model (TTM) is an excellent example and can be applied to this case study. The TTM incorporates stages of change (readiness to take action), decisional balance (benefits to and detractors from changing a behavior), self-efficacy (personal confidence in making a change), and processes of change (cognitive, affective, and behavioral activities facilitating change). The bases of the TTM are the stages of change; these are six stages that people spiral through on a path toward making and sustaining a behavioral change to promote health (see Table 1.2).

TABLE 1.2 Transtheoretical Model Stages of Change

Stage	Description
Precontemplative	Not considering change
Contemplative	Aware of but not considering change soon
Preparation	Planning to act soon
Action	Has begun to make behavioral change (recent)
Maintenance	Continued commitment to behavior (long term)
Relapse	Reverted to old behavior

Each stage offers opportunities for the nurse to provide information and support behavioral change. Encouraging people and suggesting changes to their environment that support behavioral change can increase individuals' self-efficacy and their chances of maintaining a change. This model also recognizes that people need multiple opportunities to make behavioral change before achieving success and that relapse should be expected (Prochaska et al., 2015).

Although health promotion would seem to be a practical and effective mode of health care, the major portion of health care delivery is geared toward responding to acute and chronic disease. Preventing or delaying the onset of chronic disease and adding new dimensions to the quality of life are not as easy because they take time to implement and evaluate and require personal action. These actions are more closely associated with everyday living and the lifestyles adopted by individuals, families, communities, and nations. Habits such as eating, resting, exercising, and handling anxieties appear to be transmitted from parent to child and from social group to social group as part of a cultural, not a genetic, heritage. These activities may be taught in subtle ways, but they influence behavior and have as much of an influence on health as does genetic inheritance. Although the public may not appreciate the causal relationships between behavior and health, these relationships should be apparent to health professionals. Arguably, the concept of risk is the most basic of all health concepts because health promotion and disease protection are based on this concept.

Health-promotion strategies have the potential to enhance the quality of life from birth to death. For example, good nutrition is adjusted to various developmental phases in life to account for rapid growth and development in infancy and early childhood, physiologic changes associated with adolescence, extra demands during pregnancy, and the many changes occurring in older adults. Good nutrition is known to enhance the immune system, enabling individuals to fight infections that could lead to disabling illnesses. Other individual activities are adapted to the person's needs for optimal personality development at all ages. As seen in Unit 4, much can be done on a personal or group basis, through counseling and properly directed parental education, to provide the environmental requirements for the proper personality development of children. Community participation is also an important factor in promoting individual, family, and group health (see Chapters 6–8).

Personal health promotion is usually provided through health education (see Chapter 10). An important function of nurses, physicians, and allied health professionals, health education is principally concerned with eliciting useful changes in human behavior on the basis of current research. The goal is to inculcate a sense of responsibility in individuals for their own health and a shared sense of responsibility for avoiding injury to the health of others. For example, encouraging child-rearing practices that foster normal growth and development (personal, social, and physical) addresses both the individual parent and the needs of society. Health education nurtures health-promoting habits, values, and attitudes that must be learned through practice. These must be reinforced through systematic instruction in hygiene, bodily function, physical fitness, and use of leisure time. Another goal is to understand the appropriate use of health services. For example, a semiannual visit to a dentist may teach a child better oral health habits and to visit the dentist regularly, although this is not the primary purpose of the visit. Parents, teachers, and caregivers play a vital role in health education. In addition to teaching individuals, nurses need to develop skills in group teaching and in providing education within community organizations.

Available research clearly shows an increase in longevity, a decrease in mortality and morbidity, and an improvement in the quality of life for individuals who have been involved in health-promotion activities such as physical activity and avoidance of smoking (Snedden et al., 2019). It must be emphasized that health promotion requires lifestyle change. Once a lifestyle change has been adopted, vigilance is needed to ensure that the lifestyle change is maintained and modified to fit developmental and environmental changes.

Empirical data linking risk factors, health-promotion activities, and outcomes are sufficient to drive the development of the *Healthy People 2030* objectives and to be incorporated into quality improvement measures in managed care. One of the challenges met by *Healthy People 2030* is the development of measurable outcome objectives that are based on more realistic economic models. *Healthy People 2030* has decreased the number of objectives to focus on the most important outcomes for investigation.

Health promotion is an important concept for nursing because it embodies many other concepts with which nursing is concerned. As stated earlier, much of the nursing role is involved with health teaching. Standard 5B of *Nursing: Scope and Standards of Practice* (American Nurses Association [ANA], 2015c) includes a section on the practice implementation of health teaching and health promotion. Nurses are expected to demonstrate professional role competence throughout their careers. Health education is clearly an important nursing role.

Specific Protection

This aspect of primary prevention focuses on protecting people from injury and disease, for example, by providing immunizations and reducing exposure to occupational hazards, carcinogens, and other environmental health risks. These hazards and risks include not only protection of adults from work-related injuries (e.g., back injuries in nurses, dismemberment in machinists, exposure to chemicals used in boat repair, or exposure to inhaled sawdust by carpenters) but also protection of infants and children from potential carcinogens (e.g., exposure of children to diesel emissions, damage to a fetus caused by radiation).

Primary prevention interventions are considered health protection when they emphasize shielding or defending the body (or the public) from specific causes of injury or disease. Implementing nursing interventions that prevent a specific health problem may seem easier than promoting well-being among individuals, groups, or communities because the variables are delineated more clearly in prevention than in promotion and the potential influences are less diverse.

Examples. Two examples demonstrate these differences. Immunization via vaccination against influenza and COVID-19 is recommended by the Centers for Disease Control and Prevention (CDC) and has become a regular health preservation activity for people at risk each fall (https://www.cdc.gov/flu/prevent/flushot.htm). Nurses can participate in this specific protection role by administering vaccines in clinics and offices. Another example is the creation of nut-free schools to protect hypersensitive children from life-threatening allergic reactions to peanuts and nut products. Such initiatives have largely been the result of grassroots parent organizations working with formal community organizations to adopt policies that protect the health of these children. Nurses may be involved in the parent organizations or the school or public health boards that review the proposed policies. In addition, nurses must be able to address the need to protect specific portions of the population at risk.

Secondary Prevention

Although primary prevention measures have decreased the hazards of chronic diseases such as cardiovascular disease, conditions that preclude a healthy quality of life are still prevalent. Secondary prevention ranges from providing screening activities and treating early stages of disease to limiting disability by averting or delaying the consequences of advanced disease.

Screening is secondary prevention because the principal goal is to identify individuals in an early, detectable stage of the disease process. However, screening provides an excellent opportunity to offer health teaching as a primary preventive measure. Screening activities now play an important role in the control of diseases such as heart disease, stroke, and colorectal cancer. In addition, screening activities provide early diagnosis and treatment of nutritional, behavioral, and other related problems. Nurses play an important role in screening activities because they provide clinical expertise and educationally sound health information during the screening process.

Delayed recognition of disease results in the need to limit future disability in late secondary prevention. Limiting disability is a vital role for nursing because preventive measures are primarily therapeutic and are aimed at arresting the disease and preventing further complications. The paradox here is that health education and disease prevention activities seem similar to those used in primary prevention but are applied to a person or population with an existing disease. Modifications to the teaching plan must be made on the basis of the individual's current health status and ability to modify behavior.

Tertiary Prevention

Tertiary prevention occurs when a defect or disability is permanent and irreversible. The process involves minimizing the effects of disease and disability by surveillance and maintenance activities aimed at preventing complications and deterioration. Tertiary prevention focuses on rehabilitation to help people attain and retain an optimal level of functioning regardless of their disability. The objective is to return the affected individual to a useful place in society, maximize their remaining capacities, or both. The responsibility of the nurse is to ensure that persons with disabilities receive services that enable them to live and work according to the resources that are still available to them. When a person has a stroke, rehabilitating them to the highest level of functioning and teaching lifestyle changes to prevent future strokes are examples of tertiary prevention.

Quaternary Prevention

Quaternary prevention is a concept developed by Jamoulle and colleagues (2015) that describes the potential for the overmedicalization of care recipients. The prevention of doing harm, by reducing overdiagnosis or overtreatment and the commercialization of disease, is the objective of this level of prevention. This process of prevention requires providers to make ethical and socially responsible diagnostic and treatment suggestions and include the care recipient in shared decision-making (Martin, 2018).

Levels of Prevention Strategies

In a discussion paper for the National Academy of Medicine (Hawkins et al., 2015), three program levels of prevention interventions were introduced. Universal programs are directed toward an entire population and are aimed at preventing or delaying the behavior of concern. Selective prevention strategies target specific groups that are at risk for the behavior. Indicated programs are designed to prevent risk behaviors (or symptoms) from becoming the actual behavior (or disease). These interventions or programs are focused on the primordial, primary, and secondary levels of prevention. At the level of tertiary prevention, programs focus on intervention and maintenance (Hawkins et al., 2015).

The Intersectionality of Public Health, Population Health, and Health Promotion

Public health is population-based focusing on the determinants of health for defined populations. It is grounded in social justice, centering on health promotion and disease prevention driven by the science of epidemiology, and it organizes community services (American Public Health Association, 2024). Population health refers to the outcomes (i.e., length of life, HRQoL, function) of a population that are influenced by patterns of health determinants, policies, and interventions (Kindig & Stoddart, 2003). A population is a group either defined by a geographic area or consisting of those with similarities, such as employees, ethnic groups, prisoners, or people with disabilities. It is not defined as a clinical care recipient group, such as individuals with heart failure. A clinical population focus may be an example of **population health** management or population medicine (Kindig, 2015). Because determinants of health are what drive health outcomes, they are considered in population health and public health. Determinants include medical care, public health interventions, aspects of the social and physical environment, genetics, and individual behavior (Kindig & Stoddart, 2003). Health-promotion efforts empower people to have control over their own health. These efforts involve advocating for and/or supplying support for actions and conditions that can lead to positive health practices. The WHO describes five key areas for work related to health promotion: good governance, health literacy, healthy cities, health-promoting schools, and social mobilization. **Health in All Policies** is a collaborative attempt by the CDC to consider social determinants that influence the health of communities when creating and enacting any policy (Rudolph et al., 2013). Gathering and using health information that supports healthy decisions requires health literacy. Urban planning that promotes health requires strong leadership and commitment. School health programs to promote health and prevent disease are important for children and the community. Socially mobilizing groups and communities to create sustainable resources and services that will enhance health is also an important factor of health promotion. Public health, population health, and health promotion are interwoven to meet the needs of groups of people at various ecological levels.

The COVID-19 Pandemic

An **epidemic** occurs when a disease spreads rapidly to many people, typically in one geographic region or country. An epidemic is considered a **pandemic** when large-scale social interference, economic loss, and hardship occur. The WHO declared COVID-19 a pandemic on March 11, 2020, and declared the end of the COVID-19 emergency on May 5, 2023. The COVID-19 pandemic lasted more than 3 years. Currently, COVID-19 is considered **endemic**, which means that enough people have immune protection related to vaccination to reduce the risk of COVID-19-related deaths. COVID-19 will have a constant presence in communities now; it has become normalized.

We learned during the COVID-19 pandemic that the social determinants of health severely affected COVID-19-related outcomes for groups such as the American Indian and Alaskan Native, Black, and Hispanic communities (Ndugga et al., 2022).

As a result of the pandemic, primordial prevention efforts to address social determinants of health have increased. Vaccination for COVID-19 serves as a primary prevention as well as "hands, space, and face." This is a catchphrase the United Kingdom used to cue people to the important prevention behaviors of washing your hands, staying at least 6 feet away from others, and wearing a mask. Thinking of catchy, clever, illustrative ways to communicate with the public is important in the public health environment (Bosley, 2020).

Screening for COVID-19, when a person has COVID-19 symptoms or has been around someone who has tested positive for COVID-19, is an example of secondary prevention. Tertiary and quaternary prevention are employed when someone has lingering symptoms of COVID-19, otherwise known as long COVID-19 or post–COVID-19 conditions.

Healthy People 2030 objectives were completed before the COVID-19 pandemic, but there are objectives that the Office of Disease Prevention and Health Promotion (ODPHP) has listed as the COVID-19 Custom Objective List. See Box 1.4 for examples of these objectives.

THE NURSE'S ROLE

Evolving demands are placed on the nurse and the nursing profession as a result of changes in society. Emphasis is shifting from acute, hospital-based care to preventive, **community-based care**, which is provided in health care settings

BOX 1.4 COVID-19 CUSTOM OBJECTIVE LIST

Label/Number	*Healthy People* Objective
Access to Health Services	
AHS-05 Core Objective	Reduce the proportion of persons who can't get dental care when they need it.
AHS-R02 Research Objective	Increase the use of telehealth to improve access to health services.
ECBP-D07 Developmental Objective	Increase the number of community organizations that provide prevention services.
Social Determinants of Health	
SDOH-01 Core Objective	Reduce the proportion of people living in poverty.
SDOH-R01 Research Objective	Increase the proportion of federal data sources that collect country of birth as a variable.
Health Communication	
HC/HIT-02 Core Objective	Increase the proportion of adults whose health care providers involved them in decisions as much as they wanted.
HC/HIT-R01 Research Objective	Increase the health literacy of the population.
HC/HIT-D11 Developmental Objective	Increase the proportion of adults with limited English proficiency who say their providers explain things clearly.

in the community. This demand for community-based services, with the home as a major community setting for care, is closely related to the changing demographics of the United States. Although the home and community become the existing sites for care, nurses must assume more blended roles, with a knowledge base that prepares them to practice across settings using **evidence-based practice**. Within these roles, nurses assume a more active involvement in the prevention of disease and the promotion of health. Nurses can be more independent in their practice and place a greater emphasis on promoting and maximizing health, and more than ever nurses are accountable morally, ethically, and legally for their professional behavior.

Although nurses often work with people on a one-on-one basis, they seldom work in isolation. Within the current health care system, nurses collaborate with other nurses, physicians, social workers, nutritionists, psychologists, therapists, individuals, and community groups. In this **interprofessional practice**, nurses play a variety of roles.

Advocate

As advocates, nurses help individuals obtain the resources they are seeking through the health care system, try to make the system more responsive to individual and community needs, and help people develop the skills to advocate for themselves. In the role of an advocate, the nurse strives to ensure that all persons receive high-quality, appropriate, safe, and cost-effective care. The nurse may spend a great deal of time identifying and coordinating resources for complex cases.

Care Manager

The nurse acts as a care manager to assist the individual in navigating the complexities of health care and health decision-making. Primary roles of the care manager include preventing duplication of services, maintaining quality and safety, providing education and advocacy, facilitating self-management, and reducing costs (Luther et al., 2019). Information gathered from reliable data sources enables the care manager to help individuals avoid care that is unproven, ineffective, or unsafe. Reliable sources of information on best practices, evidence-based practices, and standard protocols are available from websites sponsored by the federal government (e.g., https://www.nih.gov; https://www.cdc.gov), specialty organizations (e.g., http://www.arthritis.org; http://www.nursingworld.org; http://www.aginglifecare.org), and private foundations (e.g., http://www.rwjf.org; http://www.johnahartford.org). Successful care management depends on collaborative relationships among the care manager, other nurses, physicians, the individual and their family, the insurance provider, and other care providers who work with the individual. A key aspect of this collaborative relationship is educating and engaging the individual and family members (Witwer & Wallenstein, 2019). Without engagement, individuals assume a passive role in their health care. The wishes of the individual and the family need to be clear to the care manager as part of person-centered care provision. Facilitating communication among parties and engaging the individual in the process are two of the care manager's most important functions.

Consultant

Nurses may provide knowledge about health promotion and disease prevention to individuals and groups as consultants. Some nurses have specialized areas of expertise or advanced practice, such as in gerontology, women's health, or community/public health, and they are equipped to provide information as consultants in these areas of specialization (ANA, 2015b). A gerontologic APRN might be on a community planning board, offering advice about what types of health-promotion activities to consider when planning a new senior housing development (Smith et al., 2021). All nurses need to develop consultation skills that can be integrated into practice and allow the individual nurse to take advantage of opportunities to provide support on an individual level or for future development at the organizational level (Tabvuma et al., 2023).

Deliverer of Services

The core role of the nurse is the delivery of direct services such as health education, influenza vaccinations, and counseling in health promotion. Visible, direct delivery of nursing care is the foundation for the public image of nursing. The public demands that nurses be knowledgeable and competent in their delivery of services. This role is clearly expressed in *Nursing's Social Policy Statement* (ANA, 2015a) and in the *Code of Ethics for Nurses with Interpretive Statements* (ANA, 2015b).

Educator

Health practices in the United States are derived from the theory that health components such as good nutrition, industrial and highway safety, immunization, and specific drug therapy should be within the grasp of the total population. Even with its rich resources, society falls far short of attaining the goal of maximal health for all. The problem is not only a lack of knowledge or health literacy but also a lack of application; therefore, it is incumbent on nurses to be excellent health educators. To teach effectively, the nurse must know essential facts about how people learn and the teaching-learning process. Nurses can bridge the health literacy gap through education (see Chapter 10).

In addition to their storehouse of scientific knowledge, nurses who are committed to their teaching role know that individuals are unique in their response to efforts prompting behavioral change. Teaching may range from a chance remark by the nurse to structurally planned teaching according to individual needs. Selection of the methods most likely to succeed involves the establishment of teacher-learner goals. Health promotion and protection rely heavily on the individual's ability to use appropriate knowledge. Health education is one of the primary prevention techniques available to avoid the major causes of disability and death nowadays and is a critical role for nurses.

Healer

The role of healer requires the nurse to help individuals integrate and balance the various parts of their lives (Quinn, 2016). The concept of patient centeredness requires nurses to learn from the individual or family what is required for healing. The nurse understands that healing resides in the ability to glimpse or intuit the "interior" of an individual, to sense and identify what is important to that other person, and to incorporate the specific insight into a care plan that helps the individual to develop their own capacity to heal. It requires a mindful blending of science and subjectivity (Benner et al., 2010; Siegel, 2007). Nurses have a special ability to help people heal. The art of nursing is the extraordinary ability to manage a broad array of information to create something meaningful, sensible, and whole (see Chapter 14).

Administrator

Nurses can serve as administrators, including director positions, for public health departments. As directors, they lead health departments in establishing and accomplishing the strategic goals of the department. Nurse administrator responsibilities include reporting and responding to the local boards of health, policymaking, and ensuring compliance with state and federal public health laws. Further, they design and monitor emergency response plans and hold hearings on public health issues.

Researcher

In the current health care environment, nurses are constantly striving to understand and interpret research findings that will enhance the quality and value of individual care. To provide optimal health care, nurses need to use evidence-based findings as their foundation for clinical decision-making. When nurses or other clinicians use research findings and the best evidence possible to make decisions, the outcome is termed **evidence-based practice**. Evidence-based practice is defined as the conscientious, explicit, and judicious use of current best evidence in making decisions about the care of individuals (ANA, 2023). The practice of evidence-based nursing means integrating individual clinical expertise with the best available external clinical evidence from systematic research (ANA, 2015b).

The National Institute of Nursing Research (NINR) (2022) serves as the focal point in developing research themes for the future of the profession. The NINR supports research to establish a scientific base for the care of individuals and populations throughout the life span, from the reduction of risks of disease and disability to the management of individuals and populations during illness and recovery. The NINR has broadened its focus from individual health to the health of populations with an emphasis on high-risk, underserved, and vulnerable populations. It also prioritizes investigating systems and models of care for these and other populations. The five research foci the NINR has identified are health equity, social determinants of health, population and community health, prevention and health promotion, and systems and models of care. Notice how the *Healthy People 2030* objectives align with many of these themes.

Evidence-based practice involves searching for the best evidence with which to answer clinical research questions. Research evidence can be gathered from **quantitative studies** that describe situations, correlate different variables related to care, or test causal relationships between variables related to care. Research evidence can also be gathered from **qualitative studies** that describe phenomena or define the historical nature, cultural relevance, or philosophical basis of aspects of nursing care. **Applied research** is done to directly affect clinical practice (Burns & Grove, 2020). Sackett and colleagues (1996) stressed the use of the best evidence available to answer clinical questions and explore the next best evidence when appropriate. The next best evidence may include the individual clinical judgment that nurses acquire through clinical experience and clinical practice and other qualitative approaches to research.

Nurses need to recognize that research is important as a basis for their practice and that they need to participate in the research process. For example, both home health nurses and nurses in long-term care facilities are required to collect extensive data on the cognitive and physical functioning of individuals through the Outcome and Assessment Information Set (OASIS) and Minimum Data Set (MDS) assessment tools. These data are used as part of the quality improvement process to indicate areas for improvement in care, thereby contributing to nursing protocols. Nurses in hospital settings are asked to participate in research as part of the Magnet Hospital designation process.

The chapters of this book contain specific health-promotion research studies. Time should be taken to review these studies and explore the relationship between behavior and disease, to identify which population groups are at risk, and to discover what types of health-promotion programs work and why. Through knowledge of research, nurses can strengthen their confidence

BOX 1.5 EVIDENCE-BASED PRACTICE

Evidence-Based Programming for Older Adults

The National Council on Aging (NCOA) encourages the use of evidence-based programs to enhance health and prevent injuries and disability in older adults. Evidence-based programs are composed of interventions that have been rigorously studied and found to be helpful. These programs are translated into practice using content that has been tested. Three example programs are Self-Management Resource Center programs for chronic disease self-management education, A Matter of Balance for fall prevention, and Healthy IDEAS (Identifying Depression and Empowering Activities for Seniors) for depression management. All three of these resources have met the NCOA's evidence-based quality criteria, which include demonstrated program effectiveness through experimental or quasiexperimental research, published results, translation in at least one community site, and dissemination products that are available to the public. Once a program has been selected, it must be followed consistently to ensure that the tested interventions are properly being applied (NCOA, n.d.).

in making daily decisions about quality care (Box 1.5: Evidence-Based Practice).

IMPROVING PROSPECTS FOR HEALTH

Population Effects

Cultural and socioeconomic changes within the population unequivocally influence lay concepts of health and health promotion. Currently there are areas of the United States where the Hispanic population is larger than any other population group. By 2050, it is predicted that the majority of people in the United States will not be of White European descent (US Census Bureau, 2023). Taken together as a portent for future health-promotion strategies, these predictions about the population indicate that current knowledge of and approaches to health promotion may not meet the needs of the future US population (see Chapter 2).

In addition to changes in the ethnic and racial distribution within the population, the projected changes in age distribution will affect health-promotion practice. Considerable growth is expected in the proportion of the population that is aged 25 years or older. For example, the post–World War II baby boom will increase the number of people in the 65 years-and-older age group between 2010 and 2030 (US Census Bureau, 2020). Although there was a drop in births after 1960, this decrease has been offset by an increase in immigration, both legal and illegal. More-restrictive immigration rules related to homeland security have limited legal immigration since 2002 (US Department of Homeland Security, 2024). Analysis of these population trends and projections helps health professionals determine changing needs. In addition, analysis of the social and economic environment is necessary for the development of social policy concerning health.

Shifting Problems

The provision of personal health services must be influenced by current information regarding environmental health. Environmental pollution is a complex and increasingly hazardous problem. Diseases related to industry and technology, including asthma and trauma, remain important threats to health.

The physical and psychological stresses of a rapidly changing and fast-paced society present daily problems, such as psychosocial and spiritual poor health habits. Posttraumatic stress disorder is becoming a more common diagnosis, and suicide is on the rise (American Foundation for Suicide Prevention, 2020). Terrorism is also affecting the mental health of families (Comer et al., 2019; National Academies of Sciences, Engineering, and Medicine, 2017). Obesity, partly attributed to a lack of exercise and increasing food portion size, is a growing health issue. The ingestion of potentially toxic, nonnutritious, high-fat foods is another contributing factor (see Chapter 11). The abuse of tobacco products, drugs, and alcohol also negatively affects health.

The emphasis on treating disease through the application of complex technology not only is costly but also contributes minimally to the improvement of health. An orientation toward illness clearly focuses on the effects rather than the causes of disease. During epidemics and pandemics, which are rare but still occur, basic prevention activities are needed. Washing hands and physical distancing will help prevent the spread of these rare and lethal infectious diseases. An illness-focused model will not suffice in these cases, and following public health standards is essential. Testing, contact tracing, symptom monitoring, isolation, and treatment are all important activities that need to occur to curtail the spread of these rare infectious diseases.

A substantial change in wellness patterns is occurring. Infectious and acute diseases were the major causes of death in the early part of the 20th century, whereas chronic conditions, heart disease, cerebrovascular accident (stroke), and cancer are currently the major causes. An emphasis on the diagnosis and treatment of disease, which were highly successful in the past, is not the answer for today's needs, which are closely related to and affected by the individual's biochemical functioning, genetics, environment, and personal choices (Box 1.6: Genomics). The Patient Protection and Affordable Care Act (US Congress, 2010) was enacted to begin the process of paying for health promotion by providing insurance coverage for more people and by covering preventive health services.

Moving Toward Solutions

Solutions are neither simple nor easy, but they can be focused in two major directions: individual involvement and government involvement. The first direction concentrates on actions of the individual, especially actions related to lifestyle choices across the life span. The learning and the inherent changes that are involved require the adoption of a new set of skills by people who will need the assistance of nurses to make those changes. Approximately 40% of the US population has difficulty securing the basic necessities of housing, food, utilities, and health care. These difficulties are most prevalent among adults with lower incomes but are not limited to this group. They are experienced by families with working members and those above the poverty line (Karpman et al., 2018). Iceland and Kovach (2020) found that there is a definite link between health status and hardship. The sicker an older American is, the more likely they are to suffer hardships of food insecurity, medication reduction,

BOX 1.6 GENOMICS

Genetic research is primarily concerned with discovering, detecting, and treating illnesses related to specific abnormal genetic sequences (WHO, 2020). Genomics, as a research focus, involves the study of all human genes, which are collectively called the human genome. The study and practice of genomics are concerned with how genes express themselves and how they interact with each other and the environment to encourage or discourage disease (Allen et al., 2014). Genomic interests range from the individual level to the population-based level, similar to health-promoting activities. Genomics at the individual level is concerned with an individual's risks related to their genomic profile and environmental stimuli. At the population level, genomics is concerned with large-scale patterns of genomic risk and how that plays out in the public arena. Therefore population-based public health genomics is involved with policy development, prioritizing useful genomic information, and ensuring that genomic information is discovered and used ethically and responsibly.

Lifestyle, environment, and genetics and the interaction among the three are determining factors of disease. Currently the focus of much intervention is on lifestyle and environmental contributors to disease. Because we are just beginning to look at the genomic components of disease and how they interact with lifestyle and environment, the current scientific discussion revolves around the ethical implications of private and public genomic interventions. Current debate surrounding population genomics focuses on the public's "right not to know" (Edge & Coop, 2020). Genomic information can be used to formulate public health information and initiatives. There are potential social justice ramifications in sharing large-scale genomic information, which may accentuate discrimination and worsen stigma. If the information is too complex or difficult to comprehend, it may demotivate people from making needed positive changes. For example, if a certain health behavior is linked to a particular genomic profile, knowing this could help those who do not have the genomic profile become motivated to change their behavior, whereas those with the genomic profile might become demotivated to change their behavior. Because a combination of factors cause disease, just because a person has a certain genomic profile does not mean it is an absolute that the person will get the disease, so sharing this information incautiously may be a disservice to public health as opposed to a service. Careful consideration of the risks and benefits of sharing public genomic-related information is essential.

and difficulty paying bills. Motivational factors play a large role in influencing attitudinal change. As discussed in Chapter 10, programs for health promotion and health education are only part of the answer. Financial incentives for prevention may be another motivating factor, and health advocacy by professionals in the health field is critical. In addition, private and public action at all levels is needed to reduce social and environmental health hazards. Toxic agents in the environment, such as particles from diesel emissions, and social conditions, such as school overcrowding, can present health hazards that may not be detected for years; therefore, it is necessary for individuals and the government to play a role in mitigating such hazards.

Legislation and financing that relate to primary prevention are discussed in Chapter 3. Government activity, in the form of legislation, has increased in this area. For example, increasing activity time in schools, mandating seat belt use, and implementing taxes on gasoline use are specific areas of government intervention. Health ecology and planning are important areas for government involvement in the future. The redirection of the existing health care delivery system to place more emphasis on primary prevention is probably the most difficult and far-reaching goal; however, an emphasis on a wellness system is necessary to improve the health of the US population.

CASE STUDY

Health Assessment: Frank Thompson and Family

Frank Thompson's large brick home is located off a rural country road. A few yards away stands the small house where Frank was born at the start of the Korean War. Frank was raised knowing the odds he faced as a poor tenant farmer. He helped his father, Ben, with their small tobacco and corn crops. They were unaware that the hazardous chemicals in the pesticides they used would later affect Ben's life. As his father often reminded him, Frank had to do better than others in school so he would not be doomed to the tenant farmer's life. However, Frank's school attendance was erratic because it was interrupted by the frequent demand of tending field crops. Thin and often tired, Frank had recurrent infections. Rural health care services were insufficient or not accessible. The school nurse helped the Thompson family obtain the necessary medication for Frank's initial infection, but the family was never able to afford the penicillin that was necessary to prevent recurrent infections.

Inspired by the early work of Martin Luther King, Jr., Frank was intent on helping at home and building something better for his future. Frank managed to more than compensate for his lost time at school. He passed his college entrance examinations and was awarded one of the new equal opportunity grants, which offered him the choice of attending any of the Ivy League schools in the Northeast. Instead, he chose the prestigious public Southern University and eventually earned a Master of Business Administration degree. He married Sada, his longtime girlfriend, and the two planned their future.

With a good job in a large local sales firm, Frank built his house and started a family. He moved from being a salesman to being a division head and often traveled to regional meetings, sometimes accompanied by Sada and their three children. Frank's dream of sharing his success with his family included using part of his earnings to help his brothers and sisters with their education.

This new way of life meant Frank had little time for relaxation and frequently had to attend business luncheons and career-promoting social events. Frank kept late hours and worked long weekends. Food, alcoholic beverages, and cigarettes helped Frank relax before and after important business and social encounters; these softened the edges of hard bargaining and were status symbols.

Not surprisingly, Frank gained weight. He had a persistent cough, which was probably a result of the smoking habit that developed during the early years of his career. Frank's primary care provider, whom Frank visited regularly, said Frank's blood pressure and serum lipid levels were both higher than normal and that he had chronic bronchitis. The physician urged Frank to take the actions that Frank already recognized: reduce smoking, drinking, and intake of saturated fats and calories; get more exercise; and find ways to relax. However, Frank's

Continued

CASE STUDY—cont'd

Health Assessment: Frank Thompson and Family

life was too busy for exercise. He had to work harder because he had been promoted, but he also had to appear in control and relaxed, which was an essential characteristic for a prospective vice president. To meet these goals, Frank tended to drink and smoke more. He also refused to take medication for problems he could not see. Without the outward signs of disease, Frank believed he was out of shape but generally healthy. Then Sada noted that his chance for promotion might actually improve if he lost some weight; therefore, Frank registered for a physical fitness program that he could attend on Sunday mornings and before work during the week. At his first workout, the classic sharp pain gripped his chest, and Frank had a myocardial infarction. As a result, Frank had two stents placed in his coronary arteries.

Weeks later, Frank was convalescing at home after being released from the local hospital's coronary care facility. He was lucky to survive the heart attack, and he was also fortunate to have most of the health care services covered by his medical insurance plan; in addition, 80% of his earnings were protected by the company's disability program. (Most people in the United States do not have this protection.) Frank's insurance covered the cardiac rehabilitation program that helped him recover.

However, Frank's dreams of promotion were shattered. For many months he could go to the office only two or three times a week at most, simply to deal with routine matters. He could not travel, for business or otherwise, for a long time. He was also skeptical about his cardiac rehabilitation program because his heart attack happened during exercise.

Reflective Questions

- As a nurse, how would you explain to Frank that his heart attack was not caused by his exercise?
- How might a family approach to diet and exercise work with this family, given its structure and background?
- Are there things you do to cope with stress that may be making your health worse?

TYING IT ALL TOGETHER USING CLINICAL JUDGMENT

Recognizing and Analyzing Cues

How many problems are present in Frank's situation? The answer depends on who is asked the question and their position in relation to Frank. Each point of view focuses on different aspects of Frank's life. His physician, using a clinical model of health, might say that Frank has coronary heart disease with an acute myocardial infarction, hypertension, hyperlipidemia, chronic bronchitis, and obesity. But Frank's problems also represent an inability to meet several of the *Healthy People 2030* objectives on a personal level. Reducing illness, disability, and death related to tobacco use and reducing chronic disease risk through the consumption of healthful diets and achievement of healthy body weights are two examples. His nurse can add that he has not modified his lifestyle, even after changes were recommended. He continues to overeat, drink too much, smoke, not exercise, and live a stressful life. Frank's employer sees a man who has potential but who is now too disabled to take on new responsibilities and perhaps unable to continue performing his previous duties. Frank's children might feel that he can no longer take them on trips or play with them. His wife, Sada, knows that their plans for educating their children, and for travel and enjoyment, might need to change. The human resource personnel who manage Frank's health insurance and retirement program would say that he has an expensive disease, and the state health planner would point out that Frank's problem is only one of a growing number of disabling illnesses that result from preventable causes. A reviewer for *Healthy People 2030* might see Frank as part of the aggregated data on heart disease, indicating a continuing increase in the incidence of heart disease among Black non-Hispanic men.

To Frank, his health problems are multidimensional. His initial fear of dying, pain, dependence, and frustration decreased as he began to feel better, but Frank is haunted by his realization that he might never be able to achieve his dreams for himself and his family. Although theoretically in his prime, Frank suddenly sees himself as far older than his years, both in body and in social achievement. He believes he has reached his limit and that he will never again have the freedom to choose his future. He and his family need to evaluate their situation and make alternative plans based on asset planning.

Prioritizing and Generating Solutions

Rather than emphasizing the chronic health issues and related problems, the nurse can begin with asset planning within the family. **Asset planning** is a planning approach that, given the realities of the present, helps focus family members and their providers on the building blocks for the future. It focuses on the assets or strengths of the individual, the family, and the community, applying those assets to improve or maintain the current level of functioning.

Frank's physician and nurse can begin with the fact that Frank survived his first myocardial infarction. The coronary damage resulting from this event becomes the baseline for determining future changes in the lives of Frank and his family. Earlier, Frank's physician took a broader time perspective when he advised Frank to reduce his cigarette smoking, which was contributing to both his bronchitis and his hypertension, and to change his high-fat diet and sedentary habits, which contributed to his weight problem and his high blood pressure. These lifestyle changes now become tools for Frank's recovery and for change within his family. His cardiac event can alert his children to their own risk factors for cardiac disease.

Looking at the immediate future, Frank's employer sees the effect of the event on Frank's position within the company. Frank will have a long recovery that can be successful if he adheres to his cardiac rehabilitation program. Asset planning at this level means examining how to move Frank back into his work role without further jeopardizing his health. Frank and Sada also need to examine whether he can continue in his role given its potential effect on his health.

Frank and his family use a broader perspective than the medical personnel or the corporation. They know that to achieve the family's economic and educational goals and still spend time together they have to make decisions that will ultimately affect Frank's health. Similar to many Americans, they had been willing to live with Frank's job pressures and stressful lifestyle caused by the economy. The family members were aware of their impoverished roots and had no wish to return to them. However, they also recognize that the strength of their family, their ability to work together to achieve goals, and their faith were assets that can be used for support.

Frank's social network of friends, relatives, and church members become an additional asset. They help the family through the difficult initial weeks at home by delivering meals, taking care of the yard work and laundry, and providing companionship so Sada can shop and have time alone. As Frank recovers, they will provide support for the social and lifestyle changes that Frank and his family need to make.

The nurse-led cardiovascular rehabilitation group plays a vital role in Frank's recovery. As the physician continues to monitor Frank's cardiac status, the nurse begins the long process of working with Frank to modify his habits. He had stopped smoking while in the hospital, but with more free time than usual, he is craving to smoke again. Using an asset planning approach and Gordon's (2016) functional health patterns, the nurse identifies the changes that Frank needs to make to decrease the risk of a second heart attack. A plan is developed to help Frank begin to take control of his life through behavioral changes. These changes include relaxation techniques, diet modification, smoking cessation, and mild chair exercises. The support of the family is enlisted to reinforce the changes Frank is willing to make, because social support and environmental changes are shown to enhance personal decision-making. His employer is contacted and agrees to a plan enabling Frank to work from home via the internet while the workplace becomes smoke free. Frank becomes an asset to the workplace, serving as a spokesperson for the benefits of lifestyle change. He is enlisted to talk with other employees about stress management, exercise, weight reduction, and smoking cessation based on his personal experiences.

Health planners and public health officials used the broadest perspective in asset planning by viewing Frank as an example of a person whose potential shifted as a result of a preventable, disabling illness. The planners looked at public and private community patterns and policies that increase healthful habits and living conditions. Work schedules and workload; stress and safety in work environments; affirmative action programs for jobs and wages; availability of public transportation systems, recreational facilities, and economically accessible housing; farm price subsidies for food and tobacco crops that affect buying patterns; and excise taxes and regulation of health-damaging drugs such as alcohol and nicotine were all taken into consideration (Grzywacz & Fuqua, 2000; Rudolph et al., 2013). The asset-planning approach emphasized the positive actions that could be made at the personal, employment, community, and societal levels to minimize the effects of Frank's illness and related diseases, thereby addressing all levels of the ecological model of health.

What Was the Actual Cause of Frank's Problem?

It is not possible to separate one cause from another because heart disease is a multifactorial disease. In Frank's case the sources of illness were found in the many interrelationships in his life. Attempting to treat or change each factor as a separate entity can have only a limited effect on the improvement of overall health. Frank's health problems were numerous. In addition to a poor diet, weight gain, lack of exercise, and smoking, his hyperlipidemia, an adaptive biologic response to the pressures in his life, further debilitated him. It eventually led to clogged coronary vessels, and his responses became maladaptive. His hypertension, resulting from his diet and time-constrained lifestyle, complicated by the buildup of plaque secondary to hyperlipidemia, was also a biologic attempt to adjust to a situation that contributed to an imbalance between his personal resources and the demands of his family and the economic world. Frank's smoking was a psychosocial means to help him relieve some of the emotional pressures. It may have served this short-term purpose but only at a silently rising cost to his health. Cigarette use by persons who have hypertension or high serum cholesterol levels multiplies their risk of coronary heart disease (Zhu et al., 2019).

Evaluation of the Situation

The health status of an individual or population depends on a sustainable balance of the complex responses between physiologic, psychological, and social and environmental factors. Health was initially conceived as a biologic state, with genetic endowment as the starting point. However, health involves psychological and social aspects and is interpreted within the context of the immediate environment.

The interconnections between biophysical, psychological, and environmental causes and consequences did not end with Frank's heart attack. His heart attack was the most dramatic sign that health-damaging responses outweighed health-promoting ones. The "tip of the iceberg" analogy is frequently used to illustrate the importance of identifying individuals with subclinical symptoms. High blood lipid levels, high blood pressure, obesity, smoking, and persistent worrying were no less important than the infarction in shaping the status of Frank's health. Repairing the damage to Frank's heart without changing his lifestyle, habits, and work environment would buy only a brief amount of time before further damage would occur.

The infarction and resulting disability also permanently reshaped Frank's environment. After a few months of working full time, Frank realized that he needed to find a less stressful job. He recognized that his sales administration skills were an asset and began interviewing in the nonprofit sector. Ultimately, he landed a job at half his previous salary but with excellent benefits and a flexible work environment. His reduced income meant that his children's educational opportunities were more limited than they were before his heart attack, but his family responded by seeking tuition support from community organizations. Frank found that his contacts in both the corporate and the nonprofit sectors increased his value to his new employer. Frank's entire life, internal and external, had changed. He had learned to adapt to his health

BOX 1.7 SELECTED *HEALTHY PEOPLE 2030* OBJECTIVES

Label/Number	Objective
Access to Health Services	
AHS-04 Core Objective	Reduce the proportion of people who cannot get medical care when they need it.
AHS-R02 Research Objective	Increase the use of telehealth to improve access to health services.
Social Determinants of Health	
SDOH-01 Core Objective	Reduce the proportion of people living in poverty.
SDOH-02 Core Objective	Increase employment in working-age people.
Nutrition and Weight Status	
NWS11 Core Objective	Reduce consumption of saturated fat by people aged 2 years and over.
NWS03 Core Objective	Reduce the proportion of adults with obesity.

From: https://health.gov/healthypeople/objectives-and-data/browse-objectives.

problems and had developed a more **eudaimonistic** approach to health and life.

Frank's situation illustrates how causes and effects in life and health tend to merge into constant, inseparable interconnections between individuals and their worlds. A person's health status reflects a web of relationships that characterize that person's life. Health is not an achievement or a prize but a high-quality interaction between a person's inner and outer worlds that provides the capacity to respond to the demands of the biologic, psychological, and environmental systems of these worlds.

Which of the *Healthy People 2030* objectives listed in Box 1.7 apply to the promotion of Frank's health? Clearly, the area of heart disease and stroke is most applicable. The *Healthy People 2030* website (https://health.gov/healthypeople) has a number of objectives that relate directly to the prevention of heart disease, hypertension, and hyperlipidemia, including objectives that relate to treatment options and training the public to recognize and respond to nutrition and weight (Box 1.7: Selected *Healthy People 2030* Objectives). From the information about Frank and his experience, determine what his children should be taught on the basis of the *Healthy People 2030* objectives in this focus area.

SUMMARY

- The ways in which individuals define health and health problems are important because definitions influence attempts to improve health and care delivery.
- The view taken in this text is that a broad and longer-term perspective of health is the best guide to promoting health more effectively, even as nurses deal with individual problems on a daily basis.
- Health is a sustainable balance between internal and external forces.
- Illness represents an imbalance in which human choices (intertwined social, political, spiritual, professional, and personal choices) contribute.
- In the United States, communities may still have time to reduce the onslaught of chronic disability and shift the direction, slow the pace, and humanize the scope of economic and social life.
- To shift direction, nurses and other health professionals can work with others to inform, educate, and reeducate themselves, their colleagues, the media, and the general public using research findings and evidence-based practice methods.
- Prevention, at all levels, is important for deterring the spread of disease and illness.
- Considering patient, family, and community assets that can be accessed to encourage and maintain health is a valuable approach to health promotion.
- The responsibility of nurses as health professionals today is to see health problems in new ways and help others to do the same.

EVOLVE CHAPTER FEATURES

http://evolve.elsevier.com/Edelman/
- Study Questions

REFERENCES

Ajzen, A., & Fishbein, M. (1980). *Understanding attitudes and predicting social behavior*. Upper Saddle River, NJ: Prentice Hall.

Allen, F. M., & Warner, M. (2002). A developmental model of health and nursing. *Journal of Family Nursing, 8*(2), 96–135.

Allen, C., Senecal, K., & Avard, D. (2014). Defining the scope of public engagement: Examining the "right not to know" in public health genomics. *Public Health Genomics, 42*(1), 11–18. https://doi.org/10.1111/jlme.12114

American Foundation for Suicide Prevention. (2020). *Suicide statistics*. https://afsp.org/suicide-statistics/

American Nurses Association (ANA). (2015a). *Guide to nursing's social policy statement*. ANA Publications.

American Nurses Association (ANA). (2015b). *Code of ethics for nurses with interpretive statements*. ANA Publications.

American Nurses Association (ANA). (2015c). *Nursing: Scope and standards of practice*. ANA Publications.

American Nurses Association (ANA). (2023). *What is evidence-based practice in nursing?* https://www.nursingworld.org

American Public Health Association. (2024). *What is public health?* https://www.apha.org/what-is-public-health

Andresen, E. M., Catlin, T. K., Wyrwich, K. W., & Jackson-Thompson, J. (2003). Retest reliability of surveillance questions on health related quality of life. *Journal of Epidemiology and Community Health, 57*(5), 339–343. https://doi:10.1136/jech.57.5.339

Ardell, D. B. (2007). *What is wellness? Aging beyond belief: 69 Tips for REAL wellness*. Duluth, MN: Whole Person Associates Inc.

Badash, I., Kleinman, N. P., Barr, S., Jang, J., Rahman, S., & Qu, B. W. (2017). Redefining health: The evolution of health ideas from antiquity to the era of value-based care. *Cureus*, *9*(2), e1018. https://doi.org/10.7759/cureus.1018

Bandura, A. (1976). *Social learning theory*. Upper Saddle River, NJ: Prentice Hall.

Bandura, A. (1999). *Self-efficacy: The exercise of control*. New York, NY: W.H. Freeman.

Bandura, A. (2004). Health promotion by social cognitive means. *Health Education Behavior*, *31*(2), 143–164. https://doi.org/10.1177/1090198104263660

Barr, D., Lee, P., & Benjamin, A. (2003). Health care and health policy in a changing world. In H. Wallace (Ed.), *Health and welfare for families in the 21*st century (2nd ed.). Jones & Bartlett.

Benner, P., et al. (2010). *Educating nurses: A call for radical transformation*. San Francisco, CA: Jossey-Bass.

Bosley, S. (2020, September 9). *'Hands. Face. Space': UK government relaunch COVID-19 slogan*. The Guardian. https://www.theguardian.com/world/2020/sep/09/hands-face-space-uk-government-to-relaunch-covid-19-slogan

Bronfenbrenner, U. (1977). Toward an experimental ecology of human development. *American Psychologist*, 513–531. https://doi.org/10.1037/0003-066X.32.7.513

Burnham, J. C. (2012). The death of the sick role. *Social History of Medicine*, *25*(4), 761–776. https://doi.org/10.1093/shm/hks018

Burns, N., & Grove, S. K. (2020). *Understanding nursing research* (9th ed.). Philadelphia, PA: Saunders.

Carpentieri, J. D., Elliott, J., Brett, C. E., & Deary, I. J. (2017). Adapting to aging: Older people talk about their use of selection, optimization, and compensation to maximize well-being in the context of physical decline. *The Journals of Gerontology: Series B, Psychological Sciences and Social Sciences*, *72*(2), 351–361. https://doi.org/10.1093/geronb/gbw132

Červený, M., Kratochvílová, I., Hellerová, V., & Tóthová, V. (2022). Methods of increasing cultural competence in nurses working in clinical practice: A scoping review of literature 2011-2021. *Frontiers in Psychology*, *13*, 936181. https://doi.org/10.3389/fpsyg.2022.936181

Champion, V. L., & Skinner, C. S. (2008). The health belief model. In K. Glanz, B. Rimer, & K. Viswanath (Eds.), *Health behavior and health education: Theory, research, and practice* (4th ed.). San Francisco, CA: Jossey-Bass.

Clay, O. J., Perkins, M., Wallace, G., Crowe, M., Sawyer, P., & Brown, C. J. (2018). Associations of multimorbid medical conditions and health-related quality of life among older African American men. *Journals of Gerontology: Psychological Sciences*, *73*(2), 258–266. https://doi:10.1093/geronb/gbx090

Cohen, S. R., Sawatzky, R., Russell, L. B., Shahidi, J., Heyland, & Gadermann, A. M. (2017). Measuring the quality of life of people at the end of life: The McGill quality of life questionnaire- revised. *Palliative Medicine*, *31*(2), 120–129. https://doi.org/10.1186/s12955-020-01621-8

Comer, J. S., Furr, J. M., & Gurwitch, R. H. (2019). Terrorism exposure and the family: Where we are, and where we go next. In B. H. Fiese, M. Celano, K. Deater-Deckard, E. N. Jourlies, & M. A. Whisman (Eds.), *APA handbook of contemporary family psychology: Applications and broad impact of family psychology*. Washington, DC: American Psychological Association.

Davis, M. A., Weeks, W. B., & Coulter, I. D. (2011). A proposed conceptual model for studying the use of complementary and alternative medicine. *Alternative Therapies in Health and Medicine*, *17*(5), 32–36.

de Hond, A., Bakx, P., & Versteegh, M. (2019). Can time heal all wounds? An empirical assessment of adaptation to functional limitations in an older population. *Social Science & Medicine*, *222*, 180–187. https://doi.org/10.1016/j.socscimed.2018.12.028

Devore, R., & Kreuter, M. (1980). Update: Reinforcing the case for health promotion. *Family & Community Health*, *10*(2), 103–119.

Dunn, H. (1961). *High-level wellness*. Cincinnati, OH: R.W. Beatty.

Edge, M., & Coop, G. (2020). Attacks on genetic privacy via uploads to genealogical databases. *eLife*, *9*, e51810. https://doi.org/10.7554/eLife.51810

Endo, E. (2017). Margaret Newman's Theory of Health as Expanding Consciousness and a nursing intervention form a unitary perspective. *Asia-Pacific Journal of Oncology Nursing*, *1*(4), 50–52. https://doi.org/10.4103/2347-5625.199076

Fawcett, J., & Garity, J. (2009). *Evaluating research for evidence-based nursing practice*. Philadephia, PA: F.A. Davis.

Gehlert, S., & Ward, T. S. (2019). Theories of health behaviors. In S. Gehlert, & T. Browne (Eds.), *Handbook of health social work* (3rd ed., pp. 143–163). San Francisco, CA: Josey-Bass.

Gordon, M. (2016). *Manual of nursing diagnosis* (14th ed.). Burlington, MA: Jones & Bartlett.

Grzywacz, J. G., & Fuqua, J. (2000). The social ecology of health: Leverage points and linkages. *Behavioral Medicine (Washington, D.C.)*, *26*(3), 101–115. https://doi.org/10.1080/08964280009595758

Gyasi, R. M., & Phillips, D. R. (2018). Gender, self-rated health and functional decline among community-dwelling older adults. *Archives of Gerontology and Geriatrics*, *77*, 174–183.

Hardin, S. R., & Kaplow, R. (2017). *Synergy for clinical excellence: The AACN Synergy Model for Patient Care* (2nd ed.). Burlington, MA: Jones & Bartlett Learning.

Hawkins, J. D., Jensen, J. M., Catalano, R., Fraser, M. W., Botvin, G. J., Shapiro, V., & Stone, S. (2015). *Unleashing the power of prevention*. National Academy of Medicine. https://nam.edu/perspectives-2015-unleashing-the-power-of-prevention/

Hollingsworth, L., & Didelot, M. (2010). Illness: The redefinition of self and relationships. In I. Lang & Z. Norridge (Eds.). *Illness, bodies and contexts: Interdisciplinary perspectives* (pp. 1–13). Brill. https:// https://brill.com/display/book/edcoll/9781848880283/BP000002.xml

Iceland, J., & Kovach, C. (2020, August 11). *Poverty and the incidence of material hardship revisited*. https://www.census.gov/content/dam/Census/library/working-papers/2020/demo/sehsd-wp2020-11.pdf

Jamoulle, M., Tsoi, G., Heath, I., Mangin, D., Pezeshki, M., & Baez, M. P. (2015). Quaternary prevention: First, do not harm. *Revista Brasileira De Medicina de Familia E Coumunidade*, *10*(35), 1–3.

Johnston, Y. A., Bergen, G., Bauer, M., Parker, E. M., Wentworth, L., McFadden, M., Reome, C., & Garnett, M. (2019). Implementation of the stopping elderly accidents, deaths, and injuries initiative in primary care: An outcome evaluation. *The Gerontologist*, *59*(6), 1182–1191. https://doi.org/10.1093/geront/gny101

Karimi, M., & Brazier, J. (2016). Health, health-related quality of life, and quality of life: What is the difference? *PharmacoEconomics*, *34*, 645–649. https://doi.org/10.1007/s40273-016-0389-9

Karpman, M., Zuckerman, S., & Gonzalez, D. (2018). *Material Hardship among elderly adults and their families in 2017*. The Urban Institute. https://www.urban.org/research/publication/material-hardship-among-nonelderly-adults-and-their-families-2017

Kindig, D. (2015, April 6). *What are we talking about when we talk about population health?* Health Affairs. https://www.healthaffairs.org/do/10.1377/hblog20150406.046151/full/

Kindig, D., & Stoddart, G. (2003). What is population health? *American Journal of Public Health, 93*(3), 380–383.

Kisling, L. A., & Das, J. (2023, August 1). Prevention strategies. In *StatPearls* [Internet]. StatPearls Publishing. https://www.ncbi.nlm.nih.gov/books/NBK537222/

Leavell, H., & Clark, A. E. (1965). *Preventive medicine for the doctor in his community*. New York, NY: McGraw-Hill.

Lillard, J. W., Moses, K. A., Mahal, B. A., & George, D. J. (2022). Racial disparities in Black men with prostate cancer: A literature review. *Cancer, 128*(21), 3787–3795. https://doi.org/10.1002/cncr.34433

Luther, B., Barra, J., & Martial, M. A. (2019). Essential nursing care management and coordination roles and responsibilities: A content analysis. *Professional Case Management, 24*(5), 249–258. https://doi.org/10.1097/NCM.0000000000000355

Martins, E., Godycki-Cwirko, M., Heleno, B., & Brodersen, J. (2018). Quaternary prevention: Reviewing the concept. *European Journal of General Practice, 24*(1), 106–111. https://doi.org.10.1080/13814788.2017.1422177

McMahon, S., & Fleury, J. (2012). Wellness in older adults: A concept analysis. *Nursing Forum, 47*(1), 39–51. https://doi.org.10.1111/j.1744-6198.2011.00254.x

Mittlemark, M., & Bauer, G. F. (2017). The meanings of Salutogenesis. In M. Mittlemark, S. Sagy, M. Eriksson, G. F. Bauer, J. M. Pelikan, B. Lindstrom, & G. A. Espenes (Eds.), *The handbook of Salutogenesis* (pp. 7–14). Springer Open Source.

Murdaugh, C. L., Parsons, M. A., & Pender, N. J. (2019). *Health promotion in nursing practice* (8th ed.). Upper Saddle River, NJ: Pearson.

National Academies of Sciences, Engineering, and Medicine. (2017). *Countering violent extremism through public health practice: Proceedings of a workshop*. The National Academies Press. https://doi.org/10.17226/24638

National Center for Complementary and Integrative Health (NCCIH). (n.d.). Complementary or Integrative Health: What's in a Name? https://www.nccih.nih.gov/health/complementary-alternative-or-integrative-health-whats-in-a-name

National Council on Aging. (n.d.). *About evidence-based programs*. https://www.ncoa.org

National Heart, Lung, and Blood Institute. (2020). *Obesity education initiative. The practical guide: Identification, evaluation, and treatment of overweight and obesity in adults*. https://www.nhlbi.nih.gov/health/educational/lose_wt/index.htm

National Institute of Nursing Research (NINR). (2022). *NINR strategic plan*. https://www.ninr.nih.gov/aboutninr/ninr-mission-and-strategic-plan

Ndugga, N., Hill, L., & Artiga, S. (2022, November 17). *COVID-19 Cases and deaths, vaccinations, and treatments by race/ethnicity as of fall 2022*. Kaiser Family Foundation. https://www.kff.org/racial-equity-and-health-policy/issue-brief/covid-19-cases-and-deaths-vaccinations-and-treatments-by-race-ethnicity-as-of-fall-2022/#:~:text=While%20disparities%20in%20cases%20and,experienced%20overall%20higher%20rates%20of

Newman, M. (2003). A world of no boundaries. *Advances in Nursing Science, 26*(4), 240–245.

O'Donnell, M. (1987). Definition of health promotion. *American Journal of Health Promotion, 1*(1), 4–5.

Orchard, C. A., & Mahler, C. (2018). The association of nurse practitioner roles and practice on perceived health of residents living within subsidized housing units. *Nursing and Family Health Care, 1*(1), 1–9. https://doi.org/10.15761/NFHC.1000104

Polacsek, M., Boardman, G. H., & McCann, T. V. (2020). The influence of a successful wellness-illness transition on the experience of depression in older adults. *Issues in Mental Health Nursing, 41*(1), 31–37. https://doi.org/10.1080/01612840.2019.1673522

Prochaska, J. O., Redding, C. A., & Evers, E. E. (2015). The transtheoretical model and stages of change. In K. Glanz, & B. Rimer (Eds.), *Health behavior: Theory, research, and practice* (pp. 125–151). Hoboken, NJ: Jossey-Bass.

Quinn, J. F. (2016). Transpersonal human caring and healing. In B. M. Dossey, & L. Keegan (Eds.), *Holistic Nursing: A handbook for practice* (pp. 101–109). Burlington, MA: Jones & Bartlett.

Reed, P. G. (1983). Implications of the life-span developmental framework for well-being in adulthood and aging. *Advances in Nursing Science, 6*(1), 18–25. https://doi.org/10.1097/00012272-198310000-00006

Rogers, M. (1970). *An introduction to the theoretical basis of nursing*. Philadephia, PA: F.A. Davis.

Rudolph, L., Caplan, J., Ben-Moshe, K., & Dillon, L. (2013). *Health in all policies: A guide for state and local governments*. American Public Health Association and Public Health Institute.

Ruger, J. P., Hammonds, R., Ooms, G., Barry, D., Chapman, A, & Van Damme, W. (2015). From conceptual pluralism to practical agreement on policy: Global responsibility for global health. *BMC International Health and Human Rights, 15*, 30. https://doi.org/10.1186/s12914-015-0065-8

Sackett, D., Rosenberg, W. M., Gran, J. A., Haynes, R. B., & Richardson, W. S. (1996). Evidence based medicine: What it is and what it isn't. *British Medical Journal, 312*, 71–72.

Shelton, L. G. (2019). *The Bronfenbrenner primer*. London, UK: Routledge.

Shorey, S. (2021). Health promotion among families having a newborn baby. In G. Haugan, & M. Eriksson (Eds.), *Health promotion in health care – vital theories and research* (pp. 173–184). Springer Open Access. https://www.ncbi.nlm.nih.gov/books/NBK585667/

Siegel, D. (2007). *The mindful brain: Reflection and attunement in the cultivation of well-being*. New York, NY: W.W. Norton & Co.

Smith, J. A. (1983). *The idea of health: Implications for the nursing profession*. New York, NY: Columbia University Teachers College Press.

Smith, Y. M., & Cleveland, K. A., & Kleman, C. (2021, October 28). Understanding nurses' experiences and contributions to governing boards. *OJIN: The Online Journal of Issues in Nursing, 27*(1). https://doi.org/10.3912/OJIN.Vol27No01PPT32

Snedden, T. R., Scerpella, J., Kliethermes, S. A., Norman, R. S., Blyholder, L., Sanfilippo, J., & Heiderscheit, B. (2019). Sport and physical activity level impacts health-related quality of life among collegiate students. *American Journal of Health Promotion, 33*(5), 675–682. https://doi.org/10.1177/0890117118817715

Svalastog, A. L., Donev, D., Kristoffersen, N. J., & Gafovic, S. (2017). Concepts and definitions of health and health-related values in the knowledge landscapes of the digital society. *Croatian Medical Journal, 58*, 431–435. https://doi.org/10.3325/cmj.2017.58.431

Tabvuma, T., Stanton, R., & Happell, B. (2023). The physical health nurse consultant and mental health consumer: An important therapeutic partnership. *International Journal of Mental Health Nursing, 32*(2), 579–589. https://doi.org/10.1111/inm.13104

The Resilience Center. (2024). *The Resilience Scale*. https://www.resiliencecenter.com/products/resilience-scales-and-tools-for-research/the-original-resilience-scale/

Travis, J. W., & Ryan, R. S. (2004). *Wellness workbook: How to achieve enduring health and vitality*. Emeryville, CA: Ten Speed Press.

US Census Bureau. (2020). *65 and older population grows rapidly as baby boomers age*. https://www.census.gov/newsroom/press-releases/2020/65-older-population-grows.html

US Census Bureau. (2023). *Population projections*. https://www.census.gov/programs-surveys/popproj.html

US Congress. (2010). *About the Patient Protection and Affordable Care Act (PPACA)*. https://www.hhs.gov

US Department of Health and Human Services (USDHHS), & Office of Disease Prevention and Health Promotion. (2022). *Healthy People 2020*. Washington, DC. http://www.healthypeople.gov/2020/

US Department of Health and Human Services (USDHHS), & Public Health Service. (1986). *The 1990 health objectives for the nation: A midcourse review*. Washington, DC: US Government Printing Office, US Department of Health and Human Services.

US Department of Health and Human Services (USDHHS), & Public Health Service. (1990). *Healthy People 2000: The Surgeon General's report on health promotion and disease prevention. US Department of Health and Human Services publication no. 7955071*. Washington, DC: US Government Printing Office.

US Department of Health and Human Services (USDHHS), & Public Health Service. (1996). *Healthy People 2000 midcourse review and 1995 revisions*. Jones & Bartlett.

US Department of Health and Human Services (USDHHS), & Public Health Service. (2000). *Healthy People 2010 (conference edition, in two volumes)*. Washington, DC: US Government Printing Office.

US Department of Health, Education, and Welfare, & Public Health Service. (1979). *Healthy People*. Washington, DC: US Government Printing Office.

US Department of Homeland Security. (2024). *Enforce and administer our immigration laws*. https://www.dhs.gov/administer-immigration-laws

Westberg Institute. (2020, February 6). *Westberg Institute for Faith Community Nursing*. https://westberginstitute.org/

Witwer, S. G., & Wallenstein, D. W. (2019). Education and engagement of patients and families: The essential role of the care coordinator and transition manager RN. *AAACN ViewPoint*, *41*(1), 12–13. https://www.proquest.com/scholarly-journals/education-engagement-patients-families-essential/docview/2309781081/se-2

World Health Organization (WHO). (2004). *The World Health Organization Quality of Life (WHOQOL)-BREF*. http://www.who.int

World Health Organization (WHO). (2020). *Human genetics programme*. https://www.who.int

World Health Organization (WHO). (2023). *Constitution*. https://www.who.int/about/governance/constitution

Xu, F., Cohen, S. A., Lofgren, I. E., Greene, G. W., Delmonico, M. J., & Greaney, M. L. (2018). Relationship between diet quality, physical activity and health-related quality of life in older adults: Findings from 2007-2014 National Health and Nutrition Examination Survey. *Journal of Nutrition, Health & Aging*, *22*(9), 1072–1079. https://doi.org/10.1007/s12603-018-1050-4

Zhu, J., Nelson, K., Toth, J., & Muscat, J. E. (2019). Nicotine dependence as an independent risk factor for atherosclerosis in the National Lung Screening Trial. *BMC Public Health*, *19*, 103. https://doi.org/10.1186/s12889-019-6419-8

2

Communities at Risk and Health

Marni B. Kellogg, Kevin Chui, Sallie Beth Johnson, Frank Tudini and Sheng-Che Yen

http://evolve.elsevier.com/Edelman/

OBJECTIVES

After completing this chapter, the reader will be able to:

- Differentiate among ethnicity, ethnic group, race, and minority group.
- Describe demographic data relative to populations at risk.
- Describe health concerns and issues of people who are at higher risk.
- Discuss selected cultural factors that may have an impact on the health and well-being of people who are at higher risk.
- Contrast the folk healing system with the professional care system.
- Explain strategies for health care professionals to meet the needs of people who are at higher risk.
- Identify tools available to help meet the health care needs of immigrants.
- Describe initiatives to address the health care concerns of people who are at higher risk.

KEY TERMS

Chi
Complementary, alternative, and integrative medicine
Cultural and linguistic competence
Culturally congruent practice
Cultural humility
Cultural respect
Culture
Disabilities
Downstream factors
Ethnic groups
Ethnicity
Ethnocentric perspective
Female genital mutilation/cutting (FGM/C)
Folk healing system
Gender expression
Gender identity
Gender transition
Harm reduction
Health disparities
Health equity
Homelessness
Hot and cold concept of disease
Immigrants
Intersectionality
Jing
Lesbian, gay, bisexual, transgender, queer/questioning (one's sexual or gender identity), intersex, and asexual/aromantic/agender (LGBTQIA+)
Minority group
Nurse care systems
People first language
Professional care systems
Race
Racism
Refugees
Sexual orientation
Social determinants of health
Taoism
Transcultural nursing
Transgender
Value orientations
Values
Vulnerable populations
Yang; Yin

THINK ABOUT IT

Harm-Reduction Strategies for Individuals with Substance Use Disorder

The United States is currently facing its most severe substance use and overdose epidemic to date, further intensified by the recent global pandemic (Centers for Disease Control and Prevention [CDC], 2021). This crisis is fueled by the widespread infiltration of highly potent synthetic opioids, such as fentanyl and its analogs, as well as animal tranquilizers such as xylazine, into various types of drugs, including stimulants and counterfeit prescription pills (Substance Abuse and Mental Health Services Administration, 2023). In 2022 alone, there were over 100,000 drug-involved overdose deaths in the United States (Substance Abuse and Mental Health Services Administration, 2023). An evidence-based approach utilized in outreach programs for individuals struggling with substance use disorder is **harm reduction**. This strategy aims to preserve the health and well-being of people who use drugs by acknowledging the reality of both illicit and legal drug use while addressing the associated dangers and harms. Harm reduction fosters a collaborative relationship between practitioners and care recipients. People who use drugs are not condemned or condoned but included as partners in the creation of programs and policies benefiting them (National Harm Reduction Coalition, n.d.). Abstinence is the ultimate goal of interventions for those who use illicit drugs, but providers recognize that this may be unattainable. Therefore, harm reduction emphasizes recognizing and understanding that certain drugs pose less harm than others and that some methods of drug administration carry less risk than others (National Harm Reduction Coalition, n.d.). This practical approach maintains respect for human rights and is essential to the success of harm-reduction programs. Evidence-based interventions used in harm reduction include expanding access to naloxone for overdose prevention, distributing fentanyl test strips, providing access to medication for opioid use disorders, providing access to methadone clinics, implementing syringe service programs, and providing supervised consumption services (Ivsins et al., 2023; Nataraj et al., 2024; National Harm Reduction Coalition, n.d.). Implementing a comprehensive public health strategy, which includes enhancing access to treatment, facilitating linkage to care, and providing overdose education and harm-reduction initiatives, is crucial for reducing overdose rates and enhancing outcomes for individuals with substance use disorder (Nataraj et al., 2024).

Harm-reduction programs:

- Foster trust through consistent and reliable support services while reducing access barriers.
- Cultivate community partnerships and offer a range of services to address diverse needs.
- Provide integrated interprofessional care, including, but not limited to, education, medical care, and social services.
- Distribute opioid overdose reversal medications such as naloxone to at-risk individuals or potential responders.
- Mitigate harm related to drug use and associated behaviors to reduce the risk of infectious diseases such as HIV, viral hepatitis, and bacterial/fungal infections.
- Prevent infectious disease transmission among people who use drugs, including injection drug users, by providing sterile supplies, accurate information, and access to resources.
- Decrease overdose fatalities.
- Foster a culture of hope and recovery by involving individuals with lived experience in leadership and service planning.
- Advocate for supportive policies to reduce infectious disease and overdose risks (Substance Abuse and Mental Health Services Administration, 2023).

Despite their many benefits, harm-reduction strategies have been challenged in the United States by political opposition based on moral condemnation of drug dependence and stigmatization of persons from racial/ethnic minority groups struggling with substance use (Pyra et al., 2022).

Given the pragmatics and respect for human rights, could harm reduction effectively be implemented to help individuals with chronic illnesses such as diabetes, hypertension, or obesity, to name just a few? It's something to think about!

SOCIAL DETERMINANTS OF HEALTH AND HEALTH EQUITY

Many nonmedical factors contribute significantly to health disparities within the United States and worldwide. These factors, termed **social determinants of health**, include income, education, employment stability, working conditions, food access, housing, early childhood development, social inclusion, structural conflicts, and affordable, quality health care access (CDC, 2022c; US Department of Health and Human Services [USDHHS], n.d.; World Health Organization [WHO], n.d.-b). Social determinants of health contribute to an individual's capability to access quality health care and determine health outcomes (Hacker et al., 2022). The WHO defines social determinants of health as "the non-medical factors that influence health outcomes. They are the conditions in which people are born, grow, work, live, and age, and the wider set of forces and systems shaping the conditions of daily life. These forces and systems include economic policies and systems, development agendas, social norms, social policies, and political systems" (WHO, n.d.-b).

Focusing on the many nonmedical factors that ultimately influence health, social determinants of health are a priority focus for *Healthy People 2030* (USDHHS, n.d.-b, n.d.-c). *Healthy People 2030* directly addresses the social determinants of health by grouping them into five domains: 1) economic stability, 2) education access and quality, 3) health care access and quality, 4) neighborhood and built environment, and 5) social and community context. Box 2.1 displays the social determinants of health domains, goals, and sample objectives across topics.

Healthy People 2030 Social Determinants of Health Domains, Goals, and Sample Objectives

Although there have been many successes in improving public health over the last century, improved health outcomes have not been seen in all groups (CDC, 2023b; WHO, 2023). The CDC defines **health disparity** as "preventable differences in the burden of disease, injury, violence, or in opportunities to

BOX 2.1 *HEALTHY PEOPLE 2030*

Social Determinants of Health Domains, Goals, and Sample Objectives

Domain	Goal	Sample Objective
Economic Stability	Help people earn steady incomes that allow them to meet their health needs.	Reduce the proportion of families that spend more than 30% of income on housing.
Education Access and Quality	Increase educational opportunities and help children and adolescents do well in school.	Increase the proportion of children who participate in high-quality early childhood education programs.
Health Care Access and Quality	Increase access to comprehensive, high-quality health care services.	Increase the proportion of adults who get screened for colorectal cancer.
Neighborhood and Built Environment	Create neighborhoods and environments that promote health and safety.	Reduce the amount of toxic pollutants released into the environment.
Social and Community Context	Increase social and community support.	Reduce bullying of transgender students.

(US Department of Health and Human Services, n.d.-c)

achieve optimal health experienced by socially disadvantaged racial, ethnic, and other population groups and communities" (2017). Health disparity broadly affects an individual's ability to achieve good health. Additionally, health disparity has been documented as contributing to many conditions, including, but not limited to, cancer and heart disease, preterm births, suicide, and drug overdose fatalities, as well as health care and insurance utilization (Braveman et al., 2021b; CDC, 2023a, 2023b; USDHHS et al., 2022). See **Think About It** for an example of an intervention strategy that uses harm-reduction principles to address disparities of people who are experiencing substance use disorder.

Health equity involves enhancing opportunities for all individuals to lead their healthiest lives regardless of sex, gender, ethnicity, disability, sexual orientation, location, or socioeconomic status (CDC, 2022; WHO, n.d.-b). For more information on social determinants of health and health equity, visit the CDC's Office of Health Equity and view their informative video series: https://www.cdc.gov/healthequity/whatis/videos/index.html.

Communities at Higher Risk in the United States

Several communities within the United States are at higher risk for poor health due to health disparities. Ethnic groups and other minority groups, such as LGBTQIA+ in the United States, face challenges in accessing health care due to language and cultural differences, discrimination, racism, and lack of financial resources, among other disparities. The economic burden of health inequities, particularly for racial and ethnic minorities and individuals with lower education, is substantial, highlighting the need for continued investment in research, policies, and practices to eliminate these disparities (Horvath et al., 2023; LaVeist et al., 2023). Addressing health disparities in all groups can lower health care expenses and extend and improve people's lives (Horvath et al., 2023).

Race, Ethnicity, Ethnic Groups, Minority Groups, and Racism

Race is primarily a social construct, reflecting societal perceptions and classifications rather than biologic, anthropologic, or genetic distinctions; racial categories encompass national origin and sociocultural groupings (US Census Bureau, 2022a). The Office of Management and Budget (OMB) provides race and ethnicity guidelines for categorizing written responses to the race question (US Census Bureau, 2022a). According to the US Census Bureau, the minimal race categories for collecting data on race and ethnicity are White, Black or African American, American Indian or Alaska Native, Asian, and Native Hawaiian or other Pacific Islander (2022b). **Ethnicity** is a complex social construct that includes various dimensions, such as language, country of origin, cultural heritage, nationality, and other factors (Lam et al., 2023). Ethnicity focuses on differences in meanings, values, and living practices. Race typically refers to biologic or physical characteristics, while ethnicity encompasses cultural, linguistic, and national origins, often reflecting shared traditions and customs. **Ethnic groups** are composed of individuals who share common cultural traits (beliefs, values, and behaviors), language, religion, ancestry, or other characteristics, often passed down through generations, and who may originate from the same country or reside in the same locality (American Psychiatric Association [APA], 2018; National Institutes of Health, National Cancer Institute, n.d.). Some ethnic groups are considered minorities, although the term *minority* can refer to more than ethnicity. Minority groups are subsets of the population, which may be ethnic, racial, social, religious, or other groups, that hold varying degrees of power compared to the dominant majority (APA, 2023).

Racism is "prejudice that generally includes adverse emotional reactions to members of a group, acceptance of negative stereotypes, and racial discrimination against individuals" (APA, n.d.). Although race is not a biologic reality, racism is a social reality resulting in status ranking, exploitation, discrimination, and social and economic inequality (Braveman et al., 2021a; Markus, 2008; Omi & Winant, 2015). Racism exists when there is power of ethnic groups through racialized policing, economic exclusion, and reduced access to mainstream institutions (Ray et al., 2017). Racism adversely affects the mental and physical health of millions, perpetuating disparities in social determinants and health outcomes among racial and ethnic minority groups compared with White Americans (CDC, 2023b).

A **minority group** is usually defined as a population living within a larger social group that is disadvantaged due to poverty or loss of control over their own lives. For instance, according to data from the US Census Bureau in 2021, the overall poverty rate stood at 11.5% (Creamer et al., 2022). However, certain demographic groups exhibit disproportionately higher poverty rates: American Indian and Alaska Natives (25%), Hispanic individuals (16.9%), and Black or African American communities (17.1%). In contrast, Whites and Asians experience lower poverty rates at 8.6% each (US Census Bureau, 2023e). An increasing body of research reveals that centuries of racism within the United States have negatively affected communities of color (CDC, 2023b; Macias-Konstantopoulos et al., 2023; USDHHS et al., 2022). Racial disparity deeply permeates our society, influencing residential areas, educational opportunities, employment prospects, religious practices, and recreational activities. Consequently, racism creates disparities in accessing various social and economic advantages, including housing, education, job opportunities, and access to health care. These social determinants of health play a significant role in exacerbating disparities within communities of color. Racial disparities have led to discrepancies in health care access and variations in health care quality among different demographics, ultimately contributing to health disparities experienced by many individuals (CDC, 2022; Hacker et al., 2022).

Culture, Values, and Value Orientation

Ethnicity is evidenced in customs that reflect the socialization and cultural patterns of the group. As an element of ethnicity, **culture** refers to "the languages, customs, beliefs, rules, arts, knowledge, and collective identities and memories developed by members of all social groups that make their social environments meaningful" (American Sociological Association, 2024).

Values are beliefs about the worth of something and serve as standards that influence behavior and thinking. Cultural values are distinctive expressions within a culture that are recognized as appropriate over time; they influence actions and decisions and support self-worth and self-esteem (Andrews & Boyle et al., 2024). Cultural values are integral to the ways in which individuals employ health behaviors, maintain their health, seek care for themselves and others, and decide where to go to receive care (Andrews & Boyle et al., 2024).

Value orientations are the dominant values shared by most of a group; these values are learned through socialization and reflect a particular society's personality type. Ethnic groups have unique beliefs, values, and attitudes about culture, health, and health care services influenced by their cultural backgrounds, experiences, and traditions (Box 2.2: Health and Social Determinants/Health Equity). Incongruent beliefs and attitudes about health and health care services among ethnic groups compared with the rest of the population, particularly health care providers, are major barriers to improving the health status of ethnic group members. Health care providers must acknowledge and adapt to the cultural values of diverse populations, recognizing how this understanding can enhance compassionate and effective care delivery. Exercising **cultural respect** is crucial for health care professionals to operate effectively in evolving multicultural environments and to ensure the provision of high-quality, safe care to all.

BOX 2.2 HEALTH AND SOCIAL DETERMINANTS/HEALTH EQUITY

Female Genital Mutilation/Cutting: Changing a Cultural Tradition

Female genital mutilation/cutting (FGM/C) is the partial or total removal, or injury, of external female genitalia for nonmedical reasons. The practice, which is customary in some settings as essential for marriage, is described by four major types depending on the amount of destruction of natural vaginal and genital tissue. Globally, approximately 200 million females in 31 countries have undergone this harmful practice with no health benefit, and it often results in immediate and/or long-term physical and mental health problems (Matanda et al., 2023; Callaghan, 2023). Negative health outcomes associated with FGM/C include urinary infections, fistulas, infertility, painful menstruation or sexual intercourse, difficult childbirth, increased neonatal death, a potential increase in the risk of HIV/AIDS infection, and many psychological symptoms and disorders (Matanda et al., 2023). The US government and the governments of most nations oppose all forms of FGM/C, which is often employed on young girls. It is estimated that in 2020, 4.1 million girls were at risk globally, and this is expected to rise given that educational efforts were suspended during the COVID-19 crisis, with more girls staying home and villages suffering economic downturns (Matanda et al., 2023). FGM/C is considered a human rights violation by the World Health Organization (WHO, n.d.-a). The WHO considers FGM/C a form of cruelty and torture. One of the WHO Sustainable Development Goals is for a global community ban of the practice by 2030 (WHO, 2020; Matanda et al., 2023), which now seems unrealistic given consequences of the COVID-19 pandemic.

In the United States, FGM/C is considered a form of gender-based violence as well as child abuse (US Department of State, n.d.). It is against US law to perform FGM/C on any female or send a female out of the United States to have FGM/C performed in another country. This crime is punishable by fines and prison terms regardless of the motivation (USCIS, 2024a).

Why does a practice that violates the basic human rights of adult and young females still occur in some countries? The presence of legal sanctions contributes to the production of conflict and silence between health care providers and families who continue to practice FGM/C. Even in countries that legally prohibit FGM/C, there are reports of parents feigning a holiday or vacation to the native country to have a young daughter circumcised. In almost all cases, the young female was not informed of what was to happen.

What are the care and public health implications for health care providers? Despite the illegality of the practice, US providers will encounter young and adult females who have undergone FGM/C. In the Callaghan (2023) report, it was noted in 2019 that up to 421,000 young and adult females in the United States had undergone or were at risk for FGM/C. This risk which has increased by 12.5% to 15% in recent years is accelerated mostly by immigration into the United States. The immigrant populations principally identified are Egyptian, Somali, Ethiopian, Nigerian, Indonesian, Sudanese, or Malay and are mostly from the horn of Africa. Three countries (Egypt, Ethiopia, Somalia) accounted for about 55% of the females, and 97% of the females came from Africa (PRB, 2016). States with the highest number of adult and young females at risk for FGM/C in 2019 were Minnesota, California, New York, Texas, Washington, and Virginia. The communities were assessed as being poorer and more urban than average in the United States. About 5500 adult and young females from Dawoodi Bohra communities are known to continue the practice. The greatest risk occurs to girls before kindergarten and in elementary school. As the number of African immigrants to the United States increases, the number of adult and young females at risk for FGM/C is expected to increase even more (Callaghan, 2023).

There are many barriers to access and provision of quality of care for this population. Midwives and nurses whose area of practice is females' health are most likely to see circumcised females. Some females who have experienced FGM/C may be too embarrassed to seek any needed care due to the altered appearance of their genitalia. Many health care providers may lack experience treating females with FGM/C; some procedures can be more difficult to perform due to altered anatomical landmarks.

In the short term, FGM/C can result in pain, bleeding, infection, problems with urination, transmission of HIV/AIDS, psychological trauma, and death. In the long term, it can result in chronic infections, childbirth problems, fistulas, keloids, sexual health problems, perinatal risks, and mental health problems (WHO, n.d.-a). It is recommended that discussions of any benefits of surgical correction or intervention be done with the partner or husband present as he may be the decision-maker. This could be included in birthing instruction classes if not discussed earlier. The use of female interpreters is highly recommended to avoid embarrassment of the females. Community outreach programs including antenatal and postnatal home care are pivotal in improving outcomes for females with FGM/C. Improving the health of adult and young females is a priority for international organizations promoting gender equality and higher standards of living. Modifying legislation to decrease the FGM/C practice may be helpful in communities that are already questioning its value. However, legislation alone has to consider context, as the practice may become more secret or more underground. Other interventions in use are education of health care providers, provision of rescue centers and safe houses, raising of community awareness with particular attention to young girls and mothers, and better formal education for girls. Since many of the influences that enforce the practice are historically and philosophically based, attention to alternative rites of passage without FGM may help to increase community ownership and cultural discharge of the practice (Matanda, 2023).

The practice of FGM/C is a violation of human rights and public health issue (WHO, n.d.-a). While health care providers must care for adult and young females in a culturally sensitive manner, they must also advocate for them through education, and outreach with the goal of eliminating this unnecessary and abusive practice.

Cultural and Linguistic Competency

Cultural and linguistic competency (CLAS) entails providing health care services that respect and respond to the diverse health beliefs, practices, and needs of patients, aiming to enhance service quality for all and reduce health disparities. National CLAS Standards (Think Cultural Health), developed by the USDHHS Office of Minority Health (OMH, n.d.), offer a comprehensive framework to guide individuals and health care organizations in implementing CLAS effectively. These standards are vital for advancing health equity, improving service quality, and addressing disparities. CLAS is crucial because culture and language significantly influence individuals' health, healing, wellness beliefs, illness perceptions, health care–seeking behaviors, and attitudes toward health care providers. Providers' own cultural perspectives may also affect service delivery. CLAS competency involves being respectful of and responsive to the health beliefs and health care needs of diverse populations, promoting effective and equitable care delivery (OMH, n.d.).

In health care, there is consensus that cultural competence is a method for addressing the diverse cultural backgrounds of patients, delivering patient-centered care, and mitigating health inequalities (Lekas et al., 2020). Although there is widespread agreement in health care fields about the elements and operational definition of cultural competence, there is no large body of evidence describing care recipient compliance, health status, equity, and quality of care as a result of provider cultural competence (Andrews & Boyle et al., 2024). Currently there is less focus on cultural competence and more focus on a dynamic and reflective approach embodied by **cultural humility** (Lekas et al., 2020). This approach involves ongoing self-evaluation, recognition of power imbalances, and a commitment to addressing systemic inequalities to improve professional practice and client outcomes (Lekas et al., 2020).

Researchers have established and retested the Cultural Competence Health Practitioner Assessment (CCHPA-67), which purports to determine levels of cultural and linguistic competence (Harris-Haywood et al., 2014). The 67-item questionnaire has three domains—knowledge, adapting practice, and promoting health—and has sound clinometric properties, including reliability and validity. The CCHPA-67 can be used to examine the effectiveness of interventions to increase cultural and linguistic competence of health care practitioners and the association between their level of competence and health care outcomes.

Jongen and colleagues (2018) conducted a systematic review of 64 studies reporting on cultural competency training interventions in the United States, New Zealand, Canada, and Australia. Overall, there were dissimilarities in the definition of *cultural competence* and a wide variety of interventions and areas of focus. Outcome reports also varied, with more related to practitioner outcomes and fewer related to health care or access outcomes. Authors of the various studies agreed that more work is needed to advance the knowledge and awareness created by cultural competence training toward behavioral and practical changes that result in improved health outcomes. Several of the studies used cultural categorization in education strategies, while several used a cross-cultural method. Interestingly, none of the studies reviewed discussed practitioner bias or issues of racism.

Discrimination in health care cannot be addressed without the inclusion of these topics in cultural competence training. Jongen and colleagues (2018) suggest that, although cultural categorization is often used to teach cultural competency strategies, this may be counterproductive due to the creation of stereotyping and oversimplification of the challenges faced by **vulnerable populations** when intergroup variability is not considered. In addition, it is important to explore the effects of intersectionality on health care equity. **Intersectionality** refers to the overlapping categorization of race, sex, and gender and the resulting interdependent systems of discrimination and disadvantage. For the purpose of giving students a basic understanding of different cultural approaches to health care, we use categorization in this chapter and strive to draw attention to some important areas of intersectionality.

IMMIGRANTS/REFUGEES

Immigrants (authorized and unauthorized) and **refugees** experience health care inequities in the United States (Gelatt & Zong, 2018). In the United States, **immigrants** include all foreign-born residents. Unauthorized immigrants are those who entered the country without inspection or stayed beyond the limits of a temporary permit. The Immigration and Nationality Act originally legislated in 1954 and adjusted many times since, defines legal entry into the United States and the process for obtaining citizenship (Pew Research Center, 2024; US Citizenship and Immigration Services [USCIS], 2024b). In 2023, there were 12.68 million lawful permanent residents in the US, of which 9.04 million were eligible to naturalize (Miller & Baker, 2023). For those eligible to naturalize, the most common countries of origin included Mexico (2.39 million), China (550,000), Cuba (390,000), Dominican Republic (390,000), Philippines (350,000), India (290,000), Vietnam (230,000), El Salvador (220,000), Canada (220,000), and Korea (200,000). Most lived in California (2.2 million), followed by New York (1.15 million), Texas (980,000), Florida (880,000), and New Jersey (380,000). The majority were female (51.2%), were between the ages of 35 and 64 (57.0%), and entered the country before 2009 (66.6%) (Miller & Baker, 2023).

A **refugee** is an immigrant who is unwilling or unable to return to their country of origin due to "persecution or a well-founded fear of persecution on account of race, religion, nationality, membership in a particular social group, or political opinion" (USCIS, 2024b). After September 11, 2001, there was a sharp decline in refugee admission to fewer than 30,000 due to policy and security changes. Entries peaked again at 84,988 in 2016 followed by a sharp decline to 22,405 in 2018 (Mossaad, 2019). Refugee arrivals were suspended during parts of 2019 and 2020 due to the COVID-19 pandemic and policy changes to limit its spread, which included travel restrictions and closure of the USCIS offices to the public (Baugh, 2022). The most common countries of origin for refugees admitted from 2013 to 2022 included (in rank order): Burma, Democratic Republic of Congo, Iraq, Somalia, Bhutan, Syria, Ukraine, Iran, Eritrea, and Afghanistan (Gibson, 2023). There is some indication that net refugee levels and immigration has returned to pre-COVID levels (US Census Bureau, 2024).

The immigrant population in the United States is racially and ethnically diverse, and each immigrant group faces a unique set of disparities. Immigrants may experience a decline in economic stability and social support along with cultural and language barriers. For refugees, there is the added trauma resulting from experiences of displacement, abuse, violence, brutality, extreme poverty, and religious persecution (see Box 2.2). All these disparities lead to inequity in health care. Although some degree of medical coverage is available to immigrants who meet specific criteria, it is important to remember that many will be unable to effectively navigate the health care system due to language, cultural, and literacy barriers; lack of transportation; and fear/mistrust of the system. When the political climate and policies become more restrictive toward immigration, many immigrants may decline medical care and coverage, despite eligibility, out of fear of deportation (Kaiser Family Foundation, 2024).

Health Issues of Immigrants/Refugees

In the current political climate in the United States, health care workers have noted an increase in immigrant mental health conditions, including anxiety and depression. In addition, these families and individuals are facing increasing economic challenges due to ineligibility for medical coverage or fear of accessing available coverage. Disenrollment from Medicaid due to fear of deportation has led to gaps in care and an increased burden on nonprofit organizations and local governments (Artiga & Pham, 2019; Hill et al., 2023).

Depending upon their country of origin and individual circumstances, immigrants may face a number of acute and chronic health conditions, including infectious diseases such as tuberculosis or parasite infections, posttraumatic stress disorder, depression, diabetes, and hypertension (USDHHS, 2023).

Strategies to Reduce Health Disparities in Immigrant/Refugee Populations

The CDC has comprehensive, evidence-based guidelines for refugee health assessments. The guidelines are both general and population specific and include recommendations to a) promote and improve refugee health, b) prevent disease, and c) familiarize refugees with the US health care system. However, many health care providers who encounter newly arrived refugees lack training in population-specific illnesses, access to an interpreter, and familiarity with refugee customs and religions. These challenges, along with competing priorities during resettlement, including obtaining work and housing, often lead to suboptimal delivery of health care (Hollberg et al., n.d.). To address challenges in immigrant health care, organizations in the San Francisco Bay Area and San Diego recommend cross-sector partnerships with an emphasis on education, school-level intervention, and legal assistance. Providers suggest that a wrap-around model is most effective at meeting the multifaceted needs of immigrants (Artiga & Pham, 2019; Hill et al., 2023).

In a disaster, immigrants are one of the most vulnerable populations in the United States because of language barriers and unfamiliarity with US resources and disaster protocols. The USDHHS has published an emergency preparedness booklet in refugee languages to assist health care providers with the provision of emergency services. Numerous videos are also available for immigrants addressing health issues particular to their immigrant community. Examples include Emotional Wellness and Suicide Prevention for Bhutanese Refugees, Getting and Staying Well for Congolese Refugees, and Somali Refugee Women: Learn About Your Health. Refugees who are survivors of torture may be eligible for financial assistance in the form of grants through the Office of Refugee Resettlement (USDHHS, 2023).

FOLK HEALING AND NURSING CARE SYSTEMS

Within many cultural and/or ethnic customs and traditions, each group has a healing system that incorporates the beliefs and practices deemed essential in maintaining and restoring health. Three components of these healing systems are self-care, **nurse care systems**, and **folk healing systems** (Boyle et al., 2024). Nurse care is characterized by specialized education; advanced knowledge, skills, and abilities; responsibility; and expectation of remuneration of services provided (Boyle et al., 2024). A folk healing system embodies the beliefs, values, and treatment approaches of a particular cultural group that are products of cultural development. Folk health practices are seen in a variety of settings, including community groups, kinship groups, private homes, and healers' shrines. Unlicensed practitioners such as lay midwives, bone setters, and herbalists are part of the folk sector, as are religious practitioners such as spiritualists, Christian Scientists, and scientologists.

The choice of a health care system differs among ethnic groups and among individuals within the same group. Ethnic individuals' preference for their folk healing systems is motivated by their familiarity with the folk healer, who usually speaks the same language and is knowledgeable about the beliefs, customs, and traditions of the ethnic group. Easy access and the individual's ability to pay for the healer's services are real advantages when compared with the difficulty of getting appointments, enduring long waits, and dealing with unfamiliar institutional settings in the professional care system. Despite ongoing developments in treatments provided by **professional care systems**, many folk healing practices maintain their popularity. When folk healing practices are not effective, the individual may, as a last resort, turn to the professional care system.

The Andrews/Boyle Transcultural Interprofessional Practice (TIP) model is a model that guides the interprofessional health care team in a process that includes all of the individuals a care recipient may want to have on their health care team. Team members may include credentialed professionals, folk and religious healers, and even pets. The TIP model provides a best-practice framework for care that is evidence based, culturally competent, and culturally respectful (Andrews & Boyle, 2019). Nurses must avoid an ethnocentric perspective when working with ethnic groups. An **ethnocentric perspective**, which views other ways as inferior, unnatural, or even barbaric, can serve as a major obstacle in establishing and maintaining good working relationships with consumers of health care services. Some ethnic groups will continue to use folk remedies and healing. Therefore, nurses need to appreciate the many positive aspects of folk systems. A caring, holistic approach that incorporates family and support systems and considers the individual's viewpoint is one of the more positive aspects of folk systems. This approach is receiving recognition by the professional care system. A blend of both systems would optimize health care for ethnic Americans who also use folk systems.

ARAB AMERICANS

Arab Americans came to the United States from the Middle East and Northern Africa (MENA) regions in three immigration waves. The first wave of immigrants, who came between the late 1800s and World War I, were mostly from Greater Syria. The second wave came after the end of World War II and included many Muslims and refugees displaced by the 1948 Palestine War. The last wave occurred in the 1960s and consisted of many professionals, entrepreneurs, and skilled and semiskilled laborers (Amer, 2023).

The 2000 US census was a milestone survey because, for the first time, it recognized Arab Americans as a separate ethnic group. Anyone from the following countries was considered to be of Arab ancestry: Algeria, Bahrain, Egypt, United Arab Emirates, Iraq, Jordan, Kuwait, Lebanon, Libya, Morocco, Oman, Palestine, Qatar, Saudi Arabia, Syria, Tunisia, and Yemen.

The MENA immigrant population in the United States increased from 223,000 in 1980 to 1,167,000 in 2016 (Cumoletti & Batalova, 2018). Immigration upticks largely resulted from instability in war-torn countries such as Syria and Yemen. The Trump administration passed a series of executive orders in 2017 restricting immigration from several Muslim-majority countries, resulting in a significant reduction in MENA-region admissions. For example, Syrian arrivals fell from approximately 15,500 immigrants in 2016 to approximately 3000 in 2017 (Cumoletti & Batalova, 2018).

The largest groups (in rank order) of Arab Americans are Lebanese, Egyptians, Syrians, Iraqi, Palestinians, and Moroccans (Arab American Institute, 2024). Arab Americans live in all 50 states, but one-third of them live in California, Michigan, and New York. Approximately 94% of Arab Americans live in metropolitan areas. The top five metropolitan areas of Arab-American concentration are Los Angeles, Detroit, New York City, Chicago, and Washington, DC (Arab American Institute, 2024). Arab Americans from some countries are most highly represented in specific areas; Lebanese Americans are the majority of Arab Americans living in Rhode Island; Egyptian Americans are the largest Arab group in New Jersey; Palestinian Americans are the majority in Illinois; and Iraqi and Assyrian/Chaldean Americans concentrate in Illinois, Michigan, and California (Arab American Institute, 2024). Three major religions represented among Arab Americans are Christianity, Islam, and Judaism. More than 45% of Arab Americans have a bachelor's degree or higher, compared with 28% of Americans at large. Approximately 18% of Arab Americans have a postgraduate degree, which is nearly twice the American average (10%). Despite being better educated on average than both foreign-born and US-born residents, MENA immigrants are less likely to be employed. In 2015, 27% of MENA immigrant families lived in poverty compared with 17% of other immigrant families and 14% of US-born families. MENA immigrants were uninsured at a rate of 12% in 2016 compared with 9% of US citizens and 20% of other immigrants (Cumoletti & Batalova, 2018). Other statistical data and information on Arab Americans can be found at the website of the Arab American Institute (http://www.aaiusa.org/).

Health Care Issues of Arab Americans

Arab Americans as a group are very diverse with disparate socioeconomic profiles. For example, some MENA immigrants come from war-torn countries with a high level of poverty, and others are affluent and well educated (Abuelezam et al., 2018). In addition, Arab Americans are asked to identify as White or are reclassified as White by the US census (United States Department of Commerce, 2018), making it difficult for researchers to accurately apply ethnic and racial identifiers to this group. These issues contribute to challenges of the current literature in describing disparities and health inequities faced by Arab Americans at large (Abuelezam et al., 2018).

In a recent review including 247 studies, Abuelezam and colleagues (2018) provide an updated summary of public health literature for the Arab-American population. An important health issue on the rise among Arab-American adolescents is tobacco consumption, which is a major risk factor for many health problems affecting the respiratory and cardiovascular systems. Tobacco use has been linked to a higher rate of chronic health problems such as heart disease, hypertension, and diabetes among Arab Americans than among non–Middle Eastern Whites (Abuelezam et al., 2018). Tobacco can be consumed in many ways; however, tobacco chewing, cigarette smoking, and use of a shisha (water pipe) are the three major methods used to consume tobacco products. Arabs, both males and females, have long traditions of using a water pipe and smoking cigarettes with their friends and families and at other social gatherings. Current water pipe use has been better predicted by Arab ethnicity and a lower educational level. The water pipe seems to increase the addictive properties of tobacco and increase barriers to cessation for Arab Americans. Arab Americans have a high rate of smoking and a low cessation rate compared with non-Hispanic Whites. Abuelezam and colleagues (2018) found that smoking behaviors correlated negatively with time spent in the United States. In a cross-sectional descriptive study, Ghadban and colleagues (2019) found that having a higher perception of cancer-risk severity was predictive of willingness to cease tobacco consumption.

Hypertension is a major health problem among Arab Americans. Prevention and treatment strategies are urgently needed for this population. Tailakh and colleagues (2012) examined the awareness, treatment, and control of hypertension among Arab Americans. The prevalence of hypertension was high, with 36.5% of the sample having hypertension and 39.7% being prehypertensive. Of those with hypertension, only 67.4% were aware of their condition and only 52.2% were taking antihypertensive medication. Other significant findings included a higher prevalence in males than in females and a higher body mass index in those with hypertension compared with normotensive participants. In a subsequent study (Tailakh et al., 2016), researchers examined the relationship between acculturation, medication adherence, lifestyle behaviors, and blood pressure control among 46 Arab Americans with hypertension. Only 29.2% of the participants reported adhering to their medication regimen. Those who adhered to their medication regimen were more acculturated, were more physically active, and had better blood pressure control.

Mental health along with the role of resident status is an ongoing health concern for Arab Americans. Pampati and colleagues (2018) compared depression and anxiety levels in Arab Americans who were immigrants, refugees, or US born. All groups of Arab-American residents had high levels of depression and anxiety. Refugees had significantly higher levels of depression and anxiety than other immigrants, and refugees had significantly higher levels of depression but not anxiety than US-born residents. Residents who cited political violence or religious persecution as their reason for coming to the United States suffered the highest levels of depression and anxiety. Mental health counselors need to be aware of and consider these factors when helping Arab-American individuals. Many Arab Americans seek their immediate and extended family, community, and traditional values or cultural practices for help during a health crisis. Consequently, given the unique nature of mental illness, many Arab Americans do not receive professional mental health attention when it is needed.

Access to culturally suitable and current care is essential, yet many barriers exist that prevent Arab Americans from using professional care services. Discrimination of Muslims, or "Islamophobia," since 9/11 has further contributed to physical and mental health disparities in the United States and the United Kingdom (Karipek, 2020). Additional barriers include religious beliefs and practices; cultural norms relating to modesty; desire to uphold family reputation; gender issues, such as preference for a same-sex health care provider; use of folk remedies; and stresses of assimilation and acculturation, such as a lack of English skills. There are also barriers related to health care providers, including a lack of culturally competent services, stereotyping, and discrimination (Boyle et al., 2024).

Selected Health-Related Cultural Aspects

Arabs value the family and the ties it maintains; therefore, the extended family, a clan, and a tribe are common kinship groups. Customs center on hospitality around food, family, and friends (Boyle et al., 2024). Arab-American families are, on average, larger than non–Arab American families and smaller than families in Arab countries. According to the American Community Survey (Asi & Beaulieu, 2013), the average size of an Arab-American household was 2.93 people, compared with the national average of 2.59 people. Yemeni averaged more than 4 people per household, and Palestinian, Jordanian, and Iraqi averaged more than 3 people per household. Traditionally, more children meant more pride and economic contributors for the family. However, the cost of having large families in the United States and adaptation to American customs seems to encourage smaller families. Religion plays an important part in Arab culture, and there are dietary rules and prescribed rituals for praying and washing. In addition, Arab Americans tend to be present oriented and view the future as uncertain (Boyle et al., 2024; Callender et al., 2022).

ASIAN AMERICANS

Asian Americans represent people from over 50 countries, making their origins, cultures, lifestyles, and religions quite diverse (Fig. 2.1). For example, more than 800 languages and dialects are spoken among the Asian-American population. According to the OMB, "'Asian' refers to a person having origins in any of the original peoples of the Far East, Southeast Asia, or the Indian subcontinent," and "the Asian population includes people who indicated their race(s) as 'Asian' or reported entries such as 'Asian Indian,' 'Chinese,' 'Filipino,' 'Korean,' 'Japanese,' and 'Vietnamese' or reported other detailed Asian responses" during the last census survey (Hoeffel et al., 2012, p. 2). Based on 2020 population estimates from the US census (2020), the number of residents who identify as Asian alone is 19.9 million, or 6.0% of the total US population. The Asian-alone population grew by 35.5% between 2010 and 2020 (in 2010 the Asian-alone population was 14.7 million, or 4.8% of the population). Another 4.1 million people identify as Asian in combination with another race (US Census Bureau, 2022b). In 2020, the five largest Asian-alone groups were Asian Indian (4.4 million); Chinese, except Taiwanese (4.1 million); Filipino (3.1 million); Vietnamese (2.0 million); and Korean (1.5 million). When examining Asian alone or in any combination, Chinese, except Taiwanese, is the

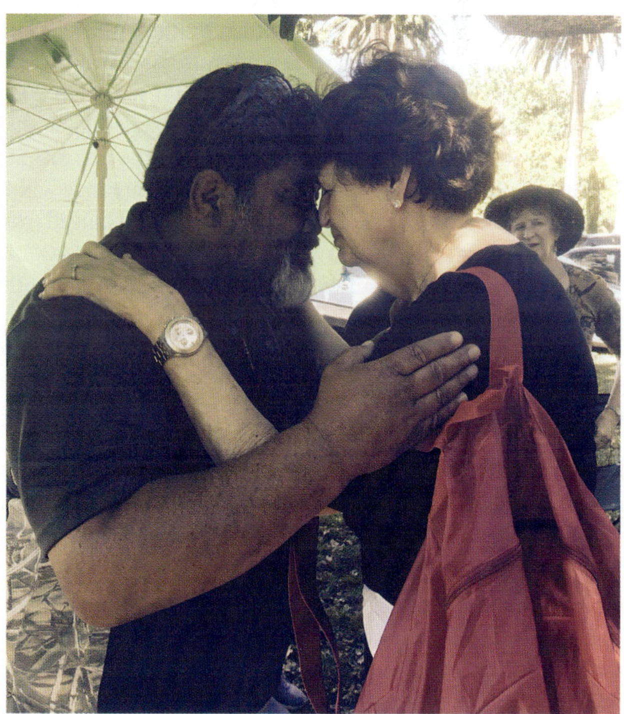

FIG. 2.1 One cultural norm of the Maori in New Zealand is to say goodbye by rubbing noses.

largest group, followed by Asian Indian, Filipino, Vietnamese, and Korean (US Census Bureau, 2023a, 2023b).

According to the Pew Research Center (Budiman & Ruiz, 2021), from 2000 to 2019 the average population growth of Asian Americans slowed—3.9% from 2000 to 2005, 3.1% from 2005 to 2010, 3.1% from 2010 to 2015, and 2.4% from 2015 to 2019—but the Asian-American population still had one of the highest growth rates of any group. During this period, the number of people reporting as Asian grew by 81%, from 10.5 million to 18.8 million, and their population is projected to exceed 27 million by 2040 and 35 million by 2060. Between 2000 and 2019, the Asian-American population increased in every state and the District of Columbia. California (5.9 million, or 14.9% of its population) is the state with the largest Asian population, followed by New York (1.7 million, or 8.8%), Texas (1.5 million, or 5.0%), New Jersey (870,000, or 9.8%), and Illinois (731,000, or 5.8%). Hawaii has the highest proportion of people that identify as Asian alone (37.2%), Asian in combination (19.4%), or Asian alone or in combination (56.6%) in the United States and is the only state with an Asian-American majority population (US Census Bureau, n.d.).

Asian Americans are often referred to as a "model minority"; this stereotype is frequently accepted because most Asian Americans are viewed as successful, resilient, hardworking, intelligent, and healthy. Education is highly valued among many Asian communities. According to reports from the US Census Bureau (2022a), Asian Americans have the highest percentage of college graduates of any racial or ethnic group. Approximately 54% of Asian American adults aged 25 and older have a bachelor's degree or higher level of education, compared with 32.5% of the total population in the United States. However, there is a wide range within the Asian population: 15% of Bhutanese have a bachelor's degree or higher, while 75% of Indians have that same level of educational attainment (Budiman & Ruiz, 2021). A look at the status of Asian Americans as a group reveals that they are doing relatively well in the United States. For instance, in 2022, the Asian median family income of $108,700 was higher than all other groups, while the national median income was $74,580 (Guzman & Kollar, 2022). Again, there was a wide range within the Asian population: the median household income ranged from $44,400 (Burmese) to $119,000 (Indian) (Budiman & Ruiz, 2021). In addition, Asian Americans were tied with White alone for the lowest poverty rate (8.6%) in 2022, while the national poverty rate was 11.5%. At the same time, the share living in poverty ranged from 6% (Indian) to 25% (Burmese and Mongolian) (Budiman & Ruiz, 2021).

Health Care Issues of Asian Americans

Health care issues of Asian Americans are related to their ethnicity, religion, and status as immigrants. Some Asian-American immigrants have carried diseases from their home countries, and they also experience new diseases in the United States because of their new lifestyle and living conditions. As a separate population, their risk of heritable disease can be studied (Box 2.3: Genomics). However, Asian Americans have among the highest life expectancies. The projected life expectancy for

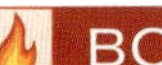

BOX 2.3 GENOMICS

Presence of the APOEε4 gene and cognitive impairment

The APOEε4 gene variant (apolipoprotein E) is an important risk for the development of Alzheimer disease and other types of cognitive impairment. A study (Jin et al., 2021) of 6160 Chinese individuals from a Chinese Longitudinal Healthy Longevity Survey commenced in 1998, with intermittent follow-up studies. Healthy lifestyle behaviors were stratified into three levels, and the behaviors categorized included smoking, alcohol consumption, diet, physical activity, and body weight. Presence of the APOEε4 gene variant (17.5% of the study population and the other more common "healthy" APOE variants) were compared with lifestyle profiles and degrees of cognitive impairment. All members of the study population were over the age of 80. No interaction between the APOEε4 gene type and lifestyle profiles was detected, probably because much of the lifestyle information was self-reported, and the body weight of the study population was less than many other country/global vulnerable comparison groups (Jin et al., 2021). However, the study pointed out that quantifying lifestyle factors and genetic risk for cognitive functioning may be valuable as more countries/global populations have larger segments of aged individuals. Care requirements are more complicated in aged individuals with memory or cognitive impairment.

Asians in 2020 was 80.7 years for both sexes, 78.4 years for males, and 82.7 years for females. The projected life expectancy for Asians in 2060 increases to 86.0 years for both sexes, 84.5 years for males, and 87.4 years for females. Despite often having less disease and better health outcomes, Asian Americans still face various factors that threaten their health. These factors include "infrequent medical visits, language and cultural barriers, and lack of health insurance" (OMH, n.d.-a, n.d.-b).

One study found that Asian Americans had the highest rate of health care–associated infections compared with other racial and ethnic groups admitted to hospitals for cardiovascular disease, pneumonia, and major surgery (Bakullari et al., 2014). Language barriers between care recipients and providers were discussed as a possible explanation for these findings. In general, Asian Americans have a range of health problems similar to those of the US population overall (Guzman & Kollar, 2022). From 2018 to 2021, cancer, heart disease, COVID-19, stroke, and unintentional injuries were the top-five leading causes of death among Asian-American adults (WISQARS, 2021). From 2016 to 2020, Asian and Pacific Islanders (290.3 per 100,000) had the lowest rate of cancer compared with all other races and ethnicities (CDC, 2023). Note that the CDC combines data from Asians and Pacific Islanders when reporting cancer statistics. The two most common new cancer cases for all races and ethnicities were breast cancer for females (127.0 per 100,000) and prostate cancer for males (110.5 per 100,000). Asian and Pacific Islander females (101.1 new cases per 100,000) were less likely to have breast cancer than White females (133.3). Asian and Pacific Islander females (11.7 deaths per 100,000) were also less likely to die from breast cancer compared with White females (19.7). Similarly, Asian and Pacific Islander males (57.0 new cases per 100,000) were less likely to have prostate cancer than White males (105.0). Asian and Pacific Islander males (8.6 deaths per 100,000) were also less likely to die from prostate cancer compared with White males (17.8) (CDC, 2023).

Asian Americans also have a high prevalence of and risk factors for chronic obstructive pulmonary disease, hepatitis B, HIV/AIDS, smoking, tuberculosis, and liver disease (OMH, n.d.-a). In general, Asian Americans have lower rates of being overweight and having hypertension and are less likely to be current cigarette users compared with White adults. In 2018, Asian cases accounted for approximately 2% of the total HIV/AIDS population in the United States, and from 2014 through 2018, the rate of diagnoses of HIV infection in adults and adolescents among Asian Americans decreased (CDC, 2020a).

Racial and ethnic minority populations, and especially Asian Americans, are disproportionately affected by tuberculous disease (CDC, 2020b). In 2019, Asian Americans had the second-highest rate (16.7 per 100,000) of tuberculosis compared with all other races (American Indian/Alaska Native = 3.4, Black = 4.3, Native Hawaiian/Pacific Islander = 17.6, and White = 0.5). On a more positive note, the rate of tuberculosis in Asian Americans has steadily decreased since 2003, when the rate was 42.2 per 100,000 (CDC, 2020b).

Disparities in the health status of Asian Americans are primarily a result of subcultures within the larger group. There are many divergent and segregated cultures within the Asian population, yet Asian ethnic groups are often classified and viewed as one homogenous, aggregate group. In 2019, approximately 57% of the Asian-American population was foreign born, which was much higher than the overall immigrant share of 14% in the United States (Budiman & Ruiz, 2021). In fact, by 2055, Asian Americans are projected to be the largest immigrant group, surpassing Hispanics (Budiman & Ruiz, 2021). Within the Asian population there is a wide range of percent foreign born, from 27% for Japanese to 85% for Bhutanese and Malaysian (Budiman & Ruiz, 2021). Furthermore, 30.9% of Asian Americans are not fluent in English, and 73.5% speak a language other than English at home. The classification and cultural barriers (such as language) limit public awareness and restrain effective and culturally and linguistically appropriate disease prevention for subgroups of the Asian American population.

Unfortunately, few studies have focused on Asian Americans, and even fewer researchers have examined individual subgroups, which has created a generalized and inaccurate picture of the experience and needs of Asian Americans in the United States. The heterogeneity of subgroups of this population and their relatively small representation in the total US population make it challenging to have sufficient and representative samples from Asian Americans. Information about health status among the different Asian subgroups is extremely limited; more studies are needed to fully understand their specific health issues.

Selected Health-Related Cultural Aspects

Asian Americans share many traditional values. A comprehensive description of traditional values in several Asian groups indicates commonalities and differences (Boyle et al., 2024). The central family and the extended family has significant influence on Asian Americans. Although family dynamics and structure differ across subgroups, the family is often the major source of functional and psychological support for Asian Americans. Usually, the interests and honor of the family are more important than those of individual family members. Older family members are typically respected and have authority that is often unquestioned. For instance, among Filipinos, calling older people by their first names is a sign of disrespect. Male friends of one's parents or grandparents are addressed as "tito" (uncle) followed by the first name. For female friends, it is "tita" (aunt). These terms, denoting respect, have been substituted for Filipino terms that do not have English translations.

In Asian-American cultures, the oldest male family member is often the decision-maker and spokesperson for the family. Maintaining harmony is an important value in Asian cultures, and avoiding conflict and direct confrontation is strongly emphasized. Authorities and professionals are usually respected in the Asian-American communities. In most cases, physicians and their recommendations are powerful and highly respected and valued. However, as a result of respect for authorities, Asian-American care recipients may avoid showing their disagreements with the recommendations of health care professionals. Health care providers should recognize that a lack of disagreement with a recommended treatment or therapy does not mean that Asian-American care recipients and their families agree with or will abide by the recommendation. However, there is a generation of Asian Americans born in the United States who do not necessarily adhere to these cultural behaviors.

The rates of psychological distress among some Asian Americans are similar to those in the general US population, but Asian Americans tend to be the least likely of all race and ethnic groups to seek mental health services. A variety of factors related to cultural values, such as the cultural impact of shame, stigma, and language barriers, may contribute to less utilization of mental health services by Asian Americans (Africa & Carrasco, 2011). Asian cultures believe that the behavior of the individual reflects on the family; therefore, mental illness or any behavior that indicates a lack of self-control is viewed as producing shame and guilt in the family. Consequently, Asian Americans may be reluctant to discuss symptoms of mental illness or depression. Although the suicide rate among the Asian American population is only half the rate of the non-Hispanic White population, among Asian Americans aged 15 to 24, it was the leading cause of death in 2017; Asian-American female students (grades 9 to 12) were 20% more likely to attempt suicide than non-Hispanic White female students (OMH, n.d.-c).

In addition to reduced access to mental health care, the culture and values of Asian Americans are associated with other health problems and risk factors that threaten health and act as barriers to accessing other health care services. For example, sexually related issues may be taboo topics and considered a private matter that should not be discussed with anyone other than the spouse. Females may feel embarrassed to discuss sex, visit physician clinics for sexually related health issues, or receive some forms of physical examinations (e.g., Papanicolaou test). Such fears have prohibited the willingness of Asian Americans to access health care services and prevented health care providers from approaching this population for interventions. For example, the reluctance to discuss sexual issues was identified as one of the key barriers making it difficult for health care providers to approach Chinese-American youths for HIV/AIDS prevention (Lee, Slaman, & Wang, 2012).

A different, but perhaps related, issue is hindrances to health research participation by Asian Americans. Although Asian Americans make up about 5% of the US population, they are underrepresented in research studies. Common barriers to participation were reported as competing demands, unintended outcomes, and lack of information about informed consent, which could be related to language barriers or a lack of translated materials or translators. A 2019 study concluded that a lack of trust by individuals of Asian descent was probably most due to language barriers (Liu et al., 2019).

Many people find the task of parenthood in a new country difficult because some of their cultural values conflict with the mainstream cultural values; for example, passivity to avoid conflict compared with assertiveness. Exposure of children to different cultures in schools and in their neighborhood facilitates their adoption of other cultural beliefs and attitudes in their socialization. In addition, the employment of immigrant females outside the home exposes their children to other caretakers. Grandparents are often the caretakers of young grandchildren.

Asian folk medicine and philosophies have a strong Chinese influence as a result of early Chinese migration throughout Asia; therefore, folk medicine practices of Filipinos, Japanese, Koreans, and Southeast Asians are all infused with Chinese principles. **Taoism** was the philosophical and theoretical foundation of Chinese medicine. The "Tao" is rooted in the idea of balancing natural processes and forces (such as yin and yang) and is closely related to Asians' activities of daily living, including traditional health practices such as acupuncture, holistic medicine, herbalism, meditation, and martial arts. According to Tao doctrine, humans are microcosms within the universe. Achieving harmony between the two is essential because the energies of both intertwine. **Yin** and **yang** are the two forces that keep innate energy, called **chi**, and sexual energy, called **jing**, in balance. **Yin** is feminine, negative, dark, and cold; **yang** is masculine, positive, light, and warm. An imbalance in energy can be caused, for instance, by yielding to strong emotions or eating an improper diet. In their interactions, humans and the universe are both susceptible to the elements of earth, fire, water, metal, and wood (Boyle et al., 2024).

Asian folk medicine uses a wide variety of herbs for healing purposes, including roots, leaves, seeds, tree bark, and parts of flowers. Some aspects of Asian folk medicine have gained popularity within the professional care system. In general, the use or nonuse of healing traditions seems to be consistent with how closely Asians identify with their heritage (Tashiro, 2006). Of these healing traditions, one of the best known is acupuncture (Boyle et al., 2024). Similar alternative treatment modalities that are slowly gaining wide acceptance include meditation, therapeutic touch, massage, imagery, relaxation, and bipolarity. Chapter 14 discusses the use of **complementary, alternative, and integrative medicine** in the United States.

NATIVE HAWAIIANS AND OTHER PACIFIC ISLANDERS

Native Hawaiians and Other Pacific Islanders (NHPIs) refers to people having Hawai'i, Guam, Samoa, or other Pacific Islands as origins (US Census Bureau, 2023b), specifically including people who "are the descendants of the original inhabitants of the Pacific regions known as Polynesia (e.g., Tonga, Samoa, and Hawai'i), Melanesia (e.g., Fiji and Vanuatu), and Micronesia (e.g., Guam and Chuuk)" (Kaholokula et al., 2019, p. 198). In addition to the state of Hawai'i, which encompasses the Hawaiian archipelago, there are inhabited US Flag Territories in the Pacific regions, including American Samoa, the Commonwealth of the Northern Mariana Islands, and Guam. Unlike states and Native American tribes, territories are not sovereign entities; instead, they are subnational administrative divisions overseen by the US government. The Pacific Island territories are part of the larger US-Affiliated Pacific Islands (USAPI). The USAPI also include the Freely Associated States of the Republic of Palau, the Republic of the Marshall Islands, and the Federated States of Micronesia, consisting of Yap, Chuuk, Pohnpei, and Kosrae; the Freely Associated States are independent, sovereign nations that share a special compact relationship with the United States (Pacific Island Health Officers Association, n.d.). The Compacts of Free Association (COFA) are international agreements that govern the relationships between the United States and the Freely Associated States, such as offering these nations economic provisions from the United States, including eligibility for some US federal programs, in exchange for providing military provisions to the United States, including operating rights in the Pacific. There are more than 500,000 inhabitants of the USAPI, living on hundreds of islands and atolls spread across the vast Pacific Ocean. The USAPI cross five time zones and are located north and south of the equator. There is much linguistic and cultural diversity in the USAPI, with more than a dozen spoken languages, but the indigenous peoples of these islands comprise a relatively small population (Pacific Island Health Officers Association, n.d.).

In the United States, approximately 1.7 million people identified as NHPI (alone or in combination) in 2018, representing approximately 0.45% of the total population (US Census Bureau, 2023d). Native Hawaiians, the indigenous population of Hawai'i, make up the majority of the NHPI population in the United States (680,353); followed by Samoans (243,682), the indigenous population of Samoa or Western Samoa; and Guamanians or Chamorros (142,516), the indigenous population of Guam (US Census Bureau, 2023). Approximately 367,000 NHPIs live in Hawaii, with California and Washington also having sizable NHPI populations (OMH, n.d.-d). Although Native Hawaiians are indigenous people, they do not have the same self-governance rights as American Indians or Alaska Natives (AIANs). In 1997, the "Asian or Pacific Islander" race category was split into two categories, "Asian" and "Native Hawaiian and Pacific Islander," and since then, federal agencies have been required to report statistics that describe the Asian American and NHPI populations separately (Galinsky et al., 2017).

According to 2017 reports from US census information, NHPIs fall behind non-Hispanic Whites in education attainment and economic measures. For example, in 2017, 89.4% of NHPIs had attained at least a high school diploma compared with 92.9% of Whites, 23.3% of NHPIs had attained at least a bachelor's degree compared with 35.8% of Whites, and 6.9% of NHPIs had attained a graduate degree compared with 13.8% of Whites (OMH, n.d.-d). Regarding economics, in 2017, the median household income for NHPIs was $60,734 compared with $65,845 for non-Hispanic White households; 15.4% of NHPIs were living at the poverty level compared with 9.6% of Whites; and the unemployment rate for NHPIs was 5.8% compared with 4.2% for Whites (OMH, n.d.-d). Many NHPIs live in the continental United States (on the mainland), and these numbers are growing. There are approximately as many Native Hawaiians living off-island as there are living in Hawai'i, and more recent figures indicate that 25% of NHPI individuals aged 25 and older had bachelor's degrees and 89.9% had high school diplomas, with military veterans accounting for 6.8% (US Census Bureau, 2023b). "Off-islander demographics have some impact on economic access to health care, yet many of cultural practices related to community and family responsibility are highly valued by Native Hawaiians [who live] in Southern California" and other parts of the country (McMullin et al., 2010, p. 54). Research on NHPI health tends to focus on NHPIs living in Hawai'i, but because as many NHPIs live off-island, their specific health needs and concerns must be considered as well, especially in states with large concentrations of NHPIs, such as California. The NHPI population is also younger; 31.2% of NHPIs are younger than 18 compared with 18.8% of the non-Hispanic White population (OMH, n.d.-d). The Native Hawaiian population is ethnically diverse and growing at a fast rate, especially the population of preschool- and school-age children.

Native Hawaiians/Pacific Islander Health Issues

Identifying specific health issues and needs of NHPIs has been limited by insufficient disaggregated data on demographics and health. Unfortunately, "in the 20 years since [the Asian and NHPI race categories were separated], the body of NHPI health statistics has hardly grown. Even the largest health surveys have struggled to obtain an adequate NHPI sample to calculate reliable NHPI statistics" (Galinsky et al., 2017, p. 3). Despite decades of work on disaggregating NHPI data, these omissions have led to NHPIs being largely missing from US public health discourse. This lack of information has also contributed to the inability of NHPIs to advocate for resources for themselves (Morey et al., 2022). To attempt to address this gap, the National Center for Health Statistics conducted the Native Hawaiian and Pacific Islander National Health Interview Survey (NHPI NHIS) in 2014 (Galinsky et al., 2017). Among its key findings, the NHPI NHIS found that NHPIs living in the United States were less likely to report excellent or very good health (61.4%) compared with the overall population (67.3%); yet there were differences in health among the NHPI detailed race groups, highlighting the diversity found in the NHPI population (Galinsky et al., 2017). Lack of resources caused by gaps in statistical data also affected the response to COVID-19 for NHPI populations (Morey et al., 2022).

Pre-Western contact, NHPIs had healthy, thriving populations. Currently, NHPIs have higher rates of obesity, smoking, and alcohol consumption compared with other ethnic groups; they also have less access to cancer prevention and control groups (OMH, n.d.-d). Leading causes of death among NHPIs are cancer, heart disease, stroke, diabetes, and unintentional injuries; other prevalent health conditions are HIV/AIDS, hepatitis B, and tuberculosis (OMH, n.d.-d). National behavioral health statistics for NHPIs are limited, but NHPI adults had similar rates of mental illness to non-Hispanic Whites in 2018, although they were significantly less likely to receive mental health treatment (OMH, n.d.-e). Despite these health disparities, the projected 2015 life expectancies at birth for NHPIs (80.7 years, with 82.5 years for females and 77.7 years for males) were slightly greater than for non-Hispanic Whites (79.8 years, with 82.0 years for females and 77.5 years for males), but both groups were less than Asian-American life expectancies (OMH, n.d.-d).

In addition to NHPIs living in the United States, severe health disparities are also experienced among the broader USAPI population. Chronic health conditions and risk behaviors prevalent in US island territories and Affiliated Pacific Islands include obesity (93.5% of American Samoan adults are overweight or obese), cardiovascular disease (56% of adults in the Commonwealth of the Northern Marianas Islands have high blood pressure), and smoking (25% of Guam adults smoke) (CDC, n.d.-a). Several complex factors have led to these disparities, including colonization and the subsequent westernization that deteriorated the cultural, social, and environmental structures and traditional practices that protected the health of the people of these islands and their environment (Pacific Island Health Officers Association, n.d.). Achieving health equity in the USAPI is particularly challenging. Barriers on these islands include their geographic isolation, stressed health infrastructures, diverse cultures, and other factors that influence policy, the economy, and political relationships (Pacific Island Health Officers Association, n.d.).

For many decades, there was a shift in the epidemiology of the Pacific from mostly infectious diseases to preventable chronic diseases. Infectious diseases decreased thriving Pacific Island populations from about 700,000 in 1778 to about 40,000 by 1900. Recent outbreaks of measles in Samoa and other places in the Pacific are reminders that close-knit island communities are at great risk. The COVID-19 pandemic upended years of infectious disease work with NHPIs (Soma & Palafox, 2020). In Hawai'i, non-Hispanic Whites and NHPIs had higher rates of COVID-19 infection. NHPIs have some of the highest rates of chronic diseases both at younger ages and with elders who have multiple chronic diseases (Samoa & Palafox, 2020). Individuals with respiratory diseases, including asthma, were at greater risk when exposed to the COVID-19 virus. NHPI adolescents and adults have some of the highest smoking rates, which makes them more susceptible to severe symptoms caused by COVID-19 (Samoa & Palafox, 2020). Again, there is a need for clearer epidemiologic information, which has been less than adequate for NHPI populations and is now even more critical given the reemergence of infectious disease. Besides reducing health inequities, social mobilization and public health approaches are required to better allocate the distribution of resources (Samoa and Palafox, 2020).

The COFA treaty and agreements permit citizens of the Freely Associated (Pacific) States to enter the United States without visas as well as to economic assistance in exchange for military access to land, water, and airspace. These documents have been under scrutiny in 2024, with a focus on the Pacific Ocean alliances. The Marshallese, who are of Micronesian origin, present a noteworthy case. Approximately one-third of the population of the Marshall Islands has migrated to the United States—mostly to Hawaii, Guam, and, to a lesser extent, Arkansas, to work in that state's poultry processing industry (Duke, 2014). This is a recent migration trend—the Marshallese population in the United States increased from 6700 in 2000 to 22,400 in 2010—and these numbers will continue to increase as several factors continue to push the Marshallese out of their homeland (Duke, 2014). One factor is the legacy of nuclear testing in Micronesia, including the Marshall Islands, by the US military in the mid-20th century (Yamada & Akiyama, 2014). This testing is arguably responsible for many of the existing health problems on the islands, including high rates of thyroid disorders, cancer, and birth defects, and it left some islands uninhabitable (Duke, 2014). Faced with rising sea levels and a lack of employment opportunities at home, the Marshallese migrate to the United States for economic and education opportunities and increased access to health care (Kaholokula et al., 2019). Unfortunately, language barriers and misunderstandings over cultural values and social organization have caused some Marshallese migrants to experience discrimination while accessing care, with reports of longer waits in emergency departments and condescending treatment by hospital staff (Duke, 2014).

Strategies to Address Health Disparities Among Native Hawaiians/Pacific Islanders

There has been limited access to culturally and linguistically appropriate care for NHPIs. In addition, many of the health disparities experienced by NHPIs have been attributed to historical trauma, including "interpersonal violence, displacement from traditional lands, cultural loss or degradation, compulsory acculturation strategies (e.g., banning of native language), and other forms of discrimination" (Kaholokula et al., 2019, p. 199). The late 1960s saw a resurgence and revival of indigenous cultures, with indigenous peoples becoming reacquainted with their cultural values, practices, and rituals; however, many Native Hawaiians remain alienated from their cultural practices and values as a result of assimilation stressors. As cultural shifts occur in the delivery of care, researchers are increasingly investigating culturally relevant interventions to support care recipient disease management, improve health outcomes, and eliminate health disparities. Examples of culturally relevant interventions include a native cultural dance program to prevent cardiovascular disease (Kaholokula et al., 2017), home-based family education programs, and cancer screening in a church setting (Mokuau et al., 2016).

Many Native Hawaiians approach health from a holistic perspective that integrates body, mind, spirit, family, community, and environment, and there is a focus on collective relationships (Mokuau et al., 2016). Effective culturally based interventions draw from the strengths of the Hawaiian culture, but not at the expense of standard practices, and include Native Hawaiians in their design, implementation, and evaluation (Mokuau, 2016). Integrating Hawaiian healing practices with Western medicine has led to the development of successful treatment plans and preventive health programs for Native Hawaiians. Native Hawaiians should be able to take an active role in planning their treatment plans and health programs. Conversely, health professionals should increase their knowledge of NHPI cultures and healing practices to provide culturally and linguistically appropriate care for these care recipients.

Talk story is a Native Hawaiian oral tradition that has had some success in culturally appropriate health interventions. Talk story is how most NHPI conversations begin, and it allows people to speak their minds and share as a group (McMullin et al., 2010). Talk story is an intergenerational tradition of oral history, and taking time to "talk story" is an important cultural value in Hawaiian communities (Sentell et al., 2019). Talk story involves carefully listening while another person tells their story to allow emotions to flow, give meaning to the story, and allow for the expression of intimate feelings. Sentell et al. (2019) tested a narrative health intervention that used care recipient stories to support Native Hawaiians' self-management of heart disease. Native Hawaiians experience disproportionately higher rates of cardiovascular disease morbidity and mortality. To address this disparity, researchers collaborated with the community to create Native Hawaiian "talk story" videos for care recipients to view. Care recipients responded positively to the videos, and they identified with the storytellers, which contributed to a sense of shared experience. This feeling prompted care recipients to share their own stories, including with providers, thereby building trust and strengthening care recipient–provider relationships in the clinical encounter. "The narrative 'talk story' intervention provided a patient-centered feasible way to communicate health issues among Native Hawaiian patients, showing promise as a culturally relevant method to reduce health disparities in chronic disease management" (Sentell et al., 2019, p. 6).

Community-based participatory research is a successful approach to eliminate health disparities.

This culturally responsive approach is often used in applied research and is the preferred approach to engage NHPI communities in health research that contributes to the development of interventions that address physical and mental health disparities (Kaholokula et al., 2019). One study that assessed diet, obesity, and psychosocial factors related to food and nutrition as a method to prevent cancer among Native Hawaiians made sure to represent the concepts aloha, mālama, maihilahila, na'auao, and ano ano hua in all aspects of the project. "The values [these researchers] tried to maintain throughout the study processes were 'aloha' having compassion and respect for all who were involved, 'mālama' caring for one another, 'maihilahila' making sure no one is shamed or wronged, 'na'auao' a sharing of wisdom or knowledge, and finally 'ano ano hua' which means seed of my seed of my seed, or ensuring future generations" (McMullin et al., 2010, p. 53). In this project, Native Hawaiian values emerged as a methodology for conducting health research with Native Hawaiians who resided, in this particular study, in Southern California (McMullin et al., 2010). Cultural values, such as the ones used in this study, can translate into practice.

LATINO/HISPANIC AMERICANS

The terms *Hispanic* and *Latino* are used interchangeably because the OMB demands federal agencies to use a "Hispanic or Latino" category to identify individuals from a specific national origin. The OMH's definition of Hispanic or Latino origin "refers to a person of Cuban, Mexican, Puerto Rican, South or Central American, or other Spanish culture or origin regardless of race" (OMH, n.d.-f). Data from the 2020 US Census Bureau show that 62.1 million people identified as Hispanic or Latino in the United States in 2020, accounting for 18.7% of the total US population and making this population the nation's largest ethnic or racial minority (US Census Bureau, 2022c). This was an increase from the 2010 US Census, when 50.5 million people, or 16.3% of the total US population, identified as Hispanic or Latino. In 2020, the largest groups were Mexicans (35.8 million), Puerto Ricans (5.6 million), Salvadorans (2.3 million), Cubans (2.2 million), and Dominicans (2.2 million). The top five states with the most Hispanics or Latinos were California (15.6 million), Texas (11.4 million), Florida (5.7 million), New York (3.9 million), and Arizona (2.2 million). The Mexican population was the largest Hispanic group in 40 states and 90% of US counties. California (39.4%) and New Mexico (47.7%) were the two states where Hispanics represented the largest racial or ethnic group. In Puerto Rico, 3.2 million (98.9%) of the total population identified as Hispanic or Latino (US Census Bureau, 2023d). A 43% increase in the Hispanic population between 2010 and 2020 made Hispanics the second fastest-growing minority group in the United States after Asians (Pew Research Center, 2022).

Approximately 71.1% of Hispanics speak a language other than English at home, and 28.4% report that they are not fluent in English (US Census Bureau, 2019c). In 2022, 20.9% of the Hispanic population had a bachelor's degree or higher, a percentage lower than all other groups. (US Census Bureau, 2023c). In 2022, the median income of Hispanics was $62,800, lower than the national median of $74,580, and their poverty rate was 16.9%, higher than the national rate of 11.5%. In 2020, Hispanic children under the age of 19 and working-age adults aged 19 to 64 had the highest uninsured rates for health coverage (Keisler-Starkey & Bunch, 2021).

Health Issues of Latino/Hispanic Americans

Latino/Hispanic Americans (LHAs) have many health issues complicated by multiple cultural, economic, political, and social factors. These factors include language and cultural barriers, a lack of access to preventive care, and a lack of health insurance. LHAs are the highest uninsured racial or ethnic group in the United States. In 2020, 24.9% of working-age adults and 9.5% of children under 19 did not have health insurance, a slight increase from 24.6% and 8.7%, respectively, in 2018 (Keisler-Starkey & Bunch, 2021). At the same time, only 49.9% of Hispanics had private insurance, the lowest rate compared with all other races and ethnicities (Whites had the highest rate at 73.9%). From 2018 to 2021, the leading causes of death among Hispanic adults included heart disease, cancer, COVID-19, unintentional injuries, and stroke (WISQARS, 2021). In 2020 and 2021, COVID-19 was the leading cause of death for Hispanic adults. Based on the 2021 National Health Interview Survey, Hispanics (52.1%) had among the lowest rates of primary COVID-19 vaccine series completion; in comparison, Asians (72.6%) had the highest rate of vaccine completion, and Whites (57.4%) had the second-highest rate. Hispanics are also significantly affected by asthma, chronic obstructive pulmonary disease, liver disease, influenza and pneumonia, suicide, and kidney disease (OMH, n.d.-f, n.d.-h). From 2015 to 2018, the overweight and obesity rates for Hispanic or Latino adults aged 20 years and older were among the highest compared with all other races and ethnicities. Their overweight or obese rate was 82.7% (highest), and their obesity rate was 45.7% (second highest). Furthermore, their overweight or obese rate increased from 78.4%, and their obesity rate increased from 42.6% in the period of 2011 to 2014. Hispanic Americans accounted for nearly 30% of HIV/AIDS infections in the United States in 2019 (OMH, n.d.-g). HIV infection rates in Hispanic males and females were 4.2 and 3.1 times higher, respectively, than their White male and female counterparts. AIDS rates in Hispanic males and females were 3.9 and 3.9 times higher, respectively, than their White male and female counterparts. Death from HIV/AIDS was almost twice as likely for Hispanic males compared with non-Hispanic White males and three times as likely for Hispanic females compared with non-Hispanic White females (OMH, n.d.-g).

Asthma was reported by 6.7% or 2.8 million Hispanic American adults aged 18 years and older in the period from 2019 to 2021, with Mexicans (5.5%) reporting a lower rate than other Hispanics (8.3%). Hispanic females (9.7%) were affected more often than males (6.2%) (CDC, 2021). Furthermore, in 2019, 70.1% of Hispanic adults with asthma had uncontrolled asthma, the highest percentage compared with other races and ethnicities (CDC, 2021).

Although cancer rates are generally lower for Hispanic Americans (339.6 per 100,000) than for non-Hispanic Whites (461.9 per 100,000), some cancers are more common for the Hispanic population (US Cancer Statistics Working Group, 2023). These include liver cancer, cervical cancer, and stomach cancer. In 2020, the rates for liver and intrahepatic bile duct (13.2 per 100,000), cervix uteri (8.9 per 100,000), and stomach (8.7 per 100,000) cancers in Hispanics of all ages were higher than the rates for all other races and ethnicities (8.5, 6.9, and 6.3 per 100,000, respectively). In 2020, Hispanic males and females (8.8 per 100,000) were more likely to die from liver and intrahepatic bile duct cancer than non-Hispanic White males and females (5.9 per 100,000). Similarly, Hispanics (4.6 per 100,000) were more likely to die from stomach cancer than Whites (2.1 per 100,000) (SEER* Explorer, 2023; OMH, n.d.-i).

Hispanic females are less likely to have had a mammogram within the past 2 years (CDC, 2018c) and less likely to have had a Papanicolaou test during the past 3 years (Agency for Healthcare

Research and Quality, 2018) compared with non-Hispanic White females. Although cardiovascular disease (104.8 per 100,000) and cancer (102.2 per 100,000) are the first- and second-leading causes of morbidity and death among LHAs, death rates in the general population are more than double (264.0 and 234.4 per 100,000 for cardiovascular disease and cancer, respectively) (Curtin, 2019). With regard to deaths as a result of COVID-19, the death rate for Hispanics (78.9 per 100,000) was slightly higher than all races and ethnicities (74.9 per 100,000).

Health disparities in Hispanics differ depending on foreign or domestic birth. LHAs born in a foreign country are more likely to develop cervical, stomach, or liver cancer but will have 48% less cancer in general compared with US-born Hispanics. Foreign-born LHAs have approximately 50% less heart disease, 29% less high blood pressure, and 45% more high total cholesterol. However, of those who have high blood pressure, 68% of Hispanics are poorly controlled compared with 54% of non-Hispanic Whites. In addition, Hispanic adults who have had blood pressure measurements within 2 years are less able to state whether their blood pressure is normal or elevated (Agency for Healthcare Research and Quality, 2022).

Migrant seasonal farm workers (MSFWs) make up a large subgroup of Hispanic Americans. MSFWs face unique health problems related to pesticide exposure, heat exposure, and food insecurity. In addition, they face a large number of musculoskeletal injuries, respiratory illnesses, skin disorders, eye injuries, and depression (Velasco-Mondragon et al., 2016).

The difficulties experienced by LHAs in receiving appropriate health care services are comparable with those of the poor and other ethnic minorities. Other barriers include the lack of racial and ethnic diversity in workforce health professionals, lack of interpreter services for Spanish-speaking people, and lack of or inadequate culturally appropriate health care resources. Many LHAs may not readily seek care because they have continued reliance on their folk system of healing. Their preference for this is logical given their lack of health insurance and perceived difficulties negotiating the health care system because of language and other sociocultural barriers.

Selected Health-Related Cultural Aspects

Each subgroup of the LHA population has distinct cultural beliefs and customs. However, a common heritage determines common similar values and beliefs. For instance, two important aspects of Hispanic culture are the emphasis on the family and the emphasis on religion (Box 2.4: Best Practice). For older Hispanic Americans, the family is a vital component of good health. The family is the most important source of support; therefore, the needs of the family supersede the needs of the individual. During times of illness and crisis, the family is there for the individual. Older family members and relatives are accorded courtesy and respect and are often consulted on important matters (Boyle et al., 2024).

Rosas and colleagues (2018) capitalized on the importance of family and community in a study exploring an intervention protocol for diabetes prevention for LHA care recipients based on the Group Lifestyle Balance (GLB) program endorsed by the CDC (2018a). Adaptations to the GLB program specific to Hispanic/Latino culture included the invitation of family members to orientation and other activities, the addition of smartphone applications to facilitate support of coaches and family members, and the provision of culturally appropriate, healthy, low-cost food at group sessions. Focus group results

BOX 2.4 BEST PRACTICE

Spiritual Practices and Health

Spirituality and its relationship with health outcomes have been the focus of considerable interest in recent years. Spirituality can be defined as an individual's sense of peace, purpose, and connection with others as well as their beliefs about the meaning of life. For many people, spirituality plays an important role in their lives. Considerable evidence has shown spiritual practice to be an important and effective coping strategy and a common approach to dealing with health problems, particularly chronic diseases such as cardiovascular disease and cancer (PDQ Supportive and Palliative Care Editorial Board, 2024).

Multiple studies confirm that hospitalized care recipients and terminally ill care recipients who receive spiritual care experience better quality of life and improved spiritual health and are more satisfied with their health care (Chen et al., 2018; Ho et al., 2018). It is recommended that spiritual care be included as part of usual care for terminally ill care recipients, with attention paid to individual needs and cultural background (Chen et al., 2018). Spiritual or religious beliefs and practices have been shown to help care recipients with cancer as well as their caregivers to cope with the disease. Spiritual practices are likely to improve coping skills and social support, promote feelings of optimism and hope, encourage healthy behavior, decrease feelings of depression and anxiety, and support a sense of relaxation (PDQ Supportive and Palliative Care Editorial Board, 2024).

Studies suggest that many care recipients would like health care providers to consider spirituality as a factor in their health care; it has been reported that 77% of people who are admitted to hospitals believe that physicians should consider the spiritual needs of care recipients, and when spiritual needs are not met, quality-of-care ratings are lower (PDQ Supportive and Palliative Care Editorial Board, 2024). Although the Joint Commission on the Accreditation of Healthcare Organizations and the American College of Physicians both emphasize the importance of provision of spiritual care, a review of the literature reveals that this is suboptimal in practice (Ho et al., 2018). A 2016 systematic review of the literature reveals that physicians speak only infrequently to care recipients about their spiritual care needs and cite lack of time and training as the most significant barriers. Most physicians prefer to refer to chaplaincy services rather than to discuss spirituality with care recipients themselves (Best et al., 2016).

A spiritual assessment may help health care providers understand how religious or spiritual beliefs will affect the way a care recipient copes with diseases and health problems. Tools used by health care providers for spiritual history-taking include the HOPE (Anandarajah & Hight, 2001) and SPIR (Frick et al., 2006). More information about widely distributed HOPE tools can be found at http://www.aafp.org/afp/2001/0101/p81.html?printable=afp. All health professions need education to give full support to patients and families managing serious illnesses. Various educational models have been proposed for education about spiritual care (Puchalski et al., 2020). This education could be part of interprofessional education for health care providers.

Palliative care practices demand special attention to spiritual care. Research priorities include assessment of spirituality, interventions, and provider education with a focus on competency (Balboni et al., 2017). A systematic review of the literature related to end-of-life care for people with cancer shows that heightened spirituality and religious beliefs are linked to increased requests for life-sustaining care and decreased use of advanced care planning (LoPresti et al., 2016). Each person may have different spiritual needs, depending on cultural and religious traditions. To better counsel and care for care recipients, health care providers should be aware of special spiritual and religious needs and the common spiritual practices used by care recipients.

revealed active engagement in the program and positive responses from care recipients, family members, and health care providers (Rosas et al., 2018). This is an example of using a **culturally congruent practice** model to tailor an existing intervention for a specific cultural group.

Some LHAs attribute the origins of disease and illness to hot and cold imbalances, spiritual or natural punishments, supernatural phenomena, or psychological causes. The **hot and cold concept of disease** was derived from the Hippocratic theory of disease and advises that illness occurs when there is an imbalance between hot and cold. This concept of hot and cold is used as a guide to categorize illnesses and select appropriate treatments. For example, an elevated body temperature is managed by giving the person a cool drink to lower the temperature. For a person who has a cold, drinking warm fluids would be considered therapeutic. The evil eye, or the *mal de ojo*, is an example of a supernatural cause of illness, and fright, or *susto*, hysteria, and nerves, or *ataque de nervios*, may be believed to have psychological causes related to strong emotions, crises, and traumatic experiences.

Many LHAs use home remedies and consult folk healers, including the curandero, spiritualist, *yerbero*, and *sabador*. Curanderos use a variety of folk remedies, including prayers, rituals, herbs, and the laying on of hands. Spiritualists use medals, amulets, and prayers to affect a cure. The *yerbero* is knowledgeable in the use of herbs, whereas the *sabador* is an expert in massage and manipulation of bones and muscles. Folk remedies are used in combination with professional care approaches. The individual's belief in the folk remedy can have positive effects on their well-being (Boyle et al., 2024). Therefore, professional care personnel should find ways to blend the two systems to the optimal benefit of LHAs and their families.

BLACK/AFRICAN AMERICANS

Black or African Americans (BAA) are people who have origins in any of the Black racial groups of Africa, and the terms *Black* and *Black or African American* are used interchangeably by the US Census Bureau (2023d). In 2021, 40.1 million BAAs lived in the United States (OMH, n.d.-j), accounting for 12.1.% of the population. Black Americans are the second-largest minority population in the United States, following the Hispanic/Latino population (OMH, n.d.-j). Most Black Americans in the United States are descendants of enslaved people brought from Africa (Waters et al., 2014), and the top states of residence are US southern states (OMH, n.d.-j). BAAs continue to experience extreme segregation and exclusion from mainstream society along with discrimination by the majority group.

In 2021, most Black Americans in the United States lived in the southern states. BAAs who live outside the South tend to be more concentrated in metropolitan areas. In 2017, the highest percentage of BAAs lived in the District of Columbia (48.8%). The county with the largest population of BAAs was Cook County, Illinois, at 1.3 million (US Census Bureau, 2019a, 2019b).

BAAs have made substantial progress in the United States in the past century. However, there are still inequities in many areas, such as in business, education, political participation, and leadership. In 2021, 19.5% of non-Hispanic Blacks were living at the poverty level compared with 10.0% of non-Hispanic Whites, and the unemployment rate for non-Hispanic Blacks was double the rate for non-Hispanic Whites. In 2017, 87.9% of non-Hispanic Blacks older than 25 had earned at least a high school diploma compared with 93.5% of non-Hispanic Whites; 24.7% of non-Hispanic Blacks had earned at least a bachelor's degree compared with 38.3% of non-Hispanic Whites (OMH, n.d.-j).

Health Issues of Black/African Americans

A complex set of social, economic, and environmental factors can be identified as contributors to the current health status of BAAs. However, poverty may be the most profound and pervasive determinant of health status. Individuals and families who are below the poverty level or lack adequate resources have limited access to health care services such as prenatal and maternal care, childhood immunizations, dental checkups, well-child care, and a wide range of other health-promoting and preventive services.

Two indices of the effects of poverty can be seen in high rates of infant mortality and maternal mortality. Despite changes in living conditions, advances in infection control, and improved standards in neonatal care, BAAs still experience high infant and maternal mortality rates. Infant mortality attributable to birth defects (IMBD) may be linked to a lack of access to or utilization of prenatal health care (Almli et al., 2020). Although rates of IMBD from 2003 to 2017 declined by 10% overall, including by 11% for non-Hispanic Black mothers, racial and ethnic disparities remain. In 2017 the IMBD rate was 35% higher for Black mothers than for White mothers (Almli et al., 2020). Between 2008 and 2017, the overall infant mortality rate dropped from 12.67 to 10.97 (number of deaths among infants aged <1 year per 1000 live births) for BAAs, but this remained 2.4 times higher than the rate for non-Hispanic Whites, which was 4.67 deaths per 1000 live births (Ely & Driscoll, 2019).

Black Americans have lower life expectancies than other races at 65 years of age. In 2017, these were 71.5 years for non-Hispanic Black males and 78.1 years for non-Hispanic Black females compared with 76.1 years for non-Hispanic White males and 81.0 years for non-Hispanic White females (CDC, 2019). Black Americans are affected disproportionately by the leading causes of death in the United States, including cancer, HIV/AIDS, obesity, diabetes, heart disease, and hypertension (OMH, n.d.-k, n.d.-l, n.d.-m, n.d.-n, n.d.-o). In 2017, although Black Americans accounted for only 13% of the US population, they accounted for 43% of new HIV/AIDS cases (CDC, n.d.-b). Severe high blood pressure is common for Black American males and females. From 2013 to 2016, 40.5% of Black American adult males and 44% of females older than age 20 had hypertension (CDC, n.d.-c). From 2006 to 2016, asthma rates rose from 12.8% to 15.7% for non-Hispanic Black children 18 years old and younger, while rates for non-Hispanic White children dropped from 8.6% to 7.1% (National Center for Health Statistics, 2018). Obesity and its contributing factors are also receiving attention. From 2013 to 2016, obesity rates for non-Hispanic Blacks aged 2 to 19 years old was 20.4% compared with non-Hispanic Whites at 14.7% (National Center for Health Statistics, 2018). During the same period, adult male obesity rates were

37.5%, and female obesity rates were 56.1% for non-Hispanic Blacks (CDC, n.d.-c).

BAAs fare worse than other racial and ethnic groups in the United States on most health indicators. Discrimination based on racism alone does not account for all inequities. Researchers suggest that discriminatory stressors have been underestimated and suggest that a focus on intersectionality with other social identities should be considered. **Gender identity**, class, age, and **sexual orientation** in combination with race and ethnicity may create significant additional discriminatory pressures resulting in health inequity (Lewis & Van Dyke, 2018).

The COVID-19 pandemic and global health crisis of 2019 to 2021 have brought BAA health disparities to the media forefront. Higher rates of heart disease, lung disease, and diabetes in BAAs leave them more susceptible to COVID-19 complications. In addition, the opportunity to work from home, maintain social distancing, and order the delivery of high-quality food (all recommended for prevention of coronavirus infection) are associated with privilege not afforded to many BAAs of lower socioeconomic status.

BAAs are dying of complications from COVID-19 at a disproportionate rate. Counties in the United States that have a majority of Black residents have infection rates three times higher than counties that are majority White. Death rates from COVID-19 are higher in Black-majority counties (Yancy, 2020). Data from Johns Hopkins University, state health departments, and American Community Survey indicate that, in Chicago, Blacks make up 32% of the population but 67% of deaths due to COVID-19. In Milwaukee County, Wisconsin, Blacks represent 26% of the population and 73% of deaths due to COVID-19. Similar statistics are seen across the country (Yancy, 2020), with people of color disproportionally affected (Artiga et al., 2020). What remains to be seen is what the US action plan will be to address the disparities that have led to the current, unacceptable reality (Yancy, 2020).

Selected Health-Related Cultural Aspects

Differences in cultural beliefs, attitudes, and practices exist between rural and urban Black Americans; however, they share some basic cultural beliefs. Black American culture is centered on the family and religion. The family, the strongest institution, provides important extended kinship bonds with grandparents, aunts, uncles, and cousins. The family is considered the strongest source of support, especially in times of crisis and illness (Chatters et al., 2018). Some family members and relatives may be consulted before BAAs seek care elsewhere.

Religion and religious behavior are an integral part of the BAA community (see Box 2.4: Best Practice). The church is a significant support system for many Black Americans; it serves many purposes beyond worship and formation. The church also serves as a place to meet where members can pass on news, take care of business, and find strength of purpose. The church provides direct social welfare service, acts as a stabilizing force in the community, facilitates citizenship training and community social action, serves as a transmitter of cultural history, provides the means for coping and surviving in a hostile world (Chatters et al., 2018), and provides counseling and community mental health services (Avent & Cashwell, 2015; Chatters et al., 2018; Hankerson & Weissman, 2012).

Many African Americans believe in the healing power of prayer (Vaughn et al., 2009). Black Americans were found to pray more for health reasons (Su & Li, 2011). The BAA church and spirituality play an important role in health issues. Religious involvement was found to have a positive effect on health behaviors (Holt et al., 2014).

Some BAAs define health as a feeling of well-being and the ability to fulfill role expectations. Diseases can be caused by natural or spiritual forces; therefore, some BAAs' approach to health care is guided by these beliefs. Family members, such as grandmothers, and community members are often consulted for traditional home remedies. Traditional interventions such as roots, herbs, potions, oils, powders, rituals, and ceremonies are still used in many Southern communities. The use of healers is also common, including the older woman who is knowledgeable about folk remedies and childcare; the spiritualist who assists with financial, personal, spiritual, or physical problems; and the voodoo priest or priestess who is knowledgeable about herbs, signs, and omens (Boyle et al., 2024).

As noted with the folk health practices of Asian and Hispanic Americans, BAAs' folk healing beliefs and practices can augment the professional care system. Some Black Americans find comfort in the support that their religious leader or traditional healer can give them. Health care providers should find an appropriate place for these modalities when caring for BAAs.

AMERICAN INDIANS/ALASKA NATIVES

American Indians or Alaska Natives (AIANs) are people who have origins in North America and South America (including Central America) and who maintain tribal affiliation or community attachment (NASEM, 2023). AIANs lived in America for thousands of years before the arrival of Europeans. AIANs are the original people of the land now occupied mainly by people of European descent. Some evidence indicates that AIANs migrated to North America via a Siberian land bridge sometime between 40,000 and 16,500 years ago. Native Americans came to be known as Indians, a label given by Columbus when he encountered the native peoples in the West Indies, which he mistook for the East Indies. This label was then extended to all the native peoples of North America and South America, from the Arctic to Tierra del Fuego. Before 1492 there were an estimated 5 million indigenous people. Columbus's discovery brought colonization and settlement by various European groups (Snipp, 2000). Thus, the ancestral lands of the Native Americans were usurped, and the people were forced to labor on farms and in mines. Thousands died of disease and hard labor or were killed in attempts to escape from slavery. Other events, such as the removal of the Southeastern tribes in 1830, the Navajos' Long March to Fort Sumner in 1864, and the massacre at Wounded Knee in 1890, caused the Native American population to dwindle to 250,000 by 1890 (Fixico et al., 2001).

In 2018 an estimated 6.9 million people in the United States identified as AIAN, an increase of approximately 800,000 people since the 2010 census (US Census Bureau, 2019c). Native Americans are concentrated in California, Oklahoma, Arizona, Texas, New York, New Mexico, Washington, North Carolina, Florida, and Michigan (Norris et al., 2012). The states with the five highest-percentage distributions of AIANs are California (13.9%), Oklahoma (9.2%), Arizona (6.8%), Texas (6.0%), and New York (4.2%). The five cities with the highest number of AIANs in 2010, in rank order, were New York, Los Angeles, Phoenix, Oklahoma City, and Anchorage. The five cities with the highest percentage of AIANs in 2010, in rank order, were Anchorage, Tula, Norma, Oklahoma City, and Billings. It is estimated that the AIAN population will increase to 10.1 million, or 2.5% of the total US population, by 2060 (US Census Bureau, 2019c).

Of the total AIAN population, 13% live on reservations or other trust lands, and approximately 60% live in metropolitan areas. In 2022, there were 324 federally recognized American Indian reservations (OMH, n.d.-p).

Disparity in education exists between AIANs and White Americans. AIANs attain degrees of associate's level or higher at a rate of 24% compared with 47% of Whites, and Alaska Natives attain degrees at a rate of 11% compared with 43% of White adults in Alaska (Del Pilar, 2018). Native Americans are making some progress in all levels of college education. However, low continuing educational attainment and low-income levels combined with higher rates of poverty are socioeconomic issues that affect the health and quality of life of this population.

Health Care Issues of American Indians/Alaska Natives

Many of the health problems of Native Americans can be linked directly to social and economic conditions such as cultural barriers, geographic isolation, inadequate sewage disposal, and low income (OMH, n.d.-p). These conditions predispose Native Americans to illnesses and health problems. Although Native Americans have responded well to prevention and treatment of infectious diseases, other health problems are closely linked with poverty and harmful lifestyle practices.

Some of the leading diseases and causes of death among AIANs are heart disease, cancer, unintentional injuries (accidents), diabetes, and stroke. A study examining trends in cancer mortality and incidence from 1999 to 2009 found less progress in cancer control for AIAN populations compared with White populations (White et al., 2014). American Indians and Alaska Natives also have a high prevalence of risk factors for mental health problems and suicide, unintentional injuries, substance abuse, obesity, sudden infant death syndrome, teenage pregnancy, liver disease, diabetes, and hepatitis (OMH, n.d.-p, n.d.-q). In 2017, the tuberculosis rate for AIANs was nearly four times higher than the rate for White Americans (OMH, n.d.-p). AIAN adults are nearly three times as likely as non-Hispanic Whites in the United States to have diabetes, and in 2016 AIANs were 2.4 times more likely to experience death due to diabetes (OMH, n.d.-s). Initiatives that encourage an active lifestyle and healthy eating habits may decrease the rate of diabetes in the AIAN population.

Arizona is the state with the third-largest AIAN population in the United States. Arizona Behavioral Risk Factor Surveillance System data from 2017 showed that AIANs consumed more sugar-sweetened beverages; were more frequently overweight or obese; and had a higher prevalence of hypertension, fair or poor health status, and leisure-time inactivity compared with White Americans. AIANs also had a lower prevalence of having a primary care physician than Whites. Having less than a high school education, being unemployed, and earning less than $15,000 per year was more prevalent among AIANs than White Americans. In 2017, AIANs reported having health care coverage at a higher rate than White Americans, but having a private physician was less prevalent. This indicates that having health care coverage did not ensure access (Adakai et al., 2018).

The health problems of Native Americans are complicated by difficult access to health care. Federally recognized tribes are provided with health and educational assistance through Indian Health Services (IHS), a government agency in the USDHHS. Since 1972, IHS has started a series of initiatives to fund health-related activities in off-reservation settings that make health care services accessible to urban AIANs. However, people insured by IHS can receive covered services only at federal hospitals and clinics funded by IHS. Because of this, many insured AIANs living in rural settings may not be able to access care (Adakai et al., 2018). Even though the IHS attempts to provide comprehensive, high-quality health care services to AIANs, quality of care and access to health services need to be improved.

The Navajo Nation had the highest COVID-19 infection rate in the United States after New York and New Jersey (National Public Radio, 2020). A high prevalence of obesity and diabetes put members of the Navajo Nation at high risk for poorer outcomes with COVID-19 infection. In Arizona, 20% of deaths due to COVID-19 were Native Americans, though they made up only 5% of the population (Public Broadcasting Service, 2020). While the Nation has been working hard to implement best practices for infection control and contact tracing, many barriers to effectiveness exist. Many people on the reservation do not have phones, and it can take hours to drive to one person's home for contact tracing (National Public Radio, 2020). Many households do not have clean, running water or electricity. Hospitals are few and far between. Per capita spending on health care for AIANs is $2834 per person, compared with $9404 per person on veterans and $12,744 per person on Medicare (US Commission on Civil Rights, 2018).

Selected Health-Related Cultural Aspects

Native Americans are generally present oriented: they emphasize events that are occurring now rather than events that will happen later. They take one day at a time, and in times of illness many may cope by hoping for improvements the next day (Boyle et al., 2024). Many Native Americans also value cooperation rather than competition. Sharing of resources, even among the poor, is an important component of this cultural value. Family and spiritual beliefs (see Box 2.4: Best Practice) are important for Native Americans. Native Americans place great value on their families and relatives. Three or more generations form an extended kinship system, which is enlarged by the membership of nonrelatives, who are included through various religious ceremonies (Boyle et al., 2024).

Despite the great diversity in the beliefs and practices of Native American groups concerning health, illness, and healing, they share a common philosophical base. Native Americans believe that optimal health exists only when a person lives in a condition with balance and harmony in the inner and outer domains of life (Grandbois, 2005). The Earth is seen as a living entity that should be treated with respect; failure to do so harms the body. Instead of viewing illness as changes in a person's physiologic state, Native Americans view it as a disparity between the person and natural forces (Grandbois, 2005). Many Native Americans believe that a person's sickness can be traced directly to that person having committed a violation against natural and spiritual laws; an individual can also inherit such a violation. The violation causes the person to have an imbalance that causes illnesses mentally, physically, emotionally, and spiritually.

Many AIANs proudly express spirituality, traditional medicinal practices, and cultural ceremonies in their lives. AIANs frequently seek traditional practitioners, who are medicine females or males known as shamans. Shamans are believed to have hypnotic powers, the gift of mind-reading, and expertise in concocting drugs, medicine, and poisons; they carry out rituals and healing ceremonies that are believed to restore the sense of balance, harmony, and unity that the acute or traumatic event has caused (Grandbois, 2005). Finding an appropriate place for the expression of traditional practices and ceremonies is an important part of providing culturally congruent health care for the AIAN population.

LESBIAN, GAY, BISEXUAL, AND TRANSGENDER PEOPLE

Based on estimates from the Williams Institute (Conron, 2019), 4.5% of the adult population in the United States identifies as lesbian, gay, bisexual, or transgender (LGBT). This population describes many individuals who may use terms describing themselves as lesbian, gay, bisexual, transgender, queer/questioning (one's sexual or gender identity), intersex, and asexual/aromantic/agender (LGBTQIA+). Among this adult population, Millennials (born 1981–1996) are more than twice as likely to identify as LGBTQ as Baby Boomers (born 1946–1964) and are 56% more likely to identify as LGBTQ as Gen Xers (born 1965–1980) (GLAAD, 2018). Twelve percent of Millennials identify as transgender or gender nonconforming (GLAAD, 2018). The LGBT adult population older than the age of 50 is estimated to increase from more than 2.4 million to more than 5 million by 2030 (Choi & Meyer, 2016).

Sexual orientation and **gender identity** are distinct, and all people have both. Sexual orientation is the romantic, emotional, or sexual attraction a person feels toward others. Gender identity is a person's concept of themselves as male, female, both, or neither, and this can be the same as or different from their sex at birth. **Gender expression** is a person's external expression of gender identity, and this can be socially conforming or nonconforming. Gender expression is often achieved through dress, hairstyle, or behavior. People who are **transgender** are people whose gender expression is culturally nonconforming with the sex they were assigned at birth. Being transgender does not indicate sexual orientation, and a person who is transgender may identify as straight, gay, lesbian, bisexual, etc. When people try to align their internal knowledge of gender identity with external appearances, they may go through **gender transition**. This can be done socially through mode of dress, hairstyle, names, and pronouns, and it can be done physically by modifying one's body through medical intervention (Human Rights Campaign, 2020).

It is important to note that people who are LGBT are not one community, but rather "are members of every community. They are diverse, come from all walks of life, and include people of all races and ethnicities, all ages, all socioeconomic statuses, and from all parts of the country" (CDC, 2018b, para. 1). Providing optimal care for LGBTQ care recipients is more about having information, a willingness to learn, and an openness to listening to care recipients, rather than being an expert in LGBTQ culture (James, 2019).

The percentage of LGBTQ people reporting discrimination based on sexual identity or gender orientation increased significantly from 44% to 55% between 2016 and 2017 (GLAAD, 2018). Tragically, LGBT children experience discrimination, violence, and abuse based on their gender orientation from an early age. According to the 2015 US Transgender Survey report, in kindergarten through 12th grade, 77% of children perceived to be transgender were mistreated; 54% were verbally harassed; 24% were physically attacked; 13% were sexually assaulted; and 17% left school because of mistreatment (National Center for Transgender Equality, 2016).

Older adults who identify as lesbian, gay, or bisexual (LGB) have unique characteristics as a population. Findings from the 2015 to 2016 California Health Interview Survey (CHIS) demonstrate that, although LGB older adults have similar educational levels and employment status as their straight counterparts, LGB older adults are more often male, more likely to live alone, and more likely to have never been married. Of those 50 to 64 years old, 30.6% of LGB adults lived alone compared with 13.6% of straight adults, and 39.8% of LGB adults older than 65 lived alone compared with 26.2% of straight older adults. Researchers did not find significant differences in health outcomes between LGB older adults and straight older adults. However, more LGB Hispanic/Latinos aged 50 to 64 lacked health insurance compared with LGB non-Hispanic/Latinos. In the age group 65 and older, LGB Hispanic/Latinos had a higher incidence of diabetes and psychological distress (Choi et al., 2018). These findings support the importance of considering intersectionality in addressing health care disparity and inequity within vulnerable populations.

LGBT Health Issues

People who are LGBT are diverse and have a variety of health issues and needs. Barriers to health care include stigma, discrimination, lack of access, and mistrust of the health care system (Martos et al., 2019). It is important to remember that before being removed from the Diagnostic and Statistical Manual of Mental Disorders in 1973, homosexuality was considered a pathology by the APA.

Approximately 152,000 adults in the United States who identify as **transgender** are enrolled in Medicaid, and less than half of these people have coverage for gender-affirming health care due to state policies and laws. An estimated 32,000 transgender individuals with Medicaid live in states that expressly ban denying coverage for gender-affirming care (Mallory & Tentindo, 2019).

Currently, transitioning care for adolescents under the age of 18 is extremely controversial and politicized, with clinics that provide this care being criticized or in some cases forbidden by law to do so.

Preexposure prophylaxis (or PrEP) refers to the use of medication to prevent HIV. PrEP is recommended to prevent HIV for all people at risk through sex or injection drug use excluding people at risk for HIV from receptive vaginal sex. Although this is a current recommended course of preventive treatment, only 4% of sexually active gay/bisexual males use PrEP, and most males between 18 and 25 who are gay/bisexual and sexually active are not tested annually for HIV as recommended by the CDC (Hammack et al., 2018). Nonuse of recommended preventive care may be indicative of inaccessibility.

Adolescents who are gender nonconforming warrant special consideration as a vulnerable population in health care. Data from the 2015 to 2016 CHIS reveal that more than 25% of children ages 12 to 17 in California are considered gender nonconforming by their peers. Although researchers found no significant difference in suicide or thoughts of suicide between gender-nonconforming youth and their peers, gender-nonconforming youth were more than two times as likely to experience psychological distress (Wilson et al., 2017). In another study that spanned multiple states (Gill & Frazer, 2016), researchers found that feminine males attempted suicide more often than nonfeminine males. Further research in the form of longitudinal studies that also assess rates of victimization and bullying are needed to better understand the mental health, counseling, educational, and support needs of LGBT youth (Wilson et al., 2017).

Females who are lesbian or bisexual face unique challenges during health care encounters that can have an effect on health outcomes. In particular, researchers have found that disclosure of sexual orientation and provider attributes play a large role in the quality of health care lesbian and bisexual (LB) females receive. In a qualitative grounded theory study, Johnson and Nemeth (2014) found that after disclosure of sexual orientation a provider's knowledge, attitudes, and communication played a large role in health care experience and resulted in females receiving timely, appropriate care compared with avoiding care and seeking answers on the Internet.

Research about the gynecologic health of LB females is severely lacking. In particular, there is a need for the use of validated tools to monitor sexual orientation in research (Robinson et al., 2017). In their systematic review and meta-analysis, Robinson and colleagues, sought to "examine differences in incidence and/or prevalence of gynecologic conditions in LB compared with heterosexual females" (p. 381). Of the 567 records searched, not one fully addressed the research question. Eleven articles were ultimately included in the study. Research methods were extremely variable, and overall findings were inconclusive. This is an area of great need considering existing myths and assumptions about risk factors for cancer and pelvic pain related to sexual orientation (Robinson et al., 2017).

During times of public health crisis, it is important to remember that **vulnerable populations** face increased risk. In an open letter to "all parties handling COVID-19 surveillance, response, treatment, and media coverage," the Gay and Lesbian Medical Association (GLMA, n.d.) and multiple other national organizations remind readers of the vulnerability of LGBT persons during the COVID-19 pandemic. The letter highlights that LGBT persons are more likely to smoke and have higher rates of HIV/AIDS and cancer than heterosexual individuals, putting them at high risk for infection and complications with COVID-19. Adding to this risk is the fact that due to discrimination and lack of understanding in many health care settings, some LGBT persons may not seek care until their situation is emergent, or they may not seek care at all (GLMA, n.d.).

Strategies to Reduce Health Disparities in LGBT Populations

One strategy to address the issue of stigma and discrimination in health care for LGBT people is the use of LGBT-specific clinics. Statistical analysis of three LGBT cohorts ($N = 1534$), stratified by age in relation to significant historical developments in US history and policy related to LGBT people, demonstrates that 13% of individuals surveyed had used LGBT-specific clinics, and 52% were interested in using such a clinic in the future. This mismatch between actual use and desired use indicates a lack of access to desired care. Individuals who had access to a usual source of health care expressed interest in future use of LGBT-specific clinics approximately half as frequently as those who did not have a usual source of care. Bisexuals were also 50% less likely to express an interest in LGBT-specific care as their gay or lesbian peers. Members of the oldest cohort were most likely to report past utilization of LGBT-specific clinics, and members of the youngest cohort were more likely to express interest in in future use. Researchers were unable to differentiate between one-time utilization and repeated utilization in this study (Martos et al., 2019).

The CDC outlined *Healthy People 2030* objectives for LGBT people centered largely on gathering more accurate population data for use in research (included in Box 2.1). This focus on increasing the amount and accuracy of survey and questionnaire data will assist researchers in population health studies aimed at reducing inequity in health care. Other *Healthy People 2030* objectives focus on improving outcomes for LGBT youth by targeting bullying, drug use, and mental health services.

HOMELESSNESS: A CONTINUING AND MULTIFACETED ISSUE

Homelessness is a lack of a regular, adequate nighttime residence, either permanent or temporary, resulting from poverty and unsafe or unstable living environments (National Coalition for the Homeless, 2023). A combination of structural and personal factors influences homelessness in the United States. A shortage of affordable housing, rising poverty rates, income inequality, insufficient public assistance, overcrowded living conditions, and inadequate housing quality force many individuals into unstable situations, increasing their risk of homelessness. (National Alliance to End Homelessness, 2024; National Coalition for the Homeless, 2023). Other contributors to the lack of consistent housing include high health care costs, domestic violence, mental illness, and substance abuse, with the latter two being particularly significant among veterans (National Alliance to End Homelessness, 2024; National Coalition for the Homeless, 2023; US Department of Housing and Urban Development or the US Government, 2023). In January 2022, over 582,000 people, or about 18 out of every 10,000 people, were experiencing homelessness in the United States (National Alliance to End Homelessness, 2024). The homeless population varies widely in age and race; almost three-quarters (72%) of people experiencing homelessness were individual adults, while 28% were families with children (National Alliance to End Homelessness, 2024). Black individuals experience more than four times the rate of homelessness compared with White individuals, while Native Hawaiian or Pacific Islanders have the highest rates, with 121 out of every 10,000 people experiencing homelessness (National Alliance to End Homelessness, 2024).

Homelessness is increasing in the United States. The most recent data show a significant rise in the number of people experiencing homelessness. Between 2022 and 2023, there was a 12% increase in homelessness nationwide, marking the most substantial yearly increase since data collection began in 2007 (US Department of Housing and Urban Development or the US Government, 2023). This issue is likely even more extensive than represented in the statistics; many studies count homeless people as individuals who are in shelters or on the streets, not taking into consideration those who live in vehicles, motels, or other hidden locations or families who are staying with family or friends (National Coalition for the Homeless, 2023). Major cities such as New York and Los Angeles, which together account for nearly a quarter of the homeless population, saw substantial increases, but even rural areas experienced a rise in homelessness (National Alliance to End Homelessness, 2024; National Coalition for the Homeless, 2023).

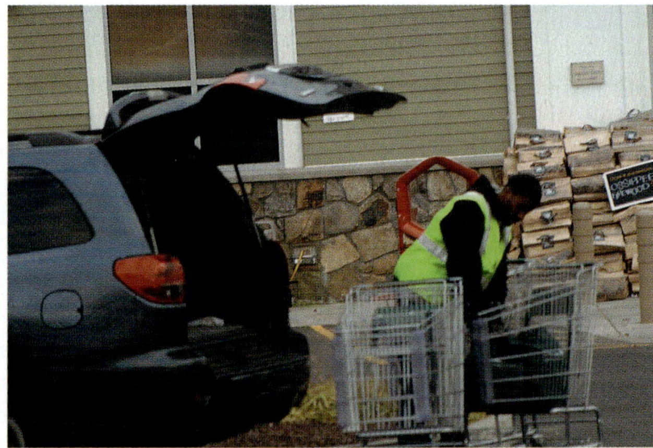

FIG. 2.2 A male works at a day labor job to earn money.

Health Issues of Homeless People and Families

Homelessness in the United States is intricately linked with health, as both a cause and an effect (Bowen et al., 2019). Rising health care costs and inadequate insurance coverage can force individuals to choose between medical expenses and housing, contributing to increased homelessness (National Health Care for the Homeless Council [NHCHC], 2019). Many individuals are just one health crisis away from losing their homes, and those experiencing homelessness often face severe health disparities (NHCHC, 2019). They are more likely to suffer from chronic conditions, mental illness, and substance abuse, and they frequently lack access to primary and preventive care crucial for maintaining health and well-being. Lack of preventive care results in higher morbidity, shorter life expectancy, and increased hospitalizations for conditions that could have been managed or prevented with proper care (NHCHC, 2019). The correlation between health issues and homelessness underscores the urgency for comprehensive solutions.

Environmental risks associated with homelessness, such as exposure to extreme weather, unsanitary living conditions, and crowded shelters, exacerbate health issues (Anderson et al., 2021; NHCHC, 2024). Homeless individuals also face high levels of violence, malnutrition, and stress, which further deteriorate their health (NHCHC, 2019). The prevalence of severe illnesses and injuries among people experiencing homelessness is significantly higher than in the general population, with rates of conditions such as heart disease, cancer, liver disease, and infectious diseases being much higher (NHCHC, 2024).

Substance abuse and mental health issues are particularly prevalent among homeless populations and are often both a cause and a consequence of homelessness. These issues complicate the ability to obtain and maintain housing and make it more challenging to adhere to treatment regimens, especially for chronic conditions such as diabetes or HIV/AIDS. The lack of stable housing makes it difficult for homeless individuals to access consistent health care, leading to higher rates of emergency department visits and hospitalizations (NHCHC, 2024). Addressing homelessness requires a comprehensive approach that includes improving access to affordable housing, health care, and supportive services to break this cycle (Fig. 2.2).

Strategies to Address Homelessness

The NHCHC is a pivotal organization that is driving initiatives to combat homelessness in the United States (2024). By collaborating with individuals who have experienced homelessness, health care providers, and policymakers, the NHCHC delivers advocacy, research, training, and clinical resources to address the intricate interplay between poor health and homelessness (NHCHC, 2024).

To combat homelessness effectively, strategies must prioritize physical and mental health considerations. Permanent supportive housing, an integral component of the "housing-first" approach, has effectively provided stability for homeless individuals (National Coalition for the Homeless, 2024). Beyond housing, initiatives should facilitate access to health care services and benefits, empower communities to offer support and resources, and enhance health literacy among homeless populations (NHCHC, 2019).

Community involvement is paramount to addressing homelessness comprehensively. Schools, religious institutions, and local governments are vital in supporting people without housing through initiatives such as providing shelter, meals, and socializing opportunities (National Alliance to End Homelessness, 2012). Collaboration and advocacy efforts at the grassroots level are essential for promoting the dignity and integration of homeless individuals into society.

Health care professionals play a pivotal role in providing tailored care to homeless individuals, which necessitates creative care planning sensitive to their unique circumstances. Given the multifaceted challenges homeless populations face, health care providers must adapt standards of care to accommodate the realities of homelessness (NHCHC, 2024).

Addressing homelessness requires a multifaceted approach encompassing housing stability, health care access, community support, and advocacy efforts. Increased awareness, community involvement, and the commitment of health care professionals are crucial in advancing toward a society where homelessness is no longer a pervasive issue.

RESPONSES TO HEALTH CHALLENGES

The Nation's Response to the Health Challenge

The National Institutes of Health has proclaimed health disparities as a major concern. It is putting significant effort into addressing and reducing health disparities involving cancer, diabetes, infant mortality, AIDS, cardiovascular illnesses, and many other diseases. In 2010 the US Congress stressed its commitment to health equity by elevating the National Center on Minority Health and Health Disparities to the National Institute on Minority Health and Health Disparities. In 2011 the USDHHS released two plans (The National Stakeholder Strategy for Achieving Health Equity and the Health and Human Services Action Plan to Reduce Racial and Ethnic Health Disparities [REACH]) to reduce health disparities (CDC, n.d.-d).

These recommendations of health-promoting practices cannot be done in silos. For example, a community health department may recommend that people increase physical activity by walking or riding bikes to work, but the planning department may not plan communities with sidewalks (Tucker, 2014). In recognition of the fact that a lack of communication within a community contributes to disparities, the Public Health Institute developed *Health in All Policies: A Guide for State and Local Governments* (Rudolph et al., 2013). *Health in All Policies* uses a complex systems approach to develop health policy aimed at achieving multisectoral action. There are many different ways to achieve cross-sector collaboration, and the guide offers multiple perspectives and examples for consideration. Nontraditional partnerships are encouraged, involving entities outside of the public health realm (Rudolph et al., 2013).

Diversifying the biomedical workforce is another USDHHS goal. The diversification of the biomedical workforce is important not only for a incorporating a broad range of researcher experiences and viewpoints but also for increasing the trust and participation of minorities in clinical trials. Increased minority participation in clinical trials will improve the health care available to minority populations. To this end, in 2018, the National Institute on Minority Health and Health Disparities developed a three-phase initiative aimed at diversifying the biomedical workforce. Phase one of the initiative included a workshop hosted by the Association of American Medical Colleges. Focus groups at the workshop identified a lack of mentorship and a lack of funds and resources as primary barriers to diversification and innovation. Phase two included development of action items, tools, and partnerships to address identified barriers and to train a diverse workforce that is representative of the population served. The third phase will focus on developing processes and target dates for producing outcomes (Newton, 2019).

Healthy People is an USDHHS initiative that began in 1979 after Surgeon General Julius Richmond published the report *Healthy People: The Surgeon General's Report on Health Promotion and Disease Prevention.* Initiatives have been established for the years 2000, 2010, 2020, and now 2030. *Healthy People* initiatives outline comprehensive, nationwide health-promotion and disease-prevention agendas. In the past 2 decades, one of *Healthy People's* primary goals has concentrated on disparities. In *Healthy People 2010,* the primary focus was not just to reduce health disparities among Americans, as with *Healthy People 2000,* but to actually eliminate health disparities. In *Healthy People 2020,* the goal was expanded further to achieve health equity, eliminate disparities, and improve the health of all groups (USDHHS, n.d.-a, n.d.-b, n.d.-c).

The framework for *Healthy People 2030* was approved by the USDHHS in June 2018. The framework is based on the Secretary's Advisory Committee on National Health Promotion and Disease Prevention Objectives for 2030. The overarching goals of *Healthy People 2030* expand the elimination of health disparities and achievement of health equity to add the attainment of health literacy for the improvement of the health and well-being of all people (USDHHS, n.d.-c). *Healthy People 2030* has an expanded vision: "a society in which all people can achieve their full potential for health and well-being across the lifespan" (USDHHS, n.d.-a, n.d.-b, n.d.-c). Specific objectives related to social determinants of health can be reviewed in Box 2.1. For more information about *Healthy People 2030* topics and objectives, visit http://www.healthypeople.gov/.

The Office of Minority Health was created in 1986 and was reauthorized by the Patient Protection and Affordable Care Act of 2010 (OMH, n.d.-r). Since its creation, the OMH has worked to improve and protect the health of racial and ethnic minority populations through the development of health policies and programs that concentrate on eliminating health disparities. The OMH also works to improve the collection, reporting, and sharing of data for ethnic and racial minority populations and to foster research and evaluation (OMH, n.d.-r). Health equity is supported through the OMH Resource Center, which disseminates research on minority health, and the National CLAS standards, which were discussed earlier in this chapter. In addition, the OMH is leading the charge to put into practice the US Department of Health and Human Services Action Plan to Reduce Racial and Ethnic Health Disparities at all levels of the USDHHS and in the communities with whom it works.

In recent years, the OMH started two initiatives to guide its efforts toward eliminating health disparities in the United States: the National Partnership for Action to End Health Disparities and the Strategic Framework for Improving Racial and Ethnic Minority Health and Eliminating Racial and Ethnic Health Disparities. Both initiatives implemented a coordinated, systems-level approach that focused on eliminating health disparities and used an evidence-based approach to notify and continually improve policies and programs. The goals of the National Partnership for Action to End Health Disparities are to enhance awareness of the importance of health disparities and actions needed to improve health outcomes for racial and ethnic minority populations, to strengthen and expand leadership for dealing with health disparities at all levels, to improve health and health care outcomes for racial and ethnic minorities and underserved populations and communities, to improve cultural and linguistic competency in delivering health services, and to improve coordination and utilization of research and evaluation outcomes. The main purpose of the Strategic Framework for Improving Racial and Ethnic Minority Health and Eliminating Racial and Ethnic Health Disparities is to direct, organize, and coordinate the systematic planning, implementation, and evaluation of efforts that are targeted at improving racial and ethnic minority health and addressing racial and ethnic health disparities. Links to ongoing OMH initiatives can be accessed at https://minorityhealth.hhs.gov/.

In 2010, the **Centers for Disease Control and Prevention** (n.d.-d) established the REACH program with the long-term aim of reducing health disparities among racial and ethnic groups. REACH provides funding and expert support to state and local health departments, community-based organizations, tribes, and universities to develop and implement programs that address health disparities. Through REACH, 31 organizations are funded by the CDC to "reduce health disparities among racial and ethnic populations with the highest burden of chronic disease, such as hypertension, heart disease, type 2 diabetes, and obesity" (CDC, n.d.-d). Information about current REACH recipients can be found at https://www.cdc.gov/reach/php/reach-2023-2028/index.html.

Nursing's Response to Vulnerable Populations and Health

The *Code of Ethics for Nurses with Interpretive Statements* (the Code) of the American Nurses Association (ANA) reinforces the profession's commitment to providing service to people regardless of background or situation (Winland-Brown et al., 2015). The Code explicitly states that nurses practice "with compassion and respect for the inherent dignity, worth, and unique attributes of every person" (Provision 1) and collaborate to "protect human rights, promote health diplomacy, and reduce health disparities" (Provision 8) (ANA, 2015a, p. v). Nurses have responsibilities to be aware of specific health needs and respond to illness in all populations. The ANA's Council on Cultural Diversity in Nursing Practice supports the work of nurses in their development of culturally and linguistically appropriate care. The organization and its leadership, through the Ethnic-Minority Fellowship Program, have played an essential role in supporting students from racial/ethnic minority groups with their graduate and doctoral work. Increasing diversity within the nursing and health professional workforce is part of a multipronged approach to addressing health disparities, improving quality of care for vulnerable populations, and increasing cultural awareness in health care delivery in the United States.

Nurses' awareness and understanding of transcultural issues have been facilitated by the works of such leaders as Leininger (1978), Giger and Davidhizar (2002), and Andrews and Boyle (2002). They, and other nurses with advanced preparation, have committed their time and energy to developing approaches and models for **transcultural nursing**. This specialty is an area of nursing study and practice that focuses on discovering and explaining cultural factors that influence the health, well-being, illness, or death of individuals or groups and seeks to provide culturally based appropriate care to people of diverse cultures with a variety of health care and spiritual beliefs (see Box 2.4: Best Practice) (Leininger, 2001). The culture care diversity and universality theory (Leininger, 2002) is a well-recognized theory used globally by many nurses, and it has significantly contributed to the establishment and advancement of transcultural nursing research, knowledge, and practice. It is essential for nurses to plan culturally tailored and competent care to mitigate health disparities and provide effective care in our rapidly changing multicultural societies, thereby delivering quality and safe care to all (Box 2.5: Quality and Safety Scenario). Wide dissemination of research findings has been made possible through the *Journal of Transcultural Nursing* and through annual conferences and other sponsored workshops for this nursing specialty.

Nursing journals and many other publications increase professionals' knowledge of health-related cultural issues. The *Minority Nurse* provides summaries of research studies, legislative updates affecting ethnic minorities, and relevant topics in education and practice. Ethnic nursing organizations also promote greater cultural understanding through their dissemination of important works by clinicians, educators, and researchers. Professional nursing organizations such as the ANA and the National League for Nursing publish culturally relevant materials to guide students, clinicians, and educators. For instance, in 2015 the ANA updated the scope and standards of nursing practice, including the addition of a new standard (Standard 8) for culturally congruent practice (ANA, 2015b).

Culturally congruent practice is the application of evidence-based nursing that is in agreement with the preferred cultural values, beliefs, worldview, and practices of the health care consumer and other stakeholders. Cultural competence represents the process by which nurses demonstrate culturally congruent practice. Nurses design and direct culturally congruent practice and services for diverse consumers to improve access, promote positive outcomes, and reduce disparities (ANA, 2015b, as cited in Marion et al., 2016, para. 7).

Culturally congruent practice has 20 associated competencies across three levels of practice: registered nursing practice (13 competencies), graduate-level nursing practice (5 competencies), and the practice of Advanced Practice Registered Nurses (2 competencies). Meeting the standard for culturally congruent practice and maintaining these competencies requires a commitment to lifelong learning and professional development, including self-assessment by nurses of their cultural beliefs and implicit biases (Marion et al., 2016). Accrediting bodies for nursing education, such as the Commission for Nursing Education Accreditation and the Commission on Collegiate Nursing

BOX 2.5 QUALITY AND SAFETY SCENARIO

Immigrants and Health Care Providers

Mr. Jade and Madam Nora have four children: Nirman (6 months), Julia (18 months), Hady (4 years), and Jamella (6 years). Mr. Jade is an economist who immigrated to the United States from Iraq 4 years ago. The family has come to the well-baby clinic because Madam Nora has been concerned about Nirman; Nirman's skin appears paler than that of her siblings, and she is also not gaining weight. Mr. Jade gives a brief summary of Nirman's situation because his wife cannot express herself in English. "My wife believes that Nirman is not growing like the rest of our children. She breastfeeds her every 2 hours, but she is not eating. My wife is upset that Nirman is not becoming bigger. My wife is exhausted, and her sister would like to come from Iraq to assist us, but she is having difficulty obtaining a visa." The vital signs are as follows: pulse 125 beats/min; respirations 22 breaths/min; blood pressure 100/70 mmHg; and rectal temperature 99.4°F. Nirman's weight is 10 lb 0 oz, and her length is 22 inches. Nirman appears pale. Madam Nora, aged 28 years, is wearing a headscarf covering her hair and a long dress. When Mr. Jade and Madam Nora are left alone, nurses can hear them arguing and raising their voices in a foreign language (Arabic), and Madam Nora appears upset. The medical history reveals a term baby female born by normal vaginal delivery with a normal birth weight. No history of vomiting, diarrhea, or fever has been reported. Pallor and jaundice are noted on physical examination. The family history reveals that both Mr. Jade and Madam Nora come from the same village, are Muslim, and are second-degree cousins. No genetic studies have been performed for the family members. Nirman's initial diagnosis was hemolytic anemia.

Nurses should consider the unique cultural background and family dynamics and functioning while providing care to this immigrant family to ensure safe and quality care. The family has an ineffective communication pattern and an inability to navigate the complexity of the health care system. Madam Nora needs to communicate with health care providers through her husband, who, in turn, is not familiar with medical terminology. Family assistance and respite for Madam Nora is lacking due to travel difficulties from Iraq. The fact that no genetic testing has been performed among family members may be attributed to unfamiliarity and the complexity of the health care system in the United States compared with the health care services in their native country. It is important for nurses to have culturally competent skills and to identify cultural beliefs that may impact how immigrant care recipients may communicate with them. Hence, effective approaches may be implemented to provide safe and quality care for this population and to mitigate health disparities.

Education, also support diversity with the inclusion of standards for maximizing diversity in the academic preparation of students pursuing bachelor's and master's degrees in nursing. The quest to deliver culturally and linguistically appropriate care has provided the impetus for nursing faculty to require transcultural courses in the nursing curriculum to facilitate awareness and understanding of cultural diversity.

In addition, major textbooks on specific clinical areas of practice often devote material to health care issues of vulnerable populations, including ethnic minorities. Discussion of specific health care problems and nursing care always includes cultural aspects. In the clinical setting, health care workers, through staff development and in-service programs, are provided with opportunities to learn and develop culturally and linguistically appropriate care approaches.

SUMMARY

- This century will continue to be a time of great challenges as the United States continues to be a nation of diverse peoples.
- Vulnerable and diverse populations share similar concerns, including health maintenance, an acceptable standard of living, and quality of life.
- Gaps and inequities are highlighted during times of crisis, such as the COVID-19 global pandemic.
- When shortcomings in our systems are brought forward during these times, opportunities for improvement become immediate and clear.
- Government, public and private industries, health care professions, and all individuals can work together to reduce health disparities and ensure a healthy nation for future generations.

CASE STUDY

An Older Immigrant Couple: Mr. and Mrs. Arahan

Mr. and Mrs. Arahan, a couple in their 70s, have been living with their oldest daughter, her husband of 15 years, and their two children, aged 12 and 14 years. They live in a middle-income neighborhood in a suburb of a metropolitan city. Mr. and Mrs. Arahan are both college educated and worked full-time while they were in their native country. In addition, Mr. Arahan, the only offspring of wealthy parents, inherited a substantial amount of money and real estate. Their daughter came to the United States as a registered nurse and met her husband, a drug company representative. The older couple moved to the United States when their daughter became a US citizen and petitioned for them as immigrants. Because the couple were facing retirement, they welcomed the opportunity to come to the United States.

The Arahans found life in the United States different from life in their home country, but their adjustment was not as difficult because both were healthy and spoke English fluently. Most of their time was spent taking care of their two grandchildren and the house. As the grandchildren grew older, the older couple found that they had more spare time. The daughter and her husband advanced in their careers and spent a great deal more time at their jobs. There were few family dinners during the week. On weekends, the daughter, her husband, and their children socialized with their own friends. The couple began to feel isolated and longed for a more active life.

Mr. and Mrs. Arahan began to think that perhaps they should return to their home country, where they still had relatives and friends. However, political and economic issues would have made it difficult for them to live there. Besides, they had become accustomed to the way of life in the United States with all the modern conveniences and abundance of goods that were difficult to obtain in their country. They also became concerned that they might not be able to tolerate the winter months and that minor health problems might worsen as they aged. They wondered who would take care of them if they became very frail and where they would live, knowing that their daughter had saved money only for their grandchildren's college education. They expressed their sentiments to their daughter, who became very concerned about how her parents were feeling.

Continued

CASE STUDY—cont'd

An Older Immigrant Couple: Mr. and Mrs. Arahan

This older couple had been attending church on a regular basis but had never been active in other church-related activities. The church bulletin announced the establishment of parish nursing with two retired registered nurses as volunteers. The couple attended the first opening of the parish clinic. Here, they met one of the registered nurses, who had a short discussion with them about the services offered. The registered nurse had spent a great deal of her working years as a community health nurse. She informed Mr. and Mrs. Arahan of her availability to help them resolve any health-related issues.

Reflective Questions

- What strategies could be suggested for this older adult couple to enhance their quality of life?
- What community resources can they use?
- What can the daughter and her family do to address the feelings of isolation of the older couple?
- What health-promotion activities can ensure a healthy lifestyle for the couple?

EVOLVE CHAPTER FEATURES

http://evolve.elsevier.com/Edelman/

- Study Questions

REFERENCES

Abuelezam, N. N., El-Sayed, A. M., & Galea, S. (2018). The health of Arab Americans in the United States: An updated comprehensive literature review. *Frontiers in Public Health*, *6*, 262. https://www.frontiersin.org/journals/public-health/articles/10.3389/fpubh.2018.00262/full

Adakai, M., Sandoval-Rosario, M., Xu, F., Aseret-Manygoats, T., Allison, M., Greenlund, K. J., & Barbour, K. E. (2018). Health disparities among American Indians/Alaska Natives – Arizona, 2017. *MMWR. Morbidity and Mortality Weekly Report*, *67*, 1314–1318. https://www.cdc.gov/mmwr/volumes/67/wr/mm6747a4.htm

Africa, J., & Carrasco, M. (2011). *Asian-American and Pacific Islander mental health: Report from a NAMI listening session*. National Alliance on Mental Health. https://www.blackradionetwork.com/

Agency for Healthcare Research and Quality. (2022). *2022 National healthcare quality and disparities report*. https://www.ahrq.gov/research/findings/nhqrdr/nhqdr22/index.html

Almli, L. M., Ely, D. M., Ailes, E. C., Abouk, R., Grosse, S. D., Isenburg, J. L., Waldron, D. B., & Reefhuis, J. (2020). Infant mortality attributable to birth defects – United States, 2003-2017. *MMWR. Morbidity and Mortality Weekly Report*, *69*, 25–29.

Amer, M. M. (2023). Arab American acculturation and ethnic identity across the life span: Sociodemographic correlates and psychological outcomes. In S. C. Nassar, K. J. Ajrouch, F. J. Dallo, & J. Hakim-Larson (Eds.), *Biopsychosocial perspectives on Arab Americans*. Springer, Cham. https://doi.org/10.1007/978-3-031-28360-4_8

American Nurses Association (ANA). (2015a). *Code of ethics for nurses with interpretive statements*. Silver Springs, MD: Author.

American Nurses Association (ANA). (2015b). *Nursing: Scope and standards of practice* (3rd ed.). Silver Springs, MD: Author.

American Psychiatric Association (APA). (2018). *APA Dictionary of Psychology "ethnic group."* https://dictionary.apa.org/ethnic-group

American Psychiatric Association (APA). (2023). *APA Dictionary of Psychology "minority group."* https://dictionary.apa.org/minority-group

American Psychiatric Association (APA). (n.d.). *Racism, bias, and discrimination*. https://www.apa.org/topics/racism-bias-discrimination

American Sociological Association. (2024). https://www.asanet.org/

Anandarajah, G., & Hight, E. (2001). Spirituality and medical practice: Using the HOPE questions as a practical tool for spiritual assessment. *American Family Physician*, *63*(1), 81.

Anderson, M. C., Hazel, A., Perkins, J., & Almquist, Z. (2021). The ecology of unsheltered homelessness: Environmental and social-network predictors of well-being among an unsheltered homeless population. *International Journal of Environmental Research and Public Health*, *18*(14), 7328. https://doi.org/10.3390/ijerph18147328

Andrews, M. M., & Boyle, J. S. (2002). Transcultural concepts in nursing care. *Journal of Transcultural Nursing*, *13*(3), 178–180.

Andrews, M. M., & Boyle, J. S. (2024). Andrews/Boyle transcultural nursing assessment guide for individuals and families. In M. M. Andrews & J. S. Boyle (Eds.), *Transcultural concepts in nursing care* (8th ed.). Philadelphia, PA: Lippincott Williams & Wilkins.

Andrews, M. M., & Boyle, J. S. (2019). The Andrews/Boyle transcultural interprofessional practice (TIP) model. *Journal of Transcultural Nursing*, *30*(4), 323–330.

Arab American Institute. (2024). https://www.aaiusa.org/

Artiga, S., & Pham, O. (2019). *Addressing health and social needs of immigrant families: Lessons from local communities*. Kaiser Family Foundation. https://www.kff.org/disparities-policy/issue-brief/addressing-health-and-social-needs-of-immigrant-families-lessons-from-local-communities/

Artiga, S., Tolbert, J., Kates, J., & Michaud, J. (2020). *Growing COVID-19 hotspots in the U.S. South and West will likely widen disparities for people of color*. Accessed May 2, 2024. https://www.kff.org/policy-watch/growing-covid-19-hotspots-in-south-and-west-likely-widen-disparities-people-of-color/

Asi, M., & Beaulieu, D. (2013). *Arab households in the United States: 2006–2010. American community survey briefs*. US Department of Commerce, Economics and Statistics Administration.

Avent, J. R., & Cashwell, C. S. (2015). The Black church: Theology and implications for counseling African Americans. *The Professional Counselor*, *5*(1), 81–90.

Awad, G. H., Abuelezam, N. N., Ajrouch, K. J., & Stiffler, M. J. (2022). Lack of Arab or Middle Eastern and North African health data undermines assessment of health disparities. *American Journal of Public Health*, *112*(2), 209–212.

Bakullari, A., Metersky, M. L., Wang, Y., Eldridge, N., Eckenrode, S., Pandolfi, M. M., Jaser, L., Galusha, D., & Moy, E. (2014).

Racial and ethnic disparities in healthcare-associated infections in the United States, 2009-2011. *Infection Control and Hospital Epidemiology*, *35*(S3), S10–S16.

Balboni, T. A., Fitchett, G., Handzo, G. F., Johnson, K. S., Koenig, H. G., Pargament, K. I., Puchalski, C. M., Sinclair, S., Taylor, E. J., & Steinhauser, K. E. (2017). State of the science of spirituality and palliative care research part II: Screening, assessment, and interventions. *Journal of Pain and Symptom Management*, *54*(3), 441–453.

Baugh, R. (2022). *Refugees and asylees: 2020*. US Department of Homeland Security. https://www.dhs.gov

Best, M., Butow, P., & Olver, I. (2016). Doctors discussing religion and spirituality: A systematic literature review. *Palliative Medicine*, *30*(4), 327–337. doi:10.1177/0269216315600912

Bowen, E., Savino, R., & Irish, A. (2019). Homelessness and health disparities: A health equity lens. In H. Larkin, A. Aykanian, & C. L. Streeter (Eds.), *Homelessness prevention and intervention in social work: Policies, programs, and practices* (pp. 57–83). Cham, Switzerland: Springer International Publishing.

Boyle, J. S., Collins, J. W., Andrews, M., & Ludwig-Beymer, P. (2024). *Transcultural concepts in nursing care* (8th ed.). Wolters Kluwer.

Braveman, P., & Dominguez, T. (2021a). Abandon "race." Focus on racism. *Frontiers in Public Health, 9*. https://doi.org/10.3389/fpubh.2021.689462

Braveman, P., Dominguez, T. P., Burke, W., Dolan, S. M., Stevenson, D. K., Jackson, F. M., Collins, J. W., Driscoll, D. A., Haley, T., Acker, J., Shaw, G. M., McCabe, E. R. B., Hay, W. W., Thornburg, K., Acevedo-Garcia, D., Cordero, J. F., Wise, P. H., Legaz, G., Rashied-Henry, K., Frost, J., Verbiest, S., & Waddell, L. (2021b). Explaining the Black-White disparity in preterm birth: A consensus statement from a multi-disciplinary scientific work group convened by the March of Dimes. *Frontiers in Reproductive Health, 3*, 684207. https://doi.org/10.3389/frph.2021.684207

Budiman, A., & Ruiz, N. G. (2021). *Asian Americans are the fastest-growing racial or ethnic group in the U.S.* Pew Research Center. https://www.pewresearch.org/short-reads/2021/04/09/asian-americans-are-the-fastest-growing-racial-or-ethnic-group-in-the-u-s/

Callaghan, S. (2023). *Female genital mutilation/cutting (FGM/C) in the United States: A study of the prevalence, distribution, and impact of FGM/C in the US, 2015-2019*. AHA Foundation. https://www.theahafoundation.org/wp-content/uploads/2023/10/AHA-FGM_C-Report-final.pdf

Callender, K. A., Ong, L. Z., & Othman, E. H. (2022). Prayers and mindfulness in relation to mental health among first-generation immigrant and refugee Muslim women in the USA: An exploratory study. *Journal of Religion and Health*, *61*(5), 3637–3654.

Centers for Disease Control and Prevention (CDC). (n.d.-a). *Chronic disease fact sheets*. https://www.cdc.gov

Centers for Disease Control and Prevention (CDC). (n.d.-b). *HIV and African Americans*. https://www.cdc.gov

Centers for Disease Control and Prevention (CDC). (n.d.-c). *Health of Black or African American non-Hispanic Population*. https://www.cdc.gov/nchs/fastats/black-health.htm

Centers for Disease Control and Prevention (CDC). (n.d.-d). *Racial and ethnic approaches to community health (REACH)*. https://www.cdc.gov/reach/php/about/?CDC_AAref_Val=https://www.cdc.gov/nccdphp/dnpao/state-local-programs/reach/index.htm

Centers for Disease Control and Prevention (CDC). (2017). *Health disparities*. https://www.cdc.gov

Centers for Disease Control and Prevention (CDC). (2018a). *Diabetes prevention recognition program: Standards and operating procedures*. https://www.cdc.gov/diabetes-prevention/media/pdfs/legacy/dprp-standards.pdf?CDC_AAref_Val=https://www.cdc.gov/diabetes/prevention/pdf/dprp-standards.pdf

Centers for Disease Control and Prevention (CDC). (2018b). *Lesbian, gay, bisexual and transgender health*. https://www.cdc.gov

Centers for Disease Control and Prevention (CDC). (2018c). *Table 33. Use of mammography among women aged 40 and over, by selected characteristics: United States, selected years 1987-2015*. https://www.cdc.gov/nchs/data/hus/2018/033.pdf

Centers for Disease Control and Prevention (CDC). (2019, June 24). United States life tables. Table A, 2017. *National Vital Statistics Reports*, *68*(7). https://www.cdc.gov/nchs/fastats/life-expectancy.htm

Centers for Disease Control and Prevention (CDC). (2020a). *HIV surveillance report, 2018 (updated)*. https://www.cdc.gov/hiv/pdf/library/reports/surveillance/cdc-hiv-surveillance-report-2018-updated-vol-31.pdf

Centers for Disease Control and Prevention (CDC). (2020b). *Reported tuberculosis in the United States, 2019*. https://www.cdc.gov

Centers for Disease Control and Prevention (CDC). (2021). *Most recent national asthma data*. https://www.cdc.gov/asthma/asthmadata/adult_prevalence_race.html

Centers for Disease Control and Prevention (CDC). (2022a). *Advancing health equity in chronic disease prevention and management*. https://www.cdc.gov/chronicdisease/healthequity/index.htm

Centers for Disease Control and Prevention (CDC). (2022b). *Health equity*. https://www.cdc.gov/healthequity/whatis/index.html

Centers for Disease Control and Prevention (CDC). (2022c). *Social determinants of health at CDC*. https://www.cdc.gov

Centers for Disease Control and Prevention (CDC). (2023a). *Cancers by age, sex, race and ethnicity*. https://gis.cdc.gov/Cancer/USCS/#/Demographics/

Centers for Disease Control and Prevention (CDC). (2023b). *Racism and health*. https://www.cdc.gov/minority-health/racism-health/index.html

Chatters, L. M., Nguyen, A. W., Taylor, R. J., & Hope, M. O. (2018). Church and family support networks and depressive symptoms among African Americans: Findings from The National Survey of American Life. *Journal of Community Psychology*, *46*(4), 403–417.

Chen, J., Lin, Y., Yan, J., Wu, Y., & Hu, R. (2018). The effects of spiritual care on quality of life and spiritual well-being among patients with terminal illness: A systematic review. *Palliative Medicine*, *32*(7), 1167–1179.

Choi, S. K., Kittle, K., & Meyer, I. H. (2018). *Aging LGB Adults in California*. The Williams Institute, UCLA School of Law. https://williamsinstitute.law.ucla.edu/publications/aging-lgbt-adults-ca/

Choi, S. K., & Meyer, I. H. (2016). *LGBT Aging: A Review of research findings, needs, and policy implications*. The Williams Institute, UCLA School of Law. https://williamsinstitute.law.ucla.edu/wp-content/uploads/LGBT-Aging-Aug-2016.pdf

Conron, K. (2019). *Adult LGBT population in the United States*. UCLA Los Angeles, CA: The Williams Institute. https://williamsinstitute.law.ucla.edu/wp-content/uploads/LGBT-Population-Estimates-March-2019.pdf

Creamer, J., Shrider, E. A., Burns, K., & Chen, F. (2022). *Poverty in the United States: 2021. Current population reports, P60-277*. Washington, DC: US Government Publishing Office. https://www.census.gov/content/dam/Census/library/publications/2022/demo/p60-277.pdf

Cumoletti, M., & Batalova, J. (2018). *Middle Eastern and North African immigrants in the United States*. Migration Policy

Institute. https://www.migrationpolicy.org/article/middle-eastern-and-north-african-immigrants-united-states

Curtin, S. C. (2019). *Trends in cancer and heart disease death rates among adults aged 45-64: United States, 1999-2017. National Vital Statistics Reports*. Centers for Disease Control and Prevention. https://www.cdc.gov/nchs/data/nvsr/nvsr68/nvsr68_05-508.pdf

Del Pilar, W. (2018). *Degree attainment for Native American adults*. The Education Trust. Retrieved January 21, 2020, from https://edtrust.org/resource/degree-attainment-for-native-american-adults/

Duke, M. R. (2014). *Marshall Islanders: Migration patterns and health-care challenges*. Migration Policy Institute. https://www.migrationpolicy.org/article/marshall-islanders-migration-patterns-and-health-care-challenges

Ely, D. M., & Driscoll, A. K. (2019). Infant mortality in the United States, 2017: Data from the period linked birth/infant death file. *National Vital Statistics Reports*, *68*(10). Centers for Disease Control and Prevention (CDC). Retrieved January 15, 2020, from https://www.cdc.gov/nchs/data/nvsr/nvsr68/nvsr68_10-508.pdf

Fixico, D., Kolata, A. L., & Neely, S. (2001). American Indian. In *The world book encyclopedia* (Vol. 10, pp. 136–185). Chicago: World Books.

Frick, E., Riedner, C., Fegg, M. J., Hauf, S., & Borasio, G. D. (2006). A clinical interview assessing cancer patients' spiritual needs and preferences. *European Journal of Cancer Care*, *15*(3), 238–243.

Galinsky, A. M., Zelaya, C. E., Simile, C., & Barnes, P. M. (2017). *Health conditions and behaviors of Native Hawaiian and Pacific Islander persons in the United States, 2014*. National Center for Health Statistics. https://www.cdc.gov/nchs/data/series/sr_03/sr03_040.pdf

Gelatt, J., & Zong, G. (2018). *Settling in: A profile of the unauthorized immigrant population in the United States*. Washington, DC: Migration Policy Institute.

Ghadban, R., Haddad, L., Thacker, L. R., An, K., Balster, R. L., & Salyer, J. (2019). Smoking behaviors in Arab Americans: Acculturation and health beliefs. *Journal of Transcultural Nursing*, *30*(2), 115–123.

Gibson, I. (2023). *Refugees and asylees: 2022*. US Department of Homeland Security. https://www.dhs.gov

Giger, J. N., & Davidhizar, R. (2002). The Giger and Davidhizar transcultural assessment model. *Journal of Transcultural Nursing*, *13*(3), 185–188.

Gill, A. M., & Frazer, M. S. (2016). *Health risk behaviors among gender expansive students: Making the case for including a measure of gender expression in population-based surveys*. Washington, DC: Advocates for Youth.

GLAAD. (2018). *Accelerating acceptance 2018. Executive summary. A survey of American acceptance and attitudes toward LGBTQ Americans*. https://www.glaad.org

GLMA. (n.d.). *Open letter about coronavirus and the LGBTQ+* communities. http://glma.org

Grandbois, D. (2005). Stigma of mental illness among American Indian and Alaska Native nations: Historical and contemporary perspectives. *Issues in Mental Health Nursing*, *26*, 1001–1024.

Guzman, G., & Kollar, M. (2023). *Income in the United States: 2022. Current population reports, P60-279*. Washington, DC: US Government Publishing Office.

Hacker, K., Auerbach, J., Ikeda, R., Philip, C., & Houry, D. (2022). Social determinants of health—an approach taken at CDC. *Journal of Public Health Management and Practice*, *28*(6), 589–594. https://doi.org/10.1097/PHH.0000000000001626

Hammack, P. L., Meyer, I. H., Krueger, E. A., Lightfoot, M., & Frost, D. M. (2018). *HIV testing and PrEP use, familiarity, and attitudes among gay and bisexual men in the US*. The Williams Institute, UCLA School of Law. https://williamsinstitute.law.ucla.edu/publications/hiv-testing-and-prep-use-us/

Hankerson, S. H., & Weissman, M. M. (2012). Church-based health programs for mental disorders among African Americans: A review. *Psychiatric Services*, *63*(3), 243–249.

Harris-Haywood, S. A., Goode, T., Gao, Y., Smith, K., Bronheim, S., Flocke, S., & Zyzanski, S. (2014). Psychometric evaluation of a cultural competency assessment instrument for health professionals. *Medical Care*, *52*(2), e7–e15.

Hill, L., Ndugga, N., & Artiga, S. (2023). *Key data on health and health care by race and ethnicity*. https://www.kff.org/racial-equity-and-health-policy/report/key-data-on-health-and-health-care-by-race-and-ethnicity/

Ho, J. Q., Nguyen, C. D., Lopes, R., Ezeji-Okoye, S. C., & Kuschner, W. G. (2018). Spiritual care in the intensive care unit: A narrative review. *Journal of Intensive Care Medicine*, *33*(5), 279–287.

Hoeffel, E. M., Rastogi, S., Kim, M. O., & Shahid, H. (2012). *The Asian population: 2010. 2010 census briefs*. US Census Bureau. https://www.census.gov

Hollberg, M. R., Pogemiller, H., & Barnett, E. D. (n.d.). *Newly arrived immigrants & refugees*. Centers for Disease Control and Prevention (CDC). https://wwwnc.cdc.gov/travel/yellowbook/2020/posttravel-evaluation/newly-arrived-immigrants-and-refugees

Holt, C. L., Roth, D. L., Clark, E. M., Debnam, K. (2014). Positive self-perceptions as a mediator of religious involvement and health behaviors in a national sample of African Americans. *Journal of Behavioral Medicine*, *37*(1), 102–112.

Horvath, T., Leoni, T., Reschenhofer, P., & Spielauer, M. (2023). Socio-economic inequality and healthcare costs over the life course—a dynamic microsimulation approach. *Public Health*, *219*, 124–130. https://doi.org/10.1016/j.puhe.2023.04.001

Human Rights Campaign. (2020). *Sexual orientation and gender identity definitions*. https://www.hrc.org/resources/sexual-orientation-and-gender-identity-terminology-and-definitions

Ivsins, A., Warnock, A., Small, W., Strike, C., Kerr, T., & Bardwell, G. (2023). A scoping review of qualitative research on barriers and facilitators to the use of supervised consumption services. *International Journal of Drug Policy*, *111*, 103910.

James, L. (2019, October 3). *LGBTQ cultural competency 101: Tools to improve patient communication, care and outcomes*. Oregon Rural Health Conference. https://www.ohsu.edu/sites/default/files/2019-10/10.3.19%201115%20am%20LGBTQ%20Cultural%20Comp%20%20JAMES.pdf

Jin, X., He, W., Zhang, Y., Gong, E., Niu, Z., Ji, J., Li, Y., Zeng, Y., & Yan, L. L. (2021). Association of *APOE* ε4 genotype and lifestyle with cognitive function among Chinese adults aged 80 years and older: A cross-sectional study. *PLOS Medicine*, *18*(6), 1003597. https://doi.org/10.1371/journal.pmed.1003597

Johnson, M. J., & Nemeth, L. S. (2014). Addressing health disparities of lesbian and bisexual women: A grounded theory study. *Women's Health Issues*, *24*(6), 635–640. https://doi.org/10.1016/j.whi.2014.08.003

Jongen, C., McCalman, J., & Bainbridge, R. (2018). Health workforce cultural competency interventions: a systematic scoping review. *BMC Health Services Research*, *18*(1). https://link-gale-com.proxy.lib.pacificu.edu:2443/apps/doc/A547114185/AONE?u=s8865459&sid=AONE&xid=9d82b1b9

Kaholokula, J. K., Look, M., Mabellos, T., Zhang, G., de Silva, M., Yoshimura, S., Solatorio, C., Wills, T., Seto, T. B., & Sinclair, K. A. (2017). Cultural dance program improves hypertension management for Native Hawaiians and Pacific Islanders: A pilot randomized trial. *Journal of Racial and Ethnic Health Disparities*, *4*(1), 35–46.

Kaholokula, J. K., Okamoto, S. K., & Yee, B. W. K. (2019). Special issue introduction: Advancing Native Hawaiian and other Pacific Islander health. *Asian American Journal of Psychology*, *10*(3), 197–205.

Karipek, A. (2020). Portrayals of Jihad: A cause of Islamophobia. *Islamophobia Studies Journal*, *5*(2), 210–255.

Kaiser Family Foundation. (2024). https://www.kff.org/

Keisler-Starkey, K., & Bunch, L. N. (2021). *Health Insurance Coverage in the United States: 2020. Current population reports, P60-274.* Washington, DC: US Government Publishing Office.

Lam, J., Aldridge, R., Blackburn, R., & Harron, K. (2023). How is ethnicity reported, described, and analysed in health research in the UK? A bibliographical review and focus group discussions with young refugees. *BMC Public Health*, *23*(1), 2025. https://doi.org/10.1186/s12889-023-16947-3

LaVeist, T. A., Pérez-Stable, E. J., Richard, P., Anderson, A., Isaac, L. A., Santiago, R., Okoh, C., Breen, N., Farhat, T., Assenov, A., & Gaskin, D. J. (2023). The economic burden of racial, ethnic, and educational health inequities in the US. *JAMA*, *329*(19), 1682. https://doi.org/10.1001/jama.2023.5965

Lee, Y. H., Salman, A., & Wang, F. (2012). Recruiting Chinese-American adolescents to HIV/AIDS related research: A lesson learned from a cross-sectional study. *Applied Nursing Research*, *25*(1), 40–46.

Leininger, M. (2001). *The theory of culture care diversity and universality*. Boston, MA: Jones and Bartlett.

Leininger, M. (2002). Culture care theory: A major contribution to advance transcultural nursing knowledge and practices. *Journal of Transcultural Nursing*, *13*(3), 189–192.

Leininger, M. M. (1978). *Transcultural nursing: Concepts, theories, and practices*. New York, NY: John Wiley.

Lekas, H. M., Pahl, K., & Fuller Lewis, C. (2020). Rethinking cultural competence: Shifting to cultural humility. *Health Services Insights*, *13*. doi:10.1177/1178632920970580

Lewis, T. T., & Van Dyke, M. E. (2018). Discrimination and the health of African Americans: The potential importance of intersectionalities. *Current Directions in Psychological Science*, *27*(3), 176–182.

Liu, Y., Elliott, A., Strelnick, H., Aguilar-Gaxiola, S., & Cottler, L. B. (2019). Asian Americans are less willing than other racial groups to participate in health research. *Journal of Clinical and Translational Science*, *3*, 90–96. doi:10.1017/cts.2019.372

LoPresti, M. A., Dement, F., & Gold, H. T. (2016). End-of-life care for people with cancer from ethnic minority groups: A systematic review. *American Journal of Hospice and Palliative Medicine*, 33(3), 291–305.

Macias-Konstantopoulos, W. L., Collins, K. A., Diaz, R., Duber, H. C., Edwards, C. D., Hsu, A. P., Ranney, M. L., Rivello, R. J., Wettstein, Z. S., & Sachs, C. J. (2023). Race, healthcare, and health disparities: A critical review and recommendations for advancing health equity. *Western Journal of Emergency Medicine*, *24*(5), 906.

Mallory, C., & Tentindo, W. (2019). *Medicaid coverage for gender-affirming care*. The Williams Institute, UCLA School of Law. https://williamsinstitute.law.ucla.edu/publications/medicaid-trans-health-care/

Marion, L., Douglas, M., Lavin, M., Barr, N., Gazaway, S., Thomas, L., & Bickford, C. (2016). Implementing the new ANA Standard 8: Culturally congruent practice. *Online Journal of Issues in Nursing*, *22*(1), 9.

Markus, H. R. (2008). Pride, prejudice, and ambivalence: Toward a unified theory of race and ethnicity. *American Psychologist*, *63*(8), 651–670. https://doi.org/10.1037/0003-066X.63.8.651

Martos, A. J., Fingerhut, A., Wilson, P. A., & Meyer, I. H. (2019). Utilization of LGBT-specific clinics and providers across three cohorts of lesbian, gay, and bisexual people in the United States. *SSM: Population Health*, *9*. https://doaj.org/article/8df57219bc6c40c69aedb19d0a214bcc

Matanda, D. J., Van Eekert, N., Croce-Galis, M., Gay, J., Middelburg, M. J., & Hardee, K. (2023). What interventions are effective to prevent or respond to female genital mutilation? A review of existing evidence from 2008–2020. *PLOS Global Public Health*, *3*(5), e0001855. https://doi.org/10.1371/journal.pgph.0001855

McMullin, J., Bone, M., Pang, J. K., Pang, V. K., & McEligot, A. (2010). Native Hawaiian voices: Enhancing the role of cultural values in community based participatory research. *Californian Journal of Health Promotion*, *8*, 52–62. Special Issue, Cancer Control.

Miller, S., & Baker, B. (2023). *Estimates of the lawful permanent resident population in the United States and the subpopulation eligible to naturalize: 2023.* US Department of Homeland Security. https://www.dhs.gov

Mokuau, N., DeLeon, P. H., Kaholokula, J. K., Soares, S., Tsark, J. U., & Haia, C. (2016). *Challenges and promise of health equity for Native Hawaiians*. National Academy of Medicine. https://nam.edu/challenges-and-promise-of-health-equity-for-native-hawaiians/

Morey, B. N., Chang, R. C., Thomas, K. B., Tulua, M. S., Penaia, C., Tran, V. D., Pierson, N., Greer, J. C., Bydalek, M., & Ponce, N. (2022). No equity without data equity: Data reporting gaps for Native Hawaiians and Pacific Islanders as structural racism. *Journal of Health Politics, Policy and Law*, *47*(2), 159–200. https://doi.org/10.1215/03616878-9517177

Mossaad, A. (2019). *Refugees and asylees: 2018*. US Department of Homeland Security. Annual flow report. https://www.dhs.gov/immigration-statistics/refugees-asylees

National Academies of Sciences, Engineering, and Medicine (NASEM). (2023). *Federal policy to advance racial, ethnic, and tribal health equity*. Washington, DC: The National Academies Press. https://doi.org/10.17226/26834

Nataraj, N., Rikard, S. M., Zhang, K., Jiang, X., Guy, G. P., Rice, K., Mattson, C. L., Gladden, R. M., Mustaquim, D. M., Illg, Z. N., Seth, P., Noonan, R. K., & Losby, J. L. (2024). Public health interventions and overdose-related outcomes among persons with opioid use disorder. *JAMA Network Open*, *7*(4), e244617. https://doi.org/10.1001/jamanetworkopen.2024.4617

National Alliance to End Homelessness. (2024). *State of homelessness: 2023 edition*. https://endhomelessness.org/homelessness-in-america/homelessness-statistics/state-of-homelessness/

National Center for Health Statistics. (2018). *Health, United States, 2017: With special feature on mortality*. Hyattsville, MD: National Center for Health Statistics. Retrieved January 21, 2020, from https://www.cdc.gov/nchs/data/hus/hus17.pdf

National Center for Transgender Equality. (2016). *The report of the 2015 U.S. transgender survey*. https://transequality.org/sites/default/files/docs/usts/USTS-Full-Report-Dec17.pdf

National Coalition for the Homeless. (2023). https://nationalhomeless.org/

National Harm Reduction Coalition. (n.d.). *Principles of harm reduction*. https://harmreduction.org/about-us/principles-of-harm-reduction/

National Health Care for the Homeless Council (NHCHC). (2019). *Homelessness & health: What's the connection?* https://nhchc.org/wp-content/uploads/2019/08/homelessness-and-health.pdf

National Health Care for the Homeless Council (NHCHC). (2024). https://nhchc.org/

National Institutes of Health, National Cancer Institute. (n.d.). *NCI dictionary of cancer terms*. https://www.cancer.gov/publications/dictionaries/cancer-terms

National Public Radio. (2020). *Navajo Nation sees high rate of COVID-19 and contact tracing is a challenge*. https://www.npr.org/2020/04/24/842945050/navajo-nation-sees-high-rate-of-covid-19-and-contact-tracing-is-a-challenge

Newton, R. (2019). Workshop addresses lack of diversity in workforce. *NIH Record*, *LXXI*(6). Retrieved January 17, 2020, from https://nihrecord.nih.gov/2019/03/22/workshop-addresses-lack-diversity-workforce

Norris, T., Vines, P. L., & Hoeffel, E. M. (2012). *The American Indian and Alaskan Native Population: 2010*. US Census Bureau. http://www.census.gov

Office of Minority Health (OMH). (n.d.-a). *Asian American Health*. https://www.minorityhealth.hhs.gov/omh/browse.aspx?lvl=3&lvlid=63

Office of Minority Health (OMH). (n.d.-b). *Cancer and Asian Americans*. https://www.minorityhealth.hhs.gov/omh/browse.aspx?lvl=4&lvlid=46

Office of Minority Health (OMH). (n.d.-c). *Mental and behavioral health – Asian Americans*. https://www.minorityhealth.hhs.gov/omh/browse.aspx?lvl=4&lvlid=54#1

Office of Minority Health (OMH). (n.d.-d). *Native Hawaiians and Pacific Islander Health*. https://www.minorityhealth.hhs.gov/omh/browse.aspx?lvl=3&lvlid=65

Office of Minority Health (OMH). (n.d.-e). *Mental and behavioral health – Native Hawaiians/Pacific Islanders*. https://www.minorityhealth.hhs.gov/omh/browse.aspx?lvl=4&lvlid=172

Office of Minority Health (OMH). (n.d.-f). *Hispanic/Latino Health*. https://www.minorityhealth.hhs.gov/hispaniclatino-health

Office of Minority Health (OMH). (n.d.-g). *HIV/AIDS and Hispanic Americans*. https://minorityhealth.hhs.gov/omh/browse.aspx?lvl=4&lvlid=66

Office of Minority Health (OMH). (n.d.-h). *Asthma and Hispanic Americans*. https://minorityhealth.hhs.gov/omh/browse.aspx?lvl=4&lvlid=60

Office of Minority Health (OMH). (n.d.-i). *Cancer and Hispanic Americans*. https://minorityhealth.hhs.gov/omh/browse.aspx?lvl=4&lvlid=61

Office of Minority Health (OMH). (n.d.-j). *Black/African American Health*. https://minorityhealth.hhs.gov/omh/browse.aspx?lvl=3&lvlid=61

Office of Minority Health (OMH). (n.d.-k). *Cancer and African Americans*. https://minorityhealth.hhs.gov/omh/browse.aspx?lvl=4&lvlid=16

Office of Minority Health (OMH). (n.d.-l). *HIV/AIDS and African Americans*. https://minorityhealth.hhs.gov/omh/browse.aspx?lvl=4&lvlid=21

Office of Minority Health (OMH). (n.d.-m). *Heart disease and African Americans*. https://minorityhealth.hhs.gov/omh/browse.aspx?lvl=4&lvlid=19

Office of Minority Health (OMH). (n.d.-n). *Stroke and African Americans*. https://minorityhealth.hhs.gov/omh/browse.aspx?lvl=4&lvlid=28

Office of Minority Health (OMH). (n.d.-o). *Diabetes and African Americans*. https://minorityhealth.hhs.gov/omh/browse.aspx?lvl=4&lvlid=18

Office of Minority Health (OMH). (n.d.-p). *American Indian/Alaska Native Health*. https://minorityhealth.hhs.gov/omh/browse.aspx?lvl=3&lvlid=62

Office of Minority Health (OMH). (n.d.-q). *Mental and Behavioral Health – American Indians/Alaska Natives*. https://minorityhealth.hhs.gov/omh/browse.aspx?lvl=4&lvlid=39#1

Office of Minority Health (OMH). (n.d.-r). *About the Office of Minority Health*. https://www.minorityhealth.hhs.gov/omh/browse.aspx?lvl=1&lvlid=1

Office of Minority Health (OMH). (n.d.-s). *Diabetes and American Indians/Alaska Natives*. https://minorityhealth.hhs.gov/omh/browse.aspx?lvl=4&lvlid=33

Omi, M., & Winant, H. (2015). *Racial formation in the United States* (3rd ed.). New York: Routledge/Taylor & Francis Group.

Pacific Island Health Officers Association. (n.d.). *USAPI Region*. https://www.pihoa.org/usapi-region/

Pampati, S., Alattar, Z., Cordoba, E., Tariq, M., & Mendes de Leon, C. (2018). Mental health outcomes among Arab refugees, immigrants, and U.S. born Arab Americans in Southeast Michigan: a cross-sectional study. *BMC Psychiatry*, *18*(1), 379.

PDQ Supportive and Palliative Care Editorial Board. *Spirituality in cancer care (PDQ®)—health professional version*. Bethesda, MD: National Cancer Institute. Updated December 12, 2023. https://www.cancer.gov/about-cancer/coping/day-to-day/faith-and-spirituality/spirituality-hp-pdq. Accessed May 1, 2024. [PMID: 26389436]

Pew Research Center. (2015). *Modern immigration wave brings 59 million to U.S., driving population growth and change through 2065: Views of immigrant's impact on U.S. society mixed*. http://www.pewhispanic.org/2015/09/28/modern-immigration-wave-brings-59-million-to-u-s-driving-population-growth-and-change-through-2065/

Pew Research Center. (2022). *Facts on Latinos in the U.S.* https://www.pewresearch.org/race-and-ethnicity/fact-sheet/latinos-in-the-us-fact-sheet/

Pew Research Center. (2024). https://www.pewresearch.org

Population Reference Bureau (PRB). (2016). *Women and girls at risk of female genital mutilation/cutting in the United States*. https://www.prb.org/us-fgmc/

Public Broadcasting Service. (2020). *Navajo Nation, hit hard by COVID-19, comes together to protect its most vulnerable*. https://www.pbs.org/newshour/show/navajo-nation-hit-hard-by-covid-19-comes-together-to-protect-its-most-vulnerable

Puchalski, C., Jafari, N., Buller, H., Haythorn, T., Jacobs, C., & Ferrell, B. (2020). Interprofessional spiritual care education curriculum: A milestone toward the provision of spiritual care. *Journal of Palliative Medicine*, *23*(6), 777–784.

Pyra, M., Taylor, B., Flanagan, E., Hotton, A., Johnson, O., Lamuda, P., Schneider, J., & Pollack, H. A. (2022). Support for evidence-informed opioid policies and interventions: The role of racial attitudes, political affiliation, and opioid stigma. *Preventive Medicine*, *158*, 107034. https://doi.org/10.1016/j.ypmed.2022.107034

Ray, V. E., Randolph, A., Underhill, M., & Luke, D. (2017). Critical race theory, Afro-pessimism, and racial progress narratives. *Sociology of Race and Ethnicity*, *3*(2), 147–158. https://doi.org/10.1177/2332649217692557

Robinson, K., Galloway, K., Bewley, S., & Meads, C. (2017). Lesbian and bisexual women's gynaecological conditions: A systematic review and exploratory meta-analysis. *BJOG: An International Journal of Obstetrics & Gynaecology, 124*(3), 381–392.

Rosas, L. G., Lv, N., Lewis, M. A., Venditti, E. M., Zavella, P., Luna, V., & Ma, J. (2018). A Latino patient-centered, evidence-based approach to diabetes prevention. *Journal of the American Board of Family Medicine: JABFM, 31*(3), 364–374.

Rudolph, L., Caplan, J., Ben-Moshe, K., & Dillon, L. (2013). *Health in all policies: A guide for state and local governments.* Washington, DC, and Oakland, CA: American Public Health Association and Public Health Institute. Retrieved January 17, 2020, from https://www.phi.org/uploads/files/Health_in_All_Policies-A_Guide_for_State_and_Local_Governments.pdf

Samoa, R. A., & Neal Palafox, M. D. (2020). COVID-19 special column: COVID-19 hits Native Hawaiian and Pacific Islander communities the hardest. *Hawai'i Journal of Health and Social Welfare, 79*(5), 143–146.

Sentell, T., Kennedy, F., Seto, T., Vawer, M., Chiriboga, G., Valdez, C., Garrett, L. M., Paloma, D., & Taira, D. (2019). Sharing the patient experience: A "talk story" intervention for heart failure management in Native Hawaiians. *Journal of Patient Experience,* 1–9.

Snipp, C. M. (2000). Selected demographic characteristics of Indians. In E. R. Rhoades (Ed.), American *Indian Health* (pp. 41–57). Baltimore, MD: Johns Hopkins University Press.

SEER*Explorer: An interactive website for SEER cancer statistics [Internet]. (2023). Surveillance Research Program, National Cancer Institute; 2023. Updated November 16, 2023; Cited January 14, 2024. https://seer.cancer.gov/statistics-network/explorer/. Data source(s): SEER Incidence Data, November 2022 Submission (1975-2020), SEER 22 registries. U.S. Mortality Data (1969-2020), National Center for Health Statistics, CDC. https://seer.cancer.gov/statistics-network/explorer/application.html?site=18&data_type=9&graph_type=2&compareBy=rate_type&chk_rate_type_1=1&chk_rate_type_2=2&chk_rate_type_3=3&sex=1&race=8&age_range=1&hdn_stage=101&advopt_precision=1&advopt_show_ci=on&hdn_view=1&advopt_show_apc=on&advopt_display=1

Substance Abuse and Mental Health Services Administration. (2023). *Harm reduction.* https://www.samhsa.gov/find-help/harm-reduction

Su, D., & Li, L. (2011). Trends in the use of complementary and alternative medicine in the United States: 2002-2007. *Journal of Health Care for the Poor and Underserved, 22,* 295–309.

Tailakh, A., Mentes, J. C., & Morisky, D. E. (2012). Prevalence, awareness, treatment, and control of hypertension among Arab Americans. *Journal of Cardiovascular Nursing, 28*(4), 1–9.

Tailakh, A. K., Evangelista, L. S., Morisky, D. E., Mentes, J. C., Pike, N. A., & Phillips, L. R. (2016). Acculturation, medication adherence, lifestyle behaviors, and blood pressure control among Arab Americans. *Journal of Transcultural Nursing, 27*(1), 57–64.

Tashiro, C. J. (2006). Identity and health in the narratives of older mixed ancestry Asian Americans. *Journal of Cultural Diversity, 13*(1), 41–49.

Tucker, C. (2014, January). Health-in-all-policies guide can help communities plan for better health. *The Nation's Health, 43*(10), 12. https://link-gale-com.proxy.lib.pacificu.edu:2443/apps/doc/A355153744/AONE?u=s8865459&sid=AONE&xid=e9404f6f

US Cancer Statistics Working Group. (2023). *US cancer statistics data visualizations tool, based on 2022 submission data (1999-2020).* US Department of Health and Human Services (USDHHS), Centers for Disease Control and Prevention (CDC), and National Cancer Institute. https://www.cdc.gov/cancer/dataviz, Released November 2023. https://gis.cdc.gov/Cancer/USCS/#/Demographics/

US Census Bureau. (2017). *American community survey 1-year estimates.* https://data.census.gov/cedsci/all?q=American%20Community%20Survey%201-Year%20Estimates&hidePreview=false&tid=ACSDT5Y2017.B26211&t=Counts,%20Estimates,%20and%20Projections&y=2017

US Census Bureau. (2018a). *Facts for features: Hispanic Heritage Month 2018.* https://www.census.gov/newsroom/facts-for-features/2018/hispanic-heritage-month.html

US Census Bureau. (2018b). *Poverty status in the past 12 months.* https://data.census.gov/cedsci/table?q=poverty&g=&hidePreview=false&table=S1701&tid=ACSST1Y2018.S1701&t=Poverty&lastDisplayedRow=35&vintage=2018. Accessed December 15, 2019.

US Census Bureau. (2019a). *American Indian and Alaska Native Heritage Month: November 2019.* https://www.census.gov/newsroom/facts-for-features/2019/aian-month.html

US Census Bureau. (2019b). *National African-American (Black) History Month: February 2019.* https://www.census.gov/newsroom/facts-for-features/2019/black-history-month.html

US Census Bureau. (2019c). *Quick facts. United States. Population estimates, July 1, 2019 (V2019).* https://www.census.gov/quickfacts/fact/table/US/PST045219

US Census Bureau. (2020). *Asian American and Pacific Islander Heritage Month: May 2020.* https://www.census.gov

US Census Bureau. (2022a). *About the topic of race.* https://www.census.gov/topics/population/race/about.html

US Census Bureau. (2022b). *20.6 million people in US identify as Asian, Native Hawaiian or Pacific Islander.* https://www.census.gov/library/stories/2022/05/aanhpi-population-diverse-geographically-dispersed.html

US Census Bureau. (2022c). *Census tables (Hispanic Latino).* https://data.census.gov/table?g=010XX00US&d=DEC+Demographic+Profile

US Census Bureau. (2023a). *Asian American, Native Hawaiian and Pacific Islander Heritage Month: May 2023.* https://www.census.gov/newsroom/facts-for-features/2023/asian-american-pacific-islander.html#:~:text=1.7%20million,the%20United%20States%20in%202021

US Census Bureau. (2023b). *Asian Indian was the largest Asian alone population group in 2020.* https://www.census.gov/library/stories/2023/09/2020-census-dhc-a-asian-population.html#:~:text=Largest%20Asian%20Alone%20Groups%20in,%2C%204%2C128%2C718%20(up%2031.6%25)

US Census Bureau. (2023c). *Census Bureau releases new educational attainment Data.* https://www.census.gov/newsroom/press-releases/2023/educational-attainment-data.html#:~:text=In%202020%2C%2037.5%25%20of%20people,difference%20is%20not%20statistically%20significant

US Census Bureau. (2023d). *Detailed races and ethnicities in the United States and Puerto Rico: 2020 Census.* https://www.census.gov/library/visualizations/interactive/detailed-race-ethnicities-2020-census.html

US Census Bureau. (2023e). *Poverty.* https://www.census.gov/topics/income-poverty/poverty.html

US Census Bureau. (2024). *Net international migration returns to pre-COVID-19 levels.* https://www.census.gov/library/stories/2022/12/net-international-migration-returns-to-pre-pandemic-levels.html

US Census Bureau. (n.d.). *State population by characteristics: 2010-2019*. https://www.census.gov/data/tables/time-series/demo/popest/2010s-state-detail.html

US Citizenship and Immigration Services (USCIS). (2024a). *Female genital mutilation or cutting (FGM/C)*. https://www.uscis.gov/FGMC#:~:text=The%20U.S.%20government%20opposes%20FGM,%2C%20and%20gender%2Dbased%20violence

US Citizenship and Immigration Services (USCIS). (2024b). *Immigration and Nationality Act*. https://www.uscis.gov/laws-and-policy/legislation/immigration-and-nationality-act

US Commission on Civil Rights. (2018). *Broken promises: Continuing federal funding shortfall for Native Americans*. https://www.usccr.gov/pubs/2018/12-20-Broken-Promises.pdf

US Department of Commerce. (2018). *Using two separate questions for race and ethnicity in 2018 end-to-end census*. 2020 Census Program Memorandum Series: 2018.02. https://www2.census.gov/programs-surveys/decennial/2020/program-management/memo-series/2020-memo-2018_02.pdf

US Department of Health and Human Services (USDHHS). (n.d.-a). *Healthy People 2030: About disparities data*. https://health.gov/healthypeople/objectives-and-data/about-disparities-data

US Department of Health and Human Services (USDHHS). (n.d.-b). *Healthy People 2030: Social determinants of health*. https://health.gov/healthypeople/objectives-and-data/social-determinants-health

US Department of Health and Human Services (USDHHS). (n.d.-c). *Healthy People 2030: Objectives and data*. https://health.gov/healthypeople/objectives-and-data/browse-objectives

US Department of Health and Human Services (USDHHS), Office of Minority Health (OMH), & Think Cultural Health. (n.d.). *National culturally and linguistically appropriate services standards*. https://thinkculturalhealth.hhs.gov/clas/standards

US Department of Health and Human Services (USDHHS). (2019). *Cultural and linguistic competency*. https://minorityhealth.hhs.gov/cultural-and-linguistic-competency. Accessed May 2, 2024.

US Department of Health and Human Services (USDHHS). (2023). *Refugee health overview*. https://www.acf.hhs.gov/orr/programs/refugee-health

US Department of Health and Human Services (USDHHS), & National Center for Health Statistics. (2022). *Health, United States, annual perspective, 2020-2021*. National Center for Health Statistics (US). https://doi.org/10.15620/cdc:122044

US Department of Housing and Urban Development or the US Government. (2023). *Housing first: A review of the evidence*. https://www.huduser.gov

US Department of State. (n.d.). *U.S. government fact sheet on female genital mutilation or cutting*. https://travel.state.gov/content/travel/en/us-visas/visa-information-resources/fact-sheet-on-female-genital-mutilation-or-cutting.html

Vaughn, L. M., Jacquez, F., & Baker, R. C. (2009). Cultural health attributions, beliefs, and practices: Effects on healthcare and medical education. *Open Medical Education Journal, 2*, 64–74.

Velasco-Mondragon, E., Jimenez, A., Palladino-Davis, A. G., Davis, D., & Escamilla-Cejudo, J. A. (2016). Hispanic health in the USA: A scoping review of the literature. *Public Health Reviews, 37*(1), 31.

Waters, M. C., Kasinitz, P., & Asad, A. L. (2014). Immigrants and African Americans. *The Annual Review of Sociology, 40*, 369–390.

White, M. C., Epsey, D. K., Swan, J., Wiggins, C. L., Eheman, C., & Kaur, J. S. (2014). Disparities in cancer mortality and incidence among American Indians and Alaska natives in the United States. *American Journal of Public Health, 104*(S3), S377–S387.

Wilson, B. D. M., Choi, S. K., Herman, J. L., Becker, T. L., & Conron, K. J. (2017). Characteristics and Mental Health of Gender Nonconforming Adolescents in California. The Williams Institute. UCLA School of Law.

Winland-Brown, J., Lachman, V. D., & Swanson, E. O. (2015). The new 'code of ethics for nurses with interpretive statements' (2015): Practical clinical application, part I. *Medsurg Nursing, 24*(4), 268–271.

WISQARS. (2021). *WISQARS leading causes of death visualization tool: Leading causes of death*. https://wisqars.cdc.gov/lcd/?o=LCD&y1=2021&y2=2021&ct=10&cc=ALL&g=00&s=0&r=3&ry=2&e=0&ar=lcd1age&at=custom&ag=lcd1age&a1=18&a2=85

World Health Organization. (n.d.-a). *Health risks of female genital mutilation*. https://www.who.int

World Health Organization (WHO). (n.d.-b). *Social determinants of health*. https://www.who.int/health-topics/social-determinants-of-health#tab=tab_1

World Health Organization. (2020). *Female genital mutilation*. https://www.who.int/health-topics/female-genital-mutilation#tab=tab_1

World Health Organization (WHO). (2023). *Public health milestones through the years*. https://www.who.int/campaigns

Yamada, S., & Akiyama, M. J. (2014). "For the good of mankind": The legacy of nuclear testing in Micronesia. *Social Medicine, 8*(2), 83–92.

Yancy, C. W. (2020, April 15). COVID-19 and African Americans. *JAMA, 323*(19), 1891–1892.

3

Health Policy and the Delivery System

Debora Elizabeth Kirsch

http://evolve.elsevier.com/Edelman/

OBJECTIVES

After completing this chapter, the reader will be able to:

- Examine key developments in the history of health care that influenced the philosophical basis of US health care and separated preventive measures from curative measures.
- Differentiate between private and public sector functions and responsibilities in the delivery of health care.
- Describe the mechanisms by which health care in the United States is financed in both the private and public sectors.
- Analyze the influence of health legislation on the health care delivery system.
- Differentiate between the purposes, benefits, and limitations of Medicare, Medicaid, and other government-sponsored programs in achieving health equity.
- Discuss the major provisions of the Patient Protection and Affordable Care Act of 2010 and its effect on improving population health.
- Compare and contrast the health care delivery system between the United States and Canada.

KEY TERMS

Accountable care organizations (ACOs)
Advanced practice nurses (APNs)
Advocate
Affordable Care Act (ACA)
Concierge care
Fee-for-service
Gatekeeper
Health insurance exchange
Health maintenance organizations (HMOs)
Health savings accounts (HSAs)
High-deductible health insurance plans (HDHPs)
Hospitalist
Indemnity insurance plans
Independent practice associations (IPAs)
Insurance
Managed care
Marketplace
Medicaid
Medicare
Nursing centers
Point-of-service (POS)
Preferred provider organizations (PPOs)
Primary care provider (PCP)

THINK ABOUT IT

The Federal Health Care Reform Law

The passage of the federal health care reform law called the Patient Protection and **Affordable Care Act (ACA)** ignited the national conversation on the expanding role of government in the various aspects of the provision of health care. Major issues in the delivery of high-quality health care to the nation include improving access to care, financing health care, and curtailing the growth of health care costs. Within the many provisions of the ACA law, a federal government mandate required most US citizens to have health insurance coverage or to pay a health care penalty when filing annual federal taxes. This federal tax penalty, also called the health care mandate or the shared responsibility payment, was legislatively reduced to zero by US Congress effective January 1, 2019, resulting in a number of individuals electing to drop coverage. Some states (Massachusetts, New Jersey, Vermont, California, Rhode Island, and the District of Columbia) have in place an individual mandate at the state level requiring eligible residents to purchase health insurance or pay a penalty (currently Vermont does not charge a financial penalty for noncompliance), similar in cost to the previous federal penalty. State legislators in other states (Connecticut, Hawai'i, Maryland, Minnesota, and Washington) are considering adding the health insurance mandate (Crail, 2024). Although health insurance coverage is an essential element in promoting the health of the individual, questions remain concerning the best legislative policy at the state and federal levels to serve the health care needs of all Americans.

- How has the ACA facilitated access to affordable, quality health care for all US citizens?
- What are the risks of an individual or family not having health insurance coverage?
- With the federal mandate to carry health insurance removed, will the overall health of the population be affected?
- How will the ACA curtail rising health care costs and deal with issues of quality and safety?
- Why is the US health care system the costliest in the world even though it falls behind in terms of life expectancy and infant mortality rates compared with other industrialized countries?
- How can the health care needs of the most vulnerable populations be best served?

The health care delivery system in the United States is a complex, multilayered entity that has the capacity to provide the newest technologic treatments and implement the most advanced and innovative health care in the world. Research findings have sparked the development of international gold standards for practicing evidence-based medical and nursing care. The market-driven, multipayer, heavily private system is distinct from any other health care delivery system in the world, employing over 21.2 million health care workers, practitioners, and health care support occupation workers and serving more than 335 million people in 2021. The US Bureau of Labor Statistics (BLS) reports that the projection of 7 of the 20 fastest-growing occupations between 2022 and 2032 are health care related (BLS, 2023). Of the 867 occupations the BLS reports on, registered nurses constitute the largest number of professionals, with more than 3.17 million jobs and an above-average median salary of $81,220 ($39.05 per hour) as of May 2022. A projected growth of 193,100 registered nurse jobs (6%) over the next decade (2022 to 2032) is predicted because of an increased emphasis on preventive care; the increased health care needs of the aging baby boomer population; the replacement of nurses who transfer from or exit the labor force or retire; and a higher prevalence of chronic conditions such as diabetes, obesity, and heart disease. Nurse practitioners, nurse anesthetists, and nurse midwives have an even higher projected job growth outlook at 38% from 2022 to 2032 (an additional 29,200 openings per year) because of an increased emphasis on preventive care and a need for increased health care services for an aging population, especially in rural geographic areas of the country. Median salary for these **advanced practice nurses (APNs)** is reported to be $125,900 per year ($60.53 per hour), with the number of jobs listed at 323,900 in 2023 (BLS, 2023). According to the BLS (2023), nurse practitioners have the largest projected job growth (44.5%) for occupations that typically require a master's degree. The US health care system is massive, but so is the cost. The rising cost of health care is consuming a growing percentage of the nation's gross domestic product (GDP). The Centers for Medicare & Medicaid Services (CMS) estimates that in 2022 national health expenditures consumed 17.4% of the nation's GDP (i.e., more than $4.5 trillion), which equates to $13,413 per person, the highest dollar amount per capita of all industrialized countries. Health spending is expected to grow 5.4% annually from 2022 to 2031, resulting in an increase in the health spending share of GDP from 18.3% in 2021 to 19.6% by 2031 ($20,425 per capita) (CMS, 2023; Keehan et al., 2023). The insured share of the population reached 92.3% in 2022 and is expected to decrease to 90.5% by 2031. The rising cost of health insurance premiums and prescription drug coverage (and other related costs, such as higher copays and deductibles) is a growing burden for individuals, families, and employers.

Despite the vast economic resources devoted to financing the health care system, the United States ranks 48th globally in terms of life expectancy at birth (80.75 years) of the 227 countries reported by the Central Intelligence Agency (CIA). Monaco ranks the highest at 89.6 years, and Afghanistan ranks the lowest at 54.1 years. Despite its mediocre global positioning, the US life expectancy ranks more than 7 years above the average world life expectancy (reported to be 73.16 years in 2023) and 24th out of the 38 member countries in the Organisation for Economic Co-operation and Development (OECD, 2024) (CIA, 2024). Within the United States, unequal access and utilization by individuals and families to components of the health care system exist both financially and geographically, especially among vulnerable populations. Although the availability and provision of health insurance is an important factor in health equity, vulnerable populations face additional obstacles, contributing to health disparities across the nation. Health disparities (a particular type of health difference that is closely linked with social, economic, and/or environmental disadvantage) adversely affect certain groups of individuals, especially vulnerable populations (Box 3.1: Vulnerable Populations at Risk for Health Disparities).

Federal, state, and local governments enact health care reform policies and laws to improve the health of communities and the greater population. In the past, health care reform consisted of incremental steps, mainly targeted at the poor (**Medicaid**) and older adult populations (**Medicare**) to improve health; however, with escalating health care costs, rising numbers of uninsured Americans, and concern for improvement in the quality and safety of care, a more substantive reform effort was taken. An expansive health care federal reform law called the Patient Protection and **Affordable Care Act** was signed into law on March 23, 2010. The federal law required the largest change in the financing of the US health care system since public Medicare and Medicaid programs were enacted in the 1960s. The law was designed to expand coverage, control cost, and improve the delivery of health care (Kaiser Family Foundation [KFF], 2013). A core goal of the ACA was to reduce the number of uninsured individuals by expanding state Medicaid programs so that more individuals and families would meet the expanded

BOX 3.1 Vulnerable Populations at Risk for Health Disparities

- Residents of rural areas
- Undocumented and other immigrants
- Socioeconomically disadvantaged
- Children, adolescents, elderly, terminally ill
- Racial and ethnic minorities
- Uninsured or underinsured individuals
- People with chronic conditions
- People with language or cultural barriers
- The physically disabled or handicapped
- Mental health patients
- People who are immunocompromised
- Alcohol or substance abusers
- People who are homeless or in poor housing
- Loweducation levels or illiteracy
- Anyone lacking health literacy
- Members of underserved communities
- People lacking food security
- Lesbian, gay, bisexual, transgender, queer (LGBT+) persons

Source: Ndugga, N., Pillai, D., & Artiga, S. (2024). *Disparities in health and health care: Five key questions and answers*. Kaiser Family Foundation. https://www.kff.org/racial-equity-and-health-policy/issue-brief/disparities-in-health-and-health-care-5-key-question-and-answers/

enrollment criteria, establishing marketplace insurance plans and subsidies for moderate-income individuals to assist with health care premium costs, banning insurance companies from discriminating against individuals on the basis of preexisting conditions, and allowing children to stay on their parents' health insurance plan until the age of 26. Implementation of the law occurred in increments, with full enactment in 2018. The law was designed to address the issues of affordability, accessibility, and financing of health care, with focused efforts on meeting the needs of vulnerable populations. Implementation of the various provisions of the ACA required substantial changes to public insurance programs, private health insurance market regulations, and other components of the health care system. Lack of bipartisan support for the original ACA, continued bipartisan disagreements over many of its provisions, a change in the political landscape of the legislature in Washington, or future actions filed in the court system may result in a repeal of the law, a dismantling of portions of the law, or additional amendments to some of the law's current and future provisions. For example, one of the first contested provisions of the ACA was the requirement for most US citizens and legal residents to either have health insurance or pay a federal tax penalty beginning in 2014. In June of 2012, the Supreme Court of the United States ruled in favor of the constitutionality of this contested provision and upheld the requirement for the individual mandate, as it was interpreted as a tax levied by the federal government. However, in 2017, under the leadership of President Donald Trump, US Congress passed a package of tax cuts setting the charge of the individual federal mandate at $0, although several states have adopted state tax penalties for individuals who do not have health insurance (Congressional Budget Office, 2022). Courts continue to argue the constitutionality of various components of the law, and other provisions may be changed in future rulings. Courts have already ruled that individual states have the option of expanding (or not expanding) the eligibility criteria of individuals qualified to enroll in a state's Medicaid program. Expanding the Medicaid program in every state would extend medical insurance coverage to a greater number of lower-income adults. However, since Medicaid is funded by federal, state, and local taxes, the increase in enrollments would mean additional tax monies would be needed to pay for each additional enrollee. As of October 2023, 41 states (including the District of Columbia) have adopted Medicaid expansion programs, and 10 states have not. As an example, in 2023, a family of four with an income of $41,400 (138% of federal poverty guidelines) or less would have been eligible for Medicaid coverage if they were living in a state that had expanded its Medicaid program. To encourage individual states to expand Medicaid coverage, additional federal tax dollars have been allotted to states that expand coverage for the first several years (KFF, 2023a; US Department of Health and Human Services [USDHHS], 2024).

Implementing the many provisions of the ACA have required organizational changes at the state level. For example, one provision allows individuals and families to purchase health insurance coverage through a public or private **health insurance exchange**. The health insurance **marketplace**, or Obamacare exchange, is for individuals and families who do not have health insurance or employer-qualifying health insurance, Medicare, Medicaid, the Children's Health Insurance Program (CHIP), or another source that provides qualifying health insurance. Exchanges are organizations that offer choices of different health plans and help individuals and families understand options and apply for coverage. Marketplace plans can also be purchased by small businesses for their employees (Small Business Health Options Program [SHOP]). As of 2024, 19 states have state-based marketplace plans, including California's Covered California, Connecticut's Access Health CT, New York's New York State of Health, and Maryland's The Maryland Health Connection. Three states—Arkansas, Georgia, and Oregon—have state-based marketplace plans but use the federal platform, and 29 other states—including Florida, Michigan, and Arizona—use a federally run health marketplace through HealthCare.gov. Consumers in a state-based marketplace apply for and enroll in coverage through marketplace websites established and maintained by the state, while consumers in a federal marketplace apply for and enroll in HealthCare.gov. Many individuals who qualify for marketplace coverage health insurance are eligible for financial assistance through premium tax credits (subsidies) based on expected income. Subsidies help individuals and families pay for premiums if their income falls within 100% to 400% of the federal poverty guidelines. The USDHHS determines poverty guidelines used for administrative purposes (adjusted each year) to determine financial eligibility for certain federal programs. The poverty guideline for an individual as of 2024 is $15,060 and increases $5380 for each additional person in the family household. Marketplace plans must cover mandated essential health benefits, which include ambulatory patient services; emergency services; hospitalization; pregnancy, maternity, and newborn care; mental health and substance abuse services; prescription drugs; laboratory services; preventive and wellness services and chronic disease management; pediatric services (including oral and vision care); and preexisting conditions, including pregnancy and preventive care. Plans must also have birth control benefits and some covered contraceptive methods. Adult vision and dental coverage are not required in the mandated essential packages, but some plans may offer these benefits, or separate dental plans may be available for a separate additional premium. Marketplace plans have deductibles, copayments, and other out-of-pocket costs for most covered services with the exception of some preventive care (HealthCare.gov, n.d.-a; KFF, 2024). Plans offered in the health insurance marketplace are presented in four metal categories: bronze, silver, gold, and platinum. The category of the metal does not indicate the quality of the health plan; rather, it designates the difference in cost between what the insurance company pays and what the individual pays. A bronze plan, for example, has the lowest monthly premium for an individual or family but higher costs if the plan is used, while a platinum plan has the highest monthly premium but the lowest cost if the plan is used. All health insurance plans must cover the mandated essential health benefits, but each plan is different, with some states opting to cover additional services (HealthCare.gov, n.d.-b). The process of selecting and applying to join a plan can be challenging for many individuals, especially for those with low literacy levels and/or limited health literacy. Despite greater health insurance coverage for many more individuals, issues for the newly insured include paying monthly premiums (if applicable), knowing how to use plan benefits effectively, finding a provider, navigating the health care system, and paying additional out-of-pocket expenses, which may include premiums, deductibles, and copays. A key responsibility of nurses is to help individuals and families overcome these barriers (see case study).

This chapter will analyze the health status of the nation compared with other countries, examine historical influences on the delivery of health care, and describe the structure and mechanisms of delivering public (Medicare and Medicaid) and private health care in the United States, the financing of the health care system, and key federal legislation (with emphasis on the provisions of the ACA of 2010) that strives to improve teamwork and communication between all these system pieces. The greatest savings in health care expenditures can be realized if individuals engage in consistent health-promotion and disease-prevention practices and avoid the costly consequences of acute and chronic disease. The ACA includes requirements for essential health benefits designed to promote health screenings and other preventive measures, with the hope that savings will be realized from early detection, decreasing hospital admissions, and unnecessary hospital readmissions. Nurses need to keep abreast of the various provisions and amendments of the law to help individuals and families navigate the health care system. Informed nurses are key players in influencing health policy as **advocates** for social justice for individuals and families.

THE HEALTH OF THE NATION

The *Health, United States* program started in 1974 with an annual report prepared by the Centers for Disease Control and Prevention (CDC) and the National Center for Health Statistics (NCHS) charged with providing trends in health statistics summarizing the health status of the nation by tracking a variety of specific, measurable health indicators. This report serves several key functions, but the main goal is to inform the public, policymakers, the president, and Congress of the trends and disparities in the nation's health to guide the development of sound health policy and allocate resources to maintain and improve the health of the nation's citizens. The *Health, United States, 2020-2021 Annual Perspective* report was based on data collected through 2019 (before the COVID-19 pandemic) with the focused theme of health disparities. The format of the report was later redesigned to publish online periodically throughout the year to better align and expand data from more than 40 data sources with trend tables and supporting topics. Reports indicated that the health of the nation improved in many areas, correlating with substantial funding of public health programs, research, provision of health care, and initiatives to support consumer education. Emerging trends indicated success in the reduction of morbidity and mortality for many diseases, better control of many widespread infectious diseases through vaccination programs, improvement in motor vehicle safety, smoking cessation measures, and reduction of cardiovascular-related deaths. Although life expectancy (projection of the average number of years an individual can expect to live at the time of birth), has slowly increased for both males and females over the previous decades, the NCHS released in November 2023 the final mortality statistics from 2021, which revealed that life expectancy fell from 77.0 years (males 74.2 years and females 79.9 years) to 76.4 years (males 73.5 years and females 79.3 years) in 2020. The primary cause (59.7%) of negative contribution (0.7 years for males and 0.6 years for females) was increases in mortality due to COVID-19 (Arias et al., 2023). Estimates released by NCHS for 2022 indicate that life expectancy rose to 77.5 years (males 74.8 years and females 80.2 years) based on available provisional mortality data in November 2023 (Arias et al., 2023). Other trends in maternal and infant mortality rates on average are declining in many geographical locations, reported on average of 5.6 per 1000 live births (significant drop from 1950, when the rate was 29.2 per 1000) but a disproportionate rise in Black and African-American mothers (10.7 in 2019) compared with White mothers (4.6 in 2019). The report also ranks the top 10 causes (by average and by age group) of death displayed in table format and links an updated online source at the CDC. For all ages, heart disease remains the number one cause of death for Americans, responsible for 26.9% (695,547) of all deaths, followed by malignant neoplasms at 23.4% (605,213), COVID-19 at 16.1% (416,893), unintentional injuries at 8.7% (224,935), cerebrovascular disease at 6.3% (162,890), and chronic lower respiratory disease at 5.5% (142,342). The other ranked causes of death were Alzheimer disease, diabetes mellitus, liver disease, and nephritis at under 5% each. For age groups greater than 1 year and under 45 years, unintended injury was the number one cause of death. Education on leading a healthy lifestyle, controlling hypertension, smoking cessation, using cholesterol-lowering medications, and participating in routine screening has contributed to better health for many Americans, but concerns about sedentary lifestyles, rising obesity trends, and chronic diseases are noted. An example of linked trend tables is data on smoking prevalence and other substance use. Recent national smoking cessation interventions for individuals aged 25 years or older are demonstrating some effectiveness, as the percentage of individuals who currently smoke cigarettes dropped to 11.5% (28.3 million smokers) in 2021 compared with 19.2% in 2010. In 2018, cigarette smoking killed more than 480,000 Americans and cost more than $600 billion in health care costs and lost productivity. The highest prevalence of current cigarette smokers in 2019 (both sexes combined) was among adults aged 25 or older with no high school diploma or GED (23.9%) and those with a high school diploma or GED as their highest level of education attainment (22.0%). Cigarette smoking rates were lowest among those with a bachelor's degree or higher (5.8%) based on the civilian noninstitutionalized population, which did not include the use of e-cigarettes. (Fig. 3.1 shows geographic differences in the United States related to high school education.) Another stark difference noted is that Black or African-American males with no high school diploma or GED have the highest rate of cigarette smoking at 35.6% (slightly down

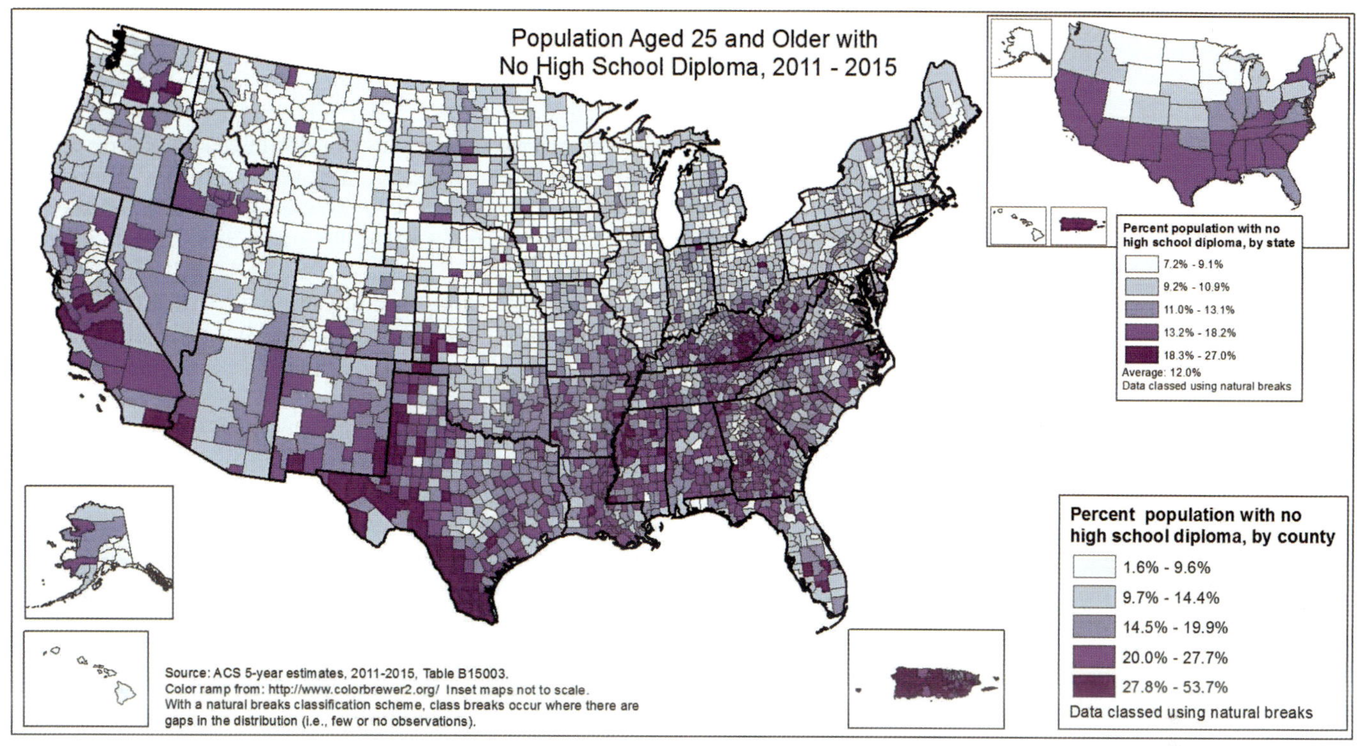

FIG. 3.1 American Community Survey on Population Aged 25 and Older with No High School Diploma 2011–2015.

from 38.2% in 2010). Although cigarette smoking may be on the decline, other substance use is a growing concern, especially among teens. Statistical findings linked to CDC trend tables report the use of various substances in the past 30 days among 12th graders, 10th graders, and 8th graders by sex and race. Data sets for 2019 reveal that while only 5.7% of 12th graders have used cigarettes in the past 30 days, 25.5% have engaged in nicotine vaping, 29.3% have consumed alcohol (14.4% binge drinking), 22.3% have used marijuana, 1% have used cocaine, 0.9% have used inhalants, and 0.7% have used ecstasy. Although they have lower numbers in all categories, 10th graders and 8th graders are engaging in these same substances and activities. Other health risks, including growing obesity rates among adults and children, remain problematic and will be discussed in later chapters. Of noted concern is the rise in the number of deaths due to suicide. Death records in 2022 (compared with 2021) revealed rates increased 3% to 9% for all age groups 35 years and older, with an average suicide death rate of 14.3 deaths per 100,000 people (23.1 male and 5.9 female). For males, the highest suicide rate occurred in the 75 years and older age group. In 2019, 70.6% of drug overdose deaths were caused by opioids (particularly heroin and fentanyl) and totaled 70,630 deaths. Drug overdose death rates among males aged 15 years and over increased from all age groups except 85 and over, with the highest increase from 25.2 per 100,000 to 56.6 for males aged 35 to 44 (NCHS, 2023). In summary, improvements in the nation's health have not been uniform, because factors affecting health outcomes are influenced by social determinants of health, which include an individual's income, race, sex, ethnicity, education level, poverty level, health insurance coverage, health status, housing, and geographic location. *Health, United States* provides health statistics and supporting evidence to guide evidence-based health policy decisions regarding optimal management of health concerns as well as to guide legislative policy and appropriations. The most effective intervention to decrease the growing cost of health care is to keep Americans healthy.

Healthy People 2030

As discussed in Chapter 1, the *Healthy People* federal initiative sets data-driven, science-based national objectives with targets to monitor and guide national health-promotion and disease-prevention efforts over the next decade to improve the health of the nation. The Secretary's Advisory Committee on National Health Promotion and Disease Prevention Objectives 2030, a division of the USDHHS, first established a framework that guided the vision of a society in which all people achieve their full potential for health and well-being across the life span. From the vision statement, objectives were developed to identify specific areas where action must be taken and targets met so as to achieve the goals during the next decade. The 359 current core objectives are tracked and periodically evaluated to determine whether the target has been met or exceeded, is improving, has seen little or no change, is getting worse, or is at a baseline. Determinations for the measurement of each objective can be found online. See Box 3.2: Healthy People 2030 *Selected Objectives* for a sample of objectives related to this health policy (Office of Disease Prevention and Health Promotion [ODPHP], 2023; USDHHS, 2020).

A health disparity as defined by *Healthy People 2030* refers to a particular type of health difference that is linked with

BOX 3.2 *HEALTHY PEOPLE 2030* SELECTED OBJECTIVES

Symbol /Number	*Healthy People 2030* SAMPLE Objectives
AHS-01	Increase the proportion of people with health insurance
AHS-03	Increase the proportion of people with prescription drug coverage
AHS-R03	Reduce the proportion of people under 65 years who are underinsured
AHS-04	Reduce the number of people who can't get medical care when they need it
ECBP-D03	Increase the proportion of work sites that offer an employee health-promotion program
TU-16	Increase Medicaid coverage of evidence-based treatment to help people quit using tobacco
ECBP-D07	Increase the number of community organizations that provide prevention services
MPS-D04	Increase the proportion of medical-surgical hospitals that report adverse drug events
PHI-R04	Monitor and understand the public health workforce: composition, enumeration, gaps, and needs
PHI-R07	Explore quality improvement as a way to increasing efficiency and effectiveness in health departments

US Department of Health and Human Services (USDHHS). [Internet]. *Healthy People 2030.* Office of Disease Prevention and Health Promotion. https://health.gov/healthypeople/objectives-and-data/browse-objectives

social, economic, and/or environmental disadvantage and that adversely affects groups of people who have systematically experienced greater obstacles to health. Health care disparity refers to differences between groups in access to and use of care, health insurance coverage, affordability, and quality of care. Groups of people who have systematically experienced greater obstacles to health on the basis of their race, color, or national origin; ethnic group; religion; socioeconomic status; gender; age; mental health; cognitive, sensory, physical, or other disability; sexual orientation or gender identity; geographical location; or other characteristics historically linked to discrimination or exclusion are vulnerable to health and health care disparities (KFF, 2023b). As will be discussed later in this chapter, the ACA demonstrated statistically significant improvements in health care coverage, access, and use in the nonelderly population (ages 0–64 years), most notably in the Hispanic population (Fig. 3.2) (Box 3.3: Health and Social Determinants/Health Equity). An expanded list of vulnerable populations at risk for health or health care disparities as discussed earlier can be found in Box 3.1: Vulnerable Populations at Risk for Health Disparities. Public health nursing as defined by the American Public Health Association is the practice of promoting and protecting the health of populations using knowledge from nursing, social, and public health sciences (American Nurses Association [ANA], 2023). The 10 essentials of public health services begin with monitoring the health status of a community to identify and solve problems; diagnosing and investigating health hazards and problems; informing, educating, and empowering people; mobilizing and developing plans to solve health problems; linking people to health services; evaluating; and researching new insights and solutions (Box 3.4: Best Practice 10 Essential Public Health Services). Community health nursing practice promotes, preserves, and maintains the health of populations through care provided to individuals, families, and groups and through the assessment of a community as a whole. (See Chapter 8 for further discussion.) *Healthy People 2030* supports the need for an effective public health infrastructure for planning, delivering, and evaluating public health, with the key components being a capable and qualified workforce, up-to-date data

2022
2021
Non-Hispanic White
93.2*
92.5
Black
88.6*
87.3
Asian
92.6
92.3
Hispanic (any race)
76.6*
74.9

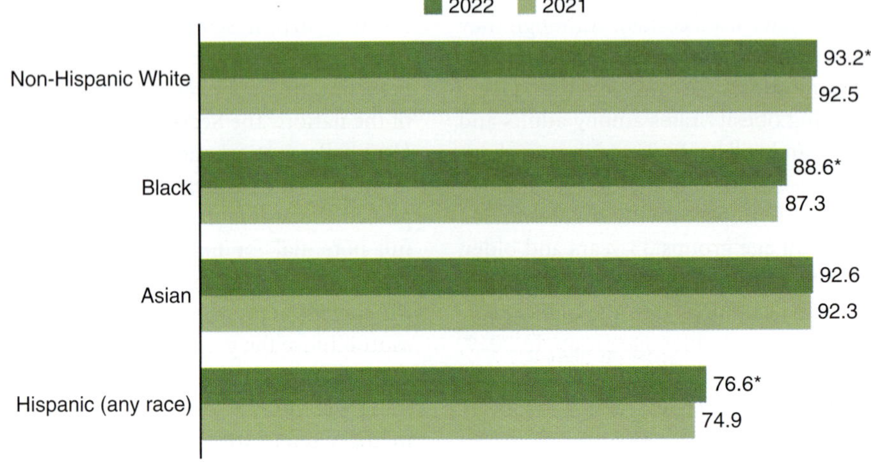

*Denotes a statistically significant difference at the 90 percent level.

Note: Information on confidentiality protection, sampling error, nonsampling error, and definitions is available at <www2.census.gov/programs-surveys/cps/techdocs/cpsmar23.pdf>.

Source: U.S. Census Bureau, Current Population Survey, 2022 and 2023 Annual Social and Economic Supplements (CPS ASEC).

FIG. 3.2 Percentage of Adults 19 to 64 years with Health Insurance by Race and Hispanic Origin: 2021 and 2022. (From US Census Bureau, Current Population Survey, 2022 and 2023 Annual Social and Economic Supplements.)

BOX 3.3 HEALTH AND SOCIAL DETERMINANTS/HEALTH EQUITY

Health and Human Services Action Plan to Reduce Racial and Ethnic Health Disparities

Community-Driven Approach to Reduce Health Disparities in the United States

Within the Centers for Medicare and Medicaid Services (CMS) is the Office of Minority Health (CMS OMH), which is responsible for working with local and federal partners to eliminate health disparities by improving the health of minority populations, including the following:

- Racial and ethnic minorities
- People with disabilities
- Members of the lesbian, gay, bisexual, and transgender community
- Individuals with limited English proficiency
- Rural communities

The *CMS Framework for Health Equity 2022–2032* defines *health equity* as the attainment of the highest level of health for all people, where everyone has a fair and just opportunity to attain their optimal health regardless of race, ethnicity, disability, sexual orientation, gender identity, socioeconomic status, geography, preferred language, or other factors that affect access to care and health outcomes (CMS OMH, 2023). Health disparities are differences in health outcomes that are closely linked with social, economic, and environmental disadvantage, which are often driven by the social conditions in which individuals live, learn, work, and play. Marked differences in social determinants, such as poverty, low socioeconomic status, and lack of access to care, exist along racial and ethnic lines, leading to poor health outcomes. The *CMS Framework for Health Equity 2022–2032* identifies five priorities to reduce health disparities:

- Priority 1: Expand the collection, reporting, and analysis of standardized data
- Priority 2: Assess causes of disparities within CMS programs, and address inequities in policies and operations to close gaps
- Priority 3: Build capacity of health care organizations and the workforce to reduce health and health care disparities
- Priority 4: Advance language access, health literacy, and the provision of culturally tailored
- Priority 5: Increase all forms of accessibility to health care services and coverage

As the demographics of the nation continue to become more diverse, nurses need to be culturally competent as one strategy for eliminating racial and ethnic disparities. Efforts to match the ethnic and racial composition of the health care workforce with the US population will contribute to addressing health disparities. Providers who speak a second language are also needed to care for people with limited English proficiency. Shortages of primary care providers in underserved areas significantly affect the health of ethnic and racial minorities. The primary care nurse practitioner is ideally suited to care for underserved populations in urban and rural areas. A capable and qualified workforce, up-to-date data and information services, and public health agencies capable of assessing and responding to public health needs are three components necessary for an effective public health infrastructure (USDHHS, 2015). Nurses can play key roles as educators and providers of care in their communities to meet the needs of vulnerable populations and close the health disparity gap.

Sources: The Centers for Medicare and Medicaid Office of Minority Health (CMS OMH). (2023). *CMS framework for health equity 2022–2032.* https://go.cms.gov/framework; US Department of Health and Human Services (USDHHS), Office of the Secretary, Office of the Assistant Secretary for Planning and Evaluation and Office of Minority Health. (2020). *HHS office of minority health 2020 update on the action plan to reduce racial and ethnic health disparities FY2020.* https:/aspe.hhs.gov

BOX 3.4 BEST PRACTICE

10 Essential Public Health Services

1. Monitor health status to identify and solve community health problems.
2. Diagnose and investigate health problems and health hazards in the community.
3. Inform, educate, and empower people concerning health issues.
4. Mobilize community partnerships and actions to identify and solve health problems.
5. Develop policies and plans that support individual and community health efforts.
6. Enforce laws and regulations that protect health and ensure safety.
7. Link people to needed personal health services and ensure the provision of health care when otherwise unavailable.
8. Ensure competent public and personal health care workforces.
9. Evaluate effectiveness, accessibility, and quality of personal and population-based health services.
10. Research for new insights and innovative solutions to health problems.

US Department of Health and Human Services (USDHHS). [Internet]. *Healthy People 2030.* Office of Disease Prevention and Health Promotion. https://health.gov/healthypeople/objectives-and-data/browse-objectives; https://www.healthypeople.gov

and information systems, and public health agencies capable of assessing and responding to public health needs.

Health Indicators of a Nation

Standard measures used to compare the health status of the population of one nation with another are actually death indicators. Although mortality-based indicators do not directly measure the health status of the living population, the data indirectly reflect the general health of a nation and are more readily available through government and world agencies. The CIA publishes the *World Factbook*, which contains summaries and comparisons of country data in specific fields. International comparisons of core health indicators (estimated for 2023) compare the average life expectancy by gender as well as the infant mortality rates of populations for 266 world entities. According to 2023 life expectancy estimates for both sexes combined, the US comparison ranking is 48th, with Monaco listed as highest in terms of life expectancy and Afghanistan as the lowest. Life expectancy between sexes, infant deaths per 1000 live births, and maternal mortality rates (deaths per 100,000 live births) are important indicators of quality of life in a country (CIA, 2024) (Table 3.1). Since the life expectancy value is based on an average, an increase in deaths that occur in the population below the average decrease the value. As discussed earlier, a higher infant mortality rate and deaths of younger people caused by homicide, opioid overdose, suicide, accidents, COVID-19 deaths, and health disparities all contribute to a lower life expectancy in the United States. Much progress has been made toward improving the global health of nations, as shown in comparing and contrasting life expectancies over several decades. In 1960, for example, life expectancy in the United States for both sexes was 69.8 years, and by 2019 it had increased to 78.5 years—a difference of almost 9 years. During the preceding 5 decades, most nations have increased life expectancy substantially for both males and females. (Table 3.2 shows select countries.) The United States and other industrialized countries have the

TABLE 3.1 International Comparisons of Core Health Indicator 2023 Estimates

	Afghanistan	Canada	France	Germany	Mexico	Sweden	United Kingdom	United States
Life expectancy at birth: males (years)	52.47	81.72	79.75	79.37	70.29	81.04	80.01	78.54
Life expectancy at birth: females (years)	55.71	86.39	85.97	84.20	76.79	84.66	84.21	82.93
Life expectancy at birth: both sexes (years)	54.05	83.99	82.79	81.72	73.46	82.8	82.05	80.75
Infant deaths per 1000 live births	103.06	4.31	3.1	3.14	12.0	2.28	3.79	5.12
Maternal mortality rate deaths/100,000 live births (Data from 2020)	620	11	8	4	59	5	10	21

Data from the Central Intelligence Agency (CIA). (2023). *The world fact book.* Retrieved October 3, 2023, from https://www.cia.gov/the-world-factbook/

TABLE 3.2 International Comparisons of Life Expectancy Rates at Birth (in Years) Over Time for 1960, 2000, and 2019

Location	Period	Male	Female	Both Sexes
Afghanistan	2019	63.3	63.2	63.2
	2000	53.7	56.1	42
	1960	31.6	31.0	31.3
Australia	2019	81.3	84.8	83.0
	2000	76.7	82.2	79.5
	1960	67.8	74	70.8
Canada	2019	80.4	84.1	82.2
	2000	76.4	81.7	79.1
	1960	68.3	74.2	71.1
China	2019	74.7	80.5	77.4
	2000	70.1	73.5	71.7
	1960	35.1	37.6	36.3
Denmark	2019	79.6	83.0	81.3
	2000	74.5	79.2	76.9
	1960	70.4	74.0	72.2
France	2019	79.8	85.1	82.5
	2000	75	82.7	78.8
	1960	67.0	73.6	70.2
India	2019	69.5	72.2	70.8
	2000	61.7	63.4	62.5
	1960	43.2	41.3	42.3
Mexico	2019	73.1	78.9	76.0
	2000	72.4	77.2	74.8
	1960	55.7	59.0	57.3
United Kingdom	2019	79.8	83.0	81.4
	2000	75.3	80.1	77.8
	1960	68.2	74.2	71.1
United States	2019	76.3	80.7	78.5
	2000	74	79.5	76.8
	1960	66.6	73.1	69.8

Data from World Health Rankings. (2023). *Country health profiles.* Retrieved October 3, 2023, from https://www.worldlifeexpectancy.com/life-expectancy-research

highest life expectancies; in stark contrast, life expectancy in developing or poorer countries lags. For example, in Afghanistan, a country with low levels of health care provisions, life expectancy in 2019 was estimated at 63.2 years, which is almost 2 decades less than industrialized countries but a vast improvement from life expectancy in 1960 of 31.3 years. India, as another example, is behind other countries with an average life expectancy of 70.8 years as of 2019, but it has made tremendous gains in increasing overall life expectancy in the last 60 years (life expectancy in 1960 for both sexes was 42.3 years) (see Table 3.2) (CIA, 2024).

Infant mortality rates compare the number of deaths of infants under 1 year old in a given year per 1000 live births in the same given year and are one of the most important indicators of the health of a nation because they are associated with factors such as maternal health, access to health care, and overall health of a society. The US infant mortality rate in 2018 was 5.7 (number of deaths of infants in the first year of life per 1000 live births) and was estimated to be 5.12 in 2023, a dramatic improvement from 29.2 reported in 1950 but higher than infant mortality rates in other developed nations (Table 3.3). Canada, the neighboring country to the north of the United States, reports an infant mortality rate of 4.31, and Mexico, to the south, has an infant mortality rate of 12.0. Globally, the infant mortality rate is listed as 30.8 deaths per 1000 live births. Outliers for an extremely high infant mortality rate are Afghanistan at 103.06, Somalia at 85.06, and the Central African Republic at 81.74. Countries at war or experiencing natural disasters, poverty, political instability, or civil unrest—for example, Ethiopia (35.8), Haiti (38.78), Iraq (19.17), Pakistan (52.73) and Iran (14.58)—all report higher infant mortality rates (CIA, 2024). Of the countries reported by the CIA, many industrialized countries report far lower infant mortality rates than the United States, with Slovenia being the lowest at 1.51, Singapore at 1.54, Japan at 1.88, Iceland at 1.63, and Finland at 2.11 deaths per 1000 births. The rationale of why the United States ranks less favorably than other industrialized nations in this health indicator is attributed to a number of factors. According to an earlier working paper from the National Bureau of Economic Research (Chen, Oster, & Williams, 2014), a lack of comparable microdata

TABLE 3.3 **Infant Mortality Rate in the United States by Race/Ethnicity, Provisional Data 2022**

Race/Ethnicity of Mother	Infant Deaths per 1000 Live Births[a]
Black, non-Hispanic	10.86
American Indian/Alaska Native, non-Hispanic	9.06
Native Hawaiian/Pacific Islander, non-Hispanic	8.50
Hispanic	4.88
White, non-Hispanic	4.52
Asian, non-Hispanic	3.5

[a]Births are categorized according to the race/ethnicity of the mother. Data from Ely, D., & Driscoll, A. (2023). *Infant mortality in the United States: Provisional data from the 2022 period linked birth/infant death file.* Centers for Disease Control and Prevention National Center for Health Statistics. NVSS Vital Statistics Rapid Release, Report 33. Retrieved November 2023, from https://www.cdc.gov/nchs/data/vsrr/vsrr033.pdf

TABLE 3.4 **Top 8 States with Highest Infant Mortality Rates Provisional Data, 2022**

Selected States	Infant Death Rate per 1000 Live Births
Mississippi	9.11
South Dakota	7.77
Arkansas	7.67
Delaware	7.49
West Virginia	7.32
Indiana	7.16
Georgia	7.07
Ohio	7.11

Data from Ely, D., & Driscoll, A. (2023). *Infant mortality in the United States: Provisional data from the 2022 period linked birth/infant death file.* Centers for Disease Control and Prevention National Center for Health Statistics. NVSS Vital Statistics Rapid Release, Report 33. Retrieved in November 2023, from https://www.cdc.gov/nchs/data/vsrr/vsrr033.pdf

sets across countries may account for about 40% of the difference in infant mortality rates between the United States and comparable countries because of the variability in the reporting of births near the threshold of fetal viability. In many European countries, infants born with very low odds of survival (under 22 weeks' gestation or a birth weight of under 500 g) are not reported in infant mortality rates, which also affects the comparison of neonatal mortality data (infant deaths within the first 28 days of life). In the United States and Canada, there is no threshold for infant weight, so low-birth-weight infant deaths are included in statistics, which inflates the infant mortality rate for both countries. When researchers adjusted 2016 US infant mortality data to exclude low-birth-weight infants (<500 g) and deaths of infants at less than 22 weeks' gestation, infant mortality rates fell a full point (from 5.9 to 4.9), but rates were still higher than other comparable countries. According to data sets from 2017, 66% of infant deaths in the United States occur within the neonatal period (first 28 days after birth), with low birth weight, short gestation, and congenital malformations cited as primary causes of death. Forty percent of infant deaths in the United States occurred within the first 24 hours of life (Peterson Center on Healthcare & Kaiser Family Foundation Partnership, 2019). Despite data-collection and reporting variations, other factors that contribute to a higher infant death rate in the United States are disparities in women's health status, geographic areas, race, ethnicity, social class, and education level. In 2022, non-Hispanic Black infants experienced the highest infant mortality rates (10.86), more than twice those of non-Hispanic White infants (4.52). Non-Hispanic American Indian or Alaska Native infants also experienced high mortality rates (9.06), significantly above the national average of 5.60 infant deaths per 1000 live births, according to provisional 2022 data. Hispanic infant mortality rates were reported at 4.88, below the national average, and Asian infants had the lowest infant mortality rate at 3.5 (see Table 3.3). Other factors considered in data sets are the mother's age and geographic locality. Infant mortality is highest among all mothers under the age of 20 (9.89 deaths per 1000 live births), and lowest for mothers aged between 30 and 34 years old (4.58 deaths per 1000 live births). Geographically, higher infant mortality rates are clustered in the south and parts of the Midwest with some outliers, while the lowest infant mortality rates are in the northeast. Mississippi has the highest infant mortality rate of 9.11, and seven other states have infant mortality rates greater than 7. Massachusetts has the lowest infant mortality rate at 3.32, and three other states—New Hampshire (3.48), New Jersey (3.57), and Rhode Island (3.90)—are under 4.0 (Table 3.4) (Ely & Driscoll, 2023). In summary, decreasing the nation's infant mortality rates will require community interventions to decrease teen pregnancies and targeted interventions for specific racial groups and geographic areas.

Historical Role of Females in Health Promotion

Nurses have a long tradition of involvement in health promotion. Florence Nightingale (born in 1820 in Florence, Italy) is credited as the founder of modern nursing. During the Crimean War in 1854, while caring for wounded soldiers in a British camp in Turkey, Nightingale fought for hospital reform by crusading for nutritious food, cleanliness, and sanitation. Within 6 months, Nightingale and her team had decreased the death rate of wounded British soldiers from 40% to 2%. She provided leadership for a group of nurses and comfort to the soldiers. Known for checking on soldiers at night, Nightingale was given the nickname the Lady with the Lamp. Her careful recordings of care outcomes quantified needed reform in health promotion (Alexander, 2019). Later, Lillian Wald, appalled by the lack of medical care in crowded dilapidated tenement housing and the living conditions of the poor in 1893, developed a settlement program in New York City that trained nurses, provided care to families, and developed education programs for the community. Wald, a leader in political activism, spearheaded organized public health in the direction of health promotion for families and communities (Rothberg, 2020). These pioneers and others set the stage for nurses' unique role in health promotion.

A SAFER SYSTEM

The health care delivery system in the United States is experiencing significant changes sparked by health care reform and recommendations from large organizations involved in forming health policy. One of the largest independent nonprofit organizations involved in health policy is the National Academies of Sciences, Engineering, and Medicine. The institute was signed into being by President Abraham Lincoln in 1863 by an act of Congress to investigate and report upon the subject of science. Since that time, the institute has evolved and is now made up of three academies: the National Academy of Sciences, the National Academy of Engineering (1964), and the National Academy of Medicine (1970). Within the academies are a multitude of program units. The National Academy of Medicine (formerly named the Institute of Medicine, or the IOM) conducts research from a systems approach, advising the nation's leaders on improving health. The Health and Medicine Division (HMD) falls under the National Academy of Medicine. Several early reports from this division were instrumental in advising Congress and others of the need to revise health policy to change the structure of health care delivery and deliver safer care. The HMD (and previous IOM) is considered the impartial evidence-based authority and provides trusted advice grounded in scientific evidence to federal agencies, Congress, state and local health authorities, nonprofit organizations, medical societies, and foundations with over 2000 publications. In 2023, 59 new publications on a wide range of pressing concerns related to health and the health care system became available. Reports can be found on the National Academy of Sciences website and downloaded at no cost (see http://nationalacademies.org). To provide safe, evidence-based care, nurses have a responsibility to be lifelong learners, to stay abreast of new scientific findings, and advocate health care policy changes that improve the health of the communities in which they practice and extend to the greater global population.

Although health care is often equated with medical care, which focuses on the treatment of illness, this chapter presents the evolution and ongoing development of a broader concept of health based on the definition given in Chapter 1.

HISTORICAL PERSPECTIVES AND THE HISTORY OF HEALTH CARE

Global Health

Established in 1948, the World Health Organization (WHO) is a specialized agency of the United Nations responsible for international public health policy. The WHO is governed by the World Health Assembly, which is composed of 194 member states and funded by assessed amounts calculated in part by countries' gross domestic products (GDPs) (the United States is a top contributor), other contributions from member states, and private donors throughout the world. The Bill and Melinda Gates Foundation in the United States has contributed millions of dollars over many years. The overarching goal of WHO is to improve equity in health, reduce health risks, promote healthy lifestyles and settings, and respond to the underlying determinants of health with the vision of a world in which all people attain the highest standard of health and well-being.

WHO and COVID-19

On December 12, 2019, officials in Wuhan, China, described a cluster of atypical pneumonia-type illnesses occurring in people seemingly connected to the Huanan Seafood Wholesale Market and not responding to treatment. They waited for 3 weeks before informing the WHO of the outbreak. The WHO determined evidence of possible human-to-human transmission of the SARS-CoV-2 virus on January 14, 2020, and 6 days later, the CDC reported the first case in the United States, triggering the activation of the CDC's Emergency Operations Center to respond to an emerging outbreak. The WHO's International Health Regulation Committee also met and decided to monitor the situation, delaying the declaration of the outbreak as a Public Health Emergency of International Concern until January 31, 2020. After more than 118,000 cases were found in 114 countries and 4291 deaths from the virus occurred, the WHO declared COVID-19 a global pandemic on March 11, 2020. Two days later, the Trump Administration declared a nationwide emergency and issued additional travel bans and other measures to prevent or slow viral transmission, but by April 10, 2020, the United States had the most reported COVID-19 cases and deaths worldwide, leading to widespread shortages of critical hospital beds, medical supplies, ventilators, and health care workforce shortages. In May of 2020, President Trump's Administration launched Operation Warp Speed, a partnership with the USDHHS, the Department of Defense, and other parties to fund pharmaceutical companies in developing and manufacturing effective vaccines against COVID-19 for widespread distribution (cutting the typical time frame of 10-plus years for development of a new vaccine to 10 months). President Trump believed that the WHO had mismanaged the coronavirus when it was first known to emerge from China and ignored credible reports of human-to-human transmission, allowing the global spread of the virus as early as December 2019. At a White House press briefing in July 2020, Trump announced that the United States would cease funding the WHO ($450 million annually) and redirect funds to other global health priorities. The number of confirmed cases in the United States at that time had surpassed 3 million, and the worldwide death toll had exceeded 1 million. Because a president lacks legal authority to withdraw from the WHO without congressional approval and withdrawal requires a 1-year notice during which dues must be paid in full, the newly elected Biden Administration halted the US withdrawal process in January 2021 and joined COVID-19 Vaccines Global Access (COVAX). During the COVID-19 pandemic, the WHO provided briefings on cases, transmission patterns, deaths, and other population-spread data to guide governments and health care professionals. In the early months of the pandemic, Pass the Message to Kick Out Corona was an example of a joint awareness campaign with WHO and key coaches and football players within International Federation of Association Football (FIFA) to educate consumers on tactics that diminish the spread of disease (Box 3.5: Evidence-Based Practice) (WHO, 2020). The principal global advisory group for vaccines and immunization is the Strategic Advisory Group of Experts (SAGE), established in 1999 to provide guidance to the WHO on global policies and strategies related to the many aspects of immunization and vaccines.

BOX 3.5 EVIDENCE-BASED PRACTICE

Football Fights COVID-19: Pass the Message to Kick Out Coronavirus

On March 23, 2020, an awareness campaign to actively spread the five steps for people to follow to protect their health and decrease transmissibility of the SARS-CoV-2 virus that causes COVID-19 was virtually launched on social media from the World Health Organization's (WHO) headquarters in Geneva, Switzerland. The virtual graphic toolkit for implementation on social media included a video published in 13 languages, called "Pass the Message to Kick Out Corona." A plea from the president of FIFA, six world-renowned coaches, and 28 male and female football athletes from around the globe made the request for everyone across the world to follow five key tactics that "tackle the spread of disease." This awareness-raising campaign reaching out to the global football community (the sport better known as soccer in the United States) outlined best practices to stop the spread of disease with a five-step plan: hands, elbow, face, distance, and feel.

The five basic protective measures described by the athletes in the video are as follows:

1. Handwashing
2. Coughing etiquette
3. Not touching your face
4. Physical distance
5. Staying home if feeling unwell

This awareness campaign intervention to help combat the spread of COVID-19 used evidence-based strategies for staying healthy and preventing or diminishing disease transmission, social media to spread information, and highly regarded figures from the football community to pass the message targeting the FIFA audience throughout the world, hoping football players and fans would heed the recommendations.

Source: World Health Organization (WHO). (2020). *Pass the message: Five steps to kicking out coronavirus.* http://www.who.int/news-room/detail/23-03-2020-pass-the-message-five-steps-to-kicking-out-coronavirus

In response to COVID-19, the 15-member SAGE developed the WHO SAGE roadmap for prioritizing uses of COVID-19 vaccines. The latest update, November 2023, addresses the evolving public health needs as the Omicron variant and its sublineages continue to circulate and provides recommendations for a global simplified vaccine schedule for high-, medium-, and low-priority-use groups (CDC, 2023; WHO, 2023).

Historical Perspectives

The complexities of the US health care system necessitate an understanding of the system as a whole before one can focus on the intermingled causative factors that have created a fragmented system of health care delivery. Many of today's problems have their roots in the decisions and directions of the past. It is not possible to identify and analyze current problems or to devise solutions without first exploring how the system developed. The relevance of the divergence between preventive and curative measures is apparent when the organization and financing of the delivery system are examined. The United States has established a system that uses two basic divisions of society to provide service: the public sector and the private sector. The merger of public health and welfare policies in the public sector is rooted in the Puritan ethic inherent in the historical development of the United States. The current focus on managed care as both an organizational strategy and a financing mechanism is highlighted in a discussion of how health care is delivered and financed.

History of Health Care

Early Influences

Historical records of early civilizations (Egyptian, Indian, Chinese, Aztec, and Greek) show that ancient peoples were concerned with disease and practiced various methods of treatment. The earliest views of health can be seen as holistic in the sense that they emerged from an integrated worldview. Primitive peoples understood illness in mystical terms: sickness and cure theories were tied to a cosmic view of life, with natural and supernatural forces often inseparable. Most religions included a person's hygiene as part of their practice. For thousands of years, epidemics were viewed as divine judgments on human wickedness, with a gradual awareness that pestilence (any epidemic disease with a high death rate) had natural causes such as climate and other aspects of the physical environment. During the Middle Ages, infectious diseases in epidemic proportions (leprosy, bubonic plague, smallpox, and tuberculosis [TB]) were the leading causes of death and led to isolation and quarantines. Clearly, health was viewed in terms of survival and absence of disease.

Industrial Influences

The population of the Western world began to increase during the 1600s, when America was first being explored. The New World had many things to offer explorers. An adequate food supply made it possible for the population to live longer, and advances in transportation made distribution of food supplies and other goods and services possible. Manufacturing advances during the 18th century, through the invention of the flush toilet and cast-iron pipe, made sanitary engineering possible, saving many lives by preventing diseases such as typhoid, paratyphoid, and gastroenteritis.

Socioeconomic Influences

Although the Elizabethan poor laws (1601) in England provided a system of relief for the poor, which included infants, the sick, older people, and laborers in workhouses, a new Poor Law was enacted in 1834 that was based on a harsher philosophy that regarded pauperism among able-bodied workers as a moral failing. If the worker did not earn a subsistence-level income, the attitude toward that worker was suspicious and punitive. These poor laws were the legal implementation of the Protestant work ethic that Puritan forebears brought to the United States. According to this view, people are held directly accountable for their state in life, and health maintenance is the responsibility of the individual. The far-reaching implications of this ethic can be seen today in the organization, financing, and delivery of health services.

Public Health Influences

Edwin Chadwick (1800–1890) is known as the father of British and American public health. Chadwick established the English Board of Health, which emphasized environmental sanitation but excluded physicians outside times of crisis. Additionally,

Chadwick was Secretary of the Poor Law Commission, which strove to improve the health of the masses for economic reasons. Chadwick's rationale was that disease among the poor was a major factor in their inability to support themselves. Therefore governmental health and welfare policies have been joined in England since the 19th century.

Lemuel Shattuck, a leader of the public health movement, began the movement in the United States using the British system as the model, with public health services and welfare combined despite the contradictory emphasis. Public health has focused on improving the health of the poor, whereas welfare has dictated subsistence at the minimal level. The influence of the Puritan ethic on the US health care system is apparent in the emphasis on the value of work and the attitude toward the poor. Today, health and welfare departments continue their contradictory approach toward the poor.

Scientific Influences

Until the 20th century, epidemics of infectious disease (plague, cholera, typhoid, smallpox, and influenza) were the most critical health problems and major causes of death and disability for Americans. Scientific advances during the 19th century by Louis Pasteur (germ theory), Robert Koch (origin of bacterial infection), Joseph Lister (antisepsis), and Paul Ehrlich (chemotherapy) expanded public health from its earlier concentration on sanitation to control of communicable diseases through a broad biologic base. In 1837, records of births, deaths, and marriages became compulsory in England and Wales, and early gathering of population health statistics in other countries called attention to death rates due to specific diseases. Lemuel Shattuck, a Massachusetts legislator, is credited for establishing a system to record births, marriages, and mortality data in the United States. Public health became an important force in decreasing death rates and increasing life expectancy through the application of bacteriology. International environmental conditions were improved by the development of systems to safeguard water, milk, and food supplies; promote sanitary sewage disposal; and monitor the quality of urban housing.

Between 1936 and 1954, the discovery and use of sulfonamides and other antibiotics to treat bacterial infections reduced the death rate to its lowest point in history, with deaths caused by primary infections reduced to 4% compared with 33% in 1886. Another decline in the death rate began after the mid-1960s and continued (with the exception of a slight increase in 1995 and the COVID-19 pandemic) with the control of many infectious diseases (Arias & Smith, 2003). As the life expectancy of the population increases, chronic diseases and comorbidities increase as well (see previous discussion on life expectancy and leading causes of death).

An effective, comprehensive public health system is imperative to enable the United States to respond to local, state, national, and global concerns, as is the case with the recent COVID-19 global pandemic. Public education, expanded testing, immunization, and contact tracing are key interventions in slowing and stopping the spread of disease. Adequate funding and installing a trained workforce in the public health system at the local, state, and national levels is warranted. The ACA established a council within the USDHHS known as the National Prevention, Health Promotion, and Public Health Council, charged with providing coordination and leadership at the federal level among 17 federal departments and agencies. The council is also charged with obtaining input from relative stakeholders to develop a plan for improving the health status of Americans and reducing the incidence of preventable disease, disability, and illness, which will require integration and coordination of all divisions (USDHHS, n.d.-a). The CDC, a large frontline agency for providing national health security, is responsible for remaining vigilant in rapidly detecting and controlling disease outbreaks in the United States and abroad. The CDC's Emergency Operations Center is the command center for monitoring and coordinating emergency responses to public health threats such as pandemics, emerging disease outbreaks, natural disasters, and bioterrorist attacks in the United States and worldwide. The CDC has responded to many global outbreaks, including the Hendra virus (1994), H5N1 bird flu (1997), Nipah virus (1999), SARS-associated coronavirus (2003), avian influenza (2006), influenza H1N1 (2009), Ebola virus (2014), and COVID-19 (2020), which all posed challenges to global public health (CDC Foundation, 2023). As a federal agency, money is tied to appropriations, restrictions, and purchasing procedures that can delay the CDC's response. The CDC Foundation is an independent public charity created by Congress that works in collaboration with the CDC and public health authorities to immediately mobilize resources. The CDC Foundation's Emergency Response Fund allows immediate flexible resources appropriated to the CDC to address and respond to emergencies both domestic and abroad. As new and ongoing threats to global health occur, the CDC is the leading source in the dispersal of science-based information to guide policy development within the United States and globally. The CDC is responsible for providing up-to-date consumer and health care professionals with information to stay abreast of current and new recommendations as scientific findings emerge. Each year, the CDC identifies top health threats to the population with a plan for focused interventions.

On January 22, 2020, the CDC reported the first case of COVID-19 in the United States; within 3 months, over 650,000 cases had been reported with over 27,000 deaths nationwide (12,000 deaths occurred in New York State alone). By May 3, 2020, the CDC had reported over 1.1 million total cases and almost 66,000 COVID-19 deaths, with over 23,000 in the hardest-hit state, New York. The CDC responded with a massive virtual campaign to slow the spread of the coronavirus, with consumer information on who is at greatest risk, how the virus spreads, how to stay protected, symptoms, what to do if sick, and other information in various languages and formats (written, video clips, sign language) (CDC, 2023). Fast facts, located and accessed on the CDC website (cdc.gov), provide selected statistics and consumer information on more than 120 health topics. The website also provides updates and links for consumers and health care professionals to stay abreast of current practices. As key members of the health care workforce, nurses are instrumental in caring for the needs of individuals, families, and communities in terms of disease prevention and health promotion, and they are essential during times of national crisis, as seen during the recent COVID-19 pandemic.

Political and Economic Influences

Political and economic considerations influence the health care system, and politics determines the decision-makers who will negotiate a desired outcome. Economics defines the resources that are distributed and the manner in which they are distributed. The effect of economics and politics on the delivery of health care is illustrated by the situation in the United States following the Great Depression. Roosevelt's New Deal had an effect on health care, specifically in the passage of the Social Security Act in 1935, which authorized grants-in-aid to individual states to improve state and local public health programs. Funds were available for categorical assistance programs, with cash grants first given to needy blind and older individuals and later to disabled people. Medical care, through subsequent amendments, was an allowable budget item, but payments were often distributed for food, shelter, or other needs. Later, the Social Security Act resulted in the development of programs such as Medicaid and Medicare.

Split Between Preventive and Curative Measures

The link between environmental health and personal medical care developed when sanitarians (people who work to maintain a clean environment) realized that their efforts alone were not sufficient to prevent and cure the diseases of the population as a whole; improvement of personal health was also necessary. Early preventive services directed toward individuals originated in medical practice rather than public health but were limited to welfare medicine (caring for individuals through state programs). Community health centers that developed in the United States before World War I limited their scope to prevention and health education and, with the exception of some prenatal clinics, were generally located in poor neighborhoods. Delivery of preventive services developed separately from clinical medicine and became associated with public health. Most physicians, educated in hospitals, were interested in individuals for whom prevention had failed and whose illnesses brought them to the hospital ward.

Despite the separation of preventive and treatment services, the benefits of prevention were eventually incorporated into clinical medicine for individuals. Preventive and early-detection measures became a part of pediatrics and obstetrics during the early part of the 20th century, when vaccines and vaginal cytology examinations became available and accepted. Later in the 20th century, internal medicine incorporated early detection of diseases such as diabetes, glaucoma, obesity, and hypertension. A shift to preventive medicine for the individual occurred, but the separate educational programs for public health and medicine still divided these areas. Not until the 1960s did the emphasis begin to turn from individual to societal values (Freyman, 1980).

This new emphasis on societal values parallels another evolution in the role of health in society. Greater governmental involvement in financing the health care delivery system has improved access to health care for many populations. Technologic developments include computerized medical records, which should improve access to care through better communication among laboratories, primary care offices, hospitals, and care delivery agencies. The Patient Protection and Affordable Care Act (PPACA) of 2010, more commonly known as the ACA, reformed certain aspects of the private health insurance industry and public health programs, extending a heavy layer of federal and state oversight.

ORGANIZATION OF THE DELIVERY SYSTEM

The health care delivery system in the United States is a mammoth system composed of a network of public and private interrelated and, in some cases, overlapping components, designed to provide health care to the American people. The structure and financing of the health care delivery system is a system of multifaceted and complex interrelationships involving providers, consumers, and settings, with both the private sector and the public sector providing services. The public sector includes voluntary and nonprofit agencies as well as official or governmental agencies. The USDHHS is the principal federal regulatory agency, whose mission is to enhance and protect the health and well-being of all Americans by providing effective health and human services and fostering sound sustained advances in the sciences underlying medicine, public health, and social services (USDHHS, n.d.-a). Delivery of services is organized on three levels in both sectors: local, state, and national. Each of the three levels consists of private providers combined with official or voluntary public agencies. The nurse is often the professional who assists the health consumer in navigating the complex delivery system; therefore, a basic understanding of the system's organization is essential.

Private Sector

Independent Practice

Traditionally, a person enters the health care delivery system by contracting directly with a health care provider for individual care on a fee-for-service basis. Free choice of the provider has been the hallmark of the American free-market system. A physician, a group of physicians (group practice), or another health care provider—as opposed to a hospital or other health care system—owns and operates the practice and provides patient care. The American Medical Association (AMA) has been surveying physicians about their practice characteristics since the 1980s. In 2012, a benchmark survey was conducted in part to capture whether a practice was physician-owned or owned by another entity. Between 2012 and 2022, a declining number of physicians (46.7%) were working in private practice compared with 60.1% in 2012, and practice size had changed with a redistribution of physicians from small (10 or fewer) to large practices. The primary reasons cited for this continuing trend of a drop in ownership are the retirement of older physicians (who tend to be owners), the lack of new physicians who choose or are unable to be owners, and issues due to payment. Motivators for selling a private practice to hospitals or health systems were the need to better negotiate higher payment rates with payers, to better manage payers' regulatory and administrative requirements, and to improve access to costly resources (Kane, 2023). In summary, a continuing shift is occurring for a growing number of physicians from traditional independent-practice ownership fee-for-service care models to employment in managed health care organizations, hospital-based specialty groups, corporate or public service settings, and academic institutions (AMA, 2023).

Private care may be delivered in numerous settings, from inpatient (hospital or extended care facility) to outpatient (ambulatory) settings. Outpatient care is defined as medical care or treatment that does not require an overnight stay in a hospital or medical facility in which room and board costs are incurred. Ambulatory settings include two major categories: care provided by owners and providers and care provided in service settings (Box 3.6: Types of Ambulatory Care Settings). These categories overlap because many providers practice in their own offices and contract with one or more managed care organizations. Individuals who receive care in a hospital who are not formally admitted are considered ambulatory or observational care. Observational care may involve an overnight (or longer) stay in a hospital, but the patient is not considered an inpatient unless the physician provides a written admission order. The distinction between outpatient (observational) and inpatient is important in determining insurance payments.

Nursing centers are nurse-managed health centers, often situated in medically underserved rural and urban areas that primarily serve vulnerable populations in the provision of primary care to individuals and families. Nursing centers trace their origin to the Henry Street Settlement for the sick and poor of New York City, founded by Lillian Wald in 1893, and another visionary, Margaret Sanger, who opened the nation's first birth control clinic. The modern movement to establish nursing centers began in 1965, when the nurse practitioner role was created, allowing nurses to provide primary care to individuals and families. Nursing centers (ambulatory care centers, family practice nursing centers, community nursing centers, and birthing centers) have provided high-quality nursing care from certified nurse midwives, nurse practitioners, and other advanced practice nurses (APNs). A number of nursing centers are academic nursing centers, established to provide nursing services to communities, learning experiences for students, and settings for faculty practice and research. The key components of a community nursing center include the following: a nurse as chief manager, a nursing staff that is accountable and responsible for care and professional practice, and nurses as the primary providers of care. Using a multidisciplinary collaboration framework, nurses have the opportunity to provide comprehensive primary care services, including a focus on wellness and health promotion, public health programs, and targeted interventions for populations with special needs. The Institute for Nursing Centers is a network of organizations whose focus is to promote and enhance the work of nursing centers by providing educational programs as well as a national repository of data for nurse-managed health centers funded by the W. K. Kellogg Foundation. Members of the Institute for Nursing Centers also provide mentoring and consultation to support colleagues in developing and advancing nursing centers (Institute for Nursing Centers, n.d.). The ACA specifically addresses nurse-managed health centers, describing them as a nurse practice arrangement managed by APNs who provide primary or wellness services to underserved or vulnerable populations.

Advanced practice nurses, an umbrella term for master's and doctoral prepared nurses who practice in the roles of nurse practitioners, clinical nurse specialists, nurse midwives, or nurse anesthetists, are well suited to provide cost-effective, quality care to individuals and their families as well as to serve economically disadvantaged and vulnerable populations. APNs not only have specialized clinical knowledge and skills at the master's or doctoral level but also have pursued an advanced curriculum that includes research and theoretical foundations to determine best practices, evaluate health policy issues, and understand the intricacies of the health care system and financial management. Nurse practitioners play a key role within the health care system and often care for vulnerable populations in rural areas and inner cities as well as practice in primary, acute, and long-term care settings.

BOX 3.6 Types of Ambulatory Care Settings

- Owner provider: Hospitals, community health agencies, managed care organizations, home health organizations, insurance agencies
- Service settings: Hospital-based clinics/centers, solo or group medical practices, ambulatory surgery and diagnostic procedure centers, telehealth service environments, university and community hospital clinics, military and settings within the Department of Veterans Affairs, nurse-managed clinics, managed care organizations, colleges and educational institutions, free-standing community facilities, care coordination organizations, walk-in clinics (some clinics are free clinics where patient-centered care can be provided for minimal or no fee—these types of clinics are an important safety net for vulnerable populations), urgent care centers, outpatient surgery centers, chemotherapy and radiation therapy centers, dialysis centers, neighborhood and community health centers, diagnostic and mobile imaging centers, occupational health centers, females' health clinics, wound care centers, fitness-wellness centers, health department clinics, nursing centers

Source: American Academy of Ambulatory Care Nursing. (2017). *The defining characteristics of ambulatory care nursing.* https://aaacn.org. Accessed November 27, 2023.

Move to Managed Care

Before the 1990s the traditional means of paying for health care was **indemnity insurance plans**. A person would choose a physician or care provider and receive care, and the provider would either bill the individual's **insurance** company or be paid on a **fee-for-service** basis. Each separate service generated a professional fee, and the provider would receive payments directly from the insurance plan; alternatively, the individual would pay the provider, file an insurance claim for each covered expense, and receive reimbursement. The provider had autonomy to treat the person without oversight from the insurance company. In a traditional fee-for-service insurance system, there are no incentives to constrain cost and care. In an effort to control costs, managed care began to regulate the use of health care. Physicians or physician groups contracted with an insurance company for a negotiated fee-for-service, usually at a discounted rate. Today, managed care plans include a network of individual providers or physician groups, and individuals who choose to seek care from health care providers within their network usually have full coverage with or without a copayment. Individuals who choose health care providers outside the managed care network may not be covered, may be covered for a lesser amount, or may have additional copayment costs and thus face greater out-of-pocket expenses. Within the network, a person has a **primary care provider** who serves as a **gatekeeper** and is the foundation of the **managed care** concept in controlling health care costs within the organization. The primary care provider may be a physician, a physician assistant, or an APN. Physician primary care providers are usually general or family practitioners, but they may also be internists, pediatricians, or obstetrician-gynecologists. Physician assistants are educated and prepared to work under the direct supervision of physicians, whereas APNs who serve as primary care providers are typically nurse practitioners or certified nurse midwives. A growing number of states have approved full-practice regulations allowing nurse practitioners (and other APNs) to provide care without the oversight or management of a physician (within scope of practice guidelines and other professional licensure requirements by a state) and to operate their own independent practices. A number of states have reduced or restricted oversight to prescribe, diagnose, and treat patients and families. The term "gatekeeper" is a common managed care term, and the primary care provider has the role of coordinating and overseeing an individual's care. The principal force behind the growth of managed care is the belief that health care costs can be controlled by managing the way in which health care is delivered and that costs can be controlled because providers of care must be careful to provide only care that is absolutely necessary. Managed care plans are arranged agreements with a group of physicians, hospitals, and other health care providers to provide care at a certain cost. The gatekeeper concept is designed to manage the individual's use of resources, to reduce self-referral to specialists, and to protect the individual from unnecessary procedures and overtreatment (Shi & Singh, 2019). Decreasing hospital admission rates, readmittance to acute care, and costly procedures, as well as limiting an individual's ability to self-refer to specialists, is designed to achieve successful containment of health care costs. An oversupply of physician specialists has occurred in some areas, and a lack of primary care providers occurs in many rural areas; thus, nurse practitioners are well suited to provide primary care. Providers of specialty care typically earn higher salaries than primary care providers, making career selection in a specialty area more attractive. Box 3.7: A Glossary of Managed Care Terms provides a glossary of key terms used in managed care.

Health Maintenance Organizations

Health maintenance organizations (HMOs) deliver comprehensive health maintenance and treatment services to a group of enrolled individuals who prepay a fixed fee. The HMO accepts responsibility for the organization, financing, and delivery of health care services for all enrolled members. Several HMO models have evolved. The traditional HMO structure was a group or staff model, in which the HMO owns the hospital and employs a group of physicians and some specialty services to provide care to its members. Salaried providers generally spent all of their time serving members of the HMO, with no financial incentive to provide more care. An example is the Kaiser Permanente health care system, which also has its own hospitals. A capitation method of payment is used in which a service provider receives a fixed amount per person (the capitation rate) and in turn agrees to provide all necessary care to each enrolled member. The employer pays a monthly or annual rate directly to the HMO. The individual may also have out-of-pocket expenses such as copayments. Staff models were described as closed panel, because employed physicians provided care only for members of the HMO. A community physician (physician or health care provider outside the HMO) could not care for a member of the HMO without prearrangement or authorization by the HMO. In an HMO plan, individuals pay low out-of-pocket expenses but must see a primary care provider first to be referred to a specialist. In a group-model HMO, the organization operates a health plan but contracts with groups of physicians and hospitals to provide care. The medical group receives a share of the capitation rate received by the HMO, and the group agrees to provide all necessary physician services for the member. The physician can be paid by salary or on a fee-for-service basis. An independent practice association HMO will be discussed later. For all types of HMOs, a fixed amount of money is available each year for health care, based on the capitation fee and the number of members enrolled (Barr, 2023). **Medicare** enrollees since the 1970s have been offered the option of enrolling in fee-for-service or HMO plans. An earlier health reform law, the Medicare Modernization Act of 2003, renamed the program to include Medicare Advantage plans.

Medicare Advantage Plans

Medicare Advantage plans are private health plans that are offered as an alternative to the traditional Medicare program and are available to 99.7% of Medicare beneficiaries (though they will not be available to Medicare beneficiaries in Alaska as of 2024). Those who enroll in a Medicare Advantage plan may have low or no additional monthly premiums (zero-premium plans), but all Medicare enrollees pay the Part B Medicare premium (standard Part B premiums are $174.70 per month per individual as of 2024, and higher brackets are up to $594.00 per month). Some Medicare Advantage plans pay a rebate toward the Part B premium (in 2024, 19% of plans offered a reduction in the Part B premium). Almost all Medicare Advantage plans include Medicare prescription drug coverage Part D. The insurer offering a Medicare Advantage plan receives federal payments (capitated monthly amount) from Medicare for each enrollee and a separate amount per enrollee if the plan offers prescription Part D coverage. For almost all insurers, Medicare Advantage plans are profitable, as the insurer is paid 106% of traditional Medicare costs ($2350 per enrollee) above their estimated cost of providing covered services, known as "the rebate." This allows Medicare Advantage plans (97% or more) to offer extra benefits not covered by traditional Medicare (vision, hearing, fitness, dental services, and others). In 2023, more than 31 million Medicare beneficiaries (51% of the eligible Medicare population) were enrolled in a Medicare Advantage plan. In 2023, 56% of Medicare Advantage enrollees were in HMOs, and 42% in local preferred provider organizations (PPOs). The Congressional Budget Office expects enrollment of Medicare

BOX 3.7 A Glossary of Managed Care Terms

Access to health care: The degree to which individuals are inhibited or facilitated in their ability to gain entry to and to receive care and services from the health care system.

Accountable care organization: A group of health care providers who give coordinated care, chronic disease management, and thereby improve the quality of care patients receive.

Beneficiary: Any person, either a subscriber or a dependent, eligible for service under a health plan.

Benefits: The dollar amount available for the cost of covered medical services.

Blue Cross/Blue Shield: A combined medical plan offered through a worker's place of employment that combines both hospital and physician coverage.

Capitation: A fixed amount of payment per individual, per year, regardless of the volume or cost of the services each client requires.

Copayments, copayments, copay: A fixed dollar payment that is made by the patient to the provider at the time of service.

Cost-sharing: Provisions of an insurance policy that require the insured to pay some portion of covered expenses (does not refer to or include the cost of the premium).

Deductible: A fixed dollar amount that the patient must pay for covered health care services before reimbursement begins from an insurance plan.

Gatekeeper: A physician or advanced practice nurse who provides primary care and who makes referrals for emergency services or specialty care.

Health care policy: Decisions, usually developed by government policymakers, for determining present and future objectives pertaining to the health care system.

Health maintenance organization (HMO): A prepaid health plan delivering comprehensive care to members through designated providers, having a fixed monthly payment for health care services, and requiring members to be in a plan for a specified period.

Indemnity: Monies paid by an insurer to a provider in a predetermined amount in the event of a covered loss by a beneficiary.

Independent practice association (IPA): An organization that physicians in private practice can join so that the organization can represent them in the negotiation of managed care contracts.

Managed care: A health care plan that integrates the financing and delivery of health care services by using arrangements with selected health care providers to provide services for covered individuals. Capitation fees generally finance plans. There are significant financial incentives for members of the plan to use the health care providers associated with the plan.

Out-of-pocket expenditures: The portion of medical expenses an individual is responsible for paying that are not reimbursed by insurance. Out-of-pocket costs include coinsurance fees, deductibles, and any amounts not covered as part of a health insurance plan.

Point-of-service (POS) plan: A plan that contains elements of both HMOs and PPOs. They resemble HMOs for in-network services in that they both require copayments and a primary care provider. Services received outside the network are usually reimbursed on a fee-for-service basis. Most plans require a referral from the primary care provider in order to see a specialist.

Preferred provider organization (PPO): A type of health plan that generally contracts with hospitals and medical providers to create a network of participating providers. The PPO provides health care services to plan members usually at discounted rates if a patient uses a provider within the network.

Primary care: Health care services that cover a range of prevention, wellness, and treatment for common illnesses.

Primary care provider: A physician or APN who provides basic and routine health care services usually in an office or clinic.

Reimbursement: Payment of services; payment of providers by a third-party insurer or government health program for health care services.

Self-insured plan: Type of plan offered by employers and other groups that directly assume the major cost of health insurance for their employees or members. The employer collects premiums from enrollees and takes the responsibility of paying employees' and dependents' medical claims.

Third-party payer: In health care finance, this is an insurance carrier, Medicare, and Medicaid or their government-contracted intermediary, managed care organization, or health plan that pays for hospital or medical bills instead of the individual.

Underinsured: People who have some type of health insurance, such as catastrophic care, but not enough insurance to cover all their health care costs.

Uninsured: Individuals or groups with no or inadequate health insurance coverage.

Utilization review: Evaluation of the necessity, appropriateness, and efficiency of the use of health care services, procedures, and facilities.

Sources: US National Library of Medicine, National Institutes of Health. *Health economics information resources: A self-study course.* Retrieved October 12, 2023, from http://www.nlm.nih.gov; HealthCare.gov. (2023). *Glossary.* Retrieved October 12, 2023, from http://www.healthcare.gov/glossary

beneficiaries choosing a Medicare Advantage plan over traditional Medicare will continue to grow. Although there are almost 4000 different Medicare Advantage plans nationwide, the number and availability of plans is specific to geographical location, with some areas having greater numbers of available plans. As of 2024, the average Medicare beneficiary will have access to 43 Medicare Advantage plans offered by multiple firms. In 2023, 73% of people enrolled in a Medicare Advantage plan had no additional monthly premium other than Medicare Part B premium and were called "zero-premium plans." Members in the traditional Medicare program have no out-of-pocket limits under Medicare Part A and Part B and thus have unlimited financial liability. Those who enroll in a Medicare Advantage plan have out-of-pocket expenses for services covered in Part A and Part B limited to no more than $8300 per year (the average was $4835 in 2023) for services received from in-network providers and $12,450 per year (average $8659) for in-network and out-of-network combined. The out-of-pocket expense amount listed does not include expenses for prescription drugs (if Part D is not included in the plan) or extra benefits not covered by the plan. The quality of a Medicare Advantage plan is rated at the contract level by a star system (one to five) with one star representing a poor rating, three stars representing an average rating, and five stars representing an excellent rating. Plans with high ratings receive higher rebate amounts from Medicare, which are then used to offer additional plan benefits not offered through traditional Medicare, such as vision, hearing, dental, and fitness plans. Some plans also offer transportation to doctor's appointments, over-the-counter medications, and adult day-care services (Medicare.gov, n.d.-c, n.d.-d). Most beneficiaries are able to choose from plans offered by eight firms or more, and all major insurers (Humana, UnitedHealthcare, Blue Cross Blue Shield, CVS Health, Cigna, and Kaiser Permanente) offered plans in more counties in 2024 than 2023. Many companies have or are developing partnerships with Walgreens, Kroger, Rite Aid, and others. Enrollment in UnitedHealthcare and Humira together account for almost half of all Medicare Advantage plans. The federal costs of Medicare Advantage plans in 2021 were $361 billion and are projected to increase to $943 billion in 2031 (Cubanski & Neuman, 2023). Individuals who decide to join a Medicare Advantage plan over selecting traditional Medicare must decide which plan best meets their needs during a time-limited open enrollment period. Medicare Advantage plans have more restrictive provider networks, require prior authorization for many health care services, and may have copays and deductibles that are higher than traditional Medicare (Freed et al., 2023). Deciphering the pros and cons of Medical Advantage plans can be overwhelming for some older adults, especially since plan benefits change from year to year, and the health care needs of an individual may change as well.

Independent Practice Associations

Independent practice associations (IPAs) are organizations composed of independent physicians in solo or group practices who provide health care services to members of an HMO in their private offices, eliminating the expense of the staff model HMO, which furnished and owned the facility in which care was provided. The HMO for a fee-for-service or a prepaid price can purchase hospital care and specialty services not within the IPA. Physicians in an IPA contract may be restricted to caring only for members enrolled in the IPA, but some contracts may allow providers to care for nonmembers as well. Other variations of the staff model and IPAs exist. In a group practice model, an HMO contracts with all physicians and specialists needed by the HMO enrollees, but physicians remain independent. Some contracts are exclusive, requiring physicians to restrict care to members of an individual HMO, and other variations allow physicians to care for members outside the HMO. In a network model, HMOs contract with individual physicians and with physician groups for both primary and specialty services. The HMO maintains control over fee arrangements (Barr, 2023).

Accountable Care Organizations

Accountable care organizations (ACOs) are key components in the ACA and a national strategy to provide high-quality coordinated care to traditional Medicare patients. ACOs in structure are similar to traditional HMOs—responsible for the quality and cost of care delivered to a defined population. Groups of primary care physicians, specialists, other health care providers, and hospitals come together and work as a team to provide coordinated quality of care, reducing duplication of services and unnecessary tests and procedures. Better communication between members of the health care team should also reduce medical errors. ACOs will have financial incentives in place to encourage providers to keep health care costs low by focusing on prevention and treatment of individuals with chronic disease out of the hospital. Performance and savings benchmarks would be in place with a financial reward system and penalties (CMS.gov, n.d.).

Concierge Medical Practices (Retainer Medicine)

Concierge care, also known as boutique medicine or platinum care, is a newer model for providing primary care in a medical practice in which a physician or group of physicians charge individuals an out-of-pocket membership fee averaging $2000 to $3500 per year (but possibly as high as $10,000 per year) in return for enhanced health care services or amenities. Most concierge physicians are family practice and internal medicine, with some specialties. Approximately 12,000 physicians operate concierge-type practices, and 80% of concierge physicians accept some forms of insurance. Amenities most often include same-day or next-day appointments for non-urgent care, 24-hour telephone/e-mail access to the physician, and routine periodic preventive examinations. Individuals electing to join a concierge practice are encouraged to have health care insurance for services used outside the practice, such as specialty care, complex diagnostics, and hospitalization. Some medical issues can be handled digitally, with patient assessments made by phone images and e-mails, avoiding the need for an office visit. Telehealth is offered in a growing number of practices, allowing distanced patient and physician contact. Physicians who provide concierge care typically care for fewer people (200 to 600 patients compared with an average load of 2000 plus), allowing physicians more time to spend with each person and enabling expanded preventive services. Concierge physicians typically treat 6 to 10 individuals per day, allowing for more time with each patient. According to a Concierge Medicine Today year-end salary poll (2017–18), the mean concierge physician salary was $260,825. Physician salaries are predominately derived from membership fees and, for those who accept insurance, from insurance companies. The average profile of a patient in a concierge practice is middle to upper-middle class (household earnings $125,000 to $250,000 annually) and living in a suburban or metropolitan area. The number of concierge medical care practices is growing slowly, and these practices are not available in all areas, and there are those who oppose a model of high-quality care that favors the affluent. The shortages of primary care providers in traditional practices limits access to primary care at a time when the ACA has increased the number of insured individuals and families. If a physician leaves a traditional practice setting and begins a concierge practice, previous patients must find a new provider, which is problematic in areas where there is a shortage of providers. Physicians who choose concierge practice over traditional primary care offices report more time off, less paperwork, the need for fewer office staff, and overall higher professional satisfaction, as they are able to spend more time with patients. Additional time allows personalized service and the ability to provide holistic care. In turn, cost savings may be realized with a reduction in chronic disease or complications of disease, a reduction in the need for emergency department visits, and a reduction in the need for hospitalization and specialty visits (Concierge Medicine Today, 2024; Kane, 2023).

Hospitalist Movement

Responding to the same impetus that spurred managed care in outpatient settings, **hospitalist** programs—supported by HMOs, hospitals, and medical groups—were formed to control hospital costs without compromising quality or satisfaction with client care. Hospitalists are physicians or APNs whose professional focus is managing the comprehensive complex care of the hospitalized patient, providing direct inpatient primary, critical, and consultative care 24 hours a day. Hospitalists engage in clinical care, teaching, research, and leadership in the field of hospital medicine and in meeting the needs of hospitalized patients with acute and chronic complex diseases. Hospitalists enhance the quality and safety of care of a patient within the hospital setting and the safe transitioning of care from the acute care hospital setting to post–acute care facilities or home. Studies have found that hospitals with a hospitalist model program have improved both the quality and the safety of care, with reduced lengths of stay, readmission rates, mortality rates, and complication rates; efficient use is made of hospital and health care resources (Society of Hospital Medicine, n.d.).

Point-of-Service Plans

Point-of-service (POS) plans evolved in response to concerns about restrictions of consumer choice in selecting providers and services. POS plans allow members, for an additional fee and higher copayment, to use providers outside the individual HMO network. Members can choose to pay for this enhanced POS or stay within the HMO network for reduced copayments. If the individual receives care from a physician or hospital not within the list of providers or hospitals, the person pays a substantial portion of the cost of care, usually as out-of-pocket expenses.

High-Deductible Health Insurance Plans

High-deductible health insurance plans (HDHPs) are structured similarly to traditional managed care plans and fee-for-service plans but have very high annual out-of-pocket deductibles of $1000 or greater for individual coverage. A growing number of employers are offering these types of plans, and for those individuals who are generally healthy, the low monthly premium is an attractive option compared with the cost of other types of employer insurance plans. Plans usually have a set annual out-of-pocket limit. Attached to these plans, an employer can offer **health savings accounts (HSAs)** or savings options. Typically, an employer will make quarterly or annual deposits into the individual's HSA, and the employee can elect to have additional funds withheld on a pretax basis to be deposited into the account, up to the annual Internal Revenue Service maximum. Individuals can withdraw money from the account at any age for health-related expenditures. The remaining money in the fund can be withdrawn at retirement without penalty. Most HDHPs are paired with in-network providers for additional savings. Office visits for sickness, laboratory tests, emergency and urgent care, and hospitalizations are covered all or in part after the deductible has been met. Until the annual deductible has been met, out-of-pocket expenses are high; individuals may decide to delay or not seek health care.

Preferred Provider Organizations

Preferred provider organizations (PPOs) are a type of managed care plan in the private sector that has a preselected list of providers who have agreed to provide health services for those individuals enrolled in the plan. Contracted providers in the PPO agree to deliver services to members for a fee-for-service pre-negotiated rate, which is usually discounted. To control costs, members must receive care exclusively from providers within the PPO or incur additional costs if a provider outside the PPO is used. Individuals are typically required to pay a copayment each time services are given. If an individual chooses to see a provider outside the PPO, they will pay additional costs. To control costs, the provider must receive preauthorization from the PPO for a member to be hospitalized or for some procedures or tests, and second opinions are usually required before major procedures or surgical operations are performed.

The KFF conducts an annual survey that reveals the distribution of the health plan type for individuals enrolled in employer health plans. Some employers, often those that are large, offer a variety of health plans to their employees. The distribution of health plan enrollment for covered workers reveals that in 2023, 47% of workers were enrolled in employer PPO plans, 29% of covered workers were enrolled in an HDHP with a savings option, 13% were enrolled in an HMO, and 10% were enrolled in a POS plan, with 1% in a conventional or indemnity plan. The survey found that 91% of all workers were employed by a firm that offered health benefits, and 79% of their employees were eligible for the health benefits offered. Only 76% of eligible employees chose to enroll, citing either cost or the fact that they were covered through another source as a factor. The average annual premiums for both single and family coverage increased 7% from the 2022 survey (KFF, 2023c).

Public Sector

The public sector contains official and voluntary public health agencies operating at the local, state, federal, and international levels. Before 1900, public health was concerned with problems related to environmental risks and infectious diseases. After the 1900s the public health agenda expanded to address the needs of children and mothers. By midcentury, treating chronic disease had also been added to the agenda. As the century progressed, public health issues came to include substance abuse, mental illness, teenage pregnancy, long-term care, epidemics of violence, HIV/AIDS, and most recently bioterrorism and disaster preparedness (Nies & McEwen, 2019).

Source of Power

The US Constitution is based on the sharing of sovereign power between federal and state governments. The powers of the federal government in relation to health are not delineated specifically in the Constitution; they are derived from its authority to tax and to spend for the general welfare and from powers delegated to it by the states. The state governor or legislature usually appoints a health commissioner or secretary of health, who directs the health agency (usually the public health department) to protect citizens from communicable diseases and environmental hazards from waste, water, and food (Nies & McEwen, 2019). State health authority is based also on the 10th Amendment, which reserves for the states, or for the people, those powers not delegated to the federal government by the US Constitution. The states then use their powers to create local governments and delegate authority to them in health matters. The US Public Health Service falls within the larger USDHHS.

Box 3.8: The Department of Health and Human Services lists the federal Public Health Service agencies within the USDHHS.

Influence of Political Philosophy

The prevailing political philosophy regarding societal health needs affects the relationship among federal, state, and local governments. Although the federal government gained power to promote health and welfare in the early 20th century by the passage of the 16th Amendment (giving it the authority to levy federal taxes), states retained sovereign power because the resources were distributed at the state and local levels. Beginning in the 1930s, however, New Deal philosophy began to displace power from the state and local governments to the federal government. Passage of the Hill-Burton Act of 1946 and establishment of what is now known as the CDC increased the federal government's power over state and local affairs. The trend toward increased federal government involvement continued during the Kennedy-Johnson era, when the government focused on societal needs and health care to an unprecedented degree. During the Nixon-Ford era, the trend began to reverse as a New Federalism movement called for less federal encroachment into states' responsibilities and greater state and local responsibility. Clearly, the federal government's role varies according to political philosophy.

During the 1980s the Reagan administration supported free-market competition among insurance plans, physicians, and hospitals to offer the best possible services with the lowest price. Reagan was adamant in his opposition to adopting national health insurance legislation for what he labeled "socialized medicine." Reagan's procompetition policies supported a decrease in federal responsibility for health care, preferring to give states power by providing block grants and control at the state level.

During the Bush administration (1989–1993), incremental steps occurred in moving new legislation toward health care reform with a system of checks and balances in place so that no single political party controlled the White House, Senate, and House of Representatives. To avoid increasing taxes, President Bush proposed a system of tax deductions or tax credits to reduce the cost of private health insurance for families not covered by Medicaid or Medicare. Bush proposed the creation of large networks of small businesses to purchase group health insurance for their employees, voluntary measures to reduce insurance paperwork, encouragement of enrollment in HMOs, and legislation to reduce medical malpractice suits. Because of an economic recession, many workers employed by small businesses did not have employer health insurance plans, and these measures would have assisted in covering working families. However, congressional Democrats refused to support the proposed reform because it did not include an expansion of federal power with a plan for universal coverage or control over the growing cost of insurance premiums.

In 1993 the Clinton administration proposed the Health Security Act to achieve universal health care coverage in the United States by mandating that all employers provide health insurance for their employees and by giving small businesses and

BOX 3.8 The Department of Health and Human Services

The Federal Public Health Service Agencies

Agency for Healthcare Research and Quality (AHRQ): Federal agency whose mission is to produce evidence to make health care safer, higher quality, more accessible, equitable, affordable, and to work within HHS and with other partners to make sure that the evidence is understood and used.

Centers for Disease Control and Prevention (CDC): Mission is to protect the public and health of the nation by providing leadership and direction in the prevention and control of disease and other preventable conditions, and to respond to public health emergencies.

Centers for Medicare & Medicaid Services (CMS): A Federal agency within the USDHHS that administers the Medicare program and works in partnership with state governments to administer the federal portion of the Medicaid program, States Children's Health Insurance Program (CHIP), some Health Insurance Marketplace plans, and related quality assurance activities with states to run the Medicaid program.

Children's Health Insurance Program (CHIP) (Title XIX and Title XXI): A joint federal and state program that provides health insurance coverage to eligible children through both Medicaid and separate CHIP programs.

Food and Drug Administration (FDA): Federal agency responsible for protecting the public by regulating the following products: drugs; medical devices; radiation-emitting products; vaccines; blood and biologics; animal and veterinary drugs, vaccines and other products; ensuring cosmetics and dietary supplements are safe and properly labeled; and regulating tobacco products.

Health Resources and Services Administration (HRSA): Primary federal agency for improving access to health care services for people who are geographically isolated, economically or medically vulnerable. Provides HRSA loan repayment and scholarship programs to health professionals.

Indian Health Service (IHS): Responsible for providing federal comprehensive and culturally appropriate public health services to American Indians and Alaska Natives (≈2.6 million individuals) who belong to 574 federally recognized tribes in 37 states. American Indians and Alaska Natives as citizens of the United States are eligible to participate in all public, private, and state health programs available to the general public and treaty rights to federal health care services through the DHIHS.

National Institutes of Health (NIH): Provides leadership, direction, and funding to programs designed to improve the health of the nation by conducting and supporting biomedical and behavioral research both within its own laboratories and clinics, as well as throughout the United States and abroad. NIH trains promising researchers and promotes collecting and sharing medical knowledge.

Office of the Inspector General: Office dedicated to fighting waste fraud and abuse and to improving the efficiency of more than 100 USDHHS programs. Provides oversight of Medicaid and Medicare, the CDC, the NIH, and the FDA. The majority of the agency's resources (approximately 1650 personnel) go toward the oversight of Medicare and Medicaid.

Substance Abuse and Mental Health Services Administration (SAMHSA): Part of the Public Health Service, improves access and reduces barriers to high-quality, effective programs and services for individuals who suffer from or are at risk for addictive or mental health illness, as well as for their families and communities. Funds mental health and substance abuse prevention and treatment services.

Source: US Department of Health and Human Services (USDHHS). (n.d.-c). *HHS agencies & offices.* https://www.hhs.gov/about/agencies/hhs-agencies-and-offices/index.html

unemployed Americans subsidies with which to purchase insurance. The plan met severe opposition from the insurance industry and the business community. Mass media advertisements by these stakeholders questioned whether HMOs would provide choice and access to health care services. Large segments of the American public, especially the 80% who had employer-based private health insurance, began to fear being forced into HMOs, which would diminish their choice of, access to, and quality of health care. The cost of a socialized, universal health care coverage system was estimated to reach trillion-dollar levels. The act was defeated in Congress, and a time of political caution followed, stalling any further movement toward universal health care. Small, incremental health reform was passed, such as the portability of health care coverage in 1996 (Health Insurance Portability and Accountability Act [HIPAA]), allowing persons to access health care throughout the United States, and the focus shifted to balancing the federal budget. Other incremental legislation included the passage of the Balanced Budget Act of 1997, which made significant reforms in Medicare, as well as the formation of a new public insurance program—CHIP. CHIP is a partnership between the federal and state governments to provide low- or no-cost health insurance to uninsured children and pregnant females whose families earn too much to qualify for Medicaid but are unable to afford private insurance coverage. Each state operates its own CHIP as a separate program, expansion of the Medicaid program, or some combination. Some states have renamed their program; for example, Georgia's program is called PeachCare for Kids, and New Mexico named its program MexiKids. CHIP must cover well-baby, well-child, dental coverage, vaccines, and benchmark-equivalent coverage of a state employee plan, HMO, or federal employees' health benefit plan. CMS determines the annual allotment for each state, and states must match funds to receive the federal funds. Funding is capped (administered in block grants to states), and Congress must act periodically to refund the program. Federal legislation is passed by Congress to fund the government for every fiscal year which begins on October 1 and ends September 30. The Bipartisan Budget Act (P.L. 115-123) was signed into law extending CHIP funding through 2027. CHIP funding has been approved to provide annual allotments that increased from $21.5 billion in federal fiscal year (FFY) 2018 to $25.9 billion in FFY 2023. In 2018, 9.6 million children were enrolled in CHIP (Medicaid.gov, n.d.-a; CMS, 2023).

Another major expansion in the role of the federal government occurred in 2003, when Congress passed the Medicare Prescription Drug Act Part D. The biggest expansion of federal oversight since Medicare and Medicaid from the 1960s came when the ACA became law.

In March 2010, President Barack Obama signed into law the ACA, also known as the PPACA or Obamacare. The primary goals of the massive health care reform act were to dramatically reduce the number of uninsured Americans, pay for coverage without adding to the national debt, slow the rising cost of health care, make affordable health insurance available to more Americans, expand the Medicaid program to cover all adults with income below 138% of the federal poverty level (FPL), and lower the costs of health care by supporting innovative medical care delivery systems (HealthCare.gov, n.d.-a; Knickman & Elbel, 2019). When first elected to office, President Obama pushed for health care reform and gained support from a strong Democratic majority in both the House of Representatives and the Senate. Before the ACA became law, bitter debates between Democratic and Republican members of the House of Representatives and the Senate occurred. Democratic control of the Senate and the House of Representatives allowed the bills to be quickly voted out of committee and introduced to the floors. In December 2009, the Senate bill passed with the support of all Democrats and no Republican senators voting in favor. In March 2010 the bill came to a vote in the House of Representatives. This time there was bipartisan support against the bill, with 178 Republicans and 34 Democrats voting against it. The bill passed by seven votes (219 vs. 212), and 2 days later the health reform act of 2010 was signed into law, and an amended version was passed in May 2010 (Office of the Legislative Council, 2010). The 974-page document is long and complex and specifies details of the many provisions and timelines for enactment (Box 3.9: Sections of the Affordable Care Act).

Trump Administration. Throughout history, health care policy and opposing views in the role of government in the health care system have occurred along the lines of political party affiliation—Democrat or Republican. Traditionally, those favoring the views of the Democratic Party support the federal government being more involved in the provision of health care, and Republicans support a system based more on private health insurance and less federal governmental involvement. Trump's Republican administration (January 2017–January 2021) followed an 8-year term of Obama's Democratic administration (2009-2017), and the new vision for health care was more choice, better care, and lower costs. One of the first changes

BOX 3.9 Sections of the Affordable Care Act

Title I
Quality, Affordable Health Care for All Americans

Title II
The Role of Public Programs

Title III
Improving the Quality and Efficiency of Health Care

Title IV
Prevention of Chronic Disease and Improving Public Health

Title V
Health Care Workforce

Title VI
Transparency and Program Integrity

Title VII
Improving Access to Innovative Medical Therapies

Title VIII
Community Living Assistance Services and Supports Act (CLASS Act)

Title IX
Revenue Provisions

Title X
Reauthorization of the Indian Health Care Improvement Act

made by the Trump Administration was the elimination of the Obamacare individual tax penalty to require health insurance coverage (see chapter introduction), along with the elimination of the medical device tax (imposing a 2.3% excise tax on certain medical devices such as magnetic resonance imaging [MRI] machines, infusion pumps, pace makers, defibrillators, and surgical equipment produced in the United States) and eliminating the Cadillac tax (employers being required to pay a 40% tax on health insurance that exceeded a certain value for each employee). Other reforms included increasing health insurance choice by promoting competition in the individual health insurance markets, allowing employers to pool together to offer more affordable quality health coverage (association plans), increased funding for Alzheimer research, the passing of "Right to Try" (giving terminally ill patients access to potentially life-saving cures), ending gag clauses preventing pharmacists from informing patients about the best prices for their prescribed medications, lowering prescription drug prices, delivering hospital and insurer price transparency, ending surprise billing, expanding telehealth services (especially in rural and underserved communities), and affirming the policy that protected patients from being denied health insurance with a preexisting condition.

President Trump's initial response on January 31, 2020, to the new outbreak of a previously unknown virus was focused on sealing US borders to prevent further entry and transmission of the virus with screening and quarantine requirements for all people entering the United States and suspending entry of those seeking asylum from Mexico or Canada. A White House COVID-19 task force was established January 27, 2020, and a number of federal emergency spending bills were signed: the Coronavirus Preparedness and Response Supplemental Appropriations Act (March 6, 2020); the Families First Coronavirus Response Act (March 18, 2020); the Coronavirus Aid, Relief, and Economic Security Act (CARES Act, March 27, 2020); and the Paycheck Protection Program and Health Care Enhancement Act (April 24, 2020). Trump also signed into law emergency relief legislation to eliminate cost-sharing for COVID-19 testing and prevention, enhanced testing capacity, and required public and private health coverage of COVID-19 diagnostic testing with no cost-sharing. States had a new optional Medicaid eligibility pathway to cover COVID-19 testing and testing-related services for uninsured individuals with 100% federally matching funds. The Army Corps of Engineers and National Guard constructed temporary hospitals and medical centers to treat the large influx of patients with COVID-19, and the Navy's two hospital ships, the USNS Mercy and USNS Comfort, were deployed to care for the growing number of patients overwhelming health care facilities, especially in the New York City area. The administration activated the Defense Production Act to direct domestic industry to expedite and expand the supply of ventilators, respirators, and other countermeasures needed to help patients and frontline workers. Federal legislation initiated Project Airbridge to procure and transport critical supplies and equipment to the United States. In June 2020 (as previously discussed), Operation Warp Speed was passed, giving pharmaceutical companies money to expedite development of effective vaccines with a goal to deliver 300 million doses of effective vaccine for COVID-19 by January 2021. In early December, the initial phases of the COVID-19 vaccination began targeting health care professionals and long-term care residents. On December 14, 2020, Sandra Lindsay, RN, MBA, DHSc, became the first registered nurse outside of clinical trials to receive a COVID-19 vaccination with the Pfizer-BioNTech COVID-19 vaccine while serving as director of nursing critical care at Long Island Jewish Medical Center in New York and later received the Presidential Medal of Freedom. December 31, 2020, marked the 1-year anniversary of the first reported COVID-19 case to the WHO (WHO, 2023; CDC, 2023).

Current Health Policy

Former vice president during the Obama administration, President Joe Biden took office in January 2021 and continued supporting the policies enacted during the COVID-19 pandemic, which the USHHS and WHO declared over effective May 11, 2023. Following the declaration of the end of the pandemic, several important laws were passed for continuation of support post-pandemic and changes in Medicare Part D. The Inflation Reduction Act passed on August 6, 2022, set a yearly cap of $2000 for 2025 on out-of-pocket prescription drug expenses in Medicare and access to recommended vaccines without cost-sharing. The American Rescue Plan Act of 2021 H.R. 1319 became law on March 11, 2021, and provided direct relief from the effect of COVID-19 with stimulus checks, increased child tax credits, extension of unemployment insurance, small business support, and other measures during the pandemic and post-pandemic recovery.

Future Health Policy

Historically there has been a lack of consensus among the major political parties and stakeholders regarding health care reform. Since the ACA became law in March 2010, a number of states, individuals, and other organizations have filed actions in state and federal courts challenging the constitutionality of the law. Since the executive branch of the federal government holds the power to change health care laws that state governments must then enact, substantial effort is needed in policy reform to prioritize both issues of access, especially to vulnerable populations, and cost containment. As future advances in science unfold, how resources are used to improve the quality and safety of patient-centered care will require ongoing adjustments in the provision and financing of health care. As discussed earlier, great strides have been made in recent decades to improve the health of the nation's population, measured by decreasing infant mortality rates and increased life expectancies for both males and females. The COVID-19 global pandemic provided gains in scientific findings in treatments, vaccinations, and other measures to meet the health care needs of the population. Nurses need to stay abreast of the political landscape and be involved in decision-making at the local, state, and federal levels to further improve population health.

Nursing's Role in Leading Change—2010 Recommendations of the Institute of Medicine

Report on the Future of Nursing. In 2008, the Robert Wood Johnson Foundation and the IOM launched a 2-year initiative to respond to the need to assess and transform the nursing profession. The IOM appointed the committee on the Robert Wood Johnson Foundation Initiative on the Future of Nursing and charged the committee with determining recommendations for an action-oriented blueprint for nursing's future. The IOM recognized that nurses play a key role in helping realize the objectives set forth in the 2010 ACA but that a number of barriers exist preventing nurses from responding effectively to rapidly changing health care settings and an evolving health care system. The committee developed the following four key messages and seven recommendations (IOM, 2010):

- Nurses practice to the full extent of their education and training.
- Nurses achieve higher levels of education and training through an improved education system that promotes seamless academic progression.
- Nurses should be full partners, with physicians and other health care professionals, in redesigning health care in the United States.
- Effective workforce planning and policymaking require better data collection and an improved information infrastructure.

A second report released in 2016, the *Assessing Progress on the Institute of Medicine Report*, highlighted progress from the 2010 initiative and developed three themes for future success: the need to build a broader coalition to increase awareness of nurses' ability to play a full role in health professions' practice, education, collaboration, and leadership; the need to make promoting diversity in the nursing workforce a priority; and the need for better data with which to assess and drive progress. *The Future of Nursing 2020-2030* reports that the workforce of nearly 4 million nurses will be challenged in new and complex ways over the next decade, requiring a diversified nursing workforce that is prepared to provide care, promote health and well-being to individuals and communities, and recommend outcomes to achieving health equity (National Academies of Sciences, Engineering, and Medicine, 2021).

Official Agencies

Official agencies are tax supported and therefore accountable to the citizens through elected or appointed officials or boards. The purpose and duties of official agencies are prescribed or mandated by law. This discussion is from the perspective of the individual gaining knowledge of or access to the health care system.

Local Level. The health department of a town, city, county, township, or district is the local health unit and is usually the first line of access and health responsibility for the population that it serves. The mayor, the board of health, or some other executive governing body appoints the chief administrator, the health officer. The local health department's role and functions usually focus on providing direct services to the public and depend on the state mandate and community resources. Local governments, but usually not health departments, have the responsibility to provide general health care services for the poor.

State Level. Public health services are organized by each state, with wide variation from one state to another. The chief administrator is usually a state health officer or commissioner appointed by the governor. One agency, typically the state health department, performs the primary responsibilities in policy, planning, and coordination of programs and services for local units under its jurisdiction.

Federal Level. The federal government assumes overall responsibility for the health protection of its citizens. Although all three branches of the federal government make health-related decisions, major policy decisions are made by the president and the president's staff (executive branch) and also by Congress (legislative branch). These two branches determine health policy. Once policy has been determined, other government agencies are responsible for oversight to ensure implementation.

The USDHHS, the main federal body concerned with the health of the nation, consists of a number of separate operating agencies (see Box 3.8: The Department of Health and Human Services, The Federal Public Health Service Agencies). Under each of the federal public health service agencies listed there are numerous other departments. USDHHS agencies that relate directly to nursing include the Health Resources and Services Administration and the National Institutes of Health (NIH). The Bureau of Health Professions, within the Health Resources and Services Administration, contains a division of nursing, which is a source for nursing education and training grants. The National Institute of Nursing Research within the NIH funds nursing research, including health-promotion and illness-prevention studies (Box 3.10: Quality and Safety, Ban of Medical Devices).

Chief Nursing Officer. The chief nursing officer (CNO) serves in the US Public Health Service and leads the Commissioned Corps of the US Public Health Service Nurse Professional Affairs. The CNO advises the Office of the Surgeon General, as the US assistant surgeon general, and the USDHHS on the recruitment, assignment, deployment, retention, and career development of nurse professionals. The CNO provides leadership to the 4500 Commissioned Corps and civilian nurses. The current CNO, Rear Admiral Jennifer Moon, was appointed on October 31, 2023 (US Public Health Service, n.d.).

Federal Emergency Management Agency. The US Department of Homeland Security is another large branch of federal agencies with numerous offices, many of which have a connection with health care. Since 2003 the Federal Emergency Management Agency (FEMA) has been part of the US Department of Homeland Security. FEMA was established in 1979 by an executive order merging many separate disaster-related services into a single entity to assist states when a disaster overwhelms a state's capacity to respond. A disaster, as defined by FEMA, includes a hurricane, earthquake, tornado, flood, fire, hazardous spill, act of nature, or act of terrorism. The role of FEMA is to support citizens and first responders to build, sustain, and improve capacity to prepare for, protect against, respond to, recover from, and mitigate all hazards. Assistance is provided to individuals, communities, and states that are determined to be eligible. In 2006 the Post-Katrina Emergency Management Reform Act created a "new FEMA" with an expanded mission and homeland security preparedness responsibilities in the areas of recovery, response, and logistics. Following the many natural disasters in 2017 (hurricanes Harvey, Irma, and Maria and wildfires in California), a new strategic plan was released with three primary goals: building a culture of preparedness, readying

BOX 3.10 QUALITY AND SAFETY

BAN on Electrical Stimulation Devices (ESDs) for Self-Injurious or Aggressive Behaviors

The US Food and Drug Administration (FDA) lists over 6000 types of medical devices sold in the United States regulated by the FDA's Center for Medical Devices and Radiological Health. The FDA protects the health of the public by monitoring reports of adverse events and other problems with medical devices and posting safety information updates on recalls, current bans, and proposed bans on their website. In 2023, 43 of the newest medical technologies and medical devices entries were cleared or approved for use, and over 60 medical devices were recalled. In 1976, the Federal Food, Drug, and Cosmetic Act became law, authorizing the FDA to ban by regulation any device intended for human use if the device presents a substantial deception or an unreasonable or substantial risk of illness or injury that could not be, or has not been, corrected or eliminated by labeling. In 1983, prosthetic hair fibers were banned, and in 2016, the FDA banned the use of most powdered medical gloves due to the risks from the use of powder to both patients and users, including acute airway inflammation because of inhalation of the powder particles, hypersensitivity and allergic reactions, and risk of granuloma and adhesion formation to patients and care workers if internal tissue is exposed to powder. Effective January 2017, all unused powdered gloves were required to be pulled from use and disposed of.

More recently in March 2020, the FDA published a final rule to ban electrical stimulation devices (ESDs) used to diminish self-injurious or aggressive behavior because they present an unreasonable and substantial risk of illness or injury that cannot be corrected or eliminated through new or updated device labeling, effective April 2020. ESDs were used on people with intellectual or developmental disabilities as aversion conditioning devices that apply a noxious electrical shock through electrodes attached to an individual's skin to condition them to stop engaging in self-injurious or aggressive behaviors. Behaviors in this vulnerable population include head-banging, hand-biting, excessive scratching, and skin-damaging behaviors, but can be more extreme and result in bleeding, fractures, eye-gouging or poking, or other injuries. ESDs were found to pose significant psychological and physical risks (pain, burns, depression, anxiety, acute stress disorder, nightmares, flashbacks, panic, rage, worsening of behaviors and others) and were used on individuals who may not be able to communicate their pain or consent. Safer treatments (using positive-reinforcement approaches and medications to suppress behaviors) and evidence from the scientific community supported the ban. In October 2023, the FDA released a proposed rule that would ban hair-straightening products (commonly known as relaxers) that contain formaldehyde or those that contain ingredients that can form formaldehyde when the product is used, such as methylene glycol. Hair straighteners are largely used by Black females, and long-term adverse health effects may increase the risk of developing uterine or other cancers. A final ruling from the FDA and possible ban is pending.

Sources: US Food and Drug Administration (FDA). (n.d.). *Medical device safety.* http://www.fda.gov/MedicalDevices/Safety/default.htm

the nation for catastrophic disasters, and reducing the complexity of FEMA. The Disaster Recovery Reform Act (DRRA) was signed into law in October 2018; this act improves disaster preparedness, response, recovery, and mitigation. The response directorate, for example, provides coordinated federal operational and logistical disaster response capability needed to save and sustain lives, minimize suffering, and protect property in a timely manner in communities overwhelmed by a disaster (FEMA, 2019; USDHHS, n.d.). Under the direction of the White House Coronavirus Task Force, FEMA, along with other federal partners working with state, local, tribal, and territorial governments, executed a whole-of-America response to fight the COVID-19 pandemic. (See fema.gov and whitehouse.gov for current information.)

Military Health Systems at the Federal Level. The Military Health System (MHS) is a unique partnership of medical educators, medical researchers, health care providers, and support personnel who are prepared to respond anytime or anywhere with comprehensive medical capability to military operations, natural disasters, and humanitarian crises around the world and to ensure world-class health care is provided to all Department of Defense active-duty members, retired US military personnel, and their dependents, including some members of the reserve component.

The Department of Veterans Affairs (VA), an independent agency directly under the president, provides integrated health care services for veterans (who did not receive a dishonorable discharge) through the Department of Defense, which sponsors health care for military personnel on active duty. The VA uses an advanced computerized information system, which allows a person's medical record to be accessed at any VA site nationally, increasing efficiency in the provision of care. For active-duty service members and retirees of the seven uniformed services, family members, survivors, and others who are registered in the defense enrollment eligibility reporting system, military health care is covered through the former Civilian Health and Medical Program of the VA. The VA health care system has the largest integrated health care system in the United States, consisting of 1321 health care facilities, including 172 VA Medical Centers and 1138 outpatient sites and serving 9 million enrolled veterans each year. The PACT Act is a new law that expands VA health care benefits for veterans exposed to burn pits, agent orange, and other toxic substances. The Act extends eligibility for VA health care for veterans with toxic exposures and veterans from the Vietnam War, Gulf War, and post-9/11 era. TRICARE is the health care program for uniformed service members, retired members, and their families, and it is available worldwide. CHAMPVA is a health care program for special enrollments of a spouse or child who is not eligible for TRICARE. The Veteran's Administration website has up-to-date information on various programs and news alerts (VA, 2023).

Wounded Warrior Care. When a soldier is severely injured, prolonged care and rehabilitation are often required before a decision can be made whether the soldier should remain on active duty. The MHS is responsible for providing clinical care to return service personnel to duty or to assist them in making the transition from MHS care to the VA health care system. Tremendous progress has been made in the rehabilitative care of injured combatants and coordination of MHS care with the VA health system. The Wounded Warrior Project provides free programs to veterans and service members who incurred a physical or mental injury, illness, or wound while serving in the military on or after September 11, 2001. The Wounded Warrior Project provides free programs and services in mental health, career counseling, and long-term rehabilitation for males and females transitioning from military to civilian life (Wounded Warriors Project, 2023).

Americans with Disabilities. Starting in 1992, health care providers, both as employers and providers of public services, were required to comply with requirements of the Americans with Disabilities Act of 1990. The act is considered the most sweeping civil rights legislation since the Civil Rights Act of 1964. The two parts that apply most directly to health care providers are the prohibition of employment discrimination and the requirements for provision of services to people with disabilities. An example of a health care provider accommodation is installing wheelchair lifts in shuttle bus systems. Despite their need for health promotion and disease prevention, individuals with disabilities face numerous problems gaining access to health-promotion programs and preventive services. The barriers are financial, social, physical, and logistical (USDHHS, 2015b).

In 1990, President George H. W. Bush signed the Patient Self-Determination Act, a law designed to increase individual involvement in decisions about life-sustaining treatment, ensuring that advance directives for health care are available to physicians at the time that medical decisions are being made and ensuring that individuals who have not prepared such documents are aware of their legal rights. As a condition of Medicare and Medicaid payment, the Patient Self-Determination Act requires health care facilities to comply with the law. The ACA has several provisions expanding the access requirements for services to people with disabilities (see Box 3.9: Sections of the Affordable Care Act).

Federal Health Information Privacy Law. Developed by the USDHHS as part of the HIPAA of 1996, federal privacy standards were enacted by Congress requiring new safeguards to protect the security and confidentiality of health information, including paper, electronic, and oral communications. Health plans, pharmacies, physicians, nurses, and other health care providers must have a written privacy procedure, provide employee training on the HIPAA, and designate a privacy officer to ensure procedures are followed. The privacy law permits disclosures without individual authorization to public health authorities authorized by law to collect and receive information for the purpose of preventing or controlling disease, injury, or disability (USDHHS, n.d.-b).

International Level. WHO, the United Nations' specialized agency for health, as previously discussed, was established in 1948. WHO comprises members from more than 190 countries, and its core functions include giving worldwide guidance in the field of health; setting global standards for health; cooperating with governments in strengthening national health programs; and developing and transferring appropriate technology, information, and standards. During the COVID-19 global pandemic, WHO provided direction in the exchange of epidemiologic clinical data and coordination measures to fight against the pandemic (WHO, 2023).

Voluntary Agencies

The voluntary (not-for-profit) health movement stems from the goodwill and humanitarian concerns that are part of the nongovernmental, free enterprise heritage of the people of the United States. Nonprofit entities that maintain a tax-free status are often powerful forces in the health field, voluntary agencies, foundations, and professional associations. The tax-free status of these organizations is challenged at times on the basis of charges that some of them serve only a limited population. Voluntary agencies are influential in promoting health affairs and research agendas at the national policy level and often have significant influence on health legislation. Their prominent role was demonstrated by the American Cancer Society's early mass media announcements about the health hazards of smoking. An example of another voluntary agency is the Alzheimer's Association, which has local chapters that provide resources for families, including publications, services, respite for caregivers, and support groups for individuals and families.

Philanthropic foundations provide valuable stimulation to the health field and operate under fewer constraints than other sources do in supporting research or training projects. Nurses interested in research or advanced clinical study that relates to the special interests of voluntary agencies or foundations may find grant monies available to support their work. For example, the John A. Hartford Foundation was established in 1929 and supports efforts to improve health care for older Americans. The foundation awards millions of dollars in grants to support research and spread evidence-based models that can improve the care of older adults. The institute has also raised the profile of geriatric nursing by creating nationally recognized awards for excellence in research and practice (John A. Hartford Foundation, n.d.). Professional associations, organized at the national level with state and local branches, are powerful political forces. Nurses can support their professional organizations in influencing the direction of health policy through membership and active participation.

The American Red Cross. The American Red Cross is a well-known volunteer-led humanitarian organization that is officially sanctioned by the federal government as a congressional charter, meaning it is not supervised by the government because it is not a governmental agency, but it is recognized officially. Founded in 1881 by Clara Barton, the International Red Cross aids victims of war and natural disasters throughout the world. There are more than 700 local American Red Cross chapters in the United States with more than 500,000 volunteers and 35,000 employees. The American Red Cross responds both to small local emergencies to help victims (such as in the case of a house fire) and to large natural disasters (such as hurricanes and earthquakes). The Red Cross is the largest supplier of blood and blood products in the United States and collects approximately 40% of the nation's donated blood. The American Red Cross also assists thousands of US service members separated from their families in maintaining communication and offers communities a range of health and safety courses. The global network of national societies relies on public donations of money, time, and blood. Local Red Cross opportunities exist, including the donation of blood and assistance with blood drives and other volunteer activities (American Red Cross, n.d.). During the COVID-19 pandemic, the American Red Cross and the US Food and Drug Administration (FDA) developed a process to identify and collect therapeutic plasma from fully recovered COVID-19 patients to treat seriously ill hospitalized patients with COVID-19. Although treatment with convalescent plasma was still experimental at the time (March 24, 2020) no treatments existed for COVID-19, and preliminary data supported the new initiative. By 2022, the virus had mutated, and convalescent plasma was authorized for use for people with weakened immune systems who were not in the hospital to lower the risk of serious COVID-19 illness (American Red Cross, 2023; Mayo Clinic Staff, 2023).

FINANCING HEALTH CARE

Costs

The health care industry is the largest service industry in the United States today and the most powerful employer in the nation. National health expenditures in the United States were greater than those in any other country, with $466 trillion (or $12,000 per person) projected to be spent in 2023, a marked increase from the $1.9 trillion spent in 2004. Under current law, projections on national health expenditures by 2031 will reach $7.01 trillion dollars, growing by an average of 5.5% per year. Predictions for 2021 forecasted that 18.2% of the GDP would be consumed for health expenditures; however, actual spending increased to 18.3% of the GDP due to the high cost of care during and following the COVID-19 pandemic. The Centers for Medicare and Medicaid anticipate that in 2031, health care spending will consume 19.6% of the GDP. Hospitals and physician services represent more than half of total health spending (Fig. 3.3: The Nation's Health Dollar, Calendar Year 2022: Where It Went).

In 2020, the amount of money spent on average per person 65 years and older was $22,356, five times higher than the amount spent per child (0–18 years of age; male children $4415 and female children $4009) and more than two times higher than the spending per working-age person (19–64 years; males $8313 and females $9989). In 2020, children 0 to 18 years old made up 23% of the population consuming 10% of health care dollars; the 19–64 age group made up 60% of the population and consumed 53% of health care dollars; and the 65 and older age group made up 17% of the population and consumed 37% of health care dollars. Health care spending on adults over 85 years in 2020 was almost $36,000, 8.5 times that per child (CMS, 2023). The OECD is a group of 38 member countries and a reliable source of comparative statistics on economic and social data; among other health statistics, it reports average health care expenditures as a share of a country's GDP. The average GDP share for health expenditures of member countries was 8.8% in 2019, before the COVID-19 pandemic. By 2021, the proportion had increased to 9.7% and was expected to fall slightly to 9.2% in 2022. The three highest-spending countries in 2022 were the United States at 16.6%, Germany at 12.7%, and France 12.1% as a percent of GDP. Countries (members and nonmembers) with the lowest share of GDP on health care expenditures were Mexico (5.5%), Turkey (4.3%), Indonesia (3.4%), India (2.9%), and China (5.7%). Switzerland and Iceland, followed by Israel and the United States, had the highest health prices, and the United States was the highest consumer of health care volume (measure of health care goods) (OECD, 2024). Although other countries spend far less per capita, life expectancy in some industrialized countries is greater and infant mortality rates are lower than in the United States, as discussed earlier in the chapter.

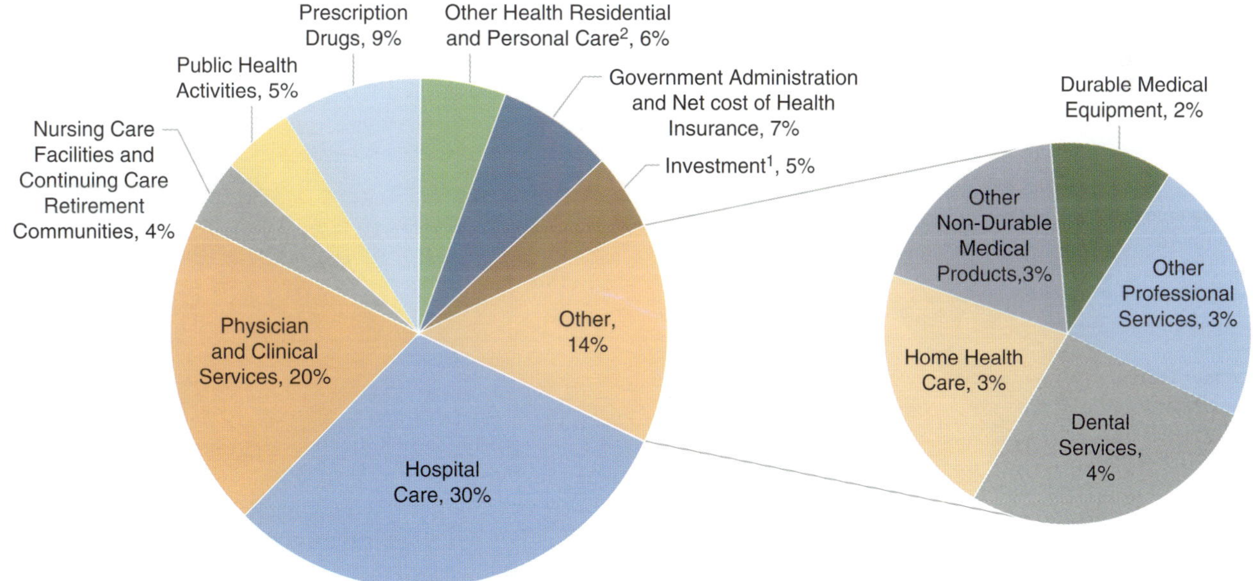

[1]Includes Noncommercial Research and Structures and Equipment.
[2]Includes expenditures for residential care facilities, ambulance providers, medical care delivered in non-traditional settings (such as community centers, senior citizens centers, schools, and military field stations), and expenditures for Home and Community Waiver programs under Medicaid.
Note: Sum of pieces may not equal 100% due to rounding.
Source: Centers for Medicare & Medicaid Services, Office of the Actuary, National Health Statistics Group.

FIG. 3.3 The Nation's Health Dollar ($4.5 Trillion), Calendar Year 2022: Where It Went. (From Centers for Medicare & Medicaid Services, Office of the Actuary, National Health Statistics Group.)

According to the Centers for Medicare and Medicaid Services' June 2023 report, the insured share of the US population is projected to have reached a historic high of 92.3% in 2022 and to have remained at that rate in 2023 due to Marketplace enrollment and continuous enrollment requirements of the Medicaid program of the Families First Coronavirus Act. By 2031, the share of the population with health insurance is projected to be 90.5%. A major goal of the ACA was to reduce the number of uninsured Americans. These figures and expenditures, although numerous, introduce the topic of health care financing.

Health care analysts predict that accelerations in health care costs will continue, putting pressure on public and private payers to finance them. Factors driving costs include general inflation; health care cost inflation; application of new and more advanced technologies; growth in the proportion of older adults; government financing of health care services, including long-term care; growth of prescription drug use and costs; misdistribution of health care providers and services; expansion of medical technology and specialty medicine; and other costs associated with providing health care. For example, diagnostic and therapeutic techniques—including computer-aided technology and noninvasive imaging (such as MRIs), cardiac surgery, organ transplantation, new medications, joint replacements (particularly hips and knees)—enhance the capabilities of medicine while increasing costs.

Sources

Ultimately, the American people pay for all health care costs. Money is transferred from consumer to provider by various mechanisms. The major sources are the government (federal, state, and local monies collected by taxes), third-party payment (private insurance), independent plans, and out-of-pocket costs, which totaled $4.3 trillion in 2021. The CMS provides statistics on the source of the nation's health care dollars and the manner in which they are spent. In 2022, the breakdown of national health spending was as follows: hospital care 30%, physician and clinical services 20%, prescription drugs 9%, government administration 7%, dental 4%, nursing care facilities 4%, home health care 3%, public health activities 5%, and other expenditures (see Fig. 3.3: The Nation's Health Dollar, Calendar Year 2022: Where It Went). In 2022 the largest percentage of the nation's health care dollars came from private health insurance (29%), Medicare, (21%), Medicaid (18%), out-of-pocket expenses by consumers (11%), and others (Fig. 3.4: The Nation's Health Dollar, Calendar Year 2022: Where It Came From). In all, some form of health insurance funds 72% of the nation's health care. As discussed earlier, keeping Americans healthy and out of the hospital would save a tremendous amount of money.

Employer Health Benefits

According to the 25th annual employer health benefits surveys conducted by the KFF, almost 153 million people rely on employer-sponsored health insurance coverage. The overall inflation rate of employer-sponsored health insurance for families has risen dramatically in the last decade. Between 2013 and 2021, health insurance premiums for family coverage have risen 5% or less each year but rose to 7% in family premiums in 2023. The average employer-sponsored health insurance annual premium in 2009 was $3515 for individuals and $13,375 for family coverage. In 2023, the average employer-sponsored

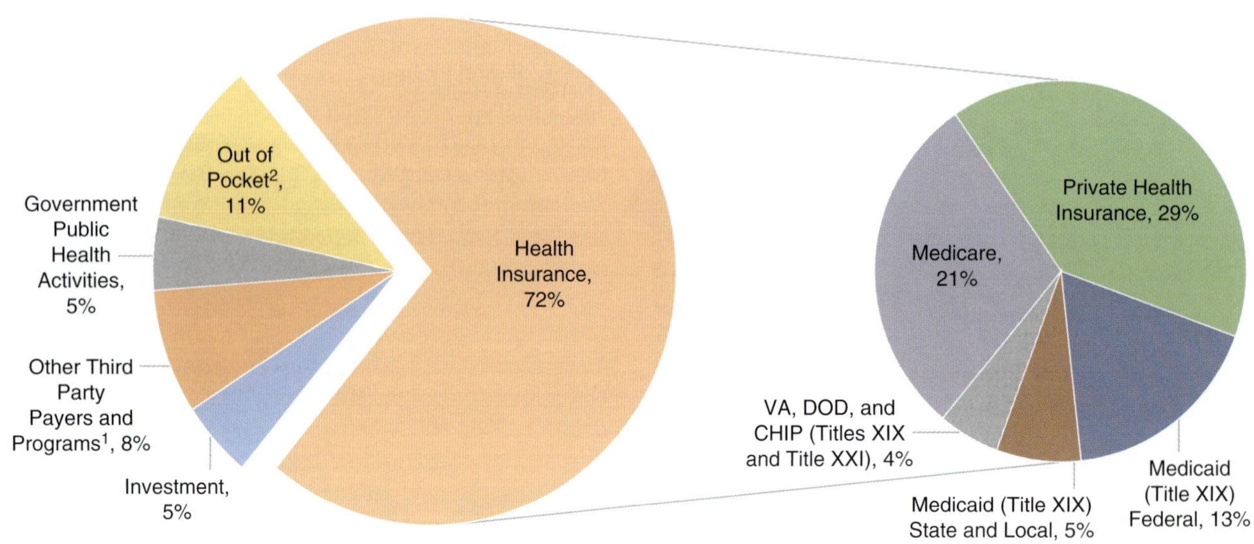

[1]Includes worksite health care, other private revenues, Indian Health Service, workers' compensation, general assistance, maternal and child health, vocational rehabilitation, Substance Abuse and Mental Health Services Administration, school health, and other federal and state and local programs.
[2]Includes co-payments, deductibles, and any amounts not covered by health insurance.
Note: Sum of pieces may not equal 100% due to rounding.
Source: Centers for Medicare & Medicaid Services, Office of the Actuary, National Health Statistics Group.

FIG. 3.4 The Nation's Health Dollar ($4.5 Trillion), Calendar Year 2022: Where It Came From. (From Centers for Medicare & Medicaid Services, Office of the Actuary, National Health Statistics Group.)

health insurance premium was $6525 for an individual and $23,968 for family coverage. Over the past 5 years, the average family premium has increased 22%. Depending on the employer and firm size, most employers pay some of the cost of the monthly premium, and the worker pays the remainder. Workers at firms with fewer than 200 workers pay on average almost $2500 more toward family premiums than those working in larger firms. Monthly premiums do not include other costs associated with using the plan, such as out-of-pocket expenses, copays, and deductibles, making it difficult for both individuals and employers to pay for higher health care premiums and for insured people to use health care. Most plans have additional out-of-pocket costs (copayments) for use of the plan for office visits, laboratory testing, and other services, such as physical therapy. Almost all plans have some sort of prescription drug coverage but may limit coverage to certain medications (a formulary of what medications are covered or denied is usually part of a prescription plan). Some plans have a tiered list of medications with differing copayments. Generic medications (if available) generally have the least additional out-of-pocket cost and are listed in the lowest-cost tier. Some plans have mail-order options for maintenance medications. Typically, a 90-day supply of a maintenance medication prescribed through this type of plan may cost the same or less than a 60-day supply at a pharmacy. Health insurance plans are also separated into different metal tiers based on the proportion of the health care cost an insurance plan covers. Catastrophic and bronze plans have the lowest monthly premium but cover the smallest portion of health care costs, with higher deductibles and copays. The highest monthly premiums are in the platinum tier and cover 90% of health care costs. Health care providers need to be aware of these variations between plans before prescribing medications, as out-of-pocket expenses may inhibit an individual from filling a prescription and following the prescribed medication plan (KFF, 2023c).

Federal and state **Medicaid** spending showed an increasing pattern of cost at $80.47 billion dollars in fiscal 2022 (October 1, 2021–September 30, 2022) or $824 billion dollars if administrative costs and US territories are included. Medicaid is the third-largest domestic program in the federal budget, and for states, Medicaid is the second-largest expenditure (elementary and secondary education is first). Although costly, the Medicaid program is essential health insurance coverage for low-income children and adults, individuals with disabilities, and seniors. Children in Medicaid account for 40% of individuals in the program but only 17% of the spending of Medicaid dollars; individuals eligible based on disability account for 11% of individuals in the program but 34% of cost. Eligible adults 65 years and older make up 10% of Medicaid enrollments and 21% of cost, and expansion adults make up 22% of enrollments and 17% of cost. Medicaid is a significant source of payment for long-term care, covering many nursing home residents. The ACA of 2010 added millions of previously ineligible individuals younger than 65 years to state Medicaid plans, diminishing the number of uninsured. Before ACA Medicaid expansion, Medicaid eligibility was limited to specific low-income groups (elderly, people with disabilities, pregnant females, and children) based on 66% to 100% of the FPL (determined each year by the federal government). For states that have opted to expand their Medicaid programs, individuals, including adults at or below 138% of the FPL ($20,120 for individuals in 2030), are now eligible to enroll in their state Medicaid program. Previously, and still in states that have not expanded their Medicaid program, the threshold of their income is measured against the FPL to determine whether eligibility requirements are met, and adults (except those listed previously) are not eligible. A state that agrees to expand its Medicaid program accepts additional federal funding to support the increase in the number of individuals enrolled in the Medicaid program and the cost of running the program. As of December 1, 2023, 41 states and the District of Columbia have expanded their Medicaid program (KFF, 2023a). This one measure has decreased the number of uninsured Americans by adding millions of newly eligible persons to the public insurance plan. States that have not expanded their Medicaid plan have higher numbers of uninsured.

Each state receives from the federal government a formula percentage of revenue to run a Medicaid program, leaving state budgets responsible for the remaining cost. Federal tax dollars must fund a minimum of 50% of a state's Medicaid cost. In 2017, 15 states—Alaska, California, Colorado (50.02%), Connecticut, Illinois (51.3%), Maryland, Massachusetts, Minnesota, New Hampshire, New Jersey, New York, North Dakota, Virginia, Washington, and Wyoming—were funded at the minimal federal level of 50% (except where noted), whereas other states—for example, Alabama (70.16%), Mississippi (74.63%), South Carolina (71.3%), West Virginia (71.8%), Kentucky (70.46%), New Mexico (71.13%), District of Columbia (70.0%), and Idaho (71.51%)—received a much greater share of the cost of their Medicaid programs from the federal government (USDHHS, 2015a). In 2021, the federal share of the costs was increased by 6.2% during the COVID-19 pandemic. States still paying the highest **state** share of Medicaid include Wyoming (38.9%), New York (35.6%), New Hampshire (35.0%), Massachusetts (35.7%), and Connecticut (35.1%). States paying the lowest share of **state** Medicaid spending include Arizona (16.4%), Kentucky (16.6%), Mississippi (14.8%), New Mexico (14.3%), Oklahoma (15.7%), and West Virginia (15.4%). The US Census Bureau estimates geographic areas that have remained in persistent poverty (Fig. 3.5), which correlates with states receiving the greatest percent of funding for Medicaid federal monies. In March 2020, at the start of the pandemic, Congress enacted the Families First Coronavirus Response Act, which included a requirement that state Medicaid programs continually enroll all individuals and families in the Medicaid program, even if they no longer met eligibility requirements. The continuous enrollment provision was phased down in 2023 and ended in December 2023. The actual numbers of affected individuals are expected to be between 5% and 17% of Medicaid individuals. The greater the percentage of federal support, the less the state has to pay with state monies. For example, when a state receives 50% of federal funding, the remaining 50% must be generated by state taxes. As the cost of the program increases and/or the number of persons enrolled in Medicaid increases, the taxpayers of the state must support the program, often through the raising of state, county, and local

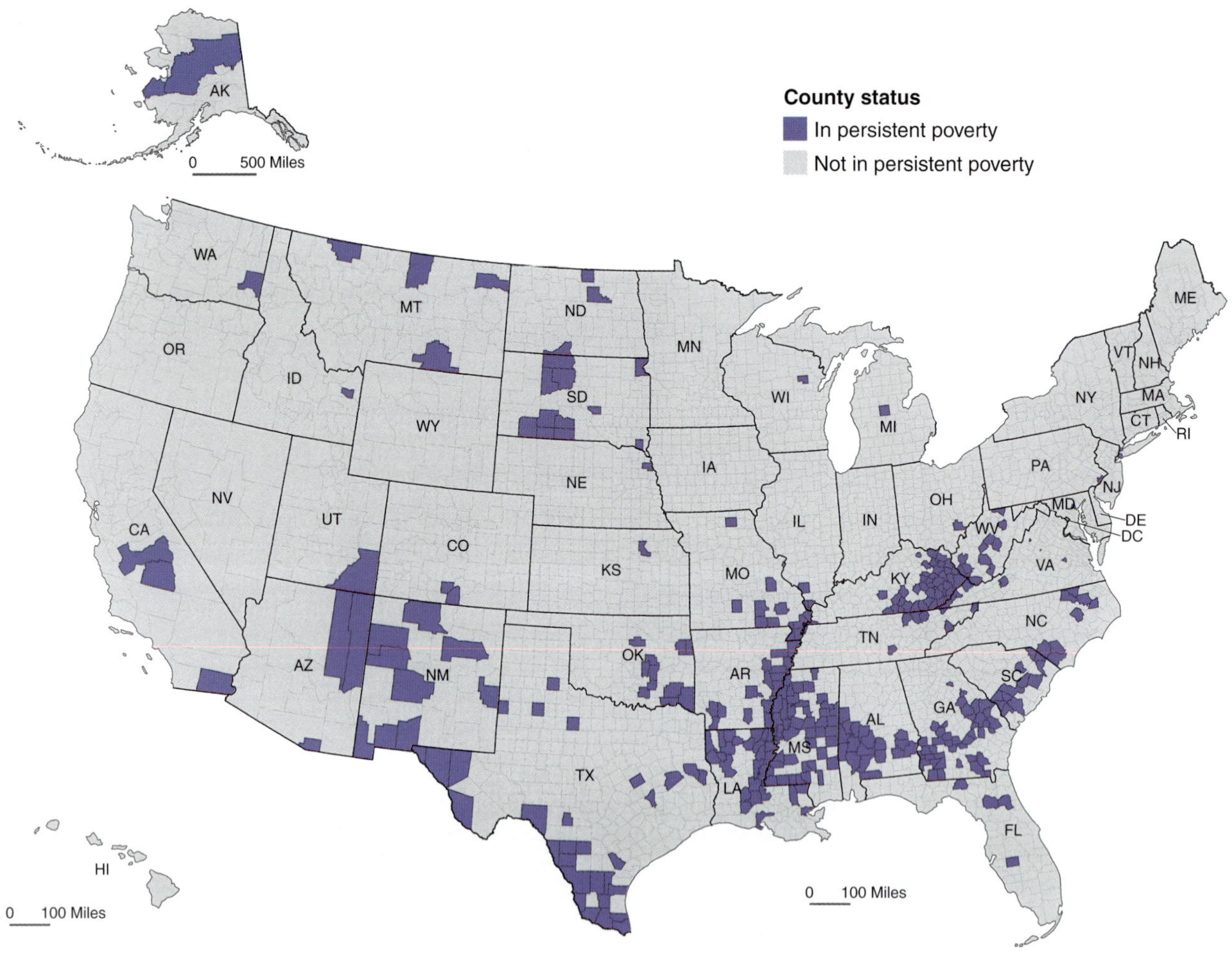

Note: In this report, a geography is considered to be in persistent poverty if it maintained a poverty rate of 20.0% or more in the 1990 and 2000 Censuses and 2005–2009 and 2015–2019 American Community Survey 5-year estimates. Other governmental agencies have alternative definitions of persistent poverty for programmatic purposes and examples of such are described in the report.

FIG. 3.5 US Census Bureau, Counties in Persistent Poverty: 1989 to 2015–2019 American Community Survey, 5-Year Estimates. (From US Census Bureau, 1990 and 2000 Censuses 2005–2009 and 2015–2019 American Community Survey, 5-Year Estimates.)

taxes. As an entitlement program, Medicaid must enroll all people who meet the state's Medicaid eligibility requirements. Many states have more lenient eligibility requirements than those set by the federal government and offer more health services than are mandated. Total spending per full-benefit enrollee varies significantly across the United States, with Nevada, for example, spending an average low of $4873 per person and North Dakota spending an average high of $10,573 in 2019. The variation in state spending occurs because there is flexibility for states in determining how the program is designed, administered, and paid for by providers, and because of large differences between eligibility groups. The ACA has addressed some of the disparities by mandating essential health benefits that all insurance plans must cover. The ACA has provisions to provide financial incentives for states that qualify to provide enhanced services to Medicaid recipients by increasing their federal matching funds. One way states have cut costs in Medicaid programs is by limiting provider payment rates and/or limiting services. These practices can jeopardize provider participation (providers willing to care for individuals enrolled in a Medicaid program) and limit access to care for Medicaid recipients. Decreasing eligibility requirements for individuals and families so they qualify for Medicaid coverage is part of the solution to reduce the number of uninsured by adding more lower-income individuals and families to the Medicaid program. States have also been required to enhance or develop efficient user-friendly systems to facilitate the enrollment process.

Mechanisms

Payment

Although some health care providers and other professionals in the private sector are paid on a fee-for-service basis, by third-party private insurance, or by public-supported insurance, most health workers, including nurses in institutional or community agencies and in the military, receive salaries or are paid by the hour regardless of the amount of care provided.

Because nurses are salaried or paid by the hour, the separation of nursing costs from all other health-related costs is difficult. The cost of acute hospital nursing care is typically incorporated in the daily room and board charge in the acute care setting. Without documentation of specific nursing costs, validating the need for skilled nursing services is difficult.

Independent nursing practice may be viewed as a logical outgrowth of seeking higher levels of professionalism. The nurse practice acts of some states encourage nurses to use their knowledge more comprehensively than many agencies sanction. Although legislation in 1997 included the reimbursement of APNs by Medicare, not all plans and provider groups include these nurses as primary care practitioners. Clearly, the nursing practice roles and prescriptive authority of APNs differ between states. Incremental steps have been taken to advance the APN role at both the federal level and the state level. Some states have passed laws for nurse practitioners to practice and prescribe medications without physician oversight. The IOM's 2010 report titled *The Future of Nursing: Leading Change, Advancing Health* and subsequent reports support nurses practicing to the full extent of their education and training.

Alternative forms of payment for APNs are salary and capitation. The salary system involves a set amount for services provided in a specified time frame. This system provides the employee with a fixed nursing income that is protected from changes in supply and demand, includes fringe benefits, and obviates fee-collection problems. The salary system's flexibility makes it easier to fill unpopular jobs or jobs in underserved areas. The disadvantages of this system include a limit on income and constraints on schedules, vacations, and peer review. A nurse in a salaried position may not be able to earn overtime, depending on the facility. Nurses who work beyond the scheduled hours are then uncompensated for additional time under a salary arrangement, which may lead to job dissatisfaction and burnout.

In the capitation system, such as in an HMO, each provider receives a flat annual fee for each participant regardless of how often services are used. Individuals who enroll in an HMO pay a fixed amount on a monthly basis whether or not they use the services; prepayment provides an incentive to provide efficient care. The objective is to keep people healthy to prevent costly services. Cost consciousness dictates that illness be treated as early as possible and in the most cost-effective setting. Capitation is simple to administer; no third-party insurance payments are present, and the HMO bears the risk of illness. Preventive primary care that avoids costly hospitalization keeps costs down, and the savings revert to the organization. On the negative side, individuals who make frequent or unnecessary visits to a provider in an HMO decrease the efficiency of the system.

Cost Containment

The government's interest in hospital treatment cost containment was exemplified by the passage of the Social Security Amendments of 1983 (Public Law 98–21), which mandates the establishment by the Health Care Financing Administration of a prospective payment system for Medicare and many health insurance companies. This system stipulates that providers be paid at preset rates based on approximately 500 diagnosis-related group categories (DRG Codes) used to classify the illness of each insured person. Rates for each diagnosis were established according to regional and national amounts based on each hospital's urban and rural cost experience. The number of hospitals in the United States in 2023 was reported to be 6129, with 919,649 staffed beds and total admissions at 34,011,386 (AHA, 2024).

Another piece of legislation that targeted cost containment was the Balanced Budget Act of 1997, which also affected Medicare. This act reduced Medicare spending by limiting provider payments, increased options in the choice of managed care plans, and made medical savings accounts an option.

The Medicare Modernization Act of 2003 promoted private managed care plans to reduce the burden on the economy of Medicare entitlements. These HMO plans, called Medicare Advantage plans, discussed previously, typically have clients who are healthier than the average Medicare client. Older adults who are enrolled in these plans pay a monthly premium and are required to choose providers within the network. If care is provided outside the network of providers, individuals must usually pay out-of-pocket costs similar to those of other HMOs discussed earlier. This can be confusing to the older person because there are many Medicare Advantage plans to choose from and the person may not realize how a Medicare Advantage plan is different from traditional Medicare coverage. Provisions have been made for enrollees to change Medicare Advantage plans or to be disenrolled during specific time frames. Providers have been lobbying for increased reimbursement because Medicare dictates reimbursement fees based on a predetermined formula (Medicare.gov, n.d.-a).

Care Management. Care management began through public programs with nurses in public health departments, social workers in public welfare systems, and caseworkers in mental health departments. In care management, an experienced health care professional, such as a nurse, social worker, or gerontologist, helps determine the nursing care that is necessary, monitors that care, and arranges for individuals to receive care in the most cost-effective and appropriate setting. Care managers are especially effective in meeting the needs of individuals recently discharged from the hospital, older adults, persons with medical conditions that are costly to treat (e.g., spinal cord injuries or high-volume diseases such as chronic illnesses), persons with complex health and social needs, and other cases requiring multiple levels of care. The care manager works collaboratively with various providers of care and families to effectively achieve a balance between cost and care. Emphasis must be on health management across the continuum of health care services. As Medicaid and Medicare managed care systems continue to develop, demand for nurses to fill the care management role will continue to grow. In addition to working within organizations, care managers can have their own independent practices. Managed care organizations rely on care management to reduce inappropriate use of services, improve quality of care, and control costs (Nies & McEwen, 2019). Basic care management services are described in Box 3.11: Care Management Services.

BOX 3.11 Care Management Services

- Assessment: Evaluating a person's physical, social, functional, psychological, financial, and spiritual needs, including the family, within a specific environment
- Care planning: Setting goals and identifying specific services to meet individual and family needs, including how to allocate resources and refer to other resources
- Geriatric care manager: Manager who develops an individualized care plan for older adults with medical, functional, and cognitive conditions to receive care and services to remain at home, avoiding costly hospitalizations and emergency department visits when possible
- Service coordination and referral: Facilitating and coordinating access to needed providers
- Care monitoring and periodic reassessments: Evaluating progress, access to and use of services, and changes in needs
- Systems advocacy: Developing or changing policies or laws at the local, state, or national level to promote or meet the needs of the population served

Managed Care Issues

Managed care options are more plentiful as states devise health care delivery systems to meet the ACA mandates. With a need to not only control costs but also to improve the functioning of the health care system to provide high-quality, evidence-based care, new systems with groups of providers delivering care in more efficient ways have evolved. The use of technology has become a valuable resource for informing consumers and employers about health care issues and allowing them to search for and compare information on various types of health care plans. Nurses can steer individuals toward appropriate websites for health-promotion and disease-oriented information and advise against misinformation and fraudulent claims. With the rapid expansion of scientific advances in health and medicine, it is not possible for the nurse to stay abreast of the growing body of research evidence without using the Internet for reliable, current, evidence-based practice. Nurses must caution consumers about the risks of relying on health advice from virtual assistant AI (such as Alexa or Siri), as not all information is accurate, complete, or up to date.

Health Insurance

Positive elements of the health care system in the United States include excellent clinicians, health care facilities, and equipment—all of which are readily available to people with health insurance and adequate finances. The US system exhibits a high degree of technologic change and innovation and excellent information, quality, and cost-accounting systems. Numerous studies have found that those who do not have health insurance or are underinsured are at risk of poorer health outcomes. The ACA has significantly decreased the number of those uninsured in states that have expanded their Medicaid programs and subsidized the cost of insurance premiums for those meeting income requirements. A high number of uninsured individuals are disproportionately low-income persons and measures as discussed previously increased the number of individuals in both private and public health plans. Public plans have in the past not addressed noncitizen foreign-born persons who have entered and are living in the United States as undocumented, though recently, some states have expanded state-funded coverage to certain groups regardless of immigration status (KFF, 2023d).

Private Health Insurance

In the private sector, the following five types of organizations provide health care insurance:

- Traditional insurance companies (including the earliest insurer, Blue Cross, and Blue Shield, a nonprofit charitable organization) and for-profit commercial insurance companies
- PPOs acting as "brokers" between insurers and health care providers
- HMOs, which are independent prepayment plans
- POS plans, which combine features of classic HMOs with personal choice characteristics of PPOs
- Self-insurance and self-funded plans, in which either the employer takes on the role of insurer or the enrollee sets up a trust account with tax savings

Individuals can purchase a health insurance plan from a state marketplace if they do not receive health care through an employer or have a federally funded policy such as Medicare or Medicaid. In 2023, over 18 million people purchased insurance through a marketplace, with various levels of subsidies provided based on income level. Each state has an option (or options) of marketplace plans.

Traditionally, private insurers charged employers or individuals annual premiums and provided services on a fee-for-service basis. Organized at the state and local levels, Blue Cross and Blue Shield generally complement each other, with Blue Cross reimbursing hospitals and Blue Shield covering physicians and other providers. After World War II, insurance companies began to provide health insurance plans in competition with Blue Cross and Blue Shield. Today, more than 900 commercial, profit-making insurance companies that offer medical coverage dominate their share of the market: Blue Cross Blue Shield operating as many independent companies, UnitedHealthcare Group, Anthem, Kaiser Permanente, Ambetter (Centene), Humana, Health Care Service Corporation, and CVS Health Core. Insurance companies are defined by the number of individuals who have enrolled in a health insurance plan with that provider (also referred to as "covered lives"). UnitedHealthcare (including all subsidiaries and divisions) is the largest health insurance company by revenue. The cost of a health care premium varies significantly by factors such as age of the person, state and county of residence, smoking or tobacco use (can pay up to a 50% higher premium), and number of people covered in a policy.

HMOs attempt to lower health care costs by emphasizing preventive rather than curative care, decreasing the progression and severity of some illnesses. Care is provided in outpatient settings when possible, and HMOs tend to use fewer services, with emphasis on the least costly means of providing a service.

POS plans enable enrollees to choose, at the POS, whether to use the plan's provider network or seek care from nonnetwork providers. Typically, network providers are paid on a capitated or discounted-fee basis, and nonnetwork providers are paid on a fee-for-service basis.

Another change in the structure of the insurance industry is the growth of self-insured or self-funded plans. Self-insurance means that an employer (or union) assumes the claims risk of its insured employees, whereas self-funding refers to paying insurance claims from an established fund, such as a bank account or trust fund.

Public Health Insurance and Assistance

Medicare. Medicare is a federal health insurance government program that pays for a variety of health care expenses for people older than 65 years, disabled individuals under 65 who are receiving Social Security disability benefits, people under 65 with end-stage renal disease requiring dialysis or a kidney transplant, or individuals living with amyotrophic lateral sclerosis (ALS, or Lou Gehrig disease). The Medicare program, also known as Title XVIII of the Social Security Amendments, began in 1966 after decades of debate and is currently operated under the administrative oversight of the CMS. Medicare is an entitlement program, meaning individuals who contributed to Medicare through taxes are "entitled" to the benefits regardless of the amount of income and assets they have. The intent of Medicare was to protect older adults against the catastrophic financial debts often incurred in managing chronic illness and to assist in the payment of health care. The total Medicare benefit payments in 2022 equaled $744.0 billion, accounting for 13% of the federal budget and 21% of the total national health spending. Medicare outlays are expected to increase to nearly $1.7 trillion in 2033. Medicare expenditures went to Medicare Advantage plans, hospital inpatient services, physician payments, other payments (such as hospice, durable medical equipment, and Part B drugs), outpatient prescription drugs, home health care, and 5% skilled nursing. Medicare spending per person increased from $5800 in 2000 to $15,700 in 2022, or by 4.6% on average. There are four parts in the Medicare plan: Medicare Part A (inpatient care in a hospital, skilled nursing after a 3-day or longer hospital admission, hospice services, and eligible home health services), Medicare Part B (physician services, outpatient medical services, durable medical equipment and preventive services), Medicare Part C (Medicare Advantage plans), and Medicare Part D (prescription drug plan) (KFF, 2023e).

Medicare Part A is financed largely through a mandatory tax of 2.9% of earnings paid by employees and their employers at 1.45% each (individuals who are self-employed pay the entire 2.9% tax on net earnings) into the Hospital Insurance Trust Fund, which accounts for 88% of Part A's revenue. Individuals who earn more than $200,000 ($250,000 or more as a couple) pay a higher payroll tax on earnings of 3.8% to fund part of the costs associated with subsidies mandated by the ACA. Part A covers inpatient care in hospitals, skilled nursing facilities (not custodial or long-term care), home health services, and hospice care. For those who are 65 years or older who have been residents of the United States for at least 5 years and have contributed to Medicare or whose spouse has contributed to Medicare for 10 years in Medicare-covered employment, there is no monthly premium for Part A, as they have paid medical taxes while employed. For those individuals who have not contributed for 10 years, premiums are prorated to the number of months (quarters of Medicare-covered employment) and in 2023 were up to $505 per month. Part A benefits are subject to a deductible ($1632 for each benefit period in 2024) and copayments, which differ depending on the number of days for each benefit period. For example, for days 1 to 60 there is zero coinsurance, for days 61 to 90 there is $408 coinsurance per day of each benefit period, and there are increased coinsurance rates for day 91 and beyond with defined limits (Medicare.gov, n.d.-b). Even if an individual does not pay a monthly premium for Part A, inpatient deductibles and coinsurance charges may be difficult for many older adults to manage as a result of fixed incomes. Medicare does not pay for private-duty nursing, TV or phone in room, or a private room unless medically necessary.

Part B is supplementary voluntary medical insurance financed through a combination of general tax revenues (72%) and 26% of premiums paid by beneficiaries. The Medicaid program pays the premium for low-income Medicaid beneficiaries. Individuals with an income of $97,000 or less (couples' income of $194,000 or less) pay $174.70 per month in 2024. People with incomes $103,000 or higher or $206,000 for couples pay a higher income–related monthly Part B premium ranging from $230.80 to $560.50 per month in 2023 based on modified adjusted gross income. Part B covers most physician visits, outpatient services, preventive services, durable medical equipment, and ambulance services. Once the deductible has been met ($240.00 in 2024), individuals typically pay 20% of the Medicare-approved amount for most physician services, in-hospital physician services, outpatient therapy, and durable medical equipment (Medicare.gov, n.d.-b).

Part C refers to the Medicare Advantage program as previously discussed. Medicare Advantage programs such as HMOs and PPOs cover all of Part A, Part B (may pay all or part of the premium), and typically Part D.

Part D is the voluntary, subsidized outpatient prescription drug benefit with additional subsidies available for low-income beneficiaries added in 2006. Part D is financed through general revenues (71%), beneficiary premiums (17%), and state payments for dually eligible people (12%). The Part D benefit is offered through private plans that contract with Medicare. There are Medicare Advantage prescription plans and stand-alone prescription plans. The Part D monthly premium differs by plan, and higher-income enrollees pay a larger share of the cost. Different plans cover different drugs and require older adults to choose a plan that best meets their needs from a plethora of choices. Older adults, especially with low education or literacy levels, or those who lack health literacy may have difficulty selecting the best plan for their individual needs (KFF, 2023f; Medicare.gov, n.d.-a).

Individuals enrolled in both Medicare and Medicaid programs (dual) are considered vulnerable populations (older adults and poor), and Medicare premiums are subsidized. Medicare benefit payments accounted for 21% of total federal spending in 2021. The financial status of Medicare can be measured by the level of assets in the trust fund compared with the level of benefit spending. If spending exceeds assets, the fund will become fully depleted. Each year the trustees predict the solvency of the trust fund (year in which funds which Part A benefits are paid) will be fully depleted. In 2023, the trustees predicted the solvency of the Medicare Hospital Insurance Fund will be depleted in 2031 and Medicare will not have sufficient funds to pay all Part A benefits. Part A trust fund solvency is affected by the economy (revenue from payroll tax contributions), health care spending trends, and number of beneficiaries. When the baby boom generation reaches Medicare eligibility age, (between 2010 and 2030), there is a declining ratio of workers per beneficiary making payroll tax contributions. Future challenges include increased costs of health care services, increased costs of technology, and increased volume and use of services attributable to population growth of older adults and increasing life expectancy. Neither Part A nor Part B of Medicare offers comprehensive coverage. Inherent in the program are deductibles; set amounts that the individual must pay for each type of service before Medicare begins to pay; and copayments, a percentage of charges paid by the individual.

Out-of-pocket expenses do not include premium payments for Part B or for supplemental private health insurance, which can add significantly to out-of-pocket expenses. A comprehensive booklet available online or through the CMS details information on enrollment, costs, and services that are covered and not covered. With some exceptions, services not covered include acupuncture, chiropractic services (unless medically necessary to correct subluxation), and custodial care (activities of daily living, such as help bathing, dressing, eating, and getting in and out of bed). Other services that are not covered include most dental care, such as cleanings, fillings, extractions, and dentures; routine eye care related to prescribing glasses and spectacles for nondiabetic individuals; routine foot care for nondiabetic individuals (cutting or removal of corns, calluses, cutting of nails); hearing aids and exams for fitting them; long-term care (if only custodial care is needed); and health care while traveling outside the United States. Items not covered, especially custodial care, contribute significantly to out-of-pocket expenses. The main population at risk, the older adult, may have limited financial resources to seek preventive health services not covered. Some low-income enrollees may qualify for Medicaid services if income requirements are met, and others may have additional benefits through private insurance (Medicare.gov, n.d.-b).

Medicaid

Medicaid is an essential health insurance program available to certain low-income individuals and families who fit into an eligibility group that is recognized by federal and state law and cover one in every five Americans. Enrolled in the Medicaid program are poor children, children with special needs, nonelderly adults with disabilities, and others as previously discussed. The Medicaid program drives state budgets in cost but is also the largest source of federal revenue to states.

Medicaid is an assistance program, managed jointly by the federal and state governments to provide partial or full payment of medical costs for individuals and families of any age who are too poor to pay for care. Medicaid legislation, Title XIX of the Social Security Amendments, came into effect in 1967. The federal government provides funds to states on a cost-sharing basis, with 50% to almost 80% from the federal government and the remainder from the state, according to the per capita income of each state, to guarantee medical services to eligible Medicaid recipients (see previous discussion on state funding of Medicaid). Some states have options to assist higher-income families with children with significant disabilities to help fill the gaps in private health insurance and limit out-of-pocket expenses.

Medicaid is an integral part of the health care system, providing health insurance coverage for 18.8% of the US population in 2022. (Medicare covered 14% in 2018.) The percentage of the population covered by Medicaid varies widely by geographic location, with a high portion of residents in persistent poverty geographic areas (see Fig. 3.5). Medicaid serves as a safety net for low-income and high-need Americans. Poverty guidelines are issued by the USDHHS and used to determine financial eligibility for the Medicaid program. The program also supports individuals and families with subsidies for insurance coverage in state-based health benefit exchanges. Individuals and families with income levels of 133% to 400% of FPLs are eligible to receive subsidies to assist in paying for health premiums. Before the ACA, states could not cover nondisabled adults without children in a Medicaid program (see previous discussion).

Additionally, Medicaid pays the Medicare premiums, deductibles, and coinsurance for certain low-income Medicare recipients. Medicaid plans are open-ended, meaning a state must admit into the program at any time all individuals who meet the criteria. A state is not allowed to cap the Medicaid budget for a fiscal year, thus making it difficult to determine exactly how much money needs to be appropriated. States administer Medicaid under federal requirements and guidelines. The ACA mandates minimal essential health benefits, and typically those that are offered in an employer's health plan are mandated, but states can provide enhanced benefits and offer a more comprehensive plan. Programs differ widely among states in terms of services covered (Medicaid.gov, n.d.-b).

The federal government, in the passage of the Deficit Reduction Act of 2005, made it harder for individuals to qualify for Medicaid nursing home benefits by increasing penalties on individuals who transferred assets for less than fair market value during the previous 5 years. Since long-term care is expensive, purchasing private long-term care insurance to cover nursing home care became an option in some states. Individuals who already have long-term care needs are not eligible, and the cost of the premium increases with an individual's age. For older individuals, the cost of the premium makes long-term care insurance unaffordable.

As part of the Balanced Budget Act of 1997, CHIP was enacted to provide health insurance coverage to children whose family income was below 200% of the FPL or whose family had an income 50% higher than the state's Medicaid eligibility threshold (Medicaid.gov, n.d.-a). Some states had expanded their CHIP eligibility to include family coverage (see the previous discussion).

Pharmaceutical Costs

The research and development of a drug before it comes onto the market takes many years, starting with the creation of numerous drug compounds. Select compounds then undergo preclinical research, which may take many years before Phase I human clinical trials begin. Phase 1 is when small groups (20–80) of healthy people or people with a disease or condition enroll in a trial lasting several months to focus on how the drug interacts with the human body, determine a safe dosage range (based on previous animal data), and assess safety. According to the FDA, approximately 70% of drugs move on to the next phase. Phase 2 follows to determine safety and side effects of the new drug, lasting from several months to 2 years and including up to several hundred volunteer participants with the disease or condition. Approximately 33% of drugs move from Phase 2 to Phase 3 trials. Phase 3 trials last 1 to 4 years, involve 300 to 3000 volunteer participants who have the disease or condition, and are designed to determine whether the drug offers a treatment benefit and if less-common side effects occur. A team at the FDA must approve the drug or device before the last Phase 4 testing can begin and may require additional studies or documentation. Only 25% to 30% of drugs that reach Phase 3 trials will continue to Phase 4. Phase 4 trials are conducted in varied populations across multiple centers and involve several thousand volunteer participants who have the disease or condition. Participants are monitored for long-term benefits and risks . If safety concerns are revealed, the drug is removed from the market. On average, the process of bringing a new drug to market costs millions of dollars and a decade or more of time, with only 12% of clinical trials successfully bringing a new drug to market. To encourage and support this process, a pharmaceutical manufacturer of a brand-name drug is granted exclusive rights to manufacture and market the drug for a period of years through a patent. Once the patent expires (usually within 10 years of the drug being on the market), other companies can manufacture generic versions of the brand-name drug, and the cost of production per unit is far less expensive because it does not include the up-front costs of years of research and development.

The spiraling cost of prescription drugs continues to add to the complexity of financing adequate health care. Newer drugs cost more to bring to market as discussed previously, and consumer demand sparked by drug advertisements, new indications for use, and increased consumer knowledge of available drugs has increased the demand for prescription medications. Increased drug cost is attributed to inflation, more days of therapy per user, a greater number of drugs per user, the cost of research and drug development, and advertising costs. As discussed earlier, Part D of Medicare is the prescription drug component of the Medicare plan.

Prescription drugs can be very expensive and drive up the cost of health care. For example, in 2021, total spending on the top 10 Medicare Part D drugs ranged from $2.6 billion for the diabetes drug Ozempic to $12.6 billion for the blood thinner Eliquis. The total gross spending in 2021 related to more than 3500 Part D prescription drug products was $215.7 billion (not including rebates paid by drug manufacturers). The top 10 selling Part D drugs cost $47.7 billion, 22% of total gross Part D spending. Some medications have a low number of users but a high price tag. For example, the oral tablet hepatitis C drug Harvoni's average cost per pill is $1175, or over $95,000 for a 12-week treatment course without insurance (or funding and before rebates) (KFF, 2023e, 2023f) (Box 3.12: Genetics and Pharmacogenetics). In 2021, Medicare covered 32% of national drug spending. The Inflation Reduction Act passed in 2022 included several provisions regarding prescription cost reductions for Medicare enrollees. Insulin cost-sharing per month was capped at $35.00, and pharmaceutical manufacturers were required to pay rebates to Medicare if prices rose higher than inflation, both effective in 2023. Effective in 2025, Medicare Part D out-of-pocket drug spending is capped at $2000 annually and requires the federal government to negotiate prices for certain high-spending drugs covered by Medicare Part D. The Medicare Drug Price Negotiation Program will negotiate 10 Part D drugs for 2023, another 15 Part D drugs in 2025, 15 from either Part B or Part D (or from both) in 2026, and 20 from either Part B or Part D (or both) in 2027 and later. Among other requirements, selected drugs must have been on the market for at least 7 years (small-molecule drugs that are chemically synthesized) or 11 years for biologics (drugs produced from living organisms). Total gross spending on the top 10 Medicare drugs ranged from $2.6 billion for Ozempic for type 2 diabetes (does not cover for off-use as a weight-loss drug) to $12.6 billion for Eliquis (a blood thinner). Also included in the top 10 are Imbruvica (cancer treatment, $3.2 billion), Humira Citrate-free pen (treatment for rheumatoid arthritis and other conditions, $2.9 billion), Jardiance, Januvia, Trulicity, Xarelto, and Revlimid (KFF, 2023d). As discussed, bringing a new drug to market requires millions of dollars and years of research before approval by the FDA, contributing to the high cost of drugs. Recent legislation will assist in curtailing rising drug costs for enrollees in the Medicare program, promoting the health of older adults.

BOX 3.12 GENOMICS

Genetics and Pharmacogenetics

The field of pharmacogenomics is rapidly expanding what is known about the influence of hereditary genetic attributes and how drugs respond in the body. A number of drugs have been found that affect certain ethnic groups and individuals in different ways. Individuals who metabolize a specific drug slowly (slow acetylators) will take longer to metabolize the drug into the active form and retain the active drug longer in the body. Slow or poor metabolizers may require a lower dose or a different choice of drug to avoid toxicity. Rapid metabolizers (fast acetylators) metabolize drugs quickly into the active form, which may then be metabolized more quickly into the inactive form, leading to therapeutic drug failure. Fast metabolizers may require no dosage adjustment or higher dosages for the dosage to be therapeutic. Other genetic variations in drug-metabolizing enzymes exist that significantly affect how a drug is metabolized. As the field of pharmacogenetics evolves, tools that determine genotyping of an individual may be used routinely to guide practitioners in the selection of therapeutic options. Optimal medication dosage and selection of drugs may personalize drug treatment regimens, preventing adverse effects and contributing to better patient outcomes. The financial and ethical aspects of the use of genotyping technology in medical decision-making will be issues to address in future health care legislation.

Source: Woo, T., & Wright, W. L. (2024). *Pharmacotherapeutics for advanced practice nurse prescribers* (6th ed.). Philadelphia: F. A. Davis.

The Uninsured: Who Are They?

The 2010 ACA reduced the number of uninsured significantly with the expansion of Medicaid, subsidies to pay premiums in health insurance exchanges, and a provision allowing children to remain on their parents' employer family insurance until the age of 26. Previously, when children reached the age of 19 and were not full-time college students, they were removed from employer family insurance plans. Even with all the new options afforded by the ACA, a number of individuals remain uninsured. The number of uninsured Americans younger than 65 years was estimated to be 30 million in 2019, up from 29 million in 2018, and 28 million in 2017. The rise in uninsured is due in part to cost, as increases in insurance premiums for lower-income individuals and families is a financial barrier. The elimination of the individual mandate penalty in 2019 that had required Americans to carry health insurance or pay a penalty added to the uninsured population. Almost half of the uninsured adults (45%) stated that the cost of health insurance coverage was too high and that they did not enroll in a health insurance plan even if it was available to them through work or a marketplace. Approximately 23% of the uninsured population are estimated to be eligible for subsidized coverage through a market plan but declined. Other factors include immigration status of an individual. Twenty-three percent of nonelderly lawfully present immigrants (including legal permanent residents, green card holders, refugees, and others authorized to live in the United States temporarily or permanently) are uninsured. Lawfully present immigrants must have "qualified status" for 5 years to be eligible for Medicaid and CHIP, though states can waive this requirement for children and pregnant femlaes. Legal immigrants within the 5-year wait can purchase coverage through the ACA marketplace and may receive subsidies with incomes in the 100% to 400% FPL. In 2017, 75% of uninsured legal immigrants were eligible under the ACA for coverage but did not enroll in a health insurance plan. Factors for this decision not to enroll included enrollment barriers such as fear, confusion about eligibility, difficulty navigating the enrollment process, and language and literacy issues. The nurse can be a key health team member in assisting this population in navigating the process. Another group, constituting 15% of the uninsured population, is eligible for Medicaid or CHIP but does not enroll. Undocumented immigrants (those who are noncitizens and are living in the United States illegally) do not qualify for Medicaid or any other public federal insurance plan. Individual states have added immigrants (both documented and undocumented) to state portions of Medicaid and other programs (Fig. 3.6: Uninsured Rates Among US Adults by Citizenship and Immigration Status, 2023). This population is extremely vulnerable because of language and cultural barriers and fear of being discovered as illegal noncitizens; therefore, they typically do not seek health care. Provisions in current law require emergency care to be provided as well as care to be provided to pregnant females regardless of alien status (KFF, 2023d). It is estimated that 7 million uninsured people are eligible for marketplace premium subsidies to assist with the cost of premiums. For about half of those who qualify, the cost of the lowest plan (a bronze plan) would have a zero-premium cost. Health care providers and nurses need to stay abreast of all of these changes to help individuals and families navigate the complexities of the financial aspects of insurance. Nurses and health care providers can assist individuals and families in both gaining

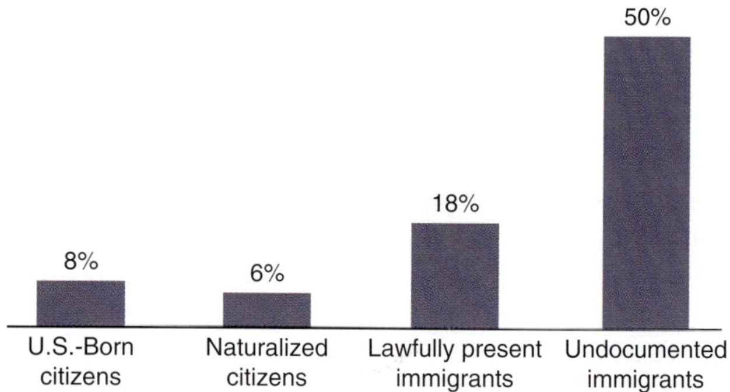

Note: Differences in uninsured rates between lawfully present immigrants, likely undocumented immigrants, and U.S.-born citizens are statistically significant at $p<0.05$.

Source: KFF/LA Times Survey of Immigrants (April 10-June 12, 2023) and KFF/LA Times Survey of Immigrants: U.S. Born Adult Comparison (June 29-July 9, 2023)

FIG. 3.6 Uninsured Rates Among US Adults by Citizenship and Immigration Status, 2023. (From KFF/LA Times Survey of Immigrants: US Born Adult Comparison [June 29–July 9, 2023].)

coverage and selecting a plan that best meets their needs. Other groups of individuals who may not have coverage are noncitizens who are legally traveling within the United States (whether for business, education, or tourism) unless they have purchased secondary travel insurance before entering the United States.

Unauthorized Immigrants

The Pew Research Center estimates that the number of unauthorized immigrants living in the United States was 10.5 million in 2017. Undocumented immigrants are not in the country lawfully and are not eligible for health insurance due to their immigration status. Unauthorized immigrants are individuals who entered the United States without valid documentation or authorization or individuals who entered the country lawfully and stayed after their visas expired. Almost 47% (4.9 million) of unauthorized immigrants are from Mexico, which represents a decline from previous years. Statistically significant increases in birth countries of undocumented immigrants between 2007 and 2017 include the Northern Triangle nations (El Salvador, Guatemala, and Honduras), India, and Venezuela. About 57% of unauthorized immigrants are located in six states: California, Texas, Florida, New York, Illinois, and New Jersey. In some states the unauthorized immigrant population declined, but in five states—Louisiana, Maryland, Massachusetts, North and South Dakota—the population grew between 2007 and 2017. Approximately 66% of unauthorized immigrants have lived in the United States for more than 10 years, with the median being 15.1 years. This means that half of unauthorized immigrants have been living in the United States for more than 15 years (Homeland Security, 2018; Pew Research Center, 2024). Immigration reform remains a contested topic, with concern about both entry into the country and how to deal with unauthorized immigrants already living in the country. The recent southern border crisis has fueled debates about border wall security and other measures to both protect US borders and care for the needs of people trying to enter (Homeland Security, 2018; Pew Research Center, 2024). According to federal law, anyone entering an emergency department must be treated regardless of the ability to pay or immigration status. However, those individuals who are in the United States illegally (undocumented immigrants) may be reluctant to seek health care for fear of legal action, being removed, or being returned. This vulnerable population is not eligible to enroll in any federally funded coverage, including Medicare, Medicaid, CHIP, or ACA Marketplace programs, but individual states can determine and provide health care in state-funded portions of programs for immigrants regardless of immigration status.

HEALTH CARE SYSTEMS OF OTHER COUNTRIES

The United States spends the highest proportion of its GDP on health care expenditures of all industrialized countries with a reported 17.3% health care share of GDP at $4.5 trillion, or $13,493 per person, as of 2022 (CMS, 2023). However, life expectancy rates are higher and infant mortality rates are lower in other industrialized countries (see previous discussion). Although each country has a different type of health plan, all share many of the same problems of the US free-market system, including rising health care costs; issues of access and affordability; workforce shortages of health care providers; increased concern over medical errors, quality of care, and safety; changing demographic population trends; escalating health care costs; and post-pandemic recovery. The Canadian health care program will be discussed as an example in comparison with the US system.

Canadian Health Care System

The Canadian health care program, called Medicare, is a group of socialized, publicly financed health insurance plans that provide health coverage to all Canadian citizens, regardless of medical history, personal income, or job status, for medically necessary hospital, physician, and dental care services when those services are performed in a hospital, without requiring the individual to pay out-of-pocket. The Canada Health Act, legislated at the federal level, determines what services must be provided, similar to the Medicaid program in the United States, but provinces and territories may provide additional services not listed in the Canada Health Act. The federal government provides health care funding to the 10 provinces and 3 territories through the Canada Health Transfer, leaving the individual province or territory responsible for the management, organization, and delivery of health services for its residents. Under the publicly funded Medicare program, services such as vision care, physical therapy, corrective lenses, home care, or prescription medicines are not covered, but separate provinces can elect to provide enhancements. The recently implemented Canadian Dental Care Plan offers publicly funded dental services to income eligible seniors, children, and the disabled, if they do not have access to private dental plans (Government of Canada, 2025). Sixty-five percent of Canadians have additional private insurance plans, mostly through employers, to supplement the Canadian health care plan for services not offered. Every Canadian citizen has the same basic primary public health insurance that is covered by the national health care plan offered through the providence of residents. For some population groups (children, seniors, social assistance recipients) the provinces and territories provide supplemental coverage. Each Canadian citizen applies for a provincial health card and, once it has been issued, the card provides access to a person's medical information and is used when the individual visits a physician or health care provider. Canadians pay for health care through a variety of federal and provincial taxes, just as US residents pay for Social Security and Medicare through payroll taxes. Because the government is the primary payer of medical bills, Canada's health care system is referred to as a single-payer arrangement. Some provinces gain additional funds through sales tax, lottery proceeds, and health premiums. Additional benefits differ among the provinces, but most provide prescription drugs to older adults and low-income clients. For Canadians with higher incomes and private supplemental insurance, private clinics are available that offer specialized services. One advantage of receiving care in a private clinic is reduced wait times and specialized services not covered by the public health plan. Canadians covered by private health insurance typically have 80% of the costs covered but pay the remainder out-of-pocket. For example, obtaining an MRI scan in a hospital may require a waiting period of months, whereas a private clinic could offer the scan much earlier (Canada.ca, 2023).

At one time, the Canadian system seemed to be an ideal model that the United States should adopt; however, increasing health care costs, timely access to health services, delays in treatment, and workforce shortages of health care providers have caused political controversy and debate in Canada. Queuing refers to a system where a person is placed on a wait list before receiving certain types of tests or surgery, allowing a person who needs more immediate care to receive priority. If care needs are determined not to be life threatening, individuals may need to wait for MRI scans, heart bypass surgery, cataract removal, or hip replacement procedures for weeks or months because those in urgent need of the procedures are higher on the list. A nonurgent elective surgery may have a 4-month wait, and a specialist referral may have a 2-month wait. Although all citizens receive the same level of public health care, private insurance allows a two-tiered system favoring Canadians with private health insurance or other financial resources to receive expedited care. If a person can pay out-of-pocket, they may elect to travel elsewhere (e.g., to the United States) to receive expedited care. A major shortage of physicians and nurses in Canada is due in part to lower reimbursement rates by the public health system as well as lower salaries, causing some health care providers to leave Canada and practice in other countries such as the United States. Over the years, the federal government has decreased contributions to the provinces and territories because of large federal budget deficits and limited fee increases to physicians for services. Regionalization of hospitals has caused access-to-care issues for those outside major cities. Health disparities for indigenous peoples, often in very rural areas, have sustained poorer health outcomes. Expansion to offer better access to home care and community-based services, inequitable access to health services in both public and private systems, and a narrow basket of services that are free at point of care are issues facing the Canadian health care system (Canada.ca, n.d.; Martin et al., 2018).

CASE STUDY

Health Teaching: Using the Internet to Increase Health Literacy

Ella, age 34, has been married to her husband Joe for 10 years and recently moved to a new area with their two children, Thomas (age 11) and Olivia (age 6). Joe just started a new sales position, and Ella works 3 to 4 days a week as a home health aide. Joe completed a 2-year college degree, and Ella took a few college courses but never finished her degree. The family is new to a primary care clinic, and Ella asks the nurse for advice in choosing a health plan that will best meet the needs of her family from several offered by Joe's employer. Ella and her husband are considering a third child in the future. Joe considers himself healthy and active, although he has had recommendations in the past to lose 30 pounds, is borderline hypertensive, and has slightly elevated blood lipid levels. He has a strong family history of coronary artery disease, and his father died from a myocardial infarction at the age of 65. Ella also struggles with a few extra pounds and often relies on fast food for quick dinners on the days she works. Both children are above the recommended BMI levels for their ages. Thomas was diagnosed with attention-deficit/hyperactivity disorder (ADHD), and Olivia has environmental allergies and asthma. Both children had a full year of remote classroom learning during the COVID-19 pandemic, and Ella developed proficiency with using the home computer and Internet to help the children with Google classroom and Zoom sessions. Ella frequently relies on social media, friends, and family members for health and parenting advice.

The nurse discusses the family's general health-promotion and protection needs and the special needs presented by the diseases that have been identified. She provides some resources for Ella to learn more about the health plans available to her and consumer-friendly health information websites. The nurse also provides websites with reliable up-to-date information for Ella to access on a variety of health topics. With the recent global pandemic of COVID-19, the nurse emphasizes the need for Ella to rely on accurate and up-to-date information sources to keep her family safe and healthy. The nurse provides Ella with information on how to access her local county health department for reliable information and alerts and emphasizes the need to seek medical information from reputable sources to dispel myths and misinformation that circulate on social media platforms.

Reflective Questions

1. What additional information does the nurse need to assess this family's needs?
2. What are the priority area teaching needs for this family?
3. What community resources might be available to Ella and her family?
4. What are some appropriate websites that Ella might find useful?

Before leaving, the nurse provides the following:

- Guidelines on choosing a health plan from the Agency for Healthcare Research and Quality (AHRQ), a federal government agency with health information for consumers: https://www.ahrq.gov/patients-consumers/patient-involvement/how-to-choose-a-health-plan.html
- Information on health plans and benefits, including several links, from the US Department of Labor: www.dol.gov/
- Information on multiple health care topics:
  Health-Care Information.org: www.health-care-information.org
  WebMD: http://webmd.com/
  MyHealthfinder: http://healthfinder.gov/
  Mayo Clinic: www.mayoclinic.com/
  Centers for Disease Control and Prevention: cdc.gov
  Johns Hopkins Medicine: hopkinsmedicine.org
  National Institutes of Health: nih.gov

SUMMARY

- The nursing workforce, composed of more than 3 million nurses, is the largest segment of the nation's health care workforce, and nurses will be key players in moving forward the objectives set forth by the 2010 ACA and *Healthy People 2030*.
- To move these agendas forward, nurses need to understand the complexity of the health care system—the structures (federal, state, and local) and financing mechanisms (public and private)—so interventions can be targeted to reduce health disparities, promote health equity, and elevate the level of health and wellness across communities and the larger population.
- The recent global COVID-19 pandemic of emphasizes the need for nurses to stay current in their delivery of health care to respond effectively to the rapidly changing needs of the population.
- Nurses require a working understanding of the complexity of the health care system to educate individuals and families about health care resources; to coordinate services; and to influence health care policy at the local, state, and national levels.

REFERENCES

Alexander, K. L. (2019). *Florence Nightingale*. National Women's History Museum. https://www.womenshistory.org/education-resources/biographies/florence-nightingale

American Red Cross. (n.d.). *About us*. https://www.redcross.org./about-us.html

American Rescue Plan Act of 2021. (2021). *H.R.1319-117*th Congress (2021-2022). Public Law No. 117-2. https://congress.gov/bill/117th-congress/

American Hospital Association (AHA). (2024). *Fast facts on U.S. hospitals, 2024*. http://www.aha.org/statistics/fast-facts-us-hospitals

American Medical Association (AMA). (2023). *Payment and delivery models*. https://www.ama-assn.org/practice-management/payment-delivery-models

American Nurses Association (ANA). (2023). *Public health nursing*. http://www.nursingworld.org

Arias, E., & Smith, B. (2003). Deaths: Preliminary data for 2001. *National Vital Statistics Reports*, *51*(5), 1–44.

Arias, E., Xu, J., & Kochanek, K. (2023). United States life tables 2021. *NVSS National Vital Statistics Reports*, *72*(12). https://www.cdc.gov/nchs/data/nvsr/nvsr72/nvsr72-12.pdf

Arias, E., Xu, J., Kochanek, K., & Tejada-Vera, B. (2023). *Provisional life estimates for 2022*. NVSS National Vital Statistics Rapid Release, Report 31. https://www.cdc.gov/nchs/data/vsrr/vsrr031.pdf

Barr, D. (2023). *Introduction to U.S. health policy: The organization, financing, and delivery of health care in America* (5th ed.). Baltimore, MD: Johns Hopkins University Press.

Bureau of Labor Statistics (BLS). (2023). *Occupational outlook handbook: Registered nurses*. http://www.bls.gov/ooh/healthcare/registered-nurses.htm

Canada.ca. (2023). *Health Canada's Departmental Plan/2023/24.* Health Canada. http://canada.ca/en/health-canada/services/health-care-systems.html

CDC Foundation. (2023). *Fighting global threats.* https://www.cdcfoundation.org/fighting-global-threats

Centers for Disease Control and Prevention (CDC). (2023). *CDC Museum COVID-19 timeline.* David J. Sencer CDC Museum: In association with the Smithsonian Institution. https://cdc.gov/museum/timeline/covid19.html

Centers for Medicare & Medicaid Services (CMS). (2023). *National health expenditure fact sheet: Historical NHE, Projected NHE, 2022-2031.* https://www.cms.gov

Central Intelligence Agency (CIA). (2024). *The world factbook.* Retrieved January 25, 2024, from https://www.cia.gov/the-world-factbook/

Chen, A., Oster, E., & Williams, H. (2014). *Why is infant mortality higher in the United States than in Europe? NBER working paper no. 20525.* http://www.nber.org

CMS.gov. (n.d.). *Accountable care organizations (ACOs): General information.* https://www.cms.gov/priorities/innovation/innovation-models/aco

Concierge Medicine Today. (2024). *Concierge medicine today's industry insights, 2024 Annual Report.* https://www.conciergemedicinetoday.net/insights

Congressional Budget Office. (2022). *Federal subsidies for health insurance coverage for people under age 65: 2022 to 2032.* https://www.cbo.gov/publication/57962

Crail, C. (2024). *Does your state require you to have health insurance?* https://www.forbes.com/advisor/health-insurance/do-you-have-to-have-health-insurance/

Cubanski, J., & Neuman, T. (2023). *What to know about Medicare spending and financing.* https://www.kff.org/medicare/issue-brief/what-to-know-about-medicare-spending-and-financing/

Ely, D., & Driscoll, A. (2023). *Infant mortality in the United States: Provisional data from the 2022 period linked birth/infant death file.* National Vital Statistics Rapid Release, Report 33. National Center for Health Statistics. Hyattsville, MD. https://doi.org/10.15620/cdc:133699

Federal Emergency Management Agency (FEMA). (2019). *Disaster recovery reform act (DRRA) annual report.* https://www.FEMA.gov/sites/default/files/2020-07/fema_DRRA-annual-report_2019.pdf

Freed, M., Damico, A., Biniek, J., & Neuman, T. (2023). *Medicare advantage 2024 spotlight: First look.* Kaiser Family Foundation (KFF). https://www.kff.org/medicare/issue-brief/medicare-advantage-2024-spotlight-first-look/

Freyman, J. G. (1980). *The American health care system: Its genesis and trajectory.* Huntington, NY: Krieger.

Government of Canada. (2025). *Canadian Dental Care Plan.* https://www.canada.ca/en/services/benefits/dental/dental-care-plan.html

HealthCare.gov. (n.d.-a). *Affordable Care Act.* https://www.healthcare.gov/glossary/affordable-care-act/

HealthCare.gov. (n.d.-b). *A quick guide to the health insurance marketplace.* https://www.healthcare.gov./quick-guide/one-page-guide-to-the-marketplace/

Homeland Security. (2018). *Population estimates: Illegal alien population residing in the United States: Jan 2015.* https://www.dhs.gov

Institute for Nursing Centers. (n.d.). *Home page.* http://www.nursingcenters.org/

Institute of Medicine (IOM). (2010). *The future of nursing: Leading change, advancing health.* https://www.ncbi.nlm.nih.gov/books/NBK209880/

John A. Hartford Foundation. (n.d.). *About us.* https://www.johnahartford.org/

Kaiser Family Foundation (KFF). (2013). *Summary of the Affordable Care Act.* http://www.kff.org/health-reform/fact-sheet/

Kaiser Family Foundation (KFF). (2023a). *Status of state Medicaid expansion decisions.* http://www.kff.org/medicaid/issue-brief/status-of-state-medicaid-expansion-decisions-interactive-map/

Kaiser Family Foundation (KFF). (2023b). *Disparities in health and health care: 5 key questions and answers.* https://www.kff.org

Kaiser Family Foundation (KFF). (2023c). *2023 employer health benefits survey: Summary of findings.* http://www.kff.org./report-section/ehbs-2023

Kaiser Family Foundation (KFF). (2023d). *Key facts on health coverage of immigrants.* http://www.kff.org/disparities-policy/fact-sheet

Kaiser Family Foundation (KFF). (2023e). *State health facts: Medicare.* http://www.kff.org/state-category/medicare

Kaiser Family Foundation (KFF). (2023f). *Medicare advantage in 2023: premiums, out-of-pocket limits, cost sharing, supplemental benefits, prior authorization, and star ratings.* https://www.kff.org

Kaiser Family Foundation (KFF). (2024). *FAQs: Health insurance marketplace and the ACA.* https://www.kff.org/faqs/faqs-health-insurance-marketplace-and-the-aca-/

Kane, C. (2023). *Recent changes in physician practice arrangements: Shifts away from private practice and toward larger practice size continues through 2022.* Economics and Health Policy Research, American Medical Association. https://www.ama-assn.org

Keehan, S., Fiore, J., Poisal, J., Cuckler, G., Sisko, A., Smith, S., Madison, A., & Rennie, K. (2023). National health expenditure projections, 2022-31: Growth to stabilize once the COVID-19 public health emergency ends. *Health Affairs, 42*(7). https://doi.org/10.1377/hlthaff.2023.00403

Knickman, R., & Elbel, B. (2019). *Jonas & Kovner's health care delivery in the United States* (12th ed.). New York: Springer Publishing Co.

Martin, D., Miller, A., Quesnel-Vallee, A., Caron, N., Vissandjee, B., & Marchildron, G. (2018). Canada's universal health-care system: Achieving its potential. *The Lancet, 391*(10131), 1718–1735. https://doi.org/10.1016/S0140-6736(18)30181-8

Mayo Clinic Staff. (2023). *Convalescent plasma therapy.* Mayo Clinic. https://mayoclinic.org

Medicaid.gov. (n.d.-a). *Children's health insurance program (CHIP).* https://medicaid.gov/chip/index.html

Medicaid.gov. (n.d.-b). *Medicaid.* https://www.medicaid.gov/medicaid/index.html

Medicare.gov. (n.d.-c). *Medicare advantage plans cover all Medicare services.* http://medicare.gov/what-medicare-covers/

Medicare.gov. (n.d.-d). *Your Medicare coverage.* http://www.medicare.gov

National Academies of Sciences, Engineering, and Medicine. (2021). *The future of nursing 2020-2030: Charting a path to achieve health equity.* Washington, DC: The National Academic Press. https://doi.org/10.17226/25982

National Center for Health Statistics (NCHS). (2023). *Health, United States, annual perspective, 2020-2021.* Hyattsville, MD: National Center for Health Statistics. https://dx.doi.org/10.15620/cdc:122044

Ndugga, N, Pillai, D., & Artiga, S. (2024). *Disparities in health and health care: 5 key questions and answers.* Kaiser Family Foundation. https://www.kff.org/racial-equity-and-health-policy/issue-brief/disparities-in-health-and-health-care-5-key-question-and-answers/

Nies, M., & McEwen, M. (2019). *Community/public health nursing: Promoting the health of populations* (7th ed.). St. Louis: Elsevier.

Office of Disease Prevention and Health Promotion (ODPHP). (2023). *Healthy People 2030*. http://healthypeople.gov

Office of the Legislative Council. (2010). Compilation of Patient Protection and Affordable Care Act as amended through May, 1, 2010. 111th Congress. PPACA Public Law 114–148.

Organisation for Economic Co-operation and Development (OECD). (2024). *OECD statistics. Health expenditures and financing*. https://stats.oecd.org/

Peterson Center on Healthcare & Kaiser Family Foundation Partnership. (2019). *Peterson-Kaiser health system tracker: What do we know about infant mortality in the U.S. and comparable countries?* http://www.healthsystemtracker.org./chart-collection/infant-mortality-u-s-compare-countries/

Pew Research Center. (2024). *Migrant encounters at the U.S.-Mexico border hit a record high at the end of 2023*. https://www.pewresearch.org/short-reads/2024/02/15/migrant-encounters-at-the-us-mexico-border-hit-a-record-high-at-the-end-of-2023/#:~:text=Migrant%20encounters%20at%20the%20U.S.,at%20the%20end%20of%202023&text=The%20U.S.%20Border%20Patrol%20had,2023%2C%20according%20to%20government%20statistics

Rothberg, E. (2020). *Lillian Wald*. National Women's History Museum. https:www.womenshistory.org/education-resources/biographies/lillian-wald

Shi, L., & Singh, D. (2019). *Essentials of the US health care system* (5th ed.). Burlington, MA: Jones & Bartlett Learning.

Society of Hospital Medicine. (n.d.). *History and mission*. http://www.hospitalmedicine.org/

US Department of Health and Human Services (USDHHS). (n.d.-a). *About HHS*. http://www.hhs.gov

US Department of Health and Human Services (USDHHS). (n.d.-b). *Health information privacy*. https://www.hhs.gov/hipaa/index.html

US Department of Health and Human Services (USDHHS). (2015a). *FY2017 federal medical assistance percentages*. Office of the Assistant Secretary for Planning and Evaluation. https://aspe.hhs.gov/reports/fy2017-federal-medical-assistance-percentages-0

US Department of Health and Human Services (USDHHS). (2015b). *Civil rights*. https://www.hhs.gov/

US Department of Health and Human Services (USDHHS). (2020). *Development of Healthy People 2030*. https://www.healthypeople.gov/2020

US Department of Health and Human Services (USDHHS). (2024). *HHS poverty guidelines for 2023*. Office of the Assistant Secretary for Planning and Evaluation. https://aspe.hhs.gov/topics/poverty-economic-mobility/poverty-guidelines

US Department of Homeland Security. (n.d.). *FEMA*. https://www.fema.gov/

US Public Health Services. (n.d.). *Leadership*. https://www.usphs.gov

Veterans Administration (VA). (2023). *Veteran's Health Administration*. https://www.va.gov

World Health Organization (WHO). (2023). *WHO roadmap on uses of COVID-19 vaccines in the context of Omicron and high population immunity*. https://www.who.int/publications/i/item/WHO-2019-nCoV-Vaccines-SAGE-Prioritization-2023.2

World Health Organization (WHO). (2020). *Pass the message: Five steps to kicking out coronavirus*. https://www.who.int/news-room/detail/23-03-2020-pass-the-message-five-steps-to-kicking-out-coronavirus

Wounded Warriors Project. (2023). *Wounded warriors project: About*. https://woundedwarriorsproject.org

4

The Therapeutic Relationship

June Andrews Horowitz and Valerie Seney

http://evolve.elsevier.com/Edelman/

OBJECTIVES

After completing this chapter, the reader will be able to:

- Evaluate values clarification as a prerequisite for effective health promotion.
- Examine the elements and process of communication.
- Analyze differences between functional and dysfunctional communication.
- Develop strategies to promote therapeutic relationships with diverse populations across clinical settings, contexts, and nursing roles.
- Synthesize knowledge of the therapeutic relationship as an essential component of health promotion.

KEY TERMS

15-minute interview
Communication process
Countertransference
Culturally competent care
Distorting
Empathy
Feedback
Health literacy
Helping or therapeutic relationship
Input
Interprofessional communication and teamwork
Loop
Metacommunication
Milieu
Motivational interviewing (MI)
Nonverbal communication
Output
Practical reflection
Process
Proxemics
Rapport
Reciprocity
Reflection
Relationship stages
Self-concept
Self-disclosure
Self-esteem
Telehealth/mhealth/ihealth
Therapeutic engagement
Therapeutic use of self
Transference
Values clarification
Verbal communication

THINK ABOUT IT

A 65-year-old male was seen regularly at the community health center for medication management for his hypertension and ongoing assessment of his psychiatric disorders. The nurse in the primary care clinic that he was seeing today was new to him. She had some information from his chart about his presenting medical conditions and homeless status. The client lived in his car in the parking lot of the local refuse center. He cooked on a burner or ate his meals at McDonald's. He showered at the local gym. The nurse who worked with him previously had tried to encourage him to apply to the local senior housing authorities to provide a more stable living situation. He continually refused to even consider these options. As the new nurse working with this individual, these are some questions you may ask yourself:

1. How can I provide care for this person if I know that his lifestyle habits are causing medical problems?
2. Given that our values are so different from a socioeconomic perspective, how can I set collaborative goals for treatment?
3. How can I develop a trusting therapeutic relationship with this client?
4. What are my feelings about interacting with this client?

The therapeutic relationship is the **milieu** (or context, setting) in which nursing care occurs. Nursing practice is shaped by the caregiver's ability to focus on the interests, concerns, and needs of the individual (Mersha et al., 2023; Peplau, 1991; Xue and Miller, 2021). Establishing a therapeutic relationship is critical to problem resolution. The nurse-person relationship comprises the key components of knowing each other; reciprocity, respect, and confidence (Riviere et al., 2019). Even in brief interactions, communicating a focus on and concern for the person is critical. A 56-year-old female who experienced an unexpected myocardial infarction recalls that the clinician who made the most effect on her sat quietly at her bedside for a few moments and made eye contact to discuss what was most important about her rehabilitation plan. What made this brief interaction memorable? It was the clinician's attention to the person who was experiencing the health crisis; it was the quiet pause from the acute care arena activity created by sitting, listening, and making eye contact; it was the clinician's focus on what was most important for the female's recovery and attention to the client as a person. Across delivery settings, the importance of the nurse-person relationship cannot be forgotten or minimized because of time constraints. As the example shared here illustrates, even episodic brief encounters can have profound effects. Moreover, in today's complex multicultural and global health care arena, nursing's concentration also extends beyond individuals to populations (De Leon et al., 2023), yet the same critical elements of the relationship remain.

Particularly in health promotion, the nurse-person relationship is the context for care. Health promotion requires sensitivity to each person's goals and values—the individual's and the nurse's. Helping a person adopt health-promoting behaviors requires more than giving information. Health promotion also requires effective communication, which is why communication is a focus area of *Healthy People 2030* (US Department of Health and Human Services, 2022) and thus a priority for nursing practice. Successful health promotion involves interpersonal skills, personal insight, accountability, mutual respect, and a supportive working milieu. Essential to this interactional process are values of clarification, communication, and the helping relationship. See Box 4.1: *Healthy People 2030* Objectives for the leading health indicators and priorities for action.

VALUES CLARIFICATION

Definition

Values are core beliefs that hold great importance in identifying the inherent worth of an object, behavior, or idea that guides action. An individual's value system is hierarchical in nature and can change over time according to the actions/decisions that they need to make (Gamage, Dehideniya, & Ekanayake, 2021). The development of values is influenced by a range of outside sources, most importantly culture. Values are intimately involved in decision-making, especially in health care. Therefore it is imperative that nurses understand their own values as they plan and deliver client-centered care. Values can also be looked at as cognitive, or those a person ascribes to verbally and intellectually. Active values, in contrast, are those a person physically acts out. Judging the power of a given value by its ability to influence action is important. For example, a nurse may claim to value the worth of all people equally but may treat individuals of various races differently and provide the most time and concern for those who are racially similar. This cognitive value has little power to shape the nurse's behavior. If the nurse treated people of all races with equal respect, the value would also be active and have great power to motivate behavior.

To engage in health promotion, the nurse must appreciate that values are culture bound and explore how culture, traditions, and practices in a multiethnic and multicultural society influence health-related values. Without this understanding, the nurse is likely to relate to individuals with a limited awareness of their assumptions and inadequate sensitivity to the uniqueness and perspective of the person, family, or community.

Values evolve; they are not static. Life events and social processes can spark a reappraisal of personal values. **Values clarification** is a method for discovering one's values and the importance of these values (Raths et al., 1978). Values clarification does not tell a person how to act, but it helps people recognize what values they hold and evaluate how those values influence their actions.

Box 4.2: The Valuing Process outlines seven steps in the valuing process. The first three steps involve a cognitive process, the next two steps involve the affective or emotional domain, and the final steps involve behavior (Raths et al., 1978; Townsend & Morgan, 2020). The nurse uses values clarification to examine personal values and their potential influence on nursing care and to help people identify their values and reflect on their connection to health-related behaviors. Box 4.3 lists suggestions for putting values clarification into action. For a values clarification exercise, try following the steps outlined in Box 4.3 in regard to a personal value. Moreover, values clarification requires exploration of both overt and covert factors that affect our perceptions and actions. The process entails shining a light on our past and current life experiences to examine the values that shape our attitudes and behavior.

Values clarification becomes a clinical aim when an individual's values lead to behaviors that conflict with the nurse's value of promoting health. For example, a nurse tells a childbirth education class consisting of pregnant females and their coaches

BOX 4.1 *HEALTHY PEOPLE 2030* OBJECTIVES

The therapeutic relationship, its development and practice, cuts across each of the proposed objectives for *Healthy People 2030* (US Department of Health and Human Services, 2022). It is especially important to provide this trusting relationship when assessing, diagnosing, and referring for care those individuals who may have mental disorders.

Access to Health Services

Increase the capacity of the primary care and behavioral health workforce to deliver high-quality, timely, and accessible patient-centered care

Increase the use of telehealth to improve access to health services

Mental Health and Mental Disorders

Increase the proportion of primary care physician office visits where adolescents and adults are screened for depression

BOX 4.2 The Valuing Process

Choosing

- Choosing freely
- Choosing from alternatives
- Choosing after careful consideration of potential outcomes of each alternative

Prizing

- Cherishing and being happy with personal beliefs and actions
- Affirming the choice in public, when appropriate

Acting

- Acting out the choice
- Repeatedly acting in some type of pattern

BOX 4.3 Techniques for Assisting Individuals to Clarify Values

Identify the Individual's Values

"What is important to you?"

"Which of the following statements sounds most like the way you think?"

"What do you value most in life?"

Use Reflection to Restate the Value and Make It Explicit

"In what you've just told me, I hear that it is very important to you that..."

"I understand that you value..."

Identify Value Conflicts or Conflicts Between Values and Actions

"What connection does this value have to your current health or illness and to the healthy behaviors, interventions, or treatments needed to maintain or restore your health?"

"How does this particular value affect your behavior and health?"

"What are some ways that you might put your values into action?"

"Are your actions consistent with your values? If not, then what might you change?"

that alcohol use poses serious risks to the fetus. After the class, one female comments, "Do you really think that having a drink once in a while is bad for the baby? I'm sick of being told that I can't do things because of the baby." In this example, an apparent conflict in values between the nurse and the individual exists. Intervention is needed to examine how this female's wish for freedom from restrictions clashes with her desire to have a healthy child. Nurses must consider their own values related to health promotion for the individual and the fetus and must weigh the importance of respecting individuals' rights to make decisions about their own health behaviors with potential risks to the fetus. Such value conflicts result in ethical dilemmas. Resolution rests on the nurse's ability to examine conflicting values and available evidence about possible outcomes when fashioning health-promotion interventions. Sharing evidence to support the clinical recommendation also helps reduce a judgmental message in the communication and opens communication for discussion about the strength of the evidence and its practical implications for health behaviors (Witteman et al., 2021).

Values and Therapeutic Use of Self

Therapeutic use of self is the application of one's cognitions, perceptions, and behaviors to create interpersonal encounters that promote health in another person, family, group, or community. Without self-awareness and clarification of values, therapeutic use of self is impaired. **Self-concept** and **self-esteem** are interrelated components of individuals' judgments and attitudes about themselves. Self-concept is a mental picture of the self—a composite view of personal characteristics, abilities, limitations, and aspirations. Self-esteem, the affective component of self-perception, refers to how individuals feel about the way that they see themselves. Internalized appraisals from others also influence self-concept and self-esteem.

Self-concept evolves throughout life. From birth, family experiences and parental identification mold the child's sense of identity. Self-esteem is learned from experience. To cultivate children's self-esteem and enable them to have a realistic perception of their strengths and weaknesses, parents should focus on positives, give feedback on abilities and limitations, and provide the child with a sense of belonging and realistic confidence. Positive, rewarding, anxiety-free interactions contribute to security, esteem, and positive self-view. Positive but realistic appraisals from significant others, especially the parents, help the young child to develop this healthy self-view. Parental resources and other systems of support are factors in one's self-esteem; social determinants of health associated with advantages and resources have demonstrated positive effects on children's development (Likhar et al., 2022; Sullivan, 1953).

The self does not develop solely in response to the reflected appraisals of others. Genetic endowment and epigenetics, experiential opportunities, and the individual's actions shape self-concept. People can accept or reject the appraisals of others and modify their behavior. The ability to control actions and evaluate outcomes of interactions allows individuals to modify and alter their views of self. As such, the self is dynamic, changing through interaction with the outside world and in response to the various maturational and situational crises of life.

The ability to examine, reflect on, and evaluate the self is a uniquely human talent. Self-awareness involves interactions between the self and the external world and the symbolic connections created by the individual. The self includes an unconscious component that is only partially accessible and influences behavior. Self-awareness is influenced by the degree to which an individual has an accurate concept of all dimensions of the self.

The goal of high self-awareness is reached through three steps. The first step is listening to oneself and paying attention to emotions, thoughts, memories, reactions, and impulses. Frequently, people ignore their feelings and thoughts because they are anxious or because they are in a hurry to accomplish some other task. Without self-reflection, people act automatically and lose some of the meaning of living. To improve the ability of self-reflection, ask questions such as the following:

- What am I feeling now?
- What emotions have I experienced today and in the past day or so? What were my thoughts?
- What events led to these thoughts and feelings?
- What actions did I take? Did my behavior fit with my thoughts and feelings, or was there a lack of harmony?
- Was I aware of my reactions at the time that they occurred?
- How have I responded in clinical situations lately?
- How did I react in response to a particularly happy, sad, or difficult situation? In what way might I alter my actions now? What feelings and reactions did I experience while interacting with this individual?

The second step is listening to and learning from others. Feedback from others that conflicts with self-image can produce anxiety. In response, the feedback is ignored or translated incorrectly to preserve self-image and reduce anxiety. However, this pattern of responding limits knowledge of the self and inhibits the ability to examine the appraisals of others, resulting in limited personal growth. Asking reflective questions enables the nurse to use feedback effectively. Helpful questions include "What feedback have I received today?" and "What is the other person trying to tell me now?" A person also can ask others directly for feedback. For example, a student nurse might ask another student how they come across. The feedback might be used to alter aspects of behavior that are ineffective or problematic before the student nurse asks a faculty member for evaluative feedback. Using clinical supervision and consultation with colleagues provides needed opportunity for reflection on practice. How the nurse comes across to the individual, family, or community is crucial to successful health promotion, making self-awareness and sensitivity to feedback essential.

The third step is **self-disclosure**; sharing aspects of the self enriches interpersonal life. Through self-reflection/self-disclosure, people come to know themselves better because they have exposed their thoughts, actions, and feelings for examination with others. Self-disclosure is an indicator of a healthy personality and a strategy for developing one (Spence et al., 2020; Townsend & Morgan, 2020). Self-disclosure by one person tends to trigger self-disclosure by another in a reciprocal pattern of interaction. Therapeutic interactions characterized by reciprocity involve a mutual exchange—a pattern of communication between the nurse and an individual, not a one-way intervention from the nurse to the individual. Traditionally, clinicians have been wary of self-disclosure because it may cross a boundary from a professional to a personal relationship. Additionally, the nurse's self-disclosure might burden the individual and shift the focus of attention from the individual to the nurse. Although these guidelines are considered so as to prevent excessive or inappropriate self-disclosure, appreciation that self-disclosure occurs within all human interactions is needed. In a study with 244 participants, Kadji and Mast (2021) found that self-disclosure made a positive effect on the therapeutic relationship or client engagement. Although the concept is still somewhat controversial, the participants in the research offered that self-disclosure increased the immediacy of the relationship with the client. This evidence supports that nurses are not blank screens, robots, or technicians when delivering care; individuals value nurses who engage in interactions as real people and who are willing to share information about themselves appropriately and thoughtfully. Seeking consultation from a colleague is helpful whenever a concern arises regarding the limits of appropriate self-disclosure.

Practical reflection (i.e., self-reflection) involves deliberating on one's own thoughts and recollections of events to understand them and to take needed corrective action. In reflection, thoughts are interpreted or analyzed. The process tends to be triggered by a seminal or meaningful event or situation, and the process results in increased understanding or awareness. These insights can then be used in the future to implement a planned approach when one is faced with a similar event or situation. Research outcomes show that self-reflection is associated with lowered practice stress and increased competence among nursing students (Alsalamah et al., 2022). The process of practical reflection dovetails with steps toward self-awareness previously described and offers complementary helpful tips. First, the nurse recalls an incident when something went wrong. Then the nurse experiences the incident again by remembering images and by privately retelling events, statements, outcomes, and associated emotions. Next, the nurse interprets the story of communication that failed by examining expectations, ideals, goals, influences, personal actions, and others' actions that occurred during the event. The last step involves honest inspection of the nurse's own role in the story. Insights gained may be applied to prevent repetition of the problem and to plan future action (Box 4.4: Components of the Self).

BOX 4.4 Components of the Self

- The public self, which is shown to others
- The semipublic self, which is seen by others but may be outside the individual's awareness
- The private self, which is known to the individual but is not revealed to others
- The inner self, which is the unconscious portion not known even to the individual because it has anxiety-provoking content

Why is it important for a nurse to clarify personal values and increase self-awareness? The nurse's values and self-understanding influence behavior. The self is the nurse's greatest tool; to use the self effectively, the nurse must be fully aware of how it functions. Thus reflection and self-awareness guide the nurse's practice framework. In addition, sensitivity to individuals' perspectives is required to build a collaborative partnership, the cornerstone of the nurse-person relationship. Helping individuals explicate their values and direct their actions accordingly toward health-related goals embodies client-centered care as defined by *Quality and Safety Education for Nurses*: "Recognize the patient or designee as the source of control and full partner in providing compassionate and coordinated care based on respect for client's preferences, values, and needs" (QSEN, 2023). In today's multicultural society, sensitivity to one's values as a health care provider and those of persons for whom we care becomes crucial to delivery of person-centered effective care (Osmancevic et al., 2023).

THE COMMUNICATION PROCESS

The **communication process** is the forum for all thought and relationships shared among people. In conjunction with the use of scientific and technologic advances, communication is an essential tool for the nurse to engage in health-promotion interventions. Communication is the foundation for any professional relationship. Nurse-client communication plays a vital role in the formation and development of the nurse-client relationship. It is the glue that connects individuals' learning and satisfaction with care (Amoah et al., 2019; Kirca & Bademli, 2019). Communication is an information exchange between individuals through shared symbols and signs and commonly understood behavior (Amoah et al., 2019). This exchange involves all the modes of behavior that an individual uses, consciously or unconsciously, to affect another person. Communication includes the spoken and written word and nonverbal communication (gestures, facial expressions, movement, body messages or signals, and artistic symbols). Furthermore, communication errors between clinical providers and individuals or their proxies as well as ineffective communication between practitioners

BOX 4.5 Use Strategies for Communicating Clearly/Enhance Health Literacy Capacity

- Greet clients warmly: Receive everyone with a welcoming smile, and maintain a friendly attitude throughout the visit.
- Make eye contact: Make appropriate eye contact throughout the interaction. Refer to Tool 10: Consider Culture, Customs, and Beliefs for further guidance on eye contact and culture.
- Listen carefully: Try not to interrupt clients when they are talking. Pay attention, and be responsive to the issues they raise and the questions they ask.
- Use plain, nonmedical language: Don't use medical words. Use common words that you would use to explain medical information to your friends or family, such as *stomach* or *belly* instead of *abdomen*.
- Use the client's words: Take note of what words the client uses to describe their illness, and use those words in your conversation.
- Slow down: Speak clearly and at a moderate pace.
- Limit and repeat content: Prioritize what needs to be discussed; limit information to three to five key points and repeat them.
- Be specific and concrete: Don't use vague and subjective terms that can be interpreted in different ways.
- Show graphics: Draw pictures, use illustrations, or demonstrate what you mean with three-dimensional models. All pictures and models should be simple, designed to demonstrate only the important concepts, without detailed anatomy.
- Demonstrate how it's done: Whether doing exercises or taking medicine, a demonstration of how to do something may be clearer than a verbal explanation.
- Invite client participation: Encourage clients to ask questions and be involved in the conversation during visits as well as to be proactive in their health care.
- Encourage questions: Refer to Tool 14: Encourage Questions for guidance on how to encourage your clients to ask questions.
- Apply teach-back: Confirm clients understand what they need to know and do by asking them to teach-back important information, such as directions. Refer to Tool 5: Use the Teach-Back Method for more guidance on how to use the teach-back method.

From The Agency for Healthcare Research and Quality (2020). *Health Literacy Universal Precautions Toolkit.*

have been identified as major sources of personal and health care delivery safety problems (Box 4.5: Use Strategies for Communicating Clearly/Enhance Health Literacy Capacity).

Communication is becoming increasingly electronic. **Telehealth**, mobile health (**mhealth**), or Internet health (**ihealth**)—the use of telecommunications and data technologies to deliver health care services, including assessment/diagnostic services, treatment, consultation, and health information across platforms—is rapidly growing as a communication/intervention system. Such electronic communication can encompass the spoken and written word, as well as nonverbal forms of communication. The use of technology to engage individuals in clinical communications is already in place, with potential for future development, and brings its own challenges (Bright and Doody, 2023). Issues of health literacy, as discussed later in this chapter, including access, technology competence, and sensory capacity (such as eyesight and hearing), influence the effectiveness of telehealth as a communication medium.

Thus clear communication is a major component of promoting an individual's, a family's, and a community's safety and quality care. Yet the format and interface differ from the modes of human communication available until the latter part of the 20th century and the 21st century, and changes will be exponential in the years to come. (For additional discussion, see Box 4.6: Best Practice.) Despite concerns about losing the "human touch" with use of technology, an advantage of technology is expanded access to care. Garnering evidence of outcomes from technology-based care is essential. Technology use and access are increasing, so we are challenged to be creative in technology use and measurement of its outcomes. Many uses of technology exist. Stern has raised interesting questions about outcomes of video-recorded versus live-streamed interaction. Evidence has suggested that interaction via live streaming activates areas of the brain involved with social recognition but that watching a recorded video does not (Denworth, 2019; Stern, 2019). Practice and clinical research implications mandate evaluation of treatment delivery on access and health outcomes, yet evidence is mounting that telehealth has many benefits, even with asynchronous delivery (Bright & Doody, 2023).

Social determinants of health can play a crucial role in access to and the effectiveness of Internet-based health information and intervention delivery. Evaluation of Internet-based health education and intervention systems, including access, is a critical goal for translation of research to practice. Moreover, Internet access via smartphones has increased rapidly across populations. Technology will not go away and likely will become even more ubiquitous. In an integrative review of the literature, current practice, and telehealth (TMH) websites, Bright and Doody (2023) discovered that TMH services offer an accessible and acceptable pathway for care delivery. Bulkes et al. (2022) compared in-person treatment delivery and telehealth treatment delivery and found that telehealth services demonstrated equal efficacy compared with face-to-face treatment encounters. Additionally, TMH services were preferred over face-to-face services among some groups.

In nursing, communication is the cornerstone of a positive nurse-person relationship. Communication refers to a set of strategies and actions that enhance reciprocity, mutual understanding, and decision-making. Focusing the clinical discussion on the individual's story rather than on a version reformulated by the provider is essential to person-centered communication. Box 4.7 highlights strategies associated with person-centered communication based on evidence from the research literature.

Considerable evidence supports the effectiveness of these strategies. Research results have shown that nurses communicate effectively when they use a person-centered approach or nurse-person relational approach consisting of their being attentive, caring, accepting, empathetic, friendly, comfortable, calm, interested, sincere, and respectful (Barker et al., 2023). Although these strategies sound simple and basic, such appraisals are noticeably absent in many instances, and their presence is essential to quality nursing care (Box 4.8: Evidence-Based Practice). Furthermore, research findings have indicated that nurses seek communication with individuals that supports openness and engagement of both the nurse and the individual to form a therapeutic alliance.

BOX 4.6 BEST PRACTICE

Telehealth/mhealth/ihealth: Therapeutic Relationships in the Age of the Internet

Technologic advances have produced rapid changes in communication. Automatic teller machines have long replaced human tellers at banks for routine transactions. Voicemail rather than a receptionist routinely answers calls, confirms appointments, and records messages electronically. An electronic response to many calls directs the caller to a series of options that may not even include speaking to a person. Email, instant messaging, and texting are ubiquitous. Information in many areas is now available via access to a computer and an Internet connection. Wireless Internet (Wi-Fi) access is increasingly used as a perk to lure customers to the local coffee spot and to ease passengers' irritation during long flight delays. Nurses use electronic records and communicate updated information via laptops and handheld devices.

In the past decade, we have witnessed exponential increases in computer and broadband penetration. Although technology disparities persist, smartphone technology ownership and access have significantly increased in the United States across all income categories (Anderson & Kumer, 2019; Statistica, 2019). Such technology access can improve work and expand capabilities. Who would prefer to use a traditional typewriter to prepare papers and documents after mastering a word-processing program? Yet many issues deserve examination as we move into the age of telehealth.

Telehealth, mhealth, or ihealth—the use of electronic information and telecommunications technologies along with data technologies to deliver health care services (including diagnostic services, treatment, consultation, and health information/education) and to support and promote long-distance clinical health care—is now omnipresent. Rather than replacing traditional care, telehealth is best understood as a complementary approach to long-distance care delivery, and faster and easily delivered contact. Telehealth typically contains costs and expands access to care, particularly for individuals who are receiving home care and those in remote areas or without good access to clinical care centers. Moreover, the concept of telehealth also encompasses remote teaching, conferencing, and consulting. The convenience of finger-tip access to services and information is highly appealing to many consumers (Bright and Doody, 2022; Tyson et al., 2019). Use of telehealth via apps for health promotion and monitoring can augment regular health assessment and health-promotion care. Additionally, the enhanced convenience and easy access to telehealth can help many overcome barriers to obtaining face-to-face care. Nurses are challenged to obtain needed skills in informatics and care delivery via technology.

Technologic advances have produced benefits; however, barriers include the need for financial investment to establish networks, inadequate and antiquated reimbursement mechanisms, potential risks to confidentiality with electronic transmission, and licensure issues when care is transmitted across state lines. However, such issues are being addressed to remove barriers (Bright and Doody, 2022). Challenges include conducting systematic evaluations of outcomes and cost effectiveness and ensuring that individuals' economic status and health literacy do not constrain access. Additionally, finding the right balance of face-to-face, synchronous, and asynchronous delivery requires generation of effectiveness and translational evidence, and skill in delivery (Bulkes et al., 2022).

Perhaps the most important threat is that care can become impersonal when face-to-face contact is replaced by contact via an electronic interface. Learning how to establish a therapeutic relationship in the age of technology is a mandate for today's nursing student population and workforce. Thus preserving core nursing values as electronic care systems are created, tested, and implemented is a crucial goal. Innovative practices to safeguard core professional values in the emerging age of telehealth include the following:

- Avoiding a "one-size-fits-all" approach through individualized or tailored algorithms and design features specific to the system's use. Moreover, clinician behaviors that facilitate a client-centered style of communication include using open-ended questions; building partnerships; sharing decision-making and information; providing counseling; and using statements of concern, agreement, and approval. This style more successfully addresses individual needs and is associated with greater client satisfaction, better psychosocial adjustment, and improved health outcomes. Adding opportunities for online questions and answers or an open electronic or telephone chat with a clinician can facilitate tailoring in this delivery approach. Text and/or email prompts can also facilitate adherence to care. Also, providing user-friendly access, providing education/instruction, and tracking/monitoring use and problems are necessary ingredients for high user satisfaction (Renzulli, 2019).
- Developing and maintaining therapeutic relationships by inviting exchanges between the nurse and the person—for example, by creating a series of layered screens that first introduce the nurse (visually and with a biography) and later invite exchanges, feedback, and sharing of experiences and stories from individuals.
- Fostering individual autonomy by building components that encourage decision-making, problem-solving, and knowledge development and that are also timely and specific to the health problem and stage of treatment or management.
- The creation of flexible technology applications that work across a variety of platforms (e.g., computer, smartphone, tablet).

Consider the following questions about telehealth:

- What effects do technologic changes have on the therapeutic relationship?
- Will face-to-face interaction become a rare occurrence? In the future, might therapeutic interactions occur primarily via technology, such as voicemail, the Internet, and video-recorded transmission? What advantages and disadvantages will appear with the increasing use of technology in nursing practice?
- What creative approaches may evolve using technology in therapeutic relationships?
- How can electronic communication systems be used in disaster preparedness to alert people at risk and direct actions to increase safety when a human-caused or natural disaster is suspected, imminent, or in progress?

Function and Process

The following are core functions of communication:

- To obtain and send messages and to retain information
- To use the information to arrive at new conclusions, to reconstruct the past, and to look forward to future events
- To begin and to modify physiologic processes
- To influence others and outside events (Xue and Miller, 2021)

Communication transmits information, both interpersonally and intrapersonally, and it provides the basis for action.

The process of communication consists of four components (Watzlawick et al., 1967). Nurses must be able to diagnose communication difficulties in any of these domains. **Input** involves taking in information from outside the individual or group. Once taken in, input must be transformed in some manner to be used. For example, symbols must be translated into words to transmit ideas. The flow and transformation of processed input refers to the way information is analyzed and stored within the individual or the way it is transmitted from person to person within a human system (group or family) before communication with the external environment occurs. The outcome of information processing, **output**, involves further exchange with the environment or the other person.

BOX 4.7 Strategies Associated with Person-Centered Communication

- Permitting people to tell their stories in their own words and chronology
- Using a conversational interviewing style
- Being friendly through humor, social conversation, and nonverbal cues such as smiling
- Eliciting people's views, perspectives, thoughts, wishes, goals, values, and expectations
- Inquiring about the nature of the person's life
- Attending to the person's needs
- Avoiding overemphasis on technical aspects of care and tasks
- Not being too busy to talk
- Responding to cues concerning emotional issues and problems
- Giving information about self-care and participation in decision-making
- Developing mutual understanding
- Creating collaborative health care plans
- Showing empathy and concern for the individual's well-being
- Connecting with individuals through humor, touch, and selective self-disclosure
- Tuning in to individuals' preferences and style
- Attending to and advocating individuals' needs
- Maintaining confidentiality

Source: Knowlton, E. K., Sternlieb, J. L., & Freedy, J. R. (2020). The clinician-patient relationship: The therapeutic value of the clinical encounter. *International Journal of Psychiatry in Medicine, 55*(1), 3–7. https://doi.org/10.1177/0091217419894472

BOX 4.8 EVIDENCE-BASED PRACTICE

Client-Reported Care Domains that Enhance the Experience of "Being Known" in an Ambulatory Cancer Care Center

This study's purpose was to explore clients' perceptions of being known in an ambulatory chemotherapy setting (Grover et al., 2018). Researchers used a qualitative descriptive design. They recruited 10 participants with various cancer diagnoses from a large cancer center in Montreal, Quebec, Canada. Audio-recorded interviews were transcribed verbatim. Textual data were coded and analyzed thematically.

Results showed that participants described their need for the staff to approach them first as individuals and secondly as persons with cancer. They also stressed the importance of "(1) feeling truly welcome in the cancer care environment, (2) being provided with person- and situation-responsive care, and (3) considering occupational and social roles that go beyond the 'sick role'" (p. 166). Mutual client-nurse disclosure also facilitated perceptions of personalized care (Grover et al., 2018).

In addition to the importance of being known, future research is needed to examine how demographic, physical/psychological, and cultural factors affect these perceptions. Furthermore, the results support the clinical importance of knowing the client. In other words, establishing a caring relationship must be a key nursing priority.

A new information exchange is triggered at this point in the cycle by the response, called feedback, a monitoring system through which the person or group controls the internal and external responses to behavior (output) and accommodates these responses appropriately. A feedback loop shows the dynamic nature of communication. Each piece of communication is both a stimulus designed to elicit a response and a response to a different stimulus.

When interpersonal communication is analyzed, two types of feedback can be identified: positive (encouraging change) and negative (encouraging homeostasis or no change). Parents' commands to a young child illustrate these types of feedback: positive, "Try that again; you almost had it," and negative, "Don't touch that; it's hot." The first statement shows the parent's attempt to encourage the child to continue new behavior; the second illustrates an effort to curtail undesired behavior. Rather than meaning "good" or "bad," *positive feedback* and *negative feedback* refer to the promotion of system change and stability, which is the process of balancing the direction, speed, and magnitude of change. Both types of feedback are needed, depending on the situation.

The situational context of communication is important. The context of communication is the setting's physical, psychosocial, and cultural dimensions. It includes the relationship between the sender and the receiver; previous experiences, feelings, values, cultural norms, age, and developmental stage; and the physical location.

Types of Communication

All human communication occurs in three forms: verbal, nonverbal, and metacommunication. Each affects the meaning and influences the interpretation of the message.

Verbal Communication

Verbal communication is the transmission of messages using words, spoken or written. As symbols for ideas, words impart meaning defined by a specific language. Communicating with language is a critical ability.

People who are deaf or hard of hearing often use sign language to communicate. Signs, similarly to spoken or written words, are used consistently to represent a particular meaning. Words may also be spelled out through finger spelling in a manner parallel to written communication. Braille assists blind and visually challenged people in reading. Touch is used to interpret markings that represent letters and words. Sign language and braille blend aspects of verbal and nonverbal communication, but both forms of communication transmit meaning through a consistent language system.

Verbal communication with people who speak a different language poses a challenge. As societies become increasingly multicultural, assistance from specially trained interpreters is essential for the provision of culturally competent care. Confidentiality issues, the complexity of health information, and the need to validate understandings and reach mutual decisions make it inappropriate to use untrained personnel or relatives to interpret what is meant simply because they are available.

The importance of language development is apparent in its three functions: informing the person of others' thoughts and feelings; stimulating the receiver of a message by triggering a response; and serving a descriptive function by imparting information and sharing observations, ideas, inferences, and memories (Watzlawick et al., 1967). The ability of verbal communication to fulfill these functions is influenced by many factors, including the communicator's social class, culture, age, milieu, and ability to receive and interpret messages.

Nonverbal Communication

Nonverbal communication or language encompasses all messages that are not spoken or written. The channels of nonverbal communication are the five senses. Movement, facial and eye expressions, gestures, touch, appearance, and vocalization or paralanguage all constitute nonverbal modes of communication (Knapp et al., 2020). Although all communication has the potential to be misunderstood, nonverbal communication is particularly subject to misunderstanding because it does not always reflect the sender's conscious intent and is highly influenced by culture. Nonverbal messages also tend to be nebulous, without specific beginnings and endings.

Body motion or kinetic behavior includes facial expression (or facies), eye movements, body movements, gestures, and posture (Knapp et al., 2020). When observing facial expression, the nurse notices the affect or emotion that is communicated. Does the person appear happy or sad; alert, distracted, or sleepy; or contented, agitated, angry, or anxious? The intensity or degree of emotion expressed should also be noted. Does the person's face express what generally is considered an excessive degree of feeling for the situation, too little, or none at all? Eyes, in conjunction with the movement of other facial muscles, move in ways that convey affect. Eye contact conveys messages of interest or trust, lack of eye contact can imply lack of interest or anxiety, and constant eye contact can send a message of hostility.

All of these nonverbal messages are culturally and situationally bound. Nonverbal behavior, particularly facial and eye expressions, is contextual. For example, in certain circumstances and cultures, avoidance of direct eye contact between some people can be a sign of respect. Yet in other situations and cultures, it can be interpreted as indicative of disinterest, avoidance, or disrespect. Therefore interpretation requires a cultural lens.

Sign language combines features of both nonverbal and verbal communication. Sign language involves nonverbal communication because, although it uses symbols that are communicated through specific signs, these are enhanced by facial expressions and body postures. However, sign language shares many aspects of verbal communication. It has syntax and grammar, words may be spelled out, and a standard meaning is assigned to specific signs to create symbolic language, just as words share common definitions.

Importance of Nonverbal Communication. Nonverbal communication has great power to transmit information about another's thoughts and feelings; therefore, careful observation is essential. Even silence can be very revealing. The significance of nonverbal communication is best captured by the axiom "actions speak louder than words." Nurses' nonverbal messages that communicate distance from a person, or signal an unfriendly or uncaring attitude, thwart development of a therapeutic relationship (Knapp et al., 2020) and thereby render health-promotion efforts unproductive.

Metacommunication

Besides verbal and nonverbal communication, a phenomenon called **metacommunication** refers to a message about the message. Watzlawick and colleagues (1967) described metacommunication as the impossibility of not communicating: that is, "one cannot not communicate. "Persons transmit a message about what is being communicated even when words are not spoken." Metacommunication is the relationship aspect of communication. In a sense, metacommunication involves reading between the lines or going past the surface content of the message to glean nuances of meaning. When the content and the relationship aspects, or metacommunication aspects, of a message are incongruent, interpreting the communication accurately may be difficult, leaving the receiver uncomfortable and confused.

Group Process

In group settings, a special type of metacommunication is called **process**. A basic principle of group theory states that all communication has content and process. Content is what is said; process is the relationship aspect of what is communicated. Group process occurs during every group encounter. Staff meetings and clinically oriented psychoeducation, therapy, and counseling groups always involve group process. For example, consider two individuals in a smoking cessation group who always support each other by agreeing with each other and offering comments or criticism to any group member who disagrees. Although this pairing between the individuals offers them some protection from anxiety that may result from self-examination and feedback, it isolates them and curtails feedback from others. Examination of this group process is an essential task. The nurse leader and participants can transform this problematic situation into a learning opportunity by identifying the pattern and pointing out the behavior after it has occurred frequently, helping the pair and other group members consider what needs are being met through this pattern, looking at each person's role in fostering this process (e.g., why other group members have failed to confront the pair), and discussing potential outcomes of changing the behavior. These steps can be applied in clinical situations when greater self-understanding is a goal.

Effectiveness of Communication

Understanding what makes communication effective improves the nurse's ability to assess needs and to intervene successfully to promote an individual's health. Steps to functional communication include firmly stating the case, clarifying the message, seeking feedback, and being receptive to feedback when it is received. Implementing these steps to functional communication between nurses and individuals, and between nurses and other care providers, is essential to ensure client safety and quality care (QSEN, 2023).

To state the case, the sender needs to make the content and the metacommunication congruent; when they conflict, the message is confusing. For example, a nurse is angry with a colleague for making statements to an administrator that undermined the nurse's plans for reconfiguring a health-promotion program in their agency. When the nurse had a chance to speak with this colleague, they exchanged pleasantries without mention of what the nurse thought about the colleague's statements to the administrator. When the colleague asked if something was bothering the nurse, the nurse responded that nothing was wrong. The colleague senses that the nurse's verbal and nonverbal communication did not match; in other words, the content of the message and the metacommunication were incongruent. The colleague was left feeling uneasy, and the nurse failed to express their thoughts or to take effective action to rectify the perceived problem with the colleague. To make the communication functional, the nurse needed to bring thoughts and feelings into awareness and reflect on the intended message. Once these steps have been accomplished, the message's content and metacommunication can be adjusted to match, and the nurse's communication is likely to be effective. This example typifies ineffective communications.

To clarify the message, the sender must give a complete message. Important features should be emphasized, and specifics of any request must be stated, not assumed. The message's importance must also be indicated. To illustrate this, a female mentions to her nurse that it is nearly June. The nurse responds that he has noticed how warm the weather is becoming. On the surface, this communication may seem functional until the intent of the female's message is considered. She meant to imply that June is the 5-year anniversary of her remission from cancer, and she hoped that her nurse would somehow know that she wanted him to comment on the significance of this anniversary. To make this communication functional, the female needed to expand the message (e.g., "My anniversary after cancer treatment is coming up") and then clarify her wish to hear a sensitive response from the nurse (e.g., "This anniversary marks the goal for you to be cancer-free" or "What will you do to celebrate?"). Additionally, she needed to show how important the message was (e.g., "I'd really like to do something special to mark this date"). If the nurse had been attuned to the metacommunication in this exchange, he could have clarified this female's intent and met her need for recognition and dialogue. For example, the nurse could have asked "Does the month of June have special significance to you?"

One technique for clarifying and qualifying messages is called the "I" statement. Use of "I" statements helps the sender state what they want, feel, think, or plan (including likes and dislikes). For example, "I felt unimportant when you forgot to recognize this anniversary" is an "I" statement that the person could have used to communicate effectively. Soliciting such "I" messages is a therapeutic technique to be encouraged.

Questions can clarify and qualify messages, depending on the type of question asked. Open-ended questions tend to elicit descriptive responses rather than one-word answers. For example, the request "Tell me what you did for exercise this week," is likely to yield a more elaborate description of a health behavior from a person than the question "Did everything go okay with your exercise plan?" However, direct questions that seek a one-word answer are useful when a specific piece of information is sought. "Did you spend 15 minutes or more walking today?" may be a better approach than "What was your activity like today?" when it is important to discuss and promote minimal exercise requirements. Also, for individuals having trouble expressing more than the simplest thoughts, asking direct questions that call for brief replies can be helpful, such as "Did you eat breakfast?" This approach is particularly useful with people who are depressed, regressed, cognitively impaired, or unable to handle complex information or communication at a particular time, or when a specific yes/no response is needed.

Seeking feedback is another element of functional communication. Consensual validation, confirming that both the sender and the receiver understand the same information, calls for the use of the clarification skills just described. In family communication, the parent, as the sender, should model this behavior for children by asking the child, as the receiver, to explain their sense of the message and how to ask the sender for further explanation. For example, "I want you to clean your room," (message from parent) can be followed by "Tell me how you think you will do that" (validating that the child and the parent agree about what the task entails). This style of seeking validation can be adapted to nurse-nurse or nurse-interprofessional exchanges between colleagues and to therapeutic interactions and is critical to effective clinical care (National Academy of Medicine, 2022). Such confirmation in communication is also essential when health-promotion interventions are being provided. Without validating that the person understands the information and its importance, and that the person has a behavior plan to follow, health-promotion efforts are likely to fail. Moreover, failure to validate understanding is a significant risk to client safety (QSEN, 2023).

Being open to feedback is also crucial. A "no questions" attitude blocks functional communication, whether in the home, classroom, work, or clinical setting. Children, students, individuals, and even other nurses may be afraid to question anyone in authority or may assume that the person should magically know what is intended or expected. For example, a person may avoid confronting a nurse who fails to explain the clinical plan and then communicates that the person should know how to follow through. Statements by the sender such as "Tell me what you think" and "What is your understanding of what I said?" are helpful in eliciting confirmation of understanding and feedback.

Receiving and sending messages involve many of the same processes. Evaluation of the intent of the message, both the content and the metacommunication, is the first step. The receiver frequently needs to seek clarification and validate understanding of the message for communication to be effective. Clarification of expectations, active exchange of information, power sharing, and negotiation will enhance the quality of nurse-person communication. The outcome is a nurse-person engagement based on trust and partnership (Palaz & Kayacan, 2023), critical ingredients of client-centered care (National Academy of Medicine, 2022; Kwame and Petrucka, 2021).

Interprofessional Communication and Teamwork

Interprofessional communication and teamwork for care design and delivery involve cross-disciplinary education and practice approaches that are now widely promoted as essential to an effective health care system (Kim et al., 2019; Schot et al., 2020). However, instruments that help students and clinicians hone their observations of teamwork behaviors have been lacking. The Jefferson Teamwork Observation Guide® is a short, easy-to-use tool, with evidence of reliability and face and predictive validity, for observation of teams in action to identify behaviors, including communications indicative of good teamwork (Lyons et al., 2016; Choice & Thomas, 2023). The Jefferson Teamwork Observation Guide is a helpful instrument for nurses to use to recognize, observe, and then implement the behaviors that constitute good teamwork and communication.

Factors in Effective Communication

Listening

Effective listening, an important part of communication, is more than passively taking in information. Effective listening is actively focusing attention on the message. Asking questions to explore what is meant helps the listener reach an accurate assessment of the message's meaning.

Many forms of nonverbal communication have been identified that, from a Western or European perspective, commonly convey that the person is listening. These nonverbal communications include direct gazing and eye contact, head nodding, orienting one's body to maintain interpersonal closeness, leaning forward, making facial expressions such as eyebrow animation and smiling, and using brief verbal statements that indicate interest, such as "Please go on" or "Tell me more about that."

Behavior that communicates a person is listening also depends on the context and intensity of the activities and the cultural norms of each person. For example, leaning close to a person might be interpreted as intrusive, yet the same behavior could be seen as a sign of support, depending on the context and perspective of those involved. Sensitivity to nuances in communication and validation of meaning can be particularly helpful strategies when the nurse and the person come from different cultural backgrounds.

Reciprocity, the patterning of similar activities within the same interval by two people, can help the nurse communicate a listening stance in an effective way. When the nurse matches nuances of the individual's type and style of behavior, the chances that the person will interpret the nurse's behavior as an indication of active listening are increased, and the likelihood of misinterpretation is reduced. Nurses can enhance the quality of their communication, even when encounters are brief, by attending to reciprocity in their interactions and by validating whether reciprocity is associated with shared interpretations of meaning.

Poor listening blocks the nurse's understanding of the person. The nurse's failure to listen may be caused by anxiety; a focus on other demands; a lack of experience, which may lead to excessive talking by the nurse; a preoccupation with personal thoughts; or a lack of practice. The importance of focusing on the individual's needs and concerns through effective listening is a recurrent theme in research concerning therapeutic interaction (Oliver et al., 2019; Townsend & Morgan, 2020) and a cornerstone of client-centered and safe care (QSEN, 2023).

Flexibility

Flexibility is a balance between control and permissiveness. In overcontrol, every message is monitored. In exaggerated permissiveness, anything can be communicated in any way. For communication to be functional, rules are needed about what is appropriate, without rigid prescriptions that inhibit meaningful interchange. For example, the guideline that nurses will not answer questions concerning intimate details of their lives sets an appropriate limit; however, this does not mean that nurses should refuse to answer any question about themselves.

Silence

Silence between people is often uncomfortable for the nurse who is somewhat insecure about what should occur during a therapeutic encounter. However, silence can be beneficial when used carefully. Although silence may appear to be an awkward lack of words, work done by Rockwell et al. (2022) has actually shown that silence is a way of being with a person: "It can be understood as a time to think, consider a response, or to express emotions" (p. 60). When one is seeking a verbal response, silence can be perceived as a lack of interest. At other times, silence allows individuals to reflect on what is being discussed or experienced, lets them know that the nurse is willing to wait until they are ready to say more, or simply provides them with comfort and support. Each situation needs evaluation and sensitivity. Rather than asking a flurry of questions to break the silence, the nurse should allow the person time to decide when to comment or make brief comments that do not demand answers, such as "It can be helpful to take time to think about what we've been discussing." Also, comments such as "Try putting your thoughts or feelings into words" and "I am here when you are ready to talk" can help the person to share these thoughts or feelings when silence is blocking rather than improving the communication.

Humor

Humor is part of being human; it relieves tension, reduces aggression, and creates a climate of sharing. Humor can block communication when it is used to avoid subjects that might be uncomfortable or when it excludes other people. Humor can also inflict emotional pain and communicate negative views or stereotypes about particular individuals or groups through teasing and jokes concerning race, ethnicity, culture, country of origin, occupation, age, sex or gender, sexual activity, or other traits that stand out or are devalued. A direct response to the latent content or message in this type of humor is an effective way to curtail its use and minimize its effect. For example, a response that shows disapproval of the latent message such as "That kind of joke makes me very uncomfortable. I don't find it funny to describe [the specific group in question] that way, and I would like you to stop" will send a clear message and likely be successful in stopping the offensive communication. In contrast, for humor to be helpful, the meaning of the humor must be understood and its purpose supportive to the individual. Humor that is self-directed often works better than humor directed at others, which can come across as deprecating and offensive. Clarification of the meaning should be used when there is doubt or concern.

Touch

Touch is an interesting means of nonverbal communication for nurses, who often touch individuals while administering care (Blondis & Jackson, 1982). The nurse's concern can be expressed by a gentle or soothing application of touch. Nevertheless, in some instances touch is inappropriate. For example, in interactions with individuals who have trauma histories or acute psychiatric disturbances, touch might be misinterpreted (Vafeiadou, et al., 2022). A female who has been raped might interpret touch during an examination as an attack. Evaluation of the context and meaning of touch to the individual is based on knowledge of that person and interpretation of feedback. Informing the individual about the purpose of touching and asking for permission and feedback are useful techniques to avoid unintended distress or misinterpretation of touching in a clinical encounter. Cultural considerations also are important (Vafeiadou, et al., 2022). For example, in some cultures or religions touching between genders is forbidden. Furthermore, while touch may be a necessary part of the medical examination, consideration should be given to gender and age differences. One study found that females tended to be more uncomfortable with a male medical professional and that comfortability with touch increased with age (Vafeiadou, et al., 2022).

Space

Space between communicators varies according to the type of communication, the setting, and the culture. Hall (1973) researched **proxemics**, the use of space between communicators, and identified four zones of space commonly used in interaction in North America; these are presented in Box 4.9: Zones of Space Common to Interaction in North America and Fig. 4.1. It is critically important for nurses to be sensitive to how spatial zones vary across cultures when caring for persons from diverse backgrounds.

BOX 4.9 Zones of Space Common to Interaction in North America

1. Intimate space: up to 18 in (45.5 cm); used for high interpersonal sensory stimulation (Fig. 4.1A)
2. Personal space: 45.5–1.2 m (18 in to 4 ft); appropriate for close relationships in which touching may be involved and good visualization is desired (Fig. 4.1B)
3. Social-consultative space: 2.7–3.6 m (9–12 ft); less intimate and personal, requiring louder verbal communication (Fig. 4.1C)
4. Public space: 3.6 m (12 ft) or more; appropriately used for formal gatherings, such as giving speeches (Fig. 4.1D)

Sources: Hall, E. (1973). *The silent language*. Garden City, NY: Doubleday/Anchor Press; Knapp, M. L., Hall, J. A., & Horgan, T. G. (2020). *Nonverbal communication in human interaction* (8th ed.). Boston: Wadsworth Cengage Learning.

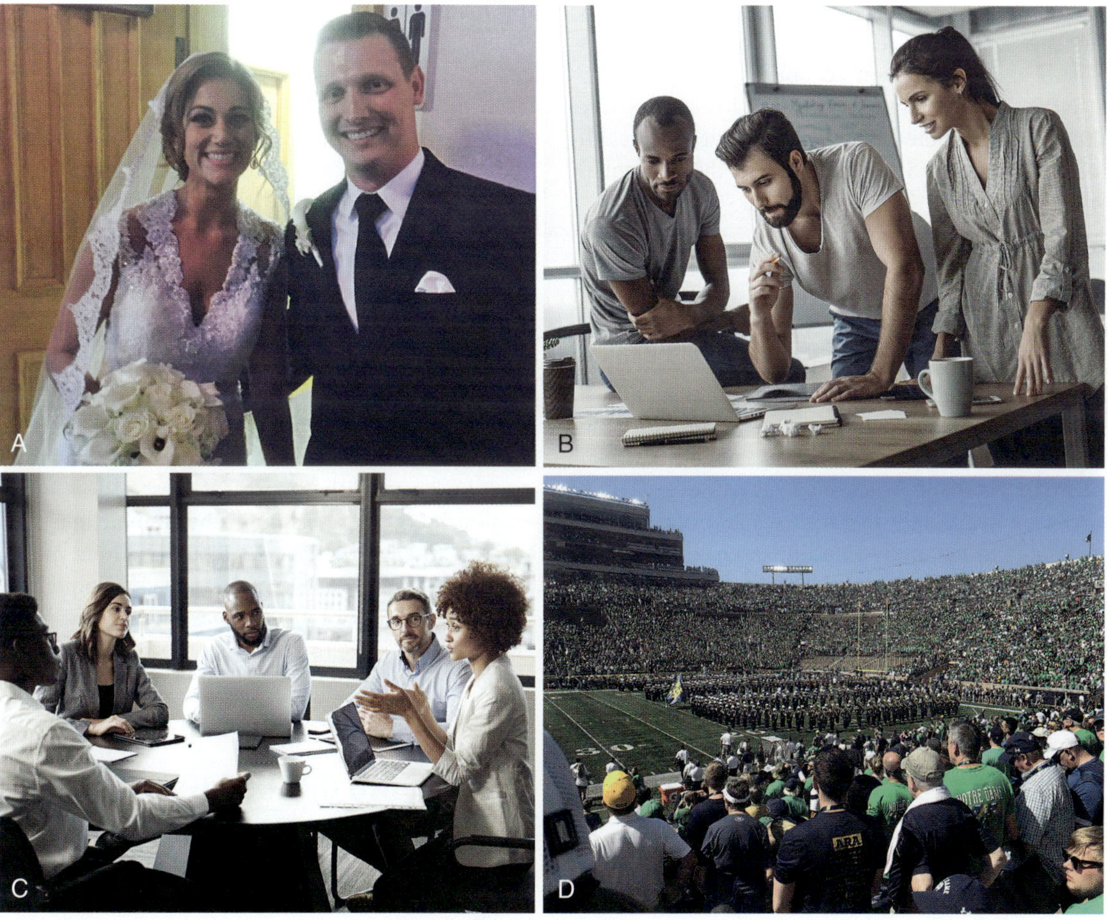

FIG. 4.1 (A) Intimate distance communication. (B) Personal distance communication. (C) Social-consultative distance communication. (D) Public distance communication. (B, From iStock.com/dima_sidelnikov; C, From iStock.com/monkeybusinessimages.)

Understanding the appropriate distance for a given type of interaction helps the nurse make nonverbal and verbal communication congruent and to avoid violating spatial norms. Awareness of cultural customs concerning distance is important in shaping communication and interpreting the behavior of others. When people from different cultures or groups communicate, there may be discomfort about the acceptable distance between them when speaking. Recognition of differences helps the nurse adjust the distance and interpret the meaning of this nonverbal communication.

Many traits and components discussed in this chapter characterize functional communication. However, communication is a subtle and intricate process. Communication cannot be reduced to a set of parts and principles; its roles and nuances are far more complex and variable. Communicating by language and symbols is a special human ability. Healthy communication enables people to move from being alone to being together—clearly one of the crucial tasks of living. Effective communication is also the foundation of the helping relationship. Moreover, effective communication is essential to providing quality care and ensuring client safety and well-being (QSEN, 2023).

Health Literacy

Clear communication improves the quality of health care encounters. **Health literacy**, the capacity to read, comprehend, and follow through on health information, is a critical component of health promotion. Yet nearly 9 out of 10 adults encounter problems using everyday health information to make good decisions about health (NIH, 2023). Literacy is essential to health safety (Bakerjian, 2023). To promote safety and combat low health literacy, nurses can encourage individuals to ask three essential questions at every health visit:

- "What is my main problem?"
- "What do I need to do?"
- "Why is it important for me to do this?"

Nurses also promote health literacy by creating a safe and comfortable environment, sitting to establish eye contact rather than standing when communicating, using visual aids and models to illustrate conditions and procedures, and verifying understanding of care instructions by having individuals then teach the content; that is, using "teach-back" as a strategy (Jared, 2019). Resources are available to help nurses and other clinicians to increase individuals' understanding of health information across health literacy levels. The Agency for Healthcare Research and Quality (2020) Health Literacy Universal Precautions Toolkit provides easily accessible and highly useful resources to promote universal health precautions; that is, steps to take when clinicians assume that all persons may have some limitations in understanding health information and accessing health services. This toolkit provides evidence-based approaches for use from assessment to intervention. The toolkit suggests fundamental communication strategies to communicate clearly (see Box 4.5: Use Strategies for Communicating Clearly/Enhance Health Literacy Capacity).

Three key factors regarding health literacy to consider are the educational level of the target audience or users; the reading/comprehension level for materials in online, verbal, or written format; and the native language of the target audience or users. A highly educated target audience generally has high health literacy because of a strong command of the native language being used. Evidence has shown that health information in use may be at a reading level above the comprehension level of most users. Recommendations include improved quality in materials and instruction, especially for those with low education/literacy skills (Larsen & Gilstad, 2023, Osborne, 2021). Furthermore, nurses need to assess comprehension of all health information and instruction, particularly of complex medical/health information. Developing materials at the fifth- or sixth-grade reading level helps ensure that comprehension is very likely across wide ranges of the target audience. Word-processing programs and online tools can evaluate the reading level of a text. Published materials are also available to aid in assessing and developing appropriate content for developing health literacy (Karami et al., 2023). These available resources enable nurses easily to determine the reading level of all health and research materials and to adjust the level by changing complex terms to more commonly used words with only one or two syllables and simplifying sentences to avoid complex constructions with multiple phrases. Finally, adjusting word usage to avoid native colloquialisms, abbreviations, and acronyms will increase understanding among persons whose native language is not being used. Moreover, advocating for development and/or revision of existing materials, and possibly for translation into the audience's native language to reach a fifth- or sixth-grade reading level, is an appropriate nursing mandate.

In the emerging age of telehealth, developing strategies for confirming understanding and individualizing methods of communicating health information is increasingly important (see Box 4.6: Best Practice). Health information and even access to appointments are steadily shifting from face-to-face interaction to access by telephone via voice prompts and Internet-based formats. Many factors involved in health literacy can impair individuals' ability to understand and respond to audio and/or visual commands. Consider the array of commands involved in the typical automated telephone system involved in ordering a prescription refill from a typical pharmacy. The individual must select from a list of options; next, multiple numbers must be keyed in that represent prescription numbers listed in small print on a prescription label and birthdays in appropriate format; finally, a variety of confirmations must be entered. Persons with auditory, visual, language comprehension, and/or cognitive limitations may not have adequate capacity to manage such common health care technologies. Therefore, technology competence becomes another component of health literacy to be considered.

THE HELPING OR THERAPEUTIC RELATIONSHIP

A helping or therapeutic relationship is a process through which one person promotes the development of another person by fostering the latter's maturation, adaptation, integration, openness, and ability to find meaning in the present situation (Mersha et al., 2023; Peplau, 1969). The therapeutic relationship emerges from purposeful encounters characterized by effective communication.

In this relationship, the nurse respects the individual's values, attends to concerns, and promotes positive change by encouraging self-expression, exploring behavior patterns and outcomes, and promoting self-help (Barker et al., 2023). The therapeutic relationship is the foundation of clinical nursing practice (Barker et al., 2023; Mersha et al., 2023)—the essential element of quality care with every individual in every situation (QSEN, 2023). Techniques, technology, interventions, and contexts differ, but the relational aspect of nursing practice produces a cohesive unity, allowing each nurse to see people holistically and as unique individuals. Although many components of the helping relationship are most germane to relationships that extend over time, the essentials of the helping relationship apply to even brief therapeutic encounters.

No perfect profile or personality of a helping person exists. However, certain traits can be nurtured without thwarting the nurse's unique personality. These characteristics enable the nurse to be an agent of therapeutic care (Peplau, 1963; Townsend & Morgan, 2020). Box 4.10 lists characteristics associated with therapeutic effectiveness.

Characteristics of the Therapeutic Relationship

No recipe is available for a successful therapeutic relationship. Techniques and concepts serve only as tools. As a nurse develops and evaluates a helping relationship, be it long term or brief in nature, the following guidelines may be useful.

Purposeful Communication

Purposeful communication means that the nurse focuses communication toward a particular goal. Social chitchat, communication without a goal, should not make up the bulk of therapeutic interaction. This does not mean that the nurse should never discuss a social topic; nonetheless, there should be some purpose. For example, discussing the weather with a somewhat disoriented older adult serves the purpose of orienting that person to the environment. Discussing the Super Bowl with an avid football fan may provide valuable assessment data and engage the person in a current topic of social interest. Goals guide the nurse in focusing communication.

BOX 4.10 Characteristics Associated with Therapeutic Effectiveness

- Self-awareness and self-reflection
- Openness
- Self-confidence and strength
- Genuineness
- Concern for the individual
- Respect for the individual
- Knowledge
- Ability to empathize
- Sensitivity
- Acceptance
- Creativity
- Ability to focus and confront

Rapport

Rapport is a harmony and an affinity between people in a relationship. By using many of the traits listed for helping a person, the nurse can establish an atmosphere in which rapport can develop. To let the person know that their concerns interest the nurse and that working together may alleviate some of their difficulties and encourage growth, it is important to be genuine, open, and concerned.

Trust

Trust is a necessary component of any helping relationship. Trust is the reliance on a person to carry out responsibilities and promises, based on a sense of safety, honesty, and reliability. Trust is an important component of partnership. The nurse promotes trust by modeling and structuring the relationship appropriately. The following strategies promote trust:

- Anticipating that the individual will do as promised
- Clearly defining the relationship parameters and expectations, particularly the purpose and specifics of time, place, and anticipated behavior
- Being consistent
- Examining behaviors that interfere with trust

Empathy

Empathy is the ability to understand another's feelings without losing personal identity and perspective. Empathic nurses draw on emotions and experiences that enable them to place themselves in the other person's situation. While the person senses increasing understanding and acceptance from the nurse, the individual's distress decreases. Results from research studies are building knowledge about the role that empathic nursing care plays in outcomes. Nurses learn behavioral approaches that enhance empathic relations with people through supervised experiential learning (Barker et al., 2023). For example, nurses do not empathize by switching the focus of the interaction to themselves or by sympathizing (e.g., "I know exactly how you feel; that happened to me once"). Rather, they use clinical and personal experience to appreciate the individual's feelings and experiences; they try to imagine themselves in the person's situation. Using personal understanding based on some shared aspect of experience such as a loss while maintaining boundaries is the essence of empathy in the helping relationship. With empathic understanding, the nurse acknowledges the affective domain of personal experiences and uses this knowledge to appreciate the person's reactions. Empathy enables the listener to share human experiences as the basis for providing care.

Goal Direction

A helping relationship is special in its goal-directed nature. Although most human relationships focus on mutual benefit, a helping relationship exists solely to meet some need or to promote the growth of the recipient. Although the nurse may benefit from the interaction, the relationship is centered on the recipient.

Goals are formulated as desired individual behaviors/outcomes. Short-term goals are likely to be achieved within 10 days to 2 weeks; all other goals are long term. All goals should be stated in measurable terms and should focus on a positive change or on the decrease of problematic behavior/health indicators. Ideally, a person works with the nurse to establish goals. However, some individuals, such as those who are seriously ill, depressed, psychotic, or cognitively impaired, may be unable to establish mutual goals. When an individual is unable to negotiate appropriate goals, the nurse establishes realistic goals and shares them to the degree possible with the person, who is free to participate or to reject efforts to reach these goals. In some circumstances where the care recipient is unable to collaborate regarding care decisions, then a family member or another designee/health care proxy may be the appropriate person for such communication.

Ethics in Communicating and Relating

Ethical decision-making is closely linked with the goal-directed nature of helping relationships. Ethical issues are present in human interactions whenever behavior may affect others, whenever actions involve conscious choices of methods and ends, and whenever actions can be evaluated in reference to standards of right and wrong (Cheraghi et al., 2023). Guidelines that may be adapted as ethical standards for interpersonal communication are highlighted in Box 4.11.

Frequently the nurse may wish to set goals that the individual does not want to reach; the nurse must remember that the problem belongs to the person, as does the choice of care alternatives. The nurse assists the individual in decision-making, with the decision based on the individual's value system. However, the nurse should not take a laissez-faire approach and avoid assisting the person. The nurse's responsibility is to help the individual to examine values, identify conflicts, and prioritize goals and desired health care outcomes. Action follows from understanding values and the best available information. Both the individual and the nurse must bring interpreted facts and personally clarified values to the interaction to establish goals. Recognizing this interplay, the nurse must clarify personal values, subsequently respect the individual's rights, and act to support and protect the integrity of the person, family, group, or community.

Ethical communication also involves safeguarding protected health information. The individual's right to privacy motivated the passage of the Health Insurance Portability and Accountability Act (HIPAA) in 1996. Individually identifiable health information is defined as the following (US Department of Health & Human Services, 2022):

> *Information protected by law includes demographic data, that relate to the individual's past, present, or future physical or mental health or condition; the provision of health care to the individual, or the past, present, or future payment for the provision of health care to the individual; and that identify the individual or for which there is a reasonable basis to believe can be used to identify the individual. Individually identifiable health information includes many common identifiers (e.g., name, address, birth date, Social Security Number).*

Sharing personal health information can be understood on the basis of "need to know" so as to care for the person. Stuart's (2013) concept of the circle of confidentiality provides a helpful guideline for nurses. Patient information may be shared among people in the circle. Members of the circle can include health care team members, health care system administrators, health care students and faculty, as well as patient consultants. To receive patient information, people outside the circle require the patient's permission. Adhering to the rules concerning protection of identifiable health information is both an ethical and a legal requirement for the nurse.

BOX 4.11 Guidelines for Ethical Interpersonal Communication

Ethical interpersonal communication involves the following:

- Being aware and open to changing concepts of self and others
- Attending to role responsibilities; individual sacrifice, when it is required to make a "good" decision; and emotions while guarding against letting emotions be the sole guide of behavior
- Sharing personal views candidly and clearly
- Communicating information accurately, with minimal loss or distortion of intended meaning
- Communicating verbal and nonverbal messages with congruent meanings
- Sharing responsibility for the consequences among communicators
- Recognizing the multicultural context of all communication
- Respecting the dignity of every person
- Avoiding coercion and use of power in communicating
- Being sensitive to gender and cultural contexts of communication and interpretation
- Building context for intercultural dialogue that is open with conditions of security and mutual respect
- Eliminating any elements of communication that denigrate, stereotype, or devalue clients
- Facilitating open and accurate communication among professional groups, professionals, staff and families, clinical care unit and department staffs or administrators, and clinical care facilities

Unethical communication involves the following:

- Purposefully deceiving
- Intentionally blocking communication—for example, changing subjects when the other person has not finished communicating, cutting a person off, or distracting others from the subject under discussion
- Scapegoating or unnecessarily condemning others
- Lying or deceiving that causes intentional or unintentional harm
- Verbally "hitting below the belt" by taking advantage of another's vulnerability
- Violating Health Insurance Portability and Accountability Act rules concerning protection of personal health information

Therapeutic Techniques

Occasionally, clinicians who are novices in establishing helping relationships assume that they are bound to "say the wrong thing" and cause terrible damage to the person or that they will learn some magical phrases and questions to create instant rapport. No nurse or other professional is so powerful that a "wrong word" will destroy the individual's self-concept or self-esteem. Even people with physical and emotional problems are resilient and have coped, at least to some degree, with a lifetime of stresses. Alternatively, no magical saying exists that the nurse can always plug into an interaction to communicate successfully. Although some techniques are often useful, they must be applied with purpose, skill, and attention to the individuality of each person and to the context of the interaction. The following techniques therefore should be viewed as guidelines, rather than prescriptions, for effective shaping of the therapeutic relationship.

Focus on the Individual

The first step to therapeutic communication is focusing on the individual and the reason that the interaction is occurring. The nurse is not the focus; the person is. Although an overly business-like style fails to communicate concern and support, delving into one's own personal life to the extent that it diverts attention from the other person's concern is also problematic. Avoiding nurse-directed conversation can be difficult; a useful rule of thumb is to answer or respond to obvious questions and to switch the focus back to clinical concerns when other questions are asked. For example:

Individual (looks at female nurse's wedding ring): "Are you married?"

Nurse: "Yes, I am."

Individual: "What does your husband do for a living?"

Nurse: "Our purpose is to talk about you, so let's get back to planning how you will manage at work."

Keeping focus on the person's concerns includes identifying the portion of the message that is clear and relevant to the purpose of the interaction, seeking validation, and helping the individual to clarify the rest of the message.

Help the Individual to Describe and Clarify Content and Meaning

Too often the nurse rushes to offer an interpretation of the nature of the problem and quickly follows up by suggesting a solution. Solving problems efficiently makes the nurse feel effective, important, and powerful; however, the person's needs may not be met. A crucial step in using the therapeutic relationship effectively is to assist the individual in describing a particular experience or concern. Description is enhanced when the nurse prompts the person to clarify the description and interpret its meaning.

Use of *who, what, where*, and *when* questions helps the person to clarify and expand the content and meaning of what is communicated. Phrases such as "tell me," "go on," "describe to me," "explain it to me," and "give me an example," are also likely to elicit description of important content and to diminish distracting generalizations and abstractions. By seeking feedback, the nurse helps the individual explain the meaning further. In clarifying the meaning, the nurse should avoid threatening, detective-like questions. Questions that begin with *why* often increase the person's anxiety because they demand reasons, conclusions, analysis, or causes (Peplau, 1964). Reformulating questions to obtain descriptive data first and then helping the individual analyze links between events, thoughts, feelings, actions, and outcomes is generally a more helpful approach.

A problem-solving approach by the nurse assists the person in describing and clarifying the content and meaning of an experience. Sequential steps help the individual explain events, change circumstances and responses that interfere with health, and solve problems (Barker et al., 2023; Peplau, 1963). This problem-solving approach can be adapted for use in health promotion to assist the person in problem-solving by working through the steps outlined in Box 4.12: Quality and Safety Scenario. These steps are a useful guideline for keeping the focus of concern on the individual and their definition of the problem. Rather than telling the person what is wrong and how to fix it, the nurse's primary goal is helping the person to describe the problem and formulate solutions in partnership. The cyclic nature of the process is illustrated in Fig. 4.2.

BOX 4.12 QUALITY AND SAFETY SCENARIO

Steps in Promoting Problem-Solving (Peplau, 1963)

Describe the Experience or Event of Concern

Helpful Verbal Nursing Strategies

"Tell me what happened."

"Describe the experience to me."

Analyze the Parts of the Experience and See the Relationships to Other Events

Helpful Verbal Nursing Strategies

"What meaning does this have for you?"

"What pattern is there?"

Formulate the Problem

Helpful Verbal Nursing Strategies

"In what way is this problematic?"

"What do you want to see changed?"

Validate the Formulation

Helpful Verbal Nursing Strategies

"Do you mean…?"

"Let me tell you what I understand you to be saying."

Use the Formulation to Identify Ways to Solve or Manage the Difficulty

Helpful Verbal Nursing Strategies

"What would you do the next time?"

"In what way has your view changed?"

"What actions are needed to solve the problem that you've identified?"

Try Out the Solutions, Judge the Outcomes, and Adjust the Plan Accordingly

Helpful Nursing Strategies

Encourage application in new situations through role-playing or through practice in appropriate settings; help the individual cycle through the preceding sequence as needed to evaluate the outcome and make adjustments to the plan.

Use Reflection

Reflection is the restatement of what the individual has said in the same or different words. This technique can involve paraphrasing or summarizing the person's main point to indicate interest and to focus the discussion. Effective use of this approach does not include frequent, parrot-like repetition of the individual's statements. Instead, reflection is the selective paraphrasing or literal repetition of the person's words to underscore the importance of what has been said, to summarize a main concern or theme, or to elicit elaborated information. In addition, to verify understanding of health information, the nurse can ask the person to restate what has been communicated. Confirmation of understanding promotes desired clinical outcomes.

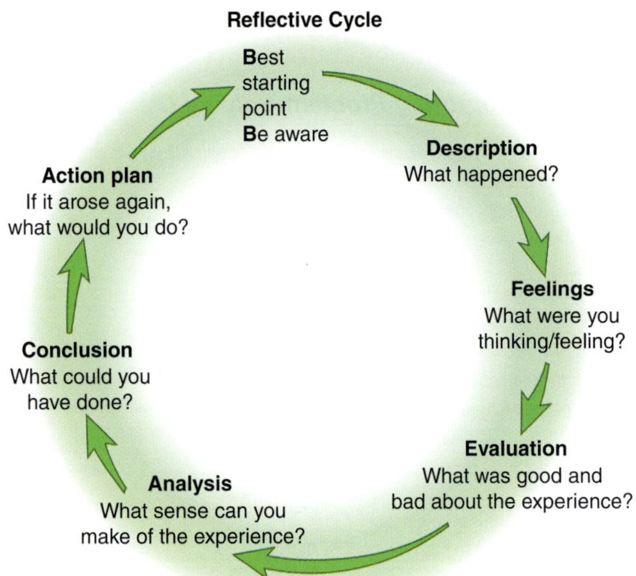

FIG. 4.2 The Process of Reflection. The reflective process is illustrated here with entry at any point to examine events, associated thoughts and feelings, and analysis with a goal of understanding the events and one's reactions/actions as well as formulating a plan for responding effectively to similar events in the future.

Use Constructive Confrontation

Confronting an individual means that the nurse points out a specific behavior and then helps the person examine the meaning, motivation, or consequence of the behavior. For example:

Nurse: "You missed your appointment for the consultation we had scheduled."

Individual: "Oh, I didn't notice the date."

Nurse: "You are usually very aware of time and appointments. What do you think was going on with you that you didn't notice the date this time?"

This type of confrontation is not an angry exchange but a purposeful way of helping the person examine personal actions and their meaning.

Use Nouns and Pronouns Correctly

Some individuals have difficulty separating themselves from others or specifying the object or subject in their language. These individuals misuse pronouns by referring to *we*, *us*, *they*, *she*, *he*, *him*, and *her* without clearly identifying the referent and by making vague statements such as "They don't like me. They told me I was useless." Others may use general nouns, such as *everyone*, *people*, *doctors*, and *nurses*, to avoid clear communication about specific persons. The nurse can clarify the meaning by asking, "Who are they?" or "Who is the person?" Additionally, the nurse must be careful to use separate pronouns when speaking of themselves and the individual, particularly when the person has disordered thinking. For example, when communicating with an individual who is confused or exhibits disordered or psychotic thinking, the nurse should say "you" and "I," rather than "us" or "we," to promote clear thinking and communication and to assist the individual in maintaining personal boundaries (Peplau, 1963).

Nevertheless, as nongendered pronouns are preferred by some persons, use of *they* rather than *he* or *she* to refer to an individual should be respected. Using a first name when possible to refer to a person rather than using a pronoun such as *they* when it could be confusing can add clarity while maintaining respect. Asking about pronoun preferences also is helpful and respectful. The nurse should be sensitive to an individual's way of speaking about themselves as important to **therapeutic engagement**.

Use Silence

Allowing a thoughtful silence at intervals helps the individual to talk at their own pace without pressure to perform for the nurse. Silence also permits time for reflection. Although silence may appear to be an awkward lack of words, it can also be thought of as a pause or a way of attending, a "presencing" for individuals who may be in too much pain to speak (Knol et al., 2020; Rockwell et al., 2022). Particularly helpful to the depressed or physically ill person, silence can reduce pressure and conserve energy. After several moments, the nurse can ask the person to share some thoughts—for example, "Try putting your thoughts into words," "Tell me what you are thinking or feeling now," or "I'll be here when you feel ready to talk."

Motivational Interviewing

Motivational interviewing (MI) is a person-centered communication approach used widely in health care and life coaching to assist individuals in making behavioral changes regarding a wide variety of lifestyle and health issues (Bischof et al., 2021; Cole et al., 2023). Key components of MI are as follows:

- Engaging—involving the individual in talking about issues, worries, and desires; establishing the basis for a trusting relationship
- Focusing—narrowing the focus to habits or patterns that individuals wish to change
- Evoking—eliciting motivation for change by increasing the sense of the importance of change, confidence, and readiness to change
- Planning—developing practical steps that the individual wants to use to create the desired changes

Nurses can seek training and use many available self-help and life-coaching resources for health promotion. For example, *The Motivational Interviewing Workbook* (Wood, 2020) is an example of a self-help book with useful tools that align nicely with MI that could be tailored to specific health care concerns. Such resources have high acceptability and can serve as helpful adjuncts to formal education and treatment/health-promotion guidance from nurses.

Current evidence supports the use of MI as an effective technique that can be taught to health professionals without advanced mental health training to promote desired behavioral change across health problems and settings. For training, use, and evaluation of MI implementation, nurses and other clinicians can use the Motivational Interviewing Skills in Health Care Encounters instrument, a reliable validated assessment tool to evaluate acquisition and use of specific MI skills and principles (Bischof et al., 2021; Cole et al., 2023).

Additional Strategies to Promote Effective Communication and Relationships

Promoting effective communication with individuals and families also involves the following fundamental elements:

- Clarifying: seeking clarity when communications are ambiguous
- Encouraging: open emotional expression of painful and positive emotions
- Fostering mutual problem-solving: using brainstorming, negotiation, goal-setting, and planning rather than being reactive

Barriers to Effective Communication

Barriers to effective communication can originate with the nurse, the individual, or the environment. Kwame & Petrucka (2021) identified barriers to therapeutic communication in the nurse-client relationship, including health care system influences (i.e., lack of knowledge/experience, all-knowing attitude, work stress), personal and behavior-related (i.e., sociodemographic factors, beliefs, world views, or educational level), and environmental (i.e., noisy or novel environment) factors.

Communication is also ineffective when some part of the communication-feedback loop breaks down. Failure to send a clear message, receive and interpret a message correctly, or provide useful feedback can interfere with communication. Diagnosing the source of the communication breakdown, taking steps to correct it, and using knowledge of the communication process and appropriate therapeutic techniques are the nurse's responsibility.

Anxiety

When the nurse or individual is highly anxious during an interaction, perception is altered and the ability to communicate effectively is curtailed sharply. Defense mechanisms, such as denial, projection, and displacement, reduce anxiety but block understanding of the true meaning of an interaction. Severe anxiety and defense mechanisms distort reality and lead to disordered communication. To enhance interpersonal communication, the nurse identifies the feeling of anxiety and its source and uses anxiety-reducing interventions.

Attitudes

Biases and stereotypes can limit the nurse's and the individual's ability to relate. When the difficulty is the individual's problem, the nurse can assist by examining those views that interfere with the person's relationships. When the problem is the nurse's, openness in a supervisory/mentoring relationship to examine personal behavior is crucial. When the nurse fails to examine their attitudes toward the person, negativity may be communicated, and perceptions of the interaction may be distorted.

Gaps Between the Nurse and the Individual

Related to attitudinal barriers, differences in sex, age, socioeconomic background, ethnicity, race, religion, or language can block functional communication between the nurse and the individual. These factors can cause differences in perception and block mutual understanding. Newly licensed nurses have attributed communication problems to differences in language proficiency among nurses, including English as a second language, as well as to problems in understanding non–English-speaking individuals (Edge & Lemetyinen, 2019). To reduce such gaps, nurses can question unclear verbal or written communications, seek clarification or assistance from translators, and explore the ways in which perceptions may differ and meanings can be clarified (Box 4.13: Health and Social Determinants/Health Equity; Communication: Cultural Competence and Cultural Humility).

Moreover, differences in understandings and meanings between faculty and student nurses, as well as between nurses and clients, can be fueled by generation gaps. Such gaps can interfere with effective development of the interpersonal skills required for therapeutic nurse-person relationships. Millennials, born from 1981 to 1996, constitute some undergraduate/prelicensure students and even more graduate nursing students. Generation Z, born after 1997 and up to 2012, now makes up much of the traditional BS/BSN undergraduate nursing student body (Pew Research Center, 2019). Evidence from the literature demonstrates that both generations benefit from deconstruction pedagogies or interactive teaching strategies such as debates, case studies, role-playing, storytelling, journaling, simulations, and audio and video webpage links rather than more traditional didactic approaches. As younger generations who have been raised with technology at their fingertips are entering nursing education, teaching approaches require ongoing change with the use of more technology and more interactive strategies. Nonetheless, our students also need to learn how to adapt their technology-mediated modes of communication to the styles and skills of older generation persons and those who may not have had the same access to technology when communicating with persons in the health care system and in professional situations. So, although faculty members need to be adept at engaging students with a variety of effective strategies, students also need to be coached to use appropriate communication approaches across situations and populations. For example, evidence supports the effectiveness of video feedback, another technologic teaching/learning strategy, to enhance the quality of communication, clinical competence, and MI skills of practicing nurses (Hong & Lee, 2022; Lee & Son 2022). Thus ongoing faculty development and testing of various teaching approaches to help students develop competence in therapeutic communication and relationships is crucial to nursing's future.

Resistance

Resistance comprises all phenomena that inhibit the flow of thoughts, feelings, and memories in an interpersonal encounter and behaviors that interfere with therapeutic goals. Resistance arises from anxiety when a person feels threatened. To reduce this anxiety, the person implements resistant behavior to divert the focus, most often in the form of avoidance, such as being late, changing the subject, forgetting, blocking, or becoming angry.

Initially, the nurse should identify the behavior, whether it is the nurse's or the individual's behavior, and then attempt to

BOX 4.13 HEALTH AND SOCIAL DETERMINANTS/HEALTH EQUITY

Communication: Cultural Competence and Cultural Humility

As health care providers, nurses might believe that they have expert knowledge about health promotion and the treatment of illness that will be beneficial to others. Therefore it seems logical that nurses would select appropriate information to share with individuals to help them maintain health and manage illness or alterations in health status. However, consider the possible influences of cultural or socioeconomic differences between the nurse and individual.

Much of the knowledge generated from nursing-related disciplines and the sciences is rooted in a Western perspective. Particularly in the United States, knowledge is developed and interpreted from the perspective of the dominant cultural group, a white, Anglo-Saxon, Christian point of view. When this perspective remains unexamined, alternative perspectives are ignored and invisible. Nurses who are members of the dominant cultural group may be well-intentioned but ineffective when they attempt to engage a person of a different cultural group in a relationship without questioning how culture influences interactions, interpretations of events and information, and beliefs and values concerning health and health care practices. Preconceived ideas about people based on some characteristic or group affiliation, such as racial or ethnic identity, religion, country of origin, sex, sexual orientation, or socioeconomic status can interfere with nurses' abilities to relate to people as individuals. At the same time, a lack of knowledge of other cultural groups and social contexts hampers nurses' understanding of the individual's point of view.

Guidelines for recognizing the cultural and social context of communication in therapeutic relationships include the following:

- Make ethnocultural assessment a critical component of every clinical evaluation.
- Allow other people to define themselves.
- Ask the person, and the family as appropriate, about cultural health care practices and traditions.
- Respect cultural practices and traditions while providing opportunity for the person to voice preferences and make choices.
- Respect the language of others and do not assume superiority in language.
- Collaborate with trained translators and health promoters (people with the same ethnic or racial background as the individuals).
- Create intercultural open dialogue based on security and mutual respect.
- Avoid use of racist, sexist, ageist, and other forms of denigrating language.
- Do not perpetuate stereotypes in communication.
- Adapt communication to the uniqueness of the individual.
- Reject humor that degrades members on the basis of sex, race, ethnicity, religion, sexual orientation, country of origin, and so forth.
- Respect the rights of others to have different practices and customs.
- Do not allow injustice to continue through silence.
- Present information clearly to all people to help them make informed choices.
- Do not judge values, traditions, and practices on the basis of their similarity to or difference from personal values, traditions, and practices, but judge them on the basis of whether they facilitate human potential.

The following are some issues for the nurse to consider:

- When the nurse works with a person from a different social/cultural background, what are common barriers to establishing a therapeutic relationship?
- In learning about different cultural groups, is there a risk of creating new stereotypes that interfere with the ability to treat people as unique individuals?
- If the nurse has little or no knowledge about a person's culture, how can the nurse provide meaningful nursing care?
- Are the two previous questions contradictory? How can the nurse meet the different challenges that they imply?
- Research measurements typically are developed from the perspective of the dominant culture. If the nurse wishes to use a standardized instrument to measure clinical or research variables among members of different cultural groups, then what questions about the instrument should the nurse ask, and what problems might the nurse encounter? What would need to be done to determine whether an instrument truly measures the same phenomenon across different populations?
- Consider the possible influences of social determinants of health, specifically cultural or other social/socioeconomic differences between the nurse and the individual. Think of an example of two people from diverse cultural or socioeconomic groups who developed a relationship. Examine how they got to know each other and what differences and similarities they uncovered. Did barriers to understanding each other exist? If so, how did they bridge these barriers? What did they learn about themselves? What did they learn about the ways that culture shapes perspective, health equity, and interactions? Think about how nurses can apply these insights to their relationships with people from cultural groups that differ from their own.
- How would a multicultural perspective change the practice?

interpret it in the context of the interaction. Exploration of possible threats in the relationship, goals, context, or a particular topic can lead to understanding the source of the resistance and finding the ability to handle these difficulties. Anxiety reduction is often a necessary step in dealing with resistant behavior.

Transference and Countertransference or Distorting

Transference is reacting to another person in an exchange as though that person were someone from the past. Another term for this process is **distorting**. Transference, although a concept from the psychoanalytic/psychodynamic tradition in psychiatry and psychiatric nursing, retains relevance today. It is best understood as a process that distorts a current relationship or interaction on the basis of past learning, expectations, and/or relationships. Transference or distorting may involve a host of feelings that generally are classified as positive (love, affection, or regard) or negative (anger, dislike, or frustration). Typical transference reactions involve an important figure from the past, such as a mother or father; however, at times transference may be more general to include all authority figures. Something about another person's characteristics, behavior, or position, in combination with individual dynamics and context, triggers this response. People in a therapeutic relationship often develop strong transference feelings toward the helping professional, arising from the interaction's intensity and the clinical provider's authoritative or nurturing role. When transference or distorting reactions interfere with the current relationship (i.e., when reactions are out of proportion to the actual situation, such as excessive anger in response to a nurse's suggestion), they require gentle probing by pointing out the reaction and asking about the associated thoughts and feelings and possible past reactions in similar circumstances (e.g., responses to authority figures). To work with a person's transference reactions effectively, the nurse first helps the person to examine feelings and thoughts about the nurse with a nondefensive or nonreactive stance. Then the nurse assists the person in comparing and contrasting the nurse with people from the person's past to reduce distortions and comprehend the present reality to move forward effectively.

Countertransference is basically the same phenomenon and involves distorting, but it is experienced by the health care professional rather than the person. The nurse experiences many feelings toward the person; these feelings are not problematic unless they remain unanalyzed and block or distort the nurse's ability to work effectively with the individual. For example, if a nurse has strong feelings about the person and thinks that the person cannot possibly function after discharge without the nurse's aid, the nurse is likely to distort the person's abilities, encourage a childlike dependency, and interfere with the person's progress. This nurse needs to examine such personal feelings to understand their source. Once understood, countertransference reactions generally cease to interfere with the relationship. Consultation for supervision with an advanced practice psychiatric nurse or other mental health expert is recommended whenever transference or countertransference (i.e., distorting) reactions are persistent and problematic.

Sensory Barriers

When the individual has sensory limitations, the nurse may need to use extra skill in communicating. Use of the other senses to send or receive messages should be attempted. Special help is often available from trained therapists and teachers; for example, many agencies have access to interpreters for deaf people, and visual aids may be useful. Nurses must be as creative as possible, learn from others who are skilled in alternative forms of communication, and make referrals as necessary. As technology evolves, new communication methods will continue to decrease these barriers. For example, voice recognition software programs help persons with visual and motor challenges communicate via text.

Failure to Address Concerns or Needs

Failure to meet the individual's needs or to recognize the individual's concerns is the most serious barrier to effective interaction. This failure can arise from inadequate assessment, lack of knowledge, inability to separate the nurse's needs from the individual's needs, and confusion between friendship and a helping relationship, including unrecognized or unresolved sexual issues. To address this dilemma, the nurse should recognize that a barrier to relating to the person exists. Using the supervisory/consultation process to determine the problem's source, the nurse should then take corrective action, such as obtaining more information or knowledge, performing a self-assessment with values clarification, and examining reactions, biases, and expectations. Nurses, particularly novice nurses and those transitioning to a new role (e.g., from staff nurse to nurse practitioner after graduate school), need to demand mentorship/clinical supervision that is not tied to performance evaluation. In other words, a supportive mentoring/supervisory relationship with a more senior nurse or another qualified clinician is a necessary ingredient in helping nurses to be effective. Cost-cutting efforts in today's health care system often neglect such needs. Yet consider the cost of a failed hire or ineffective relationships with care recipients. An argument for having professional support can be strong. Additionally, nurses can create their own cost-effective professional support systems by creating peer groups and/or engaging their own consultants with a peer group outside the work setting.

Setting

The setting of a therapeutic interaction can affect the goals and the nature of the communication. The most important aspect of any setting is that the nurse and the individual are able to attend to each other. The nurse's attention to the person helps create this atmosphere. The nurse assesses the influence of factors such as lighting, noise, temperature, comfort, physical distance, and privacy; potentially disturbing factors can be altered or controlled within the limits of the setting. Occasionally the nurse has only minimal control over the setting, as in a busy clinic, health center, inpatient unit, emergency department, or the individual's home. Although far from the ideal of a quiet, pleasant, well-lit private office, these typical clinical settings can be used effectively by creating a sense of private space. Curtains can be drawn, doors shut, and two chairs pulled to a corner to shape an environment for interaction. When possible, however, nurses seek offices or rooms to establish privacy during significant communication or when imparting important or complex health information. Home settings can be more comfortable for individuals than for nurses yet can provide invaluable context when used. The nurse can also acknowledge verbally that some aspect of the environment, such as an interruption or noise, is bothersome. This strategy shows people that the nurse recognizes possible concentration difficulties and is sharing the environment with them. Notably in today's world of virtual/online interactions, the setting may be a home or even a car. Flexibility, attending to privacy issues, and ascertaining the person's location for safety reasons are key strategies in this online age.

Stage

Therapeutic relationships follow sequential phases, which may overlap, differ in length, or involve issues that appear over time rather than in a set sequence. Orientation (introductory), working, and termination phases have been identified by researchers and clinicians (Peplau, 1991; Townsend & Morgan, 2020).

Originally these **relationship stages** were identified from clinical interactions that developed over a prolonged period. However, they can be observed in brief encounters that are effective; that is, interactions that meet individuals' needs rather than therapeutic interactions that have been reduced to little more than quick question-and-answer sessions. Whether the nurse is engaged in a long-term or short-term relationship with an individual, attention to relationship stages is important. Brief therapeutic relationships will telescope the stages; therefore, it is particularly important that the nurse focus on meeting the key demands of each relationship phase. It is important to note that individuals may move in and out of direct care episodes, while a therapeutic relationship can be maintained over a longer period. A relationship exists even when the nurse and the individual do not see each other for an extended period, and each encounter occurs within the trajectory of the relationship stages.

Orientation or Introductory Phase

The orientation or introductory phase begins when the nurse and the individual meet. This meeting typically involves some feeling of anxiety; neither party knows what to expect. When the therapeutic relationship is primarily a counseling type of

BOX 4.14 Key Topics of Discussion During the Orientation or Introductory Phase of the Therapeutic Relationship

- What to call each other
- Purpose of meeting
- Location, time, and length of meetings
- Termination date or time for review of progress through follow-up
- Confidentiality (with whom clinical data will be shared)
- Any other limits related to the particular setting

relationship, part of the nurse's role is to help structure the interaction by discussing several topics during the initial meeting and sometimes during the first few meetings. Box 4.14 lists topics appropriate to this phase. Discussion of these issues establishes a contract or pact and involves a mutual understanding of the parameters of the relationship and an agreement to work together.

The orientation stage is a critical juncture in any therapeutic relationship. Without successful transition through the orientation phase, no working alliance will exist, and the treatment goals will remain unmet. Consistency, sensitive pacing of communication, active listening, conveying concern and warmth, and paying attention to comfort and control help to establish a connection during the orientation phase. In contrast, inconsistency, unavailability, individual factors associated with trust, nurses' feelings about the other person, confrontation of delusions or strongly held views, and unrealistic expectations hamper relationships.

When the therapeutic relationship is not structured primarily as counseling with a specific number of sessions, the orientation phase may appear less distinct, and the topics noted may seem irrelevant. In this case, the nurse can adapt the suggested topics to meet the specific situation. However, except in true emergencies, initial encounters should always include introductions by name, discussion of the purpose, and presentation of a plan for ongoing care or specific follow-up.

Working Phase

The working phase of the therapeutic relationship emerges when the nurse and the individual collaborate as partners in promoting the person's health. The working phase may last for only a brief time to establish a treatment plan; may last for an established number of sessions, as in brief psychotherapy; or may extend over a longer period if the nurse is the primary care provider, care manager, or long-term caregiver in any setting or context for an individual or family. During the working phase, the relationship is the context through which change occurs. Goals are set, and the nurse and the individual work mutually toward their accomplishment. Interventions are tailored to the specific situation and health needs of the person and the family. Solving problems, coping with stressors, and gaining insight are all part of the working phase. The nurse and the individual recognize each other's uniqueness and establish trust as the first step in establishing a working relationship.

Resistant behaviors may be observed during this phase while the nurse and the individual become closer and work on potentially anxiety-producing problems. The person may pull away through the use of defense mechanisms because change can be difficult. Overcoming the resistance becomes an important nursing task.

Termination Phase

Termination marks the end of the relationship established in the therapeutic contract or negotiated in accordance with the limits of the contract. Ending a relationship can cause anxiety for both the individual and the nurse. Termination represents a loss; therefore, it can trigger feelings of sadness, frustration, and anger. Termination in this case is the loss of a relationship and the loss of future involvement, with its attendant realistic expectations or fantasies. Termination also reawakens feelings of previously unresolved losses, such as a death or divorce.

Working through any feelings related to termination is an important part of clinical care. Some individuals require the nurse's assistance to experience the feelings of loss and to connect present reactions to past real or symbolic losses. Box 4.15 lists additional interventions for use during the termination phase.

Both the nurse and the individual can learn much during termination; the process directs both participants to examine problems and progress in the relationship, feelings, and reactions. The experience also helps the nurse and the individual gain practice in ending relationships and in exploring reactions, which can be most helpful when future losses occur. Nonetheless, major gains can be accomplished with the deadline of termination. Options for follow-up or future treatment as the need determines also require exploration and planning.

Brief Interactions

Time constraints in practice are unavoidable. Although challenging, brief therapeutic encounters can be meaningful and useful. Limited time is not a valid reason to avoid interviewing or interacting with individuals. Rather, nurses can purposefully structure brief interactions to achieve specific clinical outcomes (Field et al., 2019). Box 4.16 delineates key ingredients for a 15-minute (or shorter) interview with a family (Shajani & Snell, 2019).

These guidelines for brief interactions with families can be adapted for interviews with individuals. An effective 15-minute

BOX 4.15 Interventions for Use During the Termination Phase of the Therapeutic Relationship

- Let the person know why the relationship is to be terminated.
- Remind the person of the date and how many meetings or appointments are left.
- Collaborate with other staff so that they are aware of how the person is reacting and any special needs that the person may have.
- Help the person to identify sources of support and other people with whom a relationship is possible.
- Review the gains and the remaining goals.
- Discuss the pros and cons experienced during the relationship to help the person develop a realistic appraisal.
- Make referrals for follow-up care as needed.

BOX 4.16 Key Ingredients for a 15-Minute (or Shorter) Family Interview

- Use manners to engage or reengage family members. Make an introduction by offering your name and role. Orient family members to the purpose of a brief family interview.
- Assess significant areas of internal and external structure and function (obtain information from a genogram concerning basic family composition and external support data).
- Ask family members three key questions.
- Commend the family on one or two strengths.
- Evaluate usefulness and conclude.

Source: Shajani, Z., & Snell, D. (2019). *Wright & Leahey's nurses and families: A guide to family assessment and intervention* (7th ed.). Philadelphia: F. A. Davis.

(or shorter) interview is feasible if nurses plan to introduce themselves; state the purpose of meeting; validate understanding with the person or the family; clarify parameters such as time, focus, and listening; and elicit significant individual and family data. Most important, the goal of the interaction must be realistic and clearly defined. For example, the purpose may be to elicit a family's view of the problem for which the person has sought care or to prioritize problems to be treated. Even when time is limited, the interview is structured to provide an opportunity for the person or the family to engage in dialogue as an active participant in care, and the nurse's attention is completely focused on the individual.

Circumstances also can dictate the need for immediate and instructive communications that command specific actions. For example, during a crisis, directive, clear communication is paramount. Guo, Bian, Li, Li, & Lin, 2023 documented the core competencies of disaster nursing using a scoping review of the international nursing literature. They included communication, understanding of a disaster plan, and ethics of disaster nursing. Planning in anticipation of human-caused and natural disasters is critical so as to have functional communication systems in place. Such systems will increasingly use various methods of telecommunication. After tragic events have occurred, including shootings on school and college campuses, efforts to communicate more effectively are paramount. Universities, for example, have responded by instituting systems to communicate rapidly with a large campus community. Widely deployed strategies feature instant text messaging and emailing (see Box 4.6: Best Practice).

BOX 4.17 GENOMICS

According to the Centers for Disease Control and Prevention (CDC) (2024), genetic counseling provides information about how genetic conditions might affect an individual or family. The genetic counselor or other clinician, including the nurse, collects personal and family health history. The counselor/clinician uses this information to determine how likely it is that an individual or a family member might have a genetic condition. Based on this information, the genetic counselor/clinician helps the client to decide whether a genetic test might be warranted (CDC, 2024). This process sounds straightforward, yet its human context is highly complex. The decision to have genetic testing involves existential issues about life and death, chronic illness and disability, risk for potential children, and one's personal or family members' future. Thus genetic counseling must occur within a trusting therapeutic relationship. Sensitivity to the fears and potential effect for the client and possibly their family is essential to providing effective counseling. A rushed, purely informational or coercive style by the counselor is never appropriate or therapeutic. Think about the following brief vignette and how a therapeutic relationship could have eased the parents' distress despite their understandable anxiety about a real threat to their child's health.

A 4-month-old baby girl was referred by her pediatrician for testing for a potential genetic health disorder due to lower-than-expected growth. The clinician who performed the test told the parents what to do to get the baby to "cooperate" without talking with them about their thoughts or concerns. After the sample was obtained, the parents had to wait with their baby in a busy waiting room and watch some other parents being taken to a private room to hear results while seeing other parents receive good (that is, negative) results in the waiting area. While waiting, the mother experienced severe anxiety. She knew that she would learn that their baby either did or did not have a life-threatening chronic condition. The lack of empathy shown by the clinician heightened the mother's distress even when she recalled it decades later, as did the public waiting setting and insensitive format for delivering results. This example illustrates the importance of establishing a therapeutic relationship for genetic counseling and testing even if the interaction is brief. Providing appropriate privacy is also a necessary relational component of genetic counseling and testing.

Another apt example of a typically brief interaction is genetic counseling and testing. As genetic testing increases in frequency and online testing proliferates, the "human touch" necessarily decreases. Nonetheless, the decision to have testing and the process of receiving and understanding results are best undertaken within a supportive clinical relationship (Box 4.17: Genomics).

The following case study presents a detailed scenario of a home visit and questions related to how the nurse can develop a therapeutic relationship with the person. The care plan presents a plan of care for the person, including communication interventions.

CASE STUDY

A Health-Promotion Visit: Maria Sanchez-Smith

As part of a health-promotion visit for Maria Sanchez-Smith and Thomas, her 2-week-old infant, Jessica Wong, a registered nurse, planned to conduct an infant assessment, provide breastfeeding support, teach about normal infant development and care activities, and assess Mrs. Sanchez-Smith's adaptation to motherhood and her postpartum recovery status. Before the visit, Ms. Wong reviewed the clinical information she obtained during Mrs. Sanchez-Smith's hospitalization. Mrs. Sanchez-Smith was a 34-year-old Hispanic primiparous female who had delivered a 7-pound, 10-ounce healthy boy (Thomas) after a 12-hour labor. The labor had progressed well without complications. Mrs. Sanchez-Smith received epidural anesthesia at 6-cm dilatation, and the baby was delivered vaginally. Her husband, Mark Smith, provided labor support and was present for the delivery. After a 2-day hospital stay, Mrs. Sanchez-Smith was discharged. At discharge, the infant was breastfeeding, had normal newborn examination findings, and weighed 7 pounds, 5 ounces. Ms. Wong had been impressed by both parents' preparation for the birth. They had attended childbirth classes and read several books about infant development and parenting. Ms. Sanchez-Smith

Continued

CASE STUDY—cont'd

A Health-Promotion Visit: Maria Sanchez-Smith

planned to take an 8-week maternity leave from her position as a lawyer in a large practice and had arranged for a childcare provider to come to the family's home to take care of the infant beginning 2 weeks before the end of her maternity leave. Mr. Smith had not planned to take time off from his job because he had recently been promoted to a high-level managerial position in his company that required increased travel and time at work. He was able to postpone a business trip to be present at the delivery and had sent a plane ticket to his mother-in-law so she could come and stay at their home during the first week after Mrs. Sanchez-Smith and Thomas were discharged from the hospital.

During the visit, Ms. Wong first assessed the infant. She incorporated teaching concerning normal infant development and concluded that Thomas was a healthy 2-week-old infant who was feeding well. Thomas's circumcision was healing without complications, and he had regained his birth weight.

When Ms. Wong asked how Mrs. Sanchez-Smith was doing, Mrs. Sanchez-Smith hesitated and then responded, "I'm not sure. I'm very glad that Thomas is doing well . . . but I worry sometimes that I'm not going to be able to do everything right for him. It's funny, but I've spent so many years getting an education and establishing my law career. It was hard work, but I managed to do well. Now a little infant overwhelms me. I don't know how I'll manage this." When Ms. Wong asked Mrs. Sanchez-Smith to talk more about her concerns, Mrs. Sanchez-Smith described how incompetent she felt while her mother was staying with her. "My mother could do everything so easily. I fumbled with every diaper. It felt like she criticized how I did things. When she told me about what she did when she had children, I felt pushed to do things 'her way' and not the way that I had planned. She even wanted to give him a bottle when I was trying so hard to get breastfeeding going. At least the doctor said Thomas had gained enough weight. Thomas's weight gain made me feel like I wasn't a total failure. I couldn't wait for her to go, but I fell apart after she left. I was alone. Mark is out of town until the weekend, and I couldn't get Thomas to stop crying yesterday. I thought I would scream, so I put him down in his crib and I just sat there crying. What's wrong with me? I've never felt so out of control before. I want to be a good mother, but I feel like I can't give any more right now."

In response to Ms. Wong's follow-up questions about mental status, Mrs. Sanchez-Smith described frequently feeling irritated and sad, crying a few times over the previous several days, having difficulty sleeping even when the baby was asleep, feeling fatigued, and being worried about how she would be able to go back to work in only a few weeks. Ms. Wong also inquired about the family's cultural, ethnic, and religious backgrounds. Mrs. Sanchez-Smith responded, "Interesting that you should ask. That's actually another issue right now. I'm from New Mexico and my family is Hispanic and Catholic, but I'm not a practicing Catholic now. You might guess that I'm Latina from my hyphenated name. I added my maiden name to *Smith* when I got married to honor my family. Mark is Protestant but not really religious. His family comes from New Jersey. They are very nice and were supportive when we got married. We were lucky that our families accepted us together. I have to admit, though, that we didn't really figure out what we would do about raising the baby. Mark thinks that we'd be hypocrites to have a Catholic christening. Plus, my mother told me that I'd be selfish to go back to work so soon. Can you help me? I feel like I'm going out of my mind and I don't know what to do."

This case study raises a variety of clinical concerns. As the nurse in this encounter, Ms. Wong could begin by considering the following questions.

Reflective Questions

- What are my feelings as I listen to her story and her distress? Am I aware of how my values and expectations affect my interaction with this person? How can I establish a therapeutic relationship to support Mrs. Sanchez-Smith during this stressful period?
- What is the significance of the distress symptoms that Mrs. Sanchez-Smith reported? Given that the period during which many females experience postpartum blues is passing or has passed, what is the most appropriate action for referral to obtain a thorough mental status examination for postpartum depression?
  - Who is the most appropriate health care provider to evaluate her for postpartum depression and to treat her if it is confirmed? How can I facilitate getting her the care she needs, and can I remain available to her? How can I assist Mrs. Sanchez-Smith to meet the infant's developmental needs during this stressful period?
  - Should I use a postpartum depression screening tool to help assess? What does Mrs. Sanchez-Smith's obstetrical practice use to screen for depression/anxiety symptoms? Was she screened at the hospital, as is now commonly best practice?
  - Is contacting Mrs. Sanchez-Smith's obstetrical provider the first step for follow-up?
    - How should I discuss this with Mrs. Sanchez-Smith?
    - When is her regular postpartum check-up scheduled, and might it be moved up?
  - Is return to work at 8-weeks postpartum a realistic goal? What options might be explored?
- In what ways do family dynamics, values, and expectations related to differing cultural, generational, and religious heritages contribute to the problems described? What can I do to explore these issues further? What strengths can be harnessed? Are there clergy who could be engaged for pastoral counseling? How can I engage support systems to ameliorate rather than exacerbate the difficulties? What can be done to engage both Mr. Smith and Mrs. Sanchez-Smith in a therapeutic relationship to focus on couple and parenting concerns and to involve both partners in treatment strategies?

SUMMARY

- Relating to persons has many challenges and rewards for nurses. Although some aspects of this work are predictable, each individual and family is unique and provides a chance for the nurse to learn, grow, and help in new ways.
- This chapter has provided guidelines for developing therapeutic relationships, but these guidelines do not guarantee success or an easy job. The desire and skill of the individual nurse inform best practice.
- The blend of the nurse's artistry, humanity, knowledge, skill, and ethics sparks concern and the ability to help another human being communicate effectively. These are essential components of the nurse-person relationship.
- Rising use of technology and mounting pressures for cost-effective care are here to stay. In this climate, the importance of the therapeutic relationship is underscored.
- The therapeutic relationship is the primary arena for health promotion. Values clarification, communication, and the helping relationship are its core components. For nurses, applying this knowledge to their varied roles is essential to promoting health and providing quality care.

EVOLVE CHAPTER FEATURES

http://evolve.elsevier.com/Edelman/

- Study Questions

REFERENCES

Alsalamah, Y., Albagawi, B., Babkair, L., Alsalamah, F., Itani, M. S., Tassi, A., & Fawaz, M. (2022). Perspectives of nursing students on Promoting Reflection in the Clinical Setting: A Qualitative Study. *Nursing Reports*, *12*(3), 545–555. https://doi.org.10.3390/nursrep12030053.

Agency for Healthcare Research and Quality (AHRQ). (2020). *Health literacy universal precautions toolkit*. Content last reviewed September 2020. Agency for Healthcare Research and Quality, Rockville, MD. https://www.ahrq.gov/health-literacy/improve/precautions/toolkit.html

Amoah, V. M. K., Anokye, R., Boakye, D. S., Acheampong, E., Budu-Ainooson, A., Okyere, E., Kumi-Boateng, G., Yeboah, C., & Afriyie, J. O. (2019). A qualitative assessment of perceived barriers to effective therapeutic communication among nurses and patients. *BMC Nursing*, *18*(1). https://doi.org/10.1186/s12912-019-0328-0

Anderson, M., & Kumar, M. (2019). Digital divide persists even as lower-income Americans make gains in tech adoption. *FactTank*. https://www.pewresearch.org

Bakerjian, D. (2023). *Personal health literacy*. Patient Safety Network. https://psnet.ahrq.gov/primer/personal-health-literacy

Barker, M. E., Leach, K. T., & Levett-Jones, T. (2023). Patient's views of empathic and compassionate healthcare interactions: A scoping review. *Nurse Education Today*, *131*. https://doi.org/10.1016/j.nedt.2023.105957

Bischof, G., Bischof, A., & Rumpf, H.J. (2021). Motivational Interviewing: An Evidence-Based Approach for Use in Medical Practice. *Deutsches Ärzteblatt International*, *118*(7), 109–115. https://doi.org/10.3238/arztebl.m2021.0014

Blondis, M. N., & Jackson, B. E. (1982). *Nonverbal communication with patients: Back to the human touch* (2nd ed.). New York: John Wiley & Sons.

Bright, A., & Doody, O. (2023). Mental health service users' experiences of telehealth interventions facilitated during the COVID-19 pandemic and their relevance to nursing: An integrative review. *Journal of Psychiatric & Mental Health Nursing (John Wiley & Sons, Inc.)*, *30*(6), 1114–1129. https://doi.org/10.1111/jpm.12943

Bulkes, N. Z., Davis, K., Kay, B., & Riemann, B. C. (2022). Comparing efficacy of telehealth to in-person mental health care in intensive-treatment-seeking adults. *Journal of Psychiatric Research*, *5*, 347–352. https://doi.org/10.1016/j.jpsychires.2021.11.003

Center for Disease Control and Prevention (CDC). (2024). *Genomics and precision health*. https://www.cdc.gov

Cheraghi, R., Valizadeh, L., Zamanzadeh, V., Hassankhani, H., & Jafarzadeh, A. (2023). Clarification of ethical principle of the beneficence in nursing care: an integrative review. *BMC Nursing*, *22*(1), 89. doi:10.1186/s12912-023-01246-4

Choice, E., & Thomas, S. Evaluation of Undergraduate Internship Interprofessional Experiences Using the Jefferson Teamwork Observation Guide (JTOG). *The Internet Journal of Allied Health Sciences and Practice*, *21*(3), Article 17.

Cole, S. A., Sannidhi, D., Jadotte, Y. T., & Rozanski, A. (2023). Using motivational interviewing and brief action planning for adopting and maintaining positive health behaviors. *Progress in Cardiovascular Diseases*, *77*, 86–94, ISSN 0033-0620. https://doi.org/10.1016/j.pcad.2023.02.003

De Leon, M., Solomon-Rice, P., & Soto, G. (2023). Perspectives and experiences of eight Latina mothers of young children with augmentative and alternative communication needs. *Perspectives of the ASHA Special Interest Groups*, *8*(5), 1072–1085. https://doi.org/10.1044/2023_PERSP-23-00074

Denworth, L. (2019). "Hyperscans" show how brains sync as people interact. *The Scientific American*. https://www.scientificamerican.com/article/hyperscans-show-how-brains-sync-as-people-interact/

Edge, D., & Lemetyinen, H. (2019). Psychology across cultures: Challenges and opportunities. *Psychology and Psychotherapy: Theory, Research and Practice*, *92*(2), 262–276. https://doi.org/10.1111/papt.12229

Field, C., Oviedo Ramirez, S., Juarez, P., & Castro, Y. (2019). Process for developing a culturally informed brief motivational intervention. *Addictive Behaviors*, *95*, 129–137. https://doi.org/10.1016/j.addbeh.2019.03.002

Gamage, K. A. A., Dehideniya, D. M. S. C. P. K., & Ekanayake, S.Y. (2021). The role of personal values in learning approaches and student achievements. *Behavioral Science (Basel)*, *11*(7),102. doi:10.3390/bs11070102

Grover, C., Mackasey, E., Cook, E., Tremblay, L., & Loiselle, C. G. (2018). Patient-reported care domains that enhance the experience of "being known" in an ambulatory cancer care centre. *Canadian Oncology Nursing Journal*, *28*(3), 166–177. https://doi.org/10.5737/23688076283166171

Guo, X. E., Bian, L. F., Li, Y., Li, C. Y., & Lin, Y. (2023). Common domains of nurses' competencies in public health emergencies: A scoping review. *BMC Nursing*, *22*, 490. https://doi.org/10.1186/s12912-023-01655-5

Hall, E. (1973). *The silent language*. Garden City, NY: Doubleday/Anchor Press.

Hong, S., & Lee, J. Y. (2022). Evaluation of therapeutic communication education for nursing students based on constructivist learning environments: A systematic review. *Nurse Education Today*, *119*. https://doi.org/10.1016/j.nedt.2022.105607

Jared, B. (2019). *The impact of teach-back as a patient education tool in women with inadequate maternal health literacy seeking immunizations for their children*. (2019-41129-097). ProQuest Information & Learning.

Kadji, K., & Mast, M. S. (2021). The effect of physician self-disclosure on patient self-disclosure and patient perceptions of the physician. *Patient Education & Counseling*, *104*(9), 2224–2231. https://doi.org/10.1016/j.pec.2021.02.030

Karami, M., Ashtarian, H., Rajati, M., Hamzeh, B., & Rajati, F. (2023). The effect of health literacy intervention on adherence to medication of uncontrolled hypertensive patients using the M-health. *BMC Medical Informatics & Decision Making*, *23*(1), 1–10. https://doi.org/10.1186/s12911-023-02393-z

Kim, L. Y., Giannitrapani, K. F., Huynh, A. K., Ganz, D. A., Hamilton, A. B., Yano, E. M., & Stockdale, S. E. (2019). What makes team communication effective: A qualitative analysis of interprofessional primary care team members' perspectives. *Journal of Interprofessional Care*, *33*(6), 836–838. https://doi.org/10.1080/13561820.2019.1577809

Kirca, N., & Bademli, K. (2019). Relationship between communication skills and care behaviors of nurses. *Perspectives in Psychiatric Care*, *55*(4), 624–631. https://doi.org/10.1111/ppc.12381

Knapp, M. L., Hall, J. A., & Horgan, T. G. (2020). *Nonverbal communication in human interaction* (8th ed.). Boston: Wadsworth Cengage Learning.

Knol A. S. L., Koole T., Desmet M., Vanheule S., Huiskes M. (2020). How speakers orient to the notable absence of talk: A conversation analytic perspective on silence in psychodynamic therapy. *Frontiers in Psychology*, *11*. https://doi.org/10.3389/fpsyg.2020.584927

Knowlton, E. K., Sternlieb, J. L., & Freedy, J. R. (2020). The clinician-patient relationship: The therapeutic value of the clinical encounter. *International Journal of Psychiatry in Medicine*, *55*(1), 3–7. https://doi.org/10.1177/0091217419894472

Kwame, A., & Petrucka, P. M. (2021). A literature-based study of patient-centered care and communication in nurse-patient interactions: Barriers, facilitators, and the way forward. *BMC Nursing*, *20*(1), 1–10. https://doi.org/10.1186/s12912-021-00684-2

Larsen, C. B., & Gilstad, H. (2023). Trust and distrust toward online health information in nurse–patient communication and implications for eHealth literacy. *Journal of Communication in Healthcare*, *16*(4), 412–420. https://doi.org/10.1080/17538068.2023.2279397

Lee, J., & Son, H. K. (2022). Effects of simulation problem-based learning based on Peplau's Interpersonal Relationship Model for cesarean section maternity nursing on communication skills, communication attitudes and team efficacy. *Nurse Education Today*, *113*. https://doi.org/10.1016/j.nedt.2022.105373

Likhar, A., Baghel, P., & Patil, M. (2022). Early childhood development and social determinants. *Cureus 14*(9), e29500. https://doi.org/10.7759/cureus.29500

Lyons, K. J., Giordano, C., Speakman, E., Smith, K., & Horowitz, J. A. (2016). Jefferson Teamwork Observation Guide (JTOG): An instrument to observe teamwork behaviors. *Journal of Allied Health*, *45*(1), 49–53. https://www.jstor.org/stable/48721893

Mersha, A., Abera, A., Tesfaye, T., Abera, T., Belay, A., Melaku, T., Shiferaw, M., Shibiru, S., Estifanos, W., & Wake, S. K. (2023). Therapeutic communication and its associated factors among nurses working in public hospitals of Gamo zone, southern Ethiopia: Application of Hildegard Peplau's nursing theory of interpersonal relations. *BMC Nursing*, *22*(1), 1–10. https://doi.org/10.1186/s12912-023-01526-z

National Academy of Medicine (2022). https://nam.edu/

National Institutes of Health (2023). *An introduction to health literacy*. https://www.nnlm.gov/guides/intro-health-literacy

Oliver, D., Tappana, J., Washington, K., Rolbiecki, A., Craig, K., & Ellington, L. (2019). Behind the doors of home hospice patients: A secondary qualitative analysis of hospice nurse communication with patients and families. *Palliative and Supportive Care*, *17*, 579–583.

Osborne, H. (2021). *Health literacy from A to Z: Practical ways to communicate your health message* (2nd ed.). Aviva Publishing.

Osmancevic, S., Großschädl, F. & Lohrmann, C. (2023). Cultural competence among nursing students and nurses working in acute care settings: A cross-sectional study. *BMC Health Service Research 23*, 105. https://doi.org/10.1186/s12913-023-09103-5

Palaz, S. C., & Kayacan, S. (2023). The relationship between the level of trust in nurses and nursing care quality perceptions of patients treated for Covid-19. *Scandinavian Journal of Caring Science*, *7*(2), 364–372. https://doi.org/10.1111/scs.13114

Peplau, H. E. (1963). Process and concept of learning. In S. Burd, & M. Marshall (Eds.), *Some clinical approaches to psychiatric nursing* (pp 348–352). New York: Macmillan.

Peplau, H. E. (1964). *Basic principles of patient counseling* (2nd ed.). Philadelphia: Smith Kline and French Laboratories.

Peplau, H. E. (1969). Professional closeness: As a special kind of involvement with a patient, client, or family group. *Nursing Forum*, *8*(4), 342–360.

Peplau, H. E. (1991). *Interpersonal relations in nursing*. New York: Springer.

Pew Research Center. (2019). *Defining generations: Where Millennials end and Generation Z begins*. https://www.pewresearch.org/fact-tank/2019/01/17/where-millennials-end-and-generation-z-begins/

Quality Safety and Education for Nurses (QSEN). (2023). *Patient centered care*. http://www.qsen.org/competencies/pre-licensure-ksas

Raths, L., Harmin, M., & Simon, S. (1978). *Values and teaching*. Columbus, OH: Charles E. Merrill.

Renzulli, C. (2019). Telemental health (Letter to the Editor). *Journal of the American Psychiatric Nurses Association*, *25*, 253–254.

Riviere, M., Dufoort, H., Van Hecke, A., Vandecasteele, T., Beeckman, D., & Verhaeghe, S. (2019). Core elements of the interpersonal care relationship between nurses and older patients without cognitive impairment during their stay in the hospital: A mixed-methods systematic review. *International Journal of Nursing Studies*, *92*, 154–172.

Rockwell, S. L., Woods, C. L., Lemmon, M. E., Baker, J. N., Mack, J. W., Andes, K. L., & Kaye, E. C. (2022). Silence in conversations about advancing pediatric cancer. *Frontiers in Oncology*, *12*, 894586. https://doi.org/10.3389/fonc.2022.894586

Shajani, Z., & Snell, D. (2019). *Wright & Leahey's nurses and families: A guide to family assessment and intervention* (7th ed.). Philadelphia: F. A. Davis.

Schot, E., Tummers, L., & Noordegraaf, M. (2020). Working on working together. A systematic review on how healthcare professionals contribute to interprofessional collaboration. *Journal of Interprofessional Care*, *34*(3), 332–342. https://doi.org/10.1080/13561820.2019.1636007

Spence, P. R., Lin, X., Lachlan, K. A., & Hutter, E. (2020). Listen up, I've done this before: The impact of self-disclosure on source credibility and risk message responses. *Progress in Disaster Science*, *7*, 100108. https://doi.org/10.1016/j.pdisas.2020.100108

Statistica. (2019). *Internet usage in the United States—statistics & facts*. https://www.statista.com/topics/2237/internet-usage-in-the-united-states/

Stern, G. (2019). High-tech, high touch. *Journal of American Psychiatric Nurses Association*, *25*, 410–411. https://doi.org/10.1177/1078390319869932

Stuart, G. W. (2013). *Principles and practice of psychiatric nursing* (10th ed.). St. Louis: Mosby.

Sullivan, H. S. (1953). *The interpersonal theory of psychiatry*. New York: W.W. Norton.

Townsend, M., & Morgan, K. (2020). *Psychiatric mental health nursing: Concepts of care in evidence-based practice* (9th ed.). Philadelphia, PA: F. A. Davis Co.

Tyson, L. R., Brammer, S., & McIntosh, D. (2019). Telehealth in psychiatric nursing education: Lessons from the field. *Journal of the American Psychiatric Nurses Association*, *25*, 266–271.

US Department of Health and Human Services. (2022). *Healthy People 2030 objectives*. Office of Disease Prevention and Health Promotion. https://www.healthypeople.gov

Vafeiadou, A., Bowling, N.C., Hammond, C., & Banissy, M. J. (2022). Assessing individual differences in attitudes towards touch in treatment settings: Introducing the touch & health scale. *Health Psychology Open*, *9*(2). https://doi.org/10.1177/20551029221137008

Watzlawick, P., Beavin, J. H., & Jackson, D. D. (1967). *Pragmatics of human communication: A study of interactional patterns, pathologies and paradoxes*. New York: W.W. Norton.

Witteman, H. O., Ndjaboue, R., Vaisson, G., Dansokho, S. C., Arnold, B., Bridges, J. F. P., Comeau, S., Fagerlin, A., Gavaruzzi, T., Marcoux, M., Pieterse, A., Pignone, M., Provencher, T., Racine, C., Regier, D., Rochefort-Brihay, C., Thokala, P., Weernink, M., White, D. B., & Wills, C. E. (2021). Clarifying values: An updated and expanded systematic review and meta-analysis. *Medical Decision Making*, *41*(7), 801–820. https://doi.org/10.1177/0272989X211037946

Xue, W., & Miller, C. H. (2021). Therapeutic communication within the nurse–patient relationship: A concept analysis. *International Journal of Nursing Practice (John Wiley & Sons, Inc.)*, *27*(6), 1–8. https://doi.org/10.1111/ijn.12938

5

Ethical Issues Related to Health Promotion

Yvonne M. Smith and Carolyn Cable Kleman

http://evolve.elsevier.com/Edelman/

OBJECTIVES

After completing this chapter, the reader will be able to:

- Discuss health promotion as a moral endeavor.
- Describe the relationship of health care ethics to health promotion.
- Analyze the relationships between various ethical theories and the nursing role in health promotion.
- Discuss the historical development and importance of the nursing code of ethics.
- Describe contemporary ethical issues in health promotion (e.g., genetics, genomics, culture, end-of-life decision-making).
- Analyze problems related to health promotion using an ethical decision-making framework.

KEY TERMS

Advocacy
Applied ethics
Autonomy
Beliefs
Beneficence
Civil liberties
Codes of ethics
Confidentiality
Consent
Consequentialist
Descriptive theories
Duty-based theories
Ethical dilemmas
Ethical issues
Feminist ethics
Genetic counseling
Genetics
Genomics
Genotype
Health Insurance Portability and Accountability Act (HIPAA)
Informed consent
Justice
Maleficence
Metaethics
Moral
Moral agency
Moral distress
Moral injury
Moral philosophy
Nonmaleficence
Normative theories
Paternalism
Phenotype
Practical wisdom
Preventive ethics
Privacy Rule
Social justice
Theoretical wisdom
Trust
Utilitarian theories
Value theories
Veracity
Virtue ethics

THINK ABOUT IT

Assisted Suicide or Emotional Support?

A nurse in a clinic is accountable for ongoing assessments of pain management. One of the long-term clients, Ana, has required increasing amounts of narcotics for her pain management over the last year. The nurse has known for more than a year that Ana's husband, Victor, has amyotrophic lateral sclerosis, or Lou Gehrig disease. Victor's disease adds a great deal of stress to both their lives, which has had a negative effect on Ana's physical health. The nurse assesses the emotional toll of Victor's illness as part of Ana's pain assessment. During one of these discussions, Ana asks the nurse how much of her narcotic medication her husband would need to take to end his life.

- What are the implications of providing someone, indirectly, with the means to commit suicide?
- What questions should the nurse ask Ana at this point of the conversation?
- Imagine how Ana might respond. What should the nurse say or do in response to her answers?
- What obligations, if any, does the nurse have to Victor?
- Does the nurse have a responsibility to collaborate with Victor's physician?
- What is in Ana's best interests?
- Who or what are the nurse's resources?
- Do national nursing organizations have written guidelines about assisted suicide?
- What is the law in your state?
- What should you do as the nurse?

HEALTH PROMOTION AS A MORAL ENDEAVOR

The American Nurses Association (ANA) designated 2015 as "The Year of Ethics." A highlight of the year was a revision of the Code of Ethics for Nurses with Interpretive Statements, which was the first revision since 2001. The revised code provides a succinct statement of ethical values, obligations, and duties of nurses and describes nursing's understanding of its commitment to society. The code frames how nurses provide service to society through health-promotion interventions; this care can be seen as a moral endeavor. Nurses confront moral issues in the process of attempting to enhance the well-being of a society overall, as well as in promoting and protecting health for individual members of a society. Health is considered a human good because it helps people to have a desirable quality of life and to achieve life goals. At the level of the individual, health promotion involves providing services that help people achieve their potential.

To set a higher standard of health for all people, nurses must understand the contexts of people's lives. This understanding entails consideration of a variety of factors that can affect a person's health status, such as mental, physical, spiritual, environmental, cultural, social, and genetic factors. Viewing health promotion as a moral endeavor is consistent with the intent and goals of the US government's prevention agenda for the nation as presented in *Healthy People 2030* (Office of Disease Prevention and Health Promotion [ODPHP], 2022).

The *Healthy People 2030* overarching goals are presented in the following list. For a side-by-side comparison of *Healthy People* goals from 1990 to 2030, see Table 1.1: Current and Historical Overarching Goals of *Healthy People*.

- Attain healthy, thriving lives and well-being, free of preventable disease, disability, injury, and premature death.
- Eliminate health disparities, achieve health equity, and attain health literacy to improve the health and well-being of all.
- Create social, physical, and economic environments that promote attaining full potential for health and well-being for all.
- Promote healthy development, healthy behaviors, and well-being across all life stages.
- Engage leadership, key constituents, and the public across multiple sectors to take action and design policies that improve the health and well-being of all.

The purpose of health-promotion efforts, as discussed throughout this book, is to ensure that people have access to the tools and strategies they need to live at the highest level of well-being possible. Health-promotion efforts address environmental obstacles to human health, such as pollution, marketing of harmful products, and economic disparities. Thus, health promotion is not the province of a single discipline but requires collaboration among patients, health care providers, and institutions to create a nurturing environment for achieving health goals.

This chapter focuses on understanding the health professional's moral responsibilities toward individuals and facilitating health and well-being, or the relief of suffering. Professional responsibilities are obligations incurred by disciplines that provide a service to society. For example, the Code of Ethics for Nurses with Interpretive Statements (ANA, 2015a) states that nursing addresses the "protection, promotion, and restoration of health and well-being; the prevention of illness and injury; and the alleviation of suffering, in the care of individuals, families, groups, communities, and populations" (p. vii). This document, along with the ANA's Guide to Nursing's Social Policy Statement (ANA, 2015b), describes the ethical responsibilities of US nurses. This chapter includes a link to the ANA's Code of Ethics for Nurses with Interpretive Statements. The International Council of Nurses (2021) also has a code of ethics, which is easily accessible via the Internet and serves as a standard for nurses worldwide.

Ethical issues focused on health promotion are best viewed as a subset of health care ethics that, in turn, has its roots in moral philosophy and value theory. This chapter discusses factors that can affect health promotion across the life span in diverse health care settings. The development, scope, and limits of ethical theories and perspectives are explored in relation to problems in health promotion. A basic assumption in this chapter is that the anticipation and prevention of ethical problems is a critical component of ethical professional action. A variety of real and hypothetical cases are presented to illustrate how ethical issues relate to health promotion. Strategies to aid nurses in identifying, anticipating, and addressing ethical issues are provided throughout.

The terms *ethical* and *moral* are used interchangeably throughout the chapter. Even though the two concepts are sometimes characterized differently, they have similar root meanings. The term *ethics* is derived from the Greek word *ethos*, meaning "customs, conduct, or character." The term **moral** is derived from the Latin word *mores* and originally referred to doing something from a custom or habit (Sproul, 2015).

HEALTH CARE ETHICS

Origins of Applied Ethics in Moral Philosophy

The discipline underlying ethical practice, or **applied ethics**, is **moral philosophy**. Moral philosophy is concerned with discovering or proposing what is right or wrong, or good or bad, in human action toward other humans and other entities such as animals and the environment. Singer (1993, 2023) described the crucial questions of moral philosophy as "What ought I to do? How ought I to live?" Among the tasks of moral philosophy is that of formulating theories or frameworks to guide action. Using a moral theory to propose and implement appropriate actions in troubling situations guides the decision-maker toward good actions and the avoidance of harmful actions.

The theories that emerge through philosophical inquiry about good action are called **value theories**; they are concerned with either discovering what humans seem to value (descriptive theories) or proposing what they ought to value (normative theories) to achieve predetermined goals. Value theories are based on observations of human behavior over time and in a variety of settings. **Descriptive theories** do not tell us what actions we ought to take. They are not directives; they merely tell us how people act toward each other and their environments and what they seem to believe are good or moral actions. **Normative theories**, in contrast, are concerned with ensuring good actions.

Types of Normative Ethical Theories

Normative ethical theories are reasoned explanations of the moral purpose of human interactions, or they are believed to be objective truths about good action (divinely given in the case of religious ethics). Actions that are in accord with the foundational principles of the theory are the type of right or good actions we should take given that we believe the principles (e.g., fairness and trust) are valid. What is often called the golden rule is a classic example of a normative principle. The golden rule commits us to treating other people in the manner that we would wish to be treated, given similar circumstances. Normative theories permit judgments about the value of actions on the basis of the extent to which these actions are consistent with the assumptions of the theory. The value of actions is key to decision-making and relevant for health promotion but may be overlooked by policymakers.

Consequentialist Theories

Consequentialist theories of ethics hold that the consequences or intended consequences of actions matter for determining moral worth. From the **consequentialist** perspective, any decision about intended actions or interventions must consider all knowable potential consequences. An example of a consequentialist theory is John Stuart Mill's (2019/1861) theory of utilitarianism, which identifies that actions are good insofar as they aim to yield the greatest amount of happiness or pleasure or cause the least amount of harm or pain to individuals and overall society. Mill viewed pleasure as a complex concept, but his theory is often simplified and summarized as the greatest good for the greatest number. Implications of consequentialist theories are that nurses and other health care professionals must be accountable for thorough and complete data gathering and for possessing the appropriate skills and knowledge to undertake actions that will promote good. Professional decisions can be evaluated as bad or good to the extent that those actions are in accord with the theory. In the case of utilitarianism, "right actions" would be those directed toward promoting the greatest good or causing the least harm. The propositions of the theory direct what is needed for moral action or, stated another way, for doing the right thing.

Duty-Based Theories

Other normative value theories are not as heavily weighted toward producing good consequences. For example, **duty-based theories**, such as the theory of Immanuel Kant (1724–1804) and those of various religions (Judaism, Christianity, Islam), depend more on adherence to duties than on good consequences. Individuals are viewed as having certain duties that cannot be circumvented, even if deliberately avoiding the duty would result in good outcomes. For religions, these rules are imparted in some way by a divine being.

For Kant, the capacity to reason is what guides moral action, and our ability to make rules by using reason is what separates us from other life forms. The ability to determine for ourselves a moral course of action, viewed as a categorical imperative by Kant, is identified as applying in all situations (categorical) and as being a binding command (imperative). The categorical imperative is characterized by Kant as follows: "Act only according to that maxim whereby you can at the same time will that it should become a universal law" (Kant, 1993/1785).

Kant argued that making a false promise is always wrong, even if it might produce a good outcome. It is wrong because the promise-breaker is making a moral exception for themselves. If everyone made a false promise when the immediate outcomes were likely to be positive, humans would lose their ability to trust promises, and this would make promises pointless and ineffective. Consequently, making a false promise is irrational (and therefore unethical) because one is making a promise while counting on others to act differently given the same circumstances. Questions one might ask oneself before acting include these: If I do this act, am I making a moral exception for myself? Am I counting on others to act differently than I am right now?

Another of Kant's categorical imperatives is as follows: "Act in such a way that you treat humanity, whether in your own person or in the person of another, always at the same time as an end and never simply as a means" (Kant, 1993/1785). Kant calls us all to recognize every human being as a full human being with their own ends (i.e., life and goals). To treat someone merely as a means would be to use or ignore that person for one's own purposes. For example, it would be wrong to pretend to be friends with someone just so that person could help us study for a test.

Character-Based Theories

Also referred to as **virtue ethics**, character-based approaches to ethics center on the individual agent making the decision. Aristotle (1999/350 BCE) argued that doing the right thing is all about who you are. If you are a moral person with good ethical thinking skills, you will do the right thing. So, in any given situation, one might ask, "What would a good person do in this situation?" or "If I do this, will I be the kind of person I consider good?"

Aristotle's work indicates that habits help us be moral in two ways. First, they help us put our desires in order. By always acting honestly, for instance, one will begin to form a desire for honest acts, so the habit of acting honestly makes one develop a desire to be honest. Second, habits help us learn how to be moral. The more one acts courageously, for instance, the better one becomes at it. By forming a habit of acting courageously, one is more likely to know and to perform courageous acts in any given situation.

Rather than developing hard-and-fast rules to follow, Aristotle offers general advice for making this theory easily applicable to all situations. The drawback, however, comes from the same source: Without any hard-and-fast rules to follow, it can be hard to look to virtue ethics to determine the right thing to do. Habits can help us learn behaviors that are consistent with ethics, including how to be courageous, honest, temperate, and kind. Aristotle's writings on ethics do not try to tell us what the right thing to do is in any situation. Instead, he describes using **theoretical** and **practical wisdom** to figure out what to do in any situation. **Theoretical wisdom** is scientific knowledge, and **practical wisdom** is intuitive reason (Aristotle, 1999/350 BCE). He believes that both are necessary because there is no one right way to act at all times; moral decision-making depends on the situation and the person making the decision.

Limitations of Moral Theory

Keep in mind that moral theories arise from a particular perspective or philosophy about the world. They are conceptualized as a result of this perspective and within a historical and political context. The philosophical approach that evaluates value theories or ethical perspectives for their congruence and usefulness in human decision-making across environments is called metaethics. Philosophers interested in metaethical questions investigate where our ethical principles come from and what they mean. Are they merely social inventions? Do they involve more than expressions of our individual emotions? Metaethics allows us to critique the adequacy of ethical approaches for application across a variety of practice settings and cultural environments. Additional examples of metaethical questions posed by moral philosophers include the following: Are there such things as absolute ethical truths? If so, how do we go about discovering these? If not, what foundations should we use to guide our actions? What is a valid moral theory? Should human values be congruent across settings and cultures?

Religiously based moral theories depend on the idea that good actions are those that obey the laws of a supreme being. However, because the foundational tenets of religions do not consistently mirror one another, what constitutes a moral or morally neutral action from a Jewish perspective may well be morally prohibited from a Roman Catholic perspective. Moreover, even within a religion, the tenets of its different sects or branches may not always lead to the same conclusions about good actions. Nurses and other health care professionals need to recognize the influence of religion on people's lives because their duty to provide safe, competent, compassionate, and ethical care extends to an accommodation of religious and cultural values and practices.

As a result of diverse religious and cultural values, there are divergent but strongly held views on what is good for humans. Many contemporary philosophers have argued that there can be no single approach that permits the identification or resolution of all moral problems (Rachels & Rachels, 2023; Weston, 2020). Even the golden rule can be problematic from a cross-cultural perspective. For example, I might want to be treated as an autonomous being capable of making my own decisions, but an individual from Thailand may defer to family-centered decision-making. Treating my Thai friend as I would wish to be treated would be a mistake. An understanding of cultural beliefs is necessary for good action in such cases (Box 5.1: Health and Social Determinants/Health Equity). Health care professionals wishing to engage in ethics respectful of diversity may be well served to consider the experiences of others and to reflect on their own perceptions of health care consumers and colleagues (Berlinger & Berlinger, 2017). If we fail to listen to others' stories and learn about their experiences, we are likely to be oblivious to the harm being done in health care through the unwitting oppression of minorities or people from other cultures (Halkoaho et al., 2016).

Additionally, utilitarian theories emerged from a particular era and as a result of perceived injustices in societal arrangements in England during the turmoil of the industrial revolution. Utilitarians such as Jeremy Bentham (1748–1832) and John Stuart Mill (1806–1873) sought frameworks that would permit the rectification of unjust policy decisions and the vast economic inequities within their society. For this reason, such theories tend to privilege the good of the group over the needs of individuals. In health promotion, seeking a balance between the good of the group or community and the good of the individual can be a particular challenge. Utilitarian theories, in particular, are in danger of favoring the group (the majority) over those who are in fewer numbers (the minority).

Health practitioners today should be aware that they are likely most familiar and comfortable with the ideals and morals with which they have been raised and that it is not always good to be limited by this perspective. As our society becomes increasingly complex, there are new and emergent ethical issues, such as protection of the environment, use of technology, allocation of scarce resources, and health care reform. Normative ethical theories give each of us the means to think for ourselves and reflect on what we believe is right. It is not prudent to adopt one theory to guide our actions in every situation related to health promotion. If a moral theory is applied unreflectively, it can lead to actions that are problematic for an individual or group. Health-promotion activities mandate not only a general understanding of the nature of a problem or potential problem

BOX 5.1 HEALTH AND SOCIAL DETERMINANTS/HEALTH EQUITY

Self-Reflection

An increasingly multicultural society, multiple languages spoken, and a diverse set of values present health care providers with complex assessment and planning problems. Nurses and other health professionals are charged with practicing "with compassion and respect for the inherent dignity, worth, and unique attributes of every person" (ANA, 2015a, Provision 1). It is not possible to know details about every culture as well as the unique differences of each individual, family community, and group within each culture. There are strategies, however, that a health professional can use to ensure that an individual's unique values and particular needs are the focus of health-promotion interventions.

When a particular culture is part of your population base, opportunities should be pursued for learning individual differences in beliefs, values, and needs related to that culture. To facilitate your assessment, perhaps the most important undertaking is self-reflection. The following are characteristics of individuals who seek to provide culturally sensitive care:

- Commitment to increasing knowledge and skill in sensitivity to cultural differences
- Self-awareness and awareness of one's own biases, beliefs, and values
- Awareness of the validity of different beliefs and values
- Attempts to understand the meaning behind client behavior
- Increased knowledge of the beliefs and values of other cultures
- Development of cultural skills through encounters with people from other cultures

Questions to guide self-reflection for providing culturally sensitive care include the following:

- What values and biases do I bring to the relationship?
- How has my background influenced my beliefs?
- What knowledge and experience do I have to draw upon?
- What values do I share with the client (validate with the client)?
- How comfortable am I with who I am?
- What further information do I need to facilitate culturally competent care?
- Who or what is the best resource for further information?

but also knowledge of the values, beliefs, needs, and desires of the person or population being served. In addition, it is advisable that individuals look for an action or decision supported by more than one ethical theory—such confluence means that the action or decision will be morally right from multiple perspectives or in multiple contexts.

Specific principles derived from ethical theories have proved useful because they highlight salient aspects of complex problems and help us examine implications of different proposed courses of action. Selection of pertinent principles, however, depends both on the context of the problem and on the beliefs and values of the individual or group for which action is needed. For example, imagine a female who seeks assistance in deciding whether to undergo genetic testing for the breast cancer gene BRCA2 because several members of her immediate and antecedent families have received diagnoses of breast or associated cancers. She tells her nurse practitioner that she is not sure whether it would be beneficial to be tested. The nurse practitioner, in facilitating the female's health-promotion efforts, understands that she must use clinical judgment to facilitate the female's autonomous choice. Understanding the requirements of the principle of autonomy is important in helping the female make her decision. It is not sufficient, however, to understand the meaning of autonomy and its limits; the nurse practitioner must also know something about the female's life, values, beliefs, and relationships to provide her with the information and resources necessary for her decision. If the female is screened and the results are positive for the gene, the female not only must decide her next actions but also must consider the implications of the results (e.g., how the results will affect her children or her decision to have children). Box 5.2 presents information on genetic counseling. Individual principles of importance to decision-making in health care settings are explored in this chapter. They—along with associated ethical considerations such as professional, feminist, and virtue ethics—underpin a framework of moral decision-making for health promotion that is presented at the end of this chapter.

Feminist Ethics and Caring

Feminist Ethics

Feminist perspectives on ethics derive from the feminist movement's efforts to expose and rectify injustices to females and raise awareness of the dominance of patriarchy in many ethical approaches. The feminist movement perspectives also often include problems common to all oppressed groups. Feminist ethics, emerging from feminist thought and feminist philosophy, is not another ethical theory as such; rather, it presents a viewpoint on moral problems in health care and other areas of life that have been historically neglected (Tong, 2022). As such, this viewpoint aligns well with social determinants of health and health-promotion concepts.

Feminist scholars have noted that traditional moral theories, and the principles derived from them, have failed to adequately capture the nature and origins of health care problems. Feminist critics assert that moral decision-making must include an investigation of both hidden and overt power relationships implicit in ethical problems; there is a need to understand the contexts, situations, and interrelationships of those involved, because human beings are not isolated individuals who may be viewed as totally independent of others. Hidden power imbalances in various relationships and situations are an important element in moral decision-making. Feminist ethics, then, contributes a perspective that is often missing from traditional ethical approaches and aims to change the way ethical problems are perceived and explored.

The characteristics of feminist ethics include the following (Tong, 2022):

- An understanding that human beings are inseparable from their relationships with others; relationships are the core variable of care
- A focus on care and responsibility within relationships rather than rights, rules, and an abstract system of thought
- A concern with the development of character and attitudes within the context of relationships
- A concern for the rights and equality of all persons

Feminist ethics allows for a critique of the treatment of individuals in the contexts in which they live. This approach to ethics often focuses on imbalances of power along with oppression attributable to sex, sexual orientation, ethnicity, socioeconomics, politics, and other characteristics. For example, a feminist ethicist might point out that a punitive approach to perinatal substance abuse is not associated with improved outcomes for the fetus; in fact, the fetus may be at greater risk because the possibility of such punishment makes females fearful of accessing health services.

The Ethic of Care

The feminist ethic of care is an important concept for health promotion because it focuses on the nature of nurse-person relationships and on the context of people's lives. This approach to care has found increasing acceptance in nursing as both a virtue of the nurse and a responsibility of practice in which treatment is offered on a common ground basis that will support people within their relationships. Gilligan's (1982, 2023) research, among that of others, has been instrumental in the acceptance of the concept of care as informing ethics in nursing practice. Gilligan expanded on Kohlberg's (1981, 1984) stages of moral development, which were derived from longitudinal studies of young males. These moral reasoning studies were designed around the idea that an ability to apply conceptions of justice, rules, and principles to difficult situations denoted the highest achievable level of moral development. Gilligan challenged the reliance on only males in the study of moral reasoning and implemented studies of females' experiences, discovering that females had a moral orientation based on the caring and nurturing of others. In this framework used by females, interrelationships and contexts are critically important in understanding the complexities of a given situation (Tong, 2022).

The ethic of care calls for a knowledgeable and skillful health professional to assume responsibility for the unique needs of an individual in all their complexities. Benner and colleagues (2009) define *care* as "the alleviation of vulnerability; the promotion of growth and health; the facilitation of comfort, dignity

BOX 5.2 GENOMICS

Nurses as Genetic Educators, Researchers, and Counselors

Nurses have always been important advocates for health care literacy and education. Since the International Human Genome Sequencing Consortium completed the Human Genome Project in 2003, nurses have stepped forward to gain new competencies and assume new roles related to genetics and genomics. In assuming these roles, nurses face ethical, legal, and social implications with patients and community members, which requires both basic genomic health literacy and an understanding of the expectations of the public. Research strongly suggests that people want to know their genetic testing results to better understand their health profile.

Genetics involves the study of a single gene's function. **Genomics** represents a wider view, comprising all genes in a person, including interactions of the genes with themselves and also the environment (Ponte et al., 2019). A **genotype** is a set of genes in our DNA that is responsible for a particular trait. A **phenotype** is the physical expression of that trait, which is determined by interaction between the genotype and the environment. A genotype is an inherited trait; the entire genetic information about an organism is contained in a genotype. Examples of genotypes are the genes responsible for eye and hair color. A phenotype is what you see; it is the visible expression of the results of the genes combined with the environmental influence on one's appearance or behavior. Examples of phenotypes are the visible or observable characteristics of eye and hair color.

These terms help nurses understand how the integration of genomic and genetic factors into areas such as biobehavioral research provides opportunities to understand problems that are difficult to define. For example, Lyon and colleagues (2011) noted that attempts to study fatigue have "been stymied by the lack of phenotypic clarity" (p. 274). These nurse researchers have studied genetic-genomic approaches that may increase the precision and clarity of the study of fatigue, thus enhancing understanding of mechanisms by which fatigue occurs in various health conditions. Nurses are making important contributions through integration of genetic-genomic measures into biobehavioral research. This research may lead to better prediction of risk for medical problems, as well as identification of biologic markers of symptom onset, progression, and resolution. More research is also needed in examining the relationship between individual genetic/genomic variations and outcomes of nursing interventions so that nurses can use this information to plan nursing interventions. There are potentially many nursing interventions that would be more effective if they were individually tailored to a person's genetic/genomic profile, rather than a "one-size-fits-all" approach (Munro, 2015).

The advancements made in genetic testing have created additional ethical challenges. Since 2017, there has been a sharp increase in the number of individuals seeking genetic information from companies that offer direct-to-consumer (DTC) results. Concerns about the accuracy of these testing results have arisen. Tandy-Connor and colleagues (2018) reported a 40% error rate in the identification of genetic variants in tests run by DTC laboratories. This type of error can result in the misclassification of genetic variants, providing summaries that contain false-positive or false-negative results. The DTC approach to genetic testing, though convenient for the consumer, presents challenges to the health professional who may not be qualified to interpret or contextualize the results, based on the patient's current health status, in a timely manner (Brothers & Knapp, 2018). The past decade has yielded an intensified focus on workplace wellness and the creation of programs intended to improve employee health; increase productivity, recruitment, and retention; and lower employer health care costs. Though there is disagreement on the success of these programs in meeting the intended objectives, there is widespread concern about the possibility of employers or insurance companies gaining access to employee screening results (Steck, 2018). This concern stems, in part, from the fact that approximately one-third of employees have at least one stigmatized health condition such as mental health disorders, HIV, or other sexually transmitted diseases, substance use disorders, or diabetes (Politz & Rae, 2017). The use of genetic testing in workplace wellness programs is expected to increase in the coming years (Terry, 2017). With both the use of DTC genetic testing and workplace wellness programs, concerns about the storage and use of individuals' private health data abound. The inadvertent disclosure of health data not only violates the individual's right to privacy but also puts the person at risk for harm through loss of employment and health insurance benefits. Such disclosure of private health data violates the ethical principles of confidentiality, beneficence, and nonmaleficence.

The ever-expanding discoveries in genomics challenge the nurse to be competent in genomic applications to nursing care and knowledgeable about the often-difficult ethical issues that arise with these discoveries. There is a need for nurses to attain advanced knowledge and skills related to their serving as specialized genetic counselors. For example, behavioral phenotypes have emerged as an area of specialist practice for nurses in the field of intellectual disability (Higgins & Duffy, 2006). Although many health care professionals have the skills to counsel individuals about genetic testing issues, especially in their fields of expertise, genetic counselors are an increasingly important resource and are aware of ethical issues to consider in genetic screening. Genetic counselors are master's-prepared and can obtain certification through the American Board of Genetic Counselors.

The goals of the discipline are outlined in the National Society of Genetic Counselors' Code of Ethics (National Society of Genetic Counselors, 2017). Although there is controversy about how directive or nondirective advice should be based on the ethical ideals of autonomy, counselors strive to be nondirective while at the same time tailoring information to fit the specific needs of individuals. Because advances in embryo preimplantation genetic testing and in utero fetal testing permit screening of individuals for certain characteristics or genetic diseases, the perceived need to distance the profession from this issue is understandable.

Ethical issues related to genetic counseling for screening purposes that apply both for genetic counselors and for other health care providers include the following:

- Understanding the wider context of genetic testing implications (privacy, discrimination, economics, health insurance denials, implications for family members, anxiety and apprehension, and eugenics [striving for perfection] and its associated implications for individuals and society)
- Helping people determine the risks and benefits of screening
- Helping people prepare for their future needs
- Helping people with their procreative planning
- Understanding how cultural differences affect counseling needs
- Addressing societal issues related to genetic advances, including determining research priorities, justice issues, and discrimination of the genetically disadvantaged

or a good and peaceful death," noting that care is "the dominant ethic found in [nurses'] stories of everyday practice" (p. 233).

Limits of the Ethic of Care

One problem with using care as an ethic of health-promotion practice has to do with the concern of moral predictability or certainty (Nelson, 1992), much like with Aristotle's virtue ethics. If the emphasis on the ethic of care is on relationships, and there are no criteria for right and wrong actions, how can one be assured of the morally correct action in each situation? An answer to this question could be that a morally correct action emerges as a result of judgment based on prior knowledge, experience, and an engaged relationship with the person. The process of the interaction, coupled with the character, knowledge, experience, and intent of the moral agent, is the crucial factor that achieves the moral good for an individual. A person's control of their own care is important. In a nursing setting, the action is right if the nurse incorporates this person's control into meeting their complex needs.

When the solution to one person's problems affects others, however, the rightness of the action depends on more than the one-on-one caring relationship. The problem remains one of choosing between this person's needs and the needs of others who might be affected by the actions chosen. This problem is resistant to resolution via an ethic of care alone. The problem analysis framework described later combines the ethic of care with other considerations. Both an ethic of care and the principles derived from traditional moral theory may be needed for health promotion.

The purpose of ethical inquiry in health promotion is to gain clarity on actual or potential moral issues arising in the context of health-promotion endeavors and to understand what is expected of the health-promotion agent viewed as a moral agent. Ethical inquiry will not permit the resolution of all problems, because the environments in which health-promotion efforts are conceptualized are incredibly complex. It is impossible to foresee all possible consequences of action, but ethical reasoning can facilitate appropriate and in-depth data gathering, permit the uncovering of hidden agendas and interests, and focus on the most salient aspects of a particular problem, thus enhancing professional judgment.

PROFESSIONAL RESPONSIBILITY

Professional judgment and ensuing actions are integral to the goal of providing a good for the population of concern. Nurses are educated to exercise professional judgment and take appropriate actions in a variety of situations (Smith & Caplin, 2012). Health promotion, as one example, is a moral endeavor requiring nurses to be morally sensitive, knowledgeable agents. But what are the scopes and limits of a nurse's obligations to anticipate, identify, and address morally problematic issues related to the promotion and protection of health for individuals, groups, and society? How do nurses balance their duties to individuals with their duty to society? How are individuals' freedoms (autonomy) balanced with the collective responsibilities owed to society and future generations?

Accountability to Individuals and Society

Professions

Although this section focuses on the nursing discipline's mandate to promote health, the discussion can also be applied to the responsibilities of other health professionals who assume health-promotion responsibilities. Nursing is a profession insofar as it provides a service to society and is self-governing, and its members are accountable for their actions (Grace & Uveges, 2023). A significant consequence of professional status is that members can be held accountable for their practice formally by professional licensure boards. More importantly, they are morally accountable for practicing according to their discipline's implicit or explicit code of ethics. One important characteristic of professions, especially those that provide crucial services to society, is that they have codes of ethics that provide essential elements of their promises of service to society. Codes of ethics provide a normative framework for professional actions. A professional implicitly accepts these codes on acquiring membership in the discipline. Thus, each professional should establish a personal perspective on ethical practice within the broad framework of professional codes (Corey et al., 2024).

Codes of Ethics

Codes of ethics are examples of normative ethics in that they prescribe how members of a profession ought to act, given the goals and purposes of the profession, related to individuals and society. The provisions of codes of ethics for nurses provide direction and expectations of ethical behavior. They represent the profession's promises to society. Although the public is not directly involved in the formulation of such codes and, indeed, is for the most part not even aware of their existence, the profession is responsive to the evolving needs of a given society. It can be said that codes of ethics are the tentative end results of a discipline's political process in that they are not static but result from debate and discussion over time among the profession's scholars, leaders, and members.

The current Code of Ethics for Nurses with Interpretive Statements presents a central foundation to guide nurses in their decisions and conduct (Epstein & Turner, 2015). The code establishes an ethical standard that is nonnegotiable; that is, the goals and intent of the code may not be ignored, diluted, or downplayed by individuals or institutions employing nurses in the United States (ANA, 1994). The 2015 code "addresses individual as well as collective nursing intentions and actions; it requires each nurse to demonstrate ethical competence in professional life" (ANA, 2015a, p. viii).

Codes of ethics tend to offer guidelines not only about responsibilities for ensuring quality care but also about responsibilities for recognizing and addressing barriers to service. The ANA's Code of Ethics for Nurses with Interpretive Statements proposes that "the nurse promotes, advocates for, and protects the rights, health, and safety of the patient" (ANA, 2015a, Provision 3). These actions would require a nurse to anticipate future health needs and political activity when necessary to ensure health promotion.

Professional responsibilities delineated in the Code of Ethics extend to maintaining ethical work environments. Provision 5 focuses on the nurse's duty to self and others through "promotion of health and safety, preservation of wholeness of character and integrity, maintenance of competence, and continuation of personal and professional growth" (ANA, 2015a). Provision 6 asserts that "nurses are responsible for contributing to a moral environment that demands respectful interactions among colleagues, mutual peer support, and open identification of difficult issues, which included ongoing professional development of staff in ethical problem solving" (ANA, 2015a). In a 2021 position statement, the ANA (2021) expands on Provisions 5 and 6, delineating nurses' professional responsibility to promote ethical practice environments. This position statement details resources and recommendations, encouraging nurses to "assert their moral voice" and "integrate resources for ethical practice in all settings" (ANA, 2021, p. 8).

Trust

Service professions such as nursing, medicine, and teaching are in part defined by their relationships with others. These relationships exist between the professional and those in need of services as well as between professional colleagues. The essence of these relationships is **trust** that the professional has the knowledge and skills to address the needs of the individual or group (Smith & Crowe, 2016). The potential recipients of services may lack the knowledge, confidence, or ability to anticipate or meet their own needs but trust that the professional will keep their best interests as the primary goal and will strive to meet their needs. For example, in the current health care environment in the United States, people may have trouble accessing a specialist provider because of limits imposed by their insurance coverage, the inability to afford health care insurance, or their inability to pay on their own.

Nurses are responsible not only for promoting health and healing but also for recognizing and addressing barriers to health-promotion activities. Nursing's Social Policy Statement (ANA, 2015b) provides a detailed account of the nursing discipline's responsibilities, including the social contract between society and the nursing profession, and emphasizes the nurse's responsibility to advocate changes when health care services are threatened.

Advocacy

Advocacy, as an expectation of nurses, is strongly reinforced both in the Code of Ethics for Nurses with Interpretive Statements and in innumerable scholarly articles. However, advocacy is a controversial concept. The meaning of the term *advocacy* is derived from its use in law. In legal jurisprudence, advocacy is assertive action taken on behalf of an individual, or perhaps a group viewed as an individual entity, to protect or secure that individual's rights. The individual lawyer does not have an opposing obligation to attend to social justice issues. This attention to broader questions of justice is the responsibility of other areas of the justice system.

Nurses and other health care professionals have a responsibility to speak up on behalf of people whose rights have been compromised or endangered. This is part of the nurse's role because people may not recognize either what is needed to meet their needs or when the care they are receiving is substandard. However, that is not the end of the nurse's responsibilities. They must also consider that specific actions they undertake in the name of advocacy may pose problems for other people who are relying on them for health care services.

For example, Juanita Rimmer, a nurse case manager, is helping Jim Bailey apply for services in a rehabilitation facility because he has residual hemiparesis secondary to a cerebrovascular accident. There is a waiting list at the facility, but Juanita believes it is a priority for Jim to be treated there because he lives with his frail, elderly mother, who will not be able to assist him with his activities of daily living. Because Juanita represents other people who will also benefit from rehabilitation, her decision to be an advocate for Jim must be weighed against the needs of these other people. A moral responsibility associated with advocacy in health care settings is to consider the effect of actions on others. When a nurse is advocating extra attention or specialized care for a given person, an injustice may be rendered simultaneously to other people in their care. Thus, professional advocacy requires a balancing of the health needs of the individual with the health needs of the population (Kangasniemi et al., 2015).

Advocacy is an ideal of health care professions that requires attention to vulnerable individuals, groups, and broader societal concerns. **Moral agency** is defined as the ability to carry out an action based on ethical and moral judgments (Oxford Reference, 2024). A nurse's moral agency is directed to some moral end that is enacted through relationships. Being aware of the self in relation to others helps establish the moral choice required to be an advocate for others. Understanding the interdependent nature of individual and social needs facilitates preventive and health-promotion actions on the part of nurses, from direct care of individuals to advocacy in local, national, and global policy arenas (Smith et al., 2021).

In the last decade, there has been a shift in global consciousness in both ethics and nursing, in which nursing views ethics in a much broader sense than just direct care provided to individuals (Fumincelli et al., 2019). Rather, ethics may encompass issues such as unequal care in communities composed of large minority populations or for undocumented patients. Advocacy may include political activity to address populations of concern. Preemptive and sociopolitical advocacy identifies and challenges the source of the ongoing problems. Nurses have moral obligations related to sociopolitical advocacy on behalf of their populations, and their advocacy is an essential component of the policy process (Cleveland et al., 2019). Juanita Rimmer's obligations include recognizing the problems caused by a chronic shortage of rehabilitation services. Her concerns include discovering the source of this problem and joining with others to attempt to address it at this level. Strategies for solving seemingly intractable problems of health care include collaboration with specialty nursing, medical, or client advocacy groups and communication of the issues in both professional and popular media.

Advocacy for health promotion is a concept with broad implications. It includes activities that are directed toward remedying socially based inequities or inadequacies in the health care delivery system. Advocacy can be viewed as an ethic of practice that includes all activities directed toward the person's good. Advocacy carries risks, in that addressing or facilitating the good for individuals or groups may pit nurses against their peers or against potential adversaries who do not share the same professional goals.

The nurse's role of advocacy requires that professional knowledge and judgment be applied to a variety of situations, from the relatively simple to the complex. The 2010 Institute of Medicine (currently known as the National Academy of Medicine) report, *The Future of Nursing: Leading Change, Advancing Health*, emphasized the need for nurses to exercise advocacy by practicing to the fullest extent of their education and training and engaging as full partners with physicians and other health care professionals in redesigning health in the United States (Institute of Medicine, 2010). This process requires several steps. First, potential or real problems need to be identified and analyzed, often in collaboration with others. Second, appropriate actions need to be formulated and their likely consequences considered. Third, obstacles to action should be recognized and addressed. Finally, actions are performed and evaluated. These basic steps are applied whether the object of health care or health promotion is an individual, a group, or society.

Problem-Solving: Issues, Dilemmas, Moral Distress, and Moral Injury

The nature of health care environments makes difficult decisions inevitable. However, many of the ethical problems encountered in health-promotion settings are issues rather than dilemmas. **Ethical issues** are concerns that arise but that may not require a decision to be made. **Ethical dilemmas** are those situations in which a choice must be made between two undesirable options. Weston (2020) claims that true dilemmas are actually quite rare and that one can often find additional, better options by changing the way they examine a situation.

Daniel Chambliss, a sociologist who studied nurses in acute care institutional settings, asserts that organizations such as hospitals often give rise to "practical problems, not individual dilemmas" (1996). These practical problems are nonetheless moral problems because they interfere with the goals of promoting health, well-being, or the relief of suffering. In both institutional and noninstitutional health care settings, obstacles to good care may be caused by health care system arrangements, interprofessional conflicts, and/or a lack of resources.

The goals of health promotion require that both issues and dilemmas be recognized and addressed. Neglected issues can become dilemmas. Because nurses are on the front line of providing health care, they are often the first to observe an issue with quality of care or safety. Sometimes this concern will lead the nurse to assume the whistleblower role—bringing the concern into the open in the hope of effecting change. Various studies have identified whistleblowing as key in highlighting a need for health reform (Augustine, 2022). There is considerable evidence, however, that the whistleblower may experience significant negative and harmful consequences, such as being victimized or ostracized by colleagues and administrators or losing employment (Augustine, 2022).

When a nurse is in danger of losing their position because of advocating for better conditions, a balancing of foreseeable risks and benefits to the individual or group is required. The process of decision-making in this situation can lead to moral distress. **Moral distress** occurs when a nurse knows the ethically correct action to take but feels powerless to take that action (Epstein & Delgado, 2010; Tigard, 2019). Nurses who are faced with ethical issues that seem to be irresolvable may experience guilt, frustration, and a sense of powerlessness, sometimes because they do not believe that they can adhere to their personal values. Moral distress can occur when the nurse's values and perceived obligations conflict with the needs and prevailing views of the work environment. Although generally viewed as a negative state, moral distress can serve to help nurses expand their ethical perspective. Experiences that result in moral distress can allow the nurse to develop a deeper understanding of ethical issues and their responses to the dilemma being confronted. Further, moral distress can prompt nurses to become active in the policy change process to address the moral issue (Tigard, 2019).

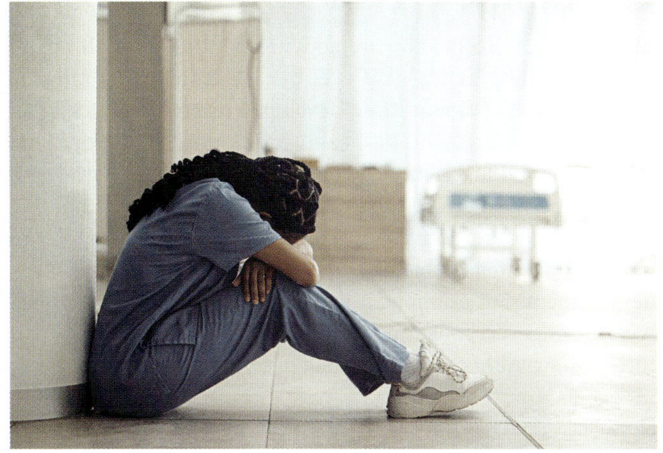

FIG. 5.1 Moral injury—an increasing risk in health care settings. (From iStock.com/Jacob Wackerhausen.)

The context of moral distress puts nurses at risk for **moral injury** (Fig. 5.1). Though this term is an emerging concept in nursing, moral injury has been studied in US veterans for over 20 years. Litz and colleagues (2009) defined *moral injury* as "lasting psychological, biological, spiritual, behavioral, and social effect of perpetrating, failing to prevent, or bearing witness to acts that transgress deeply held moral belief and expectations" (p. 698). Nurses who are frequently involved in decision-making related to matters of life and death; who work in high-stress environments such as critical, emergency, or palliative care; or who work with team members who are perceived to be incompetent are at greatest risk for moral injury, which has a negative effect on the care they provide as well as on their own mental health and quality of life (Cartolovni et al., 2021).

The recent COVID-19 pandemic created environments in which nurses experienced moral distress and moral injury. Shortages of personal protective equipment, health care professionals, medications, and equipment; the need to prioritize resources based on the likelihood of patient survival; difficulty with communication; the frequency of health care policy modifications within the agency; and the frequency at which patients died alone are a few examples of the gaps in health care and the ethical challenges nurses experienced (Cartolovni et al., 2021; Mishkin et al., 2021). The framework for making ethical decisions that is discussed later in this chapter includes considerations related to personal security along with preserving integrity. Additionally, programs such as Resilience in Stressful Events (RISE), created by the Johns Hopkins Hospital, is a resource for supporting health care professionals through training and peer support (Johns Hopkins Medical, 2024). Such programs are valuable assets to nurses who are dealing with moral distress and moral injury and to organizations that employ nurses and other health care professionals.

Preventive Ethics

Just as preventive health care activities aim to forestall health problems, the practice of **preventive ethics** aims to forestall ethical problems before they develop. Preventive ethics is an important requirement of health-promotion endeavors that includes individual action by the nurse as well as social and political activism with other nurses or professional nursing organizations. Preventive ethics requires the health promoter to envision potential problems and institute actions that halt their development. For example, it is possible to extend a dying person's life for a very long time with use of available technology and medications. Although a competent person has the right to refuse treatment, and this right is legally recognized as a result of the Patient Self-Determination Act (PSDA) of 1991, many people become incapacitated before they are able to make their wishes known. All states recognize and honor advance directives, but the legally recognized form differs from state to state (Box 5.3: Preventive Ethics: Patient Self-Determination Act and Advance Directives). It is important to think about the nurse's role in supporting individuals and their families in end-of-life decision-making. Much more work needs to be done engaging people in discussion and helping them plan for such eventualities while they are still well. Preventive ethics in this situation entails initiating communication with persons and families before a

BOX 5.3 Preventive Ethics: Patient Self-Determination Act and Advance Directives

Advance care planning is a process in which patients, their families, and their health care providers discuss the patient's goals, values, and beliefs and document how these should be reflected in future health care choices. It often cannot be predicted whether and when individuals will lose the ability to make their wishes for treatment and care known. Advance care planning is a health-promotion endeavor that can enhance an individual's quality of life, especially while they have a chronic illness (American Bar Association, 2024).

In the last 2 to 3 decades, great technologic and therapeutic advances have been made, resulting in our ability to save the lives of people experiencing catastrophic illnesses and trauma. One effect of these advances, unfortunately, is that sometimes we are successful only in prolonging the dying process. Although it is now recognized that people have a right to refuse treatment to prolong life, critically ill people may lose their ability to articulate their wishes for treatment. Advance directives are a way for people to ensure that when they become incapacitated, the care and treatment they receive matches their predetermined wishes. At their best, advance directives have the potential to ease the strain felt by loved ones as they strive to make the "right" treatment choices for a friend or relative. Advance directives also guide health professionals in their decision-making regarding the person in question (University of Missouri Center for Health Ethics, 2023).

Types of Advance Directives

There are various forms of advance directives, but the types typically recognized by state law in the United States are the living will and the durable power of attorney for health care. Living wills document patient preferences for life-sustaining treatments and resuscitation, whereas a durable power of attorney documents one's choice of a surrogate decision maker (American Bar Association, 2024). A major limitation of the living will is that it may not be applicable to every decisional dilemma the patient will actually face. Therefore, it is important to also designate a surrogate decision maker who can provide guidance to health care professionals in cases where patients are incapacitated and the living will does not apply.

The Patient Self-Determination Act (PSDA) of 1991, which was formulated in response to 2 decades of ambiguity and litigation involving right-to-die cases, represented an attempt to ensure that people's rights were honored. The PSDA required changes in public policy, public and professional education, institutional policy, and social awareness. The PSDA was intended to improve communication related to end-of-life care issues and preferences among individuals, health care providers, and proxy decision-makers. It requires institutions that receive Medicare and Medicaid funds to do the following:

- Give written information on admission to all (not just Medicare and Medicaid) persons about their rights under the law to make their own treatment decisions
- Inform people of their rights to complete state-allowed advance directives, and provide written policies about those rights
- Document when a person has an advance directive
- Not discriminate or make care conditional on the presence or absence of an advance directive
- Provide staff education about advance directives and personal rights

Although the PSDA has great potential, it serves its purpose only to the extent that it is taken seriously as a responsibility of a given institution. Institutions may fail to ensure that a qualified person is available to impart the information or to request personal preferences. It is important for those involved in health promotion to understand and address why people may be reluctant to make an advance directive and why institutions are not diligent in providing information and education. A 2017 study suggested that the percentage of older Americans who completed advance directives before their death had increased dramatically from 20% to approximately 70% over slightly more than the past decade. However, a 2020 Gallup poll revealed that only 45% of US adults had an advance directive (Jones, 2020). It is important to explore why, even in the presence of the PSDA, some people do not have advance directives.

Impediments to the Use of Advance Directives

- Discussions with health care providers about the implications of desired choices have been inadequate.
- People do not want to talk about future incapacity or death. They may have cultural prohibitions about discussing the possibility of serious illness or death.
- Past encounters with the health care system have led to distrust.
- People cannot accurately predict their future preferences, and they know too little about what constitutes life support.
- People may change their minds about what they will accept.
- The health care proxy may turn out to be a poor choice or may cause conflicts among other family members or loved ones. The person or family may ask for something that is morally unacceptable.
- Treatments may be specified to which the provider has conscientious objections.
- Documentation may be lost, misplaced, or not accessible in an emergency.
- Written instructions may be too vague and open to divergent interpretation to be useful guides.
- Even the most diligent proxy cannot always know what the person would have wanted in the absence of a detailed treatment directive.
- The proxy may make a treatment choice contrary to the person's directive.
- The proxy may make a decision with which the institution or physician disagrees.

Positive Outcomes of Use of Advance Directives

Despite impediments, research has shown that advanced care planning has resulted in the following positive outcomes:

- Higher rates of completion of advance directives
- Increased likelihood that clinicians and families understand and comply with a patient's wishes
- A reduction in hospitalization and intrusive treatments at the end of life
- Increased utilization of hospice services
- Increased likelihood that patients will die in their preferred place

problem arises. This communication is often missing both in institutional and primary care settings.

Practicing preventive ethics using a feminist ethics perspective would encourage addressing institutional practices to provide more humanistic care and addressing underlying social issues that lead people to overeat, smoke, or be inclined toward violence. For example, preventive ethics would require the investigation of why, as a society, we have trouble discussing death and dying and why we find it so hard to have a peaceful or good death. Weston (2020) notes that much of the energy used on the polarized abortion debate could be more profitably used in determining why people who do not want to be pregnant nevertheless become pregnant. Weston suggests that it would be useful to reframe the question to ask, "why pregnancy, or pregnancy at the wrong time, is so unacceptably burdensome for many women." We need to ask questions about lack of support, lack of education, poor or difficult-to-use birth control methods, resistance from spouses and lovers, lack of childcare, and so on. One strategy for identifying potential ethical problems before they occur or worsen is to examine problematic cases for their antecedents, asking fundamental questions about societal arrangements and influences on health trends.

On a local level, nurses and other health promoters need to use clinical judgment in anticipating and forecasting problems before they arise. For example, unrecognized health illiteracy may affect an individual's understanding of their rights and entitlements. *Healthy People 2030* identifies health literacy as a priority and includes six objectives focused on increasing health literacy within the population (*Healthy People 2030*, n.d.).When a nurse observes that a person and that person's family do not understand either the information given to them or the implications of following a given course of action, the nurse engages in preventive ethics by supplying that information and ensuring that it is understood. The nurse acts to prevent negative consequences that can arise from poorly understood information. Other examples of opportunities to use preventive ethics include focusing on smoking or childhood obesity. Many problems in health care occur when communication is poor or information has been provided too late for reasoned decision-making (Box 5.4: Quality and Safety Scenario).

BOX 5.4 QUALITY AND SAFETY SCENARIO

Patient-Centered Care

How Is Health Literacy Related to Ensuring Autonomy in Decision-Making for Individuals?

Autonomy is an important ethical principle for health-promotion activities. To ensure autonomy in individual decision-making, it is important to assess the individual's health literacy skills. These skills relate to a person's ability to obtain, process, and act on basic health information, which affect quality and safety in decision-making. Think about how difficult it would be for a person with low literacy skills to navigate today's complex health care system. Adequate health literacy is essential for accessing necessary health care services and for fostering effective decision-making.

In the process of implementing health-promotion activities, the nurse should first determine whether the person has adequate health literacy skills. This can be assessed with tools such as the Rapid Estimate of Adult Literacy in Medicine-Short Form or the Test of Functional Health Literacy in Adults. To ensure quality, safety, and autonomy in decision-making, the nurse must be aware of tools that help determine literacy and must have access to such tools. It is important, however, not to base an approach to health promotion solely on the results of one of these tools, which may not reveal the extent to which health recommendations may be misunderstood. The nurse should take the time to establish a rapport with the individual that includes fostering a sense of trust and openness for the person to ask important questions.

The Agency for Healthcare Research and Quality (AHRQ) has identified Health Literacy Universal Precautions and recommends their use in working with individuals who may face literacy challenges. The three recommended strategies are as follows (AHRQ, 2020):

- Simplify communications with and confirm comprehension for all patients to minimize miscommunication.
- Make the office environment and health care system easier to navigate.
- Support individuals' efforts to improve their health.

Unrecognized health literacy issues may interfere with an individual's right to autonomy in decision-making because the individual may make a decision based on inaccurate information or may automatically accept the decision of the health care provider without deciding for themselves whether the decision is appropriate for their situation. It is an ethical obligation of the nurse to make sure that effective communication is implemented. A public health approach founded on health-promotion principles can provide a useful scaffold for assessing the health literacy of persons in the community. This can help ensure that an individual is in control and is a full partner in health-promotion decisions that respect their preferences, values, and needs (*Healthy People 2030*, n.d.).

ETHICAL PRINCIPLES IN HEALTH PROMOTION

Although the tenets of nursing's codes of ethics and standards of practice provide some guidance about the nature of practice and how services will be provided, they often leave some ambiguity about the best course of action in morally troubling situations. The use of principles derived from a variety of ethical theories, along with feminist insights or an ethic of care, helps to provide further guidance in decision-making in morally problematic health situations. Beauchamp and Childress (2019) noted that ethical principles provide an important starting point for moral judgment and policy evaluation but that principles alone are not enough. In other words, principles such as autonomy, beneficence, and justice often serve as helpful starting points in teasing out the tangled elements of complex issues, but taken alone they are usually insufficient for moral problem-solving in health care environments. One must decide which principles are important to consider in each case or situation, and doing so requires an exploration of the case as discussed in the decision-making framework provided later in the chapter.

Additionally, the tenets of the Code of Ethics for Nurses with Interpretive Statements and the ANA's position statements provide guidance regarding what a nurse's moral responsibilities are in a particular type of situation. Certain tenets address the responsibilities of the nurse in improving the larger health care environment. These obligations include collaborating with others to "protect human rights, promote health diplomacy, and reduce health disparities" (ANA, 2015a, p. 31).

Autonomy as Civil Liberty

In health-promotion activities and settings, the concept of autonomy can be understood from two different perspectives.

From the vantage point of public health, the extent of individual autonomy, or freedom of action, may be limited by the duty of protecting the health and safety of the society. From this perspective there is an age-old struggle between civil rights and public safety. Moral questions ask to what degree society is justified in regulating the health and safety of society at large. There is an inevitable tension associated with curtailing civil liberties in the name of safety or health. This tension arises from perceptions that, in most Western contexts, freedom of action is a prerequisite of human flourishing.

Currently there are many indirect threats to the health and safety of our society, including, but by no means limited to, bioterrorism and the spread of viruses and drug-resistant bacteria. Actions to resolve any of these threats have the potential to impinge on civil liberties. Such actions might include surveilling citizens or requiring disclosure of disease status. Advances in genetic knowledge present the possibility of discrimination from a variety of sources. It will be difficult to maintain individual privacy, and discrimination based on class or gene profile will be made easier.

The current managed care environment, although having a stronger focus on inculcating healthy behaviors, can impinge on civil liberties. The behavior-change approach has been criticized as too paternalistic, without sufficient regard for the individual's or the group's own perceptions of what is important; this may increase the risk of failed interventions. Prioritizing behavioral change in health-promotion endeavors over the need to address underlying social concerns, such as poverty and other forms of disadvantage, may obscure a focus on the social determinants of health. Rather than focusing on behavioral change, a focus on empowerment may help a person gain control over social and economic factors that contribute to health problems (Tengland, 2016).

Autonomy as Self-Determination

A second, related sense of autonomy has to do with individual choice. Autonomy is the moral principle that underlies the concept of informed consent to treatment, interventions, and health-promotion efforts. In Western societies it is probably the most powerful moral principle underlying the treatment of individuals. This principle asserts that people have the ability to reason, and a consequence of the ability to reason is the capacity to make choices. These choices concern both one's own behavior and how one should act toward others. Although the idea that our ability to reason constitutes the essence of being human originated with Aristotle, Kant (1993/1785) developed this idea in meticulous detail in his work *Grounding for the Metaphysics of Morals*. According to Kant, people are capable of conscious desires and goals and are free agents capable of making decisions and setting goals as guided by their own reason. This principle is a salient consideration in health care settings: it underpins the health provider and promoter-person relationship and the issue of informed consent. However, there is limited agreement about the scope, limits, and strength of this principle (Beauchamp & Childress, 2019). When describing autonomy in the context of health or treatment choices, we should delineate what we mean by autonomy in the context of the problem under discussion. Feminist criticisms of an emphasis on autonomy highlight the problem that our choices necessarily affect others because we are contextual beings, inseparable from our relationships with one another.

Respect for human autonomy guides us to permit individuals to make and learn from their own mistakes. Generally, respecting autonomy requires that we permit individuals to make their own decisions, even when these decisions seem to others ill-informed. There are exceptions to this rule. Exceptions include those situations in which there is a high risk of serious injury or death and when it cannot be determined whether the person's judgment is impaired. We make exceptions to the rule of autonomy when we suspect that an individual is not able to reason adequately. A person's reasoning ability may be impaired by psychological or physical conditions or by having incorrect or incomplete information.

In health-promotion activities, respect for autonomy requires that individuals be given the information they need to make choices. Choices can be considered autonomous only if certain criteria are met. The criteria that determine whether a person is actually capable of autonomous (voluntary) choice include cognitive maturity, possession of appropriate information to permit decision-making, intact mental capacities (the ability to reason logically), the absence of internal or external coercive influences, and the ability to appreciate the risks and benefits of alternative choices. Assessing all such criteria is quite a tall order, and in one sense it may be that nobody acts totally autonomously at any given time because of the influences of entrenched beliefs and values that are derived, for the most part, from our cultural and environmental backgrounds. Some of these influences are under conscious control in the sense that we can recognize what values we hold and even revise them if they are dissonant with other values. However, some of these influences are not readily recognizable because they lie beneath the surface of consciousness and are hard to access even if we are willing to try. We all have blind spots; autonomy viewed as informed, uncoerced, and reasoned action is therefore an ideal. Many of us fall short of the ideal.

Informed Consent

Informed consent to research, treatments, or health-promotion endeavors is a process of ensuring that a person has all the appropriate information necessary to reach a decision about participation that facilitates autonomous action. Beauchamp and Childress (2019) note that informed consent occurs when a person with substantial understanding, and without substantial control by others, intentionally authorizes a professional to intervene on their behalf. The key phrase is "with substantial understanding." It is important to understand that even after a consent form has been signed, a person has the right to rescind consent considering additional information and/or changed consequences.

The components of the consent process include determining the person's competency to consent. There must be no physical or mental impairments that hinder the person in question from understanding and processing information. For example, a person with pneumonia who is febrile and confused is probably not capable of making an informed decision until the fever has been reduced and the confusion has cleared. To be substantially informed, a person must be made aware of important details of the proposed intervention, including its nature, purpose, probability of success, and important risks, and they must also understand what alternatives (if any) are available. Because this information must be tailored to meet the specific needs of an individual and such a task requires knowledge of the person, an ethic of care is important to understanding a person's unique needs. We can check understanding to a certain extent by asking the individual to articulate how the proposed intervention will facilitate their own values and goals. There must be no subtle or overt coercion by professionals or others. Finally, appropriate supports must be available to complete the proposed intervention.

Obtaining consent for any interventions, or for involvement in research, is best viewed as a process that entails ongoing assessment of the person's status and evaluation of needs for further information or support. Because individuals may not understand information well when they are in stressful situations or when the information is complex, we should assess people for and validate understanding on an ongoing basis.

The nurse's role includes ensuring that all individuals, regardless of age, make informed choices. Nurses must be aware of strategies for ensuring that older adults, who may be less able to advocate for their own health needs, participate in making informed decisions. More research is needed on ethical problems that confront nurses in caring for older adults in the community.

Adolescence is a period of transition between the dependence and vulnerability of childhood and the autonomy of adulthood. Adolescents are generally considered capable of making decisions related to health-promotion activities, and health professionals have a duty to respect those decisions, provided that doing so does not produce harm to adolescents or others (Larcher & Brierley, 2020). Most health-promotion activities do not require formal informed consent. However, it is important to integrate the underlying principles and supporting research related to informed consent to ensure that the selected health-promotion strategies fit with individuals' beliefs and values. It is also important to recognize that complex social factors may contribute to adolescents' inability to make well-thought-out decisions (Box 5.5: Evidence-Based Practice).

Exceptions to Autonomous Decision-Making

In some cases, proxy decision-making on behalf of the individual is required (Box 5.6: Proxy Decision-Making). Proxy decision-making must consider what is known about the person and must follow a path of action that is most likely to respect that individual's goals and values. The designation of proxy decision-maker is generally aligned with the individual holding durable power of attorney for health care (DPOA). At times, family members who do not hold DPOA are needed to serve as surrogate decision-makers. Researchers have found that surrogate family members who need to make decisions for loved ones, often at the end of life, find the decision-making overwhelming and extremely stressful (Sorrell, 2014; Mishkin et al., 2021). Most surrogate decision-makers have had little preparation for making these choices and worry that they are not making the right decision. Nurses should support both proxy and surrogate

BOX 5.5 EVIDENCE-BASED PRACTICE

Influences on Sexual Decision-Making of Late Adolescents

Violence has been identified by the World Health Organization as a major risk to the health and well-being of all young females. Sexual activity without clear consent is one aspect of violence against adolescents, who are still developing their values and beliefs about sexual activity and sexual norms. In a qualitative research study, Fantasia (2011) used a narrative inquiry approach to explore what influenced adolescents' decision-making related to sexual activity. The research question was "What are late adolescents' perceptions of factors that influenced their sexual decision-making?" Ten female adolescents aged 18 years and older were interviewed. They were asked to respond to the question "Please tell me, in your own words, the story of your decisions to have sex." Each participant constructed her own story without influence from the researcher.

The findings showed that in most of the sexual encounters of these adolescents, sexual consent was implied, with no consent clearly stated. The participants discussed how sexual activity eventually occurred, even when they did not want it, because of partners who used "pressure to always say yes." Inability to communicate readily with partners and the influence of alcohol were identified as contributing factors to the lack of clear consent. None of the participants expressed emotion or anger over what had occurred, and they did not label it as rape. There appeared to be an acceptance of this type of nonconsensual sexual activity.

The findings from the study provide evidence that adolescent decisions involving consent for sexual activity are complex and are influenced by myriad social factors. All individuals have a right to clearly refuse or consent to sexual activity; this is imperative for the promotion of physical, emotional, and sexual health and safety. Nurses and other health care professionals who work with adolescents need to carefully assess sexual behaviors and recognize that these young females are at risk of nonconsensual sexual activity. Sexual violence education should include information on negotiation and communication skills that will help adolescents mediate complicated interpersonal situations. Appropriate educational programs can help empower young females through opportunities for increased knowledge and self-confidence.

BOX 5.6 Proxy Decision-Making

Autonomy-Based: Person's Previously Articulated Desires

- Written
- Living will, advance directive
- Document details to various degrees what the person will or will not accept
- Substituted judgment
- Individual appoints a proxy who is expected to honor previously expressed preferences
- Informal (nonappointed significant other)

Best Interests

- Proxy chooses the actions that will give the highest overall benefit—may or may not be based on a person's previously expressed desires; a quality-of-life determination based, when possible, on knowledge about the person (Beauchamp & Childress, 2019)
- Best interests may differ from the proxy's choice; doubt about the proxy's motives possible
- Reasonable person standard
- Based on the answer to "What would a reasonable person want?"

decision-makers as they struggle with making decisions. Iverson and colleagues (2014) described what helps and hampers surrogate decision-making (Box 5.7: Best Practice).

Certain populations are considered less than fully autonomous for a variety of reasons. People with Alzheimer's disease or other physical or psychological disruptions or deficits that prevent adequate comprehension may require proxy decision makers. It is important not to assume, however, that all persons with Alzheimer's disease are incapable of providing informed consent, because many persons in the early stages of the disease are capable of making decisions related to their care (Sorrell & Cangelosi, 2009; Sorrell, 2021). Incarcerated people are restricted in their choices and may be subject to subtle or overt coercion. Children are considered less than fully autonomous because they are not developmentally mature. Additionally, in people with certain mental illnesses, such as psychoses or bipolar disorders, the capacity for decision-making may fluctuate. The President's Commission for the Study of Ethical Problems in Medicine and Biomedical and Behavioral Research (1982) was formed to study health care decision-making and noted that the minimal capacities needed for competent decision-making are "(1) Possession of a set of values and goals, (2) the ability to communicate and to understand information, and (3) the ability to reason and deliberate about one's choice." These criteria are generally accepted as a basic minimum (Beauchamp & Childress, 2019). It can be seen from these criteria that some children may be able to understand the implications of a given course of treatment, and adults with cognitive impairments may be deemed competent to make certain decisions. Competency to make autonomous choices is not an all-or-nothing capacity. Competency determinations are, as a rule, made for a given decision or task. Thus, a person may vacillate between competency and noncompetency, depending on either the task at hand (degree of difficulty) or the physical or psychological status during the period when a decision must be made.

When advocating decision-making for a cognitively impaired person, consider the risks and benefits of allowing the individual to make their own decision. The benefits in terms of self-esteem may well outweigh the risks of many choices. However, if the risk of injury is high and it is obvious that the person is not able to reason effectively, autonomous decision-making may not be feasible. In this case, nurses can collaborate with the individual, family members, and other health professionals to arrive at a decision that is best for the individual.

When children are involved, it is often the parent or guardian who provides permission to treat the child. Nevertheless, in pediatric settings it is incumbent on people involved in health-promotion endeavors or in research with minors to gain assent from the child in addition to consent from the parent or guardian (Rudd, 2019; Van Goidsenhoven & De Schauwer, 2022). The example of 5-year-old Julianna Snow illustrates how difficult these decisions can be. Julianna had an incurable neurodegenerative illness and decided that she would rather die at home than return to the hospital for a treatment that would likely lead to her death or her being sedated on a ventilator with little quality of life. Julianna's parents honored this decision, and Julianna died at home. Ethical questions were raised about whether a child of this age should be allowed to make an irreversible decision without the maturity to understand the consequences (Cohen, 2015).

For a child's assent to be meaningful, an assessment of their level of maturity and comprehension is required, and information must be provided in language and terms that are appropriate for their developmental level. Conversely, when there is conflict between the decision of the parent and that of the child, the health care provider has a duty to ensure that the parental choice is in the child's best interest. Where there is serious doubt, it may be necessary to involve the courts.

BOX 5.7 BEST PRACTICE

Surrogate Decision-Making

Most end-of-life health care decisions are made by proxy or surrogate decision-makers who are under a great deal of stress over their seriously ill family member. Both surrogates and clinicians have various degrees of preparation, knowledge, abilities, or comfort in working effectively with another in making very difficult decisions for someone else.

Iverson and colleagues (2014) explored surrogate decision-makers' challenges in making decisions related to the care of patients in critical care. They interviewed 34 designated surrogates of critically ill patients receiving care in two tertiary care institutions. Surrogates were asked to describe and reflect on their experiences of making health care decisions for others. They identified factors that added to the difficulty in decision-making:

- Stress associated with assuming a decision-making role for which they felt unprepared
- Uncertainty of patient outcomes
- Difficulty in communicating with multiple health care providers who would provide different information
- Insufficient knowledge of patients' wishes
- Conflict within the family
- Fatigue resulting from near constant vigilance in the intensive care unit

Social networks that provided access to family and/or friends were helpful in the decision-making process, as they provided surrogate decision-makers with emotional and informational support. Nurses were the preferred resource for day-to-day communication and information gathering, except when major decisions needed to be made. Most participants perceived that nurses offered compassionate communication and were able to disentangle information that was difficult to understand.

The findings of the study suggest areas where clinicians can intervene to facilitate the processes of surrogate decision-making. Stress can be minimized by improving communication between surrogate decision-makers and health care providers. Nurses are uniquely poised to intervene to improve communication and reduce surrogates' decision-making anxiety.

Confidentiality

Autonomy is also the principle underlying **confidentiality**: One expression of autonomy is the ability to maintain privacy in one's life (Yeo et al., 2020). People have the right to decide who can have access to information about them, thus limiting the negative use of personal information by others. In certain situations, the status of confidentiality between a person and others, such as clergy, is considered a privilege and as such is shielded from exposure by the legal system. In health care, confidentiality does not carry as strong a status as clergy-supplicant or lawyer-client privilege (Grace & Uveges, 2023). There may be occasions when health care providers have a duty to warn others who are unknowingly endangered. This duty was highlighted by the landmark Tarasoff case. In October 1969, Prosenjit Poddar killed Tatiana Tarasoff. Poddar, who was receiving psychiatric care, had informed his therapist 2 weeks earlier that he was going to kill a certain girl, easily identifiable as Tarasoff, on her return from Brazil. At the time his therapist tried to have him committed. The police detained Poddar briefly but determined he was rational and released him. No one warned Tatiana of the danger. The courts concluded that "once a therapist does in fact determine, or under applicable professional standards reasonably should have determined, that a person poses a serious danger of violence to others, he bears a duty to exercise reasonable care to protect the foreseeable victim of that danger" (Tarasoff v. Regents of University of California, 1976). The court recognized the difficulty of predicting the degree of danger and the importance of maintaining confidentiality but determined that when the risk is high, confidentiality should be breached.

Nurses must strive to keep the person's personal information confidential. Doing so enhances trust within the nurse-person relationship. There are strong penalties against breaching confidentiality in health care. In theory, the principle of confidentiality may be overridden only in situations in which extreme harm to self or others is imminent. In practice, this is difficult to enforce, because in medical settings, many people have access to the person's information. Insurance companies demand access to information before payment for services is made. Technology used both within and outside the health care setting can present challenges to confidentiality. Sharing information, photos, or videos on social media, for example, can reveal details that violate the principle of confidentiality and put both the individual and the nurse at risk. In most cases, the sharing of confidential patient information is unintentional or inadvertent (National Council of State Boards of Nursing, 2018a). To avoid such breaches, the National Council of State Boards of Nursing (2018b) recommends that nurses "be aware; be cognizant of feelings and behaviors; be observant of the behavior of other professionals; and always act in the best interest of the patient" (p. 11).

Challenges for privacy may occur when personnel are personally acquainted with the individual. Nurses and other health-promotion professionals may find themselves being asked by friends and relatives of the person for details about that person's health status. It can be very difficult to respond diplomatically while maintaining the person's privacy. The ethical implications of these threats to confidentiality are numerous. Thus, it is important for nurses to be aware of potential breaches of confidentiality and to advocate confidential treatment of information for those they serve.

The Privacy Rule

The **Privacy Rule** (45 Code of Federal Regulations Part 160, 164 subparts A & E) was developed as a result of the **Health Insurance Portability and Accountability Act (HIPAA)**. Its intent was to ensure that individuals' health information is properly protected while allowing for the flow of information needed to provide and promote high-quality care (including use of information about the person receiving care for research) and to protect the public's health and well-being. HIPAA was meant to protect the privacy of individually identifiable health information in the face of advances in electronic technology and to limit the ways in which "health plans, pharmacies, hospitals, clinics, nursing homes and other covered entities (any provider that conducts or conveys information in electronic form, e.g., physicians, nurse practitioners)" can use medical information (US Department of Health and Human Services [USDHHS], 2022). *Covered entities* refers to those covered by the Privacy Rule. Limitations on the use of medical information extend to any identifiable information—written, oral, or computerized. Although there are some legal guidelines about disclosure, nurses and others are responsible for using clinical judgment in deciding what level of detail to share. It is important to understand that the purpose of the rule is to protect individual rights while still facilitating important public health and epidemiologic research. Health-promotion activities include empowering people to exercise these rights. The Privacy Rule ensures that individuals are given a copy of the privacy practices at a given institution. Additionally, under the rule, individuals have the following rights:

- To access their own information
- To limit who may receive their information
- To request corrections of errors
- To receive an account of how their information has been used
- To request special confidential reporting of their information at a location of their choosing (this may be especially important for individuals at risk for intimate partner violence)
- To pursue complaints with the Department of Health and Human Services Office for Civil Rights (UHDHHS, 2022)

A rule of thumb for health professionals related to sharing information with others is to disclose only as much information as is pertinent to the situation and is necessary to provide optimal care. A decision about disclosure of a person's information requires balancing the risks of information sharing with the benefits of treatment. Although the Privacy Rule was meant to help safeguard people's rights, some commentators and researchers are finding the rule overly restrictive and worry that it might discourage important research, especially genetic research, with its far-reaching implications for individual privacy.

Adolescents: Special Considerations of Confidentiality

Adolescents often present health professionals with complex confidentiality issues. Their developmental level positions them to be caught between the independence they desire and the support they require of parents. This juxtaposition, combined with risky behavior such as alcohol and drug experimentation, defensiveness and vulnerability of the adolescent, and the desire of friends and parents to gain information about the adolescent's health status, further adds to the complexity of the concepts of autonomy and confidentiality. This complexity may create tension between the parents and the adolescent and challenges for health care professionals (Butts & Rich, 2023).

Although federal and state laws, as well as ethical considerations, generally serve to protect the privacy and autonomy of adolescents, health promotion involves more than mere protection. It involves facilitating the adolescent's health. Responsibilities include helping an adolescent grasp their authentic options and rights, facilitating interaction between the adolescent and parents or guardians, maintaining trust, and preserving confidentiality.

On the other hand, clinical judgment (which includes ethical judgment) is important in determining risk. If the risk of preserving the adolescent's privacy is high based on all pertinent and available evidence, such as the presence of sexual or physical abuse, then it may be necessary to report this information to the appropriate authorities. Mandatory reporting laws exist. Such laws are important for the general protection of a society's citizens. However, there may be rare occasions when a judgment must be made about whether upholding the legal obligation would cause more harm than good. In such circumstances there are two separate considerations. First, one must decide whether the risk to professional standing and licensure of not following the legally required path is something that the professional is willing to assume. The second consideration involves assessing the potential benefits and risks to the person resulting from a failure to report. There is no easy resolution for these types of problems. If the situation is not an emergency, it is prudent to solicit appropriate advice from a peer, a counselor, or an ethics expert or resource. In any case, it remains the professional's ethical responsibility to handle the given situation in a manner that preserves trust and provides ongoing support.

Veracity

Veracity, or devotion to the truth, is another principle that supports health-promotion activities. People whose health is in question are to varying degrees reliant on the person who possesses the knowledge and skills to bring these to bear on their behalf. The contemporary bioethics literature favors characteristics of "veracity, … candor, honesty and truthfulness" (Beauchamp & Childress, 2019, p. 327) as virtues to be nurtured in the development of health professionals. This represents a change from the paternalistic attitudes (i.e., the physician knows what is best) that prevailed early in the 20th century and up to the late 1960s.

Veracity in giving people information about their health care needs facilitates autonomous choice and enhances personal decision-making. Nurses may be tempted to withhold certain details when this is seen as serving the person's best interests or when family members demand it. It is sometimes difficult to determine how much and what types of information will best serve a person's needs. Knowledge of the person's beliefs, values, and lifestyle preferences is essential to the process of supplying adequate information to support autonomous decision-making. Withholding information or providing information that is misleading or incomprehensible in an attempt to influence someone to agree to a treatment or intervention conflicts with veracity.

Veracity has cross-cultural implications, in that some cultures have not traditionally valued truth-telling in the case of terminal illness. Decision-making about whether to honor veracity in such cases must take into consideration what is known about the culture, the particular person, the strength of their personal and cultural beliefs, and whether there is evidence about what sorts of things the person would like to know. The absence of veracity may interfere with autonomous action. In the case of terminal illness, it may deprive the person of the ability to plan the remainder of their life.

At first glance, veracity appears an easy concept to incorporate into health-promotion interventions. It may sometimes be difficult, however, in health-education endeavors aimed at changing patterns of behavior in society. Should health professionals just present the facts, or should they attempt to persuade people? What are the limits of veracity? Is it permissible to exaggerate the dangers of certain behaviors in the interests of the health of society? These questions cannot be answered within the confines of this chapter but are important to keep in mind when assessing the merits of proposed population-based interventions.

Nonmaleficence

Related to autonomy is the principle of **nonmaleficence**, which enjoins people to not harm other people. In general society, this principle constrains people from autonomous actions that are likely to harm others. For instance, a 25-year-old is allowed to drink alcohol but not to drink and drive because the latter may harm others. In health care settings, this principle prohibits clinicians from harming those for whom they provide services. For health promotion, it means that when activities are being planned on an individual or societal level, possible harms must be minimized. It is often impossible to foresee all the risks of a given course of action, but professionals who engage in health-promotion endeavors are responsible for foreseeing predictable adverse consequences and taking these potential consequences into consideration. Responsibilities include addressing social or health care policies that are discovered to have unintended effects.

Carter and colleagues (2011) illustrate how a policy designed to address obesity through use of a mass-media program can have unintended negative health effects. They describe how the program How Do You Measure Up? can carry a message to people to trim their waistlines and "turn their lives around." Although mass-media campaigns such as this one are targeted at the population level, they may also have a deeply personal and emotional effect on individuals, stigmatizing individuals who feel incapable of making changes in their lives to lose weight.

Teaching about self-esteem and fitness may help people live with obesity more healthfully. Employer incentive programs that differentiate among individuals based on their success in changing behaviors, such as smoking or weight management, also carry the possibility of discrimination. When financial benefits are provided to the most successful individuals, some individuals are disenfranchised when they face significantly greater difficulty than others in achieving desired outcomes (Madison et al., 2011). Well-designed employer incentive programs, however, can help individuals overcome barriers they face in trying to avoid disease and disability. Systematic evaluation of incentive programs will enhance understanding of how to design programs to prevent discrimination and maximize equity (Sorrell, 2015).

Unintentional harm is a possibility for actions designed to promote health. Risks can be minimized by anticipating potential negative effects and implementing measures to control them. A synthesis of reflection, critical thinking, and knowledge, along with an understanding of the details and context of a situation, is required before one embarks on a course of action aimed at facilitating a person's health or well-being. The overall discomfort encountered by the individual must be the minimum possible to achieve the primary good intended. In other words, the health care provider is accountable for their judgment and for providing those interventions that are most likely to bring about the desired result. More than just the intention not to do harm is required.

As the landscape of health care changes, concerns about the use of technology and possible maleficence have surfaced. It is unclear how current methods of knowledge development, including the use of big data, artificial intelligence, algorithms, and biologic modeling, will affect individuals and what ethical issues will arise from the use of these methods (Peirce et al., 2020). Technologies used for other purposes give rise to questions of ethics as well. Examples include the use of robotics (Tanioka, 2019), visual technologies and social media (Laholt et al., 2019), monitoring technologies (Hall et al., 2019), and electronic health records (Robichaux et al., 2019). Nurses must evaluate the use of technologies in caring for individuals and groups and be vigilant about ensuring nonmaleficence.

Nurses and other health professionals can do harm inadvertently through ignorance or incompetence, referral to a provider who is incompetent or inappropriate, or inadequate monitoring or training of those under their supervision. However, the duty of nonmaleficence does not mean that nurses are always accountable for foreseeing the consequences of their actions. For example, a course of exercise may be designed for a person who has had a thorough physical examination, but during an exercise session the person faints and fractures his arm. Further testing reveals a previously undetected cardiac anomaly that is subsequently surgically corrected. This is not **maleficence**; the main objective of the agent was therapeutic, and the event was, if not totally unforeseeable, not identified on routine preexercise testing. In this kind of case, we tend to look at the principle behind the action rather than the consequences. The clinician's duty was upheld, even though initially bad consequences were the unintended result. Both deliberate harm and harm caused by indifferent or incompetent decision-making should be considered maleficent. However, when a competent practitioner evaluates a problem thoroughly and intervenes with therapeutic intent, and nonetheless there is a partially negative outcome, such action does not violate the concept of nonmaleficence.

Beneficence

Beneficence is the quality or state of doing or producing good. As a moral principle, beneficence presents us with the duty to maximize the benefits of actions while minimizing harms. There are two related aspects of the moral principle of beneficence in health-promotion settings: actions taken to further the overall health or well-being of the society in general and actions taken to promote the good of a particular individual.

When society formulates rules designed to protect people against the negative effects of their own actions, these rules are considered beneficent. It is important to emphasize, however, that beneficence should be performed in accordance with the person's will or values and with respect for the person's autonomy (Kangasniemi et al., 2015; Keane, 2010). Sometimes rules designed to protect people are described as paternalistic because they override a person's autonomy. For example, motorcycle helmet laws and rules governing the use of therapeutic or so-called recreational drugs are paternalistic. **Paternalism** is often justified by the assertion that the persons affected will be better off or protected from harm.

The principle of beneficence, when it overrides an individual's autonomous choice so as to serve that individual's interests, is appropriate when a person lacks the capacity to make personal decisions. As such, any of the factors discussed earlier that interfere with rational decision-making may require the health care provider to beneficently override the individual's decisions. Generally, though, beneficence permits interference only when the risks of the individual's proposed actions are high. This is because autonomy is such a powerful principle in Western societies that a decision to override an autonomous choice is not taken lightly. One may be justified in preventing a person from taking an overdose of sleeping pills or jumping off a cliff because the risks of not doing so are high and, importantly, if the person succeeds there is no possibility of future autonomous actions.

Beneficence, unlike nonmaleficence, is not necessarily a moral requirement of action on the part of societal members toward each other (Grace & Uveges, 2023). Whether beneficence is viewed as a moral requirement of societal members in everyday life very much depends on philosophical beliefs and the ethical theory or perspective (if any) recognized by the person. Kant (1993/1785), for instance, distinguishes between perfect duties and imperfect duties. Perfect duties must be followed and tend to be defined in negative terms (e.g., do not lie, do not steal); imperfect duties are ones we are called to but not bound to follow (e.g., stopping to help someone who is looking for something lost on the sidewalk). An individual is not necessarily morally required to go out of their way to help someone unless the person is endangered, and assistance would mitigate the danger. In that case, failing to offer assistance could be seen as violating the principle of nonmaleficence. Also, when an individual has responsibility for vulnerable others, such as when parents must use beneficence on behalf of their children, beneficence is required.

In contrast to ordinary members of society, nurses have duties of beneficence because their professional goals involve meeting health care needs and thus are aimed at providing good. For such reasons, beneficence is a moral expectation of nurses. Beneficence is often a difficult principle to use in health-promotion settings, however, because of the dual nature of health-promotion goals—health for individuals and health for communities. As noted earlier, there is often tension between the two.

A paradox exists when we try to change unhealthy behaviors but do not address the underlying causes of those behaviors. For example, although smoking cessation programs help some people stop smoking, and restricting areas where people can smoke tends to persuade some people that it is becoming too inconvenient to continue, we also should address problems such as advertising campaigns that aim to gather new smoking recruits from among adolescents. Some advertising campaigns encourage adolescents to try flavored cigarettes through offering a variety of flavors and attractive packaging. But these tobacco cigarettes are addictive and dangerous. Education-based health-promotion programs without underlying societal changes are often doomed to fail. Thus, understanding beneficence, health professionals have obligations to address deep-rooted social problems that jeopardize health or are associated with health disparities.

Beneficence: Conflict with Autonomy

The principles of beneficence and autonomy sometimes conflict. For example, seat belt rules are ostensibly created to protect people from injury, but they take away autonomous choice. Beneficence may justify overriding the decision of a febrile, confused person who refuses to take antibiotics for treatment of pneumonia. What is the clinician's responsibility? The duties of beneficence seem to mandate medicating this person against their will, ensuring that the good of health is facilitated in violation of the principle of autonomy. The justification for this must include an assessment of the person's status related to their capacity for autonomous decision-making. Preserving a person's life so they can make autonomous decisions in the future may be required by beneficence. However, it can be argued that beneficence takes precedence over autonomy only in those cases in which the choice cannot be considered autonomous. First, there must be evidence that a choice has been made. In this case the choice was between accepting antibiotic treatment and not accepting antibiotic treatment. Second, the reasonableness (or rationality) of the decision must be discerned. It must be ascertained whether the person has really grasped the implications of refusing treatment. The reasons given for the treatment refusal, then, should illuminate gaps in information delivery or processing. Finally, it must be determined whether there are any external or internal coercion factors impinging on the decision. Perhaps the person feels they cannot afford the medicine (external), or perhaps they have a mistrust of antibiotics because of a previous experience (internal). When a decision cannot be said to be informed, the principle of beneficence directs us to decide on treatment on the basis of the person's best interests.

The conflict between beneficence and autonomy was a central focus during the COVID-19 pandemic. Individuals cited their right to autonomy as the rationale for not wearing masks in public, rebelling against quarantine recommendations, and remaining unvaccinated. Prioritizing individual autonomy over the needs of the population created many challenges for both individuals and health care organizations. These challenges were amplified when some nurses publicly supported individual autonomy over what was believed to be of benefit to all in responding to the global pandemic and the needs of individuals affected by COVID-19 (Khubchandani et al., 2022; Cartolovni et al., 2021; Mishkin et al., 2021).

Justice

Justice is an ethical principle that is of major importance in health-promotion settings. Various conceptions of justice exist, and the term is used in a variety of ways. This chapter focuses on social justice rather than criminal justice. **Social justice** refers to formal or informal systems within a society that are concerned with disparities in socioeconomic conditions that lead to poor health and fairness in the distribution of goods such as health, education, food, and shelter (Braveman, 2023; Cross et al., 2024). Justice in health care is a major commitment of nursing, and thus the discipline of nursing is becoming more focused on active engagement in social justice issues.

In democratic societies, the requirements of social justice generally include equitable distribution of the benefits and burdens of societal life. "Justice as fairness" reflects the ideas behind Rawls's (1971, 1999) *A Theory of Justice*. Rawls identifies two rules that he argues will result in a fair and just society: "First: each person is to have an equal right to the most extensive liberty compatible with a similar liberty for others. Second: social and economic inequalities are to be arranged such that they are both (a) reasonably expected to be to everyone's advantage, and (b) attached to positions and offices open to all" (Rawls, 1971, 1999). Rawls formulates these rules as a result of his hypothetical method for deciding how a society's institutions should be arranged to provide fairness. Rawls proposes that these rules of justice would emerge as a result of an average person's reasoning about what social arrangements that person would prefer if that reasoning were done from behind a "veil of ignorance"; that is, if the person did not know what their personal impediments, assets, or characteristics, such as intelligence, socioeconomic status, race, gender, or (dis)ability, were going to be. Rawls's two rules aim to balance overall good for society with respect for individual rights—in some ways, it is a balance of Mill's utilitarianism and Kant's focus on respect for persons. That is why inequalities must be open to all and must be to everyone's advantage. It is arguably fair for a judge to be paid more than a janitor because the judge's higher salary is to the advantage of all given that it leads to competition and motivates the brightest citizens to enter the profession. However, for a truly fair situation, part (b) of the second rule would also have to hold true: The pathway to becoming a judge must be open to all. Meeting part (b) would presumably require, at least, quality public education and financial support for college and law school.

Rawls's theory, although respected by ethicists, is subject to criticism on a variety of fronts. One significant criticism is that justice as fairness does not provide much guidance for some common social problems, such as abortion, welfare, and the righting of previous wrongs (e.g., affirmative action, the rights of native people), and it ignores the problems of those without legal rights, such as undocumented workers (Buchanan, 2006; Cross et al., 2024). Dinkins (2011), however, suggests that the "veil of ignorance" thought experiment described by Rawls may increase empathy in daily practice because it helps us realize that when we step out from the veil into the envisioned workplace, we could be anybody: a single mother without insurance unable to access health care for her children, an elderly female with a hoarding disorder who lives surrounded by piles and piles of decaying garbage, or a person from any other vulnerable population in our society.

An emphasis on justice in health care settings is sometimes called the "impartialist" perspective in that it considers the needs of all who fall under its umbrella. For example, within the prison system, this view of justice would mandate access to care for prisoners in need. It would not permit arbitrary obstacles to access (such as requiring good behavior or favors) that might be presented by prison officers or by other prisoners who wish to exert physical or psychological control. Justice would also require improved access to care for the poor and underprivileged, in terms of both receiving care and having access to transportation or local availability of services.

Although justice might require consideration of the special needs of a disadvantaged group, it does so impartially—that is, it does not distinguish among the particulars of individuals. Each member within the group has an equal right to whatever is proposed. In an economically and profit-driven health care system, injustices occur both at the local level and at the societal level. Because justice viewed as fairness is impartial about individual differences, that moral perspective considered alone is not a perfect tool with which to look at health care disparities and their causes.

Health disparities are a specific subset of health differences that are important for social justice because they evolve from intentional or unintentional discrimination or marginalization (Braveman, 2023). Nurses and other health professionals need to move beyond thinking about "doing no harm" to identifying and addressing adverse social influences on the health of underprivileged groups and the implications of their consequent poor health (International Council of Nursing, 2023). The combination of justice, feminist concerns about power and oppression, and the acknowledged responsibilities of nurses to promote health permit a comprehensive view of problems associated with health protection and promotion. This view incorporates an ethical approach to problems both for society and for individuals within society. Buchanan (2006) captures this necessary synthesis of perspectives well, noting "the mutually reinforcing relationships among justice, caring and responsibility" that will help nurses to "enable people to live well."

STRATEGIES FOR ETHICAL DECISION-MAKING

Locating the Source and Levels of Ethical Problems

Most health-promotion problems are moral or ethical issues in the sense that obstacles exist that prevent an individual from living life well or achieving personal goals related to health. Throughout this chapter, discussions of both the larger (societal) and the narrower (individual) perspectives have been emphasized and their relationships highlighted. Sometimes tensions between the two require mediation and may force the health promoter to decide which problem to address first. For example, a nurse at a family practice clinic is caring for a teenager who is morbidly obese. At the level of the individual, the nurse is charged with discovering the underlying causes of obesity (e.g., physical, psychological, contextual) and designing strategies with the individual to help resolve the problem. However, the nurse also has responsibilities to address the issue at the more political level with interested others.

To address health-promotion issues effectively, professionals need to possess not only disciplinary expertise and an understanding of ethical language, principles, and perspectives, but also a willingness to understand their own values and preconceptions about health and people. Understanding personal philosophy, biases, and values permits one to control these in the sense of being aware of the influences they have on our interactions with others.

Values Clarification and Reflection

Gaining confidence in moral decision-making is a slow process. The following are suggestions that will guide development related to recognizing and addressing ethical issues.

Examine Beliefs and Values

Cultivate the habit of examining how your personal values and **beliefs** relate to the human condition, justice, and responsibility. Be willing to revise your beliefs in line with your professional knowledge base, experiences, or current research findings. For example, how do beliefs that "people get what they deserve" correlate with what we know—for example, that those of lower socioeconomic status have lower levels of health and that poor health interferes with functioning and is associated with depression? How do our attitudes change when we try to place ourselves in the context of another person's life?

This is not to say that maintaining personal integrity is not important—it is. Maintaining both personal and professional integrity is essential to good practice. Integrity has to do with a sense of wholeness of the self and consistency of actions with truly examined beliefs and values. "Nurses have both personal and professional identities that are integrated and that embrace the values of the profession, merging them with personal values" (ANA, 2015a). The Code of Ethics for Nurses with Interpretive Statements validates the nurse's preservation of integrity in those situations in which they feel their personal integrity is compromised, indicating that they are justified in refusing to participate when a decision or action is objectional on moral grounds (ANA, 2015a). In contemplating refusal to provide care, however, the nurse should ensure that the decision is based on sound ethical principles, not simply on personal beliefs. When opting out of care involves risk to the individual, other arrangements must be made to safeguard individual care. A decisions not to participate in a situation cannot be made trivially because of the trust relationship and a nurse's moral accountability for their actions. The threat to the nurse's integrity must be serious, and the person's well-being must not be jeopardized by the nurse's absence. Other arrangements must be made for care of the person in such circumstances. The nurse who encounters repeated threats to integrity has a responsibility to consider changing the situation in some way. Change efforts may be directed toward institutional policy or may require that an alternative work environment be considered.

A true examination of beliefs and values requires a willingness to admit that these beliefs may not always be justifiable; they may be remnants of childhood indoctrination of various sorts. For example, one might believe that certain ethnic groups are inferior in some way or that one should not question authority.

An honest and ongoing examination of one's values and biases permits one to control these beliefs when providing care to diverse persons. Being willing to examine one's beliefs and values is thus a key part of personal and professional integrity.

Recognize the Influence of Personal Beliefs and Values

In addition to examining beliefs and values, we should also think about the influence that these characteristics have on our practice. An understanding of how personal beliefs and values are either congruent or liable to interfere with the task at hand is crucial to ethical problem-solving. In any given situation, the health professional must ask, "What are my beliefs and biases in this situation?" and "How are these likely to influence my actions?" For example, if the home health nurse believes that a below-poverty-level, depressed, obese, diabetic patient who smokes is responsible for the poor healing of their leg ulcer, the nurse may be less inclined to work with the person to discover and address the person's goals.

Reflect on Practice

A third helpful strategy is to reflect on situations afterward to discover what worked, what did not work, and what could be done differently in the future. It is often helpful to interact with peers or other experts after particularly difficult situations to discover alternative perspectives or resources for the purposes of future problem-solving. You might ask a peer or mentor to ask questions to help you think through why you made a particular decision. Or you might practice some reflective writing to help you think through your reasoning and consider whether you would act differently in the future (Dinkins & Cangelosi, 2019).

Use a Decision-Making Framework

Decision-making in health-promotion settings has inescapable moral components. As noted earlier, the nurse has a professional responsibility to further the good for individuals and society. The careful exercise of experience, skill, and knowledge is warranted when one is trying to formulate the best course of action for a given individual or group, or in resolving societal health-promotion problems. This framework is offered as a way of ensuring clarity about a particular case or situation. Because of the diverse nature of health-promotion activities, no straightforward models of decision-making can realistically be applied in all situations. Additionally, decision-making is often an ongoing process, and revisions to plans may be required in light of new information. The following are important facets of decision-making but do not necessarily occur in the order given.

Identify the Main Problem or Issue

What level of problem is this: societal, group, or individual? If the location of the problem is societal, it will also affect individuals and groups, and a decision must be made about the order of interventions. Try to determine the main ethical principle involved or whether it is a problem of conflicting principles. For example, after identifying the problem, you may determine that to provide benefit to the person, you must override the person's autonomy. Is this a social justice issue? Is it an autonomy issue? What factors led to the problem? Is there coercion or another power imbalance? If so, who has an interest in maintaining the power imbalance, and who gains the most from the imbalance? These are the questions feminist ethicists would ask.

Determine on Whom the Resolution Will Have an Affect

Who has a stake in the issue, and in how it will be resolved? Answering this question will determine whose input is crucial to the decision-making process. Who and what are important considerations (e.g., institutions, individuals, businesses, social policy)? Is this issue a result of a failure to predict the consequences of certain social policies?

Determine the Prevalent Values

What are the values held by all the different players? Are there value conflicts? The value conflicts might be individual versus social, as in the case of a person with tuberculosis who refuses to take his medicines, thus putting at risk members of his family or members of the community. Value conflicts might also be interpersonal among the health-promotion team, or they might be personal versus professional. As a general rule, more weight is assigned to the values of the individual who is most likely to be affected by a decision. It is important to consider the influence of culture on values when the issue involves health promotion for culturally diverse groups. It is also important to involve people who can help explain cultural beliefs, especially when language difficulties are present. A knowledgeable but neutral interpreter may be helpful when liaison between groups is needed.

Identify Cues and Information Gaps

Reflect on whether the decision-makers are confident about what they know and do not know, as well as what they may be overlooking. This determination is not always an easy task. Information may exist that has not yet reached our awareness, or we might fail to ask a question that would reveal important information. How can we be confident about the scope and limits of our knowledge? Clinical judgment is a good tool but is not foolproof. When doubts exist or the decision is likely to have serious or risky consequences, we need to involve knowledgeable others or try to determine the best places to gain missing information.

Formulate Possible Courses of Action and Probable Consequences

Courses of action may involve further information gathering, brainstorming, and possibly collaborating with other experts or specialists. Although further data may be needed to resolve problems at the level of individuals or small groups, it is especially necessary to enlist additional help when the issue is one that requires political action to effect policy changes. It may be necessary to recruit community members and leaders or to enlist the political power of specialty groups. Finally, a determination must be made about which proposed courses of action will be the least harmful and the most beneficial. Remember not to look just at likely consequences, however. Consider possible actions from the framework of duty and character as well.

Initiate the Selected Course of Action and Evaluate the Outcome

Does the actual outcome match the anticipated outcome? If not, was what happened unexpected? Would this outcome have been foreseeable given more data? Would you do things differently in a similar situation given what you have learned? Does the problem need to be addressed at a different level (institutional or public policy)?

Engage in Self-Reflection and Peer or Expert Group Reflection

What could you have done differently? Would consulting with others have altered your conception of the problem or your course of action? What insights can you or your peers glean from this that could be appropriate for similar situations in the future? How might continuing education opportunities help you or your peers more appropriately address similar problems in the future? Would an ethics resource (committee or consultant) be helpful in such situations? Could you use this case as a focused learning experience for your peers and collaborators?

ETHICS OF HEALTH PROMOTION: CASE EXAMPLES

Some cases of special relevance to health promotion are presented in this section. They are followed by questions that can be answered by individual readers, but they also provide a good starting point for group discussion. Try using the decision-making strategies suggested throughout the chapter as you explore these problems. It is anticipated that you will want more information than is provided. Deciding what extra information would be helpful is an important part of the exercise.

Case 1: Addressing Health Care System Problems—Elissa Needs Help

Elissa is 38 years old. She recently moved 200 miles from her home to a small town (population 6000) and separated from her abusive husband to escape his continuing threats and to be near her childhood friend. She suffers from chronic, sometimes incapacitating depression, for which she has received antidepressant medications and counseling, with temporary relief. She has been unable to work and has no private health insurance. She is eligible for the state's Medicaid program, however, and has recently discovered that Medicaid will cover her health care needs. Her friend refers her to the only primary care center in the area, where she is seen by Jill, one of the two nurse practitioners. As part of her evaluation, Jill discovers that Elissa was abused as a child and has very poor self-esteem. Elissa affirms that her childhood friend is very supportive. Jill believes that longer-term psychological counseling would benefit Elissa and facilitate her well-being, but she also knows that none of the counseling services within a 50-mile radius accepts Medicaid payment. Elissa has no transportation.

- What are Jill's options? What are her responsibilities?
- What actions might Jill pursue both on a local level and on a political level? What are her resources?
- What is the responsibility of the health-promotion disciplines in cases such as this?

Case 2: She's My Client! Lilly and "Jake" (a.k.a. Paul)

Shirley, a nurse practitioner, is at a conference when a physician colleague discusses a difficult case. One of his clients, "Jake," is HIV positive but refuses any treatment. The physician explains that Jake fears that his wife will discover and recognize the names of the medications, because he knows "these drug names are discussed on television all the time." Jake has not told his wife that he is HIV positive and has no intention of ever doing so. Jake firmly believes his condition is his private information and, for now, the couple use condoms for birth control. The physician is concerned that Jake will not tell his wife. The physician is presenting this case to colleagues to highlight the public awareness campaigns that, to some extent, have affected client privacy. He argues, "Listen to how they call out your name and the drugs at the pharmacy counter."

Shirley recognizes bits and pieces of information and comes to the painful realization that Jake is really Paul, and Paul is the husband of one of her clients, Lilly. Lilly has begun to discuss with Shirley that she wants to get pregnant soon. The town is too small for Shirley to be mistaken. Or is it?

- Is it ethical for the nurse practitioner to ask the physician if Jake is Paul?
- Is it ethical for Shirley to tell Lilly she suspects Paul is HIV positive?
- Should this information change how Shirley counsels Lilly about a pregnancy?
- What is in Lilly's best interests? Is Shirley also obligated to consider Paul's interests?
- What resources are available?

Case 3: Don't Touch My Things! Ms. Smyth and Autonomy

Ms. Smyth, 78 years old, had lived in the same home for 30 years. Never married, she cared for her disabled mother for 15 years. After her mother died, she lived alone on a small pension. She appeared to be well groomed and appropriately dressed when she left her house.

Ms. Smyth was hospitalized for a bowel obstruction, and Joe, a community health nurse, made a follow-up visit after being discharged to her home. When Joe arrived at the house, he was overcome by the smell of rotting garbage, urine, and feces. Five small dogs ran back and forth among piles of garbage and magazines, overturned furniture, and discarded appliances. There was no running water, and the bathroom was not functional. Joe had concerns about hoarding and told Ms. Smyth that her living conditions were unhealthy. Further, he stated that he would contact a community agency to help her clean her house. Ms. Smyth became very angry and said no one had the right to take her things away.

- Is it ethical for Joe to overrule Ms. Smyth's autonomy in decision-making?
- What action is in Ms. Smyth's best interests?
- What action is in the community's best interests?
- What ethical issues are involved in caring for a client with a hoarding disorder, such as that seen in Ms. Smyth's situation?

CASE STUDY

Genetic Screening Programs

A US genetic testing company has been sequencing the DNA of 20 individuals. With the individuals' consent, the results will be made available to researchers. Each donor will be offered information about genetic variations that might indicate a higher-than-average likelihood of developing a life-threatening condition.

The usefulness of genetic testing in screening for health problems is widely recognized (Huddleston, 2013; Ponte et al., 2019). Genetic tests can be used to determine risks for diseases such as Alzheimer's disease, polycystic kidney disease, bipolar disorder, Parkinson disease, and breast and ovarian cancer. There are hopes that genetic screenings of large populations will change the practice of health care from a focus on treating diseases to preventing them. Some researchers predict the complete sequencing of each human genome will provide routine data to health care providers, much like the common measurements of blood pressure, pulse, temperature, and blood counts today; however, others view traditional methods of collecting patient data, such as asking people about their family history of diabetes, their weight, and their age, as being stronger predictors of future health issues.

Reflective Questions

Apply different concepts and theories of ethics in thinking about the following questions.

- What are some of the ethical issues of these genetic analyses?
- What are the responsibilities of health care professionals in the genetic screenings of individuals and populations?
- What additional components could a nurse add to the plan of care for patients having genetic testing?

SUMMARY

- Health promotion is a vast and complex practice area; consequently, the associated ethical challenges are diverse and multileveled.
- This chapter has outlined the nature and purpose of health care ethics and related this framework to the responsibilities of health care providers in health-promotion interventions.
- Health promotion should be viewed as a moral undertaking of health care providers. After reading this chapter, students will have knowledge of some of the tools and language needed to explore ethical issues, discuss these issues with others, and address problematic issues at both the individual level and the societal level.
- Perhaps the most important factor to consider is that ethical problems manifesting themselves at the level of the individual almost always have their origins in the broader societal environment.

EVOLVE CHAPTER FEATURES

http://evolve.elsevier.com/Edelman/

- Study Questions

REFERENCES

Agency for Healthcare Research and Quality. (2020). *AHRQ health literacy universal precautions toolkit*. https://www.ahrq.gov/health-literacy/improve/precautions/index.html

American Bar Association. (2024). *Living wills, health care proxies, & advance health care directives*. https://www.americanbar.org/groups/real_property_trust_estate/resources/estate_planning/living_wills_health_care_proxies_advance_health_care_directives/

American Nurses Association (ANA). (1994). *Position statement: The nonnegotiable nature of the ANA code for nurses with interpretive statements*.

American Nurses Association (ANA). (2015a). *View the code of ethics for nurses with interpretive statements*. https://www.nursingworld.org/practice-policy/nursing-excellence/ethics/code-of-ethics-for-nurses/

American Nurses Association (ANA). (2015b). *Guide to nursing's social policy statement: Understanding the profession from social contract to social covenant*. https://www.nursingworld.org

American Nurses Association (ANA). (2021). *Position statement: nurses' professional responsibility to promote ethical practice environments*. https://www.nursingworld.org/

Aristotle. (1999). *Nicomachean ethics* (trans. T. Irwin). Indianapolis: Hackett Publishing. Original work ~350 BCE.

Augustine, L. G. (2022). Whistleblowing in healthcare for patient safety: An integrative literature review. *International Journal of Human Resource Studies*, *12*(1), 15–31. https://doi.org/10.5296/ijhrs.v12i1.19477

Beauchamp, T. L., & Childress, J. F. (2019). *Principles of biomedical ethics* (8th ed.). Oxford University Press.

Benner, P., Tanner, C. A., & Chesla, C. A. (2009). *Expertise in nursing practice: Caring, clinical judgment, and ethics* (2nd ed.). Springer.

Berlinger, N., & Berlinger, A. (2017). Culture and moral distress: What's the connection and why does it matter? *AMA Journal of Ethics*, *19*(6), 608–616. https://doi.org/10.1001/journalofethics.2017.19.6.msoc1-1706

Braveman, P. A. (2023). *The social determinants of health and health disparities*. Oxford University Press. https://doi.org/10.1093/oso/9780190624118.001.0001

Brothers, K. B., & Knapp, E. E. (2018). How should primary care physicians respond to direct-to-consumer genetic test results? *AMA Journal of Ethics*, *20*(9), 812–818. https://doi.org/10.1001/amajethics.2018.812

Buchanan, D. R. (2006). Moral reasoning as a model for health promotion. *Social Science & Medicine*, *63*(10), 2715–2726. https://doi.org/10.1016/j.socscimed.2006.07.002

Butts, J. B., & Rich, K. L. (2023). *Nursing ethics across the curriculum and into practice* (6th ed.). Jones and Bartlett Learning.

Carter, S. M., Rychetnik, L., Lloyd, B., Kerridge, I. H., Baur, L., Bauman, A., Hooker, C., & Zask, A. (2011). Evidence, ethics, and values: A framework for health promotion. *American Journal of Public Health*, *101*(3), 465–472. https://doi.org/10.2105/AJPH.2010.195545

Cartolovni, A., Stolt, M., Scott, P. A., & Suhonen, R. (2021). Moral injury in healthcare professionals: A scoping review and discussion. *Nursing Ethics, 28*(5), 590–602. https://doi.org/10.1177/0969733020966776

Chambliss, D. F. (1996). *Beyond caring: Hospitals, nurses, and the social organization of ethics*. Chicago, IL: University of Chicago Press.

Cleveland, K. A., Motter, T., & Smith, Y. (2019). Affordable care: Harnessing the power of nurses. *OJIN: The Online Journal of Issues in Nursing, 24*(2). https://www.doi.org/10.3912/OJIN.Vol27No02Man01

Cohen, E. (2015). *Heaven over hospital: Parents honor dying child's request*. CNN Health. http://www.cnn.com/2015/10/27/health/girl-chooses-heaven-over-hospital-part-2/

Corey, G., Corey, M. S., & Corey, C. (2024). *Issues and ethics in the helping professions* (11th ed.). Cengage Learning.

Cross, R., Warwick-Booth, L., & Woodall, J. (2024). *Health promotion ethics: A framework for social justice*. Routledge. https://doi.org/10.4324/9781003308317

Dinkins, C. S. (2011). Ethics: Beyond patient care: Practicing empathy in the workplace. *Online Journal of Issues in Nursing, 16*(2). https://ojin.nursingworld.org/table-of-contents/volume-16-2011/number-2-may-2011/empathy-in-the-workplace/

Dinkins, C. S., & Cangelosi, P. R. (2019). Putting Socrates back in Socratic method: Theory-based debriefing in the nursing classroom. *Nursing Philosophy, 20*(2). https://doi.org/10.1111/nup.12240

Epstein, B., & Turner, M. (2015). The nursing code of ethics: Its value, its history. *Online Journal of Issues in Nursing, 20*(2). https://doi.org/10.3912/OJIN.Vol20No02Man04

Epstein, E. G., & Delgado, S. (2010). Understanding and addressing moral distress. *Online Journal of Issues in Nursing, 15*(3). https://doi.org/10.3912/OJIN.Vol15No03Man01

Fantasia, H. C. (2011). Really not even a decision any more: Late adolescent narratives of implied sexual consent. *Journal of Forensic Nursing, 7*(3), 120–129. https://doi.org/10.1111/j.1939-3938.2011.01108.x

Fumincelli, L., Mazzo, A., Martins, J. C., & Mendes, I. A. (2019). Quality of life and ethics: A concept analysis. *Nursing Ethics, 26*(1), 61–70. https://doi.org/10.1177/0969733016689815

Gilligan, C. (1982). *In a different voice: Psychological theory and women's development*. Boston, MA: Harvard University Press.

Gilligan, C. (2023). *In a human voice*. Polity Press.

Grace, P. J., & Uveges, M. K. (2023). *Nursing ethics and professional responsibility in advanced practice* (4th ed.). Jones and Bartlett Learning.

Halkoaho, A., Pietila, A. M., Ebbesen, M., Karki, S., & Kangasniemi, M. (2016). Cultural aspects related to informed consent in health research: A systematic review. *Nursing Ethics, 23*(6), 698–712. https://doi.org/10.1177/0969733015579312

Hall, A., Wilson, C. B., Stanmore, E., & Todd, C. (2019). Moving beyond 'safety' versus 'autonomy': A qualitative exploration of the ethics of using monitoring technologies in long-term dementia care. *BMC Geriatrics, 19*, 145. https://doi.org/10.1186/s12877-019-1155-6

Healthy People 2030. (n.d.). *Health literacy in Healthy People 2030*. https://health.gov/healthypeople/priority-areas/health-literacy-healthy-people-2030

Higgins, S., & Duffy, J. (2006). Behavioral phenotypes: An emerging specialist role for nurses. *British Journal of Nursing, 15*(21), 1176–1179. https://doi.org/10.12968/bjon.2006.15.21.22376

Huddleston, K. (2013). Ethics: The challenge of ethical, legal, and social implications (ELSI) in genomic nursing. *OJIN: The Online Journal of Issues in Nursing, 19*(1). https://doi.org/10.3912/OJIN.Vol19No01EthCol01

Institute of Medicine. (2010). *The future of nursing: Leading change, advancing health*. https://pubmed.ncbi.nlm.nih.gov/24983041/

International Council of Nurses. (2023). *Position statement: Health inequities, discrimination and the nurse's role*. https://www.icn.ch/sites/default/files/2023-08/ICN%20Position%20Statement%20Health%20inequities%20discrimination%20%26%20the%20nurse%27s%20role%202023%20FINAL%2030.06_EN_1.pdf

International Council of Nurses. (2021). *The ICN code of ethics for nurses*. https://www.icn.ch/sites/default/files/2023-06/ICN_Code-of-Ethics_EN_Web.pdf

Iverson, E., Celious, A., Kennedy, C. R., Shehane, E., Eastman, A., Warren, V., Freeman, B. D. (2014). Factors affecting stress experienced by surrogate decision makers for critically ill patients: Implications for nursing practice. *Intensive and Critical Care Nursing, 30*(2), 77–85. https://doi.org/10.1016/j.iccn.2013.08.008

Johns Hopkins Medical. (2024). *Caring for the caregiver: The RISE program*. https://www.hopkinsmedicine.org/armstrong-institute/training-services/caring-for-the-caregiver#:~:text=Modeled%20on%20the%20Resilience%20in,support%20to%20individuals%20and%20groups

Jones, J. M. (2020). *Prevalence of living wills in the U.S. up slightly*. https://news.gallup.com/poll/312209/prevalence-living-wills-slightly.aspx

Kangasniemi, M., Pakkanen, P., & Korhonen, A. (2015). Professional ethics in nursing: An integrative review. *Journal of Advanced Nursing, 71*(8), 1744–1757. https://doi.org/10.1111/jan.12619

Kant, I. (1993/1785). *Grounding for the metaphysics of morals* (3rd ed.) (trans. J. W. Ellington). Indianapolis: Hackett. Original work published 1785.

Keane, M. (2010). Ethics as individual health interventions. *The American Journal of Bioethics, 10*(3), 36–38. https://doi.org/10.1080/15265160903581742

Khubchandani, J., Bustos, E., Chowdhury, S., Biswas, N., & Keller, T. (2022). COVID-19 vaccine refusal among nurses worldwide: Review of trends and predictors. *Vaccines (Basel), 10*(2), 230. https://doi.org/10.3390/vaccines10020230

Kohlberg, L. (1981). The philosophy of moral development: Moral stages and the idea of justice. In *Essays on Moral Development* (*Vol. 1*). New York, NY: Harper & Row.

Kohlberg, L. (1984). The psychology of moral development: The nature and validity of moral stages. In *Essays on Moral Development* (*Vol. 2*). New York, NY: Harper & Row.

Laholt, H., McLeod, K., Guillemin, M., Beddari, E., & Lorem, G. (2019). Ethical challenges experienced by public health nurses related to adolescents' use of visual technologies. *Nursing Ethics, 26*(6), 1822–1833. https://doi.org/10.1177/0969733018779179

Larcher, V., & Brierley, J. (2020). Children of COVID-19: Pawns, pathfinders, or partners. *Journal of Medical Ethics, 46*, 508–509. https://doi.org/10.1136/medethics-2020-106465

Litz, B. T., Stein, N., Delaney, E., Lebowitz, L., Nash, W. P., Silva, C., & Maguen, S. (2009). Moral injury and moral repair in war veterans: A preliminary model and intervention strategy. *Clinical Psychology Review, 29*(8), 695–706. https://doi.org/10.1016/j.cpr.2009.07.003

Lyon, D. E., McCain, N. L., Pickler, R. H., Munro, C., & Elswick, R. K. (2011). Advancing the biobehavioral research of fatigue with genetics and genomics. *Journal of Nursing Scholarship, 43*(3), 274–281. https://doi.org/10.1111/j.1547-5069.2011.01406.x

Madison, K. M., Volpp, K. G., & Halpern, S. D. (2011). The law, policy, and ethics of employers' use of financial incentives to improve health. *Journal of Law, Medicine & Ethics, 39*(3), 450–468. https://doi.org/10.1111/j.1748-720X.2011.00614.x

Mill, J. S. (2019/1861). Utilitarianism. In *Indianapolis: Compass Circle* (2nd ed.) Originally published 1861.

Mishkin, A. D., Allen, N., Hulkower, A., & Flicker, L. S. (2021). Increased ethical burden in surrogate decision-making during COVID-19. *The Journal of Hospital Ethics, 7*(2), 73–81.

Munro, C. L. (2015). Individual genetic and genomic variation: A new opportunity for personalized nursing interventions. *Journal of Advanced Nursing, 71*(1), 35–41. https://doi.org/10.1111/jan.12552

National Council of State Boards of Nursing. (2018a). *A nurse's guide to the use of social media*. https://www.ncsbn.org/public-files/NCSBN_SocialMedia.pdf

National Council of State Boards of Nursing. (2018b). *A nurse's guide to professional boundaries*. https://www.ncsbn.org/public-files/ProfessionalBoundaries_Complete.pdf

National Society of Genetic Counselors. (2017). *NSGC code of ethics*. https://www.nsgc.org/POLICY/Code-of-Ethics-Conflict-of-Interest/Code-of-Ethics

Nelson, H. L. (1992). Against caring. *Journal of Clinical Ethics, 3*(1), 8–20. https://uwethicsofcare.gws.wisc.edu/wp-content/uploads/2020/03/Nelson-H.-L.-1992.pdf

Office of Disease Prevention and Health Promotion. (2022). *Healthy People 2030 framework*. https://health.gov/healthypeople/about/healthy-people-2030-framework

Oxford Reference. (2024). Moral agency. In *Oxford Reference.com dictionary*. https://www.oxfordreference.com

Peirce, A. G., Elie, S., George, A., Gold, M., O'Hara, K., & Rose-Facey, W. (2020). Knowledge development, technology, and questions of nursing ethics. *Nursing Ethics, 27*(1), 77–87. https://doi.org/10.1177/0969733019840752

Politz, K., & Rae, M. (2017). *Changing rules for workplace wellness programs: Implications for sensitive health conditions. Kaiser Family Foundation*. https://www.kff.org/private-insurance/issue-brief/changing-rules-for-workplace-wellness-programs-implications-for-sensitive-health-conditions/

Ponte, A., Greenberg, S., Greendale, K., & Senier, L. (2019). Moving the needle on action around evidence-based screening for hereditary conditions: Preparing state chronic disease directors to advance precision public health. *Public Health Reports, 134*(3), 228–233. https://doi.org/10.1177/0033354919834588

President's Commission for the Study of Ethical Problems in Medicine and Biomedical and Behavioral Research. (1982). *Compensating for research injuries: The ethical and legal implications of programs to redress injured subjects*. US Government Printing Office.

Rachels, J., & Rachels, S. (2023). *The elements of moral philosophy* (10th ed.). McGraw-Hill.

Rawls, J. (1971, 1999). *A theory of justice*. Boston, MA: Harvard University.

Robichaux, C., Tietze, M., Stokes, F., & McBride, S. (2019). Reconceptualizing the electronic health record for a new decade. *Advances in Nursing Science, 12*(3), 193–205. https://doi.org/10.1097/ANS.0000000000000282

Rudd, K. (2019). Standards of practice and ethical considerations. In K. Rudd and D. Kocisko (Ed.), *Pediatric nursing: The critical components of nursing care* (2nd ed.). 11–32. F. A. Davis.

Singer, P. (1993). *A companion to ethics*. Hoboken, NJ: Wiley-Blackwell.

Singer, P. (2023). Ethics. *Online Encyclopedia Britannica*. https://www.britannica.com/topic/ethics-philosophy

Smith, Y. M., & Caplin, M. (2012). Teaching the literacy of professionalism. *Nurse Educator, 17*(3), 121–125. https://doi.org/10.1097/NNE.0b013e3182504188

Smith, Y. M., & Cleveland, K. A., & Kleman, C. (2021). Understanding nurses' experiences and contributions to governing boards. *OJIN: The Online Journal of Issues in Nursing, 27*(1). https://www.doi.org/10.3912/OJIN.Vol27No01PPT32

Smith, Y. M., & Crowe, A. R. (2016). Nurse educator perceptions of the importance of relationship in online teaching and learning. *Journal of Professional Nursing, 33*(1), 11–19. https://doi.org/10.1016/j.profnurs.2016.06.004

Sorrell, J. M. (2014). Deciding for others: Surrogates struggling with health care decisions. *Journal of Psychosocial Nursing and Mental Health Services, 52*(7), 17–21. https://doi.org/10.3928/02793695-20140603-01

Sorrell, J. M. (2015). Ethics: Employer-sponsored wellness programs for nurses: The ethics of carrots and sticks. *OJIN: The Online Journal of Issues in Nursing, 20*(1), 8. https://doi.org/10.3912/OJIN.Vol20No01EthCol01

Sorrell, J. M. (2021). Aging matters through the years: A retrospective. *Journal of Psychosocial Nursing and Mental Health Services, 59*(10), 7–11. https://doi.org/10.3928/02793695-20210908-01

Sorrell, J. M., & Cangelosi, P. R. (2009). Respecting vulnerability: Informed consent in persons with Alzheimer's disease. *Southern Online Journal of Nursing Research, 9*(4). https://snrs.org

Sproul, R. C. (2015). *The difference between ethics and morality*. Ligonier Ministries. http://www.ligonier.org

Steck, M. B. (2018). Workplace wellness programs: Educating patients and families about discrimination via disclosure of genetic information. *Clinical Journal of Oncology Nursing, 22*(5), 496–499. https://doi.org/10.1188/18.CJON.496-499

Tandy-Connor, S., Guiltinan, J., Krempely, K., LaDuca, H., Reineke, P., Gutierrez, S., Gray, P., & Davis, B. T. (2018). False-positive results released by direct-to-consumer genetic tests highlight the importance of clinical confirmation testing for appropriate patient care. *Genetics in Medicine, 20*, 1515–1521. https://doi.org/10.1038/gim.2018.38

Tanioka, T. (2019). Nursing and rehabilitative care of the elderly using humanoid robots. *The Journal of Medical Investigation, 66*, 19–23. https://doi.org/10.2152/jmi.66.19

Tarasoff v. Regents of University of California. (1976). California Supreme Court 131. https://law.justia.com

Tengland, P. A. (2016). Behavior change or empowerment: On the ethics of health-promotion goals. *Health Care Analysis, 24*, 24–46. https://doi.org/10.1007/s10728-013-0265-0

Terry, P. E. (2017). Preserving employee privacy in wellness. *American Journal of Health Promotion, 31*(4), 271–273. https://doi.org/10.1177/0890117117715043

Tigard, D. W. (2019). The positive value of moral distress. *Bioethics, 33*, 601–608. https://doi.org/10.1111/bioe.12564

Tong, R. (2022). Feminist ethics: Some thoughts about "care" and "power" for advanced practice nurses. In J. B. Butts, & K. L. Rich (Eds.), *Philosophies and Theories for Advanced Nursing Practice* (4th ed.). Jones and Bartlett Learning.

University of Missouri Center for Health Ethics. (2023). *Advanced directives and surrogate decision making*. https://medicine.missouri.edu/centers-institutes-labs/health-ethics/faq/advance-directives

US Department of Health and Human Services. (2022). *The HIPAA privacy rule*. https://www.hhs.gov/hipaa/for-professionals/privacy/index.html

Van Goidsenhoven, L., & De Schauwer, E. (2022). Relational ethics, informed consent, and informed assent in participatory research with children with complex communication needs. *Developmental Medicine and Child Neurology, 64*(11), 1323–1329. https://doi.org/10.1111/dmcn.15297

Weston, A. (2020). *A practical companion to ethics* (5th ed.). Oxford University Press.

Yeo, M., Moorhouse, A., Khan, P., & Rodney, P. (2020). *Concepts and cases in nursing ethics* (4th ed.). Broadview Press.

6 Health Promotion and the Individual

Julianne A. Walsh

http://evolve.elsevier.com/Edelman/

OBJECTIVES

After completing this chapter, the reader will be able to:

- Define the framework of functional health patterns as described by Gordon (2014).
- Describe the use of the functional health pattern framework to assess individuals throughout the life span.
- Illustrate health patterns of the functional, potentially dysfunctional, and actually dysfunctional categories of behavior.
- Identify risk factors or etiologic aspects of actual or potential dysfunctional health patterns.
- Discuss the planning, implementation, and evaluation of nursing interventions to promote the health of individuals.
- Develop specific health promotion plans based on an assessment of individuals.

KEY TERMS

Age-developmental focus
Cultural attunement
Culturally competent care
Expected outcomes
Functional focus
Functional health patterns
Health status
Individual-environmental focus
Nursing interventions
Pattern focus
Risk factors

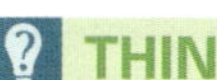

THINK ABOUT IT

Assessment of Breastfeeding Early in the Postpartum Period

In general, mothers stop breastfeeding before the recommended times. Early termination of breastfeeding peaks during the first week postpartum and again between 2 weeks and 2 months. Early assessment, then, intended to influence decision-making and maintain breastfeeding for a longer duration, may reverse these trends. Francis and Dickton (2019) conducted early assessments that included evaluation of the infant's oral cavity, physical breast assessment, and observation of infant-mother feeding behaviors. Their initial assessment shortly after birth determined the maternal feeding method intended during pregnancy and prior experience with breastfeeding. Breast care assessment included hand-expressing techniques and knowledge about comfort measures for engorgement. At 2 weeks, assessment included the infant's oral cavity, physical breast assessment, and observation of infant–mother feeding behaviors.

These assessment parameters provide indicators of breastfeeding success. Such assessments are useful strategies to guide health promotion intervention. These data support the conclusion that early feeding during the first 2-weeks postpartum with an Internationally Board-Certified Lactation Consultant (IBCLC) may increase breastfeeding at 6-weeks postpartum.

Why would a nurse tailor the assessments to individual characteristics of a population? How effectively would these assessment parameters identify primary prevention for breastfeeding in other breastfeeding populations? Could early assessment be considered an intervention in itself?

In health promotion practice, nurses assess patterns and use their assessment findings to facilitate an individual's maintenance of well-being or their progression toward wellness. Health and illness within this context reflect changing patterns of the life process. For example, generally when disorganization or ineffective coping produce fluctuations in patterns that eventually result in illness, a treatment plan is designed to alleviate the symptoms or eliminate the illness altogether. The strategies used in the assessment process previously described aim primarily to identify abnormalities. Conversely, health promotion assessment, for example in this case of ineffective coping, targets the strategies used for effective coping strategies and seeks to prevent illness (ineffective coping) in the first place. Therefore these two different assessment goals require distinctive approaches for assessment and planning. One approach is to identify assets, strengths, or characteristics of resilience in the various areas of assessment.

The framework of holistic nursing is congruent with identifying an individual's assets and using strength-based assessment. Holistic nursing provides central unifying themes that connect pattern recognition to person-environment relationships for health promotion throughout the life span. Holism emerges from each of the four American Holistic Nurses Association's (AHNA's) nursing core values of philosophy, self-care, clinical judgment, and holistic/therapeutic communication (Rosa et al., 2019). These AHNA core values require broad professional collaboration to address the needs of individuals, families, and communities and to extend globally.

In research that guides health promotion assessment in nursing, the health belief model and Pender's Health Promotion Model appear prominently in the literature, worldwide, and for a variety of health promotion health patterns (Ibrahim, Fadila, & Elmawla, 2023; Khani et al., 2020; Wilson & Nola, 2021). Asset identification or strength-based assessment are often foundational ideas presented in these and other health promotion models. In strength-based or asset assessment, nurses identify an individual's harmonious patterns of health. These self-management behavior changes of empowerment and resilience offer individuals an approach when addressing health phenomena (Jin & Peng, 2022). With the emergence of resilience interventions, Lovette and colleagues (2019) have identified the need for concept development and assessment parameters of strengths for various conditions.

Long before the current worldwide focus on health promotion and prevention, an initiative in the United States, nursing theories, such as Martha Rogers' Science of Unitary Human Beings, posited that nurses care for well individuals as well as for those who are ill (Pueyo-Garrigues et al., 2019). Rogers' theory, the science of unitary human beings, continues to serve as an underlying theory for nursing practice in many areas of nursing. For example, Karaman and Tan (2021) use Rogers' theory as a framework for Reiki therapy and breast cancer research. These authors claim that Rogers' theory complies with the philosophy and principles of Reiki practice, including how humans interact within the environment, as the application of energy-based alternative therapy methods improves fatigue and increases the quality of life of humans (Karaman & Tan, 2021). These researchers' theoretical approach forms a firm foundation for health promotion assessment and the interrelationships of Marjory Gordon's Functional Health Patterns discussed in this chapter.

In the United States, Healthy People, the national health promotion initiative, has established national goals and has provided a framework for prevention since 1979 (Ochiai et al., 2021). Healthy People continues to publish national health objectives that build on the original Healthy People initiatives that aim to identify the most significant preventable threats to health. Well before the decade comes to a close, evaluation of the previous decade begins, and experts establish a new set of science-based, national objectives to improve Americans' health for the next 10 years. *Healthy People 2030* was approved in June 2018 by a federal advisory committee composed of nonfederal, independent subject matter experts, the Committee on National Health Promotion and Disease Prevention Objectives for 2030 (US Department of Health and Human Services, [USDHHS], 2024). Before approval in 2017, the framework was reviewed by a panel of experts and open to public comment in 2017 (USDHHS, 2024). New goals and objectives for the next decade arise from the evaluation of the previous decade's outcomes. State and local communities use these objectives, leading health indicators, and data to evaluate progress toward their overall goals of attaining high-quality and longer lives, decreasing health disparities, and creating environments that promote health and improve the quality of life for all (Ochiai et al., 2021).

Many 2030 topics concern primary prevention for individuals in some way. Selected examples of how the *Healthy People 2030* objectives address these primary prevention areas for individuals are presented in Box 6.1: Healthy People 2030. Furthermore, this initiative provides current data available online for use to evaluate regional efforts toward the national goals and for the nation to progress to a healthier status for individuals, families, and communities. An array of web-based resources offers a ready supply of tools for the public to use for health promotion assessment of individuals (Ochiai et al., 2021; USDHHS, 2024). More information about these resources is available at http://HealthyPeople.gov, where you can subscribe to the Healthy People listserv and follow @GoHealthyPeople on X.

Nursing plays an integral part in the US national initiatives for health promotion and prevention. Moreover, the scope of nursing practice provides the ideal foundation for leadership globally in these initiatives aimed to promote health and prevent disease. For example, the International Council of Nurse's (ICN) definition incorporates nursing clinical judgment related to health promotion, illness prevention, and autonomous, collaborative care for people of all ages as they respond to actual or potential health concerns (ICN, 2023). Individuals, families, and communities are target populations of nurses. These elements of the definition encompass a range from individual care to design of future population health policy. The ICN's broad definition provides a foundation for nursing globally, offering a useful framework for health promotion. Nurses typically use interventions and health promotion strategies that address interactions among an individual's biophysical, psychosocial, and spiritual states and patterns with the environment. When assessing for primary prevention, the techniques also include generalized health promotion and specific protection from disease, both of which fall within the scope of nursing practice. The active process of promoting health involves protection (e.g., immunizations, occupational safety, and environmental control) along with lifestyle, value, and belief system behaviors that enhance health.

BOX 6.1 *HEALTHY PEOPLE 2030*

***Selected Examples of National Health Promotion and Disease-Prevention Proposed Objectives for Individuals from* Healthy People 2030**

Objective Number	Objective Statement
AHS-01	Increase the proportion of people with health insurance
O-01	Reduce the proportion of adults with osteoporosis
SDOH-01	Reduce the proportion of people living in poverty
NWS-01	Reduce household food insecurity and hunger
IID-02	Reduce the proportion of children who get no recommended vaccines by age 2 years

From USDHHS (2024)

This chapter addresses nursing assessment of individuals for the purpose of health promotion. In most other areas of health care, tertiary care and prevention of further disease provide the assessment focus. Tertiary care–focused assessment identifies deficits, thus excluding assessment of overall general health and wellness. Often, nursing plans are problem-oriented and reflect a focus of deficit assessment and problem-solving; however, these health promotion plans include many life processes that provide the broad base needed for nursing to address strength-based healthy responses or potential for healthy responses.

Although current US health care systems continue to use deficit assessment rather than the asset-based approach that is more appropriate for health promotion settings, movement toward including asset-based approaches is progressing in most disciplines. Mental health, social work, and nursing embrace an asset-based approach to assessment within the health promotion context. With a growing global recognition of the importance of primary prevention, organizations now may explore primary prevention assessment strategies. For example, in 2019, the American College of Cardiology (ACC) and American Heart Association (AHA) task force produced new primary prevention recommendations for atherosclerotic cardiovascular disease, including that it is reasonable to assess cardiovascular risk factors in healthy adults 20 to 39 years of age at least every 4 to 6 years. Sleep hygiene assessment and lifestyle counseling for weight loss with psychosocial intervention were also recommended (Arnett et al., 2019). Several other recommendations included patient-centered approaches, team-based care, social determinants of health assessment, and therefore primary prevention cost and benefit. Their topmost recommendation presented was to promote a healthy lifestyle throughout life (Arnett et al., 2019).

Nurses incorporate asset-based assessment into their assessment process (Bjørnsen et al., 2019). Furthermore, concentrating on strengths in specific health promotion settings provides a foundation to help individuals move toward improved health. Nurses support and enhance the ability of healthy individuals to maintain or strengthen their health.

Gordon's (2014) framework, which uses a **functional health patterns** assessment, provides the foundation for the health promotion assessment of an individual.

Functional health patterns developed by Gordon are used worldwide, providing an essential holistic framework that guides comprehensive patient assessment and offers a broad basis for assessment in most areas of nursing (De Cassia Gengo e Silva Butcher & Jones, 2021). This framework is used throughout this chapter to demonstrate assessment approaches, as well as family and community assessment (see Chapters 7 and 8). In addition, this chapter presents components of the nursing process as they relate to health promotion of the individual.

GORDON'S FUNCTIONAL HEALTH PATTERNS: ASSESSMENT OF THE INDIVIDUAL

Nursing clinical judgment is an essential critical thinking skill necessary to understand the **health status** of an individual. Table 6.1 demonstrates aspects of a complete nursing assessment. Assessment, in this case, refers to collection of data that culminates in problem identification. Effective health assessment considers not only physiologic parameters but how the human being interacts with the whole environment. Behavior patterns, beliefs, perceptions, and values form the essential components of health assessment when nurses consider the maximal health potential of the individual. Pattern recognition supports our understanding of health of individuals and is reflected in nursing theories such as those initially developed by nursing theorists such as Rogers (Karaman & Tan, 2021; Pueyo-Garrigues et al., 2019).

TABLE 6.1 Deliberate and Systematic Data Collection, Recognizing and Analyzing Cues

Components	Subjective data: Health history, including subjective reports and individual perceptions Family interviews, including historical information
	Objective data: Observations of nurse Vital signs Physical examination findings Information from health record Results of clinical testing
Function	Description of person's health status
Structure	Organization of interdependent parts describing health, function, or patterns of behavior that reflect the whole individual and environment
Process	Interview, observation, and examination
Format	Systematic but flexible; individualized to each person, nurse, and situation
Goal	Identification of areas of strengths, limitations, alterations, responses to alterations and therapies, and risks

Historically, many conceptual models in nursing have used Gordon's health-related behaviors particularly in regard to formulating a framework to guide assessment and care planning. The current expansion of electronic health records and electronic documentation from acute care, ambulatory settings, and communities requires continued emphasis on the standardization of nursing language (Herdman, Kamitsuru, & Lopes, 2021). Gordon's 11 functional health patterns interact to depict an individual's lifestyle. Using this framework, nurses combine assessment skills with subjective and objective data to construct patterns reflective of lifestyles.

Functional Health Pattern Framework

Holism and the totality of the person's interactions with the environment form the philosophical foundations of Gordon's functional health patterns. This foundation provides a context for collecting data that provide information about the entire person and most life processes. By examining functional patterns and interactions among patterns, nurses accurately determine actual or potential problems, intervene more effectively, and facilitate movement toward outcomes to promote health and well-being (Gordon, 2014). In addition to providing a framework to assess individuals, families, and communities holistically, functional health patterns provide a strong underpinning for more effective **nursing interventions** and outcomes. This stronger foundation provides a solid position from which nurses participate as decision-makers in health care systems at organizational, community, national, and international levels.

Definition

Functional health patterns view the individual as a whole being using interrelated behavioral areas. The typology of 11 patterns serves as a useful tool to collect and organize assessment data and to create a structure for validation and communication among health care providers. Each pattern described in Table 6.2 forms part of the biopsychosocial-spiritual expression of the whole person. Individual reports and nursing observations provide data to differentiate patterns. As a framework for assessment, functional health patterns provide an effective means for nurses to perceive and record complex interactions of an individual's biophysical state, psychological makeup, and environmental relationships.

Characteristics

Functional health patterns are characterized by their focus. Gordon (2014) describes five focus areas: pattern, individual-environmental, age-developmental, functional, and cultural.

Pattern focus implies that nurses explore patterns or sequences of behavior over time. Gordon's term "behavior" encompasses all forms of human behavior, including biophysical, psychological, and sociologic elements. Information collection includes exploration of these forms of behavior. Pattern and cue recognition, a cognitive process, occurs during the collection of information. Cues are identified and clustered while information is gathered.

TABLE 6.2 Typologies of 11 Functional Health Patterns

Pattern	Description
Health perception–health management pattern	Individual's perceived health and well-being and how health is managed
Nutritional-metabolic pattern	Food and fluid consumption relative to metabolic needs and indicators of local nutrient supply
Elimination pattern	Excretory function (bowel, bladder, and skin)
Activity-exercise pattern	Exercise, activity, leisure, and recreation
Sleep-rest pattern	Sleep, rest, and relaxation
Cognitive-perceptual pattern	Sensory, perceptual, and cognitive patterns
Self-perception–self-concept pattern	Self-concept pattern and perceptions of self (body comfort, body image, and feeling state); self-conception and self-esteem
Roles-relationships pattern	Role engagements and relationships
Sexuality-reproductive pattern	Person's satisfaction/dissatisfaction with sexuality and reproduction
Coping-stress tolerance pattern	General coping pattern and effectiveness in stress tolerance
Values-beliefs pattern	Values, beliefs (including spiritual), or goals that guide choices or decisions

Data from Gordon, M. (2014). Manual of nursing diagnosis 13th ed. Sudbury, MA: Jones and Bartlett.

Patterns emerge that represent historical and current behavior. Quantitative patterns such as blood pressure are readily identified, and pattern recognition is facilitated when historical baseline data are available. As the nurse incorporates a broader range of data, patterns imbedded within other patterns begin to emerge. For example, blood pressure is a pattern within both the activity pattern and the exercise pattern. Individual baseline and subsequent readings may present a pattern within expected norms. Erratic blood pressure measurements indicate an absence of pattern. The lack of pattern in this case of blood pressure would cluster within both the activity and exercise patterns. Thus functional health pattern categories, such as activity and exercise in this case, provide structures to analyze factors within a category (blood pressure: activity pattern) and to search for causal explanations, usually outside the category; for example, excessive sodium intake: nutritional pattern (Gordon, 2014).

The individual-environmental focus of Gordon's framework (2014) refers to environmental influences occurring across multiple patterns. For example, environmental influences in the functional health pattern include role relationships, family values, and societal mores. Personal preference, knowledge of food preparation, and ability to consume and retain food govern the individual's intake. Cultural and family habits, financial ability to secure food, and crop availability influence food intake. In addition, the person who secures, prepares, and serves the food controls the nutritional intake for the family. The individual's internal and external environments influence health patterns in multiple ways.

Each pattern reflects a human growth and **age-developmental focus** (Gordon, 2014). As individuals fulfill developmental tasks, complexity increases. However, these tasks provide learning opportunities for individuals to maintain and improve their health. Erikson's Stage Theory of Development considers development across the life span and extends into the realm of the older adult, providing a useful model for health promotion assessment of individuals of all ages. Erikson's framework, which organizes specific health tasks for individuals to accomplish at each developmental phase of the life cycle, continues to serve as a framework for health promotion assessment of age-appropriate development and progression through developmental milestones (Darling-Fisher, 2019; Ewing-Cooper & Merrifield, 2019; Herdman, Kamitsuru, & Lopes, 2021; Jordan & Tseris, 2018). However, Jordan and Tseris (2018) posit that Erikson's theory may not adequately capture a diversity of experiences and may exclude the developmental attainment of individuals outside the normative group such as individuals who are disabled, of lower socioeconomic status, ethnic minorities, and females.

Nevertheless, Erikson's eight stages continue to provide the traditional developmental assessment nurses generally use to plan care (Table 6.3). Each stage presents a central task or crisis that must be resolved before healthy growth can continue (Darling-Fisher, 2019; Ewing-Cooper & Merrifield, 2019). Individuals develop their sense of autonomy in early childhood and struggle with a sense of shame and doubt. When the early childhood developmental level is achieved or resolved, the child progresses toward developing initiative during the next stage.

TABLE 6.3 Relationship Between Selected Developmental Tasks and Wellness Tasks for Each Stage of the Life Cycle

Erikson's Eight Life Stages	Havighurst's Developmental Tasks	Examples of Minimal Wellness Tasks for Each Developmental Stage
1. Infancy (trust vs. basic mistrust)	Learning to walk, learning to take solid foods, learning to talk, learning to control elimination of body waste	Acquiring ability to perform psychomotor skills, learning functional definition of health, learning social and emotional responsiveness to others and to the physical environment
2. Early childhood (autonomy vs. shame and doubt)	Learning sexual difference and sexual modesty; achieving physiologic stability; forming simple concepts of social-physical reality; learning to relate emotionally to parents, siblings, and others; learning to distinguish right from wrong and developing a conscience; learning physical skills necessary for ordinary games	Learning about proper foods, exercise, and sleep; learning dental hygiene; learning injury prevention (safety belts and helmets, sunscreen, smoke detectors, poisons, firearms, and swimming); refining psychomotor and cognitive skills
3. Late childhood (initiative vs. guilt)	Building wholesome attitudes toward self as a growing organism, learning to get along with peers	Developing self-concept; learning attitudes of competition and cooperation with others; nd more mature relations with peers of both genders learning social, ethical, and moral differences and responsibilities
4. Early adolescence (industry vs. inferiority)	Learning appropriate gender identity (masculine or feminine role); developing fundamental skills in reading, writing, and calculating; developing concepts necessary for everyday living; developing conscience, morality, and scale of values; achieving personal independence; developing attitudes toward social groups and institutions	Learning that health is an important value; learning self-regulation of physiologic needs—sleep, rest, food, drink, and exercise; learning risk taking and its consequences (injury prevention)
5. Adolescence (identity vs. role confusion)	Achieving new and more mature relations with peers of both genders; achieving gender identity, accepting physique and using body effectively, achieving emotional independence from parents and other adults, achieving assurance of economic independence, selecting and preparing for occupation, preparing for marriage and family life, developing intellectual skills and concepts necessary for civic competence, desiring and achieving socially responsible behavior	Learning economic responsibility; learning social responsibility for self and others (preventing pregnancy and sexually transmitted diseases); experiencing social, emotional, and ethical commitments to others; accepting self and physical development; reconciling discrepancies between personal health concepts and observed health behaviors of others (use of alcohol, drugs, tobacco, firearms, and violence); learning to cope with life events and problems (suicide prevention); considering life goals and career plans and acquiring necessary skills to reach goals; learning importance of time to self and world
6. Early adulthood (intimacy vs. isolation)	Selecting and learning to live with a mate, starting a family, managing a home, taking on civic responsibility	Committing to mate and family responsibilities, selecting a career, incorporating health habits into lifestyle
7. Middle adulthood (generativity vs. stagnation)	Accepting and adjusting to physiologic changes, achieving adult social responsibility, maintaining economic standard of living, assisting adolescent children	Accepting aging of self and others, coping with societal pressures, recognizing importance of good health habits, reassessing life goals periodically
8. Maturity (ego integrity vs. despair)	Adjusting to decreasing physical strength and health, adjusting to retirement and reduced income, adjusting to death of spouse/life partner, establishing an explicit affiliation with own age group, establishing satisfactory physical living arrangements	Becoming aware of risks to health and adjusting lifestyle and habits to cope with risks; adjusting to loss of job, income, and family and friends through death; redefining self-concept; adjusting to changes in personal time and new physical environment; adjusting previous health habits to current physical and mental capabilities

Darling-Fisher (2019); Goodway et al. (2019); USDHHS (2024)

Both age and developmental stage provide a foundation for contemporary assessment of the individual's health status. Developmental tasks begin at birth and continue until death. By considering current epidemiologic data and recommended health behaviors, Gordon's (2020) framework continues to be useful nowadays for health promotion throughout the life span. For example, later in Unit 4, Gordon's framework provides the foundation to explore developmental tasks and their related health behaviors for health promotion.

Functional focus refers to an individual's performance level. Other disciplines plan care using functional patterns; however, assessment data collected differ among disciplines. For example, physical therapists and occupational therapists focus on physical ability to perform activities of daily living and rely on assessing independent performance of activities of daily living to develop their plans. For physicians, genitourinary function refers to frequency or voiding patterns and characteristics of urine, such as color, odor, and laboratory analysis results. Using Gordon's framework, nurses assess how the particular voiding pattern affects lifestyle, particularly how urinary frequency affects sleep patterns and the ability to perform activities such as shopping or socializing. Additional concerns might include the individual's ability to walk or climb stairs to the bathroom or to manage these activities safely at night. It has been suggested that all health disciplines should use the International Classification of Functioning, Disability and Health (ICF) to assess individuals. Relying on this classification could promote transdisciplinary communication about functional patterns (Stallinga et al., 2018). The holistic view of assessment that Gordon's framework introduced aims to address broader issues and link the patterns to decisions about interventions related to an individual's overall health and wellness (Gordon, 2014).

Culture and age, along with developmental and gender norms, are considered during assessment and influence development of health patterns. Leininger defines transcultural nursing concepts of cultural care, health, well-being, and illness patterns in different environmental contexts and under different living conditions (Gordon, 2014). **Culturally competent care** is delivered with knowledge of and sensitivity to cultural factors influencing health behavior. Complex cultural patterns transmitted from former generations contribute to an individual's health behavior. Culturally competent care respects the underlying personal and cultural reality of individuals. Given that one may never be fully competent in cultures other than one's own culture, the term "**cultural attunement**" may be more descriptive of the aim. Nurses provide more culturally attuned care when they use cultural norms, values, communication, and time patterns in reflective practice. Nurses who consider carefully the experience and perspectives of others and progress past mere social consciousness and conceptual understanding practice with attunement (Hupkens et al., 2020; Knudson-Martin et al., 2019). Socioculturally attuned practice acknowledges inequitable social structures and resources while striving to understand the unique, dynamic social identities and power structures that shape each client's individual blend of social identities (Knudson-Martin et al., 2019).

The nurse interacts with individuals, reflecting on the interaction and making changes on the basis of that reflection. For example, when one is tuning a piano, the pitch from the piano and that from the tuning fork must match. The tuning continues until the two sounds resonate. When individuals and nurses experience emotional and physiologic resonance surrounding the individual's sociocultural contexts, such as race, ethnicity, religion, and gender identity, they resonate and achieve attunement (Knudson-Martin et al., 2019).

The concept of attunement is particularly valuable when nurses are caring for people of multiple cultures, such as in an urban setting. For example, in an urban community clinic, using an advisory board or caucus of individuals from that community to serve as a cultural broker ensures that practices accurately reflect the needs and experiences of a target population of diverse cultures (Bermudez et al., 2019) Even when the individual and the nurse share ethnic or racial backgrounds, their particular heritage may be quite different. For example, many different ethnic groups speak Spanish from different countries or provinces within a country (Spain, Mexico, Puerto Rico, Cuba, Colombia, etc.) but may have different colloquialisms within their speech and different cultural values and norms. A Spanish-speaking nurse from Spain may not be culturally competent in client care for clients from Mexico. Asian clients speak a variety of languages, and cultural values differ among Asian countries. Strategies nurses can use to attune more to all clients, particularly to those whose backgrounds or ethnicity are not shared, include: acknowledging the pain of the oppression of others and having humility, reverence, mutual appreciation, and the capacity for genuine curiosity (Somma et al., 2022). Thus cultural and ethical attunement may be useful to provide better care for diverse populations (Bermudez et al., 2019; Hupkens et al., 2020).

Functional health patterns form a framework centering on health and account for cultural factors. Most nursing assessments use functional pattern assessment as a foundation to their practice. Although nursing theoretical and conceptual frameworks differ, the functional health pattern framework is embodied in most nursing conceptual models. In fact, functional health patterns provide the structure used to support nursing classification of interventions and outcome nomenclature (Gordon, 2014). Using a functional health pattern framework specific to the practice of nursing has multiple advantages, including:

- A consistent nursing language through collecting, organizing, presenting, and analyzing data to formulate nursing plans
- A flexible process that allows tailoring content for individuals and situations
- A process that is suitable for use within diverse practice areas (e.g., home, clinic, institution) for assessment of individuals (adult/children), families, or communities
- A process that supports theoretical components of nursing service, education, and research by organizing clinical knowledge using interventions and outcomes
- An incorporation of medical science data while retaining the focus on nursing knowledge and practice

The Patterns

Each pattern reflects a biopsychosocial spiritual expression of the individual's lifestyle or life processes from the perspective of both the individual and the nurse. This expression reveals how behaviors are exhibited, the role of the environment (physical surroundings, family, societal, and cultural influences), and developmental influences. The assessment of each pattern includes its status as functional (strengths/wellness), dysfunctional (actual problem), or potentially dysfunctional (risk), as well as an indication of the individual's level of satisfaction with the pattern (Gordon, 2014). Nurses expand the initial assessments to generate explanations for problems, determine remedial actions, and understand the perceived effect of these actions from the individual's perspective. The individual's knowledge of health promotion, their ability to manage health-promoting activities, and their perception of the value of health promotion play a principal role when using an asset-based approach to identify wellness plans. Each pattern is presented in this chapter along with details for nurses to use to assess individuals and determine health promotion plans using a functional health pattern framework. A discussion of nursing implications for use of the patterns in health promotion practice is included.

Health Perception–Health Management Pattern

The health perception–health management pattern involves the individual's health status and health practices used to reach the current level of health or wellness with a focus on perceived health status and meaning of health (Gordon, 2014). Assessment of this functional health pattern may reveal a pattern of skills used by the individual to promote their own health and avoid health risks. Such individuals would articulate a desire to enhance their health knowledge, participate in community programs that influence health, communicate with health providers to seek health advice, and participate fully in their own health decisions.

When eliciting this information, nurses discover areas for further exploration under other functional health patterns. For example, if the individual reports shortness of breath when mowing the lawn, the nurse stores this information for later retrieval when assessing activity and exercise patterns or cognitive-perceptual patterns.

Health perception–health management patterns affect lifestyle and ability to function even when individuals do not perceive actual health problems, are unaware of necessary health promotion in the absence of problems, do not feel capable of managing their health, or do not believe activity on their part is useless to promote health. Health-promoting activities (e.g., adequate nutrition, activity and exercise, sleep and rest), routine professional examinations, self-examinations, immunizations, and safety precautions (e.g., auto safety restraints and locked medicine cabinets) provide cues within this pattern aimed to maintain optimal quality of life.

Assessment objectives for health perception–health management consist of data about perceptions, management, and preventive health practices (Gordon, 2014). Identifying values related to health promotion can reveal potential health hazards, such as reduced stimulation, interest, or participation in recreation or leisure activities, lack of adherence to a prescribed medical or nursing regimen, or ability to manage health effectively (Herdman, Kamitsuru, & Lopes, 2021). In addition to these kinds of assessment cues, nurses identify unrealistic health and illness perceptions and expectations. One model used for health promotion assessment is the transtheoretical model, which consists of five useful stages for assessing an individual's readiness for education and change (see Chapter 10). These stages—precontemplation, contemplation, planning/preparation, action, and maintenance—have been used widely in health promotion programs for diverse populations and multiple age groups, with topics ranging from prevention of injury to nutrition education (Arshad et al., 2022; Kabak et al., 2021; Kim & Kang, 2021; Nigg et al., 2019; Wang et al., 2022).

Assessment includes the following parameters:

- Health and safety practices of the individual
- Previous patterns of adherence or compliance
- Use of the health care system
- Knowledge of health service availability
- Health-seeking behavior patterns
- Means to access health care (e.g., financial resources, health insurance, and transportation)

In addition to methods of health management, nurses explore health perceptions while asking individuals to describe their current health status, past problems, and anticipation of future problems associated with health or health care. These findings reveal beliefs about health, perceived susceptibility, self-efficacy, meaning of life, and level of knowledge of health status, taking into account the influence of culture (Hupkens et al., 2020; Somma et al., 2022; Box 6.2: Health and Social Determinants/Health Equity). Health and illness perceptions significantly influence overall direction for care planning. Health beliefs, discussed in the Values-Beliefs Pattern section, directly affect participation in care. Partnership with providers and attunement is more likely to yield better attention to self-care, particularly in cultures that value collective responsibility. In addition, individuals from cultures valuing collectivism are more likely to engage in self-care measures when their perspective of cultural patterns and social support systems within families are considered (Hupkens et al., 2020; Krys et al., 2019).

Assessing health management practices is essential. Nurses aim to identify and remedy causes for the discrepancies between provider recommendations and the individual's implementation of those recommendations. For example, an individual with high blood pressure who has failed to keep follow-up appointments, not taken medication as prescribed, and eaten foods with high sodium content should be assessed further. Branching out in the assessment, the nurse attempts to determine whether this evident nonadherence results from a conflict within the value system of the individual (health beliefs); inaccurate information; misunderstanding; inadequate ability to learn, retain, or retrieve information (knowledge deficit); denial of illness (health perception); or inability to access care and/or resources. Variables such as financial resources, transportation difficulties, nutritional preferences, daily activities (individual and family patterns), ability to read written instructions (literacy or visual acuity), and ability to manipulate numbers (numeracy) may affect the individual's behaviors.

Nutritional-Metabolic Pattern

Nutritional-metabolic patterns center on nutrient intake relative to metabolic need (Gordon, 2014). These patterns include an individual's descriptions of food and fluid consumption (history), as well as evidence of adequate nutrition (physical examination). Nurses explore an individual's satisfaction with current eating and drinking patterns, including restrictions, and their perceptions of problems associated with eating and drinking, growth and development, skin condition, and healing processes.

Intake and supply of nutrients to tissues and organs influence bodily functions and interact with lifestyle. Sufficient food and fluid intake provide energy for performance, which includes both internal physiologic functioning and external body movements. Interruption in acquisition or retention of food or fluids offsets balance and significantly alters lifestyle. In addition to an individual's nutrition and metabolism, genetic variation, specific genetic abnormalities, environmental influences, and prenatal nutrition govern growth rates.

Assessment within this pattern includes data about typical patterns of food and fluid consumption and adequacy of consumption patterns, along with perceived problems associated with nutritional intake. Nurses attend to recognizing cues for conditions of overweight, underweight, overhydration, dehydration, or difficulties in skin integrity, such as breakdown or delayed healing. Individuals may be at risk of developing these problems. Conversely, this pattern may exhibit assets or strengths that can be used to support the health promotion plan. For example, an individual's knowledge about nutritional

BOX 6.2 HEALTH AND SOCIAL DETERMINANTS/HEALTH EQUITY

Health Perspectives for Emerging Majority Groups in the United States

With the increasing percentages of individuals from multiple ethnic and racial groups, providers in the United States will provide care for a diverse population in most settings (https://online.alvernia.edu/articles/culturally-competent-nursing-care/). There is diversity among racial and ethnic groups. Cultural beliefs and language may be quite different from one group to another within the same race or ethnicity (Bermúdez et al., 2019; Hupkens et al., 2020). Individualized care attuned to ethical and cultural needs enhances health promotion rather than a stereotypical approach to care.

One resource website produced by the University of Washington for health providers takes this individualized approach. EthnoMed (http://ethnomed.org/) provides comprehensive information about cultural beliefs, medical issues, and related topics pertinent to the health care of immigrants, many of whom are refugees fleeing war-torn parts of the world. Culture Clues tip sheets for clinicians are produced by the University of Washington. Diverse cultural concepts and preferences are presented in an accessible manner. Culture Clues are available for the following cultures: Albanian, Chinese, deaf, hard of hearing, Korean, Latino, Russian, Somali, and Vietnamese. Copyright permission information for reproducing these materials is available on the website. A communication resource is available to assist with basic communication to provide patients comfort and care. With more complex communication, a qualified translator who can interpret both the language and the culture should always be used.

The EthnoMed website provides links to other cultural resources (https://ethnomed.org/cross-cultural-health/external-links) and a collection of articles about religion and cultural connections (https://ethnomed.org/cross-cultural-health/religion). A language-learning tool includes videos of native speakers saying phrases of courtesy in nine languages.

The Agency for Healthcare Research and Quality offers resources for culture, customs, and beliefs: Tool #9 (Address Language Differences) and Tool #10 (Consider Culture, Customs, and Beliefs). Tool #9 (https://www.ahrq.gov/health-literacy/quality-resources/tools/literacy-toolkit/healthlittoolkit2-tool9.html) provides guidelines for providers caring for patients who have language and sensory differences. Tool #10 (https://www.ahrq.gov/health-literacy/quality-resources/tools/literacy-toolkit/healthlittoolkit2-tool10.html) provides guidelines for providers caring for patients regarding religion, culture, beliefs, and ethnic customs that shape perceptions of health concepts and decision-making. Assessing religions, cultures, and ethnic customs connects these values to the plan of care. These guidelines are linked to Medicare reimbursement.

There is wide diversity among racial and ethnic groups. Cultural beliefs and language may be quite different from one group to another within the same race or ethnicity. For more information about these concepts see Bermúdez et al. (2019).

Agency for Healthcare Research and Quality (AHRQ) (2020, 2023); Bermúdez et al. (2019)

concepts can be used to support their strategies for weight loss or gain.

The parameters for assessment for this pattern fall into two broad categories of evaluation: nutrient intake and metabolic demand. Intake may be assessed with a 24-hour recall of food and fluid consumption; a listing of dietary restrictions, food allergies, vitamin supplements, and caffeine and alcohol ingestion (when not included in the medication history); and a schedule of eating and drinking patterns. Assessment includes screening individuals for problems associated with swallowing or chewing.

With identified problems, focused assessments include food preferences, feelings about present weight, and eating habits. Intake may be affected when individuals eat alone. Frequent dining out may indicate the need for further exploration within the nutrition area or other functional patterns. Fast food consumption may be the predominant source of nutrients. Consumption patterns may be deficient in essential vitamins or minerals. Food security may be explored. Who purchases food? Is shopping preplanned with a grocery list? Are financial resources and food budgets adequate? Is food stored properly? Who prepares food? How is food prepared (fried, broiled, steamed, boiled, or baked)?

Metabolic demands differ from individual to individual and vary within the same individual during times of illness, stress, growth, high- or low-activity levels, healing, or recovery. Developmental and environmental conditions alter metabolic demands. Appetite and reported changes in weight, skin integrity, and general healing ability are explored during the interview or health history. Individuals can report decreased tolerances for hot or cold weather.

Nurses' observations and perceptions play a vital role when they are assessing nutritional and metabolic patterns. Physical examination allows assessment of both the nutrient supply to the tissues and the metabolic needs of the individual. Objective findings serve as indicators to validate subjective reports concerning nutrient intake. Gross metabolic indicators include temperature, height, and weight. Physical examination focuses on skin, bony prominences, dentition, hair, and mucous membranes. Skin and mucous membranes, in particular, use nutrients rapidly and provide excellent indices of nutritional adequacy. Skin assessment includes assessment of color, temperature, and turgor, and evaluation of any skin lesions, areas of dryness, flaking, scaling, rashes, ecchymoses, pruritus, or edema. Mucous membranes are examined for color, integrity, moisture, and lesions. Dentition is evaluated for structure. Are teeth erupted at normal stages of development? Are teeth firmly implanted? Do dentures fit properly? In addition, decay and evidence of oral hygiene are evaluated. Healing is assessed when there is evidence of injury. The assessment may include laboratory information such as levels of fasting glucose, lipids, blood urea nitrogen, creatinine, calcium, and vitamin D.

Although problem identification occurs after assessment of all 11 functional health patterns, a problem in any one area serves as a clue to dysfunction in others. Assessment of one pattern facilitates synthesis and analysis of data collected in other functional health patterns. Nutrition and metabolism influence patterns of health management, elimination, activity, sleep, cognition, roles, and stress tolerance. The values-beliefs pattern may significantly alter all other functional patterns. Sociocultural values and ethnic backgrounds play a major role in the determination of eating patterns. Other areas to consider include eating habits, food preferences, and patterns of nutrient supply and demand across the life span. Raw fruits and vegetables may be fun "finger food" for the toddler; however, the older adult, especially one with loose dentures or arthritis of the temporomandibular joint, may find these foods intolerable. Older adults may find gastrointestinal intolerances that develop over time and were not present in their youth.

A nutritional pattern focus emphasizes educational needs. Assessment aims to demonstrate strengths in functional patterns along with disclosing dysfunctional or potentially dysfunctional patterns. Nutritional health promotion activities present a strength that provides impetus for similar activities in the other patterns. For example, if balanced nutritional intake improves functional level, individuals may extend their health-promoting behaviors to stress reduction or other behaviors. Understanding food/fluid intake and balance of body requirements helps individuals to adjust caloric intake as growth slows to prevent overweight problems during the adult years.

Elimination Pattern

Elimination patterns include those related to bowel, bladder, and skin function. Nurses determine regularity, quality, and quantity of stool through subjective reports about methods used to achieve regularity or control and any pattern changes or perceived problems. Perspiration quantity and quality determine excretory skin function (Gordon, 2014).

Elimination pattern significance differs from individual to individual. Many people view elimination patterns as a measure of health and as a sensitive indicator of proper nutrition and stress level. An individual's perceptions determine whether patterns become problematic or dysfunctional. Misconceptions about regularity exist, particularly of bowel function, and self-treatment commonly occurs to correct perceived problems.

Elimination pattern dysfunction affects interpersonal interactions (Mitchell, 2019). Lack of control affects body image (self-perception), activity level, socialization, and sleep patterns. Age, developmental levels, and cultural considerations direct the interview. Pediatric assessment includes toilet training methods, whereas adult assessment may focus on regularity and patterns of dysfunction. In addition to constipation, older adults may begin to develop urinary control problems. Females past childbearing years often develop urinary stress incontinence.

Assessment includes data about regularity and control of excreta (Gordon, 2014). Nurses investigate cues suggesting constipation patterns, diarrhea, or incontinence through focused assessment. Elimination pattern changes, pain, discomfort, and perceived problems receive attention. Data collection includes exploration of the individual's explanation of the problem, methods of self-treatment, and perceived results (Gordon, 2014). The individual is considered to have constipation if in the past month, spontaneous bowel movements occurred less than three times a week, stools were painful or hard, or fecal matter was present in the rectum (Mitchell, 2019). In addition to collection of subjective data, objective data collection may include digital rectal exam. Details of a thorough holistic assessment of constipation are beyond the scope of this chapter; however, the reader is referred to Mitchell's (2019) full holistic assessment, including details of a structured evaluation and rectal exam.

The quantity, quality (color, odor, and consistency), frequency, and regularity of stool, urine, and perspiration determine the direction of further exploration. Nurses assess excretory mode, time patterns, and control. Encouraging discussion aims to reveal more detailed information about pattern changes, perceived problems, and elimination habits. Examination includes gross screening of specimens, noting the amount, consistency, color, and odor. Skin assessment includes careful observation and description of wound/fistula drainage.

Transition from nutrition to elimination pattern assessment can occur seamlessly. Fluid intake affects elimination. Dietary fiber affects bowel elimination patterns. Skin integrity heralds concerns about urinary incontinence, leading to additional discussion of elimination patterns. Direct questions about laxatives may be necessary because of the availability of over-the-counter treatments for constipation (Mitchell, 2019). Discrepancies between dietary intake and reported bowel regularity indicate the need for further questioning (Mitchell, 2019). Laxative dependency in the form of oral supplements, suppositories, or enemas may indicate knowledge deficits in the area of bowel elimination. Health education about normal bowel function, nutritional guidelines to assist the individual in elimination, or implementation of an exercise program may significantly reduce elimination pattern dysfunction. Although overuse of laxatives is generally considered a solution for older adults to cope with constipation, young adults with bulimia and anorexia should be assessed for laxative overuse, abuse, and dependency (Mitchell, 2019). Furthermore, nurses should explore this issue with parents of children who struggle with constipation. These parents may rely on excess use of stimulant laxatives for the affected child, resulting in chronic laxative use.

Urinary frequency and urinary tract infection (UTI) require health education as well. Several approaches to prevention of UTIs in females have some evidence to support their use. Drinking 8 ounces of cranberry juice a day for 6 months to a year; low-dose prophylactic antibiotics; vaginally administered estrogen to promote growth of lactobacilli in postmenopausal females; and probiotic vaginal suppositories containing lactobacilli for premenopausal, hypoestrogenic females have each been used to prevent UTI. There is limited evidence for these strategies, except for the use of vaginally administered estrogen (Lajiness & Lajiness, 2019). In their laboratory studies using epithelial cell cultures, Kamolvit's study group found that *Lupinus mutabilis*, a South American herb with edible beans that contains phytochemicals, promoted cellular action, suggesting that *L. mutabilis* might be of some importance in this era of antibiotic resistance. The researchers concluded that future in vivo studies of *L. mutabilis* to prevent UTI are warranted (Kamolvit et al., 2018).

Presenting symptoms of UTI in both males and females include urinary urgency, urinary frequency, and nocturnal polyuria. Prolonged time between urinations is linked to UTIs (Duncan, 2019; Lajiness & Lajiness, 2019). Evidence-based practice guides the nurse in establishing a more suitable elimination routine for the individual.

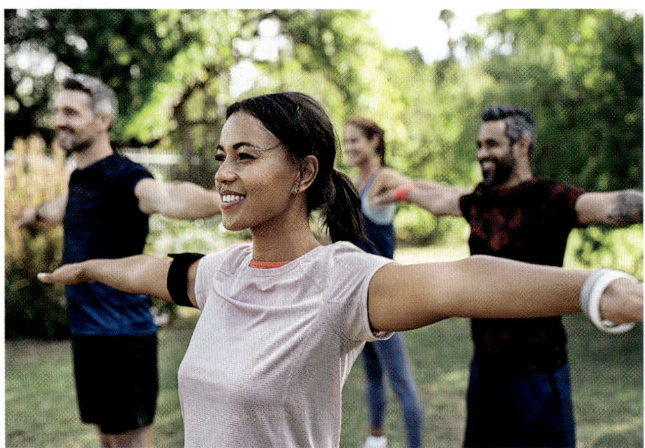

FIG. 6.1 Activity-exercise patterns provide effective indicators for commitment to health promotion and prevention. (From iStock.com/Ridofranz)

Activity-Exercise Pattern

The activity-exercise pattern centers on activity level, exercise program, and leisure activities. Parameters to explore include movement capability, activity tolerance, self-care abilities, use of assistive devices, changes in pattern, satisfaction with activity and exercise patterns, and any perceived problems (Gordon, 2014). Limitations in movement capabilities or ability to perform activities of daily living significantly alter lifestyle and may affect every other functional health pattern. Mobility and independent functioning in self-care are almost universally valued. Childrearing practices demonstrate this value: parents boast about their infant who walks early, their toilet-trained toddler, and their preschooler who dresses without assistance.

Activity-exercise patterns provide effective indicators for commitment to health promotion and prevention (Fig. 6.1). Exercise's effect on health status has been extensively documented with increased public awareness. Overweight and obesity, linked to sedentary lifestyle, have reached epidemic proportions worldwide, in both developing and industrialized areas. More than 1.9 billion adults (39%) are overweight, with 13% of the world's population and 39 million children younger than 5 years designated as obese in 2020 (World Health Organization [WHO], 2024). Worldwide obesity prevalence has tripled since 1975 (WHO, 2024).

Clear evidence continues to support that unhealthy diet and sedentary lifestyle, both modifiable risk factors, influence increased obesity and overweight, contributing to associated disorders of cardiovascular disease, diabetes, and cancer (Ebele, 2019). In their research of working adults (n = 173; 83% response rate) conducted in West Asia, Gupta and Garg (2019) reported that both unhealthy diet and physical inactivity were significantly (P <5%) associated with overweight and obesity. Increased body mass index (BMI) was associated with increases in the number of sick days, medical claims, and health care costs. Obesity and overweight were more likely as daily working hours increased in number (Gupta & Garg, 2019). The AHA identifies physical activity and diet as two modifiable risk factors promoting cardiovascular health (Tsao et al., 2022). Globally, prevalence of physical inactivity has remained relatively the same (28.5% [2001] and 27.5% [2016]). Adversely, females (8%) reported higher rates of inactivity when compared with males. Use of technology (video games, texting, and social media) has increased nationwide to greater than 3 hours/day (46.1%) since 2019. However, the long-term effects from physical inactivity due to the COVID-19 pandemic are projected to negatively affect these behavior patterns (Tsao et al., 2022). Assessments, plans, and interventions to prevent obesity have a major effect on global health and health promotion in the United States.

Activity-exercise patterns indicate energy expenditure and activity tolerance levels. Movement directly affects activities of daily living, along with control of the immediate environment. The environment contributes to mobility as well. For example, individuals living alone in high-crime areas might limit their activity for fear of harm. Factors such as inclement weather, distance from public transportation, scarce neighborhood recreation facilities, unaffordable activities, poorly maintained parks, unleashed dogs, safety concerns, illicit drug activity, lack of outdoor spaces, lack of family/significant other's support, limited time, lack of pleasure/boredom, limited confidence in exercise ability, fear of injury, fatigue, depression, parental support for minors, screen time access, and having to negotiate stairways with a cane can influence decisions about activity (Burton et al., 2019; Child et al., 2019; Cohen et al., 2019; Fazelipour & Cunningham, 2019; Garcia et al., 2019; Garland et al., 2019; Huck et al., 2019; Prochnow et al., 2019; Roth et al., 2019; Schroeder et al., 2019; Sukys et al., 2019; Wilczynska et al., 2019). Environmental barriers significantly impair exercise activity patterns for individuals with neuromuscular or perceptual disturbances. Other barriers may arise when assessment considers age or developmental stage.

For example, a qualitative study generated data from eight focus groups of older adult residents living in four-term care facilities. To address sedentary lifestyles, Poveda-López et al. (2022) concluded that a participant's attitude, knowledge, and motivation influenced older adults' self-perceived attitude toward physical exercise. Participants found that the perceived effects of exercise programs benefited their health, and routine exercise improved well-being and decreased social isolation (Poveda-López et al., 2022).

The objective of assessment within the activity-exercise pattern is to determine the pattern of activities that require energy expenditure. The components reviewed should include exercise, activity, leisure, and recreation (Gordon, 2014). The nurse seeks clues to discover strengths and weaknesses within the pattern. Decreased energy levels, perceived problems, coping strategies, changes within the patterns, and associated explanations for these changes are all important clues that require further exploration. In general, individuals with respiratory or cardiac disease warrant in-depth assessment, and focused assessment is indicated for individuals with neuromuscular, perceptual, or circulatory impairments.

The dimensions to be described and assessed within the activity-exercise pattern include daily activities, leisure activities, and exercise. Daily activities include occupation (position, hours of work or school, and amount of physical exercise versus cognitive or sedentary activities), self-care abilities (feeding, bathing, grooming, dressing, and toileting), and home-management routines (cooking, cleaning, shopping, laundry, and outdoor activities; Gordon, 2014). Problems within any of these areas require explanation. Is it a problem of energy expenditure, mobility limitations, or decreased motivation caused by depression, grieving, or incongruent values?

Exercise parameters include the type, frequency, duration, and intensity of the individual's regular exercise. Nurses assess the value the individual places on exercise as a part of determining their (i.e., the individual's) feelings about it. A 24-hour recall of the previous day's activities provides an initial picture of the pattern, whereas each major component addresses specific elements. Weekly logs provide follow-up assessment for suspected problems (Gordon, 2014). In addition to weekly logs, focused assessments include details about modes of transportation. Is a car used for transportation? If public transportation is used, how far away is the route? Are elevators or stairs used more often? Factors interfering with exercise or mobility include dyspnea, fatigue, muscle cramping, neuromuscular or perceptual deficits, chest pain, and angina. As with other patterns, feelings of satisfaction and perception of problems provide valuable indications of dysfunctional or potentially dysfunctional patterns.

Nurses evaluate subjective complaints, such as dyspnea, noting an individual's difficulty with breathing during the interview and physical examination. Examination includes objective circulatory, respiratory, and neuromuscular indicators. Assessment includes skin color, skin temperature, apical heart rate, radial heart rate, and blood pressure, as well as respiratory rate, rhythm, depth of inspiration, and effort involved. Gait, posture, and balance are evaluated during ambulation. Muscle tone, strength, coordination, and range of motion provide useful clues to validate reports of activity and exercise. Assistive devices or prostheses are evaluated for proper use, proper fit, and degree of assistance or support provided.

Information obtained during the interview is linked closely to the examination findings. Examination alone may not disclose the invaluable subjective reports of early morning pain and joint stiffness. When appropriate, the nurse can ask the individual to climb stairs or perform self-care activities under observation to assess impairment. Direct observation validates assessment findings and is a valuable technique used by health care educators and home health nurses to evaluate adequate performance of self-care activities, such as dressing, cooking, and insulin administration. Various instruments have been designed to quantify the level of ability or disability. For some individuals, a metabolic activity index, in which each activity is measured according to kilocalories of energy expended per minute, helps quantify assessment results and plan care. Developmental norms have been established for infants and toddlers. Milestones such as sitting, crawling, walking, running, and hopping determine a child's development and should be screened in children with use of standardized screening instruments (Silva et al., 2019). Careful assessment of ability, limitations, and interests helps guide the nurse in a more holistic assessment.

Problem identification is reserved for the conclusion of the assessment after all 11 patterns have been constructed. Useful clues within a pattern lead into other pattern areas; however, premature closure of a topic during the examination is avoided. At this point, only tentative plans are possible. Often, explanations of problems lie in other functional health patterns. For example, when the individual expresses an inability to perform exercise on a routine basis, barriers may be discovered in another pattern. Barriers associated with knowledge deficit, the personal or family value system, overriding priorities, or low value placed on exercise may hinder an individual's success. Is the inability to perform activities a result of general fatigue caused by inadequate or decreased sleep time associated with anxiety, nocturia, pain, or an infant waking every 3 hours for feeding? Are responsibilities associated with caring for several preschoolers and inadequate financial resources to secure a babysitter the cause? The assessment's purpose is to narrow the number of possible explanations.

Sleep-Rest Pattern

Perhaps the single most important factor assessed in the sleep-rest pattern is the perception of adequacy of sleep and relaxation. Subjective reports of fatigue or energy levels provide some indication of the individual's satisfaction. People make assumptions about the roles that sleep and rest play in preparing the individual for required or desired daily activities. This pattern becomes extremely important when sleep and rest are perceived as insufficient. Sleep serves a restorative function in most individuals. Sleep deprivation studies provide vivid demonstrations of the need for different types of sleep: light, deep, dream, and rapid eye movement sleep. Again, problems within this pattern may cause problems in other patterns. A person who has difficulty with sleep may be tense and irritable; unable to tolerate stress; more prone to infectious processes, cardiovascular disease, and excess weight gain; and less capable of taking health-promoting action. Alterations in appetite, elimination, mental health, academic achievement, interpersonal functioning activity intolerance, decision-making, memory, and driving concentration can occur (Hansen et al., 2018; Paterson et al., 2019; Scott et al., 2019; Skein et al., 2019). A higher incidence of errors, injuries, and accidents has been reported in sleep-deprived workers (Ferguson et al., 2019). Some degree of cognitive dysfunction generally occurs as well.

The objective when the nurse is assessing the sleep-rest pattern is to describe the effectiveness of the pattern from the individual's perspective (Gordon, 2014). Wide variation in sleep time (from 4 hours to more than 10 hours) does not necessarily affect functional performance; different individuals require different amounts of sleep. Extrinsic factors that may hinder effective sleep include caffeine intake patterns, screen-time patterns, early work/school schedules, stress, anxiety, long/irregular work hours, and late afternoon and evening activities.

Difficulty experienced with sleep onset, sleep interruptions, and awakening are areas of assessment to consider. The nurse evaluates disturbances such as dreaming and nightmares, sleepwalking, nocturnal enuresis, and penile tumescence. Counseling, institution of safety measures, or medical referral may be necessary. In addition to sleep, the nurse assesses rest and relaxation according to the individual's perceptions. Activities of the sedentary-isolate type, such as reading or crocheting, may be relaxing for some individuals. Passive involvement, as with television viewing, may provide the only source of relaxation for the individual. Daily naps or relaxation exercises (meditation, yoga, or breathing exercises) can be a part of this pattern.

Assessment parameters of the sleep dimension are divided into two parts: sleep quality and sleep quantity. Sleep quality includes the individual's perception of sleep adequacy, performance level, and physical and psychological state on awakening. Sleep quantity, in addition to focusing on the hours slept each day, is used to build a schedule of sleep times. The nurse assesses the individual for regularity of the time of retiring, time of awakening, and additional periods of sleep throughout the day. Sleep onset, the number of awakenings, and the reasons for awakening provide clues to problems. The dimensions of rest and relaxation include the parameters of the type, frequency or regularity, and duration. The perceived effectiveness of methods used to promote rest is assessed.

When problems exist, focused assessment that evaluates efficiency of sleep compared with actual sleeping time is warranted. Individuals are conditioned to sleep under certain circumstances, and maintaining bedtime rituals is a distinct advantage in sleep promotion. A person who expects to sleep will usually sleep if such routines are maintained. Nurses assess schedule and routine changes associated with bedtime. When assessing bedtime routines, rituals along with other aids to sleep, such as natural aids (warm milk) or medications (prescription and nonprescription), should be explored. Physical examination includes general appearance, behavior, and performance changes. As with pain, sleep is a subjective experience. Comprehensive examination, which is beyond the scope of this chapter, may be performed, including polysomnography when indicated. Research indicates that subjective reporting of sleep quality and measures of sleep time closely approximate electroencephalographic findings.

Nursing care focuses on the need to identify evidence of sleep disturbances to design appropriate interventions before sleep deprivation occurs. Frequent awakenings do not necessarily imply sleep interruption. Many individuals awaken numerous times during the night but return to sleep within seconds. These awakenings occur in older adults, who generally spend most of the night in stages of light sleep. The normal developmental pattern of aging does not include deep sleep; as a result, awakenings may not affect the sleep cycles. However, older individuals more often have trouble returning to sleep because they experience discomfort or anxiety. Biologic rhythm and peak performance time may be helpful to the nurse when he or she is planning health education and return visits. Individuals commonly refer to themselves as "morning people" or "night owls"; therefore, patterns of retiring and arising provide clues. Patterns of sleep and rest in conjunction with subjective reports of physical and mental well-being help to determine appropriate interventions.

Cognitive-Perceptual Pattern

Cognitive patterns include the ability of the individual to understand and follow directions, retain information, make decisions, solve problems, and use language appropriately. Auditory, visual, olfactory, gustatory, tactile, and kinesthetic sensations and perceptions determine perceptual and sensory patterns. Pain perception and tolerance are analyzed within this pattern area (Gordon, 2014). Capacity for independent functioning is considered a major role of thinking and perceiving. Compensation for cognitive-perceptual difficulties ensures safety. Health requires a balance between the individual and the environment. Decreased levels of cognition or perception require increased levels of environmental control. For example, mentally impaired or sensory-impaired individuals may require sheltered work environments and supervised group living arrangements.

Interrelationships among the individual, the developmental stage, and the environment contribute to several patterns. For example, the behavior patterns of a 20-year-old high school individual who never achieved a high school diploma and works in a factory may differ from those of a 20-year-old second-year nursing student. Developmental stage plays a role in cognitive and perceptual abilities as well. The individual's ability to solve problems and conceptualize as described by Piaget's theoretical framework provides data to determine the cognitive developmental stage. Jean Piaget's constructive theories widely influence current assessment of cognitive development (Silva et al., 2019). Vision and hearing achieve full potential when children reach school age, with 20/30 vision considered normal in preschoolers. As adults mature, visual acuity and the senses of hearing, touch, and even taste decline. Cognitive function must be evaluated within the context of the environment (Gordon, 2014). Environmental complexity results in different levels of functioning.

Assessing cognitive-perceptual patterns includes evaluating language capabilities, cognitive skills, and perception related to desired or required activities (Gordon, 2014). Nurses address clues indicating potential problems, particularly sensory deficits, sensory deprivation or overload, and ineffective pain management. Cognitive dysfunction may cause impaired reasoning, impaired judgment, or knowledge deficits related to health practices, as well as memory deficits.

Assessment parameters include hearing and vision test results. Changes in sensation or perception should be noted. In addition to decreased ability or acuity with regard to hearing, vision, smell, and taste, evaluation includes other perceptual disturbances, such as vertigo; increased or decreased sensitivity to heat, cold, or light touch; and visual or auditory hallucinations or illusions. Use and perceived effectiveness of assistive devices, such as hearing aids, eyeglasses, and contact lenses, is noted.

Discomfort and pain are evaluated further. Useful tools that use pain scales have been designed to record and quantify changes in pain perception; however, pain assessment in neonates, young children, and the elderly is complex because of limited language development early in life and cognitive impairment related to aforementioned assistive devices or dementia (Kappesser et al., 2019; Strand et al., 2019). Furthermore, healthy, cognitively intact older adults may consider that discomfort accompanies all normal aging, resulting in the under-reporting of pain (Kang & Demiris, 2018).

Assessment tools for these populations should include observational data, such as facial expressions, vocalizations, body movements, restlessness (agitation), rubbing, guarding, rigidity, and physical aggression (Strand et al., 2019). Examples of such tools include: Children and Infant's Postoperative Pain Scale (CHIPPS), the Neonatal Facial Coding System—Revised (NFCS-R), and Pain Assessment in Impaired Cognition (PAIC) (Kappesser et al., 2019).

The location, type, degree, and duration provide indicators of possible causes or sources. Relief measures to control pain and their effectiveness provide data as well as a focus for health education. Attitudes toward pain should be considered. For example, someone may fear that medication is a sign of weakness or that it will result in a loss of independence. For all individuals, exploring tolerance to pain is appropriate, using questions such as "Do you feel you are particularly sensitive to pain?" and "What level of pain is associated with your (cut, sprain, broken bone, or labor contractions)?"

Other areas of cognitive patterning to be explored include educational level, recent memory changes, ease or difficulty in learning, and preferred method of learning. Even when no problems are apparent or suspected, the nurse may assess these areas in more detail to determine areas of strength for use with health teaching plans.

Objective data are accumulated throughout the interview or assessment process. This data collection begins with the nurse's perceptions of the individual's general appearance: hygiene and grooming, proper use of clothing, neatness and appropriateness of dress, and indication that these are appropriate to the individual's developmental stage. Language and vocabulary use, the ability to convey an idea with words or with actions when speech is impaired or not yet developed, and grammatical correctness provide clues to cognitive functioning. Amplitude and quality of speech, affect and mood, as well as attention and concentration, are all indicative of the individual's mental status. For many individuals, this information is sufficient to relay a sense of the level of understanding, memory, and mentation. Problem-solving abilities can usually be determined when the individual is asked to relate any perceived problems, provide an explanation of the problems and/or actions taken to solve the problems, and describe the results of the actions taken. Because this is a basic assessment in each functional health pattern, the nurse already has an idea of whether thought processes are logical, coherent, and relevant for this individual.

When problems within the cognitive realm do not surface, the information is recorded as part of the objective data or findings of the physical examination. The data to be noted include language; vocabulary; attention span; grasp of ideas; level of consciousness; orientation to person, place, and time; language spoken (whether primary or secondary); and behavior during the data collection process, including posture, facial expression, and general body movements.

When a problem is apparent or suspected based on age, hereditary factors, or inconsistencies in the assessment data, a focused assessment is essential. Coma scales or functional dementia scales may be appropriate. More commonly, a Folstein Mini-Mental Status Examination (MMSE) is performed to assess orientation, attention, calculation, language (ability to name objects, repeat abstract ideas, and follow commands), and recall (immediate, short-term, and long-term memory). Abilities to read, write, and copy designs can be assessed (see Chapter 24). The examination of a sensory-perceptual pattern evaluates hearing, vision, and areas of pain at a screening level; comprehensive examinations are available and may be indicated. A full neurologic assessment is warranted when specific sensory deficits are identified during the examination.

Although completing these assessment areas may seem overwhelming, the time required is generally less than that in most other pattern areas, perhaps because more information relevant to the cognitive-perceptual patterns becomes available as each pattern is assessed. Transition into the cognitive-perceptual pattern from other patterns may be facilitated by referring to a problem already described, with a question such as "Do you generally find it easy to solve problems effectively?" The self-perception pattern follows the cognitive pattern particularly well because mental status measures include feelings and perceptions of the individual regarding self. Mood, affect, and responses to the interviewer, such as eye contact, are indications of self-esteem. Cognitive-perceptual ability greatly influences the ability to function (self-care) or manipulate (activity and exercise) within the environment.

The placement of each of the patterns in a sequence suitable to each nurse, individual, or situation has been discussed. However, when the cognitive-perceptual pattern is dysfunctional, the individual is most likely unreliable as the historian; therefore, it is wise to consider this pattern early in the assessment process. Approaching this pattern early saves valuable time and permits the identification of patterns that can be assessed more reliably. Every person has experienced temporary memory lapses at one time or another. These events alone are not a sufficient basis for judgments. Equally important is the need to assess all pattern areas before data analysis and problem identification.

Cognitive and sensory ability data guide the nurse in planning care, which is especially apparent in health teaching. Formulation of health teaching plans ideally reflects each individual's preferred method of learning. The effective plan considers the individual's demonstrated developmental level; the ability to store information, retrieve information, and compensate for deficits; and the neuromuscular and sensory levels necessary for skill development. An individually tailored plan contains mutually developed goals and short-term objectives. Although self-care might be an outcome for any person in whom diabetes mellitus has been newly diagnosed, the behaviors expected of an adult with diabetes will differ from those expected of a child.

Self-Perception–Self-Concept Pattern

The self-perception–self-concept pattern encompasses an individual's sense of their personal identity, goals, emotional patterns, and feelings about their own self-care. Self-image and sense of worth both stem from the individual's perception of personal appearance, competencies, and limitations, including self-perception and others' perceptions. Nurses assess physical, verbal, and nonverbal cues (Gordon, 2014).

The significance of the sense of self to the whole person is best exemplified by personal experiences. Individuals who feel good about their self-worth look and act differently from those who feel unable to accomplish anything worthwhile.

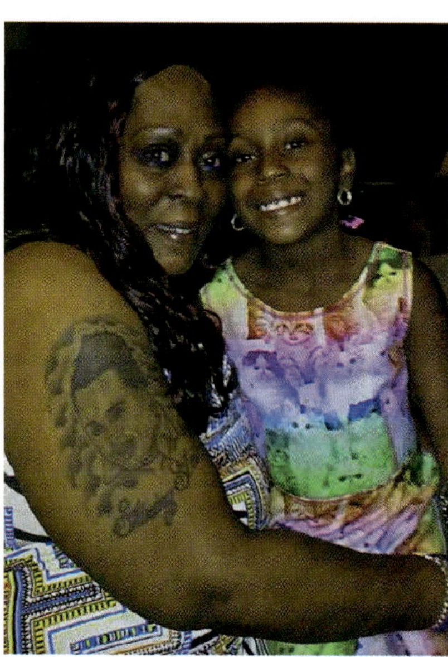

FIG. 6.2 Most people care about what others think of them; therefore, the support of significant others, such as a grandmother supporting a student grandchild, affects their self-perception–self-concept pattern.

Self-concept changes may affect patterns of eating, sleeping, and activity. Developmental level affects and is affected by this pattern (see Table 6.3). One of the tasks during the later phases of Erikson's developmental framework, described previously, is building wholesome self-esteem (Darling-Fisher, 2019; Ewing-Cooper & Merrifield, 2019; Silva et al., 2019).

Family climate and relationship patterns provide an environment to influence the self-concept pattern (see Chapter 7). Those relationship patterns closely associated to the individual, such as spouse, significant other, parents, teachers, peers, and community, affect that person's self-esteem (Fig. 6.2). Most people care about what others think of them; therefore, the support of significant others affects the self-perception–self-concept pattern (Bester, 2019; Centeio et al., 2019; Hossain & Ferreira, 2019; Silva et al., 2019).

The assessment objective in this pattern area is to describe each individual's patterns and beliefs about general self-worth and feeling states (Gordon, 2014). The nurse looks for clues that indicate identity confusion, altered body image, disturbances in self-esteem, and feelings of powerlessness. Nurses often identify anxiety, fear, and depression states that are responsive to nursing interventions.

The nurse notes the general appearance and affect of each individual, which may have been assessed as part of a formal mental status examination. Low self-esteem may be indicated by head and shoulder flexion, lack of eye contact, and mumbled or slurred speech. Anxiety or nervousness might be revealed through extraneous body movements such as foot shuffling or tapping, facial tension or grimace, rapid speech, voice quivering, twitches or tremors, and general restlessness or shifts in body position. Any of these indicators demands further exploration to determine underlying problems for each individual.

Self-concept influences each individual's understanding of themselves and life experiences, or their meaning in life (MIL), which is measured extensively with the Meaning in Life Questionnaire (MLQ), a self-report tool (Mitchell & Christian, 2019; Semma et al., 2019). The concept of MIL incorporates the belief that life is comprehensible, and existence is important. In their study of 67 pregnant females, Mitchell and Christian (2019) examined the influences of antiinflammatory cytokines, socioeconomic status, repetitive negative thinking, and MIL using the MLQ. Mitchell and Christian's (2019) data provided support that MIL contributes to biologic functioning in these females, corresponding with other research demonstrating a relationship between lower well-being and immune dysregulation. Because information gathered for this pattern is personal, sharing the information may actually facilitate the process of goal setting and intervention planning when the nurse possesses strong communication skills and a caring attitude.

Roles-Relationships Pattern

The roles-relationships pattern describes the position assumed and the associations engaged in by the individual that are connected to that position. The individual's perception is a major component of the assessment, and exploration of the pattern includes each individual's level of satisfaction with roles and relationships.

The need for relationships with other people is universal. Jhang (2019) noted the basic needs for communication, fellowship, and love in high-level wellness. The ability to communicate with other people in a meaningful way greatly affects the whole person. The understanding of health as the harmonious balance between the individual and the environment indicates the major role that relationships with others play in health. Developmental hypotheses about readiness propose that attainment of each stage is required to progress to the next stage. For example, a person can become immersed in a relationship of genuine intimacy only after self-identity has stabilized. Developmental tasks that promote family development have been identified similarly by Duvall and Miller (see Chapter 7), as noted by Amirtha and Sivakumar (2018). The emphasis within these models is on the individual's relationships within the nuclear family.

The objective of the roles-relationships pattern assessment is to describe an individual's pattern of family and shared circumstances, with the associated responsibilities. The individual's perception of satisfaction with the established relationship contributes to this assessment. Loss, change, and threat produce the major problems within this pattern. Clues indicative of impaired verbal communication, social isolation, alterations in parenting, independence-dependence conflicts, dysfunctional grieving, and potential for violence are pertinent.

Assessment focuses on family, work, and community roles and relationships. Within the family, assessment parameters include the family structure, tasks performed, social support systems, and other dynamics, such as decision-making, power, authority, division of labor, and communication patterns. Parenting or marital difficulties and family violence issues are explored. The roles of student and employee are explored to determine specific occupation or position, along with work responsibilities and work environment. Parameters such as stress, safety, and health factors should be included (see the case study and the care plan at the end of this chapter). Financial concerns, job security, and retirement plans are elicited. Activity-rest patterns elicit information about time commitments, leisure activities, and physical exercise; therefore, the assessment at this point addresses the effect of these factors on the roles-relationships pattern. Community roles and relationships indicate involvement within the neighborhood and other social groups, such as the level of socialization and the amount of social support available. The nurse asks the individual to describe their level of satisfaction with the roles and relationships within all three components (family, work or school, and community).

Threat of change, actual change, and loss are areas to be explored further. In addition, family or work roles alone may not cause stress; however, combining them may cause difficulties, as with the working or traveling parent. Life changes can affect role-relationship patterns, for example, when a new child arrives, when a child in a family develops special needs, or when a parent becomes disabled. Roles of all members of the family change and adjust to the situations. All family members must call on their coping resources when their role-relationship pattern changes.

Objective data for assessment within this pattern are usually unavailable unless the nurse makes a home visit or sees the individual in the company of significant others in some other capacity. Family interaction and communication patterns are noted whenever possible. Cognizant of meaningful relationships within the family, the nurse identifies potential problems, such as those that occur with the transition to parenthood and associated increases in routine housework, the financial stress and need for time management for parents of young children, the changing focus of stressors for parents who are now caring for adolescents and caring for their own elderly parents, and the financial stress for families with adult dependents (Amirtha & Sivakumar, 2018).

The relationships among the functional health patterns are clearly apparent in light of the developmental stages. Difficulties within the self-concept pattern and difficulties with relationships often appear together (Jhang, 2019). Relationships affect the whole person; therefore, problems within the roles-relationships pattern may be exhibited in other areas, such as sleep, appetite, and sexuality.

Sexuality-Reproductive Pattern

The sexuality-reproductive pattern describes the individual's sexual self-concept, sexual functioning, methods of intimacy, and reproductive areas. Data collection combines subjective information, nursing observations, and physical examination. Normal development and perceived satisfaction combine to provide the elements of this pattern (Gordon, 2014).

Sexuality is the behavioral expression of sexual identity. The importance of this pattern area to the individual's life and health is closely related to the self-perception and the relationship patterns. Body image, self-concept, role, and gender identity are all linked to sexual identity. This concept of sexual self and the individual's relationship pattern indicate the level and the perceived satisfaction of sexual functioning. Sexual functioning involves, but is not limited to, sexual relations with a partner. Reproductive patterns are equally significant to this pattern assessment, the whole individual, and the family and community (see Chapters 7 and 8).

As noted, individual development influences reproductive capacities, including genotype, secondary sex characteristics, genital development, phenotype, ego integrity, and the family life-cycle stage (Amirtha & Sivakumar, 2018; Hipp et al., 2019; Hossain & Ferreira, 2019; Mercurio, 2019). The environment plays a part in expression of the sexuality-reproductive pattern. Cultural and family norms may contribute to the expression of sexuality and combine with other factors, such as the family's financial stability, to influence reproductive patterns (Hipp et al., 2019).

Assessment of the sexuality-reproductive pattern is of particular importance during adolescence, a period of development where personal identity is explored (Hossain & Ferreira, 2019). For example, "sexting," defined by Steinberg and colleagues (2019) as "sending sexually explicit messages, images, or videos to a romantic partner" is often a part of adolescent behavior. In the study by Steinberg and colleagues (2019), 429 high school students (54% female) completed annual assessments of sexual behavior over a 3-year period. Findings from this study indicated that sexting in adolescence coemerges with genital contact behavior along with sexual development (Steinberg et al., 2019). Norms within society may create issues in expressions of sexuality.

During the assessment process, nurses consider the continuum of sexual identity expression, including heterosexuality, bisexuality, and transgender, gay, or lesbian sexuality. The information gathered guides the health promotion plan in those who seek guidance about their sexual identity and behavior. Sexual orientation and gender identity are linked to mortality risk in significant ways, including higher rates of suicide attempt, sexual assault, and acts of violence (Haas et al., 2019). However, items on instruments collecting demographic public health data often use self-identification items without including items that accurately collect information about sexual behavior. For example, some individuals who engage in same-sex sexual behavior or have same-sex sexual attractions do not openly identify as gay, lesbian, or bisexual (Haas et al., 2019).

One objective of assessment in this pattern is to describe behavioral problems or difficulties (Gordon, 2014). Equally important is assessing the individual's knowledge of sexual functioning and preventive health practices, such as breast and testicular self-examination, Papanicolaou tests, effective contraceptive use, and avoidance of infection. Clues are evaluated for potential or actual sexual dysfunction.

The following parameters are assessed: sexual self-concept, which may be derived from information collected in the self-perception–self-concept and the roles-relationships patterns; sexual functioning, with the nurse noting evidence of some form of intimacy, the level of sexual activity or libido, and the effect of health or illness on sexual expression; and reproductive patterns, in which the nurse collects data pertinent to health promotion factors, such as feelings related to aging, preventive practices, and knowledge of sexual functioning. For females, reproductive pattern assessment includes information about menstruation, such as onset, duration, frequency, date of last menstrual period, and discomfort during menstruation, as well as information about menopause and reproductive stage, such as pregnancy history and birth control methods.

The level of satisfaction with sexual self-concept, sexual functioning, and reproduction is explored. Difficulties such as ineffective or inappropriate sexual performance, discharges, infections, venereal disease, discomfort, and history of abuse are evaluated. Focused assessment to collect additional information is warranted with sexual dysfunction or trauma. Physical examination evaluates genital development and secondary sex characteristics. Signs of intimacy between partners, such as holding hands and hugging, are noted.

People may feel threatened by discussion of topics in this pattern; the depth of exploration is governed in part by the individual's wishes. Dialogue is encouraged; however, it could be postponed until a firm and trusting relationship is established. A clear representation of the individual's knowledge and use of preventive practices facilitates planning for health promotion. Although sex education is usually associated with school programs, information and discussion about sexuality is just as important for adults of all ages. Sex education is a key element of parenthood classes. Improved understanding of sexuality and sexual function leads to discovery and increased satisfaction.

Coping–Stress Tolerance Pattern

Gordon (2014) describes the coping-stress tolerance pattern as a depiction of general coping and the individual's ability to effectively manage stress. This pattern includes the individual's ability to process life crises and to resist disruptive factors that will influence self-integrity of ego, mode of conflict resolution, stress management, and accessibility to necessary resources (Box 6.3: Quality and Safety Scenario). The ability to manage stress effectively in life is a learned behavior. Adolescents develop their identify and gain autonomy, exposing them to unique stressors during this chaotic developmental stage (McAllister et al., 2018). Stress is a necessary part of life; without it, there is no motivation to grow. By adulthood, the healthy individual generates positive coping strategies, including support systems, cognitive restructuring, problem-solving, and emotional regulation to promote health and resilience. Vulnerability to stress may be linked to an individual's negative coping strategies, such as avoidance behavior, distraction, social withdrawal, self-criticism, blaming others, wishful thinking, and resignation (McAllister et al., 2018; Shi, 2019). Stress is exacerbated by accumulation of minor irritations. Stress is inherent not in the event but in the individual's perception of that event. One individual may experience stress from missing a bus and can think only of being 10 minutes late, whereas another will consider the same event an opportunity to spend 10 minutes reading the newspaper. This difference in perception may represent the different values used to identify sources of stress or it may represent coping strategies.

For purposes of assessing this pattern, coping, which is considered the individual behavioral response to stress, includes both problem-solving ability and use of defense mechanisms. Coping is viewed not as a single act but as a process incorporating many behaviors. The function of coping is to deal with the threat or emotional distress of an event. Coping effectiveness is assessed from the individual's perspective and from the nurse's observation of the individual's ability to function in the presence of actual or potential stressors in the environment.

The perception of stress and the ability to manage it depend on personal development, the amount of stress previously experienced, the current level of stress within the environment, and the sources of social support. For example, an older adult may experience many stresses during life and manage them effectively. Coping may be hindered by stressors related to aging, such as physical incapacitation, fixed income, fear of illness/injury, and lack of transportation. In addition, this person may no longer have a social support system, which has been associated with promotion of health; individuals who maintain an optimistic outlook on life seem to better cope with these stressors that accompany normal aging (Lee et al., 2019).

Determining an individual's stress tolerance and past coping patterns becomes the objective of assessment for this functional pattern. Clues to difficulties in managing past and current stressors and changes in the effectiveness of a coping pattern help to determine personal coping capacity. The following assessment parameters are included: the coping task, including the physical, psychological, and socioeconomic stimuli with which the individual must cope; coping style, or the tendency to use a specific style, such as approach-oriented, avoidance-oriented, or nonspecific; coping strategies, including specifics; and coping effectiveness. Coping strategy may be divided into information-seeking, direct action (fight or flight), inhibition of action, or use of social support. Individual resources include the variety of coping mechanisms used by the individual, the flexibility of these mechanisms, and the health promotion value associated with each of them.

Stress tolerance patterns elicit the amount of stress effectively processed in the past. Use of anticipatory coping is assessed

BOX 6.3 QUALITY AND SAFETY SCENARIO

Improving the quality of health promotion was explored in six primary health centers in Australia (Turner et al., 2019). These centers served Australian Indigenous people. The researchers reported that their qualitative data indicated that community participation was an important contextual factor in five of the six services. Interaction and relationship-building occurred with collaborative sharing of participants' viewpoints. These researchers concluded that participation of the Australian Indigenous people will result in more effective continuous quality-improvement processes.

The findings suggest that quality-improvement projects can improve the delivery of evidence-based health promotion by engaging those served in planning. This study attempted to engage the community members in a systems approach to quality improvement.

along with whether the individual knows how to cope but does not cope (production deficit) or simply does not know how to cope (skill deficit). Other indicators of value within this pattern are discussed in the section Self-Perception–Self-Concept Pattern. Objective data of concern include physical signs of restlessness, irritability, and nervousness, such as increased heart rate, blood pressure, and perspiration. Evidence of coping ability and tolerance to stress are found in every other functional health pattern. Stress affects the other patterns, thereby resulting in health problems such as insomnia, weight loss, and poor concentration (Gordon, 2014; Herdman, Kamitsuru, & Lopes, 2021).

Health promotion uses early intervention to reduce stress. Coping patterns and stress tolerance from past experiences may uncover unhealthy coping behaviors, such as smoking and alcohol consumption, that need to be replaced by alternative coping strategies. Healthy coping behaviors involving optimism, such as humor, need to be supported. Stress-reduction workshops would be helpful for most of the population because the future undoubtedly holds stressful events, some of which may be overwhelming without coping strategies. Increasingly, evidence supports that optimism and humor support healthy lifestyles. Box 6.4: Best Practice explores the use of humor in practice. Evidence for the use of humor in practice indicates it is an innovative way to support and promote health.

Evidence-based stress management strategies include social engineering strategies, such as time management, critical thinking, decision-making, and planned change; personality engineering strategies, such as assertiveness training, effective communication, social/interpersonal relationships, resilience strategies, and cognitive rehearsal; achieving altered states of consciousness, such as through meditation, self-awareness, mindfulness, and relaxation; using biofeedback; learning effective communication; maintaining social and interpersonal relationship support; dealing with trauma or loss and learning how to maintain resilience; and learning problem-solving skills (Arshad et al., 2022; Ochiai et al., 2021; Shi, 2019). Planning based on the assessment of all functional health patterns to help determine a coping pattern should include these kinds of strategies.

Values-Beliefs Pattern

The values-beliefs pattern describes values, including the individual's spiritual values, beliefs, and goals. This pattern includes perceptions of what is right, what is good, and any conflicts that beliefs or values impart. Each of the 11 patterns addresses the value systems of individuals, their family, and society. Individual beliefs or values develop over time and govern life through personal experiences, family support, and societal influences (Lee et al., 2019). Though most longevity studies focus primarily on biological factors, Lee and colleagues (2019) report that psychosocial factors, particularly optimism, are also a factor. Their analyses included 69,744 females from the Nurses' Health Study (NHS) and 1429 males from the Veterans Affairs (VA) Normative Aging Study (NAS), two highly valued longitudinal studies that collected data over 10 and 30 years, respectively (Lee et al., 2019). The objective in assessing this pattern is to determine the basis for health-related decisions and actions (Gordon, 2014). Individuals engage in preventive health behavior when a threat to wellness or health status exists. Several other health belief models expand on this concept by including other motivations, such as personal values and environmental influences. Clues to conflict within the individual's value system or between the person's value system and that of the family or society are explored.

BOX 6.4 BEST PRACTICE

Humor in Practice

Research studies provide evidence that humor improves health and well-being. Optimism and longevity have been linked (Lee et al., 2019). Emerging innovations in health care aim to incorporate humor strategies into practice to promote enhanced health. Many online strategies are available; however, scant research provides evidence for specific strategies using humor to promote health. Baisley and Grunberg (2019) created a humor workshop training model to teach professionals how to use humor in practice. They reported that their study produced a valid and feasible humor workshop training model. They conclude that their findings support the use of continued humor training with a focus on assessment of health outcomes from the training.

In their meta-analysis of 37 articles, Schneider et al. (2018) explored the evidence regarding habitual humor styles and mental health. They concluded that humor styles present a complex multidimensional effect on mental health. Their analysis showed that the style of humor emphasizing self-enhancement was particularly promising as a strategy in mental health. Determination of humor styles used by individuals, then, takes on an important role during health promotion assessment. These finding suggest using humor as a self-regulator when coping with challenges enhances mental health. Learning to assess humor and develop strategies to enhance this coping technique are innovative ways for a nurse to foster health promotion.

The Association for Applied and Therapeutic Humor (AATH) is a nonprofit international professional organization that provides cutting-edge resources, products, television shows, and seminars using humor as a strategy. This member-driven organization provides a supportive community to promote expertise and healthy humor. The Joy of Stress, one television program, earned a nomination for a regional Emmy award. The Humor Academy (https://aath.memberclicks.net/humor-academy) aligns its learning levels with the mission of the AATH, "to serve as a community of professionals who study, practice and promote healthy humor." Each year's learning program consists of a preconference intensive day, monthly conference calls, and homework that lead to eligibility and certification by the AATH board as a Certified Humor Professional.

Contact information:

Association for Applied and Therapeutic Humor
220 East State Street FL. G
Rockford, IL 61104
E-mail: info@aath.org
Executive Director: Kathy Velasco
Managing Director: Michele St. Clair
Website: https://aath.memberclicks.net/
Telephone: 815-708-6587

Baisley & Grunberg (2019); Lee et al. (2019); Schneider et al. (2018)

The dimensions of assessment include the individual's values, beliefs, or goals that guide choices or decisions that are related to health. The nurse collects information while exploring each pattern, while summarizing, clarifying, and securing additional information. Specifically, values and beliefs about self, relationships, and society are appraised. The individual's beliefs, goals, and purposes of life are reviewed, along with any conflicts, perceived philosophies, and philosophies of the family, culture, and society. Sources of strength, such as a higher being or significant individual practices, are explored, including religious beliefs and preferences. Past goals and expectations are assessed through the individual's satisfaction. The nurse must identify the individual's goals and expectations concerning health, clarifying them to help the individual achieve them. Providers design health promotion interventions based on the individual's value system and health beliefs (Lee et al., 2019). The brevity of this discussion is not an indication of the importance that the values-beliefs pattern plays in the assessment of the individual. Individual values play a role in all the patterns.

FOSTERING INDIVIDUAL HEALTH PROMOTION

Nursing clinical judgment—the systematic approach to reduce or eliminate the individual's health problem—is accomplished in several steps, the first being the collection of necessary data. With the individual, the nurse analyzes the data, establishes a plan, projects outcomes, prescribes interventions, and evaluates effectiveness. Periodic reassessment, reordering of priorities, revising goals, and modifying plans continue as part of the process toward outcome attainment (Ladwig et al., 2019).

Collection and Analysis of Data

Assessment is a systematic technique used to learn as much as possible about the individual. The main purpose of this data collection from new individuals is to establish the existence of any health problems and to clarify an individual's health goals. Data collection includes biographical data, such as age, sex, and the purpose of the visit. Assessment of the previously outlined 11 functional health patterns follows. Next, subjective findings, observations, nursing perceptions, and physical examination findings are recorded. These data collection and assessment elements provide the foundation required to form an analysis and plans.

Problem Identification

As the concept of problem identification evolves, a careful examination and analysis of the facts provides a basis for nursing intervention. When developing health promotion plans, the nurse identifies individual, family, and community responses to actual or potential life processes (Gordon, 2014; Ladwig et al., 2019). These identified life processes form the basis for selecting nursing interventions aimed to achieve outcomes for which the nurse is accountable (Gordon, 2014). Box 6.5: Evidence-Based Practice discusses how this nursing classification system compares with a nonnursing system.

BOX 6.5 EVIDENCE-BASED PRACTICE

Stress Management Strategies and the Nurse

Stress is viewed as a global epidemic that can significantly affect an individual's health. The American Institute of Stress (AIS) contends that 120,000 individuals die each year as a direct result of stress. Additionally, the rising cost of health care due to work-related stress is estimated at $190 billion (AIS, 2024). Stress among nurses is one of the most under-represented yet profound consequences directly related to this profession (American Nurses Association [ANA], 2024). As job-related stress increases among essential health care workers (American Heart Association [AHA], 2024), a gap exists related to self-care measures essential for combating stress (AIS, 2023; ANA, 2024). Evidence suggests that stress management strategies are critical to achieving overall health and wellness (AHA, 2024; AIS, 2024; ANA, 2024). New programs, for example, Healthy Nurse, Healthy Nation™ (HNHN), have been developed by the ANA as a social movement designed to transform the health of the nation's 4 million registered nurses. This initiative is free and may support evidence-based health promotion programs. To find out more about such programs, nurses can join at https://www.hnhn.org.

AHA (2024); AIS (2024); ANA (2024)

The meaning of any problem must be clearly defined and identified. The concept of problem as used in this text refers to Gordon's (2014) proposition that a health problem is defined as a dysfunctional pattern and that nursing's major contribution to health care is in preventing and treating such a pattern. A pattern is dysfunctional when it represents a deviation from established norms or from the individual's previous condition or goals. Normative behavior is further discussed in Unit 4. A dysfunctional pattern is a problem when it generates therapeutic concern on the part of the individual, others, or the nurse and when it is amenable to nursing therapies.

When analyzing patterns, nurses propose several hypotheses for functional or dysfunctional labeling. At the completion of the assessment, conclusions must be drawn. The possibility exists that all patterns are functional, that some are functional, and that others are dysfunctional or potentially dysfunctional. "Functional" refers to wellness and optimal health. Dysfunctional patterns, indicating some health problems, may be present in the absence of disease; that is, nursing care may be needed for health promotion and health maintenance, not health restoration. The case history of Frank Thompson in Chapter 1 effectively illustrates the multiple nursing care needs of an individual who is not ill. In potentially dysfunctional patterns, sufficient evidence exists or enough **risk factors** are present to indicate that a dysfunctional pattern will likely occur without intervention. Systematic data collection and analysis aim for early identification of potential problems.

Contributing Etiologic Factors

To plan care, the nurse must first determine what has caused the actual or potential health problem or its contributing etiologic factors. The etiologic factors of most dysfunctional patterns lie within another pattern or patterns. Although cause is never an absolute within human sciences, the projection of outcomes or goals must be based on probable causes. Interventions then focus on mediating or resolving the probable causes. Most often, many factors are involved, and problems are said to relate to rather than be a result of these factors. Potential problems are not actual problems but risk states. Nursing intervention is directed toward risk reduction through education (classes or brochures) to improve nutrition, prevent accidents, and so forth. Risk estimate theory and potential health problems are developed further in Chapters 7 and 8 and Unit 4.

Recognizing and Analyzing Variables

Accurate analysis, even when comprehensive data are unavailable, is governed predominately by nurses' clinical knowledge. Expertise improves effectiveness of analysis when nursing is performed as a scientific process. Nurses gather information, interpret it based on normative values, organize group information on the basis of healthy findings, identify the problem, and then plan appropriate goals and interventions. Difficulties occur when norms are unavailable, as occurs frequently in the psychosocial assessment components. Use of the 11 interdependent functional health patterns helps solve these difficulties. By focusing on each of these areas, nurses find it easier to recognize whether problems exist. Changes within the pattern are signs of dysfunction or unhealthy but stabilized behavior. For example, a 2-year-old child who is still not walking illustrates an indicator of dysfunction. Developmental milestones are major factors in activity patterns of infants, toddlers, and children.

The use of physiologic parameters to assess development clearly demonstrates the idea of a stabilized dysfunctional pattern; however, equal attention must be given to psychological development. For instance, the developmental patterns of a 26-year-old male who lives with his mother and gives no indication of independent decision-making should be evaluated. In contrast to health promotion assessment, acute situations and emergencies rely on quick assessment of major problems, giving priority to problems based on hierarchy of needs. Full nursing assessment may be postponed temporarily.

Planning Care and Generating Solutions

Planning is the proposal of treatment to assist the individual toward the goal or expected outcome of optimal health. The individual's goals provide the basis for planning. Clear goals are critical to development of an effective plan of care. The nursing process identifies the following purposes of the planning phase: to assign priority to the problems; to specify the behavioral outcomes or goals with the individual, including the expected time of achievement; to differentiate individual problems that can be resolved by nursing intervention into those that can be handled by the individual or family members and those that should be referred to other members of the health team; to designate specific actions, the frequency of these actions, and the short-, intermediate-, and long-term results; and to list the individual's problems and nursing actions (frequency and **expected outcomes** or goals) on the nursing care plan or blueprint for action (Herdman, Kamitsuru, & Lopes, 2021). This plan provides the direction for individual and nursing activities and is the guide for the evaluation. Research involving evidence and outcomes should guide nurses to increase the effectiveness of their care.

Taking Action and Implementation

Implementation comprises actions designed to achieve outcomes/goals identified in the planning phase; it is the enactment of the nursing care plan that elicits behaviors described in the proposed individual outcome. The selection of nursing action depends on factors such as the desired individual outcome, the characteristics of the issues, the research base associated with the intervention, the feasibility of implementing the intervention, the acceptability of the intervention to the individual, and the capability of the nurse. These interventions may be classified as independent or interdisciplinary (Ladwig et al., 2019).

As discussed in Unit 1, a critical component of effective communication is the accurate interpretation of the individual's information. This feedback process continues throughout all phases of the nursing process; the nurse continues to collect data to modify the plan as needed and does not blindly implement the care plan. As discussed in Unit 3, the most frequently used nursing interventions in health promotion are screening, education, counseling, and crisis intervention. All of these interventions require strong communication abilities from the nurse. Checklists and screening instruments may be used to document nursing assessment and help to ensure transmission of reliable and quality information for client-centered care. Implementation requires transdisciplinary collaboration in the analysis and plan. Computerized data entry, information systems, and electronic medical records may facilitate communication; however, ongoing interaction with other health care providers is essential for collaboration.

Evaluation of Outcomes

The process of analyzing cues experienced by the individual occurs in the evaluation of the outcomes phase of the clinical judgment model (National Council of State Boards of Nursing [NCSBN], 2024; Tanner, 2006), with the nurse examining the reasoning patterns in the evaluation of the effectiveness of the intervention. Clinical judgment requires more than analyzing cues; it involves collecting data to formulate decisions, prioritization of actions, and taking action to improve an individual's health.

As discussed, the health issues and goals guide the evaluation of the nursing care plan. Many variables influence outcomes: the interventions prescribed by the health care providers, the health care providers themselves, the environment in which the care is received, motivation, the individual's genetic structure, and the individual's significant others (Box 6.6: Genomics). Families and clients are partners in the process of client-centered care (Herdman, Kamitsuru, & Lopes, 2021).

BOX 6.6 GENOMICS

The Healthy People 2030 goals to improve health and prevent harm through valid and useful genomic tools in clinical and public health practices have two associated objectives, both of which are linked to health promotion assessment of the individual.

1. Increase the proportion of females with a family history of breast and/or ovarian cancer who receive genetic counseling
   Females with a family history of breast and/or ovarian cancer face multiple decisions that encompass both a cognitive and an emotional component. Risk estimates, disease course, family/reproductive plans, potential interventions, and timelines should be discussed. Open dialogue should include numerical risk, past experiences with cancer and deaths in the family, whether the woman has children, anxiety, depression, and general risk aversion. Treatment option discussion should include the types of breast cancers that develop in *BRCA1* and *BRCA2* carriers, the role of age at diagnosis, risk-reducing medications, surveillance, and surgical options (mastectomy and salpingo-oopherectomy). Information presented clearly with time and emotional support as factors in decisions is essential. The efficacy of risk-reducing mastectomy has been supported in large-scale studies; however, the efficacy and side effects of salpingo-oopherectomy are less well established. Moreover, physical and psychosexual adverse effects may accompany these approaches. A genetic counselor who specializes in these disorders is the preferred provider to provide individualized care based on the specific gene mutation.
2. Increase the proportion of persons with newly diagnosed colorectal cancer (CRC) who receive genetic testing to identify Lynch syndrome (or familial colorectal cancer syndromes)
   The estimated lifetime risk of CRC in those with Lynch syndrome is 60% to 80%. Those with Lynch syndrome are at increased risk of developing ovarian cancer and may have moderately increased risks of breast cancer. The criteria (Amsterdam II) to determine which individuals should be screened for Lynch syndrome include:
   - Three biologic relatives with CRC or another Lynch-associated cancer (endometrial, ovarian, upper urinary tract, small bowel) who are linked through a first-degree relative
   - At least two consecutive generations affected
   - One cancer diagnosis when younger than 50 years

Individuals who meet the criteria but choose to forego genetic screening should receive aggressive surveillance with colonoscopy every 1 to 2 years starting at the age of 20 to 25 years. Failure to identify at-risk individuals is common, and aggressive screening is often not completed.

One potential barrier is provider lack of knowledge regarding recommended screening guidelines. Nurses who promote health should be aware of these screening criteria.

(Samadder et al. 2019a; Samadder et al.2019b)

CASE STUDY

Readiness for Enhanced Health Literacy: Perla

Perla is a 67-year-old female who visits you at the community health center. She has a history of breast cancer, with her last visit to the oncologist 1 year ago without recurrence since her initial diagnosis 20 years ago. She is conscientious about her oncology follow-up appointments. Her spouse died many years ago. She lives alone and cares for a 95-year-old female full time who lives alone across town. Her only son, who visits on holidays, lives 300 miles way. Her sisters live nearby, and she visits them regularly. One sister, who lives alone, has early dementia. Recently, Perla came to the clinic for treatment of an upper respiratory tract infection with early signs of bronchitis. Today, she arrives for her follow-up appointment.

Perla tells you that she was afraid to use the bronchodilator inhaler that you prescribed, because it was expensive and she was concerned that she would become addicted and need it all of the time. She waited several days before filling the prescription. When you explored these concerns further, she mentioned that she did not understand the inhaler materials that came from the pharmacy and expressed a desire to be able to communicate more effectively with the pharmacy, clinic staff, and you in the future about her plan of care.

Today, her lungs are clear. She says she has no nasal congestion and feels back to her "normal self." She has no other acute health issues at this time.

Reflective Questions

- What health promotion strategies should the nurse consider?
- Describe other individuals you know who have expressed a desire to enhance their health knowledge and literacy.

Actions to Enhance Health Literacy

- Take time to be present and available to listen to the individual.
- Convey a nonjudgmental attitude.
- Encourage the individual to verbalize feelings.
- Review patient medication information thoroughly.
- Provide contact information for the resources available (clinic staff, pharmacist).
- Consider role play to facilitate taking assertive action to ask questions in the future.

SUMMARY

- Data relevant to the health promotion activities of the individual focus primarily on the assessment of the current health status so that the nurse can identify problem areas or areas of dysfunction within the individual's health and lifestyle patterns.
- This process is a fundamental first step and precedes all other components of clinical judgment. Without a clear picture of the problem, nursing activities are fruitless.
- Gordon's (2014) functional health pattern framework provides guidance for the individual assessment.
- The focus of each pattern includes the age-developmental influences exerted, cultural and environmental roles played, functional ability displayed, and behavioral patterns specific to each individual.
- The interaction between internal mechanisms and the environment is assessed through these 11 functional health patterns.
- When assessing each pattern, the nurse must understand the pattern definition, the significance of the pattern to the whole individual, the developmental influences, the environmental role, the assessment objectives, the assessment parameters and indicators, and the nursing implications.
- Assessment is essential to all components of clinical judgment in health promotion for the individual.

EVOLVE CHAPTER FEATURES

http://evolve.elsevier.com/Edelman/

- Study Questions

REFERENCES

Agency for Health Care and Quality [AHRQ]. (2020). *Health literacy universal precautions toolkit*. https://www.ahrq.gov/health-literacy/improve/precautions/index.html

Agency for Health Care and Quality [AHRQ]. (2023). *Health literacy universal precautions toolkit, 2nd ed., address language differences: tool # 9*. https://www.ahrq.gov

American Institute of Stress. (2024). *Stress effects*. https://www.stress.org/stress-effects. Accessed February 6, 2024.

American Heart Association [AHA]. (2024). Essential advice for stressed-out essential workers. https://www.heart.org/en/news/2020/04/24/essential-advice-for-stressed-out-essential-workers. Accessed February 6, 2024.

American Nurses Association [ANA]. (2024). *Combating stress*. https://www.nursingworld.org/practice-policy/work-environment/health-safety/combating-stress/. Accessed February 6, 2024.

Amirtha, R., & Sivakumar, V. J. (2018). Does family life cycle stage influence e-shopping acceptance by Indian women? An examination using the technology acceptance model. *Behaviour & Information Technology*, *37*(3), 267–294. https://doi.org/10.1080/0144929x.2018.1434560

Arnett, D. K., Blumenthal, R. S., Albert, M. A., Buroker, A. B., Goldberger, Z. D., & Hahn, E. J. (2019). 2019 ACC/AHA guideline on the primary prevention of cardiovascular disease: Executive summary: A report of the American College of Cardiology/American Heart Association Task Force on Clinical Practice Guidelines. *Journal of the American College of Cardiology*, *74*(10), 1376–1414. https://doi.org/10.1161/cir.0000000000000724

Arshad, R., Hamid, A., & Shahid, S. (2022). The design of persuasive prompts to induce behavioural change through an mHealth application for people with depression. *Behaviour & Information Technology*, *41*(12), 2497–2513. https://doi.org/10.1080/0144929x.2021.2006787

Baisley, M. C., & Grunberg, N. E. (2019). Bringing humor theory into practice: An interdisciplinary approach to online humor training. *New Ideas in Psychology*, *55*, 24–34. https://doi.org/10.1016/j.newideapsych.2019.04.006

Bermúdez, J. M., Muruthi, B., Zak-Hunter, L. M., Stinson, M. A., Seponski, D. M., & Boe, J. L. (2019). "Thank you for including us!": Introducing a community-based collaborative approach to translating clinic materials. *Journal of Marital and Family Therapy*, *45*(2), 309–322. https://doi.org/10.1111/jmft.12317

Bester, G. (2019). Stress experienced by adolescents in school: The importance of personality and interpersonal relationships. *Journal of Child & Adolescent Mental Health*, *31*(1), 25–37. https://doi.org/10.2989/17280583.2019.1580586

Bjørnsen, H. N., Espnes, G. A., Eilertsen, M. E. B., Ringdal, R., & Moksnes, U. K. (2019). The relationship between positive mental health literacy and mental well-being among adolescents: Implications for school health services. *Journal of School Nursing*, *35*(2), 107–116. https://doi.org/10.1177/1059840517732125

Burton, C., Doyle, E., Humber, K., Rouxel, C., Worner, S., Colman, R., et al. (2019). The biopsychosocial barriers and enablers to being physically active following childbirth: A systematic literature review. *Physical Therapy Reviews*, 1–13. https://doi.org/10.1080/10833196.2019.1632049

Centeio, E. E., Somers, C. L., Moore, E. W. G., Garn, A., Kulik, N., & Martin, J. (2019). Considering physical well-being, self-perceptions, and support variables in understanding youth academic achievement. *The Journal of Early Adolescence*, *31*(1), 25–37. https://doi.org/10.1177/0272431619833493

Child, S. T., Kaczynski, A. T., Fair, M. L., Stowe, E. W., Hughey, S. M., Boeckermann, L., et al. (2019). We need a safe, walkable way to connect our sisters and brothers: A qualitative study of opportunities and challenges for neighborhood-based physical activity among residents of low-income African-American communities. *Ethnicity & Health*, *24*(4), 353–364. https://doi.org/10.1080/13557858.2017.1351923

Cohen, D. A., Han, B., Park, S., Williamson, S., & Derose, K. P. (2019). Park use and park-based physical activity in low-income neighborhoods. *Journal of Aging and Physical Activity*, *27*(3), 334–342. https://doi.org/10.1123/japa.2018-0032

Darling-Fisher, C. S. (2019). Application of the modified Erikson psychosocial stage inventory: 25 years in review. *Western Journal of Nursing Research*, *41*(3), 431–458. https://doi.org/10.1177/0193945918770457

De Cassia Gengo e Silva Butcher, R., & Jones, D. A. (2021). An integrative review of comprehensive nursing assessment tools developed based on Gordon's eleven functional health patterns. *International Journal of Nursing Knowledge*, *34*(4), 294–307. https://doi.org/10.1111/2047-3095.12321

Duncan, D. (2019). Alternative to antibiotics for managing asymptomatic and non-symptomatic bacteriuria in older persons: A review. *British Journal of Community Nursing*, *24*(3), 116–119. https://doi.org/10.12968/bjcn.2019.24.3.116

Ebele, N. (2019). Noncommunicable diseases prevention in low-and middle-income countries: An overview of Health in All Policies (HiAP). *PeerJ Preprints*, *7*, e27962v1. https://doi.org/10.7287/peerj.preprints.27962v1

Ewing-Cooper, A., & Merrifield, K. (2019). *Voices of the global community*. National Academic Advising Association (NACADA). The Global Community of Academic Advising.

Fazelipour, M., & Cunningham, F. (2019). Barriers and facilitators to the implementation of brief interventions targeting smoking, nutrition, and physical activity for indigenous populations: a narrative review. *International Journal for Equity in Health*, *18*(1), 169. https://doi.org/10.1186/s12939-019-1059-2

Ferguson, S. A., Appleton, S. L., Reynolds, A. C., Gill, T. K., Taylor, A. W., & McEvoy, R. D. (2019). Making errors at work due to sleepiness or sleep problems is not confined to non-standard work hours: Results of the 2016 Sleep Health Foundation national survey. *Chronobiology International*, *36*(6), 758–769. https://doi.org/10.1080/07420528.2019.1578969

Francis, J., & Dickton, D. (2019). Preventive health application to increase breastfeeding. *Journal of Women's Health*, *28*(10), 1344–1349. https://doi.org/10.1089/jwh.2018.7477

Garcia, A. S., Takahashi, S., Anderson-Knott, M., & Dev, D. (2019). Determinants of physical activity for Latino and White middle school-aged children. *Journal of School Health*, *89*(1), 3–10. https://doi.org/10.1111/josh.12706

Garland, M., Wilbur, J., Semanik, P., & Fogg, L. (2019). Correlates of physical activity during pregnancy: A systematic review with implications for evidence-based practice. *Worldviews on Evidence-Based Nursing*, *16*(4), 310–318. https://doi.org/10.1111/wvn.12391

Goodway, J. D., Ozmun, J. C., & Gallahue, D. L. (2019). *Understanding motor development: Infants, children, adolescents, adults*. Jones & Bartlett Publishers.

Gordon, M. (2014). *Manual of nursing diagnosis* (13th ed.). Sudbury, MA: Jones & Bartlett.

Gupta, H., & Garg, S. (2019). Obesity and overweight: Their impact on individual and corporate health. *Journal of Public Health, 28*, 211–218. https://doi.org/10.1007/s10389-019-01053-9

Haas, A. P., Lane, A. D., Blosnich, J. R., Butcher, B. A., & Mortali, M. G. (2019). Collecting sexual orientation and gender identity information at death. *American Journal of Public Health, 109*(2), 255–259. https://doi.org/10.2105/ajph.2018.304829

Hansen, L. P., Kinskey, C., Koffel, E., Polusny, M., Ferguson, J., & Schmer-Galunder, S. (2018). Sleep patterns and problems among Army National Guard soldiers. *Military Medicine, 183*(11–12), e396–e401. https://doi.org/10.1093/milmed/usy107

Herdman, H. T., Kamitsuru, S., & Lopes, C. (Eds.), (2021). *NANDA international nursing diagnoses: Definitions & classification 2021-2023*. Thieme. https://doi.org/10.1055/b-006-161179

Hipp, S. L., Chung-Do, J., & McFarlane, E. (2019). Systematic review of interventions for reproductive life planning. *Journal of Obstetric, Gynecologic & Neonatal Nursing, 48*(2), 131–139. https://doi.org/10.1016/j.jogn.2018.12.007

Hossain, F., & Ferreira, N. (2019). Impact of social context on the self-concept of gay and lesbian youth: A systematic review. *Global Psychiatry, 2*(1), 51–78. https://doi.org/10.2478/gp-2019-0006

Huck, G., Mahr, M., Morrison, B., Finnicum, C., & Umucu, E. (2019). Barriers to physical activity among assertive community treatment participants: A mixed-methods analysis. *Journal of Applied Rehabilitation Counseling, 50*(2), 102–117. https://doi.org/10.1891/0047-2220.50.2.102

Hupkens, S., Goumans, M., Derkx, P., & Machielse, A. (2020). Nurse's attunement to patient's meaning in life: A qualitative study of experiences of Dutch adults ageing in place. *BMC Nursing, 19*(41), 1–13. https://doi.org/10.21203/rs.3.rs-19312/v2

Ibrahim, F. M., Fadila, D. E., & Elmawla, A. D. (2023). Older adults' acceptance of the COVID-19 vaccines: Application of the health belief model. *Nursing Open, 10*(10), 6989–7002. https://doi.org/10.1002/nop2.1954

International Council of Nurses. (2023). *Definition of nursing*. https://www.icn.ch/nursing-policy/nursing-definitions. Accessed February 6, 2024.

Jhang, F. H. (2019). Effects of changes in family social capital on the self-rated health and family life satisfaction of older adults in Taiwan: A longitudinal study. *Geriatrics & Gerontology International, 19*(3), 228–232. https://doi.org/10.1111/ggi.13599

Jin, Y., & Peng, Y. (2022). The development of a situation-specific nurse-led culturally tailored self-management theory for Chinese patients with heart failure. *Journal of Transcultural Nursing, 33*(1), 6–15. https://doi.org/10.1177/10436596211023973

Jordan, K., & Tseris, E. (2018). Locating, understanding and celebrating disability: Revisiting Erikson's "stages". *Feminism & Psychology, 28*(3), 427–444. https://doi.org/10.1177/0959353517705400

Kabak, V. Y., Gursen, C., Aytar, A., Akbayrak, T., & Duger, T. (2021). Physical activity level, exercise behavior, barriers, and preferences of patients with breast cancer-related lymphedema. *Supportive Care in Cancer, 29*(7), 3593–3602. https://doi.org/10.1007/s00520-020-05858-3

Kamolvit, W., Nilsén, V., Zambrana, S., Mohanty, S., Gonzales, E., Östenson, C. G., et al. (2018). Lupinus mutabilis edible beans protect against bacterial infection in uroepithelial cells. *Evidence-Based Complementary and Alternative Medicine*, 1–8. https://doi.org/10.1155/2018/1098015

Kang, Y., & Demiris, G. (2018). Self-report pain assessment tools for cognitively intact older adults: Integrative review. *International Journal of Older People Nursing, 13*(2), e12170. https://doi.org/10.1111/opn.12170

Kappesser, J., Kamper, E., de Laffolie, J., Faas, D., Ehrhardt, H., Franck, L. S., et al. (2019). Pain-specific reactions or indicators of a general stress response? Investigating the discriminant validity of five well-established neonatal pain assessment tools. *The Clinical Journal of Pain, 35*(2), 101–110. https://doi.org/10.1097/ajp.0000000000000660

Karaman, S., & Tan, M. (2021). Effect of Reiki therapy on quality of life and fatigue levels of breast cancer patients receiving chemotherapy. *Cancer Nursing, 44*(6), E652–E658. https://doi.org/10.1097/ncc.0000000000000970

Khani, F., Pashaeypoor, S., Nikpeyma, N., & Kazemnejad, A. (2020). Effect of lifestyle education based on Pender model on health promoting behaviors in HIV positive individuals: A randomized clinical trial study. *Nursing Practice Today, 7*(1), 45–52. https://doi. org/10.18502/npt.v7i1.2299

Kim, Y., & Kang, S. (2021). Effects of a weight control intervention based on the transtheoretical model on physical activity and psychological variables in middle-aged obese women. *Journal of Women and Aging, 33*(5), 556–568. https://doi.org/10.1080/08952841.2020.1728183

Knudson-Martin, C., McDowell, T., & Bermudez, J. M. (2019). From knowing to doing: Guidelines for socioculturally attuned family therapy. *Journal of Marital and Family Therapy, 45*(1), 47–60. https://doi.org/10.1111/jmft.12299

Krys, K., Zelenski, J. M., Capaldi, C. A., Park, J., van Tilburg, W., van Osch, Y., et al. (2019). Putting the "We" into well-being: Using collectivism-themed measures of well-being attenuates well-being's association with individualism. *Asian Journal of Social Psychology, 22*(3), 256–267. https://doi.org/10.1111/ajsp.12364

Ladwig, G. B., Ackley, B. J., & Makic, M. B. (2019). *Mosby's guide to nursing diagnosis e-book*. Elsevier Health Sciences.

Lajiness, B., & Lajiness, M. J. (2019). 50 years of urinary tract infections and treatments-Has much changed? *Urologic Nursing, 39*(5). https://doi.org/10.7257/1053-816x.2019.39.5.235

Lee, L. O., James, P., Zevon, E. S., Kim, E. S., Trudel-Fitzgerald, C., Spiro, A., et al. (2019). Optimism is associated with exceptional longevity in 2 epidemiologic cohorts of men and women. *Proceedings of the National Academy of Sciences, 116*(37), 18357–18362. https://doi.org/10.1073/pnas.1900712116

LoVette, A., Kuo, C., & Harrison, A. (2019). Strength-based interventions for HIV prevention and sexual risk reduction among girls and young women: A resilience-focused systematic review. *Global Public Health*, 1–25. https://doi.org/10.1080/17441692.2019.1602157

McAllister, M., Knight, B. A., Hasking, P., Withyman, C., & Dawkins, J. (2018). Building resilience in regional youth: Impacts of a universal mental health promotion programme. *International Journal of Mental Health Nursing, 27*(3), 1044–1054. https://doi.org/10.1111/inm.12412

Mercurio, A. (2019). Integrating sexuality and gender identity into the reproductive life plan. *Journal of Women's Health, 28*(1), 107–108. https://doi.org/10.1089/jwh.2018.7341

Mitchell, A. (2019). Carrying out a holistic assessment of a patient with constipation. *British Journal of Nursing, 28*(4), 230–232. https://doi.org/10.12968/bjon.2019.28.4.230

Mitchell, A. M., & Christian, L. M. (2019). Repetitive negative thinking, meaning in life, and serum cytokine levels in pregnant women: Varying associations by socioeconomic status. *Journal of Behavioral Medicine*, 1–13. https://doi.org/10.1007/s10865-019-00023-6

NACADA. Resources. https://nacada.ksu.edu/Resources/Academic-Advising-Today/View-Articles/The-Eight-Crises-of-College-Students-Advising-with-Erikson-Across-a-Students-Academic-Lifespan.aspx. Accessed February 6, 2024.

National Council of State Boards of Nursing. (2024). *Clinical judgment measurement model: a framework to measure clinical judgment & decision making*. https://nclex.com. Accessed February 28, 2024.

Nigg, C. R., Harmon, B., Jiang, Y., Ginis, K. A. M., Motl, R. W., & Dishman, R. K. (2019). Temporal sequencing of physical activity change constructs within the transtheoretical model. *Psychology of Sport and Exercise*, *45*, 101557. https://doi.org/10.1016/j.psychsport.2019.101557

Ochiai, E., Kigenvi, T., Sondik, E., Pronk, N., Kleinman, D. V., Blakey, C., et al. (2021). Healthy People 2030 leading health indicators and overall health and well-being measures: Opportunities to assess and improve the health and well-being of the nation. *Journal of Public Health Management and Practice*, *27*(6), S235–S241. https://doi.org/10.1097/phh.0000000000001424

Paterson, J. L., Reynolds, A. C., Duncan, M., Vandelanotte, C., & Ferguson, S. A. (2019). Barriers and enablers to modifying sleep behavior in adolescents and young adults: A qualitative investigation. *Behavioral Sleep Medicine*, *17*(1), 1–11. https://doi.org/10.1080/15402002.2016.1266489

Poveda-López, S., Montilla-Herrador, J., Gacto-Sanchez, M., Romero-Galisteo, R. P., & Lillo-Navarro, C. (2022). Wishes and perceptions about exercise programs in exercising institutionalized older adults living in long-term care institutions: A qualitative study. *Geriatric Nursing*, *43*, 167–174. https://doi.org/10.1016/j.gerinurse.2021.11.013

Prochnow, T., Ylitalo, K. R., Sharkey, J., & Meyer, R. U. M. (2019). Perceived physical activity barriers of Mexican-heritage sibling dyads. *American Journal of Health Behavior*, *43*(4), 781–794. https://doi.org/10.5993/ajhb.43.4.11

Pueyo-Garrigues, M., Whitehead, D., Pardavila-Belio, M. I., Canga-Armayor, A., Pueyo-Garrigues, S., & Canga-Armayor, N. (2019). Health education: A Rogerian concept analysis to translate theory into practice. *International Journal of Nursing Studies*, 131–138. https://doi.org/10.1016/j.ijnurstu.2019.03.005

Rosa, W. E., Dossey, B. M., Watson, J., Beck, D. M., & Upvall, M. J. (2019). The United Nations Sustainable Development Goals: The ethic and ethos of holistic nursing. *Journal of Holistic Nursing*, *37*(4), 381–393. https://doi.org/10.1177/0898010119841723

Roth, S. E., Gill, M., Chan-Golston, A. M., Rice, L. N., Crespi, C. M., Koniak-Griffin, D., et al. (2019). Physical activity correlates in middle school adolescents: Perceived benefits and barriers and their determinants. *The Journal of School Nursing*, *35*(5), 348–358. https://doi.org/10.1177/1059840518780300

Samadder, N. J., Baffy, N., Giridhar, K. V., Couch, F. J., & Riegert-Johnson, D. (2019a). Hereditary cancer syndromes: a primer on diagnosis and management, part 2: gastrointestinal cancer syndromes. *Mayo Clinic Proceedings*, *94*(6), 1099–1116. https://doi.org/10.1016/j.mayocp.2019.01.042

Samadder, N. J., Giridhar, K. V., Baffy, N., Riegert-Johnson, D., & Couch, F. J. (2019b). Hereditary cancer syndromes: a primer on diagnosis and management, part 1: breast-ovarian cancer syndromes. *Mayo Clinic Proceedings*, *94*(6), 1084–1098. https://doi.org/10.1016/j.mayocp.2019.02.017

Schneider, M., Voracek, M., & Tran, U. S. (2018). "A joke a day keeps the doctor away?" Meta-analytical evidence of differential associations of habitual humor styles with mental health. *Scandinavian Journal of Psychology*, *59*(3), 289–300. https://doi.org/10.1111/sjop.12432

Schroeder, K., Klusaritz, H., Dupuis, R., Bolick, A., Graves, A., Lipman, T. H., et al. (2019). Reconciling opposing perceptions of access to physical activity in a gentrifying urban neighborhood. *Public Health Nursing*, *36*, 461–468. https://doi.org/10.1111/phn.12602.

Scott, H., Biello, S. M., & Woods, H. C. (2019). Identifying drivers for bedtime social media use despite sleep costs: The adolescent perspective. *Journal of the National Sleep Foundation*, *5*(6), 539–545. https://doi.org/10.1016/j.sleh.2019.07.006

Semma, B., Henri, M., Luo, W., & Thompson, C. G. (2019). Reliability generalization of the meaning in life questionnaire subscales. *Journal of Psychoeducational Assessment*, *37*(7), 837–851. https://doi.org/10.1177/0734282918800739

Shi, W. (2019). Health information seeking versus avoiding: How do college students respond to stress-related information? *American Journal of Health Behavior*, *43*(2), 437–448. https://doi.org/10.5993/ajhb.43.2.18

Silva, M. A. D., Mendonça Filho, E. J. D., & Bandeira, D. R. (2019). Development of the dimensional inventory of child development assessment (IDADI). *Psico-USF*, *24*(1), 11–26. https://doi.org/10.1590/1413-82712019240102

Skein, M., Harrison, T., & Clarke, D. (2019). Sleep characteristics, sources of perceived stress and coping strategies in adolescent athletes. *Journal of Sleep Research*, *28*(4), e12791. https://doi.org/10.1111/jsr.12791

Somma, A., Gialdi, G., Frau, C., Barranca, M., & Fossati, A. (2022). COVID-19 pandemic preventive behaviors and causal beliefs among Italian community dwelling adults. *Journal of Health Psychology*, *27*(3), 601–611. https://doi.org/10.1177/1359105320962243

Stallinga, H. A., Dijkstra, P. U., ten Napel, H., Roodbol, G., Peters, J. W., Heerkens, Y. F., et al. (2018). Perceived usefulness of the International Classification of Functioning, Disability and Health (ICF) increases after a short training: A randomized controlled trial in Master of Advanced Nursing practice students. *Nurse Education in Practice*, *33*, 55–62. https://doi.org/10.1016/j.nepr.2018.08.004

Steinberg, D. B., Simon, V. A., Victor, B. G., Kernsmith, P. D., & Smith-Darden, J. P. (2019). Onset trajectories of sexting and other sexual behaviors across high school: A longitudinal growth mixture modeling approach. *Archives of Sexual Behavior*, *48*(8), 2321–2331. https://doi.org/10.1007/s10508-019-1414-9

Strand, L. I., Gundrosen, K. F., Lein, R. K., Laekeman, M., Lobbezoo, F., Defrin, R., et al. (2019). Body movements as pain indicators in older people with cognitive impairment: A systematic review. *European Journal of Pain*, *23*(4), 669–685. https://doi.org/10.1002/ejp.1344

Sukys, S., Cesnaitiene, V. J., Emeljanovas, A., Mieziene, B., Valantine, I., & Ossowski, Z. M. (2019). Reasons and barriers for university students' leisure-time physical activity: Moderating effect of health education. *Perceptual and Motor Skills*, *126*(6), 1084–1100. https://doi.org/10.1177/0031512519869089

Tanner, C. (2006). Thinking like a nurse: A research-based model of clinical judgment in nursing. *Journal of Nursing Education*, *45*(6), 204–211. https://doi.org/10.3928/01484834-20060601-04

The American Institute of Stress. *Stress effects*. https://www.stress.org. Accessed February 6, 2024.

Tsao, C. W., Aday, A. W., Almarzooq, Z. I., Alonso, A., Beaton, A. Z., Bittencourt, M. S., et al. (2022). Heart disease and stroke statistics – 2022 update: A report from the American Heart Association. *Circulation*, *145*(8), e153–e639. https://www.ahajournals.org/doi/full/10.1161/CIR.0000000000001052

Turner, N.N., Taylor, J., Larkins, S., Carlisle, K., Thompson, S., & Carter, M., et al. (2019). Conceptualizing the association between community participation and CQI in aboriginal and Torres strait islander PHC services. *Qualitative Health Research*, 29(13), 1904–1915. https://doi.org/10.1177/1049732319843107

US Department of Health and Human Services, [USDHHS]. *Healthy people 2030*. https://health.gov/healthypeople. Accessed February 16, 2024.

Wang, L. H., Liu, Y., Tan, H., & Huang, S. (2022). Transtheoretical model-based mobile health application for PCOS. *Reproductive Health*, *19*(1), 1–10. https://doi.org/10.1186/s12978-022-01422-w

Wilczynska, M., Lubans, D. R., Paolini, S., & Plotnikoff, R. C. (2019). Mediating effects of the 'eCoFit' physical activity intervention for adults at risk of, or diagnosed with, type 2 diabetes. *International Journal of Behavioral Medicine*, *26*(5), 512–521. https://doi.org/10.1007/s12529-019-09800-8

Wilson, J. C., & Nola, J. (2021). *Pender: Health promotion model. Nursing theorists and their work E-book* (9th ed., pp. 323–338). Elsevier.

World Health Organization. (2024). *Obesity and overweight. Fact sheet no 311 January 2015*. http://www.who.int/mediacentre/factsheets/fs311/en/. Accessed October 6, 2023. @Normal:

7

Health Promotion and the Family

Julianne A. Walsh

http://evolve.elsevier.com/Edelman/

OBJECTIVES

After completing this chapter, the reader will be able to:

- Describe various theoretical approaches to the study of families.
- Assess families throughout the life span using the functional health pattern framework.
- Describe examples of the clinical data to collect in each health pattern during each family developmental phase.
- Provide examples of behavioral changes (functional, potentially dysfunctional, and actually dysfunctional) within the health patterns of families.
- Describe developmental and cultural characteristics of the family to consider when identifying risk factors or etiologic factors of potential or actual dysfunctional health patterns.
- Plan, implement, and evaluate nursing interventions in health promotion with families.
- Evaluate a specific health-promotion plan based on family assessment, contributing risks and etiologic factors.

KEY TERMS

Cultural competence
Developmental theory
Ecomap; Family
Family developmental tasks
Family function
Family health status
Family nursing plans
Family nursing interventions
Family pattern
Family resilience
Family risk factors
Family strengths
Family structure
Family theory
Genogram
Risk-factor theory
Systems theory

THINK ABOUT IT

Caring for Older Adults

Adult family members, who may have health problems of their own, find themselves caring for their older adult parents as well as their grandchildren. The number of Americans living in homes with two or more adult generations, or grandparents caring for grandchildren under age 25, is growing (Murphy, 2019). This population, known as the "sandwich generation," is expected to become more prevalent in the coming years. An increasing number of parents of children older than 18 years provide financial support or care for grandchildren younger than 18 years, along with caring for an older parent aged more than 65 years (Murphy, 2019; US Census, 2024).

- What are the implications of this growing situation for individuals? For families? For communities? For the nation?
- How will this trend affect individual lives personally and professionally?
- How does multigenerational caring affect family finances?

A family consists of a group of interacting individuals related by blood, marriage, cohabitation, or adoption who interdependently perform relevant functions by fulfilling expected roles. Relevant family functions include practices and values placed on health. Family health practices, whether effective or ineffective, encompass activities performed by individuals or families as a whole to promote health and prevent disease. How well families complete developmental tasks and how well families, including individuals within a family, generate health-promoting behaviors determine a family's potential for enhancement of family health practices.

How family members relate to one another influences their behavior, which is demonstrated in the family's structural, functional, communicational, and developmental patterns (Shakarami, 2019). Families provide the structure for many health-promotion practices; therefore, family assessment

TABLE 7.1 Variety of Family Structures

Configuration	Positions in Family
Single parent (separated, divorced, or widowed)	Mother or father, sons(s), daughter(s)
Unmarried single parent (never married)	Mother or father, sons(s), daughter(s)
Unmarried cohabitating couple	Two adults living together in a long-term relationship that resembles marriage
Unmarried parents	Two adults, sons(s), daughter(s)
Commune family	Mothers, fathers, adults, shared son(s), daughters(s) living together
Stepparents	Adults with son(s), daughter(s) from previous marriage
Adoptive family	Adults who provide a permanent home to son(s) and/or daughter(s) through a legal process
Family of choice	Adults with selected partners and family members
Married couple	Two cohabitating adults living in a recognized legal union
Same-sex couple	Two persons of the same sex sharing an intimate, romantic, or sexual relationship
Married parents	Mother and father, son(s), daughter(s)
Nuclear family	Mother and father, son(s), daughter(s)
Gay, lesbian, transgender family	Adults and children living together with one or more members of the group who identifies as gay, lesbian, or transgender
Immigrant family	Adults and children living together with one or more members of the group who is foreign born
Biracial or multiracial family	Mother, father, adults, or children include two or more races
Transracial family	Mother, father, adults, or children include at least one member who is born of one race and decides to represent themselves as another race
Blended family	Mother, father, adults, or children represent members of from previous unions
Joint-custody family	Adults living with children who are legally awarded to both biologic parents
Conditionally separate families	A family member is separated from the family but remains a significant member of the family (military service, incarceration, distant employment, hospitalization)
Extended family	Significant family members beyond the nuclear family that may include grandparents, aunts, uncles, and other adults who live nearby or in one household
Foster family	Adults, serving as state-certified caregivers for children placed into a ward, group home, or private home
Grandparent(s)	Grandchildren, son(s) and/or daughter(s) Grandmother and/or grandfather

Terms from Senkowski, V., Bhochhibhoya, S., Bernard, R., Zingg, T., & Maness, S. B. (2019). Assessing the variation of measurement of family structure in studies of adolescent risk behaviors: A systematic review. *Vulnerable Children and Youth Studies, 4*(14), 287–311. https://doi.org/10.1080/17450128.2019.1614708

informs health-promotion and disease-prevention planning. Within families, children and adults are nurtured, provided for, and taught about health values by word and by example. Family members first learn to make choices to promote health within the family structure (Table 7.1). Appreciating how families make decisions and encouraging family participation in all aspects of care from acute care to health promotion helps families and individuals acquire new behaviors (Nickbakht et al., 2019).

Families influence children's lifestyle choices. *Healthy People 2030* views families in the United States as a means of providing important opportunities for health promotion and disease prevention (US Department of Health and Human Services [USDHHS], 2023). Through family planning, parents assume the responsibility of caring for their children. Prenatal care and breastfeeding give infants a healthy start. Nutritious diets support physical growth and development. Children first observe and learn behaviors within their family. Patterns of nutrition, activity, oral hygiene, and coping develop at early ages, supported by the example of family members. Patterns of alcohol consumption and tobacco use are similarly established within families. Learning about human development fosters a healthy self-concept, including positive awareness of the family member's sexuality. Promoting self-esteem and reinforcing positive behaviors strengthen the health of children. Primary care providers support positive behaviors by offering family members scientifically sound health-promotion and clinical preventive services, such as anticipatory guidance for developmental tasks, immunizations, screening for early detection, and appropriate counseling.

This chapter uses **family theory**, **systems theory**, **developmental theory**, and **risk-factor theory** to guide the nursing process with families. The 11 functional health patterns described in Chapter 6 establish the structure for interview questions during data collection. The analysis phase of the nursing process categorizes these data within stages of family development, and nursing plans are formulated from the analysis. **Family health status** is considered functional, potentially dysfunctional (potential problem), or dysfunctional (actual problem) (Gordon, 2014). The planning phase begins when family goals and objectives are stated. The family, the nurse, or another health professional facilitates implementation. Later in this chapter, four types of interventions for health promotion and disease prevention are discussed: increasing knowledge and skills, increasing strengths, decreasing exposure to risks, and decreasing susceptibility. Nurses assume various roles throughout the stages of family development, and these roles are presented. Evaluation of a family plan considers outcomes that are specific, objective, and measurable and that rely on the family's subjective interpretation of concerns and probability of success, as well as that at the population level (Kokorelias et al., 2019).

NURSING CLINICAL JUDGMENT AND THE FAMILY

Purpose of Clinical Judgment

Promoting the health of families includes nursing clinical judgment and decision-making related to the family as a group and the interactions among family members. The National Center on Parent, Family, and Community Engagement (NCPFCE) views the entire family as the participant that guides assessment from a holistic framework (USDHHS, 2022). Partnerships with families begin with an assessment (USDHHS, 2022). The home is a natural environment for health-promotion encounters, although the process may occur in other settings as well. Different age groups (infants, children, and older adults) are likely to be present in the home. Nurses observe physical surroundings firsthand during home visits. For example, household safety hazards are observed directly. Nurses monitor family-unit rituals, roles, and interpersonal interactions. Generally, the nurse contacts the family and establishes an appointment time for visiting the family. Including each family member in the visit provides a broad perspective. During visits, the process of nursing clinical judgment and decision-making develops mutually with families; it is not a treatment done for the family. Families collaborate with nursing in all phases. Guidelines for home visits are presented in Box 7.1.

Comprehensive family assessment provides the foundation to promote family health (USDHHS, 2022). Several factors influence family assessment, such as nurses' perceptions about family constitution, theoretical knowledge, norms, standards, and communication abilities during visits. In addition to factors that pertain to the nurse, familial factors influence assessments. These factors include family cooperation, mutual agreement to work toward goals, and family ability to recognize the relevance of health-promotion plans. Useful health-promotion family assessments involve listening to families; engaging in participatory dialogue; recognizing patterns; and assessing family potential for active, positive change (USDHHS, 2022).

The assessment phase of the nursing process seeks and identifies information from the family about health-promotion and disease-prevention activities. To obtain this information, nurses follow family progress through developmental tasks and identify strengths in the family's ability to generate behaviors associated with disease prevention. The approaches considered in this chapter include the developmental framework, strength-based assessment, and the risk-factor estimate. Developmental phases

BOX 7.1 Guidelines for Home Visits to Promote Health and Prevent Disease

Planning the Visit

- Make arrangements with the family.
- Study information regarding the family from agency records, referral forms, family history, cultural background, and other sources.
- Prepare material to bring (instruction sheets, business cards, agency forms, computer, etc.).
- Notify agency personnel of location and time of home visit.
- Contact family and state the purpose of the visit.
- Obtain appropriate supplies and teaching aids for visits.

Making the Visit

- Offer an introduction and explain the purpose of the visit.
- Set the tone (warm introduction; thank family for participating).
- Establish rapport to develop a caring relationship.
- Show respect. Include all family members in the discussion; allow family input.
- Identify the family's request for assistance.
- Understand the situation from the family's perspective.
- Identify appropriate activities for health promotion and disease prevention.
- Identify how the home visit is to be financed when needed.
- Make a contract with the family that states specific goals and objectives that the family wants to reach.
- Ask about other people/animals. Consider taking a buddy. Check gasoline and tire pressure.
- Identify and respond to health and home safety issues. Wear a name tag.
- Identify family strengths; establish mutual goals.
- Provide information and share resources; request feedback from family and answer questions.
- Terminate the visit with specific instructions and information about the next visit: when it will occur, what will happen, who will be present, and what the family plans to accomplish before then.

Ending and Summarizing the Visit

- Discuss next steps.
- Provide business cards and contact information.
- Closure and goodbye.
- Carry through promptly on agreements made. Record notes promptly with additional follow-up items and required reports. Provide copies of documents to family.

Evaluating the Visit

- Is there a sense of trust from the family members—mutual goal setting?
- Were reciprocal relationships developed?
- Did family members participate actively in the planning?
- Was family involvement in the plan of care evident?
- Are service provisions individualized and valuable for each family member?
- Has the family's physiologic and physical health improved?
- Did family members contribute autonomously?
- Did the family perceive that goals and plan were important?
- Did the provider consider family preferences, goals, and values joint decision-making?
- Were the recommended resources available?

Terms from Southern Oregon Head Start (SOHS). (2024). *Our programs.* https://www.socfc.org/programs/; Tøien, M., Torunn Bjørk, I., & Fagerstrom, L. (2020). 'A longitudinal room of possibilities' – Perspectives on the benefits of long-term preventive home visits: A qualitative study of nurses' experiences. *Nordic Journal of Nursing Research, 40*(1), 6–14.

for families as proposed by Duvall and Miller (1985), strength-based assessment using standardized tools (e.g., The Family Adaptability and Cohesion Scale-I [FACES] or Structured Assessment of Protective Factors for Violence Risk [SAPROF]), and risk-factor estimates delineated by *Healthy People 2030* can be used to guide nurses through the steps of the nursing process when they are working with families (Duvall, 1988; Duvall & Miller, 1985; Kashiwagi et al., 2018; Priest et al., 2018).

The Nurse's Role

Nurses collaborate with families using a systems perspective to understand family interaction, family norms, family expectations, effectiveness of family communication, family decision-making, and family coping mechanisms. The nurse's role in health promotion and disease prevention includes the following tasks:

- Learn family attitudes and behaviors toward health promotion and disease prevention.
- Act as a role model for the family.
- Collaborate with the family to assess, enhance, and evaluate family health practices.
- Assist the family in growth and development behaviors.
- Assist the family in identifying risk-taking behaviors.
- Assist the family in decision-making about lifestyle choices.
- Provide reinforcement for positive health-behavior practices.
- Provide health information to the family.
- Assist the family in learning behaviors to promote health and prevent disease.
- Assist the family in problem-solving and decision-making about health promotion.
- Serve as a liaison for referral/collaboration between community resources and the family.

Nurses use family theoretical frameworks to guide, observe, and classify situations. Nursing roles for families in various stages of development are presented in Table 7.2.

FAMILY THEORIES AND FRAMEWORKS

Family theory stems from a variety of interrelated disciplines (Lerner et al., 2019). Family systems theory explains patterns of living among the individuals who make up family systems. In systems theory, behaviors and family members' responses influence patterns. Meanings and values provide the vital elements of motivation and energy for family systems. Every family has its unique culture, value structure, and history. Values provide a means for interpreting events and information, passing from one generation to the next. Values usually change slowly over time. Families process information and energy exchange with the environment through values. For example, holiday food traditions may be changed slightly by a daughter-in-law, whose own daughter may then adjust the traditional recipe within her own nuclear family.

System boundaries separate family systems from their environment and control information flow. The family acts as an internal manager that influences and defines interactions and relationships among its members and with those outside the family system. The family forms a unified whole rather than the sum of its parts—an integrated system of interdependent functions, structures, and relationships. For example, one drug-dependent individual's health behavior influences the entire family unit.

Living systems are open systems. As living systems, families experience constant exchanges of energy and information with the environment. Change in one part or member of the family results in change in the family as a whole. For example, loss of a family member through death changes roles and relationships among all family members. Change requires adaptation of every family member as roles and functions assume new meanings. Changes families make are incorporated into the system.

Within family systems, issues can be clarified by family processes, communication interaction among family members, and family group values. Health-promotion research contains well-documented links to family function, relationships, mental health issues, parent-child relationships, and spirituality. Furthermore, systems theory connects family systems with health providers and the community (Badanta et al., 2022; Lerner et al., 2019). In Bowen's family systems theory, individuals' behavior and family members belong to interdependent systems. This interdependence contributes to differences from one family to another (Handley et al., 2019; Palombi, 2018). When individual family members exhibit behaviors that differ from the learned family pattern, differentiation of self occurs. Interaction among family members and the transmission of these interaction patterns from one generation to the next provide an evolutionary framework for the family systems approach (Palombi, 2018).

The framework for Pender's health-promotion model recognizes the family as the unit of assessment and intervention because families develop self-care and dependent-care competencies, foster resilience among family members, provide resources, and promote healthy individuation within cohesive family structures (Murdaugh et al., 2020). Furthermore, because the family often provides the structure for implementation of health promotion, family assessment becomes an integral tool for fostering health and healthy behaviors (Murdaugh et al., 2020).

The Family From a Developmental Perspective

Building on Erikson's (1998) theory of psychosocial development, Duvall and Miller (1985) identified stages of the family life cycle and critical **family developmental tasks**. Although Duvall's classification has been criticized for its middle-class homogeneity and lack of diversity in family forms, this conceptual model supports the anticipation of family events and has formed the basis for many contemporary developmental models (Aeby et al., 2019; Handayani et al., 2019). Knowing a family's composition, interrelationships, and particular life cycle helps nurses predict the overall **family pattern**. Box 7.2 lists characteristics of healthy families (Roygardner et al., 2019; Search Institute, 2023). From Duvall's perspective, most families complete these basic family tasks. Each family performs these tasks in a unique expression of its personality. Progression through the stages occurs in a linear fashion; however, regression may occur, and families may complete tasks in more than one stage at a time (Duvall & Miller, 1985; Handayani et al., 2019). Specific tasks arise as growth responsibilities during family development.

TABLE 7.2 **Possible Nurse's Roles in Health Promotion and Disease Prevention Through Stages of Family Development**

Stage	Possible Nursing Role
Couple	Counselor for sexual and role adjustment Teacher of and counselor for family planning Teacher of parenting skills Coordinator for genetic counseling Facilitator in interpersonal relationships
Childbearing family	Monitor of prenatal care and referrer for problems of pregnancy Counselor for prenatal nutrition Counselor for prenatal maternal habits Counselor for genetic services Emotional support for amniocentesis if scheduled Counselor on breastfeeding Coordinator with pediatric services Referrer to social services Assistant in adjustment to prenatal role Supervisor of immunizations Counselor for family nutrition Counselor for managing more limited resources with the additional family member Counselor for parenting regarding food, protection, developmental stimulation, and emotional support Counselor for parenting regarding engaging and interacting with babies (hugging; calming; and comfort with reading, singing and playing) Facilitator of parents' role as responsive caregivers Facilitator of parents' role of developing behavior regulation skills Counselor for helping parents manage frustrations and challenges
Family with preschool or school-age children	Monitor and facilitator of early childhood development; referrer when indicated Teacher of first aid and emergency measures Coordinator with pediatric services Counselor for nutrition and exercise/activity Teacher about dental hygiene Counselor for environmental safety in home Facilitator of parent-child interaction Counselor for the teaching role of parents Counselor for managing a more complex and busy family lifestyle Facilitator of parents' abilities to be present, responsive, and able to guide children from a distance as families grow Facilitator for encouraging consistency, routines, healthy lifestyle activities, independence, relationships with friends, and family rituals Teacher of how to translate children's broader experiences away from home and participate in activities outside the home
Family with adolescents	Facilitator for positive family interpersonal relationships Teacher of risk factors to health Teacher of problem-solving issues regarding alcohol, smoking, diet, and exercise Facilitator of interpersonal skills with adolescents and parents, balancing freedom and responsibility Facilitator of open communication among all family members Direct supporter of, counselor on, or referrer to mental health resources Counselor for puberty, relationships, growing up, avoidance of sexually transmitted infections, avoidance of unintended pregnancy, and informed family planning Referrer for sexually transmitted infections Facilitator for parents' interests beyond nuclear family
Family with young or middle-aged adults	Participant in community organizations involved in disease control Teacher of problem-solving issues regarding lifestyle and habits Participant in community organization involved in environmental control Case finder in home and community Screener for hypertension, Pap test, breast examination, mental health, and dental care Counselor on menopausal transition
Family with older adults	Facilitator of interpersonal relationships among family members Referrer for work and social activities, nutritional programs, homemakers' services, and nursing home Monitor of exercise, nutrition, preventive services, and medications Supervisor of immunization Counselor on safety in home Counselor on bereavement

Wording from Handayani, A., Setiawan, A., & Yulianti, P.D. (2019). Individual adaptation based on family development stage. *Advances in Social Science, Education and Humanities Research, 287*. https://web.archive.org/web/20190426165648/https://download.atlantis-press.com/article/55912207.pdf; The University of Nebraska. (2012). *Families across the lifespan: The normal, to-be-expected, satisfactions and challenges couples and families experience.* http://extensionpublications.unl.edu/assets/pdf/g2124.pdf

BOX 7.2 Characteristics and Indicators of Healthy Families

Nurturing RELATIONSHIPS

- Maintains trust traditions and shares quality time
- Maintains caring communications wherein members listen to one another

Establishing CONSISTENCY

- Maintains intentional activities that promote health patterns of nutrition, hygiene, rest, physical activity, and sexuality
- Intentionally promotes safety and injury prevention, health protection, disease prevention, smoking and alcohol or substance abuse, and/or violence
- Establishes intentional patterns to promote mental health: interacting, communicating, and expressing affection, aggression, sexuality, and similar interactions

Maintaining TRUST

- Nurtures a caring, trusting environment where family members strive to improve and attain their personal goals
- Maintains morale and motivation, rewarding achievement, meeting personal and family crises, setting attainable goals, and developing family traditions, loyalties, and values

ADAPTING to challenges in growth

- Expresses care during crises and respect each member of the group
- Promotes strategies to make decisions about health and illness

Connecting to COMMUNITY

- Ensures that family table time and conversation occur regularly
- Ensures that members have a voice in decision-making and progress toward self-regulation
- Ensures that members act as interactive caregivers across the life span to socialize children and adolescents, participate in the community, and support members as they age

Modified from Search Institute. (2023). *A snapshot of developmental relationships between parents and youth.* https://www.search-institute.org/wp-content/uploads/2017/12/Snapshot-of-Parent-Youth-Relationships-2017-final.pdf

Failure to accomplish a developmental task leads to negative consequences. For example, intimate partner violence or child abuse or neglect may result in intervention by police, welfare, health department, or other agencies. Life cycle tasks build upon one another. Success at one stage is dependent on success at an earlier stage. Early failure may lead to developmental difficulties at later stages.

As families enter each new developmental stage, transition occurs. Families move through new stages as a result of events that range from marriage (heterosexual, homosexual), gay and lesbian relationships, childbirth, single-led families, joint custody, and remarried families, to adolescents maturing into young adults and leaving the home and the aging years.

Each new developmental stage requires adaptation with new responsibilities. Concurrently, developmental stages provide opportunities for families to realize their potential. Nurses anticipate change through analysis of progress through each stage. Each new stage presents opportunities for health promotion and intervention. Family developmental stages, although reflective of traditional nuclear families and extended family networks, apply to nontraditional family configurations (Kiwanuka et al., 2019; Senkowski et al., 2019). A family systems approach addresses the interaction of these multiple family configurations. For example, couples may marry and bring children from a previous marriage to a blended family that works toward achieving developmental tasks of couples along with family stages for the children (Eickmeyer et al., 2019). Both the couple and their children possess values and beliefs from the past that must integrate within the present union. Childless couples present developmental tasks that are different from those proposed for couples with children. One family conceptual model proposed by Gunn and Eberhardt (2019) illustrates multiple connections: interdependence among family systems, shared environments, and parenting styles influence the development of hypertension.

Nurses collect data to determine progress toward family developmental task attainment during the family assessment. Multiple tools that focus on assessment of family assets and social network resources are currently available. Use of assessment tools that include gathering factors that strengthen and protect families, such as the American Family Strength Inventory (https://digitalcommons.unl.edu/cgi/viewcontent.cgi?article51052&context5extensionhist), intends to build on strengths at particular developmental stages to promote healthy family environments. Assessment of family developmental stages entails use of guidelines to analyze progress toward developmental tasks, family growth, and health-promotion needs.

The Family from a Structural-Functional Perspective

Families consist of both structural and functional components. **Family structure** refers to family composition, including roles and relationships, whereas **family function** consists of processes within systems as information and energy exchange occurs between families and their environment. Changing family structures in the United States have been influenced by increased social acceptance of single parenting, premarital cohabitation, same-sex parenting, adoption, and cohabitation of stepfamilies resulting in a lack of consistency regarding how the dynamic complex concept of family structure is viewed (Senkowski et al., 2019).

The Family from a Risk-Factor Perspective

Family risk factors can be inferred from lifestyle; biologic factors; environmental factors; social, psychological, cultural, and spiritual dimensions; and the health care system. As outlined in the Frank Thompson case study in Chapter 1, lifestyle habits such as overeating, drug dependency, high sugar and cholesterol intake, and smoking influence health outcomes. Biologic risk factors may include the elements of genetic inheritance, congenital malformation, and mental retardation. Family structure and function have consistently been linked to adolescent risk behaviors (Senkowski et al., 2019). To fully explore environmental risk factors that influence family function, nurses explore work pressures; peer pressure; stress; anxieties; tensions; and air, noise, or water pollution. Social and psychological dimensions such as crowding, isolation, or rapid and accelerated rates of change are areas to consider when nurses are assessing family risk factors. Cultural and spiritual aspects may include traditions of preventing illness, such as daily prayer and meditation practices. Finally, health care system factors such as overuse, underuse, inappropriate use, or accessibility are considered in the family risk assessment.

To reduce risk factors, nurses help families focus on influencing health behaviors of their members (Box 7.3: Evidence-Based Practice). Society glamorizes many hazardous behaviors through advertising and mass media promotions that minimize negative health consequences. Families influence their members to weigh the consequences of risk-taking behavior. Awareness of risk factors may prompt families to reduce modifiable risk factors. Healthy behavior, including use of preventive health care services, is a significant area of family responsibility.

Traditionally, epidemiology has used levels and trends of mortality and morbidity rates as indirect evidence of health. Data such as infant mortality rates, stillbirth rates, and leading causes of death have long been used as indicators of collective community health. Healthy family functioning links the family life cycle stages with specific risk factors. Epidemiology often describes a disease association in terms of risk. Health risks can be physiologic or psychological. Physiologic risks arise from genetic background, whereas psychological risks include those related to low self-image. Parent-child connectedness is linked with risk for depression, anxiety, and substance use (Fosco et al., 2019). Risks arise from environmental considerations, including the physical environment and socioeconomic condition (Gunn & Eberhardt, 2019). Risk-factor theory considers families a pivotal part of the environment and an important support system used to decrease health risks for individuals. As young family members mature developmentally and seek more independence from the family, peers may influence risk to compete with family values.

Risk estimates calculate differences between two groups: one with the risk factor and one without. The frequency of deaths, illnesses, or injuries with some specific risk factor compared with those for another group without the risk factor, or the population as a whole, determines the risk estimate. Some diseases (e.g., sickle cell anemia in Black-American families of sub-Saharan African descent and Tay-Sachs disease in families of Ashkenazi Jewish descent) occur more frequently in certain families and can be identified by carrier screening (Elander, 2019; Fan et al., 2018). Other recessive genetic disorders (e.g., cystic fibrosis and Gaucher disease) have decreased in incidence with prenatal carrier screening with genetic counseling in couples with suspect family histories (Fan et al., 2018). In a randomized trial, Fan and colleagues (2018) compared two groups: a pretest computer genetics education module group that required no provider counseling (n = 26) and a group that received in-person genetic counseling (n = 28). There were no statistically significant differences between the two groups in postinterventional genetics knowledge, perceived genetic risk, and anxiety, indicating that the computer module could be used; however, postintervention satisfaction scores were generally higher in the in-person genetic counseling group than in the computer module group, indicating that in-person genetic counseling may be preferable for some patients. Using this technology may be appropriate for populations where provider access is lacking. These researchers concluded that their computer module may not be ideal for all populations, but it might be of some use where provider access is limited. Other diseases such as iron-deficiency anemia may not be attributed to a specific genetic background.

BOX 7.3 EVIDENCE-BASED PRACTICE

What are the best strategies for families to use to address the multiple risk behaviors in their children? MacArthur et al. (2018) conducted a systematic review of 424 research articles gleaned from over 34,000 titles using 11 databases and multiple manual searches of reference. Most of the studies included used universal school-based interventions (40%) and were conducted in the United States (79%). Additionally, four common behaviors—(1) alcohol use (55 studies), (2) drug use (53 studies), (3) behavior (53 studies), and (4) tobacco use (42 studies)—were examined.

Researchers reported that for multiple risk behaviors, universal school-based interventions demonstrated moderate-quality evidence in relation to tobacco and alcohol use, indicating that targeting numerous risk behaviors using school-level interventions may be effective in decreasing tobacco and alcohol use. In addition, researchers reported moderate-quality evidence for using universal school-based interventions for multiple risk behaviors to increase participation in physical activity. The findings support using multiple risk behavior universal school-based interventions on three or more risk behaviors. Evidence for family-level interventions was limited due to the number of studies (n = 4) that included family-level interventions. MacArthur et al. (2018) concluded that universal school-based interventions are most effective when targeting multiple risk behaviors.

The review by MacArthur et al. (2018) highlighted a gap in the current research, with a lack of evidence supporting the effectiveness of family-level interventions for the risk behaviors studied. This underscores the need for further research to explore the impact of family-level interventions and to establish a solid evidence base for their use in families.

A partner systematic review and metaanalysis by Tinner et al. (2022) of the MacArthur et al. (2018) study (n = 66) concluded that there is insufficient evidence to support universally targeted interventions preventing multiple risk behaviors within the 8-to 25-year-old age group and that further research is needed to determine effective strategies.

The probabilities of risk could change depending on the family's activities in health promotion and disease prevention. Stages of family development are used to classify risk factors. Age-specific developmental stages, along with their associated age-specific health risks, are given in Table 7.3, which displays periods during which families become most sensitive to certain problems, with corresponding key times for health promotion and disease prevention. The risk behaviors highlighted include tobacco and alcohol use, faulty nutrition, overuse of medications, fast driving, stress, and relentless pressure to achieve. Habits learned in family settings support development of individual lifestyle behaviors. In fact, five habits—nutrition, smoking, exercise, alcohol use, and stress—affect at least 7 of the 10 leading causes of death listed in *Healthy People 2030* (USDHHS, 2023). See Box 7.4 for selected objectives related to families.

GORDON'S FUNCTIONAL HEALTH PATTERNS: ASSESSMENT OF THE FAMILY

Gordon's (2014) 11 functional health patterns help organize basic family assessment information. Patterns form the standardized format for family assessment using a systems approach with emphasis on developmental stages and risk factors. Assessment

TABLE 7.3 Family Stage: Specific Risk Factors and Related Health Problems

Stage	Risk Factors	Health Problems
Beginning childbearing	Lack of knowledge of family planning Adolescent marriage Lack of knowledge concerning sexual and marital roles and adjustments Low-birth-weight infant Lack of prenatal care Unmarried status First pregnancy before age 16 years or after age 35 years History of hypertension and infections during pregnancy Rubella, syphilis, gonorrhea, and acquired immunodeficiency syndrome (AIDS) Genetic factors Lack of safety in home	Premature baby in family Birth defects Birth injuries Accidents Sudden infant death syndrome (SIDS) Sterility Pelvic inflammatory disease Fetal alcohol syndrome Mental retardation Injuries Birth defects Underweight
Family with school-age children	Working parents with inappropriate use of resources for childcare Generational pattern of using social agencies as a way of life Multiple closely spaced children Low family self-esteem Children used as scapegoats for parental frustration Repeated infections, accidents, or hospitalizations Parents immature, dependent, and unable to handle responsibility Unrecognized or unattended health problems Strong beliefs about physical punishment Toxic substances unguarded in the home	Behavior disturbances Speech and vision problems Communicable diseases Dental caries School problems Learning disabilities Injuries Chronic diseases Homicide Violence
Family with adolescents	Health disparities Lifestyle and behavior patterns leading to chronic disease Lack of problem-solving skills Family values of aggressiveness, competition, rigidity, and inflexibility Daredevil risk-taking attitudes Conflicts between parents and children Pressure to live up to family expectations	Violent deaths Unwanted pregnancies Sexually transmitted diseases
Family with middle-aged adults	Hypertension Smoking High cholesterol levels Genetic predisposition Use of oral contraceptives Geographical area or occupation Residence	Cardiovascular disease, principally coronary artery disease and cerebrovascular accident (stroke) Diabetes Accidents Homicide Abnormal fetus Mental illness Periodontal disease and loss of teeth
Family with older adults	Age Drug interactions Metabolic disorders Pituitary malfunctions Cushing syndrome Hypercalcemia Chronic illness Retirement Loss of spouse Past environments and lifestyle Lack of prevention for death	Mental confusion Reduced vision Hearing impairment Hypertension Acute illness Infectious disease Influenza Pneumonia Injuries such as burns and falls Death without dignity

Terms from https://health.gov/healthypeople
Risks of poverty, abuse, neglect, substance abuse, poor nutrition, denial behavior, and socioeconomic status affect all ages. Depression, suicide, cancer, overweight, obesity, sedentary lifestyles, and respiratory distress syndrome affect most age groups. Therefore, these items have been excluded from the table.

BOX 7.4 *HEALTHY PEOPLE 2030*

Selected Examples of National Health-Promotion and Disease-Prevention Objectives for Families

DH-D01	Reduce anxiety and depression in family caregivers of people with disabilities
EMC-02	Increase the proportion of children whose family read to them at least 4 days per week
FP-01	Reduce the proportion of unintended pregnancies
FP-03	Reduce pregnancies in adolescents
FP-08	Increase the proportion of adolescents who get formal sex education before age 18 years
FP-11	Increase the proportion of adolescent females at risk for unintended pregnancy who use effective birth control
FP-D01	Increase the proportion of publicly funded clinics that offer the full range of reversible birth control
HC/HIT-04	Increase the proportion of adults who talk to friends or family about their health
SDOH-04	Reduce the proportion of families that spend more than 30% of income in housing

From US Department of Health and Human Services (USDHHS). (2023). *Healthy People 2030: Browse objectives by topic.* https://health.gov/healthypeople/objectives-and-data/browse-objectives

includes evaluation of dysfunctional patterns within families, with corresponding details in one or more of the other interdependent patterns (see Chapter 6).

The presence of risk factors predicts potential dysfunction. Developmental risk and risk arising from dysfunctional health patterns increase whole family risk (see Table 7.3). Zapolski and colleagues (2019) interpret risk states of the family as potential problems for the individual as well. To formulate nursing plans, nurses identify problems along with their associated and etiologic factors. Influencing factors may precede or occur concurrently with the problem and are used to plan care. Interventions aim to modify influencing factors to promote positive change.

Family history begins with the health perception–health management pattern. Exploring issues within this pattern first provides an overview to help locate where problems exist in other patterns and to determine which problems require more thorough assessment. Interviewing from the family's perspective helps families define situations. The roles-relationships pattern defines family structure and function. The remaining nine patterns address lifestyle indicators.

Health Perception–Health Management Pattern

Characteristics of family health perceptions, health management, and preventive practices emerge with assessment of the health perception–health management pattern. The National Survey of Children's Health (http://www.childhealthdata.org/) and other data sources contribute additional information to help identify health-promoting behaviors of families. Data collected in the Survey of Children's Health include information about the frequency of family meals, attendance at religious services, characteristics of parental relationships with children, parents' coping abilities while raising children, and methods for handling family disagreements. The intent of the survey is to provide a data source to explore research questions related to *Healthy People 2030* and the variables correlated with drug use. However, such data have been associated with eating disorders and risk behaviors other than drug use. These assessment indicators provide data to guide the remaining functional health pattern assessment. Patterns overlap, and findings in one pattern may encourage further assessment in another pattern. The following are some research questions that concern family health promotion:

- What are the chief concerns of parents and other adults in the household about their children's development, learning, and behavior?
- How do children's health status and the health practices of the adults (physical activity and smoking behavior) compare?
- What health-related behaviors, such as eating three meals a day at regular times, eating breakfast every day, exercising for a minimum of 2 or 3 days a week, sleeping for 7 to 8 hours each night, and abstaining from smoking, are practiced by the family?
- How safe are homes, schools, and neighborhoods from the perspective of the family?

Health practices differ from family to family. Families identify and perform health-maintenance activities based on their beliefs about health. Exploration during the assessment includes the following areas:

- What is the family's philosophy of health? Does each family member hold similar beliefs? Do family members practice what they believe?
- In what negative behaviors or lifestyle practices, such as smoking, alcohol, and drug abuse, do the family engage?
- What chronic disease risk behaviors are exhibited within the family?
- Are risk factors present for infections, such as lack of recommended immunizations, lack of knowledge of transmittable diseases, and poor personal hygiene?
- Are risk factors for bodily injury, accidents, or substance abuse present in the home?
- Do older adult members know what medications they are taking and the reasons for their using them?
- Does the family discard outdated medications or those not used?
- What unattended health problems exist?
- Is there a history of repeated infections and hospitalization?
- Does the home lack developmental stimulation, or is it overstimulating?
- Where does the family obtain health and illness care?
- Is the family engaged in a dental program?
- How does the family describe previous experiences with nurses and other health care professionals?

Nutritional-Metabolic Pattern

The nutritional-metabolic pattern depicts characteristics of the family's typical food and fluid consumption and metabolism (Gordon, 2014). Included in it are growth and development patterns, pregnancy-related nutritional patterns, and the family's eating patterns. Risk factors for obesity, diabetes, anorexia, and bulimia are identified.

Dietary habits, learned within the family context, involve behavioral patterns central to daily life. Keeping a diary of intake for a week is a useful strategy for assessing family food and fluid intake patterns. Assessment notes both meals shared with the whole family and additional consumption by individuals. Recent research provides evidence that family meal sharing is associated with healthier eating habits and improved well-being (Utter et al., 2019). For example, Utter and colleagues (2019) provided nine families with meal plans, recipes, and ingredients for five meals weekly for 4 weeks. Frequency of family meals increased, and families reported improvements both to nutrition and to mental well-being. This small pilot study reduced household food insecurity and supported the idea that strategies to increase family meal frequency may affect the family holistically.

Exploration during nutrition pattern assessment includes the following areas:

- What kinds of foods are typically consumed?
- Who eats together at mealtimes?
- How is food viewed (reward/punishment)?
- Is there adequate storage and refrigeration?
- How is food purchased?
- How is food prepared?
- Who prepares food?

Elimination Pattern

The elimination pattern describes characteristics of regularity and control of the family's excretory functions (Gordon, 2014). Bowel and bladder function and environmental factors such as waste disposal in the home, neighborhood, and community that influence family life are considered in this pattern. Questions are phrased according to the age-specific developmental stage of the family. For example, when the nurse is attempting to determine whether there is a problem in the preschool stage, it would be appropriate to ask whether the child is being toilet trained. In families with adolescents, the nurse may ask how often individuals have bowel movements and whether there have been any changes from usual patterns. The nurse may ask older adult members whether they have any problems with constipation. Issues that particularly concern older adults include constipation, diarrhea, polyuria, and incontinence, as well as use of antacids and constipation-relieving agents and strategies. The nurse evaluates whether use of these strategies is appropriate or possibly contributing to poor health.

Activity-Exercise Pattern

The activity-exercise pattern represents family characteristics that require energy expenditure (Gordon, 2014). The nurse reviews daily activities, exercise, and leisure activities. Families create settings for individual members to be physically active, sedentary, or apathetic toward physical activity. The quantity of sedentary activities, such as television and video game screen time, is explored.

Exploration during assessment of this pattern includes the following areas:

- How does the family exhibit its beliefs about regular exercise and physical fitness being necessary for good health?
- What types of daily activities include physical exercise, and who does what with whom?
- What television viewing habits do the children exhibit?
- How are other screen-viewing activities (computers, video games) incorporated into daily routines?
- How often do children exercise?
- How are these activity and exercise factors related to children's health?
- What does the family do to have fun (Fig. 7.1)?

Sleep-Rest Pattern

Rest habits characterize the sleep-rest pattern (Gordon, 2014). Without the restorative function of sleep, individuals exhibit decreased performance, bad temper, and decreased stress tolerance, and they may rely on alcohol or other substances to induce sleep. Regular, sufficient sleep patterns are linked to better mental status, including learning and decision-making. Most families have sleeping patterns, although in some families these patterns may not be readily apparent. It is important to elicit data about sleep and rest from the family's perspective.

Assessment of the sleep-rest pattern includes the following considerations:

- What are the usual sleeping habits of the family?

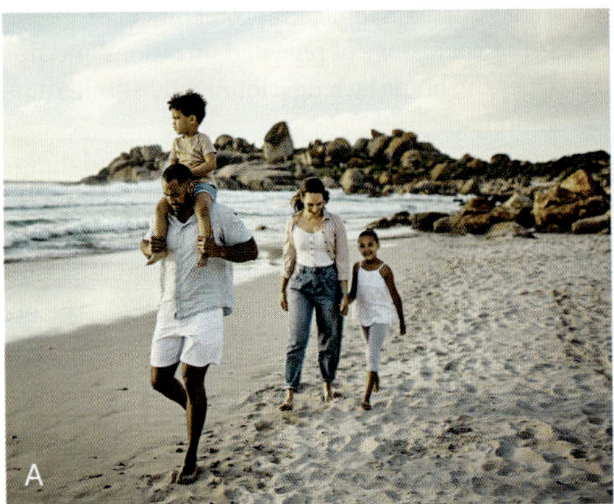
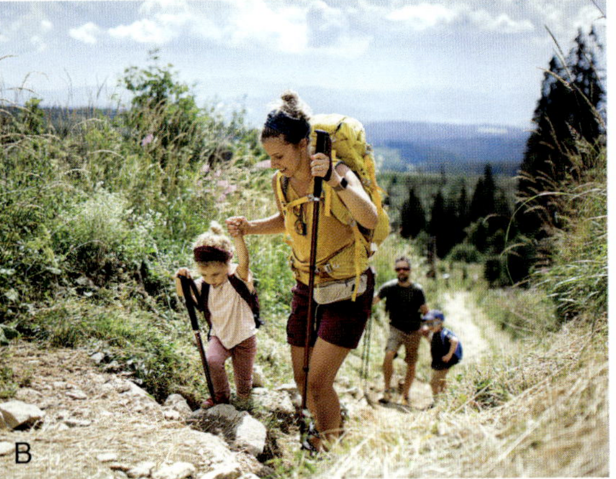

FIG. 7.1 Family outings can be (A) leisurely and restful or (B) adventurous and exciting. (A, From iStock.com/Halfpoint; B, From iStock/com/pixdeluxe.)

- How suitable are they to the age and health status of the family members?
- What are the usual hours established for sleeping?
- Who decides when and how children go to sleep?
- Do family members take naps or have other regular means of resting or relaxing?
- How early does the family rise? What are the patterns related to bedtime and rising?
- Do all family members have the same general sleep-rest pattern?
- Is there a family member with sleep disruption?

Cognitive-Perceptual Pattern

The cognitive-perceptual pattern identifies characteristics of language, cognitive skills, and perception that influence desired or required family activities (Gordon, 2014). Specifically, this pattern concerns how families access information to make decisions, how concrete or abstract the thought processes are, and whether the decisions focus on present or future issues. Decision-making in families is associated with power in family functioning. Highly educated families usually have greater repertoires for problem-solving. Power and ability to solve problems are linked to leadership; family leaders must be acknowledged if nursing interventions are to be implemented.

Cognitive-perceptual pattern assessment includes the following:

- How does the family access and interpret information, especially about health (e.g., newspaper, books, computer, television, or radio)?
- What are the usual family reading patterns and strategies used for ongoing learning (e.g., continuing education programs)?
- What kinds of materials does the family read to the children?
- How does the family usually make decisions about health promotion and disease prevention?
- How do family members contribute to the decision-making process?
- How knowledgeable is the family about risk factors and developmental milestones?
- How are choices made regarding lifestyle?
- How knowledgeable are family members about correct information or recognizing misinformation?
- How do family members acquire information?
- How accurate are the information sources used to make health-promotion choices?
- How do family members describe whether their health behavior is constructive or destructive?
- How do family members recognize signs and symptoms of deteriorating health?
- How do family members decide when medical attention is necessary?
- Who makes the decisions about when to seek health care?
- What factors contribute to delays from the time of onset to the time of treatment?
- How long do families wait before seeking care?
- What are some of the cues that signal to families that care is needed?
- How is professional care accessed?
- What type of health care is generally used health maintenance for immunizations (well-childcare or emergency/urgent care facilities)?
- How are decisions made about the use of over-the-counter medications or the use of alternative or traditional health practices?

Self-Perception–Self-Concept Pattern

The self-perception–self-concept pattern identifies characteristics that describe the family's self-worth and feeling states (Gordon, 2014). Rapport between the family members and the nurse facilitates disclosure. Families have perceptions and concepts about their image, their status in the community, and their competencies as a family unit. Families manifest these perceptions through shared aspirations, values, expectations, fears, successes, and failures. Relationships in families determine the amount of sharing that occurs. Situations affecting one member influence perceptions of the entire family group. How each member describes the family often gives clues to the family self-concept.

Exploration during assessment includes the following considerations:

- How is this family similar to or different from other families?
- How does this family perceive itself to be similar to and different from other families?
- What special assets does each member contribute to the family?
- What changes would each member like to see occur in the family?
- What kinds of feelings do family members have for one another?
- Describe the general tone of feelings in the family. Is the tone indifferent, secretive, angry, or open?
- How does the family think it assimilates into the neighborhood and community?
- How does the family handle stress and crisis situations?
- How does the family experience change in the way they feel about their family?
- How does the family describe the events that led to a change?

Roles-Relationships Pattern

The roles-relationships pattern identifies characteristics of family roles and relationships (Gordon, 2014). Both structural and functional aspects of the family are assessed. Structural aspects of families include each member's name, age, sex, education, occupation, and role in the family. Traditionally, families have been described as nuclear and extended. The traditional nuclear family consists of husband, wife, and children, with an extended family that would include aunts, uncles, cousins, and grandparents. Today there are many varieties of nuclear and extended families. Senkowski and colleagues (2019) describe various contemporary family structures: traditional nuclear family, extended families, single-parent families, stepfamilies, cohabiting families, gay and lesbian families, grandparent-headed families, foster families, and fragmentary families. Traditional nuclear family structure has been influenced by societal changes, such as the women's movement, employment of mothers, divorce, remarriage, immigration, and, in extreme cases, war (Denov & Shevell, 2019). Exploration of family origin and genetic heritage completes family identification data collection. Cultural practices differ from family to family, and the notion of health, illness, sickness, and care may or may not reflect the family's genetic heritage; therefore, it is important to explore the diversity of cultural and ethnic practices during the family assessment (Kumar et al., 2019).

The American Academy of Pediatrics (APA) regards the family as the most enduring link to health for children. The APA policy statement on Effective Discipline to Raise Healthy Children reinforces the importance of the pediatric provider as a source of anticipatory guidance for families concerning their children (Sege et al., 2018). Trends in family structure and function influence how pediatric providers approach family health guidance.

For example, the American Community Survey tables from 2018 to 2022 reflect that out of the 125,736,353 households in the United States, 23,110,031 have children under the age of 18; 2,862,821 of children under age 18 live with both parents; 6,284,441 live with a single mother; and 1,563,417 live with a single father (US Census Bureau [USCB], 2024). Households with stay-at-home mothers far outnumber those households with stay-at-home fathers. Of children under 18 years of age who do not live with a parent, 2,243,607 live with one or both grandparents (USCB, 2024). The burden to these grandparents is complex and includes multiple factors, such as age, disability, and financial constraints. Many of these grandparents remain in the labor force (USCB, 2024). Ohio State University (2020) describes the demographic patterns that illustrate a clear relationship between increased rate of opioid prescribing and a higher number of grandparents caring for their grandchildren in the United States. Furthermore, the percentage of young adults aged 15 years and over who have never married is 37.0% of males and 31.2% of females. As the median age of marriage continues to rise, with fewer young adults choosing marriage, the percentage of married young adults aged 18 to 34 has dropped 30 points compared with first-marriage rates 40 years ago (USCB, 2024).

Although the official poverty rate in 2022 was 11.7%, with 37.9 million people in poverty, neither the rate nor the number in poverty was significantly different from 2021 (USCB, 2024). The reasons are complex, from low unemployment rates to states taking an active role in addressing poverty—even while the federal government withdraws programs and changes the way poverty is calculated, which decreases the official rate without improving economic security. Families living slightly higher than the poverty level, then, may lose other benefits because of criteria changes without appearing in the federal poverty data. This slight increase in their income could result in food insecurity (USCB, 2024).

These low-income families are likely to live in low-income communities, resulting in developmental deficits in their children in social competence, self-regulation, and behavioral control (Justice et al., 2019). In their study, Justice and colleagues (2019) used family caregiver well-being to evaluate how parent-child interactions in toddlers, who live in low-income households, react to language. These researchers reported that that family poverty conditions measured in 322 families' mother–child dyads influenced language skills in these toddlers (Justice et al., 2019). These data indicate the need to assess for family structure and poverty-related factors to determine those families at risk and effectively intervene (Figs. 7.1–7.3). Family structure and function influence family stability and pose a challenge to the nurse in health promotion and disease prevention.

Divorce involves a complex transition that requires the disintegration of one family structure and reorganization to another with remarriage. How couples cope during any situational crisis, such as divorce, influences long-term individual and family adjustment. See the case study at the end of this chapter for the presentation of a family in a situational crisis managing Lewy body dementia (LBD) in a parent. Developmental levels of children, individual temperaments of children, and quality of environmental support in families with children all contribute to family response to crises. For example, in their study using family-based treatment, Hayes and colleagues (2019) reported that when the family (n = 181) adjusted home environment by increasing healthy foods and decreasing use of electronics, weight, dietary behaviors, and screen time improved. Family system factors, such as family meal routines and distress during meals, interact with the biologic risk of obesity.

A **family resilience** framework may be useful to promote strategies for prevention efforts aimed at strengthening families as they face life challenges (Chavez, 2023). Family resilience theories describe how some families, during difficult times, experience changes that reveal useful strengths and abilities for personal interaction and growth. In their qualitative study of the experiences of 11 couples caring for a child with autism spectrum disorder, Sim et al. (2019) reported that these couples' overall attitudes reflected a sense of a solid connection with each other to address the burden to their family. Their strong relationship, shared values, and collaboration provided a source of resilience.

Family disruption has been associated with substance abuse and psychosocial maladjustment in adolescents and young adults. Family supports are associated with adherence, and substance abuse may decrease healthy social support systems. Moreover, both family dissolution and family disruption may be associated with substance abuse, alcohol consumption, and externalizing behaviors such as theft, property destruction, fighting, and assault (Zapolskiet al., 2019). The current literature provides support for the importance of the roles-relationships patterns in the development of health-promoting behaviors (Gordon, 2014; Zapolski et al., 2019).

Family organization influences performance of health-promotion and disease-prevention functions. For example, a single parent without an extended family network may be in need of more community resources to help raise children. A two-parent family living near its extended family may need less support to raise children, but family members may need to know about growth and developmental stages as well as immunization schedules. Individuals may experience a variety of family structures in one lifetime. A person may be part of a nuclear family as an infant, a single-parent family after the parents have divorced, a stepparent family after the mother or father has remarried, and an unmarried couple family when the person is one of two adults who share a household. The person brings the values and beliefs about health promotion and disease prevention that were practiced in previous unions to each new family configuration. Divergent values may result in conflicting expectations unless the new union forms a set of integrated values and beliefs. The current trend away from the nuclear family with the extended family may influence the general direction of the health care system and the strategies used to promote health with other family configurations.

Certain health-promotion issues are of particular concern to the nurse while they assess family health promotion and disease prevention. Violence is a health problem that threatens the integrity of all families. Violent injuries continue to increase at a steady rate in the United States (Lawless et al., 2018). Often pregnancy-associated suicides involve intimate partner conflict attributable to the suicide, and pregnancy-related homicides are a leading cause of death during pregnancy (Burnett et al., 2019). Furthermore, bullying contributes to violence issues that pertain to families and peers. Students who self-identify as lesbian, gay, bisexual, or transgender (LGBT) continue to feel unsafe in their school and home environments (Berry, 2018). Bullying is addressed in the *Healthy People 2030* objective of reducing bullying of sexual minority (gay, lesbian, bisexual, or not sure) high school students. The role of family dysfunction and support is linked to bullying behavior. Furthermore, bullying within families among siblings can occur (Nocentini et al., 2019).

Family violence includes child abuse, spousal abuse, and elder abuse, with females being victimized more often during pregnancy. Death from trauma in pregnancy is often associated with domestic violence (Tibbott et al., 2021). Health promotion and violence prevention require a complex set of skills. Nurses use approaches to reduce violence-related injuries and deaths by acquiring the role of advocate and helping to eliminate victim blaming. Explorations to assess families for health promotion and violence prevention may include the following:

- What formal positions and roles does each of the family members fulfill?
- What roles are considered acceptable and consistent within the family's expectations?
- What kind of flexibility in roles occurs when needed?
- What informal roles exist? Who plays informal roles and with what consistency?
- What purpose do the informal roles serve?
- How are the family's social support networks associated with health and development?
- Who were the role models for the couples or single people as parents?
- Who were the role models for marital partners, and what were their characteristics?
- How does the family manage daily living? How are the household tasks divided?
- How are problems handled? How are problems with children handled?
- Who is employed outside the home?
- Who takes care of the children when both parents are employed outside the home?
- How does the family care for its ill members? How does it care for its older adult members?
- Are behaviors appropriate for family stages of development?
- Is decision-making allocated to the appropriate members?
- Does the family respond appropriately to its members' developmental needs?
- Is there fair distribution of tasks among family members?
- Is the family's emotional climate conducive to growth and development?
- Is there a connection between family and community crime?

In their study of the effect of connectedness to alcohol and smoking behaviors, Cambron and colleagues (2018) reported that adolescents (n = 808) in their study involving fifth- to ninth-grade students (49% female) were more likely to engage in alcohol use and smoking behaviors if they experienced family dysfunction with permissive alcohol/smoking use and if their associations included deviant peers. This study highlights the importance of family relationships in early adolescent alcohol and smoking behaviors. Another study of 283 male participants (10 to 24 years old) residing in an urban area (Culyba et al., 2018) reported that family connectedness protects youth from violence. The findings suggest that family connectedness ameliorates direct involvement in violent behavior. These studies both indicate that nurses working with families should encourage parents to maintain open communication within the family and that parents should enlist additional support from their extended family members, peers, and the community as a larger network of positive influence for their children.

When this initial assessment reveals possible neglect, abuse, or violence, further assessment is warranted, with a branched assessment that may include the following assessment parameters and questions:

- What cues are present to indicate substance abuse?
- Who are the significant adult members of the household? (Determine the presence of a boyfriend/girlfriend.)

Nursing planning stems from a thorough assessment. High-quality evidence-based intervention is based on this systematic approach to assessment. For example, quality intervention for victims of intimate partner violence can be planned in advance to promote the safety and well-being of the victims (Box 7.5: Quality and Safety Scenario).

Genogram

A **genogram**, or family diagram, represents the family on the basis of identification data that depict each member of the family, with connections between the generations. This useful technique gathers data on at least three generations, including the current generation; their parents, grandparents, aunts, and uncles; and their children. The genogram explores clues within family histories contributing to health problems. Fig. 7.2 depicts accepted genogram symbols, with a sample genogram of the fictional Graham family portrayed in Fig. 7.3 (Stanhope & Lancaster, 2024). The Graham family genogram shows a variety of family structures, including changes resulting from marriage, divorce, death, and childbearing. This information highlights family health patterns to use for anticipatory health guidance—for example, in the case of the Graham family, hypertension,

BOX 7.5 QUALITY AND SAFETY SCENARIO

Domestic Violence: Intimate Partner Violence

If the person is still in the relationship:

- Think of a safe place to go if an argument occurs—avoid rooms with no exits (bathroom) or rooms with weapons (kitchen).
- Think about and make a list of safe people to contact.
- Keep a cell phone with you at all times.
- Memorize all important numbers.
- Establish a "code word" or "sign" so that family, friends, teachers, or coworkers know when to call for help.
- Think about what to say to the partner if they become violent.
- Remind the individual that they have the right to live without fear and violence.

If the person has left the relationship:

- Change the phone number.
- Screen calls.
- Save and document all contacts, messages, injuries, or other incidents involving the batterer.
- Change locks, if the batterer has a key.
- Avoid staying alone.
- Plan how to get away if confronted by an abusive partner.
- If a meeting is necessary, have it in a public place.
- Vary the routine.
- Notify school and work contacts.
- Call a shelter.

If the individual is leaving the relationship or thinking of leaving, that person should take important papers and documents to facilitate application for benefits or take legal action. Important papers include Social Security cards and birth certificates for self and children, marriage license, leases or deeds, checkbook, charge cards, bank statements and charge account statements, insurance policies, proof of income (pay stubs or W-2s), and any documentation of past incidents of abuse (e.g., photos, police reports, medical records).

The National Coalition Against Domestic Violence (NCADV) provides information to health care providers, a network of shelters, and counseling programs. NCADV also operates an anonymous national hotline, 1-800-799-SAFE (7233) or 1-800-3224 (TTY), and a website with a chat line (https://www.thehotline.org/help/). The National Domestic Violence Hotline PO Box 90249 Austin, Texas 78709; Administrative Line: 737-225-3150

Adapted from National Coalition Against Domestic Violence (NCADV). (2023). *Voice of victims, home for advocates: National coalition against domestic violence.* http://www.ncadv.org

type 2 diabetes, cancer, and hypercholesterolemia. Family histories provide a unique perspective of family risk of inherited diseases as well as family environmental contribution (Murdaugh et al., 2020). Although My Family Health Portrait (https://phgkb.cdc.gov/FHH/html/index.html) takes a more traditional approach to family history, encouraging families to visit the website helps them explore their own family history. Resources for this continuously evolving topic of genomics can be found at the National Human Genome Research Institute (http://www.genome.gov/HealthProfessionals/), and online genetics education resources can be found at the National Institute of Health's National Genetics Research Institute (http://www.genome.gov/10000464). Box 7.6 explores how family assessment incorporates genomics.

Ecomap

The **ecomap**, which is similar to the genogram, uses pictorial techniques to document family organizational patterns with visual clarity. A genogram is constructed for a family or household. It begins with a circle in the center of the page. Outside the circle, smaller circles are drawn and labeled with the names of significant people, agencies, and institutions in the family's social environment. Lines are drawn from the family household to each circle. Solid lines indicate strong relationships. Dotted lines reflect fragile or tenuous relationships. Slashed lines signify stressful relationships. Arrows can be drawn parallel to the lines to indicate the direction of the energy flow or resources (Stanhope & Lancaster, 2019). Fig. 7.4 shows an ecomap for the fictional Graham family. Both the genogram and the ecomap provide useful information and can be incorporated into family systems assessment (Libbon et al., 2019). The ecomap helps overcome the issues of the genogram encountered when one is assessing nontraditional families. The ecomap uses a functional rather than a structural approach to the assessment of family roles and functions. Health-promotion nursing relevance cannot be underestimated. Nurses who maintain competency position themselves to determine the most accurate risk profiles and family risk assessment.

Sexuality-Reproductive Pattern

Sexuality is the expression of sexual identity. The sexuality-reproductive pattern describes sexuality fulfillment (Gordon, 2014), including behavioral patterns of reproduction. This pattern includes perceptions of satisfaction or disturbances in sexuality, sexual relationships, reproduction (including contraception), and developmental changes throughout the life span, such as menarche and menopause. The sexuality-reproductive pattern addresses transmission of information within the family about sexuality, as well as sexuality for the couple, including their sexual relationship, perception of problems, manner in which problems are handled, and actions taken to solve problems (Gordon, 2014). Information transmission during childhood is an important area to explore to better understand how issues related to sexuality and gender identity are addressed within the family (Gordon, 2014).

Topics to explore during the assessment may include the following areas:

- How do the adults in the family communicate their needs to one another?
- How do family members commit to, love, and care for one another, as well as fulfill their obligations and responsibilities toward one another?
- How do the adults in the family view marriage, parenthood, and their relationship as lovers?
- How does the family address family planning and birth control?
- How do family members participate in the choice of family planning and contraceptives used?

When needed, complete pregnancy histories include sexual practices and partners, the number and ages of children, the number and outcome of pregnancies (live births, miscarriages,

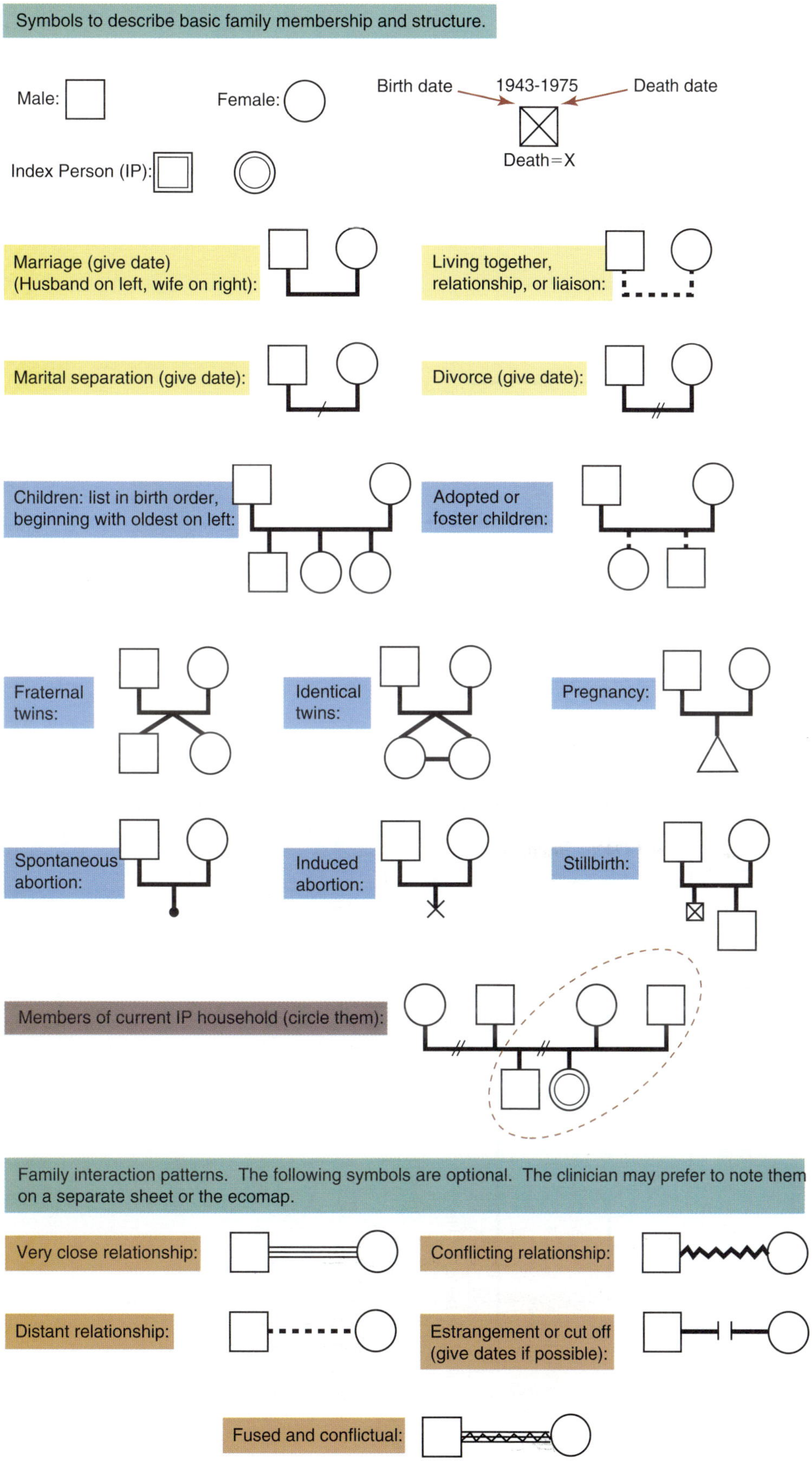

FIG. 7.2 Genogram symbols. (From McGoldrick et al. [2020].)

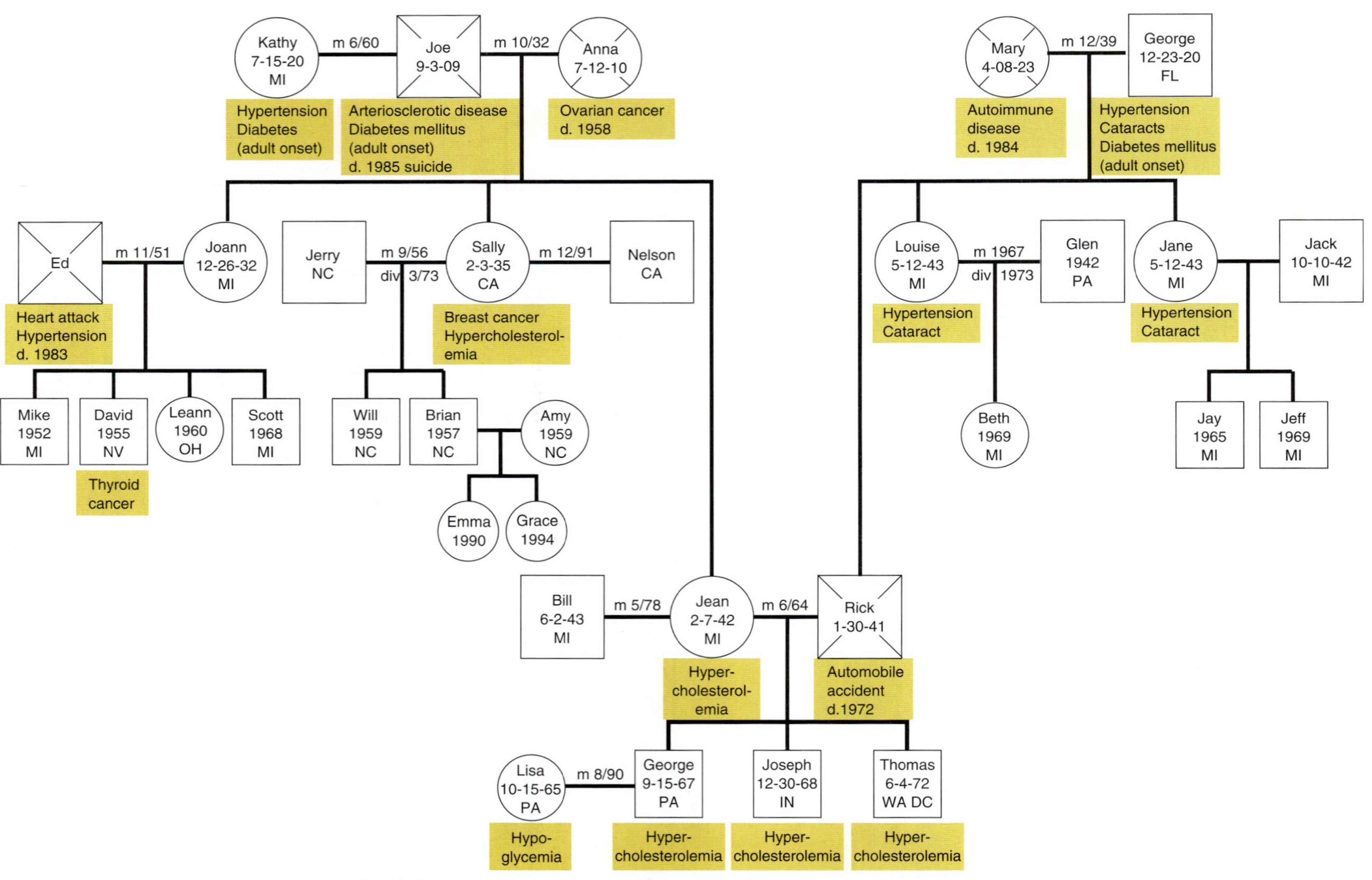

FIG. 7.3 Genogram of the Graham family. (From Stanhope & Lancaster [2024].)

BOX 7.6

Genomics and Family Assessment

Family assessment is the first line of assessment for genetic testing. Family assessment encompasses both genetic and environmental risks shared among family members. Family assessment provides the foundation for the complex process of genetic assessment, which includes nondirective genetic counseling to facilitate the balance of risk versus benefit (Li et al., 2019; National Academy of Medicine [NAM], 2022). Thanksgiving Day, a day in the United States when families customarily gather, has been designated as Family History Day for a family history initiative. Family History Day sets aside Thanksgiving Day each year as a time when family members can discuss their health history (https://nationaltoday.com/national-family-health-history-day/).

Multiple tools facilitate gathering and sharing information to use within electronic health record (EHR) environment. These tools aim to improve effectiveness of the family history while decreasing disease burden and cost. Li et al. (2019) describe four commonly used electronic tools along with their features, limitations, and a URL to access each tool. Their description includes how to incorporate family history into routine intake histories. They state that accurate family history identifies families at risk for genetic disorders, and they report highlights from the following four tools: My Family Health Portrait (https://www.genome.gov/For-Patients-and-Families/Family-Health-History), Family Health Link (https://ceo.osu.edu/technologies/family-healthlink-health-risk-assessment-tool), ItRunsInMyFamily (https://itrunsinmyfamily.com/), and Progeny Clinical (https://www.progenygenetics.com/clinical/).

Evidence supports the conclusion that accurate family assessments contribute to multiple genomic interventions. A number of conditions have been identified as tier 1 disorders. Tier 1 designation indicates that family health history supports implementation of genomic evidence into practice. Tier 1 disorders have evidence-based disease interventions that result in capability to limit the disease or its risk. Currently the following genetic disorders that rely on accurate family assessment are classified as tier 1: hereditary breast and ovarian cancer; Lynch syndrome; and familial hypercholesterolemia (CDC, 2021). Adding family health history to meaningful use standards for EHRs may decrease the gaps between the evidence and how it is implemented in practice. Promoting the importance of family assessment through education and policy may facilitate identification of at-risk families (CDC, 2021).

spontaneous/therapeutic abortions), and the birth control methods used. Nurses observe the comfort levels the adults demonstrate when discussing their own sexuality or note if an adult seems uninformed when discussing sexual subjects with children. Because of the effect that sexual relationships within the family have on children, exploring the variety of sexual practices within heterosexual, homosexual, and bisexual relationships in the family is an important part of health-promotion assessment (Hockenberry et al., 2023). The onset of the use of electronic health records in many settings provides an opportunity to systematically assess and intervene to provide best practices and eliminate disparities in these populations (Ehrenfeld et al., 2019).

Coping–Stress Tolerance Pattern

The coping–stress tolerance pattern helps depict the family's adaptation to both internal and external pressures (Gordon, 2014). On a daily basis, family members generate energy to face evolving needs. Society continually compels families to adapt to new situations. Survival and growth depend on coping mechanisms as families face external demands required to move from one developmental stage to the next. The family's ability to cope with demands of everyday living determines family success. Family relationships support coping or generate more stress. Life events, such as divorce, moving, or developmental stages of the life cycle, and economic hardships, such as loss of a job, provoke stress and mobilize family coping strategies. Exploration of coping and stress tolerance includes the following assessment areas:

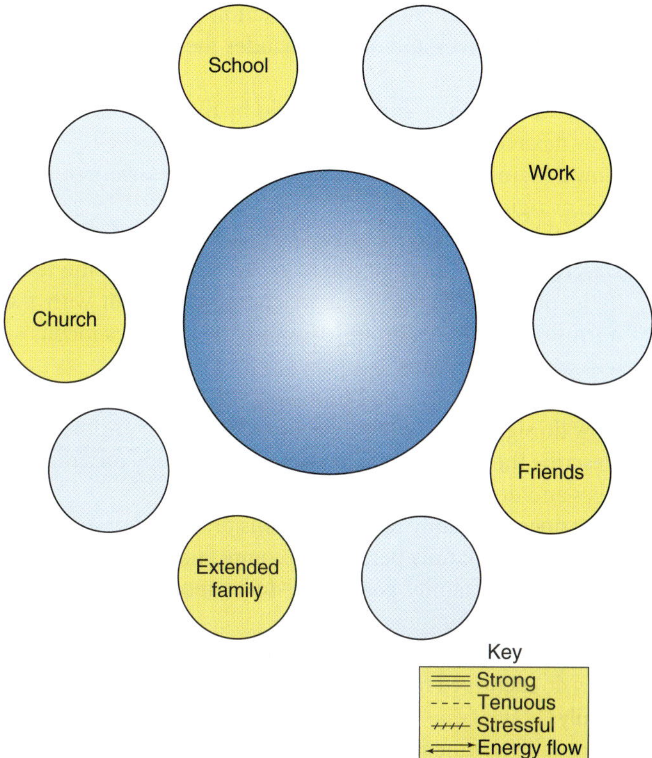

FIG. 7.4 Ecomap of the Graham family. (From Stanhope & Lancaster [2024]; Kaakinen et al. [2018].)

- How does the family cope with stressful life events?
- What experiences have family members had with substance abuse?
- What strengths does the family have and use to counterbalance the stresses?
- What stressful family situations are experienced?
- How does the family view the association between stress and children's health and development?
- How does the family make appraisals of the situations, and are they realistic?
- Describe the family's resources. How do family members use knowledge or links to family networks or community resources?
- What kinds of dysfunctional adaptive strategies, such as substance abuse or violence, are used?

Values-Beliefs Pattern

The values-beliefs pattern characterizes the family's perspective and attitudes about life meanings, values, beliefs, and spirituality and the way these issues affect behavior (Gordon, 2014). Assessment and intervention are based on these attitudes. Assessment of this pattern enhances the interpretation of family behavior. Exploration of values and beliefs includes the following assessment areas:

- What are the values and beliefs held by the family?
- How flexible are rules?
- How do family members interact (calm, aggressive, competitive, or rigid)?
- How do family members view spirituality?
- Describe the cultural or ethnic group with which the family identifies. What family practices are consistent with the norms of that ethnic group? How are the practices inconsistent with these norms?
- What are the family's traditions and practices?
- How do significant cultural beliefs affect health or illness?
- Describe the role that religion plays in the family on a regular basis and during times of stress.
- How does the family rely on religious practices?
- How does the family perceive its competency during crisis?
- What are the family goals, and do members perceive that they are attaining these goals?
- How are value conflicts demonstrated within the family?
- How do identified family values affect the health status of the family?

Spirituality, defined as life purpose and connection with others, affects health. The metaphysical and transcendental phenomenon of spirituality, as well as the religious and nonreligious systems of belief within families, should be assessed (Badanta et al., 2022; Williams-Reade et al., 2019). How well families communicate their unconditional love and forgiveness for injury or betrayal may contribute to physical symptoms within families. Clearly, spirituality and social skills promote health and prevent disease.

Data collected in the 11 functional patterns reveal ideas about family health-promotion and disease-prevention practices. Risks to healthy family functioning may be identified in each pattern. Risk factors may be found in more than one area. For example, passive smoke from one family member's cigarettes may be identified as an environmental risk factor in the home. However, the family's reaction to passive smoking determines the family members' perceived susceptibility, their perceived severity of the problem, and whether they will make a change in the environment to promote family health. The pattern indicates high risk if chronic asthma is described during the family history. In this situation, several other pattern areas support the finding. The nurse determines each risk behavior along with its effects on the others.

ENVIRONMENTAL FACTORS

The environment influences family health and well-being. The home, neighborhood, and community constitute the family environment. Assessment includes exploration of the following home environment areas (Fig. 7.5):

- What type of dwelling is it (condominium, single dwelling, low-income apartment, or temporary shelter)?
- How has the family acquired the home (purchase, rental)?

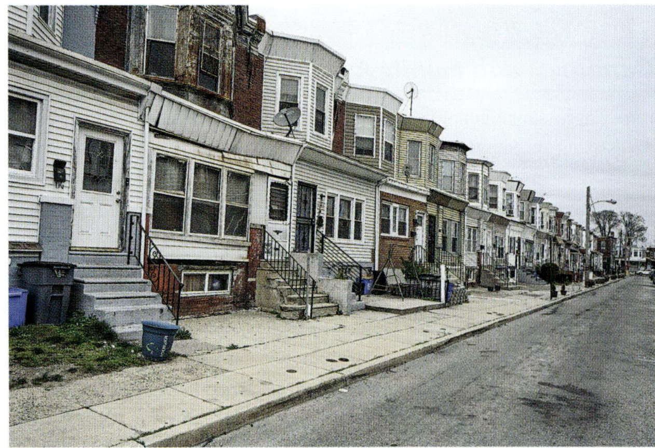

FIG. 7.5 Assessment of the home includes environmental assessment of the areas around the living quarters. (From iStock.com/Olga Kaya.)

- What is the condition of the home (interior/exterior: glass, trash, broken stairs, peeling paint, inadequate insulation, inadequate lighting on stairs, or broken fixtures)?
- Are the number and type of rooms adequate for the size of the family?
- How satisfactory are the furnishings to meet the needs of the family (enough chairs and beds, and a kitchen table)?
- How comfortable is the temperature (warm in winter and cool in summer, insulated)?
- How adequate is lighting for reading, sewing, and other activities?
- How adequate is the water supply (sufficient/clean/fluoridated/polluted)?
- Does the family have access to a telephone, and are emergency numbers available?
- How safe are the kitchen sanitation and refrigeration capabilities?
- How adequate are bathroom sanitation facilities, water supply, toilet, and towels and soap?
- Are the sleeping arrangements adequate for family members considering age, sex, relationships, and spatial needs?
- How adequate is the plan for escape in an emergency (smoke detectors/escape route/plan inside the home)?
- What are the arrangements for and knowledge of first aid (directions posted for poisons, burns, lacerations, and other first-aid needs)?
- What signs of rats, mice, or cockroaches are present inside or outside the home?
- What are the family's impressions about the home?
- How do the family members describe the adequacy of their living space for privacy, their own interests, and status?
- How are substances stored in the home (out of reach of children)?
- How is safety ensured in the home?
- What safety issues are evident?

Although Chapter 8 explores strategies for community assessment, the family environment sits within the community.

While focused on the family environment, areas to explore for neighborhood assessment include the following:

- What is the condition of the dwellings and streets (maintenance/deterioration)?
- How and when is the garbage collected?
- What is the incidence of violent crime, burglaries, and automobile accidents?
- What kinds of industry are nearby, and do they produce air pollution or toxic waste?
- What are the social class and ethnic characteristics of the neighborhood?
- What are the occupations and interests of the families in the neighborhood?
- What is the population density?
- How available and accessible is public transportation?
- Why is public transportation not used if it is available?

And exploration during family assessment includes some of the following resource considerations:

- What resources, such as schools, church, transportation, shopping, and recreational facilities, are available for family use?
- How accessible are the health facilities, such as physician's office, clinic, hospital, gym, swimming pool, natural food store, and weight-reduction clinic?

By driving or walking around the area, the nurse can obtain neighborhood and community data. Other sources of information include the family, health professionals, teachers, nearby business owners, and others who work in the area. Official resources, such as reports from the US Census Bureau (http://www.census.gov/) or statistics from city or state health departments and libraries, are helpful in describing a neighborhood and community.

NURSING PROCESS

Nursing Analysis

Analyzing Cues and Data

After completing the data collection, the nurse and the family analyze the data. Several approaches are used to analyze health data, including systems theory, developmental theory, and risk-estimate theory. A systems approach categorizes families as open or closed, with permeable or rigid boundaries determining both structural and functional components of family systems.

Developmental theory approaches families from the perspective of tasks and progression through cycles. Nurses analyze data to identify accomplishment of family life cycle stages and family tasks needed to function successfully. Family developmental needs are determined considering the wide variety of family structures and functions in society. Although most family models are based on nuclear family structures, additional family structures should be explored as indicated by current population trends (Kiwanuka et al., 2019; Senkowski et al., 2019). The stages of family development guide the baseline data analysis. Gaps, missing data, or conflicting information are identified and clarified.

Couple Family. The first stage of family development begins when adults define themselves as a family regardless of legal status. When individuals move from their family of origin to a new couple relationship, adaptation to role expectations of a partner becomes a developmental task for each individual. Establishing a mutually satisfying adult relationship that converges with the kinship network is one family developmental task. Adjustment for couples includes learning how to weave together two personalities, two life histories, and two aspirations of growth. Decisions in this stage include whether adults are gainfully employed, how money is managed, where they live, how they socialize with friends and other family members, patterns of sexual activities, and whether the couple has decided to have children. Determining how to divide household tasks of cooking, washing, cleaning, and shopping occurs either consciously or subconsciously.

Developmental tasks that integrate health practices and habits into the couple's lifestyle require consideration during analysis. Health behavior constitutes particular actions that promote health and prevent disease. Examples of health-promotion and disease-prevention activities may include maintaining well-balanced rest, exercise, diet, and contraception; attending smoking-cessation classes; wearing seat belts; and directing activities toward self-actualization. Each individual brings values and beliefs to the relationship. Practices from the family of origin and values from personal experiences combine to form the adult beliefs of the individual. Achieving mutually satisfying relationships depends on couples' conflict management. Strategies that stem from congruent value systems facilitate couples' adjustment. When couples use divergent strategies, problem-solving tends to be less effective.

Childbearing Family. Decisions about adding children to the family commit couples to more complex long-term responsibility. Family development and primary health needs change to focus on additional members. To analyze the learning needs of couples with a pregnant member, nurses consider aspects of decisions and motivations involved with the pregnancy. With single-parent families (usually mothers) becoming increasingly common through divorce, death, adoption, or the choice to have a child out of wedlock, analysis of family function addresses these diverse family structures (Hadfield et al., 2018; Senkowski et al., 2019).

Attitudes and practices in society regarding sexuality have influenced the incidence of sexually transmitted diseases, such as genital herpes, gonorrhea, and syphilis. Acquired immunodeficiency syndrome (AIDS), first described in 1981, poses a threat to the family and society, in addition to affected individuals. Human immunodeficiency virus (HIV) is transmitted through heterosexual, homosexual, or oral sexual intercourse, as well as through direct contact with infected blood, shared needles during intravenous drug use, and perinatal transfer from infected mothers to their infants. Prevention of HIV transmission requires abstinence from and modification of relevant behaviors.

Risk factors associated with sexuality include lack of knowledge of safe sexual practices, the reproductive system, and personal hygiene; lack of prenatal care; pregnancy before age 16 years; pregnancy after age 35 years; a history of hypertension or infection during pregnancy; and unplanned or unwanted pregnancy.

Risk factors for premature pregnancies and unsatisfying marriage consist of ignorance about, or values regarding, family planning; adolescent age; and sexuality and role adjustment problems. In unplanned pregnancies, adolescent parents put themselves and their developing child at risk. Lack of knowledge of prenatal care, childbirth, and childrearing practices compounds the risks for both the mother and the child. Parents who are unable to perform parenting roles risk an unsatisfying relationship and inappropriate developmental growth for this beginning stage of the family life cycle. If couples decide to remain childless, learning needs include information about contraception.

The birth or adoption of a child begins a new family unit. Family members adjust to new roles as the unit expands in function and responsibility. As described more fully in the section **Formulating Family Nursing Plans**, parents' history as a dyad and their experiences in other groups, particularly their families of origin, influence the development of the triad (Box 7.7: Health and Social Determinants/Health Equity). Accommodating new members disrupts family equilibrium. As a group, families explore ways to meet each other's needs, to minimize differences, and to work together. First-time parents often feel a lack of emotional support during the first several months of parenthood. Some, but not all, new parents have available family leave policies that may facilitate this transition. Without a family network or friends, the first days after the birth or adoption may be difficult. Parents may care for the child proficiently but may need assistance to grow in the parenting role. If parents are both employed outside the home, they may encounter difficulty with the routines of baby care and being confined to the house more for childcare. Anxiety about the adequacy of income may cause parents to increase their work hours to increase their income. Exhaustion for both parents is common from working full time while providing childcare as the infant develops. Single parents, usually mothers, carry these same burdens alone. Family structure changes from divorce or other disruptions affect children's welfare and have a cumulative effect (Hadfield et al., 2018). Emotional support may be limited, particularly if one has not found satisfaction in parenthood. The families of origin or other support systems, such as self-help groups, neighbors, or friends, assist family members as they struggle to adapt to a new member. Nurses facilitate processes within families of origin, families of choice, or other support systems to promote health in the newly formed family unit.

Some parents thrive during the period when an infant needs almost constant care and nurturing. These parents find support in a network of family and friends. Couples who find satisfaction in parenthood seem to realize that parental influence begins at

BOX 7.7 HEALTH AND SOCIAL DETERMINANTS/HEALTH EQUITY

Diversity-informed practice recognizes that race, ethnicity, class, gender, sexuality, ableism, age, xenophobia, and homophobia are important attributes in families. Strategies health-promotion providers use to care for diverse family populations include preparing safe and inclusive spaces and reflecting their own awareness of diversity, equity, and inclusion that arise in families they serve. Mindfulness techniques have been reported to reduce bias and generate a more open dialogue to provide perceptive and attuned health promotion for families.

The Diversity-Informed Tenets for Work With Infants, Children, and Families (https://diversityinformedtenets.org/the-tenets/english/) address the impact of social forces of race, ethnicity, class, gender, sexuality, ableism, age, xenophobia, and homophobia on the welfare of families. These tenets were developed to connect principles of diversity, equity, and inclusion into the infant and early childhood mental health field.

The tenets begin with the claim that an essential component of diversity-informed practice is the capacity for providers to reflect on their own experiences with families and make adjustments in their approaches based on this self-reflection. The diversity-informed provider remains open to family members' insights. To remain a valuable resource, professionals assess and appreciate layers of meaning within each family's context. Cultivating self-awareness is a crucial strategy for professionals who collaborate with families in diverse communities. Specific family cultural practices may indicate socio-cultural connections to religious, ethnic, tribal, socioeconomic, or national cultural identifications.

The 10 tenets listed below focus on the concepts of self-awareness for professionals; services for infants, children, and families; allocation of resources; and advocacy toward diversity, inclusion, and equity in institutions.

1. Families receive better diversity-informed, culturally attuned services when providers practice self-awareness. Providers aim to improve their care of families by reflecting on their own culture, values and beliefs, and the impact of racism, classism, sexism, ableism, homophobia, xenophobia, and other systems of oppression on their life and the lives of the families they serve.
2. Families deserve welcoming, protecting, and nurturing services wherever they live in the world.
3. Discriminatory practices harm families. Professionals acknowledge privilege where they hold it, and they use it strategically to combat racism, classism, sexism, ableism, homophobia, xenophobia, and other systems of oppression against families.
4. Family knowledge and sources of strength and healing are respected even when different from mainstream Western health care.
5. Diverse family structures are respected, and contributions of all family members are recognized, including second mothers, fathers, kin and felt family, adoptive parents, foster parents, and early care and educational providers.
6. The power of language is acknowledged. Family communication may sever or bond relationships. Inclusive interaction, both verbal and nonverbal, supports families.
7. Use of native or preferred language promotes family health.
8. Diversity-informed providers act to allocate resources that improve access and ameliorate disparity and inequity.
9. Family services provide diversity of care settings with equitable access for historically and currently marginalized individuals and groups.
10. Just and equitable policy and legislation agendas for families include input from diversity-informed providers.

From Clark, R., Gehl, M., Heffron, M. C., Kerr, M., Soliman, S., Shahmoon-Shanok, R., & Thomas, K. (2019). Mindful practices to enhance diversity-informed reflective supervision and leadership. *Zero to Three, 39*(11), 18–27; Thomas, K., Noroña, C. R., & St John, M. S. (2019). Cross-sector allies together in the struggle for social justice: Diversity-informed tenets for work with infants, children, and families. *Zero to Three, 39*(3), 44–54. https://www.irvingharrisfdn.org/wp-content/uploads/2019/01/Thomas-Norona-St.-John-January-2019-Tenents-2nd-Edition.pdf birth and is the single most important factor in the child's physical, emotional, and cognitive development. The parents' ability to assume responsibility depends on a complex array of factors: their own maturity; how they were nurtured as children; their conceptions about self, culture, social class, and religion; their relationship with each other; their values and philosophy of life; their perceptions of and experiences with children and other adults; and the life stresses they have experienced.

In analyzing the needs of childrearing families, nurses consider many factors, including providing for physical health, economic support, and nurturing actions that are vital to learning and social development of children. In analyzing couples' needs during this stage, nurses recognize the importance of interactions among the triad. Observing decision-making helps nurses determine family functioning, member roles, and effectiveness of family members. Risks associated with role relationships include working parents with insufficient resources for childcare, abuse or neglect of children, multiple closely spaced children, low family self-esteem, children used as scapegoats for parental frustration, immature parents who are dependent and unable to handle responsibility, and strong beliefs about physical punishment or obedience.

Family With Toddlers/Preschool Children. Families may have more than one child, each growing and developing at an individual pace. Preschool children place great demands on families. Families adjust to each new member with space and equipment for expansion. The needs and interests of preschool children influence home environments. Nurses assess the quality of the home environment for whether children have healthy amounts of stimulation-promoting opportunities. Safety balanced with exploration by the child results in health-promoting home environments. Rather than removing children from the kitchen or garden, finding ways to include them in a cooking or planting activity provides learning experiences. Other environmental influences affecting the child's rate and style of development include religious practices, ethnic background, education, and discipline techniques.

Evidence increasingly demonstrates the link between environment and health. Home environments that contain contaminated air, water, or food increase health risks. For example, lead poisoning, a preventable disease that continues to affect thousands of children, often results from lead paint and other factors in the home, such as water. Although restrictions exist in the United States to limit lead-based paint to exteriors, many homes have interiors coated with lead paint. Generally, lead in water is attributed to poor infrastructure in the home plumbing or the city. As a result, poorer neighborhoods are at higher risk of lead poisoning from their water sources (Wheeler et al., 2019). For example, families in Flint, Michigan, experienced increased lead in the water coming into their homes when the local government changed their water source. In 2016, 3 years after a water crisis in Flint began, Day and colleagues (2019) surveyed Flint's citizens (n = 208) to explore information sources during the crisis. These researchers reported that minority and vulnerable populations were affected more by the water crisis than other populations. The US Environmental Protection Agency (2023) contends that 9.2 million lead service lines remain nationally, mostly in low-income neighborhoods. Under President Biden, the Bipartisan Infrastructure Law invested $15 billion to deliver the necessary resources for lead pipe removal. The incidence of elevated blood lead levels is generally highest in neighborhoods with poor families (Wheeler et al., 2019). Both homes and automobiles are considered possible sources of exposure to the poisonous agent carbon monoxide. Nurses review data for home safety, including storage of dangerous materials, such as detergents, insecticides, and medications.

Health-promotion needs for young children include proper foods, adequate exercise and sleep, and dental hygiene. Parents teach children through modeling and use of positive reinforcement. Family developmental tasks include adjusting to fatigue resulting from parenting demands. Nurses explore alternatives to relieve parents. Parents need time for themselves, individually and as a couple (e.g., to exercise, to socialize), while knowing their children are safe with a responsible person. Economic restraints may limit relaxation time away from the children. Sharing childcare with friends and the family provides one source of support for new parents.

Family With School-Age Children. A family with children in school may have reached its maximal size in numbers and interrelationships. The parents' major problem during this stage is the dichotomy between pursuing self-interests and finding fulfillment in producing the next generation. Family developmental tasks revolve around goals of reorganization to prepare for the expanding world of school-age children. School achievement becomes a critical task for socialization. Viewing social and educational goals from the perspective of family culture and parents' defined goals becomes particularly important during this developmental stage. For example, many opportunities for health education exist in schools, including influencing healthy beliefs and behaviors. However, school health programs focus on problems such as tobacco and substance abuse, with messages aimed at problems and crises rather than healthy behaviors. Families influence health at home and in school both by teaching children ways to assess and manage risky situations and by describing the benefits to expect when healthy behaviors are practiced.

As children's activities broaden away from the home, another important developmental task for both the parent and the child becomes "letting go." Parents become involved in community groups such as the parent-teacher association, scout groups, sports teams, and other volunteer organizations. Encouraging children to join in family discussions to learn about their heritage can foster understanding of self within the family network (Fig. 7.6). Children exposed to unsafe home environments are at risk of behavior disturbances, school problems, and learning disabilities. Parents who cannot manage their children in growth-promoting ways soon experience energy depletion and may turn to dysfunctional relief from parenting (e.g., drug and alcohol abuse).

Family With Adolescents. Parents with adolescent children may experience a late pregnancy, resulting in care for an infant while other children in the family are in school. A new family member at this stage may be a source of joy or frustration

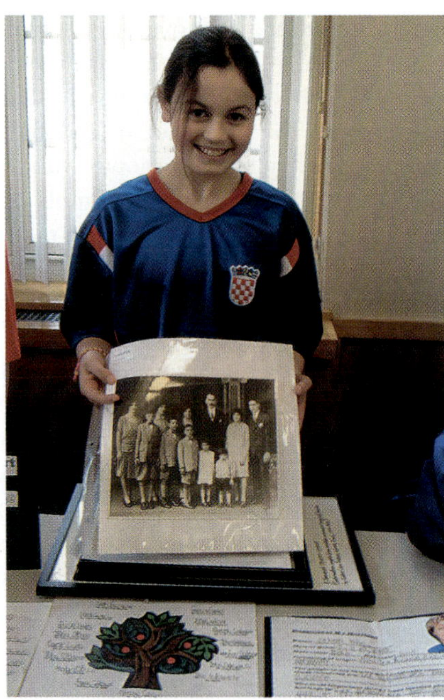

FIG. 7.6 School-age female learns about her family heritage and presents this information through a school project.

for the family. The overall goal with adolescent members is to loosen family ties to allow greater responsibility and freedom in preparation for releasing young adults. Although each member of the family strives to achieve individual developmental tasks in the midst of social pressures, the family as a whole has tasks to accomplish. Strengthening the marital relationship to build a foundation for future family stages is a critical task during this time.

Open communication is often difficult during this stage, partly because of the differing developmental tasks of adolescents and adults. Adolescents seek their own identity, and adults attempt to facilitate adolescent decision-making processes. Choices about values and lifestyles may differ. Adolescents may challenge family values and standards. Although parents maintain some authority, adolescents tackle their own desires and needs. Adolescents want to do what their friends do, have their own cars, and make their own money to spend in ways that they see fit. Parents who give adolescent members opportunities to experience social, emotional, and ethical situations with others are providing learning opportunities to enhance their sense of autonomy and responsibility. As adolescents become mature and emancipated, families face balancing freedom with responsibility. Health problems in this age group include violent deaths, including suicide, injuries, and alcohol and drug abuse. Contributing risk factors involve lack of problem-solving skills, family values of aggressiveness and competition, socioeconomic factors, peer relationships, rigid and inflexible family values, daredevil risk-taking attitudes, and conflicts between parents and children. Environmental risk–related violent deaths and injuries are influenced by the highway system, automobile manufacturers, and the legislation of standards of safety. Families rely on public health officials and nurses' efforts as advocates to reduce environmental risks.

Families support adolescents in this stage of development by including them in decision-making and ensuring that they experience the positive and negative consequences of their choices. Family values of winning at all costs, aggressiveness, and competition may need to be explored during this period. Adolescents may discard these values if they are no longer applicable. Considerable change in adolescent values produces conflict and poses a threat to family cohesiveness. Families may place pressure on adolescents to conform to family values. In matters of life and death—for example, regarding driving rules—parents must stay firm.

Families with adolescents experience identity crises for the adolescent, the adults, and the family as a whole. Adolescents move from childhood to adulthood while adults progress beyond parenthood. Adolescents struggle to find independent identities that remain connected to their family. Adults, in midlife, must resolve their own adolescent fantasies to move toward an identity for their remaining life.

Family With Young Adults. Families with young adults act as a launching center when children begin to leave home. As children leave home, parents relinquish their parenting roles of many years to return to the marital dyad. The couple builds a new life together while maintaining relationships with aging parents, children, grandchildren, and in-laws. Couples focus on redefining relationships during this stage. As children develop, they no longer need a primary caregiver, often their mother, in the same way as during childhood. When mothers/caregivers devote years to raising children, their role and purpose within the family changes as children develop. Transition from a life with children as the priority to new or renewed interests (e.g., career, community service) may require assistance and support from the entire family. Careers at this stage may become more stable. Developmental tasks at this stage for the family's adults require focus on future prospects. In addition to individual changes occurring at this stage, families with young adults may experience other pressures. Aging parents and adult children may require financial or emotional support. Financial and emotional responsibilities to other family members may hinder the couple's ability to focus on relationships during this developmental phase. Health-promoting activities to focus on during this stage include coping with pressures of social roles and occupational responsibilities, maintaining health tasks to promote healthy aging, and reassessing life goals.

Family With Middle-Aged Adults. Families consisting of only two members are able to enhance self-concept and support their relationship during middle age. Usually children have left home, and adults experience a sense of freedom and well-being. Some relationships, by this stage, have reached a level of security, stability, and ability to meet each other's needs. Parenting pressures diminish, allowing parents to enjoy the accomplishments of their children and grandchildren. Couples have acquired a network of friends. Long-time acquaintances seek participation from the couple in neighborhood rituals and events. Economic security and personal self-esteem may be at a peak.

In contrast, some relationships falter at this time. Departed children create a quiet house with less activity, known as the "empty nest." When individuals are unprepared for this stage, they might seek opportunities to enhance self-concept from outside of the family. With parenting roles now complete, adults may develop feelings of inadequacy or begin new relationships, start new families, or resort to substance abuse. In addition, this life phase may include becoming grandparents, parenting grandchildren, coping with the needs of middle-aged children, and caring for older adults (children, siblings, or parents).

Health tasks in this developmental stage require new awareness of susceptibility or vulnerability to health problems. Couples adjust their lifestyle and habits to cope with health risks. Losses promote health problems, and at this stage couples begin to cope with deaths among family and friends, along with declining income. If either member has developed physical or mental illness, the other adjusts to the resultant physical and mental impairments, redefining self-concept.

Middle-aged families face a host of risk factors leading to three prevalent causes of death: heart disease, cancer, and cerebrovascular accident (stroke). Family lifestyle may decrease risks by placing a high value on being physically active, refraining from smoking, maintaining adequate and sound nutritional habits, and consuming moderate amounts of alcohol. Lifestyle habits that are transmitted through role modeling have a greater influence on the younger members of the family than any verbal edict. Middle-aged members positively influence their health if they are able to choose environments low in water and air pollution and free from crippling stress factors such as excessive noise, traffic, and overcrowding. Family members can apply pressure on key members of the community to decrease risks in the environment.

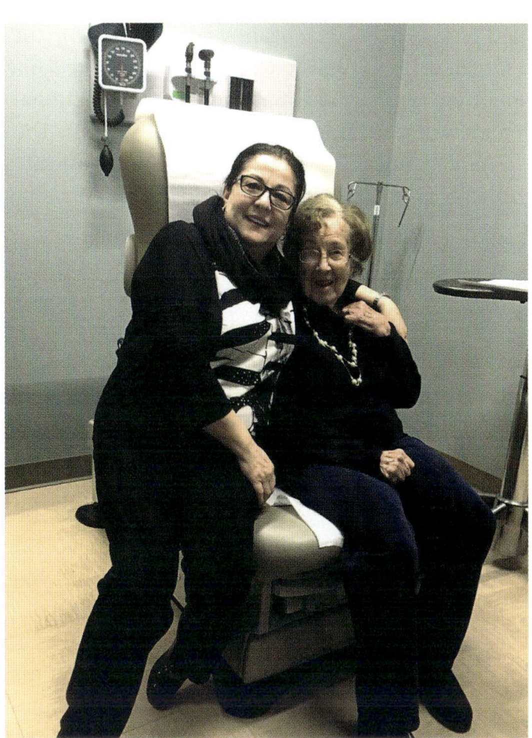

FIG. 7.7 As with all people, older adults hope for well-being that allows highest-capacity functioning. Medicare now covers yearly wellness visits. More details at https://www.medicare.gov/coverage/yearly-wellness-visits

Family With Older Adults. Retirement affects many aspects of life for couples, along with each individual in the family and their relationships with others. Besides decreased work hours, retirement means reduction in income and fixed incomes for most people. These limited funds may make purchasing choices (e.g., food, utilities, insurance, medications, transportation) difficult (Lloyd, 2019). Adjusting living standards to retirement income and being able to supplement this income with wage-earning activity is one task of the family with older adults. Other tasks during this stage include ensuring a safe and comfortable home environment, preparing for end of life, and adjusting to the loss of a spouse and finding meaning in the grief process.

Families provide intergenerational connectedness for elders that may enhance interpersonal relationships and support developmental tasks (Giraudeau & Bailly, 2019). In their systematic review of 11 articles about intergenerational programs, Giraudeau and Bailly (2019) noted that some studies reported improved health and quality of life for older adults.

Health promotion aims to maintain functional ability, limit the effects of disabling conditions, and maintain quality of life. Older adults may fear becoming helpless, feeling useless, and being incapable of caring for themselves. When analyzing risk factors in the aging family, nurses look for the couple's ability to function well enough to carry out normal roles and responsibilities. As with all people, older adults hope for a state of well-being that will allow them to function at their highest capacity physically, psychologically, socially, and spiritually (Fig. 7.7). Many older adults remain in their own homes, and most of these individuals are vigorous and completely independent. Assuming that most older adults prefer to remain in their own homes, assessment of the family for this age group should consider predictors of independence or those factors that indicate a need for institutionalized care such as assisted living, adult day care, or nursing homes. In her interviews (~300 hours) with 20 older females in southern Louisiana, Hedman (2019) found that disruption of health care services, decreased social support, cognitive impairment, declining health, limited income or poverty, and threat of eviction contributed to stressors in these females. During these disruptions, families relied on spirituality, psychological strengths, relationships, family support, friendships, access to senior activities/grocery store/café contacts, and home services. Increased incidence of falls, limited access to assistance, diminished cognitive function, and both high and low body mass index significantly increase the likelihood of institutionalization. These findings highlight the importance of assessing fall risk, social support networks, cognitive function, and body weight in families with older adults. Many researchers use deficits in physical and psychological functioning to predict long-term care entry, as mentioned previously. Factors such as falls, number of health conditions, self-rated health, social interaction, difficulty with activities of daily living, psychiatric problems, cognitive decline, and living alone are considered typical predictors of entry to long-term care. Davodi and colleagues (2023) conducted a randomized control trial to determine the effectiveness of a health-promotion intervention program in reducing complications associated with aging and promoting active, healthy aging (n = 60). The World Health Organization (WHO) defines *active healthy aging* as the "process of developing and maintaining the functional ability that enables well-being in older age" (WHO, 2020). The results of this study confirm that interventions supporting health-enhancement approaches can effectively promote active aging in older adults (Davodi et al., 2023).

Ego integrity (the union of all previous phases of the life cycle) is the challenge in this stage and demands successful aging through continued activity. Having gone through the various stages of family development, the couple accepts what they have done as their own. At this time, they may need family or professional support to pursue other interests or maintain former activities to feel needed and useful.

Families join nurses to analyze information together, comparing the family's data with documented norms of health promotion and disease prevention in older adults. Norms or expected values can be derived from the family's baseline information of 11 functional pattern areas, knowledge of growth and development for all age groups and the family as a whole, risk-factor estimates, and population norms. Population norms specify normal ranges for these groups. For example, age is associated with various risk factors; some disorders are so common that they are referred to as diseases of the older person. In certain diseases, such as lung cancer, there is a long period of exposure. Risk increases with cumulative exposure; therefore, the incidence and prevalence of diseases increase with age.

Sexuality Because of the popular perception that older adults are asexual, their sexual concerns may be disregarded (Gewirtz-Meydan et al., 2019). General population norms for values, beliefs, self-perception, or role relationships may be less available than physical population norms. Cultural, ethnic, and religious factors contribute to values and beliefs about health. Family baseline information provides important comparative criteria for analysis. Family records provide useful information when available. The first contact assessment provides baseline information for subsequent comparison and evaluation of progress. Whether the family perceives situations to be problematic should be considered in the analysis phase. Nurse and family perceptions about problems may differ.

Formulating Family Nursing Plans. Writing a **family nursing plan** helps families promote health throughout the life cycle and prevents disease by decreasing risk-taking behaviors. Nurses derive plans from assessed validated data. A concise summary statement of a problem or potential problem provides direction for outcomes and interventions by identifying negative health states and factors to change to alleviate or prevent the problem (see Chapter 6). Describing health and validating potential or actual health problems with families facilitates cooperation. Assessment and negotiation continue until agreement occurs and a plan for resolution develops.

Cultural competence, attunement, and respect for familial beliefs forms a foundation for the nursing process of assessing, planning, intervening, and evaluating (see Chapter 2). With changing trends in families and shifts in heritage within society, cultural competence and cultural attunement become priorities for family assessment and nurses (Nickbakht et al., 2019).

Knudson-Martin and colleagues (2019) define *sociocultural attunement* (SCA) as "an awareness and responsiveness to the intersections of societal context, culture, and power in client experience and positioned to promote equity" (p. 47). Societal context includes but is not limited to ethnicity, gender, race, religion, poverty, and sexual orientation.

Cultural values, such as those connected to nutrition, influence most health-promotion practices. As globalization occurs, diversity will expand, and competent care for indigenous populations and migrating populations will be needed (Edge & Lemetyinen, 2019). Although it seems that cultural competence should improve health-promotion strategies for all families, particularly families from within vulnerable populations, evidence-based support is reported as low to moderate (Edge & Lemetyinen, 2019). To develop providers' cultural competency for global mental health, Edge and Lemetyinen (2019) recommend preparation to enhance provider/client collaboration using face-to-face supervised contact and/or computerized simulation with expert patient-centered providers' guidance. Rigorous training would include experiential learning activities that promote knowledgeable use of interpretation and translation services, methods to modify communication approaches, and exploration of culturally specific explanatory models of health disorders. Culturally competent providers realize that prescriptive tailored interventions must evolve for each family and that no one strategy works for every family. Culturally attuned family care includes strength-based approaches that guide communities toward improving the health promotion of their own families (Edge & Lemetyinen, 2019).

Planning With the Family

Intervention planning stems from complete assessment and analysis. The plan's purpose aims for behavioral change in families to promote health or prevent dysfunction. As in the assessment phase, family members play an active role in the planning process. Family responsibility for personal health status enhances the success of behavioral change outcomes. The planning process involves several steps, with the nurse and family identifying the following:

- Order of priority for problems or potential problems
- Items that can be handled by the nurse and the family and items that must be referred to others
- Actions and expected outcomes

The nursing plan provides direction for implementation and a framework for evaluation (see the case study at the end of this chapter).

As mentioned, a family's health status can be delineated as functional, potentially dysfunctional, or dysfunctional. Functional family health status warrants verification by the nurse with a plan for periodic reevaluation that is formulated jointly. Plans to continue healthy living behaviors are reinforced. The nurse provides specific information requested by the family, such as immunization schedules, growth and development milestones, and recommended dietary allowances. In working with healthy families, the nurse controls the assessment and analysis phases of the nursing process. If health status is judged to be functional, then planning health-education materials, scheduling periodic examinations, and providing accessibility to the nurse remain professional responsibilities. Implementation and evaluation of health-promotion activities become family responsibilities.

In health-promotion and disease-prevention settings, life-threatening situations rarely occur; however, when such situations do occur, they become the highest priority for intervention. For other identified potential or actual problems, the nurse relies on the family to decide which problem or potential problem to approach. After the ordering of priorities has been established, the family and nurse determine who will work on the problem. Problems or potential problems to be resolved by the nurse are identified separately from those requiring referral or family intervention. Problems for the family to handle or those the family is already addressing are considered strengths and are acknowledged and supported by the nurse. For example, when there is consistency among values and actions, physical fitness, weight management, and ability to cope with stress, the family is already taking informed and responsible action in these areas. The extent to which family members can provide their own health promotion and disease prevention will depend on their knowledge, skills, motivation, and orientation toward health.

Problems that need medical, legal, or social attention are referred to appropriate agencies. The nurse should have a directory of resources in the community for when referrals are needed. Nursing intervention requires clearly stated actions that are purposeful, moral, capable of being accomplished, and adapted to the particular life situation, beliefs, and expectations of the family.

Generate Solutions

Goals are statements describing desired outcomes. Family outcome statements include expected family behaviors, circumstances for exhibited behaviors, and criteria for determining performance. Health-promotion goals reflect a desire to function at a higher level of health and to grow beyond maintaining health or preventing disease.

Action and Implementation With the Family

The implementation phase is dynamic. As the nurse and family work together, adaptation and revision of plans occur as new information unfolds. **Family nursing interventions** aim to assist families in performing functions that members cannot perform for themselves. In health promotion and disease prevention, nurses assist families in improving their capacity to act on their own behalf. Such family involvement would include the following (Park et al., 2018):

- Family education
- Family participation in care activities
- Sharing clinical status, progress, and prognosis
- Shared family decision-making
- Family support programs

Park's study group reported their findings from a systematic review of 17 family-centered care intervention studies. These researchers reported that strategies used with family members affected stress, anxiety, and depression positively. Improved levels of satisfaction and interaction with providers were described.

The Patient Protection and Affordable Care Act (2010) was a landmark law that addressed and reformed some of these health care issues as more robust insurance became available to individuals and families. Although the Patient Protection and Affordable Care Act (PL 111-148) became law on March 23, 2010, and was amended by the Health Care and Education Reconciliation Act of 2010 (PL 111–152), the statute was brought before the US Supreme Court beginning March 26, 2012, as unconstitutional, citing four major arguments (requiring the individual mandate, applying the Anti-Injunction Act, lacking a severability clause, and expanding Medicaid). The Supreme Court ruled in favor of the statute in June 2012. The Patient Protection and Affordable Care Act profoundly altered the US health care system (Crowley & Bornstein, 2019). Based on their evaluation of the effect of the act, the American College of Physicians (ACP) identified at least three resulting improvements in health care family coverage: better coverage for preexisting conditions, more accessible health insurance and preventive services, and Medicaid expansion. In their position paper, the ACP prescribed strategies to improve eligibility for subsidies, to stabilize the marketplaces, to acquire sustained funding, to increase enrollment, to extend the Medicaid expansion to all states, and to create a public insurance option to rival the existing options (Crowley & Bornstein, 2019).

Health promotion and disease prevention may not be part of a family's life experiences, giving nurses the task of addressing attitudes and values to expand options for family health promotion. Four types of nursing interventions are frequent in health-promotion and disease-prevention planning: increasing knowledge and skills, enhancing strengths, limiting exposure, and decreasing susceptibility. Increasing knowledge and skills to improve family capacity for health-promotion and disease-prevention behavior may be the primary strategy. Use of this strategy helps families make informed choices about healthful lifestyle behaviors and eliminate harmful environmental influences that affect health. Improved knowledge aims to create awareness as the nurse and family work together to uncover actual or potential problems. Nurses recognize particular families that are at risk and move toward motivating and supporting behavioral change in these families. Box 7.8 presents an example of one program that provides education and support to people with cancer and their families.

Family strengths or forces that contribute to family unity and solidarity foster the development of inherent family potential (Hanson et al., 2019). These factors include the following:

- Physical, emotional, and spiritual factors
- Healthy childrearing practices and discipline
- Meaningful and clear communication
- Support, security, and encouragement
- Growth-producing relationships and experiences
- Responsible community relationships
- Growth with and through children
- Self-help and acceptance of help
- Flexibility in family functions and roles
- Mutual respect for individuality
- Crisis as a means for growth
- Family unity and loyalty and intrafamily cooperation
- Adaptability of family strengths

 BOX 7.8 **BEST PRACTICE**

Cancer Support Community and Gilda's Club

The Cancer Support Community and Gilda's Club support individuals affected by cancer in 190 locations worldwide, offering free personalized cancer support and navigation services for patients and families. Comedian Gilda Radner attended the Wellness Community during her battle with ovarian cancer and shared her experiences in her book *It's Always Something*. After her death, Joel Siegel and Mandy Patinkin began Gilda's Club, opening the first clubhouse in New York in 1991 with the support of her spouse, Gene Wilder. Emphasis is placed on the family to acknowledge that no person with cancer makes the journey alone. Weekly support groups help family members support one another, explore new ways of coping with the stresses of cancer, and learn ways to become the most effective partners possible with their health care teams. These two organizations have partnered to continue their vision with the Cancer Support Community to "ensure that all people affected by cancer are empowered by knowledge and strengthened by action and sustained by community" (Cancer Support Community, 2024).

These communities now offer a wide variety of award-winning digital and educational resources (Gentle Strength and Stretch, Meditation and Guided Imagery, Nutrition Matters, Nutrition and the Immune System, Nutrition at Midlife: Preventing Heart Disease and Osteoporosis, tai chi, yoga, mindfulness, and feng shui). Social events are organized (comfort food, potluck dinner, couples networking groups, single networking groups, and family and friends networking groups). Cutting-edge research continues at all levels of government policy development. Although chapters generally do not charge for their services, donations are appreciated and are necessary to help serve thousands of people with cancer and their families.

Contact Information
Cancer Support Community: Gilda's Club
Email: help@cancersupportcommunity.org
Website: http://cancersupportcommunity.org
Toll-free helpline 888-793-9355

In recent years, a shift of family health care from an illness or problem and deficiency focus to a strength-based focus has occurred (Crandall et al., 2019; Hanson et al., 2019; Kiwanuka et al., 2019; Search Institute, 2023). Multiple models in nursing view families as systems and base their assessment and nursing processes on strengths rather than deficits. These models of nursing provide the framework for assessing and planning care using family strengths and resources (Kiwanuka et al., 2019). Family members develop and maintain health-promoting behaviors by using commitment, appreciation, affection, positive communication, time together, a sense of spiritual well-being, and ability to cope with stress and crisis. Multiple assessment tools are available for nurses to use to generate discussion among family members about their strengths. Both Crandall et al. (2019) and Park et al. (2018) describe the importance of corresponding nursing interventions to support and further develop the family dynamics of socialization, support, and nurturance.

Families with significant strengths may need to learn new, unfamiliar skills for mastering a specific technique, such as meditation, and to apply new tools for decision-making. These families rarely require ongoing supervision or support of sustained interventions aimed at changing their coping patterns, communication, or role behavior. Assisting functional families can simply involve providing information in understandable terms and offering opportunities to ask questions and clarify information. Unit 3 contains individual chapters devoted to many of the strategies commonly used in health-promotion intervention, such as health teaching and counseling.

Decreasing exposure to risk factors may include enhancing parents' ability to assess their behavior and adjust it to their child's temperament. Parents with limited literacy may need assistance to learn to respond constructively to their child's communication attempts. Health promotion includes teaching parents to avoid exposure to risks—for example, to use adequate restraints in automobiles, to protect their toddler from wandering into dangerous streets, and to supervise children to avoid falls and hazardous materials.

Although no substitute can be found for continuous supervision of a child, homes can be made safer if common hazards are moved out of children's reach. This effort includes storing all cleaning solutions and medications beyond children's reach; erecting barriers in front of exposed heaters, high windows, and stairways; keeping pots and pans turned inward on the stove; fencing in a yard or a swimming pool; and teaching children to avoid dangerous areas. Becoming aware of peeling paint and toxic substances that parents might carry home from the job on their clothing can also protect the child.

Decreasing susceptibility means educating families about prevention principles. Families who realize how diseases are spread are better able to avoid transmission from person to person; through air, water, and food; and by insects and the rodents on which insects live. Health promotion involves emphasizing the role of personal hygiene and cleanliness to avoid infection. Families who know signs and symptoms that require medical attention and how to treat minor illnesses are better able to maintain healthy environments.

Murdaugh and colleagues (2020) cite research that demonstrates how perceived susceptibility predicts preventive behavior. Perceived susceptibility is the family's estimated subjective probability that a specific health problem will be encountered. Family members' perceptions of health risks and their susceptibility to them will determine how they change their behavior. If the overweight family believes obesity is a threat to the health of the family, the family members are more likely to react positively to the changes suggested by the nurse than if they perceive no health threat. Nurses who introduce threats as motivators to action are morally obligated to reduce these threats by meaningful and purposeful interventions. Table 7.2 lists various nursing roles used in the implementation stage.

Evaluation With the Family

The purpose of evaluation is to determine how the family has responded to the planned interventions and whether these interventions were successful. Goals and objectives that are stated in specific behavioral terms will make evaluation much easier than when they are given in general terms. The criteria used to evaluate interventions, such as weight change, increased lung capacity from an exercise program, and lower pulse rate as a result of relaxation exercises, are simple to measure. Other results of health promotion and disease prevention are not as easy to measure but must be considered in the evaluation step of the nursing process. When considering factors such as values, beliefs, self-perceptions, or role relationships, the nurse may base the evaluation on whether the family indicates that the interventions were successful. Additionally, the family's baseline data are used as comparative criteria in evaluation. The nurse reassesses the situation and compares the new information with the information from the original assessment to determine whether change has occurred.

The following five measures of family functioning can be used to determine the effectiveness of interventions: changes in interaction patterns, effective communication, ability to express emotions, responsiveness to needs of members as individuals, and problem-solving ability. Using these measures, the nurse returns to the original assessment of the family's functioning and compares current observations with previous data. These characteristics of family functioning continue to provide a useful framework even today, with widely diverse family structures becoming more common and the prevalence of nuclear families decreasing (Hadfield et al., 2018; Senkowski et al., 2019).

When, during the planning phase of the nursing process, the nurse has identified the criteria (norms and standards) for the desired outcomes, these outcomes are the basis of evaluation. Data from the family that describe the behavior of family members relative to the desired outcomes determine whether the nursing care was successful. With the criteria stated, the goals and objectives outline how the family can demonstrate a successful outcome and the behavioral change expected to result from nursing intervention. The more objective and measurable the desired outcome is, the more reliable the results of evaluation will be.

After the goals and objectives have been reached, the problem no longer exists. If evaluation shows the nursing actions did not achieve the goals or objectives, the nurse must review the nursing process to determine whether there were gaps in the assessment data, errors in analysis, or alternative interventions that might have been considered. Additionally, the nurse should review the process with the family to determine whether the family members have contributed to outcome failure. Finally, the agency employing the nurse may be another factor; if intervention is costly or a shortage of staff exists, then health promotion and disease prevention may have low priority.

CASE STUDY

Family Member with Lewy Body Dementia (LBD): Roberto and Marianne

Roberto and Marianne have been married for 40 years. Their grown children live thousands of miles away. Roberto's mother lives with the couple. She has lived with them for more than 5 years and was recently diagnosed with LBD, the second most common type of progressive dementia after Alzheimer disease. Lewy bodies are protein deposits that develop in brain nerve cells, affecting thinking, memory, and movement (motor control). Roberto, an only child, promised his mother, Loretta, long ago that he would care for her as she aged.

Marianne is the primary caregiver for Loretta, who is no longer able to recognize her loved ones. Marianne is unable to continue with social activities or her previous activities at her church. Traveling to visit their children has been curtailed. The couple is reluctant to have friends visit, because their home is now organized for the care of Loretta, who is in a hospital bed in their family gathering area. The couple shares responsibilities for Loretta; Roberto maintains responsibility for finances, health visits, and much of the cooking. Marianne provides physical care and hygiene. The couple is always tired, and they often fall asleep before finishing all of the household and caregiving tasks. Their sleeping patterns are disrupted, and they are unable to plan even a few days into the future.

Reflective Questions

- How is the couples' sense of role performance affected in this current situation?
- How might this current situation influence the couple's health?
- How might this current situation affect the entire family's relationship?

FAMILY DEALING WITH LEWY BODY DEMENTIA: ROBERTO AND MARIANNE

Health Promotion Issue: Roles-Relationships Pattern

Planned Health-Promotion Strategies

- Identify indicators of increased stress or depression in the family (e.g., anger, fatigue, irritability, withdrawal from friends/socials, sleep/weight changes).
- Jointly prepare a pragmatic approach for the family that accounts for Loretta's deteriorating condition.
- Jointly reevaluate the plan regularly.
- Include Loretta to the level of her ability in all aspects of the plan and daily activities.
- Encourage family members to seek respite care, adult day care, family/friend relief from responsibilities.
- Encourage family members to maintain a healthy lifestyle with respect to nutrition, exercise, social activities, LBD, dementia, or caregiver support groups.
- Encourage family members to create an atmosphere of nonjudgmental open communication and request assistance from each other.
- Help the family members learn to accept help if offered.
- Encourage Roberto and Marianne to communicate regularly with their children to alleviate any sense of guilt about the importance of their role from a distance or the costs of caregiving/travel.
- Support Loretta, Roberto, Marianne, and their children as they accommodate Loretta's decline and adapt their expectations.
- Facilitate discussion about the wide range of emotions, from joy to burden, that will be experienced while caring for Loretta.
- Advise Roberto and Marianne to seek care for their fatigue and sleep difficulties.
- Help Roberto and Marianne assess their strengths and limitations, as well as the evolving roles for both of them, Loretta, and their children.
- Encourage the family to approach their new roles realistically and to seek help as needed.
- Help each family member recognize that the pace of their progress in this journey may vary from the pace of other family members. Help them aim for

Continued

their own balance, which should include a future focus as well as the creation of a loving atmosphere in the present.
- Help Roberto and Marianne establish routines that include sharing simple activities with Loretta (e.g., listening to music, spending time outdoors, watching a favorite television show together, physical touch).
- Help Roberto and Marianne develop strategies for the acceptance of Loretta's diagnosis, recognizing that their progress toward acceptance may range from denial to the supportive acquisition of new roles and responsibilities.
- Refer Roberto and Marianne to the most current resources for LBD disease support services (e.g., Well Spouse, https://wellspouse.org/; Respite Care, www.archrespite.org/respitelocator) (National Institute on Aging [NIH], 2018).
- Refer Roberto and Marianne to the Lewy Body Dementia Association (http://www.lbda.org/) and the Dementia Society (https://www.dementiasociety.org/).
- Help Roberto and Marianne learn more about LBD so that they can inform health providers who may not be as familiar with LBD.
- Educate Roberto and Marianne to monitor for sensitivities Loretta may develop to antipsychotic medication.
- Advise Roberto and Marianne to involve Loretta's neurologist as new medications are considered.
- Gather materials from the Lewy Body Dementia Association (http://www.lbda.org/) to learn more about LBD and to have these materials available for new caregivers and health providers, families and friends.
- Help Roberto, Marianne, and their children prepare for emergencies by keeping Loretta's health documents—health insurance cards, medication list, health history, health care advance directives (https://www.nia.nih.gov/health/advance-care-planning-healthcare-directives), and allergies/adverse responses to medications—current.
- Complete a medical alert card for Loretta (https://www.ibda.org/).
- Maintain current contact information for physicians, services used, family members, and friends.
- Help Roberto and Marianne prepare for visits from family or friends who may not understand the symptoms and care responsibilities associated with LBD.
- Help Roberto and Marianne set into motion plans for preparation for the unpredictable death trajectory for an individual with LBD.

SUMMARY

- Learning about health promotion and disease prevention begins at birth, with the family providing the stimulus for incorporating health in the value system of its members.
- From a systems perspective, the family has both structure and function; relevant functions include values and practices related to health.
- The effective execution of health-related functions involves the family's progression through its developmental tasks and its ability to generate low risk-producing behaviors associated with disease prevention.
- Developmental and risk-estimate theories can be applied effectively to the nursing process with the family.
- The nurse uses functional patterns (an inherent part of both theories) to collect data for assessment.
- After organizing information on family life cycle stages for analysis with the family, the nurse plans, implements, and evaluates the interventions used to promote health and prevent disease in the family.

EVOLVE CHAPTER FEATURES

http://evolve.elsevier.com/Edelman/
- Study Questions

REFERENCES

Aeby, G., Gauthier, J. A., & Widmer, E. D. (2019). Beyond the nuclear family: Personal networks in light of work-family trajectories. *Advances in Life Course Research*, *39*, 51–60. https://doi.org/10.1016/J.ALCR.2018.11.002

Badanta, B., Rivilla-Garcia, E., Lucchetti, G., & de Diego-Cordero, R. (2022). The influence of spirituality and religion on critical care nursing: An integrative review. *Nursing in Critical Care*, *27*, 348–366. https://doi.org/10.1111/nicc.12645

Berry, K. (2018). LGBT bullying in school: A troubling relational story. *Communication Education*, *67*(4), 502–513. https://doi.org/10.1080/03634523.2018.1506137

Burnett, C., Crowder, J., Bacchus, L. J., Schminkey, D., Bullock, L., Sharps, P., & Campbell, J. (2019). "It doesn't freak us out the way it used to": An evaluation of the domestic violence enhanced home visitation program to inform practice and policy screening for IPV. *Journal of Interpersonal Violence*, *36*, 13-14. https://doi.org/10.1177/0886260519827161

Cambron, C., Kosterman, R., Catalano, R. F., Guttmannova, K., & Hawkins, J. D. (2018). Neighborhood, family, and peer factors associated with early adolescent smoking and alcohol use. *Journal of Youth and Adolescence*, *47*(2), 369–382. https://doi.org/10.1007/s10964-017-0728-y

Centers for Disease Control and Prevention (CDC). (2021). *Genomics and precision health*. https://blogs.cdc.gov/genomics/2012/08/23/evidence-matters-in-genomic-medicine-round-2/

Chavez, S. (2023). *The strengthening families movement: Looking back and looking ahead*. Washington, DC: Center for the Study of Social Policy. https://cssp.org/2019/01/looking-back-at-the-strengthening-families-movement/

Clark, R., Gehl, M., Heffron, M. C., Kerr, M., Soliman, S., Shahmoon-Shanok, R., & Thomas, K. (2019). Mindful practices to enhance diversity-informed reflective supervision and leadership. *Zero to Three*, *39*(11), 18–27. https://www.zerotothree.org/resource/journal/mindful-practices-to-enhance-diversity-informed-reflective-supervision-and-leadership/

Crandall, A., Novilla, L. K. B., Hanson, C. L., Barnes, M. D., & Novilla, M. L. B. (2019). The public health family impact checklist: A tool to help practitioners think family. *Frontiers in Public Health*, *7*, 331. https://doi.org/10.3389/fpubh.2019.00331

Crowley, R. A., & Bornstein, S. S. (2019). Improving the Patient Protection and Affordable Care Act's insurance coverage provisions: A position paper from the American College of

Physicians. *Annals of Internal Medicine, 170*(9), 651–653. https://doi.org/10.7326/m18-3401

Culyba, A. J., Miller, E., Ginsburg, K. R., Branas, C. C., Guo, W., Fein, J. A., Richmond, T. S., Halpern-Felsher, B. L., & Wiebe, D. J. (2018). Adult connection in assault injury prevention among male youth in low-resource urban environments. *Journal of Urban Health, 95*(3), 361–371. https://doi.org/10.1007/s11524-018-0260-8

Davodi, S. R., Zendehtalab, H. R., Zare, M., & Behnam Vashani, H. R. (2023). Effect of health promotion interventions in active aging in the elderly: A randomized controlled trial. *International Journal of Community Based Nursing & Midwifery, 11*(1), 34–43. https://doi.org/10.30476/IJCBNM.2022.96246.2117

Day, A. M., O'Shay-Wallace, S., Seeger, M. W., & McElmurry, S. P. (2019). Informational sources, social media use, and race in the Flint, Michigan, water crisis. *Communication Studies, 70*(3), 352–376. https://doi.org/10.1080/10510974.2019.1567566

Denov, M., & Shevell, M. C. (2019). Social work practice with war-affected children and families: The importance of family, culture, arts, and participatory approaches. *Journal of Family Social Work, 22*(1), 1–16. https://doi.org/10.1080/10522158.2019.1546809

Duvall, E., & Miller, B. (1985). *Marriage and family development* (7th ed.). New York: Harper Collins.

Duvall, E. M. (1988). Family development's first forty years. *Family Relations, 37*, 127–134.

Edge, D., & Lemetyinen, H. (2019). Psychology across cultures: Challenges and opportunities. *Psychology and Psychotherapy: Theory, Research and Practice, 92*(2), 261–276. https://doi.org/10.1111/papt.12229

Eickmeyer, K. J., Guzzo, K. B., Manning, W. D., & Brown, S. L. (2019). A research note on income pooling in partnerships: Incorporating nonresident children. *Journal of Family Issues, 40*(18), 2922–2943. https://doi.org/10.1177/0192513x19868270

Ehrenfeld, J. M., Gottlieb, K. G., Beach, L. B., Monahan, S. E., & Fabbri, D. (2019). Development of a natural language processing algorithm to identify and evaluate transgender patients in electronic health record system. *Ethnicity & Disease, 29*(2), 441–450. https://pmc.ncbi.nlm.nih.gov/articles/PMC6604788/

Elander, J. (2019). Sickle cell disease. In C. D. Llewellyn, S. Ayers, C. McManus, S. Newman, K. J. Petrie, T. A. Revenson, & J. Weinman (Eds.), *Cambridge handbook of psychology, health and medicine* (3rd ed., pp. 585–587). Cambridge: Cambridge University Press. https://doi.org/10.1017/9781316783269

Erikson, E. H. (1998). *The life cycle completed*. New York: W. W. Norton.

Fan, C. W., Castonguay, L., Rummell, S., Lévesque, S., Mitchell, J. J., & Sillon, G. (2018). Online module for carrier screening in Ashkenazi Jewish individuals compared with in-person genetics education: A randomized controlled trial. *Journal of Genetic Counseling, 27*(2), 426–438. https://doi.org/10.1007/s10897-017-0133-4

Fosco, G. M., Mak, H. W., Ramos, A., LoBraico, E., & Lippold, M. (2019). Exploring the promise of assessing dynamic characteristics of the family for predicting adolescent risk outcomes. *Journal of Child Psychology and Psychiatry, 60*(8), 848–856. https://doi.org/10.1111/jcpp.13052

Cancer support community: Gilda's club. (2024). *About us*. https://www.cancersupportcommunity.org/about-us

Giraudeau, C., & Bailly, N. (2019). Intergenerational programs: What can school-age children and older people expect from them? A systematic review. *European Journal of Ageing, 16*, 363–376. https://doi.org/10.1007/s10433-018-00497-4

Gewirtz-Meydan, A., Hafford-Letchfield, T., Ayalon, L., Benyamini, Y., Biermann, V., Coffey, A., Jackson, J., Phelan, A., Voß, P., Geiger Zeman, M., & Zeman, Z. (2019). How do older people discuss their own sexuality? A systematic review of qualitative research studies. *Culture, Health & Sexuality, 21*(3), 293–308. https://doi.org/10.1080/13691058.2018.1465203

Gordon, M. (2014). *Manual of nursing diagnosis* (14th ed.). Jones & Bartlett.

Gunn, H. E., & Eberhardt, K. R. (2019). Family dynamics in sleep health and hypertension. *Current Hypertension Reports, 21*(5), 39. https://doi.org/10.1007/s11906-019-0944-9

Hadfield, K., Amos, M., Ungar, M., Gosselin, J., & Ganong, L. (2018). Do changes to family structure affect child and family outcomes? A systematic review of the instability hypothesis. *Journal of Family Theory & Review, 10*(1), 87–110. https://doi.org/10.1111/jftr.12243

Handayani, A., Setiawan, A., & Yulianti, P. D. (2019). Individual adaptation based on family development stage. *Advances in Social Science, Education and Humanities Research, 287*. https://web.archive.org/web/20190426165648/https://download.atlantis-press.com/article/55912207.pdf

Handley, V. A., Bradshaw, S. D., Milstead, K. A., & Bean, R. A. (2019). Exploring similarity and stability of differentiation in relationships: A dyadic study of Bowen's theory. *Journal of Marital and Family Therapy, 45*(4), 592–605. https://doi.org/10.1111/jmft.12370

Hanson, C. L., Crandall, A., Barnes, M. D., Magnusson, M., Novilla, L. B., & King, J. (2019). Family-focused public health: Supporting homes and families in policy and practice. *Frontier Public Health, 7*, 59. https://doi.org/10.3389/fpubh.2019.00059

Hayes, J. F., Balantekin, K. N., Conlon, R. P. K., Brown, M. L., Stein, R. I., Welch R. R., Perri, M. G., Schechtman, K. B., Epstein, L. H., Wilfley, D. E., & Saelens, B. E. (2019). Home and neighbourhood built environment features in family-based treatment for childhood obesity. *Pediatric Obesity, 14*(3), e12477. https://doi.org/10.1111/ijpo.12477

Hedman, K. (2019). Strengths and support of older people affected by precarity in South Louisiana. *International Journal of Older People Nursing, 14*(2), e12232. https://doi.org/10.1111/opn.12232

Hockenberry, M. J., Duffy, E.A., & Gibbs, K. (2023). *Wong's nursing care of infants and children* (12th ed.). St. Louis: Mosby.

Justice, L. M., Jiang, H., Purtell, K. M., Schmeer, K., Boone, K., Bates, R., & Salsberry, P. J. (2019). Conditions of poverty, parent–child interactions, and toddlers' early language skills in low-income families. *Maternal and Child Health Journal, 23*(7), 971–978. https://doi.org/10.1007/s10995-018-02726-9

Kaakinen, J. R., Padgett-Coehlo, D., Steele, R., & Robinson, M. (2018). *Family health care nursing: Theory, practice, and research* (6th ed.). Philadelphia: FA Davis.

Kashiwagi, H., Kikuchi, A., Koyama, M., Saito, D., & Hirabayashi, N. (2018). Strength-based assessment for future violence risk: A retrospective validation study of the Structured Assessment of PROtective Factors for violence risk (SAPROF) Japanese version in forensic psychiatric inpatients. *Annals of General Psychiatry, 17*(1), 5. https://doi.org/10.1186/s12991-018-0175-5

Kiwanuka, F., Rad, S. A., & Alemayehu, Y. H. (2019). Enhancing patient and family-centered care: A three-step strengths-based model. *International Journal of Caring Sciences, 12*(1), 584–590. https://internationaljournalofcaringsciences.org/docs/65_kiwanuka12_1.pdf

Knudson-Martin, C., McDowell, T., & Bermudez, J. M. (2019). From knowing to doing: Guidelines for socioculturally attuned family therapy. *Journal of Marital and Family Therapy, 45*(1), 47–60. https://doi.org/10.1111/jmft.12299

Kokorelias, K. M., Gignac, M. A., Naglie, G., & Cameron, J. I. (2019). Towards a universal model of family centered care: A scoping review. *BMC Health Services Research*, *19*(1), 564. https://doi.org/10.1186/s12913-019-4394-5

Kumar, R., Bhattacharya, S., Sharma, N., & Thiyagarajan, A. (2019). Cultural competence in family practice and primary care setting. *Journal of Family Medicine and Primary Care*, *8*(1), 1–4. https://doi.org/10.4103/jfmpc.jfmpc_393_18

Lawless, R. A., Moore, E. E., Cohen, M. J., Moore, H. B., & Sauaia, A. (2018). US national trends in violent and unintentional injuries, 2000 to 2016. *JAMA Surgery*, *153*(12), 1154–1158. https://doi.org/10.1001/jamasurg.2018.2496

Lerner, R. M., Lerner, J. V., & Chase, P. A. (2019). Toward enhancing the role of idiographic-based analyses in describing, explaining, and optimizing the study of human development: The sample case of adolescent family relationships. *Journal of Family Theory & Review*, *4*(11), 495. https://doi.org/10.1111/jftr.12347

Li, W., Murray, M. F., & Giovanni, M. A. (2019). Obtaining a genetic family history using computer-based tools. *Current Protocols in Human Genetics*, *100*(1), e72. https://doi.org/10.1002/cphg.72

Libbon, R., Triana, J., Heru, A., & Berman, E. (2019). Family skills for the resident toolbox: The 10-min genogram, ecomap, and prescribing homework. *Academic Psychiatry*, *43*(4), 435–439. https://doi.org/10.1007/s40596-019-01054-6

Lloyd, J. L. (2019). From farms to food deserts: Food insecurity and older rural Americans. *Generations*, *43*(2), 24–32. https://www.jstor.org/stable/26760111?seq=1

MacArthur, G., Caldwell, D. M., Redmore, J., Watkins, S. H., Kipping, R., White, J. Chittleborough, C., Langford, R., Er, V., Lingam, R., Pasch, K., Gunnell, D., Hickman, M., & Campbell, R. (2018). Individual-, family-, and school-level interventions targeting multiple risk behaviours in young people. *Cochrane Database of Systematic Reviews*, *10*(10), CD009927. https://doi.org/10.1002/14651858.cd009927.pub2

McGoldrick, M., Gerson, R., & Petry, S. (2020). Genograms: Assessment and treatment (4th ed.). W.W. Norton and Company.

Murdaugh, C., Parsons, M. A., & Pender, N. J. (2020). Health promotion in nursing practice (7th ed.). Upper Saddle River, NJ: Pearson.

Murphy, M. L. (2019). How the “sandwich generation” affects retirement: Insight into this demographic trend can help CPAs advise clients. *Journal of Accountancy*, *227*(4), 44. https://www.journalofaccountancy.com/issues/2019/may/retirement-sandwich-generation-trend.html

National Academy of Medicine (NAM). (2022). *A proposed approach for implementing genomics-based screening programs for healthy adults*. https://nam.edu/wp-content/uploads/2018/11/Considering-Genomic-Screening-Programs.pdf

National Coalition Against Domestic Violence (NCADV). (2023). *Voice of victims, home for advocates: National coalition against domestic violence*. http://www.ncadv.org

National Institutes of Health (NIH). (2018). How to care for a person with Lewy body dementia. National Institute on Aging. https://www.nia.nih.gov/health/how-care-person-lewy-body-dementia

Nickbakht, M., Meyer, C., Scarinci, N., & Beswick, R. (2019). A qualitative investigation of families' needs in the transition to early intervention after diagnosis of hearing loss. *Child: Care, Health and Development*, *5*(45), 670–680. https://doi.org/10.1111/cch.12697

Nocentini, A., Fiorentini, G., Di Paola, L., & Menesini, E. (2019). Parents, family characteristics and bullying behavior: A systematic review. *Aggression and Violent Behavior*, *45*(2), 41–50. https://doi.org/10.1016/j.avb.2018.07.010

Palombi, M. (2018). From Gestalt therapy to family systems: How theoretical frameworks inform clinical applications. *Australian and New Zealand Journal of Family Therapy*, *39*(4), 514–527. https://doi.org/10.1002/anzf.1334

Park, M., Lee, M., Jeong, H., Jeong, M., & Go, Y. (2018). Patient- and family-centered care interventions for improving the quality of health care: A review of systematic reviews. *International Journal of Nursing Studies*, *87*, 69–83. https://doi.org/10.1016/j.ijnurstu.2018.07.006

Priest, J. B., Parker, E. O., & Woods, S. B. (2018). Do the constructs of the FACES IV change based on definitions of “family?” A measurement invariance test. *Journal of Marital and Family Therapy*, *44*(2), 336–352. https://doi.org/10.1111/jmft.12257

Roygardner, D., Palusci, V. J., & Hughes, K. N. (2019). Advancing prevention zones: Implementing community-based strategies to prevent child maltreatment and promote healthy families. *International Journal on Child Maltreatment: Research, Policy and Practice*, *3*, 81–91. https://doi.org/10.1007/s42448-019-00039-0

Search Institute. (2023). *A snapshot of developmental relationships between parents and youth*. https://www.search-institute.org/wp-content/uploads/2017/12/Snapshot-of-Parent-Youth-Relationships-2017-final.pdf

Sege, R. D., Siegel, B. S., Council on Child Abuse And Neglect, & Committee on Psychosocial Aspects of Child and Family Health. (2018). Effective discipline to raise healthy children. *Pediatrics*, *142*(6). https://doi.org/10.1542/peds.2018-3609

Senkowski, V., Bhochhibhoya, S., Bernard, R., Zingg, T., & Maness, S. B. (2019). Assessing the variation of measurement of family structure in studies of adolescent risk behaviors: A systematic review. *Vulnerable Children and Youth Studies*, *4*(14), 287–311. https://doi.org/10.1080/17450128.2019.1614708

Shakarami, S., Veisani, Y., Kamali, K., Mostafavi, S. A., Mohammadi, M. R., Mohamadian, F., Ahmadi, N., Fararouei, M., & Delpisheh, A. (2019). The association between parents' lifestyles and common psychiatry disorders in children and adolescents: A population-based study. *Shiraz E-Medical Journal*, *5*, e81486. https://doi.org/10.5812/semj.81486

Sim, A., Cordier, R., Vaz, S., & Falkmer, T. (2019). “We are in this together”: Experiences of relationship satisfaction in couples raising a child with autism spectrum disorder. *Research in Autism Spectrum Disorders*, *58*, 39–51. https://doi.org/10.1016/j.rasd.2018.11.011

Stanhope, M., & Lancaster, J. (2024). *Public health nursing* (11th ed.). Elsevier.

Southern Oregon Head Start (SOHS). (2024). *Our programs*. https://www.socfc.org/programs/

The Ohio State University College of Social Work. (2020). *States with high opioid prescribing rates have higher rates of grandparents responsible for grandchildren*. https://u.osu.edu/ohiostart/2020/01/14/grandparents-raising-grandchildren-opioid-prescribing-rate-matters/

The University of Nebraska. (2012). *Families across the lifespan: The normal, to-be-expected, satisfactions and challenges couples and families experience*. https://www.familyconsumersciences.com/wp-content/uploads/family-life-cycle-info.pdf

Thomas, K., Noroña, C. R., & St John, M. S. (2019). Cross-sector allies together in the struggle for social justice: Diversity-informed tenets for work with infants, children, and families. *Zero to Three*, *39*(3), 44–54. https://www.irvingharrisfdn.org/

Tibbott, J., Di Carlofelice, M., Menon, R., & Ciantar, E. (2021). Trauma and pregnancy. *The Obstetrician & Gynaecologist*, *23*, 258–264. https://doi.org/10.1111/tog.12769

Tinner, L., Palmer, J. C., Lloyd, E. C., Caldwell, D. M., MacArthur, G. J., Dias, K., Langford, R., Redmore, J., Wittkop, L., Watkins, S. H.,

Hickman, M., & Campbell, R. (2022). Individual-, family- and school-based interventions to prevent multiple risk behaviours relating to alcohol, tobacco and drug use in young people aged 8-25 years: A systematic review and meta-analysis. *BMC Public Health, 22*(1111), 1–17. https://doi.org/10.1186/s12889-022-13072-5

Tøien, M., Torunn Bjørk, I., & Fagerstrom, L. (2020). 'A longitudinal room of possibilities' – Perspectives on the benefits of long-term preventive home visits: A qualitative study of nurses' experiences. *Nordic Journal of Nursing Research, 40*(1), 6–14. https://doi.org/10.1177/2057158519856495

US Census Bureau (USCB). (2024). *Selected social characteristics in the United States – Table DP02.* https://data.census.gov/cedsci/table?q=single%20parents&hidePreview=false&tid=ACSDP1Y2018.DP02)

US Department of Health and Human Services (USDHHS). (2022). *National center on parent, family, and community engagement (NCPFCE).* https://eclkc.ohs.acf.hhs.gov/about-us/article/national-center-parent-family-community-engagement-ncpfce

US Department of Health and Human Services (USDHHS). (2023). *Healthy People 2030.* https://health.gov/healthypeople

US Environmental Protection Agency (EPA). (2023). *Ground water and drinking water: Identifying funding sources for lead service line replacement.* https://www.epa.gov/ground-water-and-drinking-water/identifying-funding-sources-lead-service-line-replacement#:~:text=Bipartisan%20Infrastructure%20Law%20(BIL)&text=The%20Bipartisan%20Infrastructure%20Law%20will,towards%20LSLR%20through%20the%20DWSRF

Utter, J., Denny, S., Farrant, B., & Cribb, S. (2019). Feasibility of a family meal intervention to address nutrition, emotional wellbeing, and food insecurity of families with adolescents. *Journal of Nutrition Education and Behavior, 7*(51), 885–892. https://doi.org/10.1016/j.jneb.2019.03.015

Wheeler, D. C., Jones, R. M., Schootman, M., & Nelson, E. J. (2019). Explaining variation in elevated blood lead levels among children in Minnesota using neighborhood socioeconomic variables. *Science of The Total Environment, 650*, 970–977. https://doi.org/10.1016/j.scitotenv.2018.09.088

Williams-Reade, J. M., Lobo, E., & Gutierrez, G. (2019). Integrating spirituality into MFT training: A reflexive curriculum and qualitative evaluation. *Journal of Marital and Family Therapy, 45*(2), 219–232. https://doi.org/10.1111/jmft.12314

World Health Organization (WHO). (2020). *Healthy ageing and functional ability.* https://www.who.int/news-room/questions-and-answers/item/healthy-ageing-and-functional-ability

Zapolski, T., Clifton, R. L., Banks, D. E., Hershberger, A., & Aalsma, M. (2019). Family and peer influences on substance attitudes and use among juvenile justice-involved youth. *Journal of Child and Family Studies, 2*(28), 447–456. https://doi.org/10.1007/s10826-018-1268-0 Edelman 7-5

8

Health Promotion and the Community

Julianne A. Walsh

http://evolve.elsevier.com/Edelman/

OBJECTIVES

After completing this chapter, the reader will be able to:

- Describe the functional health patterns and explain how they are used for data collection to assess communities.
- Evaluate community characteristics that indicate risk.
- Explain methods of community data collection and sources of information.
- Describe a method of planned change for the community.
- Discuss the planning, implementation, and evaluation of nursing interventions in health promotion with communities.
- Develop a health-promotion plan based on community assessment, available resources, and other contributing factors.

KEY TERMS

Advocate	Community risk factors	Measurement data
Ambient	Demography	Observation data
Community	Developmental theory	Policy decision-making
Community evaluation	Focus groups	Risk-factor theory
Community health promotion	Function of a community	Structure of a community
Community mutual goal setting	Interview data	Systems theory
Community nursing intervention	Key informants	Windshield survey
Community outcomes	Lobbying	
Community pattern	Lobbyist	

THINK ABOUT IT

Teenagers: Drinking and Driving

In a small rural community, seven teenagers have died in alcohol-related car accidents within the past 3 months. An alcohol and drug education program is taught during the first year at the local high school. Driver's education classes are not available, because the school cannot afford the program. Parents within this community are extremely concerned. A group of concerned parents have gathered with the superintendent of schools, the principal of their only high school, and the school nurse to brainstorm about how to provide primary prevention programs throughout the grades to promote health, including health related to alcohol and substances that students will encounter as they develop from elementary grades to high school graduation.

What other information should be gathered?

What health-promotion ideas could be recommended based on the information provided?

In the last few decades, several social trends in the United States have increased public interest in health promotion and disease prevention. The *Healthy People 2030* initiative shifts the focus of health care from reactive to proactive, with its emphasis on disease prevention and health promotion. By identifying national health objectives as population-specific risks to good health, this venture guides community strategies to promote health, thereby reducing disease risk factors. Box 8.1: *Healthy People 2030* highlights an emphasis within the environmental and community context.

Healthy People 2030 has three types of objectives: core, developmental, and research. Core objectives contain data sources of national importance; most objectives are core objectives. Core objectives emphasize gathering effective, evidence-based data about interventions that enable attaining health equity while achieving the associated Healthy People 2030 objective. Developmental objectives represent high-priority areas with accepted evidence-based interventions but without current reliable baseline data sources. Research objectives address valuable topics with limited data sources, high health/economic burden, or disproportionate health outcomes. There are 23 leading health indicators (LHI) that cut across lifespan topic areas. Nurses can follow the most current progress of Healthy People 2030 programs at the following website: https://health.gov/healthypeople/objectives-and-data/browse-objectives.

Another social trend creating interest for health promotion is the changing population of the United States (see Chapter 2).

BOX 8.1 *HEALTHY PEOPLE 2030*

Objectives Related to Health Promotion and The Community

AH-10	Reduce the rate of minors and young adults committing violent crimes
C-07	Increase the proportion of adults who get screened for colorectal cancer
D-D01	Increase the proportion of eligible people completing CDC-recognized type 2 diabetes prevention programs
EH-05	Reduce health and environmental risks from hazardous sites
EH-08	Reduce the exposure to lead
FS-D06	Reduce the number of norovirus outbreaks
GH-D03	Increase laboratory diagnostic testing capacity, surveillance, and reporting globally
HC/HIT-R01	Increase the health literacy of the population
HC/HIT-R05	Increase the proportion of adults with broadband internet
LGBT-01	Increase the number of national surveys that collect data on lesbian, gay, and bisexual populations
LGBT-02	Increase the number of national surveys that collect data on transgender populations
SDOH-01	Reduce the proportion of people living in poverty

CDC, Centers for Disease Control.
From the U.S. Department of Health and Human Services. *Healthy People 2030 Objectives and Data.* Accessed January 31, 2024; US Department of Health and Human Services. [Internet]. Healthy People 2030. Office of Disease Prevention and Health Promotion. Retrieved from https://health.gov/healthypeople/objectives-and-data

The Centers for Disease Control (CDC) (2024) contends the US population life expectancy at birth rate has decreased from 77 years in 2020 to 76.4 years in 2021, suggesting the lowest levels since 1996. Contributing factors include accidental injury, COVID-19, and drug overdose deaths. In addition, heart and liver disease and suicide are on the rise.

With these demographic changes, disability, chronic disorders, and access to health care resources will take a predominant role in health promotion assessment of the community. Older adults tend to have more chronic diseases and consume larger proportions of health care resources than people in other age groups. This aging population will use more home services than previous generations because of increased life span and concurrent health issues (including altered levels of functioning). Moreover, with poverty levels, slower economic growth, and long-term financial shortfalls, there is continued concern regarding the financial viability of Medicare and Social Security as expenditures are rising (The New York Times, 2024; Fig. 8.1).

The term "**community**" is used in various contexts with various meanings, depending on the frame of reference. Nursing generally adopts a broad sense of community that includes the concepts of groups of people that share social relationships, generally live within the same geographic location, and share common interests (Stanhope & Lancaster, 2025). A broad definition of community encompasses a wide variety of settings, such as schools, workplaces, and the international community.

In the nation's schools, nurses serve youth and provide access to community resources. School nurses collect meaningful assessment data to improve health promotion within their school community. Linking school nurses with communities can increase access to resources to improve health-promoting behaviors. Partnering to share data and health promotion strategies benefits both the schools and the community at large (Wolfe et al., 2019). People are integral to any concept of community; human beings give each community shape, character, and form. The diversity within a community and the diversity among various communities contribute to the health of that community. Community-based participatory strategies aim to effectively blend the needs of the people with the available resources (Barceló et al., 2019; Kumar et al., 2019; Martinez-Bianchi et al., 2019; Roygardner et al., 2019). Individual health is reflected in each community through each person's contribution to its statistical rates and cultural and psychological makeup. Conversely, the context of the community is reflected in the individual through similar modes of expression (Pender et al., 2020).

This chapter focuses on the application of nursing clinical judgment to the community with independent, interdependent, and dependent nursing activities with an emphasis on assessment. Globalization affects all communities. Swift methods of travel and internet communication affect community health (Lockwood, 2019). Communities globally are exposed to emerging infectious diseases, such as the COVID-19 outbreak in 2019, Zika virus disease, Ebola fever, severe acute respiratory syndrome coronavirus (SARS), Middle East respiratory syndrome coronavirus (MERS), human immunodeficiency virus (HIV), acquired immunodeficiency syndrome (AIDS), and pandemics of tuberculosis and influenza. For example, in January 2020, The World Health Organization (WHO) declared a global emergency for a novel coronavirus, designated as "COVID-19." This coronavirus emerged in Wuhan, China, at the close of 2019. It is the third coronavirus in the last 10 years to appear. The last two, MERS and SARS, were able to be contained more quickly than COVID-19.

Because of its potential affect on countries with fewer resources than China, containment of COVID-19 surfaced as the predominant concern, thus precipitating the global emergency designation, Public Health Emergency of International Concern (PHEIC), soon after the disease first surfaced (WHO, 2020). This PHEIC designation aims to limit the outbreak, to encourage global transparency regarding transmission and scientific findings, to aim for collaboration to enhance worldwide preparedness, and to mobilize resources for regions of the world that may need additional support. Critical to these aims is a rapid response from global, national, and local health organizations.

Strategies ensued to minimize deaths and the economic effect of COVID-19 transmission (Anderson et al., 2020). By March 11, 2020, when WHO declared COVID-19 a pandemic, transmission was widespread in Italy, Iran, South Korea, and Japan, and multiple other countries were experiencing new cases (WHO, 2020). Quarantine, social distancing, and isolation helped to contain COVID-19 in China. Some other countries that experienced SARS responded to COVID-19 with these same strict tactics (Anderson et al., 2020; Ferguson et al., 2020).

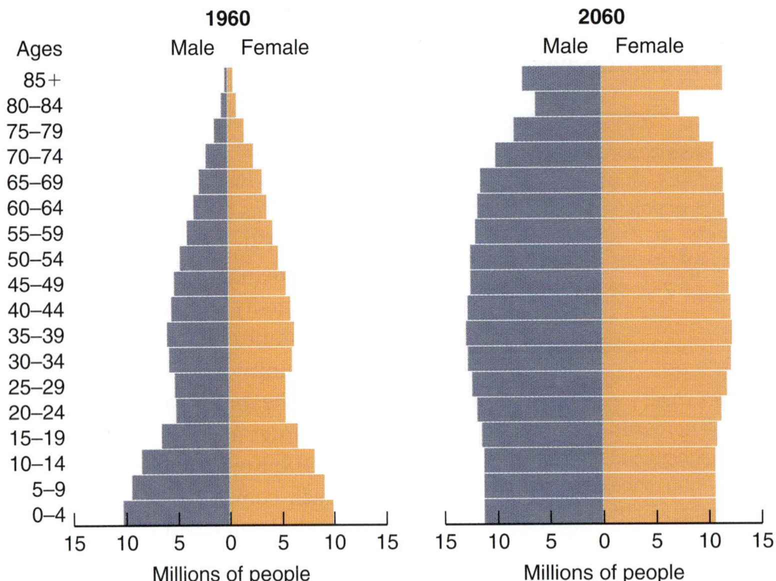

FIG. 8.1 Age and gender structure of the population of the United States: 1960 to 2060. (From US Census [2018]. *From Pyramid to Pillar: A Century of Change, Population of the U.S.* Retrieved from https://www.census.gov/library/visualizations/2018/comm/century-of-change.html [Accessed February 4, 2025].)

When epidemics or pandemics occur, nurses assess typical elements of transmission, such as the mean number of cases resulting from a primary infection, whether symptoms appear before infectiousness, the number of asymptomatic cases, and the duration of the infectious period. COVID-19 provides a model where these four elements were uncertain as it traveled in the early stages of transmission. For COVID-19, personal response may play a larger role than enactment of administrative rules (Anderson et al., 2020; Ferguson et al., 2020). Clearly, such a response requires community nurses with expertise in communication, marketing, and community-based partnerships. Globally, immunization treatment is one of the most cost-effective public health interventions. Successful public health strategies and immunization programs require effective communication to increase vaccine confidence. Because of new technology and rigorous research studies, there was an unprecedented rapid development of COVID-19 vaccines, thereby creating an uptake in vaccine-hesitant populations (Breckenridge et al., 2022; Weinstein et al., 2024). Policy makers and regulators must be mindful of vaccine hesitancy when developing such strategies. For more information about COVID-19, refer to Chapter 25.

Nurses can follow such outbreaks and participate in limiting transmission through agency websites such as WHO's emerging diseases website (https://www.whoint/emergencies/disease-outbreak-news) and the CDC outbreaks website (https://www.cdc.gov/). Often, local city and state health departments will offer the ability to subscribe to emergency response email/texts for health professionals and community members.

Health disparities worldwide are linked to poverty, lack of industrialization, limited educational opportunities, inadequate food access, poor maternal health, violence, and social disruption (United States Department of Agriculture [USDA], 2024). Even in developed countries with health resources, disparity occurs. Health may be different in urban versus rural geographical areas. In the past 40 years, poverty rates between rural and urban areas have narrowed from a 4.5 to a 3.1 percentage point average difference; however, regional differences exist. Poverty clusters, particularly in the southern regions of the United States, create barriers that extend beyond the individual to the community at large, contributing to health disorders, crime, school dropout, unemployment, food insecurity, and housing issues. These factors compound the cycle of poverty for these communities (USDA, 2024). Furthermore, poverty exists in all parts of the country. Because Hispanic populations tend to experience poverty at higher rates than non-Hispanic Whites, poverty increased in Hispanic populations in the United States during the 1990s and 2000s, in the associated regions of growth such as California, Nevada, Arizona, Colorado, North Carolina, and Georgia (USDA, 2024).

Poverty rates set by the US government do not account for regional cost-of-living differences. For example, urban cost of living that is higher than rural cost of living will skew the actual poverty level. These differences shift in either direction. The current measure of poverty level ignores variations in regional, urban, or rural resources such as health care, schooling, communication networks, noise, and pollution (USDA, 2024). The Consumer Expenditure Survey generates a more comprehensive measure, the Supplemental Poverty Measure (SPM), which adds tax payments and work expenses, along with basic need expenditures, and adjusts for geographic differences.

In his 2019 report on poverty for the Marguerite Casey Foundation, Abramsky (2019) describes a variety of reasons for the declining poverty rates. In 2018, the poverty rate (11.8%) was actually lower than before the 2008 Great Recession (Abramsky, 2019). Many states attack the problems related to poverty with strategies such as instituting a higher minimum wage, the

Earned Income Tax Credit, paid family leave programs, loan-free higher education, and interest-rate limits. States implementing antipoverty measures lower poverty levels to nearly half of those of states who choose not to implement these programs. About three million people lost Supplemental Nutrition Assistance Program (SNAP) eligibility. The hunger of these people is not reflected in traditional poverty estimates. The working poor who do not qualify for government benefits may still be too poor to achieve economic or food security (Abramsky, 2019). The American Rescue Plan and the extension of the Child Tax Credit (pandemic relief funds) supported a decline in poverty due to successful governmental interventions (Trisi, 2023). However, with the shutdown of programs, poverty levels could increase.

Methods of data collection and sources of information about communities differ from individual sources. **Systems theory**, **developmental theory**, and **risk-factor theory** guide nursing clinical judgment. Developmental theory refers to a variety of explanations of phases of human development—physical, psychosocial, cognitive, and spiritual dimensions—based on descriptive research studies. Similarly, risk-factor theory identifies human characteristics and behaviors that increase the likelihood of the manifestation of health problems. Diverse communities require comprehensive assessment techniques that gather information about the unique characteristics of the population (e.g., cultural health practices or herbal remedies).

Gordon's (2014) Functional Health Patterns provide the assessment framework for this chapter. Although other community assessment strategies exist, Gordon's patterns are useful to align community assessment findings with those of families and individuals to plan health promotion. An example of a data collection guide pattern is presented to facilitate the comprehension, synthesis, and application of **observation data**, **interview data**, **focus groups**, and **measurement data**.

THE NURSE'S ROLE

Community Health Nursing

Community health nursing combines nursing practice and public health concepts to promote the health of populations without limitation to any particular individual or group of individuals (Stanhope & Lancaster, 2025).

Nursing concerns address community responses to existing and potential health-related issues, including health-supportive actions such as monitoring and educating population groups. Nurses provide educational resources to at-risk communities to help them develop health-oriented skills, attitudes, and behaviors.

Competencies nurses generally use patient-centered focus, interpersonal communication, organizational skill, critical thinking, clinical judgment, safety issues, accountability, quality, and decision-making for community nursing assessment (West et al., 2018; Young & Thompson, 2018). Additional competencies pertinent to a quality community assessment include leadership, emotional intelligence, community-centered focus, interprofessional collaboration, ability to foster partnerships with multiple agencies/groups, cultural consciousness, cultural competence, self-reflection, ethical values, respect for community diversity/preferences/needs, and informatics. Clearly, competencies sit within a dynamic global environment that shifts with the fast-paced changes in health care (Di Leonardi et al., 2020; Lambert et al., 2018; Liu & Aungsuroch, 2018; West et al., 2018; Young & Thompson, 2018). Although other nursing specialties may use these additional competencies, a predominant skill that may be used in other nursing specialties is community assessment.

Community nurses develop essential relationships and partnerships aimed at accomplishing the community's health-related missions. Complex and dynamic communities, with their increasing public involvement in health and health policy, highlight the importance of human interactions inherent in nurses' responses to potential health problems, needs, and expectations. For example, active participation in environmental issues, such as decreasing control of toxic substances, provides an avenue for nurses to promote healthy environments by influencing policy. Concern about harmful effects of environmental contaminants includes decreased fertility in females, demasculinization of males exposed to plastics, and premature maturation of the reproductive tract with a trend toward earlier sexual maturation.

Community nursing practice, therefore, requires a broad knowledge base derived from the natural, behavioral, and humanistic sciences, with application of intellectual, interpersonal, and technical skills using the nursing process.

Influencing Health Policy

The primary responsibility of the nurse is to the individual, family, group, or community served. A significant portion of the nurse's role is to **advocate** for justice in health care delivery. Nurses need to be aware of issues that affect the health of the American people and understand how to influence necessary change.

Influencing policy requires local, state, federal, and global health partnerships and collaborations (Klopper et al., 2020). Nurses, who comprise the majority of health care professionals, fortify health care when they participate in policy initiatives. Aging, health inequity, migrant/refugee health, HIV/AIDS, tuberculosis, and emerging infections are all areas where nurses are well equipped to serve as primary advocates to shape health care policy for the future. One organization, The Global Advisory Panel on the Future of Nursing and Midwifery (GAPFON) supports a global initiative to serve as a catalyst to give voice to those individuals, such as nurses, who have previously been disregarded (Klopper et al., 2020).

Nurses' first-hand knowledge of situations can influence policy through narratives. For example, in their systematic review of how policy is influenced by narratives, Fadlallah and colleagues (2019) report their findings from 18 studies. Two particular narratives described in this systematic review highlight how nursing influences policy. During the early days of the emerging infections of HIV and hepatitis C, the president of the Massachusetts Nurses' Association presented her personal story about contracting both HIV and hepatitis C from a needlestick during the time she served as an emergency department nurse. Her testimony to Massachusetts state house legislators became a catalyst. This nurse's initiative to introduce a needlestick bill began its progression through the Massachusetts legislature the next day. The nurse, Karen Daley, who spent more than 25 years as a front-line caregiver, spearheaded this policy initiative and actively engaged on state, national, and international levels. Daley has traveled across the United States, Europe, Australia, and Asia to advocate for sharps injury prevention. In recognition of her integral role in its passage, Daley was among those invited to the Oval Office to witness President Clinton sign the "Needlestick Safety Prevention Act" into law on November 6, 2000.

Another example occurred in England, where nurses shared patient stories during transition from one area to another and from nursing preoperative visits. These stories led to a number of patient-centered quality improvements within the National Health Service's quality improvement projects.

As health care delivery advocates, nurses address environmental issues. Health and the environment are integrally connected; therefore, when engaging in community planning and policy, nurses promote the health potential of the communities served. Involvement that includes attention to policy decisions and political action affects broader aspects of environmental, biophysical, and socioeconomic conditions of homes, schools, workplaces, communities, and health care delivery. For example, Barraclough and colleagues (2019) established a baseline for environmental stability in their assessment of dialysis centers. Data were gathered from their Green Dialysis Survey of 71 of 83 dialysis centers in Victoria, Australia. These authors describe opportunities to improve environmentally sustainable infrastructure:

- Use low-energy lighting with motion sensors.
- Use computer/copier automatic settings to hibernate.
- Set thermostats appropriately with staff access.
- Keep heating and cooling off when not in use.
- Use green or renewable electricity options.
- Address recovery and reuse of reverse osmosis water.
- Use water-saving toilets/taps, recycle general and clinical waste.
- Recycle polyvinylchloride (PVC).
- Address environmental sustainability during the procurement phase.
- Reduce unnecessary paper copies.
- Use double-sided copies/email.
- Use recycled/sustainably sourced paper.

These nurses' ideas depict clear guidelines for nurses to shape future policy to provide environmentally sustainable dialysis health care in Victoria, Australia. Strategies to ensure these guidelines are met require active participation in policy development as nurses are well positioned to advocate for climate change.

By virtue of their numbers, nurses, who constitute the largest group of health care providers worldwide, have tremendous potential to influence decision-making. Participation in **policy decision-making** requires that nurses take a proactive stance to determine needs before a problem arises. Policy development change and health-related decision-making occur on many levels, from within the nurse's agency or work group to the community, state, and national levels. Laws—rules enforced by a ruling authority by which society is governed—and regulations—agency or department rules developed to implement laws—define the services offered. The nurse examines underlying rationales for existing or planned policy to determine their current relevance.

At the US national level, the Alliance of Nurses for Healthy Environments (ANHE) (2024) has created a website called the "Knowledge Network" to facilitate nurses' participation and competence in environmental health issues. This organization contributes by promoting collaboration and partnerships to advance environmental health. Moreover, the scope of practice for community and public health nursing (C/PHN) expects these competencies. To extend ideas from a project into a sustainable change, collaborations must negotiate partnership expectations, develop confidence in each other, aim to cooperate, and eradicate power differentials (Campbell et al., 2020; Rosa et al., 2019; Stanhope & Lancaster, 2025). In their systematic evaluation, Campbell and colleagues (2020) reviewed and revised the eight principles of competencies for C/PHN identified by the Quad Council of Public Health Nursing Organization. Nurses use such principles and practice guidelines to shape their practice. Rosa and colleagues (2019) offer the American Nurses Association, Public Health Nursing: Scope and Standards for Practice as an example of practice standards that demonstrate that nurses' practice expectations prepare them to engage in global initiatives such as the United Nations' (UN) Sustainable Development Goals (SDGs).

Politics influences change and provides an arena for nursing to participate in shaping the future of health care. Political involvement may include voting, communicating with local representatives, supporting candidates, contributing time or financial support, and running for city, county, state, or national office. Voting, after nurses have become well informed on current issues and candidates, and serving on local and state committees are important ways for nurses to be actively involved. At the institutional level, clinical decisions influence policy, as do management issues. Nurses use their education and experience to communicate, collaborate, and apply change theory to influence policy.

Progress to expand practicing Advanced Practice Nurses' (APNs) authority in the United States demonstrates how nurses influence legislative change. In one recent example, described by Smith and colleagues (2020), Virginia APNs used an incremental approach to move closer to full practice authority (FPA) with the passage of House Bill 793 (HB793): Nurse practitioners; practice agreements. In Virginia, APNs identified access to care as a problem related to APNs' limited scope of practice. Access to care and limited-scope problems were addressed over the years by incremental legislative actions. Collaborations continue with legislators, American Association of Nurse Practitioners (AANP), various other nursing organizations, hospital associations, the American Association for Retired People (AARP), major regional health systems, and the Medical Society of Virginia. Virginia APNs used outcome evidence to communicate their stance and neutralize opposing claims. These actions by Virginia nurses help to inform those states classified as reduced/restricted APN scope of practice, who continue to advance to join the 27 states plus the District of Columbia and Guam that are designated with FPA for APNs.

Clearly, knowing local representatives, informing them about health care issues, and advising them as to their constituents' needs are ways nurses become involved. Legislators are influenced by information received and by the sources of that information. Nurses have a wealth of knowledge about health care. The process of seeking to influence legislators' views and votes is called "**lobbying**." When an individual is employed to lobby, they are known as a "**lobbyist**" and are required to register as the representative of a special interest group. The American Nurse Association [ANA] located in Washington, DC, employs nurse lobbyists, as do many states. Individual nurses, however, can support colleagues who represent nursing's interests and who run for political office. The ANA Nurses Strategic Action Team (N-STAT) network is an organized grassroots effort by nurses to help elect endorsed candidates and to inform legislators about policy issues of concern to nurses. When nurses join N-STAT, they receive alerts and updates detailing specific legislative issues. Financial contributions to Nurses for Political Action Coalition, the ANA's political arm, increase the power base of nurses. Membership in professional and community groups provides nurses with the collective voice to influence legislators.

Communicating with legislators is essential and can be done by phone, writing a letter, personal visits, or email correspondence. Legislators have staffs of experts in various areas, and each legislator is assigned to committees. To understand the US legislative process, follow the progress of a bill. Thousands of bills are introduced at both the state level and the federal level and must be passed within 2 years or the bill will die by default. Once a bill has been introduced, it is referred to committee, and the committee chairperson determines which bills will be considered. Hearings are then held on the considered bills. When hearings have finished in committee, a bill is "reported out" at the federal level to the floor of the Senate or House of Representatives for a vote. Both the Senate and the House of Representatives must pass identical versions of the bill and, once passed by both chambers, it is forwarded to the president for signing. If signed, it is enacted into law (https://www.usa.gov/how-laws-are-made#item-213608). It is essential for nurses to lobby, to inform legislators of new issues, and to give expert testimony on introduced bills. Nurses who are politically aware extend the collective nursing voice to its full potential.

Nurses have multiple professional organizations that extend their collective voice. With high membership dues, nurses likely join only a few groups and may gravitate toward their specialty organization. Without a single national organization with the majority of nurses as members, nursing's voice is diluted. When organizations promote an issue, the collective voice of the group rather than the voice of the individual sends a more powerful message to influence policymakers. Without a collective voice, nursing's influence on shaping health care policy is weakened.

To strengthen nursing's collective voice, the ANA emphasizes collaboration with its state constituent organizations, specialty organizations, and nonnursing health organizations. Advancing nurses' political participation contributes to the ANA's ability to expand nurses' agendas (https://www.nursingworld.org/practice-policy/advocacy/).

Engaging students in these strategies early in legislative processes will help to provide more well-informed practicing nurses. Well-informed, empowered professional nurses play significant roles in supporting legislative initiatives that promote and protect the health of the public. Other ways for nurses to be involved in policy change are to support candidates and run for office. Volunteering during campaigns to help a specific candidate or to encourage voter registration and voting are ways that nurses can influence policy. Many nurses now represent their local constituencies and have increasing visibility at the state and national levels. For example, three nurses currently serve in the United States 118th Congress (http://www.nursingworld.org/MainMenuCategories/Policy-Advocacy/Federal/Nurses-in-Congress).

Community nurses' roles include the interaction of independent, interdependent, and dependent functions. Independent functions include analyzing and recognizing cues, prioritizing, taking action, generating solutions, and evaluating communities for health promotion and health education. Interdependent functions include collaboration with community members and interdisciplinary teamwork functions that are crucial to effective community health. Dependent functions include implementing therapeutic plans of team members.

Community health promotion includes all the following (US Department of Health and Human Services [USDHHS], 2024):

- Community participation, with representatives from multiple community sectors, including government, education, business, faith organizations, health care, media, voluntary agencies, and the public
- Assessment guided by a community-planning model to determine health problems, resources, perceptions, and priorities for action
- Targeted and measurable objectives to address health outcomes, risk factors, public awareness, services, and protection
- Comprehensive, multifaceted, culturally relevant interventions that have multiple targets for change
- Monitoring and evaluation of the objectives and strategies used

NURSING CLINICAL JUDGMENT AND THE COMMUNITY

Community nursing stems from a theoretical foundation that recognizes the effect of systems on health. General systems theory (described in Chapter 7) provides a foundation for how community nurses assess, plan, and evaluate (Stanhope & Lancaster, 2025). Because nursing theories often address self-care and individual-environment interaction, nurses are well prepared to function in this setting. Public health theory uses a population focus with risk identification to assess communities. Assessing aggregates is therefore an important part of community nursing assessment. For example, Parasuraman and de la Cruz (2019) used aggregate data from 95 National Healthy Start grantees to describe the high-risk populations served. Their aggregate data revealed potential areas for strategic planning to bridge gaps in access and utilization of services for National Healthy Start.

Nursing community assessment and clinical judgment address each community as unique and provide the rationale for the assessment. Community nurses use comprehensive and rigorous needs-assessment approaches that include all aspects of the community. In strength-based approaches and Gordon's (2014) functional pattern approach, positive factors play a consistent role in information gathering.

Gordon's (2014) health-related patterns provide a useful guide to collect observation, interview, and measurement data. Health-related patterns depend on community settings, assessment focus, and the preference of each community. Assessing all pattern areas provides a basic data set to analyze and use for comparison during evaluation (see Chapter 6).

Risk factors and development influence health patterns. For example, health concerns may occur in one pattern area, such as the increased age-related factor of teenage pregnancy (sexuality-reproductive pattern). Data from other areas may reveal that parental opposition (values-beliefs pattern) tends to restrict sex education and limit sex education in schools (coping–stress tolerance pattern). Attempting to restrict sex education or "ignoring" it in school and primary care may place the community at risk of unwanted pregnancy in its young people of childbearing age. Factors from several pattern areas may form clusters of risk for certain groups (see Chapter 6).

Methods of Data Collection

Nurses obtain assessment data through observation, interviews (including focus groups), and measurement. In community assessment, these three methods are often used in various combinations to ensure the validity of the information. Obtaining data through observation—often referred to as the "**windshield survey** approach to assessment"—includes the use of the senses (sight, touch, hearing, smell, and taste) to determine community appearances. These appearances include the types and condition of residential dwellings and their people and physical and biologic characteristics, such as animal and plant life, temperature, transportation, sounds, and odors. Some communities have a characteristic "flavor." A community's physical characteristics influence health. What type of space is available? What does the air feel and smell like? What does the water taste like? Children need space to run and play; young and middle-aged adults require space for recreation and exercise. What spatial barriers exist? Where is this space located in relation to traffic and schools? Kaczynski et al.'s (2018) research group, for example, used windshield surveys in 130 communities to determine whether certain neighborhood qualities were linked to youth physical activity. Community nurses obtain abundant subjective data by simply walking or riding around a community. Data obtained by observation provide important clues about the community, its actual or potential health problems, and its strengths.

Technologic advances such as the use of geographical information systems (GIS) and earth observation (EO) enhance nurses' abilities to assess communities. These advances provide a cost-effective approach to view community features such as vacant properties, illegal dumping, parks, tree canopy, aggravated assaults, and theft, for assessment of neighborhood irritants, neighborhood safety, walkability, pollen, and other environmental characteristics. The intensity of various area determinants such as recreational areas, proximity of health and other urban services, transportation flow, and pollution factors and their influence on health decisions are readily explored with GIS and EO. When combined with other assessment tools (survey, census, and large data sets, for instance), GIS and EO improve the precision of observation data collection (Thomson et al., 2019). Analysis of observation data generates hypotheses to explore further with use of interview, focus group, and measurement data.

Interview data, the most common source of information from people, include verbal statements from community residents, key community officials, health care personnel, and various community agency staff. **Key informants** provide useful ways to learn how members perceive their community. Key community leaders often provide important information about community health concerns, necessary health resources, and community strengths, along with particular health beliefs and community health goals. Community residents provide useful information about their perceptions of health, health concerns, and needs, as well as their perceptions of the availability, accessibility, and acceptability of health services. Health agency personnel provide data about health resources, the population served, availability, and perceptions of concerns and needs. Developing a basic set of questions in advance enhances the relevance of interview data.

Ideally, community partners collaborate to assess, plan, intervene, and evaluate using participatory approaches. In their comprehensive meta-review of community-engaged literature from 2005 to 2018, Ortiz's (2020) research group delineated the most commonly used concepts of community-based participatory approaches. Community-based participatory approaches described in these 100 reviews generally aimed to ameliorate health and social inequities by addressing the community context, partnering processes, collaborations, shared decision-making, trust, empowerment, reciprocity and outcomes, and social justice. Community-based participatory approaches continue to show promise for addressing community assessment, planning, intervention, and evaluation (Ortiz et al., 2020). For example, Duran et al.'s (2019) study group reported that productive community-based activities were generally guided by a community-based conceptual model, particularly in the areas of community context and collaboration strategies. Their findings generated useful recommendations to enhance community participation, such as sharing power, clarifying values, improving community capacity, and adopting action plans together. These useful recommendations depend on the ability of individuals and groups who differ from each other in culture, identity, research ability, and academic/community roles to progress toward mutually identified outcomes.

Community nurses who have expertise in building partnerships use community partnership models to conduct assessment, planning, the choosing of effective strategies, and evaluation (Table 8.1). In fact, current public health curricula should include community-based participatory research (CBPR) to address developing science, policy, and public

TABLE 8.1 Implementation of Community Health Plans with Objectives and Rationale

Goal: North High School population will have reduced incidence (at least 20%) of fatal motor vehicle accidents related to alcohol use and abuse by December.

Objective	Plans	Rationale
1. Community will have access to information about incidence of fatal motor vehicle accidents and drunken driving arrests of its high school population for the past 5 years by March	Interview local police about the incidence of fatal automobile accidents and substance abuse in the community. Interview parents of deceased high school students, students, teachers, physicians, clergy, and emergency department personnel about the incidence of the problem and suggested measures for decreasing the incidence; suggest that interviews be broadcast over the high school radio station. Have several people write to the community newspaper, commenting on the broadcast and the problem.	Unfreezing: For change to occur, the community has to become dissatisfied with the status quo and sense a need for change. Empiric-rational strategy: People are rational; discussion of facts can result in support for change. Important elements for preventing the problem include educating the public and having key community leaders discuss their views; concern lends credibility and is necessary for action. People tend to listen to those with informal power. Keeping the issue before the community can raise consciousness.
2. Community will take action to inform the population at risk about responsible drinking and driving by June	Suggest to the school principal and the school board the creation of a task force of community residents to plan a health program on individual responsibility and alcohol use in high school. Conduct focus group discussions with the task force and develop collaborative group goals and strategies. The task force should include teachers, students, parents, clergy, police, nurses, and physicians. The task force will examine ways to determine and teach content, integrate it into the curriculum, and recommend that community members, such as a nurse, be involved in teaching content.	Changing: Moving to a new level; community involvement will influence acceptability of changes. Community residents like to be involved in decision-making. It is important to establish trust and collaboration among community groups; this opens communication channels between adolescents and the health community. Community involvement facilitates acceptance of change.
3. Community will implement an educational program for its high school population related to use of alcohol and individual responsibility	Implement educational plans. Possible topics: Dispelling myths Knowing yourself Peer pressure Thinking about "The 3 Fs" (Family, Friends, and Future) Alcohol and other substances No phones Safe driving lessons	Refreezing: Moving to level of change brought about by community forces. Educational strategies built around the concept of individual responsibility are essential elements in promoting health of young adults.

From The Royal Canadian Mounted Police Centre for Youth Crime Prevention Accessed on January 31st, 2024 from (http://www.rcmp-grc.gc.ca/cycp-cpcj/id-cfa/lp-pl/index-eng.htm) State of Virginia; Safe Driving Lesson Plan (Driver Education | Virginia Department of Education; Accessed on January 31st, 2024 from https://www.quitalcohol.com/resource/organizations-fight-drinking-driving.

health concerns (Stanhope & Lancaster, 2025). The increased use of community-based participatory strategies has produced multiple resources for review. For example, the University of New Mexico Health Science Center, Center for Participatory Research houses many useful resources at their website (https://cpr.unm.edu/). This website provides a CBPR model that can be viewed at the following URL: https://hsc.unm.edu/population-health/research-centers/center-participatory-research/cbpr-community-engagement/cbpr-model.html

Additionally, a curriculum for CBPR can found at the Community-Campus Partnerships for Health website: https://www.ccphealth.org/cbpr-curriculum/.

Brockie and colleagues (2019) provide a useful delineation of the process they used to initiate a community-based partnership between universities and the Fort Belknap Indian Reservation in the Northern Plains region of Montana. The initial process of the partnership recognized the challenges this reservation experiences with health disparities, given limited resources and the resulting differences in outcomes. Addressing the historical context of oppression, prejudice, attempted annihilation, and geographic isolation was vital to the success of the community's projects. Mutual trust and collaboration strengthened the partnerships, resulting in joint goal setting, efficient use of resources, and delineation of boundaries for participants. These researchers describe their initial experience fully to facilitate the expansion of such partnerships to other communities (Brockie et al., 2019). These authors provide examples of how strategies initiated by engaged community members empower community partners and enhance the ability to transfer evidence-based strategies into their unique communities.

Measurement data use instruments to quantify data during information collection. Measurement data include population statistics, pollution indices, morbidity and mortality rates, census statistics, and epidemiologic data. These data can be accessed by the internet or locally in community libraries; health departments; environmental protection agencies; schools; police and fire departments; local health system agencies; and town, city, or state planning offices. Publicly supported agencies share their information, and community nurses readily use such data.

Sources of Community Information

Census information available from http://www.census.gov and found in libraries and public agencies is the most complete source for population information. Because the US Census is completed once every 10 years at the beginning of a decade, data for most communities become less accurate as the decade progresses. Community agencies and local planning commissions, project statistics, and developmental trends reflect ways in how nurses understand population patterns and dynamics. Many communities and states have databases available for public use.

Environmental measurement data can be obtained from the local branch of the US Environmental Protection Agency. Generally, local health departments monitor water, food, and sanitation systems. Nurses may be called on to facilitate safeguarding of natural resources to protect communities from industrial toxins. As private well water testing is not regulated in the United States, residents using well water should regularly test their water. Community health nurses can participate in interventions to promote testing to ensure the safety of water used in homes.

Concerns about water safety arise in communities within regions with active hydraulic fracturing, particularly with those residents who rely on well water for household use (Turley & Caretta, 2020). Hydraulic fracturing, a technique used to process liquid natural gas (LNG), provides great increases in national energy sources for the United States. However, water combined with chemicals used in LNG production forms contaminated hydraulic fracturing fluid, chemicals, and sedimentary radioactivity. Residents wonder whether these substances affect groundwater purity.

The Appalachian region's LNG production rose from 2% to 40% of the national LNG production during the early part of the 21st century. This rise in production created an increase in hydraulic fracturing fluid, which contains water, chemicals, and sedimentary radioactivity influencing water security (Turley & Caretta, 2020). Hydraulic fracturing in this region affects residents' perception of their communities' water security (water access, quality, and emotional aspects). Turley and Caretta (2020) studied aspects of water security of one Appalachian region in rural Northwestern West Virginia where 150,000 residents rely on groundwater for household use and hydraulic fracturing is widespread.

Turley and Carretta (2020) conducted 30 interviews with participants, most of whom relied on household groundwater and interacted with oil/gas companies, contractors, and regulators. These researchers focused on the affective aspect of water security, that is, the participants' subjective experiences regarding LNG production and water quality. Turley and Carretta (2020) describe participants' experiences of feeling uncertainty, marginalization, and exclusion from water-testing result reports. These researchers' interviews revealed that private water testing was financially prohibitive for most of the participants.

Community nurses in this setting could intervene using an integrated knowledge-to-action method. This method would include strategies including community outreach, home visits, and environmental home assessment planning. These strategies use community partnerships and home visits for informing the public and developing resources for citizens to test water in their private wells. Possible long-term public health initiatives for involvement of community health nurses in such environmental initiatives include training that include awareness, testing, and treatment; low-cost or no-cost convenient testing stations; and mandatory regulated enforced testing at the point of property transfer or when new wells are constructed.

Other sources to date include health departments, along with school nurses and administrators. Town, city, or county administrators provide information about land use, boundaries, housing conditions, utilities, and community services. Community newspapers supply information about community dynamics, health-related concerns, cultural activities, and community decision-making. The documentation techniques for community observation, interview, and measurement data are similar to those used for individuals and families. A triple-column format that separates the data obtained with each method facilitates recording.

COMMUNITY FROM VARIOUS PERSPECTIVES

Community From a Systems Perspective

Systems theory provides an overall framework to connect and integrate community data. Using systems, the nurse examines how the parts of a community interact with each other and with the entire community. Systems consist of interrelated, interacting parts or components within boundaries that filter both the type and the rate of input and output (Stanhope & Lancaster, 2025). Similar to how families form systems (see Chapter 7), communities viewed as systems have both structure and function. Assessment of communities includes exploration of aspects of the population within specific geographic areas.

Structure

The **structure of a community** system or subsystem consists of a formal or informal arrangement of parts, including both animate and inanimate properties. Nursing, which operates within the context of the health system, can be considered within the context of community systems. Fig. 8.2 displays the arrangement of the strong connections of family, individuals, and health delivery in a community system (Dietz et al., 2017). The broad macrosystem includes societal ideologies, population health, policy, social norms, and culture that shape the larger part of the system. The outer sphere encompasses numerous subsystems, such as training, education, and health equity (Dietz et al., 2017).

Communities' structural parts form the subsystems, each of which is in itself a system. Health agencies, schools, fire departments, and governmental bodies are examples of structural

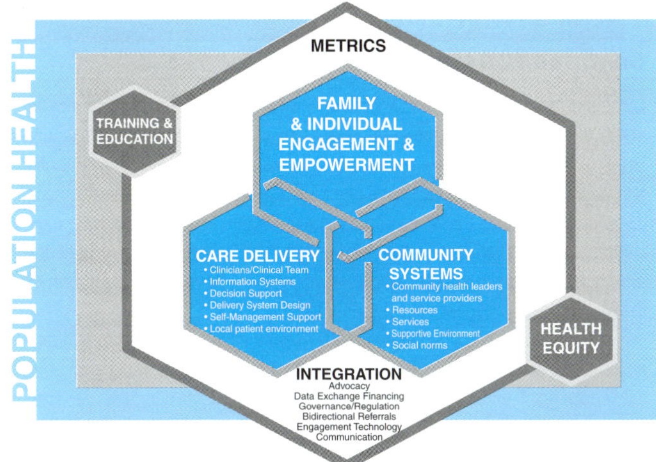

FIG. 8.2 Clinical-community integration model. (From Dietz, W. H., Belay, B., Bradley, D., Kahan, S., Muth, N. D., Sanchez, E., & Solomon, L. [2017]. A model framework that integrates community and clinical systems for the prevention and management of obesity and other chronic diseases. Washington DC: National Academy of Medicine. Accessed on February 1st, 2024 from https://doi.org/10.31478/201701b.)

parts. Bronfenbrenner's bioecological theory continues to be used in contemporary contexts (Kim et al., 2018). The subsystems, such as individuals, family, school, and community, lie within overarching macrosystems. These systems and subsystems interact and change over time within a social context. For example, in their study of bullying, Kim et al.'s (2018) research group explored influences related to systems—family relationships, gender, friendships, school environment, and development—using Bronfenbrenner's Bioecological Systems Theory as an underlying framework. In this study, microsystems included family and friendships. The researchers identified the macrosystems, although they were not measured, as values and policies of the larger society.

In their study, 374 female participants were randomly selected from five middle schools (7th-9th grade) in Korea. Consistent with similar studies, the microsystem factor of stress, particulary family and school stress, rose with the rate of rising bullying perpetration. This study illustrates how systems assessment provides valuable information about the interaction of systems in the arrangement and organization of the five specific middle-school communities. The authors suggest further studies should examine macrosystem, mesosystem, and exosystem factors for a better understanding of adolescent's bullying perpetration.

Community leadership provides direction for both health-promotion and health-protection activities; therefore, community assessment includes exploration of various community systems as they relate to health. The practice of viewing community structure as a population (collection of people) and considering the arrangement of the community's health care parts (existing health services) play an important role in the assessment process.

The study of populations is referred to as "**demography**." A population is a group defined as an aggregate of people who share similar personal or environmental characteristics. Demography provides information about population characteristics—such as numbers and racial composition, along with the distribution of age, sex, marital status, nationality, language, religious affiliations, education, and occupation. Demographic data provide a basis for analysis and a means to identify groups who may have a high risk of health concerns. Such information provides direction for health strategies. For example, examination of the age distribution over several years reveals important population shifts, with associated needs for additional health-promotion activities. The increasing numbers of individuals older than 65 years require changes in community health priorities that reflect this group's needs. Comparing population characteristics statistically enables nurses to make inferences about the community. Comparisons are made among three systems: the town, which is a part of the county; the county, which is a part of the larger system; and the state. Comparisons between affluent and poor communities, rural and urban communities, and diverse and homogeneous communities may provide important information for planning.

Function

The **function of a community** refers to the process of dynamic change, with adaptation in the system's parts and the ways that community systems and subsystems interact. Decision-making and allocation of health-promotion and health-protection resources are important considerations for community assessment. As health educators, nurses interact with communities to promote health. Community health promotion involves a complex array of responsibilities. Nurses act as advocates using proactive planning and collaboration with other disciplines and agencies. As a community liaison, the nurse establishes priorities for programming; matches resources with needs determined by a community needs assessment; empowers community members; and facilitates social, environmental, and political change. These multifaceted functions require expertise in communication and interpersonal relations that involve a deliberate approach. By using such an intentional process, while maintaining the community's vision, nurses can produce effective change.

Interaction

Through dynamic interaction with the environment, systems exchange matter, energy, and information (in communication forms such as verbal and behavioral) to make decisions. Interaction contributes to community systems' survival ability and protects and promotes the health of community members. Through environmental interactions, community systems use adaptation mechanisms. Nurses determine how communities apply these mechanisms toward health services. For example, policy that removes soft drink and candy sales from schools must consider lost revenue from these unhealthy but lucrative structures within the school system.

Various health-related patterns emerge from these interactions. For example, certain human-activity patterns negatively alter natural environmental patterns, which in turn influence human health patterns. Gordon's (2014) assessment framework focuses on 11 health-related functional patterns that assume community and environment interaction from a systems perspective.

Community From a Developmental Perspective

A framework based on developmental theory can be used to identify existing or potential health problems for particular age groups in communities. Community nurses, focusing on the total community population, use a developmental, age-correlated approach to identify health-promotion and health-protection activities.

Nurses identify age-related risks at each life stage, taking steps to maximize wellness and health promotion as a lifelong concern (USDHHS, 2024). For example, adolescent single mothers of infants, at risk both emotionally and physically for medical problems, require parenting skills. Accidents are the greatest threat to children's health; therefore, accident-prevention activities become a priority for communities with a young population and with adolescent mothers. Age-related risk factors (see Chapters 6 and 7) associated with individuals and families can be extended to include community groups, based on the demographics of the community.

Community From a Risk-Factor Perspective

Risk factors associated with disease, illness, and death rates, although not causally associated with them, predict the likelihood of a particular adverse health condition in communities of interest (USDHHS, 2024). Risk factors include a combination of demographic, psychological, physiologic, and environmental characteristics (or they may include a single characteristic). The influence of various risk factors differs from person to person and from group to group because of genetic composition, geographic location, lifestyle patterns, resources, socioeconomic status, education level, and community, neighborhood, or environmental variation (Box 8.2: Genomics). For example, age, sex, race, geographic location, consumption pattern, and lack of health services may be considered risk factors, because one or more may contribute to disease or death and place the population sharing them at risk (Box 8.3: Evidence-Based Practice). Some groups may be at high risk from a single risk factor, such as insufficient immunizations or exposure to asbestos. A combined potential for adverse health effects exists when many risk factors are present, because they interact in multiple ways and synergistically influence each other.

Communities therefore experience substantial variability in health conditions with regard to both incidence and susceptibility. Risk-factor theory views health and disease as multifactorial, with cause attributed to no single risk factor. For example, risk factors such as air pollution, smoking, and forms of radiation in various combinations may be related to high rates of lung cancer, emphysema, and bronchitis in a community. The potential to control risk factors and to provide relevant health-related resources forms the basis for health-promotion and health-protection activities.

BOX 8.2 GENOMICS

Community Assessment

Combinations of genetic, individual, and environmental factors interact to affect the risk of and/or protection from many chronic disorders, such as diabetes, Alzheimer's disease, cardiovascular disease, and depression. Genetic modifications at both the individual level and the community level affect these disorders. Moreover, these disorders modify genetic expression in both individuals and communities. Exchanges between the environment and genetics alter manifestations of these complex disorders. In contrast, manifestation of the disorder alters the environment and genetics.

The wide scope of community genetics spans all disciplines in health and addresses genetic screening, genetic literacy, and education, along with ethical, legal, social, and economic issues. As sequencing costs decrease, capacity for new therapy should increase for communities (Schmidtke & Cornel, 2020). For example, carrier screening for autosomal recessive disorders (e.g., sickle cell, cystic fibrosis, and Tay Sachs) is widely performed. Carrier screening commonly focuses on target populations for these disorders. Universal carrier screening, proposed by Rowe and Wright's (2020) research group, would include multiple recessive conditions and offer an option for a broader screening; however, established evidence and public health capacity hinder this expansion.

Expansion of the latest genome editing tools can permit the production of evidence for evolutionary propositions such as the "thrifty gene hypothesis" by including under-represented communities. Individuals of European descent (95%) predominate in the current genetic trials in the United States (Fox et al., 2020). Using these new tools becomes particularly meaningful when exploring genetic predisposition disorders such as diabetes, which affects large numbers of under-represented communities (Fox et al., 2020).

Several researchers have begun to prepare the way for expansion by exploring utilization of genetic services in community settings. Miller et al.'s (2020) research team surveyed 108 high-risk patients about their potential use of genetic services. The majority (78%) were interested in using the services and intended (75.0%) to use the services if offered. Cancer risk influenced 63% to 70.6% of responses. Apprehension (37%) and cost (39.6%) were viewed as obstacles to seeking screening (Miller et al., 2020).

One study explored the feasibility of collecting saliva samples from a group of individuals of Pacific Island (PI) descent from Southern California using a community-based participatory approach (Kwan et al., 2020). In this study, samples were collected by trained and trusted PI community leaders from the partner sites. The participants' ($n = 214$) interest in assisting the development of science and their community guided their decision. These current projects highlight the need to approach community genetics from an evidence-based, ethical, and community-based participatory perspective.

GORDON'S FUNCTIONAL HEALTH PATTERNS: ASSESSMENT OF THE COMMUNITY

A variety of functional health pattern assessments are used with communities. Nurses use Gordon's (2014) Functional Health Reference Assessment as exemplified in this chapter or other assessments described in the literature.

Health Perception–Health Management Pattern

The health perception–health management pattern identifies data about community health status, health-promotion and disease-prevention practices, and community members' perceptions of health (Gordon, 2014). Residents may perceive a substance abuse problem in adolescents or a high rate

BOX 8.3 EVIDENCE-BASED PRACTICE

Viewpoints From Grandchildren, Grandparents Caring for Them, and Community Informants About Housing

Polvere and colleagues (2018) used a qualitative study design to explore the housing needs in five communities of the US state of New York. These communities reflected urban, rural, and suburban environments throughout the state. As with other communities in the United States, more African American participants cared for their grandchildren than other racial or ethnic participants. In this study, the percentage of African American grandparent caregivers was about 10% higher than the African American population in the state.

In this study, the researchers used focus groups with grandparents ($n = 46$) and the children ($n = 34$) who lived with them, along with interviews with 17 key informants. The grandparents' ages ranged from 46 to 88 (average age 66) and children ranged from elementary school age to college, with most in middle school or high school. Housing arrangements included renting (68%), owning (30%), and shelters (2%).

These participants indicated that lack of resources contributes to their inability to escape unacceptable, dangerous accommodations. Aging grandparents face possible family role identity changes, decreases in abilities needed to care for children, and ineligibility for government programs. Polvere and colleagues (2018) highlight the overarching issues of poverty and financial burden among the aging population and how those factors contribute to added stress for grandparents caring for children. This study concurs with other research about grandparents in caregiving situations and the role resources play in the ability to care adequately for their children's offspring. Moreover, the study gives voice to grandchildren's perspectives on their housing needs.

of unwanted pregnancies, breast cancer, or sexually transmitted disease as concerns. Community health nurses provide data to address perceived health issues and mutually develop community health management plans. For example, national data provide evidence for the extent of the perceived health issue of increases in their community's illegal substance use. The National Institute on Drug Abuse (https://www.drugabuse.gov/related-topics/trends-statistics) identified that the United States suffers greater than $700 billion each year from crime, loss of work productivity, and health care related to the top areas of abuse: tobacco, alcohol, and prescription opioids (Dickerson et al., 2020).

Responding to complexities of the prescription opioid abuse epidemic requires a multifaceted approach. Because opioid analgesics maintain an important role in therapeutic management of pain, regulating availability rather than banning the substance as illicit plays a role in the response. As the opioid crisis has evolved, fatalities have increased in the presence of a decrease in opioid prescriptions. These fatalities seem linked to a change in use of opioids: the shift is to combining opioids with psychostimulants and/or synthetic opioids such as fentanyl (Volkow & Blanco, 2021). Community partners compare these national data and trends with local data to determine public health issues to pursue.

Valuable information can be elicited by nurses conducting focus group discussions and by interviewing key community members about their health concerns and issues. Mortality and morbidity statistics and other public health information sources provide measurement data.

Nutritional-Metabolic Pattern

The nutritional-metabolic pattern identifies data relevant to community consumption habits as reflected in accessibility and availability of food stores and subsidized food programs for infants, children, and older adults. Community well-being, which depends on adequate dietary habits, food intake, and supply of nutrients, is influenced by culture, the presence or absence of kitchen facilities, and adequate plumbing.

Community assessment includes the collection of data by driving or walking through the community while using all five senses; it provides information about grocery stores, fast-food establishments, ethnic shopping facilities, and street corner vendors. Even affluent and developed countries contain areas without adequate access to food, or "food deserts," places where fresh food is not available. Income and food insecurity are highly correlated. The USDA contends that 10.2% of the population is classified as food insecure. For low-income households, this number approaches 26.5% (https://www.ers.usda.gov/topics/food-nutrition-assistance/). Movements to respond to food insecurity and access have evolved, promoting strategies such as backyard gardening, community gardening, community-supported agriculture, and local markets (Aptekar & Myers, 2020). Government programs, private soup kitchens, and food donations by houses of worship provide information about nutritional patterns of communities.

Elimination Pattern

The elimination pattern identifies environmental factors, including exposure to pollutants in the community through contaminated soil, water, and air, and the food chain. This pattern further classifies environmental factors into two broad categories—physical and biologic. Alterations in environmental processes threaten the health and integrity of communities, necessitating health-promotion and health-protection activities. For example, humans eliminate endocrine-disrupting chemicals, pharmaceuticals, and personal care products into the environment (Ohoro et al., 2019). Antibiotics and hormones from animals and fish contaminate the environment. Groundwater, drinking water, surface water, and treatment plant effluents can be affected. Furthermore, some contaminants transform into contaminants that are more toxic than the original substance.

Physical agents include geologic, geographic, climatic, and meteorologic aspects of the community. Acute respiratory disease and aggravated asthmatic episodes place certain population groups at risk when the air quality is poor. For example, Liévanos (2019) reported that individuals in Black and Hispanic neighborhoods in the San Joaquin Valley of California were more likely exposed to pollutants than those in White neighborhoods. In this same study, neighborhoods with predominantly Black residents experienced more asthma-related emergency department visits and delivery of low birth-weight infants. Schools located in high-pollution or high-traffic areas expose children to polluted air. Furthermore, home cooking devices, particularly those used inside the home, can expose families to polluted air (Coker et al., 2020). Use of solid-fuel combustion such as wood or coal for cooking inside produces polluted home air and may result in increased respiratory risk and lower intelligence quotient (IQ) levels in children (Benka-Coker et al., 2020; Brabhukumr et al., 2020; Coker et al., 2020; Estévez-García et al., 2020). Community health nurses can use the WHO Clean Household Energy Solutions Toolkit (CHEST) to plan interventions (WHO, 2024). Depending on resources, community collaborations, and partnerships, the community health nurse may use a variety of possible interventions to eliminate home air pollution from solid-fuel cooking indoors. These interventions include simple chimney stoves with adequate exhaust, stoves with fan-assisted combustion, and/or clean fuel (WHO, 2024).

The geographic locations of communities and major waterways, highways, or mountains located within communities act as barriers to access health facilities. Inaccessibility of health care services hinder health in at-risk groups. Knowledge of climatic conditions provides clues to susceptibility to illness resulting from temperature or humidity in certain populations.

Biologic agents include living things—such as plants, animals and their waste products, disease agents, microbial pathogens, and toxic substances—that can be hazardous to health. For example, Lyme disease, viral hepatitis, pneumonia, influenza, and the large number of diseases associated with childhood continue to be threats to community health. Observation, focus groups, and interviews with key community members reveal information concerning elimination patterns. The Environmental Protection Agency (http://www.epa.gov/) and the CDC (http://www.cdc.gov/) provide excellent resources for community health nurses.

Activity-Exercise Pattern

The activity-exercise pattern identifies physical activities and recreational options within communities. Science and technology have increasingly influenced productivity while simultaneously reducing or eliminating physical work. Consequently, physical activity no longer occurs during the workday for most community members, leaving leisure time as the only time for physical activity. Physiologic evidence demonstrates that physical activity improves many biologic measures associated with health and psychological functioning. Regular physical activity and musculoskeletal fitness are important for healthy, independent living as people grow older. Physical activity reduces the risk of many diseases, including obesity, heart disease, hypertension, cancer, osteoporosis, and diabetes mellitus.

Observation, focus groups, and interviews provide clues to a community's ability to provide cultural and recreational activities (Fig. 8.3). Furthermore, noting whether the community has evidence of recreational facilities or is a "built community" with physical activity options (such as bike/walking trails), assessing transportation options, and observing community development that encourages walking should be included in the community assessment of the activity-exercise pattern.

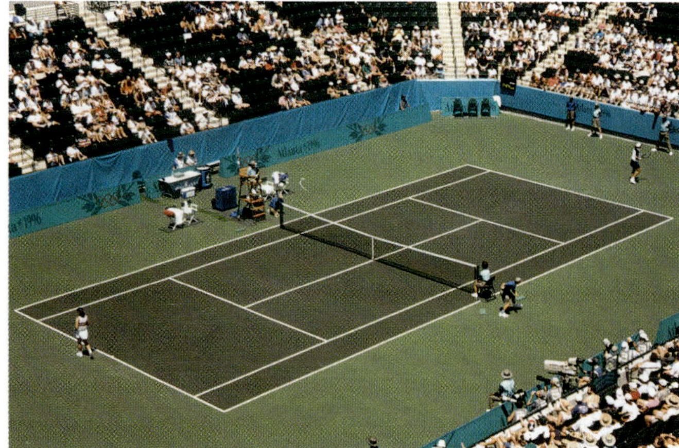

FIG. 8.3 The activity-exercise pattern identifies a community's physical activities and recreational options.

Sleep-Rest Pattern

The sleep-rest pattern identifies a community's rhythm of sleeping, resting, and relaxing. Some towns never close, with stores, traffic flow, and recreational facilities operating during both day and night hours. This ongoing activity produces unpleasant disturbances, such as unwanted noise that may be harmful to community well-being. Excessive noise from highways or airplanes produces physiologic or psychological problems eliciting responses ranging from mild irritation to pain or permanent hearing loss. Although noise cannot be eliminated, efforts to minimize and control it are possible. Observation, focus groups, and interviews provide clues to this pattern.

Cognitive-Perceptual Pattern

The cognitive-perceptual pattern identifies information about problem-solving and decision-making within communities. Systems depend on decision-making and resource allocation processes for survival. Communities require functional decision-making bodies to ensure adherence to rules and attainment of goals. Individual patterns and environmental patterns connect with important implications for community health. Community assessment includes appraisal of interaction with the environment, as in the participatory processes of community-based system dynamics. The effectiveness of the strategies used depends on a collaborative evolution and long-term commitment of the nurse in the community (Duran et al., 2019).

One strategy, bargaining, offers communities a plan to exchange resources for health service. For example, a community that owns a mammography machine but has no primary care facility might negotiate with another community to provide mammography in return for primary care services. Strategies using outside authority (legal bureaucratic methods) ensure compliance through rules and structures. In this case, states may mandate that communities maintain certain health standards. For example, a law may require all school children to be immunized against specific diseases before they enter public school. Cooperative strategies promote health when members share common goals (Duran et al., 2019). For example, community residents may unite to oppose a chemical landfill that is a health hazard.

Convincing people to comply because they hold some loyalty in the situation or relationship is another method that mobilizes communities. For example, community residents might expend a great deal of effort and money to retain a particular health clinic because of loyalty to the agency. Identifying decision-making patterns used by communities provides clues about health priorities and values, as well as matches and mismatches between existing circumstances, health goals, and planning strategies. Data can best be obtained by observation, focus groups, and interviews.

Self-Perception–Self-Concept Pattern

The self-perception–self-concept pattern identifies self-worth and personal identity of communities. Characteristics such as image, status, and perceived competency with problem-solving indicate community self-concept. Housing conditions, buildings, and cleanliness reflect community image. School systems, crime rates, accidents, and opinions about whether the community is considered a good place to live suggest community perception of self-worth. Competency with social and political issues as well as community spirit create positive self-evaluation. Community pride facilitates development of innovative health programs. Emotional tone (fear, depression, or positive emotional outlook) relates to findings in other pattern areas. For example, tensions in the cognitive-perceptual pattern (conflict between groups concerning health issues) may explain a general feeling of fear among the residents. Data are obtained through observation, focus groups, and interviews.

Roles-Relationships Pattern

The roles-relationships pattern identifies communication styles along with formal and informal relationships. Of particular concern are roles and relationships affecting community ability to realize health potential. Patterns of crime, racial incidents, and social networks form indices of human relationships in communities. Publicizing health promotion becomes more effective when patterns of official communication are used. Health program success depends on support from prominent community members. Community members involved in health programs help identify other key community leaders. Use of media and other mass information programs improves communication, the flow of health information, and the number of community members reached. Interviews, television, the internet, and newspapers are examples of ways to obtain and convey information.

Sexuality-Reproductive Pattern

The sexuality-reproductive pattern identifies reproductive data of communities, which is reflected in live birth statistics, mothers' ages, ethnicity, and marital status. This information provides clues to the health-promotion needs of a particular community group. Premature infant rates, low birth-weight infants, and abortion rates, as well as neonatal, infant, and maternal death rates, reflect reproductive patterns of communities. Such information identifies at-risk groups on the basis of particular characteristics associated with these rates. Mismatches between existing health services, health education, and community health statistics indicate health concerns. Availability of sex education in schools, the levels of spousal and child abuse, and the number of sex-related crimes indicate health-promotion issues. Minutes of meetings, health records, statistical data, and public documents provide sources for these data; in addition, throughout 2020 and 2021, provision for sexual and reproductive health care was disrupted in the United States, with limited access to reproductive health services (Vussel et al., 2022).

Coping–Stress Tolerance Pattern

The coping–stress tolerance pattern identifies the community's ability to cope or adapt. Communities respond to stress in different ways, some of which might threaten their integrity. Community responses reveal the group coping patterns. Communities develop abilities to exchange goods, services, goals, values, and ideals to survive and to promote community health. Community efforts to obtain goods from the environment, contain goods within the environment, retain goods within the community, and dispose of goods play significant roles in influencing health. Examples of resources that communities obtain from the environment to promote health include local, state, or federal funding; health services; health-related workforce personnel; new knowledge; and technologic advances.

Some communities obtain abundant health care services; however, primary services often remain inadequate or nonexistent. Lack of available health services, or lack of ability to obtain them, characterizes community health need. Examples of problems communities may attempt to control include sex-related crimes, diseases, substance abuse, industry, hazardous waste in the water supply, and noxious chemicals in the air.

Community coping patterns aim to retain certain health-protection services, such as immunization services for children and adequate health facilities. Coping efforts may include strict zoning laws and housing codes or certain values such as sex education within the home. Expendable goods of communities include industrial and human waste. Data can be obtained through minutes of meetings, public documents, health surveys, statistical data, and health records.

Values-Beliefs Pattern

The values-beliefs pattern identifies the community values and beliefs. Such information provides clues for health-promotion and health-protection efforts valued by the community. Values underlie decisions about community health education and tax support for schools, hypertension screening for the public, disease-prevention programs, and well-child clinics. Traditions, norms, and cultural and ethnic groups share values and beliefs in communities. Data can be obtained through focus groups and through interviews with key community members and health-related personnel.

ANALYSIS WITH THE COMMUNITY

Analysis refers to data categorization and pattern determination. Data synthesis and organization occur to ascertain patterns of health activities and trends. An example of a clinical scenario about a particular community is presented in the Case Study and care plan at the end of this chapter. Decision-making and clinical judgment are essential during the analysis phase. Table 8.2 presents an example of one way to organize community data using Prochaska's Stages of Change (Pender et al., 2020).

TABLE 8.2 Stages of Change

Stages	Interventions
Precontemplation	Provide information (identify risk factors) Raise doubts about current behaviors and future outcomes
Contemplation	Discuss risks of not changing Discuss benefits of changing
Planning or preparation	Help plan phases of change Help implement phases of change
Action	Help develop strategies to prevent relapse, emphasizing self-efficacy Offer encouragement
Maintenance	Highlight past successes and future benefits

Modified from Pender, N. J., Murdaugh, C. L., & Parsons, M. A. (2020). Health promotion in nursing practice (8th ed.). Upper Saddle River, NJ: Pearson.

Organization of Data

Charts, figures, and tables graphically display population distributions, morbidity and mortality data, and vital statistics to pinpoint significant community concerns about actual or potential health problems along with health-related responses to these concerns. Another valuable organizational technique—mapping—facilitates data analysis. For example, a series of maps gathered with use of technology such as GIS display data that change over time. Analysis of several variables occurs simultaneously. Overlap of the locations of environmental hazards, densely populated areas, health-promotion services, and major highways becomes apparent. Poor environmental conditions; the distribution of illness, disease, and death rates; and accessibility of health-protection and health-promotion activities for the population appear at a glance with dotted scatter maps. Use of maps requires knowledge about the community's population base.

Less-populated rural areas with fewer health facilities or fewer neonatal deaths in a community with fewer females of childbearing age are examples of how population statistics influence interpretation of mapping techniques. Use of theoretical frameworks for community health and Gordon's (2014) 11 pattern areas facilitate analysis of community data. Several guidelines, presented next, help community nurses analyze population data. Analysis often supports the need for further data collection.

Guidelines for Data Analysis

Check for Missing Data

The complexity, size, and number of community characteristics prohibit the gathering of all possible facts about the health-related pattern areas; however, missing or insufficient data that indicate areas for further assessment should be identified. Additional assessment may determine specific approaches or a particular **community mutual goal setting**. Examples of missing data in community assessment include pollution indices, links between health resources and population groups, accessibility to resources, and morbidity statistics. Dates for census data used should be noted.

The nurse examines community data for incongruities and conflicting information. For example, a key community official might deny the existence of pollutants in the water supply, whereas newspaper reports of health department water analysis findings indicate otherwise. The nurse evaluates such inconsistencies before identifying existing or potential health concerns.

Identify Patterns

Clues about a **community pattern** emerge from subjective and objective data gathered. During this stage, community nurses make decisions, begin to formulate hypotheses (ideas and tentative judgments about possible health concerns), identify community groups that might be at risk, and establish probable causes or relationships. Ideas generated from this activity direct the search for additional clues in the data to confirm, reject, or revise hypotheses. Judgments about hypotheses continue to support patterns in the data.

To narrow the huge list of possible community health-promotion and health-protection concerns, community nurses formulate broad problem statements based on the health-related pattern areas (Gordon, 2014). For example, the community nurse differentiates among elimination problems (e.g., noxious chemicals), coping and stress-tolerance problems, and health perception–health management problems (e.g., high teenage mortality rate from motor vehicle accidents). Developing these general categories facilitates analysis.

Apply Theories, Models, Norms, and Standards

Analysis of community data requires extensive knowledge of developmental and age-related risks, as well as theories and concepts of nursing, public health, and epidemiology. Such a broad foundation enables nurses to identify additional clues in health-related patterns that contribute to community intervention. Developmental approaches form a basis to identify groups with potential health concerns. Age groups differ in susceptibility; therefore, nurses examine community resources directed toward highly susceptible groups. For example, community data that show increases in the number of live births among older females indicate a need for health-promotion services for this group. If community data show increasing numbers of aging citizens, nurses explore the availability and accessibility of existing health services for this older group.

Analysis of data for common personal or environmental characteristics occurs. For example, select groups may be at risk on the basis of a shared health concern, such as substance abuse, lack of immunizations, unsafe housing conditions, high exposure to asbestos or noxious chemicals, or inadequate health services. Shared characteristics, such as recent immigration status or ethnicity, provide clues to susceptibility and the need for screening activities. For example, male populations warrant screening for prostate cancer. Additionally, community literacy contributes to health-promotion activity development methods used by nurses to establish educational programs. A low literacy level limits the ability to use all available resources.

Environmental information is readily available on the internet. Databases and search engines provide useful information about environmental hazards and other environmental problems in communities. Prevention of disease worldwide depends on the dissemination of global environmental health information (USDHHS, 2024). Analysis of data relies on standards developed nationally or globally. For example, community data regarding air quality can be compared with state or national ambient air quality standards to determine health. In this context, the term "**ambient**" refers to outside air in a town, city, or other defined region. In the United States, air-monitoring stations are generally located in urban and rural areas within each state. One source for air quality information is the CHARTing Health Information for Texas, which is maintained by the University of Texas Health Science Center at Houston School of Public Health. The goal of this center is to serve as a resource in Texas for publicly available data to use for analysis and research. Data and links to other sites are continually monitored and updated (University of Texas Health Science Center at Houston, 2019). Current information about community resources enables more effective strategies to prevent risk factors and avoid health problems. Internet access facilitates identification of gaps in health-promotion and health-protection services.

Identify Strengths and Health Concerns

Interpretation of community data occurs with regard to community concerns, community strengths, and feasibility studies. Community nurses make judgments and inferences about community health, community responses to health situations, and population needs. One approach assumes health concerns exist unless assessment data indicate otherwise (Gordon, 2014). Other systems of assessment base decisions on community strengths. With the problem-focused assessment of health concerns, nurses make judgments based on summarized data using the nursing process, which results in one or more of the following determinations:

- No problem exists, but providing health-promotion or health-protection services may address a potential health concern. For example, providing health education in a high school could offset a potential for increased sexually transmitted disease in the high school population.
- A problem exists but is recognized by community members or health-related professionals with effective strategies for problem-solving, for example, flu or COVID immunizations.
- A problem exists that the community recognizes, but resources are inadequate or the community has not responded. Assistance is needed, for example, with the problem of highway traffic noise.
- A problem exists that the community recognizes but cannot cope with at this time, such as a lack of fluoridated water systems. Dentists, nurses, and nutritionists could be assigned to assist the community in resolving actual problems of dental caries.
- A problem or potential health concern exists that needs further study, for example, lack of sidewalks near schools.

Use of strength-based approaches to assessment emphasizes strengths and integrates health-promotion and health-protection activities into a person's plans. For example, a community may have nutritional feeding programs for older adults, females, and children that are underutilized. Community members may not use them because communication is inadequate. Examples of community strengths and concerns are shown in Table 8.3.

Identify Causes and Risk Factors

Data are examined for factors or characteristics that contribute to identified potential and existing health-related concerns. Nurses make inferences about population groups and identify risk factors. Identification of risk factors guides community nursing actions. Some risk factors signify immediate health concerns, such as a polluted water supply, whereas other risk factors indicate potential problems, such as lack of knowledge of childhood disease prevention. Nurses consider whether **community risk factors** can be altered, eliminated, or regulated through nursing actions. Nurses modify risk factors, when possible by using strategies such as health education (Box 8.4: Health and Social Determinants/Health Equity).

Community Analysis

Community assessment, as previously described, culminates in analysis. The following components are included in the community planning process: community situations or states within a population or population group; data collection using some combination of observation, focus groups, interview, and measurement; a framework; existing or potential health concerns; risk factors related to health concerns; and potential solutions through nursing actions (Gordon, 2014). Box 8.5: Quality and Safety Scenario and Box 8.6: Best Practice provide an overview of how workplace violence contributes to quality and safety and how leaders might intervene to prevent or defuse violence.

Community problem structuring facilitates communication among community health professionals, team members, and community members through the use of clear and concise nomenclature with development of categories using both inductive and deductive reasoning specific to community nursing (Stanhope & Lancaster, 2025).

Structural aspects include those related to the population, such as the demographic characteristics of groups with similar

TABLE 8.3 Examples of Community Strengths and Concerns

Strengths	Concerns
Well-child clinic available	Unavailable
Meal program accessible to older adults	Inaccessible
Sex education in schools acceptable	Unacceptable
Family planning services accessible	Inaccessible
Fluoridated water system	Nonfluorinated water system
Open communication	Miscommunication
Interagency cooperation	Dysfunctional transactions
Adequate kitchen and plumbing facilities	Inadequate
High interest of key leaders in health promotion	Lack of interest

BOX 8.4 HEALTH AND SOCIAL DETERMINANTS/HEALTH EQUITY

Addressing Health Equity in the Design of Health Promotion Interventions

Health promotion strategies for culturally diverse populations present a number of challenges. In fact, one NIH funding mechanism, Interventions for Health Promotion and Disease Prevention in Native American (NA) Populations, was designed to address challenges encountered by the US NA community. This mechanism funded programs to develop and test strategies addressing health issues disproportionate in these populations, and 21 of these studies were explored for their success (Dickerson et al., 2020).

These 21 studies often relied on CBPR approaches to design their ultimate implementations to garner culturally appropriate knowledge and viewpoints from the community. They used theories of the community along with Western frameworks. Although the researchers were attuned to cultural needs, their measures remained consistent with Western data collection methods to facilitate comparison with other data sets. Furthermore, these studies adapted evidence-based strategies using formative methods during the study development.

For example, 1 of the 21 studies used Intertribal Talking Circles to garner culturally appropriate views from the community representatives and Caring Contacts to intervene with suicide prevention (Walters et al., 2020). This same study used the Yup'ik concept of Qungasvik (Tools of Life) to address alcohol and suicide risk prevention in their community's youth population. This toolbox is available at the following URL: http://www.qungasvik.org/preview/. The toolbox incorporates local adaptation of cultural activities that include both Native Alaska and postcolonial strategies using Yup'ik change theory that is capable of fusing with Western change approaches. Another example is the use of a wood stove intervention where the ecological knowledge of the communities' cultural leaders was used to design three short films with partnering communities.

These studies illustrate how community nurses might approach diverse populations to facilitate health promotion and health improvement. Creatively addressing impediments to promote health in diverse communities involves:

- Garnering culturally appropriate knowledge and viewpoints from the community
- Using theories from the community along with Western frameworks
- Adhering to Western methods of data collection
- Adapting evidence-based strategies to the community's cultural beliefs and practices

CBPR, Community-based participatory research; *NA,* Native American; *NIH,* National Institutes of Health

characteristics (preschool children, adolescents, or a high school population). Functional aspects include those related to the psychosocial, physiologic, or spiritual health patterns, such as decision-making (cognitive-perceptual pattern) or communication links among health care resources (roles-relationships pattern). Functional health patterns guide data collection about health concerns and risk factors. Structural and functional aspects of the community provide a framework for plans (see Chapter 6).

PLANNING WITH THE COMMUNITY

Community health planning begins with analysis. Nurses design goals to resolve existing or potential health concerns. For example, high rates of childhood diseases in the community require goals aimed at decreasing rates. Identification of specific or potential health concerns with planned actions to achieve desired **community outcomes** provides the framework and data for **community evaluation**.

Purposes

The following are major purposes of the planning phase:

- Prioritization of problems and identification of interventions and plans through assessment
- Differentiation of problems resolved through nursing actions from those best resolved by others
- Identification of immediate, intermediate, and long-term goals, as well as behavioral objectives oriented to the community derived from the goals and specific actions to achieve objectives
- Formalization of a community nursing care plan (see the care plan at the end of this chapter) that includes written problems, actions, and expected behavioral outcomes

The planning phase culminates in a nursing plan that provides the framework for evaluation. Once developed, the plan is implemented. The costs associated with the delivery of health services and personnel, as well as the financial resources available, influence the priorities for implementation. Community values and the nurse's philosophy about people, health, the community, and nursing influence implementation. High-priority issues often include infectious agents, sexually transmitted disease, alcohol and drug use, smoking, inadequate nutrition, inadequate infant and childcare, high death rate from motor vehicle accidents, texting while driving, heroin overdose, and unwanted teenage pregnancies.

Community participation in health planning facilitates effective assignment of priorities. As health service recipients, community members strive for reasonably priced, high-quality services. Residents aim to acquire appropriate benefits for the needs and concerns of the population. Communication and the rationale for designating priorities help to resolve differences in opinion.

During the planning phase, nurses determine those problems most amenable to **community nursing intervention**, behavior implemented by the nurse to fulfill a health goal of the community. Community nurses differentiate problems nursing can resolve from those health concerns that could best be managed by community members, referred to health-related professionals, or handled with community support. Nurses refer problems related to the presence of rodents, poor sanitation conditions, or the absence of community recreational facilities to appropriate community leaders or agencies.

Community nurses focus on determining goals, developing measurable behavioral objectives, and designating actions to achieve expected outcomes. Nurses describe specific behaviors intended to reach projected outcomes. Evaluation includes appraisal of the effectiveness of nursing actions. Health planning emphasizes promoting and protecting population health; therefore, problems, solutions, and actions are defined at the group level. Community nurses plan and implement health plans for groups, such as school-age children, and facilitate development of health-promotion services for all residents. Nurses frequently act as change agents by taking responsibility for influencing health patterns and behavior. Decisions about health interventions stem

BOX 8.5 QUALITY AND SAFETY SCENARIO

Workplace Violence

Targets for violent acts may be places where people work to support their families. Workplace violence was once considered to consist of isolated, unplanned incidents that fell under the jurisdiction of the federal Occupational Safety and Health Administration (OSHA). Currently, workplace violence prevention and preparation often include external threats of terrorism. Furthermore, post–COVID-19, evidence suggests increased prevalence rates of anxiety, depression, and insomnia among health care providers as identified factors that could increase violence within the workplace (Jahan et al., 2021). The following are some recommendations to minimize workplace violence:

- Encourage public awareness campaigns.
- Develop workplace policies and plans.
- Adopt a zero-tolerance workplace violence policy.
- Apply preventive law enforcement policies.
- Perform background checks on employees.
- Study government agencies that make workplace violence a priority.
- Provide proper training for employees, supervisors, and managers about warning signs of violent behavior.
- Encourage a workplace culture that facilitates health relationships, creative problem-solving, and voicing concerns, while discouraging a hostile environment.
- Expect nonautocratic leadership styles.
- Prevent/minimize negative coworker behavior.
- Encourage social support (listening, recognition) for employees to succeed at their work.
- Implement strategies to minimize absenteeism, turnover, and low performance.
- Implement strategies to encourage participatory management.
- Ensure protection of the abused person when domestic violence or stalking occurs in the workplace.
- Develop and distribute clear and comprehensive legal and legislative guidelines.
- Evaluate programs and strategies after they have been implemented.
- Suggestions for approaches include the following strategies:
- Educational efforts should reflect cooperative efforts by government agencies, major corporations, unions, and advocacy groups, with OSHA acting as a facilitator and coordinator.
- Multidisciplinary no-threats/no-violence policies and prevention plans should be enacted.
- Violence prevention training should occur regularly and include practicing the plan.
- The work space and policies should provide a physically secure work environment.
- Preventive measures should be established, including documenting incidents, planning antiviolence strategies, and conducting threat assessments.
- Systems should be developed for the monitoring of incidents of workplace violence.
- Resource lists should be maintained and include social services, mental health, legal, and other agencies that provide assistance.
- Training programs should extend community policing concepts to workplace violence. Government or private organizations should develop training materials for small employers. Employers should keep the abuser out of the workplace (e.g., screening telephone calls, making the victim's work space physically more secure, instructing security guards or receptionists).
- Employers should provide resources for emotional, financial, and legal counseling. Clear, comprehensive, and uniform legal guidelines should be distributed widely.
- Incentives for employers should be identified and instituted.

COVID-19, Coronavirus disease 2019; *OSHA,* Occupational Safety and Health Administration.
Modified from Occupational Safety and Health Administration. (n.d.). Workplace Violence. Retrieved from https://www.osha.gov/SLTC/workplaceviolence/index.html (Accessed January 16, 2024)

BOX 8.6 BEST PRACTICE

Engaging Communities with Health Innovation

One innovative method for promoting empathy-driven, human-centered community engagement is called "Design Thinking" (van der Westhuizen et al., 2020). Design Thinking relies on comprehending and responding to the affective components of the experiences of others, including an ability to accept uncertainty while creating solutions.

The Design Thinking process includes inspiration (problem identification and motivations), ideation (idea testing), and implementation (forming concrete action plans).

A qualitative study of students partnering with community stakeholders to design a strategy for health promotion was used to explore the use of Design Thinking. Medication compliance in an elderly community in South Africa was the focus of their project. Students met with residents and both shared their backgrounds and roles played in the community. This sharing included aspects of identity that emphasized the unique skill set of the team, such as technical writer or candlemaker, rather than academic titles. The aim during this "entry" phase is to establish trust and allow each participant to participate fully.

In the next phase of ideation, ideas and models are launched with participation of the entire team along the way. The community stakeholders, however, hold the primary place for formalizing the ideas. The aim is to coconstruct the models with ongoing participation in development of the ideas, rather than merely requesting input from the community on a final model presented by the academics/professionals.

Design Thinking includes the aim for the end users to own the strategy adopted. Community participants at times may be reluctant to voice concerns about a strategy. Expecting and encouraging community stakeholders to challenge ideas during the process creates a more accurate perspective of the community.

Clearly, Design Thinking creates an innovative method to engage communities with academic agencies. The complex skill sets for implementing Design Thinking include experiential learning and a knowledge of the community and its specific needs. Promoting active participation in a trusting, sharing environment during design development establishes an environment for mutual planning and implementing of community health promotion programs. Ownership of the project may facilitate sustainability of the models designed.

from community nurses' appreciation of human behavior and principles of planned change.

Planned Change

Planned change results from efforts by individuals or groups and involves fundamental shifts in behavior (Pender et al., 2020). Individuals act as agents of their own health conditions. Community health objectives often depend on active decisions by groups of individuals to change their lifestyles or community resources that influence health. Efforts to influence and reinforce changes in community health behavior (transportation, childcare, resources, housing) become the central focus of effective community risk-reduction programs (Stanhope & Lancaster, 2025).

Studies attempt to explain why some groups of people effectively participate in certain health programs or make lifestyle changes whereas others do not. Early work by Rosenstock, who developed the health belief model, has evolved to models such as those by Pender and Prochaska, which are used to explain and change health-promotion behaviors (Pender et al., 2020). These models identify critical concepts for understanding how individuals change their health behavior. Rosenstock's model includes the following four steps:

- Perceiving behavior as a health threat in terms of susceptibility and seriousness
- Believing the behavior is a threat to their personal health
- Taking action to adopt preventive health behaviors
- Reinforcing the new behavior

In Rosenstock's model, community members take a passive role at first and then transition from passive to active between the second and third steps (belief to action). Ultimately, to improve community health through risk reduction programs, community members assume more responsibility for their own health, become more active in adopting healthy lifestyles, and monitor resources in the community to achieve healthy behaviors. In planning health-promotion activities, nurses consider effective strategies to motivate and support community transition from a passive to an active state.

Plans guide nursing actions. Nurses make additions and changes on the basis of community problems, resources, and problem resolution to maintain a viable plan. Table 8.1 provides one example of a community-oriented, health-promotion plan based on the goals recommended by the surgeon general's report about health promotion and disease prevention. The report's general goal generates several specific objectives. Nursing analysis guides the direction of the objectives, including the risk factors to be addressed. Examples of various rationales in Table 8.1 show how nurses incorporate important concepts of planned change into community-based health-promotion plans.

Communicating plans to other health professionals, community members, and key officials remains an essential aspect of planning. Unification of care systems and linkages through shared data entry, computerized documentation, and electronic medical records contributes to more streamlined and transparent communication and collaboration. Local newspapers, local bulletins, and school correspondence to parents provide avenues to communicate with the community about health-promotion plans. Other community-based actions, such as those for nursing involvement in prevention of alcohol abuse in the community, can be used. The various plans are categorized according to the health patterns to show that a community problem can be approached from multiple directions. Feasible plans that are well formulated facilitate implementation (USDHHS, 2024)

IMPLEMENTATION WITH THE COMMUNITY

Implementation of the nursing process begins on the basis of the health-promotion and health-protection plans. In collaboration with community members or other health team members, the nurse tests feasibility and implements the plan. Involving key community members in the assessment and planning process is crucial for success. To ensure involvement, activities must be accessible. For example, schedule meetings in accessible areas, offer childcare services, and provide light refreshments. Identify clearly what the community perceives as health-promotion needs. Maintain open communication—clear and correct information at regular intervals.

Intellectual, interpersonal, and technical skills of the community members facilitate the collaborative contribution. Community nurses often prepare community members with the technical skills for community engagement and empowerment. Success depends on the overcoming of expected resistance to change. Resistance to new health-promotion and health-protection activities, however, provides useful feedback to improve planning. People generally resist change to defend values that appear to be threatened by the change. Collaborating with communities initially facilitates change during the implementation phase. Table 8.4 lists factors that deter community participation. Informed nurses collaborate with community members throughout the process.

Community nurses implement health-promotion and health-protection plans in multiple community settings (schools, industry, public and private health agencies, and ambulatory care settings) where population groups experience relatively good health. Nursing-led community centers provide nursing faculty, staff, and students with unique opportunities to assess health and to plan, implement, and evaluate care (including holistic health promotion and primary health care) for individuals, families, and communities with unmet health care needs

TABLE 8.4 Potential Sources of Resistance to Health-Promotion Programs, With Agent Responses

Source of Resistance	Response
Lack of communication about implementation of program	Communicate through social media, internet, community newsletter, newspapers, high school radio station, electronic billboards, and posters
Misinformation regarding time and place of healthy activity	Disseminate valid information
Fear of unknown	Inform and encourage
Need for security	Clarify intentions and methods
No desired need to change behaviors	Demonstrate opportunity for change
Cultural or religious beliefs or vested interests threatened	Enlist key community leaders in planning change
Inaccessibility	Focus activities near the largest target population and in an area accessible by public transportation

Adapted from Dwyer, K. (2019). Managing resistance to change: Engaging and shaping. IQ: The RIM Quarterly, 35(1), 47. Retrieved from: Managing resistance to change: Engaging and shaping | IQ : THE RIMPA QUARTERLY (informit.org) (Accessed January 16, 2024)

(Sheffield, 2019). Community assessment includes observation of reciprocal interaction between the individual and his or her environment, which is similar to those techniques used for individual and family health promotion assessment (see Chapters 6 and 7, respectively). Community assessment commonly uses factors related to self-efficacy and Bandura's Social Learning Theory to explain relationships between human behavior and the environment. The complexity of health actions differs from one community to another. Community advisory boards play a critical role in community planning. As plans evolve, nurses learn more about the community and their own responses, strengths, limitations, and abilities to cope or adapt (Freda et al., 2018). Although implementation takes an action focus, it also includes assessment, planning, and evaluation activities to monitor actions taken to resolve, reduce, eliminate, or control the health concern.

EVALUATION WITH THE COMMUNITY

During the evaluation phase of the process, community nurses learn whether planned actions achieved desired outcomes. Communities and nurses determine progression toward goal achievement through methods that expand collaborations (Freda et al., 2018). Nurses may take overall responsibility for the process; however, collaborating with community members and health team members produces the most valid results. For example, if implemented plans intend to reduce the incidence of fatal motor vehicle accidents, nurses may guide the process to obtain community indicators and outcomes data, requisite community actions, and expected outcomes achieved from joint collaboration with community stakeholders.

Nursing plans, which include goals and interventions, provide the evaluation framework. With a community focus, mutual goal setting and the related objectives define the evaluation, considering how the community responded to planned actions. For example, if childhood disease rate reduction is expected to result from certain actions, community responses before the actions are compared with those after the actions. Comparison determines the level of effectiveness (complete, partially effective, or ineffective) of the nursing actions to achieve the goal.

Community nurses approach the dynamic process of evaluation in a purposeful, goal-directed manner (Stanhope & Lancaster, 2025; USDHHS, 2024). Determining the effectiveness of nursing actions evaluates the degree to which goals are achieved. The frequency of evaluation depends on the situations, changes expected, and objectives. For example, an individual who is bleeding may need evaluation at frequent intervals, whereas behavioral changes in community groups occur slowly and require long-term evaluation methods. Evaluation intervals differ depending on immediate, intermediate, and long-range goals. Units of evaluation for a community project include outcomes at the individual level and aggregate level (family, neighborhood, city, and/or region). The evaluation process continues until community goals are realized.

Evaluation results indicate the need for reassessment, revision, or modification of plans. Community nurses reassess situations, plan new approaches, and implement and evaluate revised plans, creating the continual cycle of the nursing process. Self-evaluation determines strengths and weaknesses as well as ways the nursing plan could have been more effective or efficient. The quality of community health-promotion and health-protection efforts depends on the professional qualities of those providing the services along with effective use of the nursing process.

Workable, cost-effective programs of community health promotion are needed. Nurses play an important role in providing evidence to support effective community health plans. Historically, documentation of effective health-promotion activities has been limited (Pender et al., 2020). Effectiveness is determined through research studies that include analyses and outcomes evaluation of home-based and community-centered nursing interventions designed to meet the needs of high-risk families, geographical communities, and vulnerable populations. For example, Walters et al.'s (2020) community-based participatory research team created, initiated, and evaluated health promotion strategies in partnership with five Native communities. The projects included one intervention to address risks associated with residential wood smoke and another intervention using intertribal talking circles to address abuse prevention and intervention (see Box 8.4). Such evidence-based practice and research helps garner support for community health-promotion programs. The Healthy People 2030 objectives include examples of national and state partnerships establishing health objectives and sustaining the initiatives (USDHHS, 2024).

CASE STUDY

Community Efforts to Decrease Adolescent Pregnancy Rates

The community health nurse is facilitating a grassroots community group that is determined to decrease the adolescent pregnancy rate in the city. The community population hovers around 100,000. The community lies on the Mexican border of the United States. The population is predominantly Mexican American, and there is a high poverty rate and less-than-adequate females' health care.

The schools offer health courses twice between seventh grade and 12th grade. The only formal sex education provided occurs within the context of these two health courses. A community group that has researched the problem has decided to use a social marketing approach because of community controversy and resistance.

Most of the materials reviewed do not address the cultural needs of the region. Many of the Spanish language materials use Spanish from countries other than Mexico. The situations posed in the audiovisual materials show people whom adolescents will perceive as different from themselves.

Reflective Questions

- How could the community group approach its goal to decrease the adolescent pregnancy rate in a manner that will be culturally competent?
- How might the community group approach this issue without the support of the school district?

Community Efforts to Decrease Adolescent Unwanted Pregnancy Rates

- Assess demographic variables associated with unwanted pregnancy in adolescents, nationally, regionally, and locally.
- Include adolescents in assessment, data collection, and planning.
- Implement community engagement techniques for collaboration with the grassroots group and other stakeholders to design, develop, and adapt relevant health interventions.
- Identify stakeholders: adolescents, teachers, school psychologists, counselors, school nurses, parent/teacher groups, youth groups, churches, social service organizations, and local businesses/corporations.
- Consider creating social groups and peer support groups for adolescents to partner with other stakeholders to foster attributes, attitudes, and information acquisition about sexuality.
- Consider using social media to broadcast targeted health messages to reach large numbers of community members, both adults and adolescents.
- Consider creating centers where adolescents have access to information and health care related to sexual activity and pregnancy.
- Create a community contact list for adolescents with information about human sexuality courses and health care related to pregnancy and reproductive health services.
- Maintain documentation of strategies/programs implemented to enhance the evaluation process and determine the effectiveness of the programs (Ackley & Ladwig, 2022).

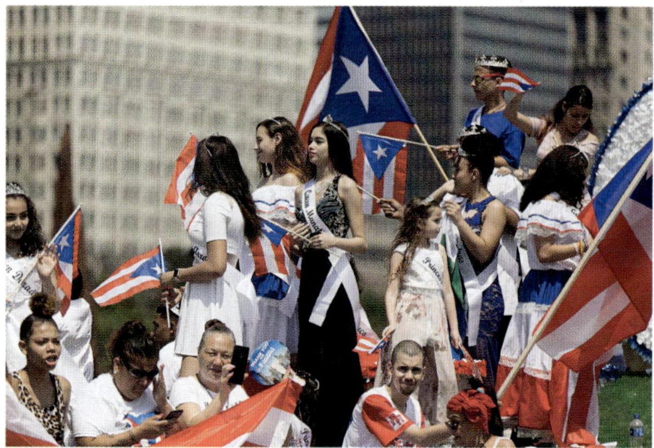

FIG. 8.4 Communities come together for the enjoyment of one of their traditional holidays. (From iStockphoto/Roberto Galan)

SUMMARY

- Risk factors, injury, and disease are not inevitable events experienced equally among a community's members. Effective community nurses understand the dynamic and complex nature of communities (Fig. 8.4).
- Nurses use various theoretical frameworks to assess health-related patterns, health concerns, and health-action potential and to implement the nursing process within communities.
- Collection and analysis of community data identify susceptible subpopulations.
- Planning contributes to the development of effective and efficient health-promotion and health-protection services.
- The nursing process enhances the efficacy of planning activities.
- Many communities experience obvious deficiencies in health services that warrant health planning action.
- Community nurses play a significant role in health planning directed toward reducing the risks associated with disease, premature death, and injury as well as health promotion among community members.
- Nurses use principles of planned change to increase community awareness of health, promote healthy behaviors, and encourage participation in preventive health services.
- The complexity differs from one community or geographic area to another. Community nurses connect health-promotion actions to specific community phenomena, providing scientific evidence to support nursing actions in the community.

EVOLVE CHAPTER FEATURES

http://evolve.elsevier.com/Edelman/
- Study Questions

REFERENCES

Abramsky, S. (2019). *Tackling poverty in America means grasping reality*. Seattle, WA: Marguerite Casey Foundation. https://www.caseygrants.org. Accessed January 16, 2024.

Ackley, B. J., & Ladwig, G. B. (2022). *Nursing diagnosis handbook-e-book: An evidence-based guide to planning care* (13th ed.). St. Louis, MO: Elsevier Health Sciences.

Alliance of Nurses for Healthy Environments (ANHE). (2024). *Knowledge network*. https://envirn.org/?s=knowledge+network. Accessed January 16, 2024.

American Nurses Association. (2024). *Legislative and Political Advocacy for Nurses*. https://www.nursingworld.org/practice-policy/advocacy. Accessed January 16, 2024.

Anderson, R. M., Heesterbeek, H., Klinkenberg, D., & Hollingsworth, T. D. (2020). How will country-based mitigation measures influence the course of the COVID-19 epidemic? *The Lancet*, *395*(10228), 931–934.

Aptekar, S., & Myers, J. S. (2020). The tale of two community gardens: Green aesthetics versus food justice in the Big Apple. *Agric Hum Values*, *37*, 779–792. https://doi.org/10.1007/s10460-019-10011-w

Barceló, N. E., Lopez, A., Tang, L., Nunez, M. G. A., Jones, F., Miranda, J., et al. (2019). Community engagement and planning versus resources for services for implementing depression quality improvement: exploratory analysis for Black and Latino Adults. *Ethnicity & Disease*, *29*(2), 277. https://ethndis.org/archive/files/ethndis-29-277.pdf

Barraclough, K. A., Gleeson, A., Holt, S. G., & Agar, J. W. (2019). Green dialysis survey: Establishing a baseline for environmental sustainability across dialysis facilities in Victoria, Australia. *Nephrology*, *24*(1), 88–93. https://doi.org/10.1111/nep.13191

Benka-Coker, M. L., Peel, J. L., Volckens, J., Good, N., Bilsback, K. R., L'Orange, C., et al. (2020). Kitchen concentrations of fine particulate matter and particle number concentration in households using biomass cookstoves in rural Honduras. *Environmental Pollution*, *258*, 113697. https://doi.org/10.1016/j.envpol.2019.113697

Brabhukumr, A., Malhi, P., Ravindra, K., & Lakshmi, P. V. M. (2020). Exposure to household air pollution during first 3 years of life and IQ level among 6–8-year-old children in India: A cross-sectional study. *Science of The Total Environment*, *709*, 135110. https://doi.org/10.1016/j.scitotenv.2019.135110

Breckenridge, L. A., Burns, D., & Nye, C. (2022). The use of motivational interviewing to overcome COVID-19 vaccine hesitancy in primary care settings. *Public Health Nursing*, *39*, 618–623. https://doi.org/10.1111/phn.13003

Brockie, T., Azar, K., Wallen, G., Solis, M. O. H., Adams, K., & Kub, J. (2019). A conceptual model for establishing collaborative partnerships between universities and Native American communities. *Nurse Researcher*, *27*(1), 27–32. https://doi.org/10.7748/nr.2019.e1613

Campbell, L. A., Harmon, M. J., Joyce, B. L., & Little, S. H. (2020). Quad council coalition community/public health nursing competencies: building consensus through collaboration. *Public Health Nursing*, *37*(1), 96–112. https://doi.org/10.1111/phn.12666

Centers for Disease Control and Prevention (CDC). (2024). *National Center for Health Statistics*. https://www.cdc.gov/nchs/pressroom/nchs_press_releases/2022/20221222.htm. Accessed January 20, 2024.

Coker, E., Katamba, A., Kizito, S., Eskenazi, B., & Davis, J. L. (2020). Household air pollution profiles associated with persistent childhood cough in urban Uganda. *Environment International*, *136*, 105471. https://doi.org/10.1016/j.envint.2020.105471 https://doi.org/10.1007/s40615-022-01431-2

Dickerson, D., Baldwin, J. A., Belcourt, A., Belone, L., Gittelsohn, J., Kaholokula, J. K. A., et al. (2020). Encompassing cultural contexts within scientific research methodologies in the development of health promotion interventions. *Prevention Science*, *21*(S1), 33–42. https://doi.org/10.1007/s11121-018-0926-1

Dietz, W. H., Belay, B., Bradley, D., Kahan, S., Muth, N. D., Sanchez, E., et al. (2017). A model framework that integrates community and clinical systems for the prevention and management of obesity and other chronic diseases. *NAM Perspectives*. Washington, DC: National Academy of Medicine. https://doi.org/10.31478/201701b

Di Leonardi, B. C., Hagler, D., Marshall, D. R., Stobinski, J. X., & Welsh, S. S. (2020). From competence to continuing competency. *The Journal of Continuing Education in Nursing*, *51*(1), 15–24. https://doi.org/10.3928/00220124-20191217-05

Duran, B., Oetzel, J., Magarati, M., Parker, M., Zhou, C., Roubideaux, Y., et al. (2019). Toward health equity: A national study of promising practices in community-based participatory research. *Progress in Community Health Partnerships: Research, Education, and Action*, *13*(4), 337–352. https://doi.org/10.1353/cpr.2019.0067

Dwyer, K. (2019). Managing resistance to change: Engaging and shaping. *IQ: The RIM Quarterly*, *35*(1), 47.

Estévez-García, J. A., Schilmann, A., Riojas-Rodríguez, H., Berrueta, V., Blanco, S., Villaseñor-Lozano, C. G., et al. (2020). Women exposure to household air pollution after an improved cookstove program in rural San Luis Potosi, Mexico. *Science of the Total Environment*, *702*, 134456. https://doi.org/10.1016/j.scitotenv.2019.134456

Fadlallah, R., El-Jardali, F., Nomier, M., Hemadi, N., Arif, K., Langlois, E. V., et al. (2019). Using narratives to impact health policy-making: A systematic review. *Health Research Policy and Systems*, *17*(1), 26. https://doi.org/10.1186/s12961-019-0423-4

Ferguson, N. G.,Ainslie, B., Bhatia, B., et al. (2020). Impact of non-pharmaceutical interventions (NPIs) to reduce COVID19 mortality and healthcare demand imperial college COVID-19 response team. https://www.imperial.ac.uk. Accessed January 16, 2024.

Fox, K., Rallapalli, K. L., & Komor, A. C. (2020). Rewriting human history and empowering indigenous communities with genome editing tools. *Genes*, *11*(1), 88. https://doi.org/10.3390/genes11010088

Freda, B., Kozick, D., & Spencer, A. (2018). *Partnerships for health: lessons for bridging community-based organizations and health care organizations*. https://www.issuelab.org/resources/29899/29899.pdf. Accessed January 16, 2024.

Gordon, M. (2014). *Manual of nursing diagnosis* (14th ed.). Sudbury, MA: Jones & Bartlett.

Jahan, I., Ullah, I., Griffiths, M. D., & Mamun, M. A. (2021). COVID-19 suicide and its causative factors among the healthcare professionals: Case study evidence from press reports. *Perspectives in Psychiatric Care*, *1*(57), 1707–1711. https://doi.org/10.1111/ppc.12739

Kaczynski, A. T., Besenyi, G. M., Child, S., Morgan Hughey, S., Colabianchi, N., McIver, K. L., et al. (2018). Relationship of objective street quality attributes with youth physical activity: Findings from the healthy communities study. *Pediatric Obesity*, *13*, 7–13. https://doi.org/10.1111/ijpo.12429

Kim, Y. J., Seay, K. D., Moon, S. S., Lee, J. H., & Kim, J. K. (2018). Types of stressors and bullying perpetration among female adolescents in Korea. *Journal of Human Behavior in the Social Environment*, *28*(7), 936–947. https://doi.org/10.1080/10911359.2018.1485603

Klopper, H. C., Madigan, E., Vlasich, C., Albien, A., Ricciardi, R., Catrambone, C., et al. (2020). Advancement of global health: Recommendations from the global advisory panel on the future of nursing & midwifery (GAPFON®). *Journal of Advanced Nursing*, *76*(2), 741–748. https://doi.org/10.1111/jan.14254

Kumar, R., Bhattacharya, S., Sharma, N., & Thiyagarajan, A. (2019). Cultural competence in family practice and primary care setting. *Journal of Family Medicine and Primary Care*, *8*(1), 1. https://doi.org/10.4103/jfmpc.jfmpc_393_18

Kwan, P. P., Sabado-Liwag, M., Tan, N., Pike, J. R., Custodio, H., LaBreche, A., et al. (2020). A community-based approach to biospecimen collection among Pacific Islanders. *Health Promotion Practice*, *21*(1), 97–105. https://doi.org/10.1177/1524839918786222

Lambert, A. W., Johnson, T. L., Fox, M. W., & Hsuan Wang, C. (2018). Enhancing community education through innovative teaching strategies in a baccalaureate nursing program. *Journal of Nursing Education*, *57*(4), 240–244. https://doi.org/10.3928/01484834-20180322-10

Liévanos, R. S. (2019). Racialized structural vulnerability: Neighborhood racial composition, concentrated disadvantage, and fine particulate matter in California. *International Journal of Environmental Research and Public Health*, *16*(17), 3196. https://doi.org/10.3390/ijerph16173196

Liu, Y., & Aungsuroch, Y. (2018). Current literature review of registered nurses' competency in the global community. *Journal of Nursing Scholarship*, *50*(2), 191–199. https://doi.org/10.1111/jnu.12361

Lockwood, C. J. (2019). Coping in the age of acceleration. *Contemporary OB/GYN*, *64*(8), 3–6.

Martinez-Bianchi, V., Frank, B., Edgoose, J., Michener, L., Weida, J., Rodriguez, M., et al. (2019). Addressing family medicine's capacity to improve health equity through collaboration, accountability and coalition-building. *Family Medicine*, *51*(2), 198–203. https://doi.org/10.22454/fammed.2019.921819

Miller, I., Greenberg, S., Yashar, B. M., et al. (2020). Improving access to cancer genetic services: perspectives of high-risk clients in a community-based setting. *Journal of Community Genetics*, *11*, 119–123. https://doi.org/10.1007/s12687-019-00420-z

Occupational Safety and Health Administration. (n.d.) *Workplace violence*. https://www.osha.gov/SLTC/workplaceviolence/index.html. Accessed January 16, 2024.

Ohoro, C. R., Adeniji, A. O., Okoh, A. I., & Okoh, O. O. (2019). Distribution and chemical analysis of pharmaceuticals and personal care products (PPCPs) in the environmental systems: a review. *International Journal of Environmental Research and Public Health, 16*(17), 3026. https://doi.org/10.3390/ijerph16173026

Ortiz, K., Nash, J., Shea, L., Oetzel, J., Garoutte, J., Sanchez-Youngman, S., et al. (2020). Partnerships, processes, and outcomes: a health equity–focused scoping meta-review of community-engaged scholarship. *Annual Review of Public Health, 41*, 171–199. https://doi.org/10.1146/annurev-publhealth-040119-094220

Parasuraman, S. R., & de la Cruz, D. (2019). Evaluation of the implementation of the healthy start program: findings from the 2016 National Healthy Start Program Survey. *Maternal and Child Health Journal, 23*(2), 220–227. https://doi.org/10.1007/s10995-018-2640-9

Pender, N. J., Murdaugh, C. L., & Parsons, M. A. (2020). *Health promotion in nursing practice* (8th ed.). Upper Saddle River, NJ: Pearson.

Polvere, L., Barnes, C., & Lee, E. (2018). Housing needs of grandparent caregivers: Grandparent, youth, and professional perspectives. *Journal of Gerontological Social Work, 61*(5), 549–566. https://doi.org/10.1080/01634372.2018.1454566

Rosa, W. E., Upvall, M. J., & Leffers, J. M. (2019). Partnerships for the goals: the keystone of sustainable development attainment. *Public Health Nursing, 3*(36), 255–256. https://doi.org/10.1111/phn.12616

Rowe, C. A., & Wright, C. F. (2020). Expanded universal carrier screening and its implementation within a publicly funded healthcare service. *Journal of Community Genetics, 11*(1), 21–38. https://doi.org/10.1007/s12687-019-00443-6

Roygardner, D., Palusci, V. J., & Hughes, K. N. (2019). Advancing prevention zones: implementing community-based strategies to prevent child maltreatment and promote healthy families. *International Journal on Child Maltreatment: Research, Policy and Practice, 3*(4), 1–11. https://doi.org/10.1007/s42448-019-00039-0

Schmidtke, J., & Cornel, M. C. (2020). A new decade of community genetics: old and new challenges. *Journal of Community Genetics, 11*(1), 1–3. https://doi.org/10.1007/s12687-019-00448-1

Sheffield, A. J. (2019). Improving access to health: a business plan approach to creating a sustainable nurse-led community clinic. *Nursing Economics, 37*(6), 306–316.

Smith, S., Buchanan, H., & Cloutier, R. (2020). Virginia NP scope of practice: a legislative case study. *The Nurse Practitioner, 2*(45), 33–37. https://doi.org/10.1097/01.npr.0000651120.61281.12

Stanhope, M., & Lancaster, J. (2025). *Public health nursing* (11th ed.). St. Louis: Elsevier.

State of Virginia. (n.d.). *Safe driving lesson plan (driver education | Virginia Department of Education).* https://www.quitalcohol.com/resource/organizations-fight-drinking-driving. Accessed January 31, 2024.

The New York Times. (2023). *Social Security and Medicare funds still face long-term shortfalls, report says.* https://www.nytimes.com. Accessed on January 30, 2024

The Royal Canadian Mounted Police Centre for Youth Crime Prevention. (n.d.). *Impaired driving lesson plan (grades 11 &12).* http://www.rcmp-grc.gc.ca/cycp-cpcj/id-cfa/lp-pl/index-eng.htm. Accessed January 31, 2024.

Thomson, D.R., Linard, C., Vanhuysse, S., Steele, J. E., Shimoni, M., Siri, J., et al. (2019). Extending data for urban health decision-making: a menu of new and potential neighborhood-level health determinants datasets in LMICs. *Journal of Urban Health, 96*, 514–536. https://doi.org/10.1007/s11524-019-00363-3

Trisi, D. (2023). *Government's pandemic response turned a would-be poverty surge into a record poverty decline.* Center on Budget and Policy Priorities. https://www.cbpp.org/sites/default/files/8-29-23pov.pdf

Turley, B., & Caretta, M. A. (2020). Household water security: an analysis of water affect in the context of hydraulic fracturing in west Virginia, Appalachia. *Water, 12*(1), 147. https://doi.org/10.3390/w12010147

United States Department of Agriculture (USDA). (2024). *Rural poverty & well-being. Rural economy and population.* https://www.ers.usda.gov/topics/food-nutrition-assistance/. Accessed January 16, 2024.

University of Texas Health Science Center at Houston. (2019). *CHARTing health information for Texas.* https://libguides.sph.uth.tmc.edu/charting_health. Accessed January 16, 2024.

US Census. (2018). *From pyramid to pillar: a century of change, population of the U.S.* https://www.census.gov/library/visualizations/2018/comm/century-of-change.html. Accessed January 16, 2024.

US Department of Health and Human Services (USDHHS). (2024). *Healthy people 2030.* https://health.gov/healthypeople. Accessed January 16, 2024.

van der Westhuizen, D., Conrad, N., Douglas, T. S., & Mutsvangwa, T. (2020). Engaging communities on health innovation: experiences in implementing design thinking. *International Quarterly of Community Health Education, 41*(1), 101–114. https://doi.org/10.1177/0272684x19900880

Volkow, N. D., & Blanco, C. (2021). The changing opioid crisis: development, challenges and opportunities. *Molecular Psychiatry, 26*(1), 218–233. https://pubmed.ncbi.nlm.nih.gov/32020048/

Vussel, A. V., Castillo, P. W., Kirstein, M., Mueller, J., & Kavanaugh, M. (2022). Disruptions and opportunities in sexual and reproductive health care: how COVID-19 impacted service provision in three US states. *Perspectives on Sexual and Reproductive Health, 54*, 188–197. https://doi.org/10.1363/psrh.12213

Walters, K. L., Johnson-Jennings, M., Stroud, S., Rasmus, S., Charles, B., John, S., et al. (2020). Growing from our roots: strategies for developing culturally grounded health promotion interventions in American Indian, Alaska Native, and Native Hawaiian communities. *Prevention Science, 21*(1), 54–64. https://doi.org/10.1007/s11121-018-0952-z

Weinstein, N., Schwarz, K., Chan, I., Kobau, R., Alexander, R., Kollar, L., et al. (2024). COVID-19 vaccine hesitancy among US adults: safety and effectiveness perceptions and messaging to increase vaccine confidence and intent to vaccinate. *Public Health Reports, 139*(1), 102–111. https://doi.org/10.1177/00333549231204419

West, A., Gagliardi, L., Gatewood, A., Higman, S., Daniels, J., O'Neill, K., et al. (2018). Randomized trial of a training program to improve home visitor communication around sensitive topics. *Maternal and Child Health Journal, 22*(1), 70–78. https://doi.org/10.1007/s10995-018-2531-0

Wolfe, L. C., Maughan, E. D., & Bergren, M. D. (2019). Introducing the 3S (student–school nurse–school community) model. *NASN School Nurse, 34*(1), 30–34. https://doi.org/10.1177/1942602x18814233

World Health Organization (WHO). (2005). *Statement on the second meeting of the International Health Regulations (2005). Emergency committee regarding the outbreak of novel coronavirus (2019-nCoV) Geneva Switzerland.* https://www.who.int. Accessed January 30, 2024.

World Health Organization (WHO). (2020). *Virtual press conference on COVID-19 – 11 March 2020.* https://www.who.int. Accessed February 21, 2024.

World Health Organization (WHO). (2024). *Clean Household Energy Solutions Toolkit (CHEST).* https://www.who.int/publications/i/item/WHO-HEP-ECH-AQH-2022.8. Accessed November 4, 2024.

Young, C., & Thompson, H. (2018). The role of the district nurse in Northern Ireland. *British Journal of Community Nursing, 23*(7), 328–333. https://doi.org/10.12968/bjcn.2018.23.7.328

9

Screening and Health Promotion

Elizabeth Connelly Kudzma

http://evolve.elsevier.com/Edelman/

OBJECTIVES

After completing this chapter, the reader will be able to:

- Discuss screening and its application in secondary prevention and health promotion.
- Analyze criteria to determine whether a disease has evidence-based guidelines for screening.
- Identify health care, economic, and ethical implications related to the screening process.
- Discuss how collaborative community and national partnerships and policies assist in the development and implementation of screening programs.
- Describe elements of the nursing role applicable to the screening process.

KEY TERMS

Asymptomatic pathogenesis
Community assessment
Community resources
Cost-benefit ratio analysis
Cost-effectiveness analysis
Cost-efficiency analysis
Disability-adjusted life year
Efficacy
Efficiency
Epidemiology
False negative test results
False positive test results
Group or mass screening
Iatrogenic
Incidence
Individual screening
Interobserver reliability
Interprofessional education
Intraobserver reliability
Key community individuals
Lead agency
Morbidity
Mortality
Multiple test screening
National Prevention Strategy
One-test disease-specific screening
Prevalence
Primary Prevention
Quality-adjusted life year
Quality of life
Quantity of life
Racial and Ethnic Approaches to Community Health (REACH)
Reliability
Secondary prevention; Sensitivity
Significance
Specificity
Stakeholders
Target community
US Preventive Services Task Force (USPSTF)
Validity

THINK ABOUT IT

Screening Starts Even Before Birth: Next Generation Screening

New parents are familiar with required screening tests performed on babies very shortly after birth. Testing with dried blood spot (DBS) technology allows treatment and lifetime monitoring before the serious signs associated with disease occur. Early in the 20th century, when educators started to investigate the concepts of intelligence quotient (IQ), "cretin" was a medical/educational category used to describe a lower level of intelligence. We now recognize that cretinism manifests as neonatal hypothyroidism. Early treatment of the baby with thyroid hormone prevents mental deficiency. The incidence of neonatal hypothyroidism was more common in mountainous inland areas away from sea salt sources of iodine. It is rare in the modern world because of the screening of all infants at birth (blood tests measure levels of thyroid-stimulating hormone and thyroxine). This disorder and others (e.g., phenylketonuria [PKU]) are health screenings' modern success stories. DBS sampling is mandated by state governmental regulations that list specific tests, and it is most useful for the detection of metabolic disorders (Freeman et al., 2018; Moat, George & Carling, 2020; Givler & Givler, 2023). Even before birth, newer uses of maternal ultrasound on the pregnant uterus may identify mothers most at risk for preterm birth due to thinner uterine walls with a structurally inferior cervix (Schaffer, 2019). Some screened fetal problems may even be treated with intrauterine fetal surgery. Screening tests affecting babies are becoming more common, more numerous, and less invasive.

More recently DNA tests have been developed to screen an individual's DNA for genes associated with diseases or population subgroups (Ramos & Weissman, 2018; Moat, George & Carling, 2020). DNA testing examines a person's genetic code to provide information about genealogy or ancestry that may be helpful in assessing a person's risk of disease. Personalized DNA testing kits are available to help consumers discover their risks of developing disorders (such as Alzheimer disease, diabetes, and breast cancer). Screening options that may be novel but unproven raise new questions about media information provided to the public, the politics involved, specific information requested from health providers (Ramos & Weissman, 2018), and the reliability and validity of screening methods and associated necessary counseling.

Home-screening test kits came to the forefront during the COVID-19 pandemic. Immediately after genomic analysis of the virus was established, scientists begin to develop COVID-19 screening test kits to identify the virus and/or antibodies created when a person has come into contact with the virus. In addition, between 2020 and 2022, local COVID-19 testing sites were set up to screen for the virus and to allow the start of early treatment for more severe disease, especially in older adults or adults with other comorbidities (https://www.hhs.gov/coronavirus/community-based-testing-sites/index.html). Although we often think of screening for the purposes of diagnosis, there is a wide range of screening tests (e.g., cholesterol, blood pressure, congenital disease, illicit drug use), so this chapter will focus on the use of screening devices for health promotion and some chronic diseases. But the recent coronavirus pandemic refocuses attention that many screening tests were originally developed to diagnose infectious diseases (e.g., tuberculosis) (Forsythe et al., 2020; Vessey & Betz, 2020; Givler & Givler, 2023).

- Why has the newborn period been identified as an important time to require screening tests?
- Each government regulates a list of mandated screening for newborns and other conditions. Do you know what your government/state/ministry of health requires?
- The availability and feasibility of detection and screening tests is constantly changing. How are new screening tests evaluated and added to the mandated requirements?
- What characteristics of screening tests make for accurate testing?
- How is the margin of error further defined for screening tests/instruments? What aspects of screening program development should nurses participate in? Assessment, data analysis, implementation, evaluation of health outcomes? For infectious disease, contact tracing, preventing, containing, and mitigating the spread?

Clinical and community preventive services are vital to health promotion and disease prevention. Identified as such, they have become one of the four strategic directions of the National Prevention Strategy (safe community environments, elimination of health disparities, clinical and preventive services, empowered people). Originally, preventive services were overseen by the Centers for Disease Control and Prevention (CDC) to distribute to the states, with the hope that the CDC would be able to manage unfragmented, flexible national services (Chait & Glied, 2018). Screening is an important component of clinical preventive services because it is a valuable tool for health care professionals to identify acute and chronic conditions and risk factors before the condition becomes costly both in financial terms and for quality of life. This is particularly important as the health care paradigm shifts from medical and volume-based delivery to a health-promotion and value-based model of care. In Chapter 1, preventive strategies are described as primordial, primary, secondary, and tertiary. Although health education about screening is usually categorized as part of the rubric of **primary prevention**, the actual process of screening may also be part of **secondary prevention**. Some testing may also be part of tertiary prevention to follow disease recurrence.

Detection and preventive services are effective in reducing death and disability and are cost-effective or even cost-saving. A wide range of detection/screening tests can be combined with counseling, immunizations, or medications used to prevent disease. These measures find health problems early and provide individuals (and sometimes the overall population) with the information needed to make good health decisions. Although most preventive screening services may be traditionally delivered in clinical settings, some can be delivered within communities, work sites, schools, residential treatment centers, or homes (Chait & Glied, 2018).

The importance of accurate detection and screening tests has been clearly demonstrated while the world grapples with strategies to counter the coronavirus pandemic. For acute infectious illnesses, the appropriate screening or detection test "enables mapmaking: quantifying the size and sources of an infection and tracking its movements. For an individual patient, it enables plan-making: assessing whether you've been infected and should be isolated, and tracing whom you've put at risk. In the later stages of a pandemic, the ability to test on a wide scale allows agencies to concentrate on hot spots" (Mukherjee, 2020a, p. 26).

For all screening modalities, accurate detection and screening is important for both acute and more chronic diseases. This chapter will focus primarily on screening for chronic disease and prevention, but the recent onset of coronavirus (and rapid testing at the point-of-care for hospital admissions) illustrates that the principles of screening apply to both acute and chronic conditions.

Screening Goals. The primary goal of screening is to detect risk factors and conditions early to prevent or treat them and deter their progression. An important assumption underlying many uses of screening is that detection early in the asymptomatic period allows treatment at a time when the eventual course of the disease can be altered. Similarly, identifying risk factors assists in identifying the populations needing screening and focuses attention on necessary behavioral change before disease develops. Screening strategies for many chronic conditions are based on the principle that the selected disease is preceded by a period of **asymptomatic pathogenesis** or latency (disease development before symptoms first appear), when risk factors predisposing a person to the disease are building toward full manifestation of the disease (Fig. 9.1). Screening takes advantage of the prepathogenic/preclinical state and the early pathogenic/clinical state—thereby identifying risks relating to disease in the earliest and most treatable stages.

Screening strategies at the beginning or front end are essential to the core of the health-promotion metaphor and effort at the back end. This is an adaptation of the upstream/downstream

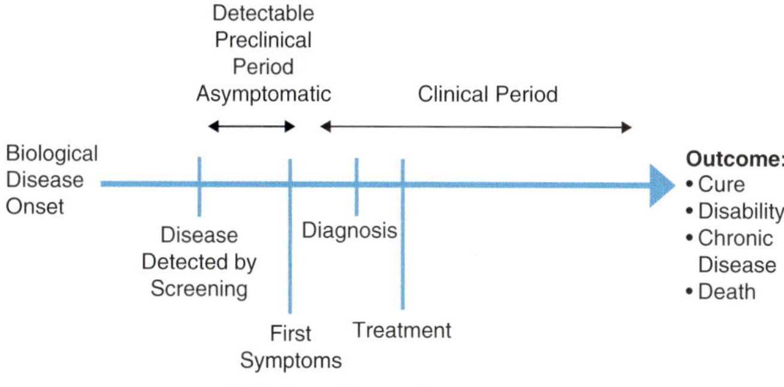

FIG. 9.1 Screening periods.

health care treatment narrative process. If health care providers are so preoccupied with managing the acute care (ill or dying) of those affected drowning downstream, they have little time, energy, or money to focus on why individuals become ill and fall into the river upstream. Screening tests are essential to focus attention on what is happening upstream at the source to better identify valid determinants and risks to health status. During the coronavirus pandemic, the identification of infected individuals or those who have overcome the infection is essential to lowering the number of infected individuals who would seek hospital services and overwhelm hospital units. Use of valid, accurate tests is fundamental to modeling how infection or other health status measures relate to planning for future care (Kisling & Das, 2023).

Administration of accurate and targeted screening tests, some of which might be simple and inexpensive when compared with the burden of disease, provides value in improved quality of care and decreased health care costs. Screening can be a diagnostic measure, but it is usually not curative in itself. It tends to be a preliminary step to identify individuals at the beginning who need more diagnostic workup or counseling to prevent further development of the condition or disease and to ameliorate adverse disease outcomes. More importantly, it is a step toward empowering individuals to make more informed choices about their health and health behaviors.

A second, but equally important, objective of screening is to reduce the costs of managing the disease by avoiding more intensive interventions later. In the case of infectious disease, it may allow for early isolation and mitigation, and prevent others in the population from coming in contact with the pathogen. A cost-conscious approach to health care mandates that health care professionals at all levels acquire a basic understanding of the screening process and its application. Unfortunately, some initial screening and the application of screening processes may involve complicated decision-making and is entangled in issues of social policy, state regulations, communication and media information, and personal choice.

ADVANTAGES AND DISADVANTAGES OF SCREENING

Advantages

The concept of health screening is complicated. Some screenings are simple and performed at home (blood pressure, heart rate, weight, oxygen saturation, COVID-19 infection), and nurses are involved in promoting and educating people about their use. For many screening tests, there are extensive statistics and economic/financial literature. This chapter will focus more on the **efficacy** and **efficiency** of clinical, procedural, and laboratory-based tests. In general, health screening tests offer several advantages. Although some screening procedures are simple and relatively inexpensive, others are expensive and may not be cost-effective. The simplicity of some screening procedures decreases the time and cost of the health care personnel involved, especially when compared with the cost of treating the disease after symptoms appear, and enables less-skilled technicians to administer the test.

A second advantage is the ability to apply the screening process to both individuals and larger populations. In an **individual screening** program, one person is tested by a health professional who has selected the individual as high risk (e.g., the individual is elderly and has prior hypertension or the person is elderly and resides in a skilled nursing facility). The practitioner can make this decision independently, the health care agency can define a specific policy, or legislative bodies can require the screening by law. As another example, newborn screening is a public health program for infants after birth to detect conditions that are treatable but may not be clinically evident in the infant. Metabolic conditions, such as hypothyroidism and PKU, are included in screening programs in all states (Dubay & Zach, 2023; US National Library of Medicine, 2020). From the old to the very young, a wide range of populations may be targeted for testing.

PKU is a rare genetic disorder that causes the level of an amino acid, phenylalanine, to build up because of a metabolizing enzyme defect. Children who are identified as having PKU can be placed on a phenylalanine-restricted diet and medication to avoid the worst complications of PKU-related disease (neurologic problems, delayed development, and intellectual disability/mental retardation). Lead screening for children is an essential component of later well-child visits. Children younger than 6 years are at greatest risk, and once exposure has occurred, it is difficult to reverse toxic effects (CDC, 2021a).

Group or mass screening occurs when a target population is selected on the basis of an increased incidence of a condition or a recognized element of high risk within an identified group. For example, the target population may be invited to a central location on a designated day to be tested for the selected disorders (elevated levels of lipids and cholesterol, hypertension, osteoporosis, elevated blood glucose level).

A third advantage is the ability to provide one-test disease-specific screening or multiple test screenings. A **one-test disease-specific screening** is the administration of a single test that searches for a characteristic that indicates a high risk of developing a disorder. An example of this is blood pressure screening to evaluate hypertension. **Multiple test screening** involves the administration of two or more tests to detect more than one disease. In some cases, one sample can be used to evaluate an individual for several conditions, saving time and money and making the process efficient and economical. For example, a blood sample can be assessed for a number of components, including glucose and cholesterol levels. The combination of the relatively low-cost screening test and flexibility makes screenings adaptable to all levels within the health care delivery system. Other multiple test screenings of importance are for substance abuse, mental health disorders and depression, and sexually transmitted infections (STIs).

A final advantage of public health screening is that it creates an opportunity for providing health education and science literacy (see Chapter 10) to a group of individuals who may not otherwise receive it. In some situations, it is possible to establish a clinical relationship during the screening process that leads to preventive visits and includes educating people about healthy lifestyles, risk reduction, developmental needs, activities of daily living, and preventive self-care. Many of today's chronic illnesses are a result of individual health behaviors. Awareness is the first step in prevention. If better awareness is combined with health-education and health-promotion tools, individuals have a better opportunity to manage their own risks. Promoting the advantages of potential teachable health-promotion moments should never be overlooked.

The recommended 6-month dental screening is an example. Although the individual is at the dentist's office to be screened for cavities and to have teeth cleaned to avoid gum disease, the hygienist provides education and reminders on the correct way and the necessity to brush and floss teeth correctly, and a check is provided for oral cancer (ADA, 2022). Another example is the recommended counseling and coaching for smokers. It is not enough to simply screen an individual with the question, "Do you use tobacco?" Readiness to quit also should be determined and combined with cessation treatment assistance—for example, finding safe substitutes for cigarettes (CDC, 2021b). Nurses who are familiar with community resources can then refer individuals to smoking cessation programs that fit with the person's preferences, lifestyle, and values.

Disadvantages

The primary disadvantages of screening stem largely from uncertainties in scientific evidence, which sets normal testing ranges and therefore also ranges of error for screening tests. When effectiveness depends on the screening program's ability to distinguish those who probably have the disease from those who do not, any margin of error can result in serious consequences. Some individuals who do not have the condition will be referred for further tests, and some who do have the disease will not get needed referrals. Those incorrectly referred (**false positive**) suffer needless anxiety and unnecessary medical interventions, some of which can be harmful, while awaiting more definitive diagnosis (e.g., high levels of prostate-specific antigen [PSA]). False positive osteoporosis screening results can lead to unnecessary bone-building medication treatment that may have adverse effects. Some prenatal screening tests for quite rare disorders and the predictive value might be questionable (Gregg et al., 2021). For example, carrier screening might be recommended for cystic fibrosis and spinal muscular atrophy. Mammography screening for breast microcalcifications identifies a significant number of females (who may be false positives) who later undergo medically invasive breast biopsies. Females or individuals with false-positive results bear the burden of the follow-up visits, lost time, inconvenience, and the cost of follow-up interventions to determine whether the disease is actually present.

The effects on those whose diseases have been overlooked (**false negative**) are even more important. For example, in maternal serum sampling for fetal DNA (cell-free DNA testing), false negative reports have occurred with twin pregnancies and cell mosaicism (possession of normal and abnormal cells) in either the baby or the placenta. The use of maternal serum sampling for fetal DNA has largely replaced the use of amniotic fluid sampling to reduce the risk of miscarriage at the increased risk of less-accurate results (Pös et al., 2019), and the health care provider must choose between various screening tests depending on what is known about test reliability and false positive or false negative results (Rose et al., 2020). Individuals receiving false negative results have a false assurance of health that will be broken eventually when a disease illness becomes obvious; they lose the opportunity to receive earlier treatment that could prevent irreversible damage. The coronavirus situation in 2020 exposed the many challenges associated with developing early accurate tests (including home tests) and distribution to target populations. The difficulty of balancing the benefits to some populations or regions against the burdens to others can create ethical issues underlying many screening programs. The significance of advantages and disadvantages of screening tests can vary; therefore, it should be assessed for each screening program, disease, and population.

SELECTION OF A SCREENED DISEASE

The selection of a screened disease goes beyond examination of any disease alone. The selection process must also encompass fewer tangible factors, such as the emotional effect (for example, HIV infection) and the financial effect (cancer, a disease requiring substantial insurance coverage) of the disease's detection on the screened population. Even after data have been gathered and the critical issues have been reviewed, the final decision of whether to screen individuals must often be reached with incomplete evidence or with choices that raise ethical issues on an epidemiologic and a personal level.

The potential uncertainties confounding the decision to screen individuals emphasize the need to conduct an analysis of available material to obtain a decision that is as objective and scientific as possible. Consideration of the following questions may provide a basis for designating a disease as screenable or not screenable:

- Does the significance of the disorder warrant its consideration as an individual or community problem?
- Can the disease or condition be accurately detected by screening?
- How invasive is the testing procedure?
- What are the short- and long-range health benefits? For example, can the disease be treated with some certainty? Does early treatment lead to better outcomes?
- What are the tangible and intangible costs?
- Are there other issues to consider?

As simplistic as these questions may appear, the answers or lack of answers, in addition to individual preferences, may expose complex issues that determine whether a well-informed decision can be made on screening.

Significance of the Disease for Screening

Epidemiology is the "method used to find the causes of health outcomes and diseases in populations. In epidemiology, the patient is the community and individuals are viewed collectively. By definition, epidemiology is the study (scientific, systematic, and data driven) of the distribution (frequency, pattern) and determinants (causes, risk factors) of health-related states and events (not just diseases) in specified populations (neighborhood, school, city, state, country, global)" (CDC, 2018).

Health information on morbidity and mortality may be used to identify the most important diseases affecting community populations. The term **morbidity** refers to a diseased state or disability from any cause; however, the view of morbidity can be broader, including a range or degree of the illness that affects the person. **Mortality** statistics (deaths) in a given population can be easier to use as end outcome indices as long as statistical collection measures are accurate.

The **significance** of a disease refers to the level of priority assigned to the disease as a public health concern. Although the opinions of political and public interest groups may influence this evaluation, significance is generally determined by incidence and prevalence, and by the quantity (severity) and quality of life affected by the disorder (CDC, 2018). The media may also have a role in defining a public health problem that should be screened for or addressed, as the media provides a site for relaying stories about the effect of disease and potential screening and testing recommendations. During the significant COVID-19 epidemic, the increase in social media and coverage of day-to-day updates incited fear about lockdowns, quarantine periods, misinformation, and unproven cures and medicines (Anwar et al., 2020). The COVID-19 pandemic of coronavirus has focused global media attention on the spread, acuity, and mortality of the virus and apparent mortality differentials for different age groups, especially the elderly (Mukherjee, 2020b), which in some cases led to an increase in domestic and elderly abuse (Anwar et al., 2020). To date, there are many unanswered questions about the coronavirus infection, including questions related to its origin, extent, and length of time for transmission; its ability to infect animals; and the evolving spectrum of immunity (Vessey & Betz, 2020; Wang et al., 2020).

Key factors in assessing the need for screening criteria are quantifying measures of disease frequency. The two measures most used in epidemiology are incidence and prevalence (CDC, 2018; Rector & Stanley, 2021). **Incidence** indicates the rate of a new population problem and estimates the risk of an individual developing a disease or condition during a specific period or over a lifetime. **Prevalence** is the proportion of a given population with the disease or condition at any one point in time. It provides the best estimate of whether a person is likely to become ill during a specific period. In short, incidence refers to new cases, and prevalence refers to all cases within a set period. Chronic conditions are usually measured by their prevalence (generally existing, e.g., hypertension), whereas acute conditions are assessed by their incidence (rate of new occurrences, e.g., acute COVID-19). Both are used in assessing the need for community services and screenings and help develop the criteria for evidence-based practice screening guidelines, including the age at which screening should be performed, the frequency and manner of screening, and the person who should perform the screening. A first step in assessing screening feasibility is evaluation of disease significance to decide whether the disorder warrants the time, effort, and financial resources that must be allocated. For example, there has been a significant decline in the incidence of late-stage colorectal cancer in the United States since 1987, and some but not all of this decline can be attributed to screening (Givler & Givler, 2023). The greater the physical and psychological harm experienced by the population, the greater the urgency to designate the condition/disease as a priority health problem is. The recent global spread of the coronavirus, its lethality in the population over 75, and its capacity to overload hospitals and intensive care units, infect health care providers, and disrupt economic systems provided extreme urgency for testing measures to understand how acute disease caused by this virus affects individuals within the population.

Quality of Life Estimates. Estimating the **quality of life** affected by a disease presents problems but is also a necessary step. The perception of quality of life is subjective, and individual evaluations may differ. For example, not all people equally perceive the disability resulting from a disease; some may adjust and cope, whereas others may not. Those who do not may be more likely to say that the quality of their lives is significantly lower than that of other people.

Two epidemiologic measures are used to estimate quality of life. A **quality-adjusted life year** (QALY) is a measurement of quality of life. It is defined as perfect health minus the **disability-adjusted life year** (DALY). The QALY assumes that 1 year of excellent health is 1 QALY (1 year of life times 1 utility value equals 1 QALY). It also assumes that 1 year spent in a less-perfect state of health or with disease (or comorbidities) is worth less. A determination of the QALY value involves multiplication of the utility value associated with a state of health by the number of years lived in that state of health. Following this thinking, half a year lived in excellent health is 0.5 QALY (0.5 year of life times 1 utility value), which is the same as 1 full year of life lived in a disease state (immobile, fractured hip assuming half utility value) (1 year times 0.5 utility value). There is controversy over the application and use of QALYs. Some report that the QALYs are not client focused, could be used in rationing health care, and may be viewed as impersonal and dehumanizing (Neumann & Cohen, 2018; Moreno-Ternero et al., 2023).

A second measure used to measure quality of life, the DALY, refers to a year spent in less-than-healthy life. It gauges the burden of disease and measures the gap between the current health status and excellent health status. It also accounts for life lost and life quality diminished through disability. The QALY and DALY measures may both be used and considered interchangeable depending on whether the outcome of the screening measure is intended to maximize health or minimize disability. The differences between the two tend to be modest with little effect on resource allocation (Augustovski et al., 2018; Feng et al., 2019; Neumann & Cohen, 2018).

There is currently greater focus on quantifying measurements of health outcomes so as to weigh the costs of screening, treatment, and effects on populations. The QALY incorporates morbidity and mortality in a single arithmetic measure. It allows computation, estimation, and comparisons of screening decisions. However, the estimation of formulas associated with utility and disability (DALYs) is difficult and emphasizes disease over health. QALYs assist in analyzing the gap between strict treatment decisions and their economic costs, informing public health decision-making (Augustovski et al., 2018). A newer distributed framework for evaluation of population health is health-adjusted life years (HALYs) which combines quality of life, and health disability into aggregated HALYs giving greater importance to the length of years of healthy life (Givler & Givler, 2023).

Measures of the **quantity of life** or length of life affected by health, particularly by disease, are more readily obtainable. In addition to prevalence and incidence rates, disease-specific mortality rates present different aspects of the disease for analysis. Disease-specific mortality may be linked to the severity of an incident occurring or the long-term health burden cost associated with management of the disease. There is some evidence that mandatory screening of athletes reduces the incidence of sudden cardiac death in athletes who are supposedly young and fit; however, the cost of comprehensive cardiac screening is high and controversial (Dhutia & MacLachlan, 2018), yet a death in a young athletically fit person can be a sudden, untoward, severe event. With other disorders, the prevalence may not be high, but the problem requires disproportionate amounts spent on maintenance or management after the condition is fully expressed. For neonatal PKU, a case undetected and managed at birth means a lifetime burden of suboptimal development and neurologic disease management.

Detection

With the relative significance of the disease established, the next step is to determine whether health professionals can screen individuals for the disease. Are there well-documented diagnostic criteria for the disorder? Is there a valid and reliable screening instrument? Are sufficient community resources and treatment modalities available to support a screening program?

Diagnostic Criteria

Detection of a disease requires knowledge of the characteristics that indicate its presence or, as in screening, its early pathogenic, asymptomatic state, and it is often based on risk factors such as heredity, age, sex, and family history. For example, certain screening tests may be recommended for males or females (Womenshealth.gov). Selected disease diagnostic criteria should be well documented and defined and not merely accepted as commonly used indicators. The effect of uncertainty in detecting disease is amplified when the application of the screening design is considered. Some diseases, such as sickle cell anemia or PKU, are defined by the presence or absence of a single, isolated gene or enzyme. Individuals have or do not have the risk factor or the disease, a binary condition (Mukherjee, 2020b). Other conditions, such as high blood glucose levels (diabetes) and blood lipid levels, are measured according to numerical values for which a normal range has been set. The usual ranges for these screening tests may be provided as standard values. Screening tests should only be recommended on the basis of strong evidence (Givler & Givler, 2023).

While this discussion has focused more on health conditions that can be detected through laboratory testing, it is also important to mention that there are behavioral screening measures which, if detected, may lead to social, mental, or physical interventions. An example of this is screening for adverse childhood experiences (ACEs). There is compelling evidence that exposure to childhood trauma affects the quality of later life; as the number of ACEs increases, there is greater likelihood of subsequent conditions such as cancer, depression, diabetes, alcoholism, and heart disease. An ACEs quiz of 10 questions asks adults about childhood trauma. Five of the questions relate to the person, and the other five relate to family members or those in close contact during childhood. This quiz screens for childhood trauma, such as if a child has witnessed abuse of his mother or sibling or has lived with a parent who has a substance disorder. A high ACE score would place the person at greater risk for experiencing later poor health outcomes (CDC, 2023a; ACESTooHigh.com, 2023).

Screening Measures

The next step is to determine whether methods exist to detect the disease during an early stage. If screening measures are available, an analysis should determine whether any of them fulfill the requirements for the screening process: available, easy to administer, safe with minimal discomfort, cost-effective, and accurate. Ultimately the decision to use a screening test will depend on how well the measure can distinguish those individuals who probably do not have and will not develop the condition from those who are likely to develop the condition. The variables that aid in a screening instrument's evaluation include reliability, validity, and reproducibility, which are a measure of the accuracy of the instrument.

Reliability is an assessment of the reproducibility of the test's results when different individuals with the same level of skill perform the test during different periods and under different conditions. The instrument or measure should yield consistent or stable results over time. If the same result emerges when two individuals perform the test, **interobserver reliability** is shown. If the same individual is able to reproduce the results several times, **intraobserver reliability** is demonstrated.

From this information, health professionals can determine the amount of training required for health care professionals, technicians, or personnel who administer the test. For example, if interobserver reliability is low, additional training might be required to work toward a more consistent method of screening test delivery. This is frequently necessary in blood pressure cuff hypertension screening or in weight measurements, where the measurement device may not function properly. If intraobserver reliability is low, the health professional might surmise that the instrument, and not the individual, is at fault. Retesting is almost always indicated for measurement outliers. Some screening measures are of necessity more qualitative, and intraobserver reliability may be very important in the case of substance abuse or mental health/depression screening. Finally, for a screening test to be valid, which is the next requirement, it must first be reliable, but reliability is only a necessary condition and is not entirely sufficient for validity.

Validity reflects the accuracy or truthfulness of the test or instrument itself. In a controlled setting, one evaluates validity by testing the instrument on a group of individuals who have positive or negative results. A valid test correctly distinguishes individuals who have preclinical disease from those without preclinical disease. The ideal result is to have the instrument identify 100% of the diseased individuals (positive reactions) and 100% of the nondiseased individuals (negative reactions).

There are also ranges of measurement for disease reliability and validity. Perfectly accurate categorization of validity rarely occurs in practice; therefore, the measure of validity has been divided into two components that quantify the margin of error in screening instruments. **Sensitivity** measures the first component. This refers to the proportion of people with a condition who correctly test positive when screened. If a test has good sensitivity, the number of individuals with the disease who are missed through inaccurate categorization as false negatives will be low. Conversely, a test with poor sensitivity will overlook individuals with the condition, and there will be a large number of false negative test results—individuals who actually have the condition but are told they are disease-free or have tested negative for the disease.

Specificity is the second component. Specificity measures the test's ability to recognize negative reactions or individuals in which disease is absent. A test with excellent specificity will rarely produce a positive result if the disease is not present. A test with poor specificity could result in false positive test results. Individuals with false positive test results are told that they have a disease or condition when in actuality they do not. Specific epidemiologic formulas are used to measure both sensitivity and specificity.

In a perfect world, tests would be highly sensitive and highly specific; however, that is usually not the case, and some balance is reached between the two ideal visions. For some tests, there may also be an indeterminate zone in which the individual does not test strictly negative or positive. In these tests, the numerical cutoff may be subject to interpretation or a more arbitrary decision. A cutoff decision may be made so that the screening instrument is less likely to miss actual cases of disease at the cost of erroneously identifying cases of disease (false positives) that will need more diagnostic work, which may be expensive and invasive.

Consider the issues in population health when using a newly developed screening test with low specificity and moderate sensitivity. Low specificity means few true negative test results and more false positive test results. This is the current situation with mammography screening (Mao et al., 2023). The nurse and other health professionals (also health advocacy groups such as those involved in breast cancer awareness) must then consider the cost, inconvenience, and psychological stress experienced by the people with false positive results during the period after their incorrect screening test, the unnecessary additional referrals, and the ability of the existing follow-up services to meet these needs. With only moderate sensitivity, a number of false negative results could occur, which may ignore individuals who could benefit from treatment.

Medical, economic, political, and ethical issues are involved; that is, should a screening program be implemented when it is known that the tests may involve avoidable harms such as additional biopsies and excessive treatment? The use of mammography screening became a special case for inclusion under the US Affordable Care Act (ACA) coverage, as this legislation requires coverage for repetitive preventive services with a certainty of moderate or substantial benefit (Duffy et al., 2021; Morrell et al., 2023) and poorer states may have less access to preventive care. In screening for coronavirus, the states have taken the leadership role in finding test kits, mandating state laboratories that can process and analyze the findings of the test, and making geographical sites for testing available (Forsythe et al., 2020).

A broader issue concerns larger health fair screening programs, for example, where a targeted population such as older adults is sought for a mass screening. The efficiency and efficacy of such programs must be analyzed. The following are examples of questions that address efficiency and efficacy: Is the targeted population prepared in an appropriate way before engaging in the screening tests? Are the health care practitioners who are administering the test educated (and certified) according to the standard protocols of test administration? Are health care providers following the latest screening evidence? Are follow-up measures and appropriate referral access instituted in the program? There are times when an elder lacks the cognitive ability or finances to follow-up on positive screening results. Patients and health care providers may overestimate the benefits and underestimate the harm of screening and associated treatment. Answers to these questions challenge health care providers in the development, implementation, and follow-up processes identified so that screening efficiency and efficacy is enhanced.

Several for-profit genomic and biotechnology companies have marketed genetic tests (Box 9.1: Genomics) to identify

BOX 9.1 GENOMICS

New Norms: Noninvasive Prenatal Testing (NIPT) for Fetal Chromosome Abnormalities

Prenatal screening on maternal blood samples is the norm and is reducing the need for invasive amniocentesis testing. Noninvasive prenatal testing (NIPT) has consistently shown fewer false positives and more true positives; this would indicate that this testing has high specificity and high sensitivity (Johnston et al., 2023). These maternal blood tests on fetal-free DNA can determine whether the fetus has a chromosomal abnormality (e.g., Down syndrome—chromosome 21—or other chromosomal abnormalities, such as on chromosome 13, 18, X, or Y). If the finding is abnormal, amniocentesis is used to confirm the original result. NIPT can also be ordered as early as 10 weeks' gestation and therefore greatly reduces the need for invasive testing. The ease of using NIPT also leads to its potential use for early sex determination so could involve ethical issues in populations that might use sex selection to increase the birth of male babies. Asian countries such as India and China regulate NIPT closely to discourage sex selection.

The uses of fetal genomic testing on maternal blood samples are just beginning to be realized and may lead to diagnoses and in directions that were not expected given the original purpose of the screening (Johnston et al., 2023).

genes and ancestry associated with risk factors and diseases. A number are available on the Internet. Various companies report that DNA analysis can provide at least 30-plus trait reports and 2000 geographic regions, a DNA relative finder, health predisposition reports, carrier risks, some drug responses, and disease risk (e.g., Parkinson disease, cholesterol levels, pres ence of diabetes). A more advanced assessment through the same company includes wellness reports, heart health reports, drug metabolism reports, and skin cancer susceptibility, among other important health information. This is only one example of online companies selling such individual DNA assessments. Newer applications of maternal ultrasound on the pregnant uterus may identify mothers most at risk for preterm birth due to thinner uterine walls with a structurally inferior cervix (Schaffer, 2019). Many of these screening tests are becoming more common and less expensive.

Crow (2019) reported that the US Food and Drug Administration (FDA) may be cautious in its oversight of consumer genetic testing/genomics, as it is requiring stricter disclosure of information to consumers. Consumer DNA testing has been criticized by the FDA for making what the administration views as overreaching health diagnostic claims (Crow, 2019). Consumer-available tests can involve concerns of standardization, cost, privacy, and failure to make reports fully understandable. Comprehensive research on screening tests significantly influences the efficacy of the entire process. When available, data on the reliability and validity of individual tests and screening programs in general provide valuable information to evaluate, anticipate, and ideally control these influences, enabling the program to work effectively toward its established goal and positive health care outcomes.

Primary Care, Lead Agency, and Community Screening Resources

Screening is often done in an outpatient primary care setting. As funding for traditional public health nursing roles is declining, the responsibility for screening often falls to nurses in more traditional and advanced practice roles. Implementing a screening program depends on the availability of appropriate **community resources**, such as funds, health care workers, and follow-up services, including access, referrals, treatment sources, and administrative personnel. Nurses can provide structure and design for screening programs, as seamless organization of a program is essential to success. Knowledge of a disease's characteristics and an effective screening instrument are useless without financial and organized human support to use them. Many screening programs are by necessity complex, requiring collaborative efforts for health agency partner development.

A **lead agency** or group may be identified to oversee the development of the community health program. The origins of the lead agency range from a community service organization to local public health departments responding to regulations or a mandate at the state or federal level. Regardless of its origin, the agency must perform a self-evaluation to compare its level of expertise with what is required to supervise the process of the screening effort. Early identification of the lead agency, along with potential partnerships, allows the effective use of talents and the division of labor.

Some screening programs may involve complicated legal issues; for example, states have policies about HIV testing and privacy and identification of individuals. HIV screening and testing is highly recommended in high-risk individuals—those who have injected steroids or drugs, those who have unprotected sex (especially males who have sex with men), and those who have other STIs or comorbidities (e.g., hepatitis C [HCV]). Current recommendations for HCV now include screening for the virus for all adults between ages 18 and 79 (US Preventive Services Task Force [USPSTF], 2020) (https://www.uspreventiveservicestaskforce.org/uspstf/recommendation/hepatitis-c-screening).

HIV testing kits may be ordered online with screening performed at home. This consumer-controlled home screening may protect individual identity, ensure confidentiality, and motivate individuals who might be afraid to access provider screening in clinics or hospitals. OraQuick (http://www.oraquick.com), the only FDA-approved home test for HIV screening, has sold millions of test kits. OraQuick requires a fluid specimen from the mouth at the upper and lower gums and gives preliminary results in 20 minutes. Their website provides specifics about the kits and provides a 24-hour resource support hotline for questions on directions or results.

For the lead agency to develop and oversee the development of any community health program, such as the delivery of a screening program, partnerships and coalitions are essential. The agency must contact and organize necessary stakeholders. **Stakeholders** are individuals or groups who have a legitimate interest in an issue. Examples of stakeholders may include key community individuals; hospitals; health and social service agencies, such as primary health care centers; and community organizations, including houses of worship, community centers, schools, transportation agencies, and volunteer organizations. **Key community individuals** are those people who are considered leaders within the community. The primary rule is to never assume that what is appropriate and effective for one community will be appropriate and effective for another.

Stakeholders and partners along with nurses can perform **community assessments** together. A community assessment is a systematic method of data collection that provides a detailed account, first identifying need and subsequently determining the type, quantity, and quality of resources. Review of demographic data, vital statistics, and morbidity and mortality data may delineate the assessed need. Resources might come from an eclectic variety of support sources, including government entities such as public health departments, social services, and even safety and transportation in the case of car seat safety screenings. Schools, private businesses, churches, and places of social gatherings might provide resource support, either in screening support or in the actual administration of the screening.

After the assessment has been completed, the data analysis will reveal the **target community** or high-risk population, the available health care resources, and the health needs of the high-risk population. The identified partners collaborate, review, and analyze the data, leading to the development of health-improvement strategies (in this case a screening program), with methods of

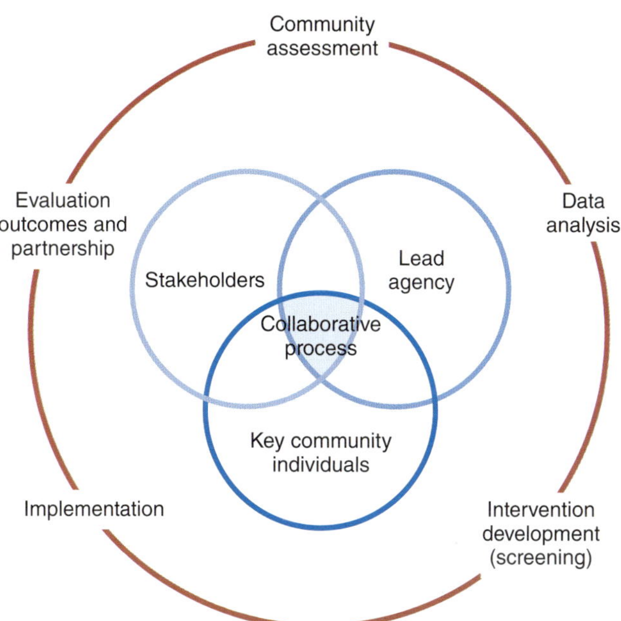

FIG. 9.2 Collaborative partnership: Community health program development.

implementation to move the target population smoothly through the screening process. Finally, monitoring and evaluating outcomes is essential to determine the effectiveness of the program and the achievement of the stated goals. Evaluation includes monitoring of the entire process, including the successful workings of the partnership. Fig. 9.2 presents one model of a collaborative partnership: community health program development. Population health nursing is an important component of this partnership.

The constraints affecting the operation of a screening program include financial concerns, political issues, cultural constraints, follow-up and referral services, and accessible treatment facilities. All partners are aware that responses from the target community are affected partly by their experience with other screening programs, such as the means used to inform them, the accessibility of the location, the availability of transportation, the convenience of the program's hours, and the cultural sensitivity of the delivery and design of the program. A preventive health nursing approach identifies the necessary community resources and defines how these resources interact and may be mobilized to achieve maximal benefits and positive outcomes. Financial support of a screening program is a constraint that can influence all points in the system. Although some programs are delivered entirely on a voluntary basis, organizers of others must submit grant proposals to local, state, or federal departments when consideration of medical and economic ethics is involved. Planners must look beyond the screening day and investigate financial resources for follow-up care and treatment.

In addition to financial accessibility, follow-up services need to be accessible in terms of convenient locations and opening hours. For example, an evening clinic may reach those who are reluctant or financially unable to miss work. Nurse practitioner clinics facilitate access to preventive health services at convenient times for various population groups. An efficient referral system links the follow-up resources to the screening program, providing continuity of care. A process should be devised to encourage the participant to take positive action on the referral. Public health nurses will facilitate this process with a variety of communication techniques, such as emails, telephone or in-person counseling, mailings, and home visits. Community outreach navigation nurses, employed by hospitals and insurance companies, follow-up on individuals with particular conditions that are either chronic or harder to treat. Given that all services needed may not be available within a service catchment area, referrals to clinics and hospitals out of state may be facilitated.

Another example is that a college of health sciences organizes a health fair that includes screening. This creates opportunities for **interprofessional education** and practice and has been highlighted as important by the World Health Organization (Wei et al., 2022; Rutherford-Hemming, 2018). Nursing students and medical students could manage physical assessments and laboratory screenings. Pharmacist students screen individuals for medical use of inappropriate or contraindicated medications. Social worker students may assess individuals for mental health issues. There is a plan for continuation of care if disease issues and risks are identified—for example, for individuals needing immediate referrals for hypertension control, the college may agree to assist in referrals to providers who will donate time to assist in this effort.

Should Screening for the Disease Be Done?

After it has been determined that the disease is significant and can be screened for, organizing the screening activity is the next step. Screening for a particular disorder and ultimately treating those with the early-identified disorder improve the chances of a favorable outcome in comparison with those whose disorder is not found until signs and symptoms become evident. Therefore several questions must be considered. If a test accurately identifies a condition in the early stages, is there any benefit to the individual? Are there effective treatment modalities for the condition? To summarize, can the screening test be used to prevent identified disease for which early treatment is curative, shortens a period of disability, increases life span, or improves quality of life? Recommendations for a wide variety of screening tests are on governmental websites. The **US Preventive Services Task Force** may recommend for (or against) routine screening for many health conditions and diseases (USPSTF, 2023) (https://www.uspreventiveservicestaskforce.org/uspstf/). There is a frequently updated listing of screening recommendations on the USPSTF website. For example, the USPSTF recommends against PSA screening for prostate cancer in males 70 and older (rating D). PSA screening was rated as grade D (not recommended) because evidence indicated that the balance of harms from early treatment (urinary incontinence, bowel control, erectile dysfunction) outweighed the benefits of early diagnosis. This was further modified. For males 55 to 69 years, the decision to screen should be made individually (rating C) after discussion of potential harms and benefits. For some recommendations there may also be subrecommendations recognizing varying clinical decisions in higher-risk populations or age groups. For example, prostate screening may be recommended for African American males and males with a family history of prostate cancer.

For females aged 50 to 74 years, mammography is recommended (rating B). However, for females at average risk aged 40 to 49 years, the decision to begin mammography screening is individual (rating C). There is a new recommendation in process (2023) that females receive screening every other year starting at age 40. Recommendations for mammography screening have changed several times within the last decade because of high rates of false positive test results, overdiagnosis, many normal/benign biopsy specimens, and overtreatment (USPSTF, 2023). Finding testing or screening sites and necessary follow-up appointments may be difficult for females with work or childcare responsibilities.

In 2022, the recommendation for the use of low-dose aspirin for primary prevention of cardiovascular disease (CVD) in adults ages 40 to 59 who have a greater CVD risk was that it should be an individual decision (grade C), but the USPSTF recommended against low-dose aspirin in adults 60 or older (grade D). Low-dose aspirin recommendations have changed frequently. For all the latest information on screening activities, the CDC maintains an updated website (sexually transmitted diseases, HIV, hepatitis) for individuals to enter their ZIP codes and find local testing and clinic sites (https://gettested.cdc.gov/).

It is necessary for the health care provider to remain aware of or check for the best evidence on changes in screening guidelines. Screening may be based on the disease's asymptomatic period; therefore, adequate information must exist concerning the optimal time for screening, specific intervention during this time, and knowledge regarding the effect of early detection and treatment on the prognosis. Without this knowledge, health care professionals are unable to explain how the outcomes of those with early-detected disease differ from the outcomes of those with undetected disease, and they cannot support the health benefits derived from the screening program.

Follow-up is critical to determine whether the intervention strategies prescribed are in fact happening. Should screening be done if there is no potential follow-up in terms of medical or social services? A prescribed follow-up regimen may be very broad and include a wide variety of interventional strategies, such as diet, exercise, and drug therapy. Follow-up services may include an evaluation and review of the literature that discusses evidence-based practice pertaining to a particular drug, as well as the identification of intervention characteristics that impair follow-up, such as cost, inconvenience, or side effects. Consideration must also be given to those factors that enhance follow-up. For example, nurses can provide ongoing counseling and education about medications and assist individuals in lifestyle transformations that include health-promoting behaviors.

The safety of a potential intervention is a concern when the widespread application of further medical interventions or invasive diagnostic tests after a screening program is considered. Risks or harmful side effects can be costly in terms of human health and the increased medical care required to correct **iatrogenic** or interventional effects (e.g., additional surgical procedures or emotional distress). As an example, Jordana, who is 54 years old and has a low risk of breast cancer, attends a community clinic and wants more information about the optimal interval between breast cancer screenings. She has heard that there are disagreements between US government studies (USPSTF), the American Cancer Society, and other sources of credible medical advice. The nurse, using an evidence-based practice model, helps Jordana find or review the most recent and best sources of information that would answer her question (e.g., American Cancer Society, https://www.cancer.org/; American Heart Association, https://www.heart.org/) (USPSTF, 2023). In addition to the scientific literature, the nurse locates consumer information for Jordana. In this case, the nurse assists the female in making informed health choices about her screening tests.

The bottom line is that to be effective, a high-quality, cost-effective, research/evidence-based screening tool or technique must identify a real or potential "problem." Screening must provide real and workable "solutions" in which the tangible and intangible costs of the screening are less than the risk of the disease and result in measurable health benefits.

ETHICAL CONSIDERATIONS FOR SCREENING

Improving health is considered just and morally consistent with values endorsed throughout the care delivery system. Screening activities are separate from interventions offered for established disease (e.g., myocardial infarction). Rather than treating those who have established disease, a screening program invites ostensibly well individuals to be tested to determine their disease risk and the need for follow-up. This request for voluntary participation implies an expectation of a health benefit, although at this stage little may be announced about specifics of testing, cost, or what participant must do. Screening programs need to clarify expectations and inform participants as contingent issues occur. Screening participants need to know whether the ultimate benefit is preventive, ameliorative, or curative and whether future activities may be needed to secure a healthy outcome.

Borderline Cases and Cutoff Points

A screening program measurement is often based on a numerical value, so a question often arises about the use of cutoff points for the screening instrument and borderline cases. The goal of a screening program—identifying an individual as having high risk or not having high risk—may depend on clearly established evidence-based numerical values. For many conditions, cutoff points and standard ranges are used. For test outcomes above the designated range, the person is disease positive; below this point, the individual is disease negative. Consequently, readjusting cutoff points or laboratory values can become a highly controversial issue, as the cutoff point controls the percentage of positive and negative results. If the disease were potentially life-threatening, an increase in false positive results (lower cutoff point) could be preferred to missing individuals who may have the disease. In addition, if a disease is relatively benign in terms of potential stigmatization, anxiety, and problems with treatment, lowering the cutoff point could again be safe and ethical. For example, at the individual level, a change in the cutoff point on blood pressures from 130/90 to 120/80 means that a larger portion of the adult population would fall outside the guidelines and might need additional lifestyle or drug treatment (Reboussin, et al., 2019). This also can be a global issue, as cutoff points for laboratory tests and toxic exposure values may vary between countries.

Examples of problems related to identifying cutoff points and borderline cases are very common in community nursing practice. Blood pressure control is a common health problem in which a variance of 5 mmHg to 10 mmHg can make the difference in identifying a person as having a high risk of hypertension. Lipid and cholesterol level cutoffs and ratios are always subject to further examination. Limits for toxic chemicals and products of manufacturing in the environment are constantly becoming identified; for example, there is evidence that microplastics and heavy metals in the environment are toxic to humans and animals. Recommendations change as new evidence emerges. When involved with screening, more sophisticated approaches may discriminate between borderline cases that should be referred and ones that should not. Research and use of current evidence are essential when selecting diseases or conditions for screening.

Economic Costs and Ethics

In the past, the tendency was to disregard the cost of promoting a healthy, disease-free, or disease-controlled status; this results in a philosophical stance that all care should be given to all people at all costs. There is now a fuller recognition that enormous costs are involved with many screening programs. Allocating community funds to one large screening event may result in a lack of funds for other projects. Populations benefiting from a screening test will be balanced by those suffering in terms of decreases in service of other medical or social needs.

Initial operational costs must be considered, including buying or renting screening equipment and floor space and engaging professionals or technicians to administer the tests and interpret the results. These costs are encountered a second time when individuals are referred for further evaluation. Consumer costs include follow-up visits, treatments, and lost time and income. Given the combined operational and consumer costs, several questions are raised: Do the costs result in improved health outcomes? Are the benefits worth the necessary expenditures? These answers are influenced partly by the values (other than monetary) attributed to the benefit. Saving lives in a young population may be judged as more valuable than screening older populations with chronic illnesses. Communities or states may set targets for their own screening programs. However, a strictly economic approach may eliminate the intangible variables and require the use of more objective data for decision-making.

When program designs are reviewed, three main approaches are often used to evaluate the economic resources affected: cost-benefit ratio, cost-effectiveness, and cost-efficiency analyses. The current relevance and use of such concepts require a basic understanding of their roles in the selection of a condition for screening. They tend to be separate methods and most frequently are used independently of one another.

Cost-Benefit Ratio

A **cost-benefit ratio economic analysis** is sometimes performed first because it allows for the comparison of various outcomes in monetary terms. This comparison is necessary in health planning when the initial consideration is dependent on whether the expected health outcome (e.g., reduction in the incidences of cardiovascular disease, decrease in infant mortality, or reduction of the detection of a visual problem) will be most beneficial to the community at the most reasonable cost. The cost of the screening versus the cost of long-term care management may be weighed. For example, what is the cost-benefit ratio of blood pressure screenings, compared with the medical and financial cost of a stroke caused by undiagnosed hypertension, to the individual, the community, and the health care system? The cost of screening is often weighed against other factors, such as the cost and feasibility of vaccination programs, as in the case of screening individuals for cancers associated with the human papilloma virus (Chesson et al., 2019). Resources are available on the CDC site for some diseases, health issues, and lifestyle changes (CDC, 2024, https://www.cdc.gov/diabetes-prevention/employers-insurers/cost-calculator-tools.html).

Cost-Effectiveness

If the reduction of cardiovascular disease is chosen as the desired outcome, the next step is a **cost-effectiveness analysis**, which determines the optimal use of resources to reach a predetermined, constant endpoint or the desired health outcome. The screening benefit remains the same; the best method of getting to the target outcome is the focus of the investigation. For example, for reduction of cardiovascular disease, various methods might be used. These methods include screening individuals for hypertension and cholesterol, performing electrocardiograms on all individuals aged 25 years or older who are admitted to the hospital, screening young athletes for cardiovascular disease (Petek & Baggish, 2020), sponsoring an antismoking campaign, or providing nutrition counseling. Implementation of all these options would be ideal, but with limited resources some choices are made.

Cost Efficiency

The last approach to help bring economic resources into perspective is a **cost-efficiency analysis**. The purpose is to be efficient and budget a limited amount of money toward achieving as much of the desired outcome as possible. The funds are the focus, not the health benefit.

SELECTION OF SCREENABLE POPULATIONS

The selection of a screenable population is as important as the selection of a screenable disease and is often based on incidence and prevalence data. The objective is to identify a high-risk group that, when tested, will yield a significant number of diseased individuals. With a well-planned selection approach, the efforts and cost of screening the population are minimized, and the health benefit is maximized. The main criterion used to define an appropriate population is the definitive presence of risk factors related to the disorder. Within community settings, nurses can ensure a thorough examination of possible risk factors, including both person-dependent and environment-dependent factors (see Box 9.2: Evidence-Based Practice).

BOX 9.2 EVIDENCE-BASED PRACTICE

Population-Based Research Optimizing Screening Through Personalized Regimens

The National Cancer Institute created the collaborative Population-Based Research Optimizing Screening Through Personalized Regimens (PROSPR) (National Cancer Institute, 2023) to support research on the community-based screening processes to include experiences and outcomes for breast, colon, and cervical cancer. This effort started a decade ago and was funded through 2024. The collaborative sharing of research has had several stages. The overall aim was to develop coordination between the research practices conducted at multiple sites. It reviewed recruitment, screening, diagnosis, referral, and treatment rates. It focuseed on research translation and implementation, addressing issues such as the controversy regarding breast cancer screening and mammography by studying the comparative effectiveness and outcomes of existing and emerging research. In September 2011, the National Cancer Institute initially funded seven research centers and one statistical site as part of this integrated research screening program. New programs supported by the Affordable Care Act will support the development of other evidence-based health-promotion and disease-prevention activities.

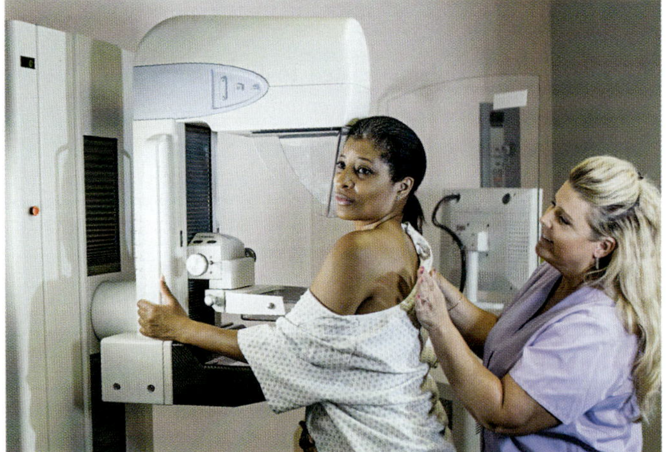

FIG. 9.3 Mammography screening. (From iStock.com/kali9.)

Person-Dependent Factors

A person's age is important because of age-dependent changes in the levels of risk factors throughout the population. For example, the risk of many cancers increases as a person grows older (Bottazzi et al., 2018; Laconi et al., 2020). A high priority is placed on screening vulnerable populations, especially females, infants, and children, as the outcomes obtained affect long-range growth and development patterns. However, as the average life span increases, the effects of risk factors in young, middle-aged, and older adults are becoming more apparent, making certain prevalent and costly chronic conditions equally important to control. The middle-aged adult population may be screened for hypertension, diabetes, breast cancer, glaucoma, and heart disease; this population requires earlier screening, as some of these disease conditions are becoming apparent in early adulthood and even teenage years. Older adults may be screened for cognitive decline, although screening for the asymptomatic elderly is controversial because of a lack of effective dementia treatment. Routine genetic screening for various markers, such as beta-amyloid and APOE-e4, is under investigation, along with other research studies (Alzheimer's Association, 2023). Although children may be at no greater risk than adults for contracting coronavirus, older adults bear much of the intense disease burden and almost all the associated mortality (Vessey and Betz, 2020).

Sex has obvious implications for screening programs. For example, females are tested frequently for two reproductive-related conditions: breast cancer and cervical cancer (Fig. 9.3). Current screening test recommendations for females are available at Womenshealth.gov (https://www.womenshealth.gov/search/node?keys=screening+for+women).

Selecting screening tests for a population from a particular ethnic or racial group also may be appropriate, as some disorders/unhealthy conditions occur more frequently in certain racial or ethnic groups. In 2015 to 2016, Hispanic (47%) and non-Hispanic Black adults (46.8%) reported a higher prevalence of obesity than White adults (37.9%) (CDC, 2023b). In 2011 to 2014, diabetes was more prevalent in non-Hispanic Black adults (18%) and Hispanic adults (16.8%) than in non-Hispanic White adults (9.6%) (CDC, 2023b). Since 1999, **Racial and Ethnic Approaches to Community Health** (REACH) communities have used participatory approaches to identify and disseminate strategies for addressing health disparities. Nurses can lobby and advocate for specific groups to have more targeted screenings, particularly in communities that have large ethnic or racial minority populations (Box 9.3: Health and Social Determinants/Health Equity).

Income level has been associated repeatedly with population-specific health disparities. Chronic conditions are more likely to be diagnosed in low-income Americans than in high-income Americans. Physical illness and disparities for depression, high blood pressure, diabetes, and obesity are more prevalent in lower-income populations, so these populations are at greater risk (Cohen et al., 2018). In addition to a greater likelihood of not having adequate health insurance, low-income Americans can least afford necessary preventive care, effective treatment, and health education (Cohen et al., 2018).

Personal behavioral characteristics related to lifestyle may suggest the need to screen a particular individual or group. When health care practitioners review lifestyle, they are looking at daily habits that affect health and wellness, such as nutrition, fitness level, tobacco use, alcohol and drug use, sexual practices, stress management, adequate rest, immunizations, periodic examinations, use of seat belts, and other safety factors. Engaging in some of these behaviors while avoiding others is essential for living a healthy life. Therefore screening for personal behavioral characteristics that are considered risky assesses the likelihood of a longer, disease-free life. After risky behaviors are eliminated, the development of substitute healthy behaviors via programming and transformation of lifestyle is crucial. Health care providers have a responsibility to educate and empower individuals about the next step in the evaluation of their potential condition once screening has been completed. Those being screened have a responsibility to seek treatment and follow-up services and to ultimately engage in behavioral

BOX 9.3 HEALTH AND SOCIAL DETERMINANTS/HEALTH EQUITY

Eliminating Health Disparities Among Ethnic Groups

Population diversity is acknowledged as a strength of the United States, but it is apparent that disparities exist among the various immigrant, racial, and ethnic groups in the attainment and maintenance of health. The minority populations of the United States include Black Americans, Hispanics, Asian/Pacific Islanders, American Indians, and Alaska Natives. These categories along with immigration oversimplify the reality of the multicultural nature of assessing health status, screening, and planning to improve health. Specific racial groupings are not absolute because there are subgroups within each, and separate population group numbers rise and fall.

These disparities and factors, such as access to care, need to be taken into consideration when planning screening programs. To plan, implement, and evaluate a screening program that targets a specific population, the provider must have an awareness of the target population that includes components such as lifestyle, socioeconomic characteristics, education, heredity, environmental factors, values, religious and cultural beliefs, communication style, and language. Partnering with key individuals and organizations in the community through the entire process is important for any screening program to be successful, as the following example scenario illustrates.

As an example, public health officials in a town located in the Midwest might be concerned about the health status of a new immigrant population. Recent census data indicate that the number of immigrants has grown; these immigrants are drawn to the area by better lifestyle and full employment in industrial plants. The census data also reveal that this population is primarily young adults, male and female. The town officials are aware that most of the males and females work shifts side-by-side on lines in the packing plant, often with overtime hours.

Based on these data, hospital officials decide to plan a health and screening day for this population. The hospital distributes flyers in the community in the primary native language of the target population. The day of the screening arrives, and the number of participants is very low. The hospital officials are very concerned. They had good intentions. They do not know what to do next.

- What critical actions did the hospital officials perform that might be considered positive in the planning of the health and screening day?
- What critical actions did the hospital officials not perform that might have contributed to the poor turnout at the health and screening function?
- What might the hospital officials consider in their planning for the next health and screening day?
- How might they engage the community, community leaders, and target population in planning the health and screening day?
- What local community agencies and groups might be invited to participate as partners when the health and screening day is being planned and implemented?
- Can you identify any creative ways to bring the health and screening day to the targeted population, making the program more accessible?

change toward a healthy lifestyle if the screening techniques are to serve a purpose.

Regional and rural disparities exist and include many of the previously mentioned disparities. These disparities are of great concern, but identifying causes can be difficult. Research is being done on interrelationships between the determinants of health to include biology and genetics, individual behaviors, the social environment, the physical environment, and health services (access and quality). The REACH program (http://www.cdc.gov/reach) addresses the factors and is demonstrating success by empowering residents to "plan and carry out local, culturally appropriate programs to address a wide range of health issues among African Americans, American Indians, Hispanics/Latinos, Asian Americans, Alaska Natives, and Pacific islanders" (CDC, 2023b). Appropriate screening is integrated into the REACH program, which aims to reduce health disparities among racial and ethnic populations with the highest burden of chronic disease.

Environment-Dependent Factors

The area of environmental health and protection has expanded over the years and is becoming more complex. Environmental health and protection have been defined as the science that is concerned with elements of the environment that influence people's health and well-being. These factors include conditions of the workplace, home, and communities, including chemical, physical, and psychological forces (Rector & Stanley, 2021). Workplace designs that may be considered include indoor and outdoor air pollution; water pollution; safe drinking water; noise pollution; radiation exposure; biologic pollutants; hazardous waste management and disposal of garbage; vector and pesticide control; deforestation, wetlands destruction, and desertification; energy depletion; inadequate housing; contaminated food and foods with toxic additives; safety at the work site and in the community; and psychological hazards (Rector & Stanley, 2021; Seller et al., 2019).

In occupational health, a legitimate population for screening includes those in high-risk work areas, where harmful chemicals, airborne particles, or high-decibel machinery puts the workers at risk of cancer, respiratory conditions, or auditory problems. For example, nail salons were recently mandated to require mechanical ventilation and exhaust (Seller et al., 2019). At the other extreme is the sedentary executive work life, where the lack of exercise is prevalent, placing the worker at risk of obesity and obesity-related conditions such as diabetes. The recent introduction of the coronavirus globally increases testing of health care workers and others providing essential services to determine who is immune and can work safely. The use of occupational health nurses to provide individual and mass screening for such problems, in addition to routinely recommended screening, is recognized as integral to promoting better occupational health practices.

National Guidance and Health Care Reform

Healthy People 2030

Many national organizations are guiding and promoting evidence-based care and screening. The *Healthy People* programs, for each decade, have been establishing benchmarks and monitoring progress on goals and objectives to promote health care delivery partnerships, guide individuals toward making empowered health decisions, and assess the efficacy of preventive programs (HealthyPeople.gov, 2023). The most current version of *Healthy People 2030* includes guidelines for implementing community programs that support its goals and objectives, including screening. The content on the site is often rearranged for easier retrieval of information. For examples of more specific objectives related to screening, see Box 9.4 for *Healthy People 2030* objectives related to screening.

BOX 9.4 HEALTHY PEOPLE 2030 OBJECTIVES RELATED TO SCREENING

Symbol	*Healthy People 2030* Objectives
BDBS-D01	Increase the proportion of persons who donate blood
C-01	Reduce the overall cancer death rate
C-09	Increase the proportion of females who get screened for cervical cancer
C-07	Increase the proportion of adults who get screened for colorectal cancer
C-05	Increase the proportion of females who get screened for a breast cancer
C-11	Increase the proportion of cancer survivors who are living 5 years or longer after diagnosis
EH-01	Reduce the number of days people are exposed to unhealthy air
EH-04	Reduce blood lead levels in children aged 1–5 years
MICH-17	Increase the proportion of children who receive a developmental screening
MHMD-08	Increase the proportion of primary care physician office visits where adolescents and adults are screened for depression
V-01	Increase the proportion of children aged 3–5 years who receive vision screening
HDS-06	Reduce cholesterol in adults

From US Department of Health and Human Services. *Healthy People 2030 objectives.* Office of Disease Prevention and Health Promotion. https://health.gov/healthypeople;
HealthyPeople.gov. (2023). *Healthy People 2030.* Washington, DC: US Department of Health and Human Services, Office of Disease Prevention and Health Promotion. https://health.gov/healthypeople

Recommended Screenings of the US Preventive Services Task Force

Also, more specifically, the USPSTF and the Agency for Healthcare Research and Quality of the Department of Health and Human Services identify specific population recommendations in the Recommendations for Primary Care Practice. There are recommendations A through D, which evolve as new scientific evidence becomes available, so this chapter will not provide details on specific recommended screenings (USPSTF, 2023). Boxes 9.5 and 9.6 list the recommended preventive screening services for adults and children covered by the ACA and required of marketplace insurance health plans in the United States. These lists are continually revised and updated.

The US Affordable Care Act and Prevention Incentives

The passing of the ACA in 2010 and adjustments to it since have shifted the focus of public health movements toward prevention and health promotion. One result is that standard preventive services are required to be covered by health insurance plans, and more preventive services have been outlined for Medicare recipients. Medicare now covers annual wellness visits that incorporate a personalized prevention plan based on an individual's age and health status; these visits can be conducted by a variety of practitioners, including nurse practitioners, clinical nurse specialists, and certified nurse midwives (Center for Medicare Advocacy, 2023).

Among other more recent incentives, Medicare has also enhanced Medicare Advantage programs, which may provide additional services such as in-home care, pharmacy, vision, and dental. During the fall enrollment period, there are many commercials for Medicare Advantage programs; elders have to choose according to which services they are more likely to use. In addition, websites are available to help elders identify preventive services, quality insurance plans that best cover their individual needs, and any necessary follow-up.

BOX 9.5 Screening and Preventive Services for Adults (Examples)

- Abdominal aortic aneurysm one-time screening for males of specified ages who have smoked
- Alcohol misuse screening/counseling
- Aspirin for prevention of cardiovascular disease
- Blood pressure screening
- Colorectal cancer screening
- Depression screening for adults
- Diabetes mellitus (type 2) screening
- Hepatitis B and C screening
- HIV infection screening
- Obesity screening and counseling
- Sexually transmitted infection prevention counseling
- Statin preventive medication
- Syphilis infection screening for pregnant females
- Tobacco use screening
- Tuberculosis screening

From US Centers for Medicare and Medicaid Services. (2023). *Preventive care for adults and children.* https://healthcare.gov.

BOX 9.6 Screening and Preventive Services for Children (Examples)

- Alcohol, tobacco, and drug misuse
- Autism screening
- Behavioral assessments
- Bilirubin concentration screening
- Blood pressure screening for children at various ages
- Blood lead levels
- Cervical dysplasia screening
- Child maltreatment
- Depression screening
- Developmental screening
- Fluoride chemoprevention and varnish
- Gonorrhea preventive medication for newborns
- Hearing screening
- Height, weight, and body mass index screening
- Hematocrit or hemoglobin screening for children
- Hepatitis B screening
- HIV screening
- High blood pressure screening in children
- Hyperbilirubinemia screening in infants
- Hypothyroidism screening
- Immunizations
- Iron supplements
- Obesity screening and counseling
- Phenylketonuria screening
- Sexually transmitted infection prevention, counseling, and screening
- Speech and language delay screening
- Vision screening
- Well-baby and well-child visits

From US Centers for Medicare and Medicaid Services. (2023). *Preventive care for adults and children.* https://healthcare.gov.

National Prevention Strategy

In addition to increasing the funded coverage of preventive services and screenings, the ACA also created the National Prevention Council, comprising "17 heads of departments, agencies, and offices across the Federal government who are committed to promoting prevention and wellness. The Council provides the leadership necessary to engage not only the federal government but a diverse array of stakeholders, including state and local policymakers, business leaders, individuals, their families and communities, to champion the policies and programs needed to ensure the health of Americans prospers" (Fig. 9.4; National Prevention Council, 2011) (Box 9.7: Best Practice).

The National Prevention Strategy launched in June 2011 and is still active, with ongoing webinars in 2023 and 2024. The strategy "recognizes that good health comes not just from receiving quality medical care, but also from clean air and water, safe outdoor spaces for physical activity, safe work sites, healthy foods, violence-free environments, and healthy homes. Prevention should be woven into all aspects of our lives, including where and how we live, learn, work and play. Everyone—businesses, educators, health care institutions, government, communities and every single American—has a role in creating a healthier nation" (Box 9.8: Quality/Safety Scenario) (https://prevention.nih.gov/education-training/prevention-focus-webinars).

BOX 9.7 BEST PRACTICE

Informatics, Technology, Electronic Medical Records, and Newborn Screening

Health information technology will allow professionals to better assess and manage quality health care with the streamlining of efficient and effective information. State and federal sites list information about newborn screening and long-term follow-up. The results of newborn screening may include normal values and out-of-range values. Access to digital medical records allows for the sharing of results and follow-up findings between clinicians, testing laboratories, and health delivery providers.

- How does access to newborn electronic screening results benefit the clinician? How does it benefit the person seeking care? How does it benefit public health?
- Where else do you think health care could benefit from similar abilities?
- What do you think is necessary for this to happen (think about differences in data collection requirements)?
- How can privacy concerns be addressed?

Examples of websites that have information on newborn screening:

March of Dimes (2020). *Newborn screening tests for your baby.* https://www.marchofdimes.org/find-support/topics/parenthood/newborn-screening-tests-your-baby

US National Library of Medicine. (2023). *What's new on Medline Plus.* https://medlineplus.gov/whatsnew/

US National Library of Medicine. (2018). *Newborn screening coding and terminology guide.* https://lhncbc.nlm.nih.gov/newbornscreeningcodes/

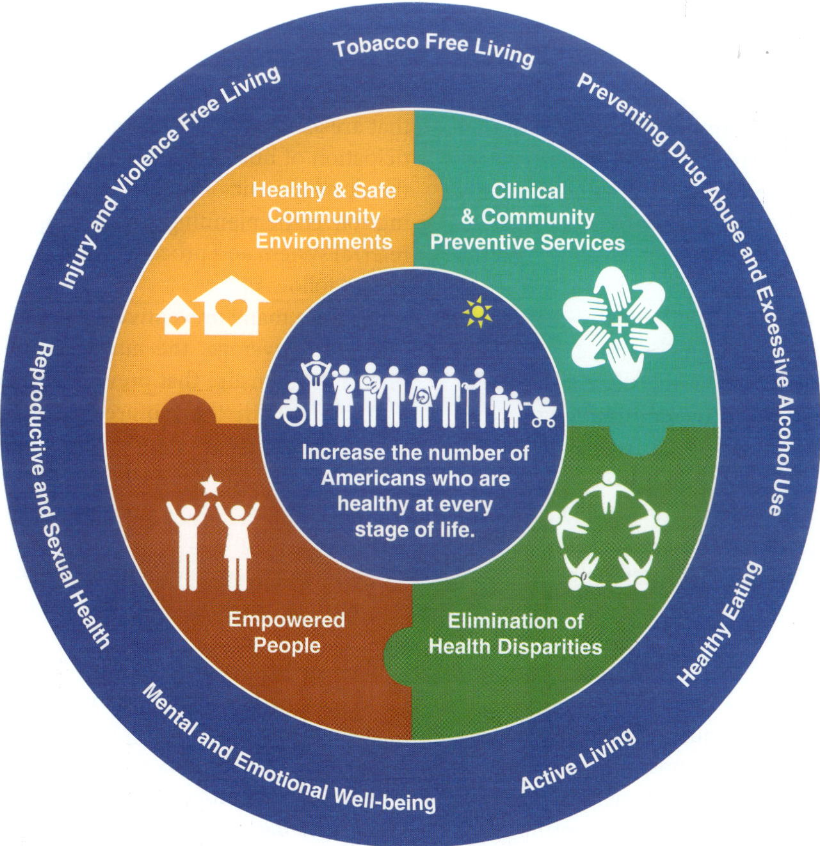

FIG. 9.4 America's plan for better health and wellness. (From National Prevention Council. (2011). *National Prevention Strategy: America's plan for better health and wellness.* Washington, DC: US Department of Health and Human Services, Office of the Surgeon General. https://www.hhs.gov/sites/default/files/disease-prevention-wellness-report.pdf. https://www.cdc.gov/public-health-gateway/php/communications-resources/national-health-initiatives-strategies-action-plans.html?CDC_AAref_Val=, https://www.cdc.gov/publichealthgateway/strategy/index.html.)

BOX 9.8 QUALITY AND SAFETY SCENARIO

Using Health-Promotion Models

A health care provider's responsibility is to assess, plan, implement, and evaluate a screening program. Part of this responsibility includes teaching individuals, families, and populations about the importance of participating in these programs and ultimately engaging in safe behaviors promoting health. Two models that may be helpful in care delivery are Pender's health promotion model (Pender et al., 2019) emphasizing health behavior, and a theory called salutogenesis (Seah et al., 2022), which emphasizes health assets and resources helping people to control and manage their health. Pender's model is a useful guide for practice and focuses on the interrelationship among behavior-specific cognition and affective factors and individual characteristics and experiences that motivate individuals to engage in behaviors that promote health and decrease unsafe habits and practices. The health care provider may find that the application of this model in practice influences the relationship between the provider and the individual in a positive way, influencing health behavioral changes. Salutogenesis emphasizes a positive approach to achieving health by focusing on the individual's sense of health coherence attained within the environment and strongly involves health literary. Health is more of a resource for everyday life rather than a goal to be obtained. Analysis of health-related cues obtained by accurate assessment and interview is important. Ultimately the use of health-promotion models facilitates identification of the best choices to implement selected interventions to assist individuals in achieving positive health outcomes.

Examples of health-promotion analysis and cueing questions are as follows:

- How do you define health?
- What does health mean to you?
- Describe your health now.
- Do the choices you make and the actions you take affect your health?
- Can you give examples of when choices and actions created a positive change in health for you?
- Can you give examples of when choices and actions created a negative or unsafe change in health for you?
- What factors facilitated choices and actions that created a positive change in health?
- What factors created barriers to choices and actions that led to a negative or unsafe change in health?
- Are there any supportive personal influences in your life that would assist you in choices and actions that would create a positive change in your health (e.g., family, friends, health care providers)?
- Are there any supportive situational influences, such as more than one plan of action, pertaining to the health change available to you?

The four National Prevention Strategy ongoing directions are as follows:

- Healthy and safe community environments: Create, sustain, and recognize communities that promote health and wellness through prevention
- Clinical and community preventive services: Ensure that prevention-focused health care and community prevention efforts are available, integrated, and mutually reinforcing
- Empowered people: Support people in making healthy choices
- Elimination of health disparities: Eliminate disparities, improving the quality of life for all Americans

Under the second strategic direction, the strategy identifies six recommendations, including a focus on improving cardiovascular health, incorporating screenings, using payments and reimbursement to encourage clinical preventive services, and reducing access barriers to community preventive services. There are four broad goals and seven priority areas for improving health and wellness of Americans (National Prevention Council, 2011) (see Fig. 9.4).

THE NURSE'S ROLE

As one of the important stakeholders, nurses play a role in every aspect of the screening program development process, including assessment, data analysis, planning, implementation, evaluation of health outcomes, and evaluation of process (including the workings of the partnership; see Fig. 9.2). One aspect of this health process is the development and implementation of screening programs for targeted groups. As nurses employ higher decision-making skills based on advanced education and expertise, they will face more complicated questions, such as "Should this condition be screened for or not?" In the role of decision maker and planner, the nurse is responsible for reviewing all issues concerned with screening individuals for an appropriate disease, including the criteria specific to the disease, the medical and economic ethics, and the community resources that are affected. If the choice is to screen individuals, the participation of nurses and other partnering groups is essential in the development of a plan. The last step integral to the nursing role is the planning and development of an active, efficient referral system and process to enhance continuity of care and to ensure follow-up.

Because many preventive care services are provided through insurance coverage, the nurse collaborates with other health providers to ensure that preventive services (see Boxes 9.5 and 9.6), along with the required education and counseling, are available through primary care or community services such as a primary care clinic, a person-centered medical home, a community health center, or even the work site. These services may include the following:

- Blood pressure, diabetes, and cholesterol tests
- Cancer screenings, including mammograms and colonoscopies
- Counseling on topics such as quitting smoking, losing weight, eating healthily, treating depression, and reducing alcohol use
- Routine vaccinations against diseases
- Flu and pneumonia immunizations
- Counseling, screening, and administering vaccines to ensure healthy pregnancies
- Regular well-baby and well-child visits, from birth to age 21 years

Nurses have long been responsible for screening individuals and educating people about healthy lifestyles and decreased risks as part of the ordinary primary care assessment process. Questions concerning nutrition, coping, and self-care are all assessment or screening questions, leading to moments of opportunity or "teachable moments" for health promotion. These evaluation activities are invaluable for gauging risk and potential areas for education and screening. Teaching individuals the meaning and limitation of screening test results is an important element of this role, as is informing them of their part in obtaining implied benefits.

Nursing staff, at all levels, are important in terms of applying preventive services to include screening and education. The concept of the person-centered medical home encourages the use of each member of the primary health care team to the highest level of their professional and licensing abilities. The combined nursing roles of health educator and screener mean that the nurse continues to educate individuals about risk factors and teach them ways to alter and reduce risks generally through lifestyle changes, such as proper nutrition, exercise, and stress management, and by limiting the use of alcohol, drugs, and tobacco. The role of educator is essential in the screening process because nurses provide individuals with the information necessary for choices they will make regarding healthy behavioral change. The nurse is actually practicing primary prevention interventions, but this is done in coordination with a secondary preventive role.

RACIAL AND ETHNIC APPROACHES TO COMMUNITY HEALTH

Another excellent resource is the CDC REACH website (https://www.cdc.gov/nccdphp/dnpao/state-local-programs/reach/index.htm). This program supports effective community-level programs to reduce health disparities in minority communities across the United States. Data from the REACH 2019 Risk Factor Survey, focusing on breast and cervical cancer prevention, cardiovascular health, and diabetes management, have shown that changing health behaviors in minority communities has improved health and reduced community disparities (see Box 9.9).

BOX 9.9 Racial and Ethnic Approaches to Community Health (REACH)—US Keys to Success

Trust: Build a Culture of Collaboration With Communities that Is Based on Trust and Ethics

- Empowerment: Give individuals and communities the knowledge and tools needed to create change by seeking and demanding better health, building on local resources and values.
- Culture and history: Design health initiatives that are grounded in the unique historical and cultural context of diverse racial and ethnic minority communities in the United States.
- Focus on causes: Assess and focus on the underlying causes of poor community health and implement solutions that will stay embedded in the community infrastructure.
- Community investment and expertise: Recognize and invest in local community expertise and motivate communities to mobilize and organize existing resources.
- Trusted organizations: Enlist organizations within the community that are valued by community members, including groups with a primary mission unrelated to health.
- Community leaders: Help community leaders and key organizations forge unique partnerships and act as catalysts for change in the community.
- Ownership: Develop a collective outlook to promote shared interest in a healthy future through widespread community engagement and leadership.
- Sustainability: Make changes to organizations, community environments, and policies to help ensure that health improvements are long lasting and community activities and programs are self-sustaining.
- Hope: Foster optimism, pride, and a promising vision for a healthier future (CDC, 2023b).

CASE STUDY

Screening

Ethel C. is an 82-year-old White widow. Six years ago, she moved from her house into an elderly housing one-bedroom apartment where she lives alone. Her primary insurance is Medicare. She maintains her apartment and does her errands without assistance, all of which she is very proud. She reports that occasionally she has fallen, probably because of some degree of decreasing vision, especially when moving from direct sunlight into shadows and when walking at night. She has been told that she might need surgery for cataracts in the near future. The only medications she takes are an analgesic for pain management of osteoarthritis, an antihypertensive agent, and a daily vitamin and cranberry supplement. Her antihypertensive medication has recently been changed. She has questions about Medicare coverage and the Medicare Advantage plans that are highly promoted on television.

She will have her annual "check-up" with nurse practitioner (NP) Kelly, who is part of a new practice of "integrative medicine." The collaborative practice of registered nurses, NPs, and physicians emphasizes the role of prevention, including screenings. While Kelly is assessing Mrs. C.'s health status, she is also reflecting on how to better care for the practice's ever-enlarging older adult population. Kelly has access to a large referral group that includes medical specialists.

Recognizing and Analyzing Cues Using Reflective Questions

- What data will nurse practitioner Kelly collect to assess Ethel's health? Why?
- What cues and risk factors would Kelly evaluate? Why?
- What screening tests or referrals to other practitioners might Kelly suggest? Why? Propose several possible nursing solutions and activities for Ethel. What possible etiologic factors from Ethel, her family, and her community might be involved?
- Compare and contrast different (individual, family, and community) approaches to health promotion, emphasizing screening and cost-effectiveness.

Potential Solutions and Actions

- Promote attitudes of openness to new health information.
- For elevated blood pressure readings, repeat blood pressure screening on three different visits.
- Develop a more detailed activity/experience log with special attention to physical safety (falls) and vision problems.
- Explore nutritional and activity strategies that are appealing to each individual.
- Begin the new program of activities slowly.
- Follow up on additional risk factors.
- Offer or provide information on community resources to support goals and interventions.

SUMMARY

- Screening is the administration of measures or tests to distinguish individuals who may have a condition from those who probably do not have it.
- Screening is an effective, efficient tool in preventive health care if used for conditions applicable to a screening model and directed toward an appropriate at-risk population.
- Implementing screening programs requires coordination and planning and provides numerous opportunities for nursing intervention and care delivery within the currently evolving health care environment, which is emphasizing prevention activities.
- Nurses can provide individuals, communities, and populations with valuable preventive, health-promotion, and health-education support in the care of healthy individuals and populations.

EVOLVE CHAPTER FEATURES

http://evolve.elsevier.com/Edelman/

- Study Questions

REFERENCES

ACESTooHigh.com. (2023). *What ACEs/PCEs do you have?* https://acestoohigh.com/got-your-ace-score/

Alzheimer's Association. (2023). *Alzheimer's & dementia/research.* http://www.alz.org

American Dental Association (ADA). (2022). *Oral home care.* https:/www.ada.org

Anwar, A., Malik, M., Raees, V., & Anwar, A. (2020). Role of mass media and public health communications in the COVID-19 pandemic. *Cureus, 12*(9), e10453. https://doi.org/10.7759/cureus.10453

Augustovski, F., Colantoio, L. D., Galante, J., Bardach, A., Caporale, J., Zarate, V., Chuang, L. H., Pichon-Riviere, A., & Kind, P. (2018). Measuring the benefits of healthcare: DALYs and QALYs - Does the choice of measure matter? *International Journal of Health Policy Management, 792*, 120–136.

Bottazzi, B., Riboli, E., & Mantovani, A. (2018). Aging, inflammation and cancer. *Seminars in Immunology, 40*, 74–82.

Center for Medicare Advocacy. (2023). *Medicare coverage for prevention and wellness.* http://www.medicareadvocacy.org

Centers for Disease Control and Prevention (CDC). (2018). *Introduction to epidemiology.* https://www.cdc.gov/training-publichealth101/php/training/introduction-to-epidemiology.html?CDC_AAref_Val=https://www.cdc.gov/training/publichealth101/epidemiology.html

Centers for Disease Control and Prevention (CDC). (2024). *Calculate benefits and cost of covering the lifestyle change program.* https://www.cdc.gov/diabetes-prevention/employers-insurers/cost-calculator-tools.html. https://www.cdc.gov

Centers for Disease Control and Prevention (CDC). (2021a). *Blood lead levels in children.* National Center for Environmental Health, Division of Environmental Health Science and Practice. https://www.cdc.gov/nceh/lead/prevention/blood-lead-levels.htm

Centers for Disease Control and Prevention (CDC). (2021b). *Smoking and health.* cdc.gov/tobacco/about/osh/index.htm

Centers for Disease Control and Prevention (CDC). (2023a). *About adverse childhood experiences.* https://www.cdc.gov/violenceprevention/aces/index.html

Centers for Disease Control and Prevention (CDC). (2023b). *Racial and ethnic approaches to community health: About REACH* 2023. https://www.cdc.gov

Chait, N., & Glied, S. (2018). Promoting prevention under the Affordable Care Act. *Annual Review of Public Health, 39*, 507–524.

Chesson, H. W., Meites, E., Ekwueme, D. U., Saraiya, M., & Markowitz, L. E. (2019). Updated medical care cost estimates for HPV-associated cancers: Implications for cost-effectiveness analyses of HPV vaccination in the United States. *Human Vaccines & Immunotherapeutics, 15*(7–8), 1942–1948.

Cohen, C. G., Ramey, D. M., Cooksey, E. C., & Williams, D. R. (2018). Racial disparities in health among nonpoor African Americans and Hispanics: The role of acute and chronic discrimination. *Social Science & Medicine, 199*, 167–180.

Crow, D. (2019). A new wave of genomics for all. *Cell, 177*(1), 5–7.

Dhutia, H., & MacLachlan, H. (2018). Cardiac screening of young athletes: A practical approach to sudden cardiac death prevention. *Current Treatment Options in Cardiovascular Medicine, 20*(10), 85.

Dubay, K. S., & Zach, T. L. (2023). *Newborn screening.* [Updated 2023 May 1]. In *StatPearls [Internet]*. Treasure Island, FL: StatPearls Publishing. https://www.ncbi.nlm.nih.gov/books/NBK558983

Duffy, S. W., Tabár, L., Yen, A. M., Dean, P. B., Smith, R. A., Jonsson, H., Törnberg, S., Chiu, S. Y., Chen, S. L., Jen, G. H., Ku, M. M., Hsu, C. Y., Ahlgren, J., Maroni, R., Holmberg, L., & Chen, T. H. (2021). Beneficial effect of consecutive screening mammography examinations on mortality from breast cancer. *Radiology, 299*(3), 541–547.

Feng, X., Ollendorf, D. A., Kim, D. D., Cohen, J. T., & Neumann, P. J. (2019). Using QALYs versus DALYS to measure cost-effectiveness: Does it matter? *Value in Health, 22*(2), S36.

Forsythe, S., Cohen, J., Neumann, P., Bertozzi, S. M., & Kinghorn, A. (2020). The economic and public health imperatives around making potential coronavirus disease-2019 treatments available and affordable. *Value in Health, 23*(11), 1427–1431. https://doi.org/10.1016/j.jval.2020.04.1824

Freeman, J. D., Rosman, L. M., Ratcliff, J. D., Strickland, P. T., Graham, D. R., & Silbergeld, E. K. (2018). State of the science in dried blood spots. *Clinical Chemistry, 64*(4), 656–679.

Givler, D. N., & Givler, A. (2023). *Health screening.* [Updated 2023 February 19]. In: *StatPearls [Internet]*. Treasure Island, FL: StatPearls Publishing. https://www.ncbi.nlm.nih.gov/books/NBK436014/

Gregg, A. R., Aarabi, M., Klugman, S., Leach, N. T., Bashford, M. T., Goldwaser, T., Chen, E., Sparks, T. N., Reddi, H. V., Rajkovic, A., Dungan, J. S., & ACMG Professional Practice and Guidelines Committee. (2021). Screening for autosomal recessive and X-linked conditions during pregnancy and preconception. *Genetics in Medicine, 23*(10):1793–1806.

HealthyPeople.gov. (2023). *Healthy People 2030.* http://healthypeople.gov

Johnston, M., Warton, C., Pertile, M. D., Taylor-Sands, M., Delatycki, M. B., Hui, L., Savulescu, J., Mills, C. (2023). Ethical issues associated with prenatal screening using non-invasive prenatal testing for sex chromosome aneuploidy. *Prenatal Diagnosis*, *43*(2), 226–234. https://doi.org/10.1002/pd.6217

Kisling, L. A., & Das, J. M. (2023). *Prevention strategies*. In: *StatPearls [Internet]*. Treasure Island, FL: StatPearls Publishing. https://www.ncbi.nlm.nih.gov/books/NBK537222

Laconi, E., Marongiu, F., & DeGregori, J. (2020). Cancer as a disease of old age: Changing mutational and microenvironmental landscapes. *British Journal of Cancer*, *122*, 943–952. https://doi.org/10.1038/s41416-019-0721-1

Moat, S. J., George, R. S., & Carling, R. S. (2020). Use of dried blood spot specimens to monitor patients with inherited metabolic disorders. *International Journal of Neonatal Screen*, *6*(2), 26. https://doi.org/10.3390/ijns6020026

Mao, X., Wei, W., Humphreys, K., Eriksson, M., Holowko, N., Strand, F., Hall, P., & Czene, K. L. (2023). Factors associated with false-positive recalls in mammography screening. *Journal of the National Comprehensive Cancer Network: JNCCN*, *21*(2), 143–152. https://doi.org/10.6004/jnccn.2022.7081

Moreno-Ternero, J. D., Platz, T. T., & Østerdal, L. P. (2023). QALYs, DALYs, and HALYs: A unifying framework for the evaluation of population health. *Journal of Health Economics*, *87*, 102714. https://doi.org/10.1016/j.jhealeco.2022.102714

Morrell, B. L., Morrell, M. B., Ball, J. A., Ochoa, A. C., & Seewaldt, V. L. (2023). Disparities in the use of screening breast magnetic resonance imaging persist in Louisiana after the Affordable Care Act: A question of access, policy, institutional support, or something else? *Cancer*, *129*(6), 829–833. https://doi.org/10.1002/cncr.34605

Mukherjee, S. (2020a). After the storm. *The New Yorker*, *4*, 24–31.

Mukherjee, S. (2020b). The one and the many. *The New Yorker*, *6*, 18–22.

National Cancer Institute. (2023). *PROSPR: Population-based Research Optimizing Screening Through Personalized Regimens*. https://healthcaredelivery.cancer.gov/prospr

National Institutes of Health (NIH). (2025). Office of Disease Prevention, Prevention in Focus Webinars. https://prevention.nih.gov/education-training/prevention-focus-webinars

National Prevention Council. (2011). *National Prevention Strategy: America's plan for better health and wellness*. Washington, DC: US Department of Health and Human Services, Office of the Surgeon General. https://www.hhs.gov/sites/default/files/disease-prevention-wellness-report.pdf

Neumann, P. J., & Cohen, J. T. (2018). QALYs in 2018—Advantages and concerns. *JAMA*, *319*(24), 2473–2474. https://jamanetwork.com/journals/jama/fullarticle/2682917

Pender, N., Murdaugh, C., & Parsons, M. A. (2019). *Health promotion in nursing practice* (8th ed.). New York: Pearson.

Petek, B. J., & Baggish, A. L. (2020). Pre-participation cardiovascular screening in young competitive athletes. *Current Emergency and Hospital Medicine Reports*, *8*(3), 77–89. https://doi.org/10.1007/s40138-020-00214-5

Pös, O., Budiš, J., & Szemes, T. (2019). Recent trends in prenatal genetic screening and testing. *F1000 Faculty Rev-764*. https://doi.org/10.12688/f1000research.16837.1.

Ramos, E., & Weissman, S. M. (2018). The dawn of consumer-directed testing. *American Journal of Medical Genetics*, *178*(1), 89–97.

Rector, C., & Stanley, M. J. (2021). *Community health and public health nursing* (10th ed.). Philadelphia: Wolters Kluwer.

Reboussin, D. M., Carey, R. M., & Whelton, P. K. (2019). Evidence supporting the blood pressure treatment goal of less than 130/80 mm Hg. *Hypertension*, *73*, 972–974. https://doi.org/10.1161/HYPERTENSIONAHA.119.12804

Rose, N. C., Kaimal, A. J., & Dugoff, L. (2020). Screening for fetal chromosomal abnormalities. ACOG Practice Bulletin #226. *Obstetrics & Gynecology*, *136*(4), e48–e69. https://doi.org/10.1097/AOG.0000000000004084

Rutherford-Hemming, T. (2018). State of interprofessional education in nursing: A systematic review. *Nurse Educator*, *43*(1), 9–13.

Schaffer, A. (2019). *The science of pregnancy* (pp. 12–17). MIT News.

Seah, B., Tan, G. R., Eriksson, M., Wang, W., & Ramazanu, S. (2022). Re-orienting healthcare for healthy living communities: A qualitative exploration of nursing students utilising the salutogenic theory for community health practice. *Nurse Education Today*, *119*, 105545. https://doi.org/10.1016/j.nedt.2022.105545

Seller, S. L., Roelofs, C., Shoemaker, P. A., Nguyen, N. H., & Nguyen, T. D. (2019). Improving Boston nail salon indoor air quality through local public health regulation, 2007–2019. *American Journal of Public Health*, *109*(12), 1711–1713. https://ajph.aphapublications.org/doi/10.2105/AJPH.2019.305329

US National Library of Medicine. (2020). *What disorders are included in newborn screening?* https://ghr.nlm.nih.gov/primer/newbornscreening/nbsdisorders

US Preventive Services Task Force (USPSTF). (2023). *USPSTF A and B recommendations and primary care recommendations*. https://www.uspreventiveservicestaskforce.org/; https://www.uspreventiveservicestaskforce.org/Page/Name/recommendations

Vessey, J. A., & Betz, C. L. (2020). Everything old is new again: COVID-19 and public health. *Journal of Pediatric Nursing*, *52*, A7–A8.

Wang, C., Horby, P. W., Hayden, F. G., & Gao, G. F. (2020). A novel coronavirus outbreak of global health concern. *Lancet*, *395*(10223), 470–473.

Wei, H., Horns, P., Sears, S. F., Huang, K., Smith, C. M., & Wei, T. L. (2022). A systematic meta-review of systematic reviews about interprofessional collaboration: Facilitators, barriers, and outcomes. *Journal of Interprofessional Care*, *36*(5), 735–749. https://doi.org/10.1080/13561820.2021.1973975

10

Health Education

Jody Spiess and Stephanie Dribben

http://evolve.elsevier.com/Edelman/

OBJECTIVES

After completing this chapter, the reader will be able to:

- Analyze the goals of **health education**.
- Discuss learning principles that affect health education.
- Apply teaching and learning concepts to teaching.
- Describe selected theoretical models used in health education to influence the **behavior change** process.
- Explain the steps in preparing a health teaching plan.
- Propose learning strategies appropriate to each learning domain.
- Discuss the importance of evaluating the educational process.

KEY TERMS

Behavior change
Ecological model
Empowerment
Health behaviors
Health belief model
Health counseling
Health disparities
Health education
Health literacy
Health promotion
Plain language
Quality and safety
Self-efficacy
Social cognitive theory
Social justice
Social marketing
Teach-back method
Transtheoretical model or "stages of change"
Universal precautions

THINK ABOUT IT

The Challenges of Health Education

The goal of **health promotion** and prevention is to keep populations healthy. Effective health interventions should empower and engage individuals and communities to increase control over their health. Part of this goal includes creating an environment that makes it easier for individuals and communities to make healthy changes and choices. Childhood obesity has become a significant concern in the United States. Looking at the issue through a health promotion and prevention lens will allow nurses to develop or initiate appropriate interventions to reduce the risk of childhood obesity and its associated chronic diseases. Reflect on the following scenario. Vincent is a 13-year-old Black American who lives with his grandma and two younger siblings. The family resides in a low-income housing complex in a high-risk, high-crime neighborhood. Vincent is responsible for feeding himself and his siblings after school. His grandma works two jobs to take care of her grandkids and has to leave much of the after-school responsibilities to Vincent. She leaves frozen meals for him to heat up in the microwave or cash for the dollar menu at the local fast-food restaurant. The kids come home from school, lock the doors, and do homework before dinner. After dinner, they watch Netflix, play video games, and snack on dollar-store candy. There are not many locally accessible neighborhood food stores. When assessing the family for the risk of obesity, the nurse should consider the following initial assessment steps:

- What is the body mass index (BMI) of each family member based on height and weight?
- Determine percentile by plotting BMI on growth chart.
- Obtain a focused family history, including the health literacy level of Vincent's grandma.
- When choosing interventions to keep the family healthy or to address obesity concerns, the nurse should consider the following domains and questions:
- Individual food intake
  - What is the individual intake of snacks, meals, and beverages each day?
  - What is the recommended calorie intake for each individual?
  - How many calories are from processed foods?
- Individual activity
  - What is the amount of daily activity for the individual?
  - Do they meet the recommended 60 minutes of activity per day?
  - Does any of this activity happen at home? School?
- Food environment
  - What are the prices and availability of healthy options at school and in the neighborhood?
  - What are the portion sizes at the local fast-food restaurants?
- Physical activity environment
  - Does the environment around the school and housing complex support active living?
  - Is the environment safe?

Other questions to consider are these: What effect does social marketing have on the problem? What effect does the health literacy of Vincent's grandma have on the problem? How could this information be used to decrease the risks associated with the problem? The collected information will help nurses select an intervention that will address the individual and community barriers to health.

Health education is a vital component in promoting individual and community health. Individual behaviors such as diet, physical activity level, and substance abuse play a significant role in health outcomes.

Individual lifestyle changes may help in managing chronic disease; however, lifestyle changes should not be viewed as only primary prevention. Chronic diseases related to health behaviors are the major causes of poor health, disability, and death and contribute considerably to health care costs. One effective way to begin a lifestyle change is through health education. Nurses can use a population health approach to educate their clients on ways to remain healthy, identify illness early, and decrease the level of disability caused by disease, which will also reduce health care costs (Niederhauser, 2020). Population health looks at factors beyond the cause of disease to risks that may have been at play years before the occurrence (Riegelman, 2020).

Health education to promote positive behavior change, along with policies and programs that address the social determinants of health, can reduce the rates of chronic illness and disability in the United States. The *Healthy People 2030* national health update adds challenges and improvements from lessons learned that emphasize priorities for improving the health of individuals, groups, and communities in the United States. These priorities involve promoting positive health behaviors, increasing health literacy, and reducing health disparities (US Department of Health and Human Services [USDHHS], n.d.). Achievement of these objectives provides challenges and opportunities for health promotion (Box 10.1: *Healthy People 2030*).

Although many health goals are affected by individual lifestyle practices, health is influenced significantly by social, economic, physical, and political factors. The *Healthy People 2030* vision for health promotion includes a commitment to providing an environment where all populations can achieve their full potential throughout their lives, which includes health literacy and health equity (USDHHS, n.d.).

Nursing, with its unique contributions to health care, is a professional resource that can help facilitate these changes through health education strategies. Nurses, in partnership with other health care professionals, can be the link between the updated vision of *Healthy People 2030* and the people who need to hear its messages and act on them (USDHHS, n.d.).

BOX 10.1 SAMPLE OBJECTIVES *HEALTHY PEOPLE 2030*

Symbol	*Healthy People 2030* Objective
ECBP-D03	Increase the proportion of worksites that offer employee health-promotion program(s) to their employees
ECBP-D06	Increase the number of community-based organizations providing population-based primary prevention services
HC/HIT-D01	Increase the number of state health departments that use social marketing in health promotion programs
HC/HIT-R01	Increase the health literacy of the population
HC/HIT-04	Increase the proportion of adults who talk to friends or family about their health
HC/HIT-03	Increase the proportion of adults whose health care providers involved them in decisions as much as they wanted
HC/HIT-01	Increase the proportion of adults whose health care provider checked their understanding
HC/HIT-02	Decrease the proportion of adults who report poor communication with their health care provider
HC/HIT-D11	Increase the proportion of adults with limited English proficiency who say their providers explain things clearly
HC/HIT-D10	Increase the proportion of people who say their online medical record is easy to understand

From *Healthy People 2030* by the US Department of Health and Human Services. (n.d.). https://health.gov/healthypeople

NURSING AND HEALTH EDUCATION

Nurses as educators play a key role in improving the health of the nation. Educating people is an integral part of the nurse's role in every practice setting—schools, communities, work sites, health care delivery sites, and homes. **Health education** involves not only providing relevant information but also facilitating health-related **behavior changes**. The nurse, using health education principles, can assist people in achieving their health goals in a way that is consistent with their personal lifestyles, values, and beliefs.

Nursing: Scope and Standards of Practice (American Nurses Association, 2021) describes health teaching and health promotion as primary nursing responsibilities. These responsibilities include educating people about healthy lifestyles, developmental needs, activities of daily living, preventive self-care, and risk management in addition to coping, adaptability, and resiliency. *Nursing's Social Policy Statement* and the *Code of Ethics for Nurses* also establish health teaching and health promotion as a primary nursing responsibility in the context of individual self-determination (ANA, 2015; Fowler, 2015). The responsibility to teach individuals is balanced by their right to receive information about their health status, their risks, and ways to reduce their risks. The nurse provides health teaching and **health counseling** based on individual interests and decisions that enable individuals to make informed decisions about their health.

Nurses usually function as health care coordinators for individuals in their care. Depending on the interests and needs of a person, nurses establish a partnership to guide the individual in the selection and use of relevant health services. Health education principles provide the nurse with strategies and tools for assessing an individual's readiness for health teaching, with technical information, and with help promoting healthy behaviors in their daily life. These strategies also help the nurse facilitate behavior change while satisfying the person's right to relevant health information and the freedom for people to make decisions about their own health. Health education encourages self-care, self-empowerment, and, ultimately, less dependence on the health care system.

Nurses have long been involved in public health education, taking on the full-time role of coordinating the educational services provided by a health agency or institution. As a health educator, the nurse may use marketing strategies to enhance the effectiveness of health education programs that are focused on certain target populations. The health education specialist helps other nurses and health professionals improve their skills in developing and delivering teaching plans.

Definition

Health education is "any combination of planned learning experiences in which theory and evidence-based practices are used to provide equitable opportunities for the acquisition of knowledge, attitudes, and skills needed to adapt, adopt, and maintain healthy behaviors" (Videto & Dennis, 2021). This process involves several key components. First, health education involves the use of teaching-learning strategies. Second, learners maintain voluntary control over the decision to make changes in their actions. Third, health education focuses on behavior changes that have been found to improve health status.

Health education facilitates the development of health knowledge, skills, and attitudes through the application of theories or models. Commonly used theories of individual and community behavior change will be discussed later in this chapter. In general, health education strategies help to ensure that individuals, as consumers of health services, are satisfied and have received the health information that is most relevant to their health risks. From a public health perspective, **health education** programs are intended not only to enhance individuals' abilities to make positive lifestyle changes but also to support social and political actions that promote health and quality of life in communities.

The following scenario is an example of a therapeutic situation in which a health education approach may be used to meet an individual's health needs.

Sada Thompson, a 21-year-old university senior, visits university health services because she wants to change her method of birth control. She has experienced side effects from the birth control pill that she has been taking for the past year and knows little about other options. She has recently started dating John after breaking up with Steven 3 months ago. Having decided to be sexually active with John, Sada is feeling uncertain about what she needs to do to take care of herself and how to discuss this uncertainty with John. She is aware of all the talk about HIV on campus, and she knows that John is popular and has dated several other females in school, which concerns her.

Sada needs to learn new information, she may need to acquire new skills, and she needs to clarify any feelings or attitudes that affect her decision to use a new birth control method and ensure her continued safety. After recording her health assessment history and arranging for a gynecologic examination and laboratory tests, the nurse develops a teaching plan. Selecting one or more strategies for helping Sada review all the birth control options, the nurse establishes an environment in which Sada can choose to try a new method or request a change in her prescription for oral contraceptives. Together they identify actions Sada can take to use the method properly. They also anticipate and identify ways Sada can solve problems of adjusting to the new method.

The nurse answers Sada's immediate questions about safe sex, gives her several pamphlets written for college students about this topic, and suggests that she participate in the peer counseling night on sexually transmitted diseases that will be held on campus in 2 weeks. The peer counseling hotline number and drop-in hours are given to Sada. The nurse explains that the students who provide peer counseling are trained to help other students talk about and deal with this important issue. The nurse invites Sada to call or come back to the office for additional help, information, or problem-solving discussion.

This example illustrates that educational interventions, in addition to direct health services, are necessary to meet the individual's goals. Although health care providers and nurses prefer that people choose to take actions that will promote health and not detract from it, the individual determines the at-home application of health recommendations.

Goals

The goal of health education is to help individuals, families, and communities achieve, through their own actions and initiative, optimal states of health. Health education facilitates voluntary actions to promote health and improve quality of life. Another important goal of health education is to improve health literacy. **Health literacy** is about people being able to find, understand, and use health information and services (USDHHS, 2022). *Healthy People 2010* and *Healthy People 2020* defined *health literacy* as "the degree to which individuals have the capacity to obtain, process, and understand basic health information and services needed to make appropriate health decisions." However, *Healthy People 2030* distinguishes between personal health literacy and organizational health literacy with the following definitions:

- **Personal health literacy** is the degree to which individuals have the ability to find, understand, and use information and services to inform health-related decisions and actions for themselves and others.
- **Organizational health literacy** is the degree to which organizations equitably enable individuals to find, understand, and use information and services to information health-related decisions and actions for themselves and others.

The new definitions encompass a public health perspective, acknowledging that health literacy is dependent on the context in which people operate and that organizations and professionals have a duty to equitably address health literacy. This duty extends to nurses, who are expected to address problems patients face at the individual and societal levels, including issues related to health equity and health disparities (Fowler, 2015). The new definitions also emphasize the ability to use rather than to simply understand health information and focus on making well-informed rather than "appropriate" decisions. The nurse facilitates informed decision-making by providing the individual with understandable, accurate, and complete information and by helping the individual weigh the options, benefits, and burdens related to health care (ANA, 2015).

The 2003 National Assessment of Adult Literacy classic landmark study showed that only 12% of US adults had proficient health literacy (Kutner et al., 2006). More than one-third of US adults have only basic or below basic health literacy. This means they would have difficulty with common health tasks, such as following directions on a prescription drug label or adhering to a childhood immunization schedule using a standard chart. Although the study results showed that half of adults without a high school education had below basic health literacy skills, even high school and college graduates can have limited health literacy. The more vulnerable members of our communities—those with lower education levels, those who are racial/ethnic minorities, the uninsured and publicly insured, and the elderly—have the lowest levels of health literacy.

Nurses are uniquely positioned to assess and improve health literacy and health outcomes. Low health literacy may not always be apparent, and measurement may not be practical in the health care setting. Individuals with higher levels of education and health literacy may not always understand health information due to emotional stress or other challenges. By implementing a **universal precautions** approach to health literacy that assumes all persons are at risk of not understanding, nurses can take on a lead role in improving oral, written, and environmental communication (Barton et al., 2018). Using **plain language** and common everyday words, except when technical words are necessary, helps ensure clear, effective communication in each nurse-patient-family interaction regardless of perceived level of health literacy. Nurses should use the **teach-back method** to evaluate the effectiveness of teaching with all patients:

- Show and explain how to do something.
- Check understanding by asking the learner to explain in their own words what they were taught. Take responsibility for their understanding by stating that you want to be sure that you did a good job explaining.
- If the person does not understand clearly, explain a second time using a different approach, and check again (Agency for Healthcare Research and Quality, 2020). See Box 10.2 for guidelines for effective communication.

Addressing health literacy and providing culturally sensitive health education are critical to reducing health disparities and achieving health equity. **Health equity** is the ability for people to achieve their highest level of health, whereas **health disparities** are systematic, potentially avoidable health differences that adversely affect socially, economically, and/or environmentally disadvantaged groups. The groups affected are those with characteristics such as race/ethnicity, skin color, language, or nationality; socioeconomic resources or position; sex, sexual orientation, or gender identity; age; physical, mental, or emotional disability or illness; geography; or other characteristics that have been linked historically to discrimination or marginalization (Ndugga & Artiga, 2023). Nurses have an obligation to advocate for those affected by health inequities and to speak up against social injustices such as discrimination, racism, and poverty. Nurses serving in the community, particularly public health nurses, frequently work at the individual and family levels to address social needs and at the community and population levels to address the social determinants of health (National Academies of Sciences, Engineering, and Medicine, 2021). At the population level, interventions often target individuals with specific health risks, such as HIV and substance use disorder, or those with complex health conditions or in complex social situations. Reducing health disparities can also be accomplished through community organizing, coalition building, and policy development.

Person-centered care is an essential component of **quality and safety**, whether health promotion is directed toward an individual, family, or community. In the planning and implementation of health education programs, essential components include showing respect for values and cultural, ethnic, and social diversity; empowering and actively involving the learners; promoting physical and emotional comfort; communicating in

BOX 10.2 Clear Messages

Engage the Learner

- Know and respect your audience (gender, race/ethnicity, location, beliefs, culture, literacy skills, and current knowledge about the topic).
- Use language they use and with which they feel comfortable. Use a qualified translator when needed.
- Focus on what they want or need to know/do. State what to do rather than what not to do.
- Address them directly by using pronouns ("you"), active verbs, and present tense: "Wash your hands before you eat."
- Use plain language (familiar, simple, short [1–2 syllable] words and short sentences).
- Limit technical terms and define when necessary.
- Encourage questions and listen carefully.

Organization

- Present information in logical order.
- Give the most important information first.
- Be specific and concrete.
- Limit the number of messages, repeat when necessary, and skip "nice to know" details.

Written Materials

- Left justify text, leave right margin ragged.
- Use size 12–14 sans serif font.
- Use upper- and lower-case letters, not all caps.
- Highlight important information.
- Break information into chunks using headings.

Visuals

- Show what to do rather than what not to do.
- Use simple, instructive images familiar to your audience.
- Use a brief caption with the key message.

Evaluation

- Use teach-back to check understanding.
- Pretest any written materials or visuals with the intended audience.

Adapted from Agency for Healthcare Research and Quality. (2020). *AHRQ health literacy universal precautions toolkit, 2nd edition.* http://www.ahrq.gov/professionals/quality-patient-safety/quality-resources/tools/literacy-toolkit/index.html. Centers for Disease Control and Prevention (CDC), US Department of Health and Human Services. (2019). *CDC Clear Communication Index: A Tool for Developing and Assessing CDC Public Communication Products* https://www.cdc.gov/ccindex/

ways that are appropriate to health literacy and sociocultural background; and seeking continual self-improvement in effective education (Quality and Safety Education for Nurses, 2022). Use of person-centered health education strategies can significantly affect the outcomes of health care recipients (Box 10.3: Quality and Safety Scenario).

Changes in health behaviors that are related to health education help prevent disease and disability. Two main objectives of health education and health counseling are to change health behaviors and to improve health status. Information alone does not change behavior.

BOX 10.3 QUALITY AND SAFETY SCENARIO

A Community-Based Person-Centered Health-Promotion Program

The Nurse-Family Partnership (NFP) program is an evidence-based, person-centered community health program that focuses on improving pregnancy outcomes, child health and development, and economic self-sufficiency in socially and economically disadvantaged first-time mothers and their children (NFP, 2023).

The theories that guide the program include human ecology, attachment, and self-efficacy. Human ecology theory recognizes that many factors in the environment influence human development. For example, partner and family relationships as well as the dynamic of the neighborhood can influence mothers and babies. Attachment theory acknowledges that physical and emotional attachment is critical to child development. Teaching skills to first-time mothers is essential to nurturing the mother-baby relationship. Self-efficacy reflects confidence in the ability to exert control over one's motivation, behavior, and environment. Helping mothers recognize their potential is essential to building a strong sense of self and family.

As part of the program, specifically trained registered nurses make one-on-one in-home visits with expectant mothers. The visits start during pregnancy and may continue through the child's second birthday. The length and frequency of visits throughout the program is tailored to the mother's needs. NFP (2023) goals include the following (para. 3):

1. Improve pregnancy outcomes by partnering with moms to engage in good preventive health practices, including receiving thorough prenatal care from their health care providers, improving their diets, and reducing use of habit-forming substances.
2. Improve child health and development by helping families provide responsible and competent care.
3. Improve the economic self-sufficiency of the family by supporting parents in developing a vision for their own future, planning additional pregnancies, continuing their education, and finding work.

The NFP program started in New York in 1977 and has since expanded throughout the United States and globally, including in regions throughout Canada, Australia, and Europe. In Australia, Massi et al. (2023) have found that the program fosters access to health and social services, cultural connection, and peer support for first-time mothers who are having a First Nation baby, all of which have contributed to self-efficacy.

Through the National Service Office, the NFP is committed to advocacy through "evidence-based policy solutions that improve the health and well-being of families and promoting economic mobility for communities" (NFP, 2024, para. 1). **Social justice** refers to fair treatment, equal access to goods and resources, and the right to self-determination and cultural expression for all people. By addressing social justice and social determinants of health through individualized care and public policy, the NFP improves health outcomes and promotes equity for vulnerable families.

Health education encourages positive, informed changes in lifestyle behaviors that prevent acute and chronic disease, decrease disability, and enhance wellness. Another goal of health education that may foster successful changes in health behavior is **empowerment**. Empowerment can occur at the individual, organization, or group level, and empowerment at one level frequently influences other levels (Cottrell et al., 2023). At the individual level, those who believe they can make a difference in their health and who are involved in decision-making are more likely to make changes.

Health education and health counseling are mutually supportive activities. Health educators often use one-to-one and group counseling techniques as strategies for active health learning. Counselors may refer people to health education resources or assist them in acquiring information pertinent to solving a health problem. The following example helps illustrate the goals of health education. The general principles of learning found in Box 10.4: How to Facilitate Learning are fundamental to the planning of successful health education programs.

Kate Hanson, aged 22 years, visits the local family health center for fatigue and symptoms similar to influenza. During the assessment with the nurse, Kate discloses that she has missed her last two periods.

The physical examination findings, the laboratory test findings, and the health assessment pattern confirm Kate's suspicions of pregnancy. Psychosocial evaluation reveals that Kate works part-time as a secretary for a temporary agency and lives in an apartment with her recently unemployed husband, Jim. Further interviewing reveals that Kate has minimal knowledge of prenatal care; she has a diet of take-out food that is high in fat, sodium, and sugar, with infrequent consumption of fresh fruits or vegetables; and she has three or four beers on the weekends. Kate has never taken vitamin supplements; she leads a sedentary lifestyle; and she is obviously overwhelmed by the news that she is pregnant.

The nurse first takes steps to create a safe and trusting atmosphere in which Kate can feel free to share her concerns and apprehensions. When Kate expresses concerns about telling her husband about the pregnancy, the nurse discusses this with her.

BOX 10.4 How to Facilitate Learning

- Use methods that stimulate a variety of senses.
- Involve the person actively in the learning process.
- Establish a comfortable, appropriate learning environment.
- Assess the readiness of the learner, which may be affected by physical, social, emotional, and financial factors.
- Make the information relevant by connecting with the existing needs and interests of the learner.
- Use repetition. Review and reinforce concepts several times in a variety of ways.
- Make the learning encounter positive. Structure it to achieve progress that is recognizable by the individual, and provide frequent, positive feedback.
- Start with what is known and proceed to what is unknown, moving from simple to complex.
- Apply the concepts to several settings to facilitate generalization.
- Pace the learning appropriately for the individual.

Kate is then taught the importance of taking a multivitamin with an iron supplement daily, discontinuing the consumption of alcohol, checking with her physician before taking medications, and making time for more rest during the day. Sensing that this is all that can be accomplished at this time, the nurse gives Kate two pamphlets on prenatal care and makes an appointment for her to return in 1 week with her husband. Kate acknowledges that she understands the instructions, and the nurse documents the teaching and recommendations in Kate's medical record.

During the next visit, the nurse meets Kate and Jim, explores the meaning of the pregnancy in their lives, and helps them identify actions they will need to take. The recommendations that were made during Kate's first visit are reviewed and reinforced. The nurse then details specifics of dietary changes, reinforces the need for proper rest and exercise, and helps the couple solve problems while they adjust to these new responsibilities. Most importantly, the nurse gives them information on the clinic's weekly prenatal classes and explains that because the classes are partially covered by local community funding, the charge is minimal. The classes provide information about physical changes, psychosocial changes, and nutritional needs during pregnancy, the labor and delivery period, and the newborn and postpartum periods. A nurse practitioner conducts the classes at the clinic, which are given in a group format to facilitate social support and problem-solving among expectant parents.

The nurse gives Kate and Jim several other pamphlets to read at home, makes a clinic appointment for Kate in a couple of weeks, and encourages her to call if she has questions or concerns in the interim. A schedule of the prenatal classes is reviewed, and a date for the next session is made. The couple is encouraged to meet with the social worker to explore their financial needs and options because Jim was recently laid off. Kate and Jim acknowledge that they understand what they need to do, and the nurse documents what was taught and discussed in Kate's health care record.

This example illustrates the goal of **health education**: to help individuals achieve optimal health and well-being through their actions and initiative. Through health education, individuals can learn to make informed decisions about personal and family health practices and to use health services in the community. The couple in this example receives educational assistance from the nurse that will promote better health and well-being for Kate and their baby.

Learning Assumptions

Chapters 16 to 24 in this text address the factors one should consider when teaching different age groups and the learners' respective characteristics to consider when one is developing a teaching plan. The nurse considers the developmental stage, cognitive level, and interests of the individual. The level of information to be conveyed and the skills and abilities of the individual will guide the methods and resources used.

Family Health Teaching

The family plays an important role in health and illness. When an individual is sick, the effect is felt by the entire family and the community in which the family resides. Therefore, it is important that families are included in decision-making and education (Webb, 2020). Because the family is the unit within which health values, health habits, and health risk perceptions are developed, organized, and performed, the individual's health, understanding, and intervening with the family are essential to promoting health and reducing health risks in individuals and communities (Webb, 2020). Skills in family interviewing and assessment are valuable tools for nurses. Family health assessment and health teaching are closely related. The family assessment model in Chapter 7 provides a comprehensive approach to identifying problems, strengths, and health education needs. The goal is to help family members achieve optimal states of health while guiding them through problem-solving and decision-making. This process empowers them to believe they can make a difference in their own health.

In clarifying the health teaching needs of a family, the nurse might reflect on the following questions: Who is in this family? What health-related tasks are they performing? How are they functioning and how are they meeting each other's needs? How well are they communicating? What does this family need to know? What do they need to know now? What do they think they need to know? How can they learn what they need to know?

The nurse works with the family to set a broad health-promotion goal and then directs health teaching toward a more specific area. It is essential that the family agrees with the goal and teaching needs. As the family participates in the assessment interview, perhaps members can identify their own health teaching needs. Health teaching includes all family members, with learning activities appropriate for each individual. The general teaching goal will be the same for all members, but the approaches and specific goals for each member or subsystem will be different. Children, adolescents, and elderly members pose special challenges to the nurse, who may be more comfortable teaching young or middle-aged adults (Fig. 10.1).

Health Behavior Change

Health behaviors are any activities that affect a person's health. The process of health education directs people toward voluntary changes of their health behaviors to enhance health, prevent

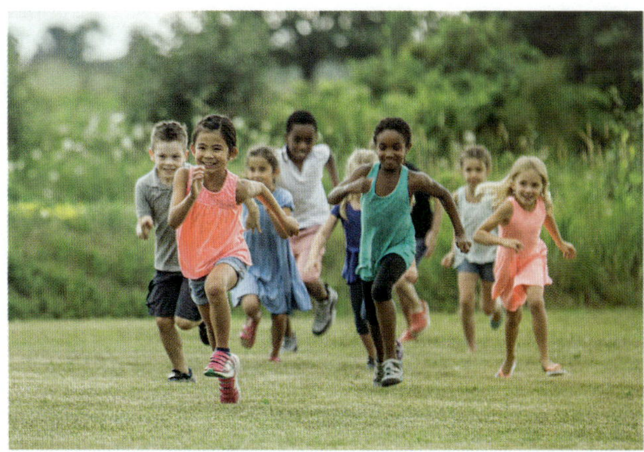

FIG. 10.1 School-aged children running together. (From iStock.com/FatCamera)

disease, and detect and control the symptoms of a disease. Viewing health behavior through an **ecological model**, the nurse recognizes the complex interaction of individuals with their environment and the multiple influences of the individual, family, and community on health behavior. This section examines the use of commonly used models of individual health behavior change. Community and group models in health education planning are addressed later in this chapter.

Individual models of health behavior help explain the factors that influence and interfere with positive health behaviors. In addition, they contribute to an understanding of how educational intervention supports behavior change. The goal of health education is to motivate clients to seek ways to change their behavior. Internal motivators such as beliefs, attitudes, and values are powerful and are more likely than external motivators to result in successful behavior change (Botchwey et al., 2020).

Identifying and teaching people about lifestyle behaviors that need to change is only the first step in the process of assisting individuals in moving from knowledge to action. Nurses apply concepts from the health belief model, social learning theory, and the transtheoretical model (TTM) in subsequent steps to formulate an action plan that meets the needs and capabilities of each person in making healthy behavior changes.

Health Belief Model

The **health belief model** is a paradigm used to predict and explain health behavior. The following components of the health belief model provide guidelines for nurses to analyze factors that contribute to a person's perceived state of health or risk of disease and to the individual's probability of making an appropriate plan of action (Simons-Morton & Lodyga, 2023):

- Individual perceptions of susceptibility to a health condition or disease
- Perceived seriousness of the disease
- Cues that promote action (feelings or media responses)
- Modifying factors, such as age, sex, race, socioeconomic status, and knowledge
- Perceived benefits of health action
- Perceived barriers to the health action
- Perceived readiness to perform the action

Application of components of the health belief model generates data to assist nurses in choosing effective educational strategies. The nurse then determines the most appropriate interventions for a particular person through collaboration with the individual.

Social Cognitive Theory

Social cognitive theory is another model that adds to the understanding of the determinants of health behavior. The theory proposes that individuals learn from both themselves and from the observed actions of others (Botchwey et al., 2020). Bandura (1997) emphasizes the influence of self-efficacy, or efficacy beliefs, on health behavior. **Self-efficacy** refers to an individual's belief in being personally capable of performing the behavior required to influence their own health (see the case study at the end of this chapter). Social cognitive theory also describes the roles of reinforcement and observational learning in explaining health behavior change. Modeling, or providing opportunities for imitating the behavior of others, can be used to demonstrate the desired behavior.

Transtheoretical Model of Change

The **transtheoretical model, or "stages of change model,"** is useful for determining where a person is in relation to making a behavior change (Prochaska & DiClemente, 1984). According to the TTM, health-related behavior change progresses through the following five stages regardless of whether an individual is quitting or adopting a behavior (Cotrell et al., 2023):

- Precontemplation: The person is not thinking about or considering quitting or adopting a behavior change within the next 6 months (not intending to make changes).
- Contemplation: The person is seriously considering making a specific behavior change within the next 6 months (considering a change).
- Planning or preparation: The person who has made a behavior change is seriously thinking about making a change within the next month (making small or sporadic changes).
- Action: The person has made a behavior change, and it has persisted for 6 months (actively engaged in behavior change).
- Maintenance: The period beginning 6 months after the action has started and continuing indefinitely (sustaining the change over time).

The TTM is useful in determining the person's readiness for learning in relation to changing a behavior so that health education or behavior change interventions can be matched to the stage. Self-efficacy is a key construct in this model. This model also acknowledges the importance of continuing intervention to maintaining behavior change in the long term. The TTM has been used by health professionals in planning interventions with a wide variety of people at risk.

Regardless of the quality of nurses' assessment methods and educational strategies, experience in the area of health education indicates that people do not always make the choices recommended to them by health professionals or adhere to the healthy changes. Naturally, health professionals want people to choose the recommended course of action, but each individual has the right to choose not to follow advice. Enlisting the individual's partnership or cooperation achieves better results.

Attempts to influence a person's behavior through education are not always successful. Attempting to persuade people to change their behavior to something that might make them, their friends, and their family healthier can be discouraging and sometimes futile. An individual's values, beliefs, and life stresses may present obstacles to these changes. Effective health education requires an understanding of the influential factors affecting the individual's decision-making (values, beliefs, attitudes, life stresses, religion, previous experiences with the health care system, and life goals). Another key factor in the ability to comply with health education is financial constraints. The individual may not have the resources to pay for a proper diet or may not have a safe, convenient place to exercise.

Many health professionals tend to view a person's cooperation with the health care regimen as a single choice when this cooperation actually involves many choices every day. For example, following a low-fat, low-cholesterol diet involves making constant, and often inconvenient, choices throughout the day. The expectation is that people will do this every day for the rest of their lives, even when the nurse cannot guarantee health as a result.

Ultimately, the nurse needs to respect a person's right to choose. However, nurses can increase an individual's motivation and capabilities to change by involving the individual in planning and goal setting, providing information that is understandable and acceptable, and assisting the person in developing new skills.

After clarifying behaviors that a person is willing to change, the nurse can use the following framework for developing interventions for behavior change:

- Assess the behavior.
- Educate the person about the need for and benefits of change.
- Motivate the person using personalized messages.
- Assess and increase the person's self-efficacy.
- Assess and offer resources to decrease barriers to change.
- Assist the person with goal setting to modify behavior.
- Practice the skills needed to change behavior.
- Plan ways to monitor and maintain the behavior change.

Theories of health behavior change are at the heart of health education. The theories presented in this section help nurses to assess an individual's stage in the behavior change process and to develop appropriate teaching plans. The goals of the teaching plans and the strategies selected will differ depending on the factors affecting the individual's readiness to learn and to change.

Ethics

Applying principles of respect, autonomy, justice, and beneficence, nurses have an active role as advocates in empowering people to make informed decisions about their health. The nurse works as a partner, facilitator, and resource for individuals and families. Although the focus of health education may be on the behavior change process, the nurse needs to exercise caution in using tools of persuasion in communication with people because of the potential for manipulation and coercion (Burkhardt & Nathaniel, 2020).

Choices about health care practices belong to individuals, not health care providers. All competent people have the right to autonomous choice. Nurses should respect decisions made by individuals and their families, even when the choice is not what the nurse might personally do or suggest. The nurse and the family should work together on a plan that incorporates these individual and family values and beliefs (Burkhardt & Nathaniel, 2020). When health promotion focuses on individual behavior, disregarding other social factors that may contribute significantly to the problem, this can inadvertently lead to victim blaming. A plan or intervention should take into consideration all environmental and societal factors. Although individuals and families are empowered to take charge of their health, certain social determinants may create barriers. Nurses can examine these barriers and make a plan that is feasible and will lead to positive health outcomes.

The role of the nurse is to facilitate a communicative environment in which people can exercise their right to make informed, free choices. Individuals need to participate in the decision-making process when their lives may be influenced by a change.

Although each person's state of health affects family members and the community, individuals are responsible for their own health maintenance. Health professionals need to accept and welcome individual differences in meeting this responsibility. By selecting interventions that create an environment of open communication and risk-taking, individuals can better develop the problem-solving skills to direct their own growth and development.

Genomics and Health Education

Advances in genetics and genomics present new opportunities and responsibilities for nurses in health education. Nurses should consider the effect of genomics on individuals and families and maintain knowledge of the relationship between genomics, genetics, and health (Fleming & Riper, 2022). Routine use of genetic and genomic technologies requires nurses to incorporate information about and implications of the technologies into educational programs for vulnerable individuals, families, and populations. Although an increasingly wide range of situations include the need for the nurse to be prepared to discuss genetics and genomics, the primary focus for nursing is health promotion, symptom management, and disease prevention. Box 10.5: Genomics describes the components of a genetic/genomic nursing assessment.

Diversity and Health Teaching

The increasing racial and ethnic diversity of the US population, as well as the challenge to eliminate disparities in the health status of people of diverse backgrounds, demands that nurses provide culturally appropriate health education and health promotion. The events of 2020 further highlighted the need for health care providers to do their part in improving the health outcomes of marginalized populations with the COVID-19 pandemic and numerous killings of persons of color (Kalevor, Kurts-Uveges, & Meyer, 2022). Individuals' cultural groups influence their beliefs about health, perceptions of disease and

BOX 10.5 GENOMICS

Components of a Genetic/Genomic Nursing Assessment

A genetic nursing assessment includes the following information (Fleming & VanRiper, 2022):

- Health history of family members
- Three-generation pedigree using standardized symbols
- Reproductive history
- Ethnic background of family members (as described by the family)
- Documentation of variations in growth and development of family members
- Individual member and family understanding of causes of health problems that occur in more than one family member
- Identification of questions family members have about potential genetic risk factors in the family
- Identification of communication preferences for genetic health information within the family

illness, help-seeking behaviors, and attitudes toward health providers and play a role in their use of traditional and complementary healing practices. To be effective, health education efforts must include consideration of these cultural influences. Nurses should familiarize themselves with each individual's or family's beliefs in building a trusting relationship.

An innovative way to learn about people with diverse cultural health backgrounds is to listen to educational podcasts. This experience provides a way to walk in someone else's shoes by the simple act of listening. See Box 10.6 for podcast experience instructions.

Nurses also need to provide a nonjudgmental environment for the lesbian, gay, bisexual, and transgender community. This involves using inclusive language (e.g., preferred pronouns), not making assumptions, and understanding that this population has unique needs and barriers. This population and the social stigma that surrounds them often prevents them from seeking health care. The unique challenges the LGBTQ population faces are higher rates of mental health issues, including suicidal thoughts and suicide (Gross et al., 2020).

The health professional should assess cultural beliefs that influence social and health practices and promote educational interventions that are appropriate, acceptable, and satisfying to the individual. **Social marketing** processes and the diffusion of innovations model discussed in the next section can help in identifying characteristics, interests, and concerns of target populations.

When teaching people of different cultural, racial, and ethnic groups, the nurse endeavors to provide culturally sensitive education. Nurses can improve care by self-reflection and examination of their own implicit bias, which can ultimately lead to self-improvement and positive change (Kalevor, Kurts-Uveges, & Meyer, 2022). The Robert Wood Johnson Foundation offers a framework to guide health care professionals in creating a culture of health (Box 10.7: Health Equity/Health and Social Determinants).

BOX 10.6 BEST PRACTICE

Promoting Health, One Episode at a Time

An innovative teaching and learning activity peer-reviewed and published on the Association of Community Health Nurse Educator's webpage aims to use a podcast to educate students (Strickland & Jones, 2021). The students will then apply the health education from the podcast to their own lives, discern ways to apply the health-promotion techniques from the episode to the broader community, and identify resources in the community for improved health and wellness.

The instructions for the assignment are as follows:

Download a podcast platform to your smart device (e.g., iHeartRadio, Google Podcasts, Overcast, Spotify, Apple Podcasts, Apple iTunes, Pandora).

Search for "Nurse Narrative."

Listen to the assigned episode.

Prepare to participate in the discussion post, classroom discussion, or community engagement experience with the episode in mind.

Evaluate student learning through reflection questions such as the following:

1. What types of approaches might you use to identify the needs of Dr. Marie Charles's community? (Quad Council Public Health Nursing Competency Domain 1: Assessment and Analytic Skills, 1A9)
2. Describe the implications and potential effect of public health programs and policies on individuals, families, and groups within Dr. Marie Charles's community. (Quad Council Public Health Nursing Competency Domain 2: Policy Development/Program Planning Skills, 2A2)
3. How does Dr. Marie Charles's discussion of the Haitian culture inform your approach toward communicating with individuals, the community, and stakeholders within her specific neighborhood? (Quad Council Public Health Nursing Competency Domain 3: Communication Skills, 3A2 and 3A3)
4. Consider what it means to deliver culturally responsible public health nursing services for individuals, families, and groups. (Quad Council Public Health Nursing Competency Domain 4: Cultural Competency Skills, 4A3)

This could occur through a live discussion or through a reflective journal entry. Course leaders may also divide the class into separate teams who listen to different episodes and then discuss them together.

Through this podcast and innovative teaching strategy, listeners have been reached in 6 continents, 30 countries/territories, 684 cities, with over 5,949 downloads worldwide. The reach is significant. The authors are working to develop more evaluation strategies as time progresses. Part of knowing the podcast's effect and measuring its success is incorporating it into nursing schools' syllabi and teaching engagements (Strickland & Jones, 2021).

Data from Quad Council Coalition Competency Review Task Force. (2018). *Community/public health nursing competencies.* http://www.quadcouncilphn.org/wpcontent/uploads/2018/05/QCC-C-PHN-COMPETENCIES-Approved_2018.05.04_Final002.pdf

COMMUNITY AND GROUP HEALTH EDUCATION

When nurses begin to teach groups of people, they automatically enter a program planning and administrative process. When an organization wants to offer an ongoing health education program for a target population, social marketing provides a strategy for reaching members of the group and implementing a service that will satisfy these members as consumers. Principles of **social marketing** and health education strategies are combined to promote population-based changes in behavior to improve health. Concepts from community group health behavior change models and health education strategies are combined to promote population-based changes to improve health.

Social Marketing

"In social marketing, service users are viewed as customers who need to be understood so they can become actively engaged in health promotion interventions, rather than remaining passive recipients of such interventions" (Woods, 2022). Social marketing provides a strategy for reaching members of the group and implementing a service that will satisfy these members as consumers. One of the first social marketing campaigns to be used was targeted at family planning, and since then, social marketing has been used successfully to promote health education and understand health behavior (Riegelman, 2020). Social marketing models can be used by nurses to create health-promotion plans and interventions that increase the likelihood of positive health outcomes (Woods, 2022).

Social marketing communication reaches beyond the individual level to influence social conditions, policy, legislation, and normative group behavior. This is done through a variety of methods, including mass media and social media. Key attributes of a social marketing approach are the offering of benefits and the reduction of barriers to influence the target group's behavior.

BOX 10.7 HEALTH EQUITY/HEALTH AND SOCIAL DETERMINANTS

Building a Culture of Health in Health Education

The Robert Wood Johnson Foundation has a vision of creating a culture of health across the nation. A culture of health framework has been developed to assist in carrying out this vision. The social determinants of health are complex factors that affect our health. Where we live, our support system, and our socioeconomic status are some examples of these factors. According to the Robert Wood Johnson Foundation, "When we work together to create opportunities that improve health equity for everyone, we're building a culture of health." The framework provides an agenda for the nation to work toward health equity. Nurses play a large role in creating a culture of health when promoting health and providing health education to individuals, groups, and communities. Following this framework provides nurses and other health care professionals with guidelines for cultivating an equitable environment. The framework includes four focus areas, with topics under each, that were developed by using the 10 principles for a culture of health.

10 Principles for a Culture of Health

1. Every individual, family, and community are seen as deserving of health and well-being.
2. America's national narrative acknowledges that health and well-being is affected by injustice, systemic racism, and inequities in social and economic conditions.
3. All families—no matter who they are, where they live, or how much money they make—should have the resources they need to help their children grow up healthy.
4. Public policy and decision-making in the private industry is guided by the goal of ensuring everyone has a fair and just opportunity for health and well-being.
5. Health data, research, and measures prioritize collecting information by race, age, ethnicity, sex, geographic region, and other relevant factors to advance health equity for all.
6. Health is considered a shared responsibility within our society.
7. Everyone, no matter their background, has access to the resources they need to create conditions that support good health and well-being.
8. Health care, public health, and social services work together to fully address the goals and needs of the people they serve.
9. Communities, regardless of income or geography, have the power, agency, and resources to create and implement their own solutions to the unique health issues facing them.
10. No one is excluded.

Focus Areas and Topics

Focus area 1: Health systems – Bringing key health systems together around a shared goal of better health for all

Topics: Health care quality and value, health care coverage and access, public and community health

Focus area 2: Healthy communities – Supporting initiatives that help communities reach their greatest health potential

Topics: Equitable community development, health disparities, social determinants of health

Focus area 3: Healthy children and families – Supporting research and programs that expand our understanding of growing up healthy

Topics: Economic inclusion for family well-being, valuing caregivers and families

Focus area 4: Leadership for better health – Helping leaders address health challenges across the nation

Topics: Health leadership development, nurses and nursing

From Robert Wood Johnson Foundation (2023). *Building a culture of health*. https://www.rwjf.org/content/rwjf/en/cultureofhealth/taking-action.html

Social marketers attempt to modify the attractiveness of specific behavioral options to favor one choice over competing alternatives. Making the healthy choice the easy choice, while gearing it toward the desires of a population, is key (Riegelman, 2020). Social marketing strategies can be used in designing programs for health promotion (substance abuse, obesity), injury prevention (seat belt wearing, gun storage), and environmental protection (pesticides, water conservation) and should address several questions, including the following: What is the goal? Who has power over the goal? To whom do individuals listen? How can you get the message across to them? How can you effectively put forward the message (Riegelman, 2020)? Any information about the target population that is generated by social marketing strategies will improve the nurse's ability to develop effective educational interventions.

Another model commonly used in community health-education planning is the diffusion of innovations model (Rogers, 2003), which explains how an idea or product is adopted and spreads through a social system. In public health, diffusion of innovations is used to address the factors that support or inhibit the adoption of effective, evidence-based interventions to improve community health. Practical application of the model involves understanding the target population and recognizing the importance of their readiness to accept an innovation, and it will inform the methods and strategies to be implemented (Bensley & Brookins-Fisher, 2023).

Creating a Teaching Plan

Preparation for teaching a group program, such as a seminar or course, begins after the marketing and administrative plans are well underway. These activities ensure that there are enough participants for the program and that a structure for developing the teaching plan—program objectives, available time, human and material resources, and so on—is provided. When the marketing and administrative functions have been provided by others, and when educational strategies are developed for one person at a time, the nurse can concentrate their efforts on developing the teaching plan.

A health teaching plan may emphasize a phase of the behavior change process that is related to the individual's or group's health-promotion needs or problems. The written teaching plan represents a package of educational services provided to a consumer or student. The plan is written from the learner's point of view.

The process of generating a teaching plan helps the nurse to recognize and use methods of learning that involve the individual as an active participant. The plan includes a list of specific actions or abilities that the person may perform at intervals during and at the end of the educational intervention. Teaching plans help nurses clarify these outcomes. The purpose of a written plan is to direct a teaching-learning session to achieve the desired outcomes. Table 10.1 shows the outline and examples of the components of a 20-minute teaching plan for an individual.

Analysis and Assessment

Assessment, the first step in the process, involves analyzing the characteristics of the learner and identifying their learning

TABLE 10.1 Teaching Plan

Objectives	Content Outline	Methods of Teaching	Time Allotted	Instructional Materials	Evaluation Methods
Following a 20-minute teaching session, the learner will be able to:					
List at least three examples of types of exercise that can be done outside work. (Cognitive)	Examples of simple, everyday ways to increase exercise (e.g., take stairs rather than elevator)	1:1 instruction	5 minutes	"Physical Activity" poster showing practical ways to increase activity	Question and answers
Recognize barriers that interfere with remaining active. (Affective)	Common barriers and ways to deal with them	Discussion	5 minutes	CDC website article: "Make Your Workout Work for You"	Describes barriers and ways to avoid interference
Demonstrate four exercises that can be completed inside the home. (Psychomotor)	How to perform sit-ups, lunges, wall sits, and using stairs	Demonstration/return demonstration	10 minutes	Space for performing exercises	Demonstrates correct performance of each exercise

needs. The following characteristics of the learner are important for the nurse to identify and consider in planning; they are listed as individual factors and environmental factors (National Council of State Boards of Nursing, 2019).

Individual Factors:

- Knowledge
- Skills
- Specialty
- Characteristics
- Prior experience
- Level of experience

Environmental Factors:

- Environment
- Client observation
- Resources
- Medical records
- Consequences and risks
- Time pressure
- Task complexity
- Cultural consideration

The reader is encouraged to refer to the chapters (see Unit 4) about individual development.

Assessment of the learner can be accomplished by one answering the following five questions:

- What are the characteristics and learning capabilities of the individual?
- What are the learner's needs for health promotion, risk reduction, or health problems?
- What does the person already know, and what skills can the person already perform that are relevant to their health needs?
- Is the learner motivated to change any unhealthy behaviors?
- What are the barriers to and facilitators of health **behavior change**?

When preparing a teaching plan for one person in a primary care setting, the nurse may learn background information about the individual from that person's record and agency reports that include descriptions of the person's population group. Nurses often agree to teach health classes that others have organized. In this case the nurse asks for project reports that provide marketing and needs-assessment information about the students who are expected to attend the classes.

Determining Expected Learning Outcomes

To determine the expected learning outcomes of a health-education intervention, the nurse answers the following questions:

- What broad public health and social goals guide the proposed educational program?
- What are the participant's learning goals?
- What does the learner need to know, do, and believe to progress through the behavior change process?

Program Goals

The program goals of a health education project reflect the desire to facilitate improvement in some health problem or social living condition. Program goals can be broad and long range or specific and measurable. The SMART framework is an effective tool for developing goals that are clear, realistic, and meaningful (CDC, 2022). The following guidelines and questions can be used to inform goal development and evaluate achievement of those goals (CDC, 2022; Weiss et al., 2023):

- Specific: What are the goals? Who is the audience? Are the goals clear and agreeable to all involved? Decide on the main goals, and establish the who, what, when, where, and why of how the goals will be achieved.
- Measurable: How will progress and success be measured? What data will be used to determine whether the goal has been met?
- Achievable/Attainable: Can the goals be achieved with the skills, resources, and time available? If so, how? What are the existing barriers?
- Relevant: Do the goals align with those of the individual, community, and/or organization? Will the steps in the action plan have an effect on the specified goals and intended audience? A relevant goal is consistent with identified needs, is done at the right time, and is worthwhile.
- Time-bound: What is the deadline for accomplishing each goal? Develop a reasonable time frame, and set deadlines or time limits for achievement of the specified goals.

Learning Goals

Learning goals are best established when the student and the nurse work together. These goals reflect the health behavior or health status change that the person will have achieved by the end of an educational intervention. Learning goals relate to the program goals.

Learning Objectives

Learning objectives indicate the steps to be taken by the individual toward meeting the learning goal and may involve the development of knowledge, a skill, or a change in attitude. Objectives are most useful when stated in behavioral terms and when they contain the following components: the learner and a precise action verb that indicates what the learner will be able to do, the conditions under which the task is performed, and the level of performance expected (Bastable & Capacci, 2021). Learning objectives guide the selection of content and methods and help narrow the focus of a teaching plan to more achievable steps; they also aid in setting standards of performance and suggesting evaluation strategies.

Selecting Content

To select appropriate content for a health education program, the nurse considers what information, skills, and attitudes need to be taught and the level of learning to be achieved.

Three Domains of Learning

Content is commonly divided into three domains: cognitive, psychomotor, and affective. Cognitive learning refers to the development of new facts or concepts and to building on or applying knowledge to new situations. Psychomotor learning involves developing physical skills, from simple to complex actions. Affective learning alludes to the recognition of values, religious and spiritual beliefs, family interaction patterns and relationships, and personal attitudes that affect decisions and problem-solving progress.

To learn or change a health behavior, a person may need to acquire new information, practice physical techniques, and clarify the ways in which the new behavior may affect their relationships with others. The nurse's role is to select a combination of content from the three domains that is appropriate to meet the behavioral objective. To find samples of content for a teaching plan, the nurse researches resource materials, such as books, teaching guides, journal articles, pamphlets, and flyers created by nonprofit agencies and professional organizations. The nurse is careful about providing materials with technical vocabulary that is too complex for the audience.

Examples of Learning Objectives

In writing learning objectives, the nurse selects action verbs from the taxonomies previously mentioned that indicate observable learning. Table 10.2 provides examples of objectives in each domain of learning. The first objective listed for each domain is incorrect because the verb does not indicate observable learning. The second example for each domain is measurable because the verb used (indicated in boldface type) allows the learning to be observed.

TABLE 10.2 Examples of Nonmeasurable and Measurable Teaching Objectives

Domain	Objectives
Cognitive	Not measurable: Dan will understand the correct food choices for following a low-fat diet Measurable: Dan will correctly select low-fat foods from the options provided
Affective	Not measurable: Dan will demonstrate the importance of weight loss Measurable: Dan will verbalize the importance of weight loss
Psychomotor	Not measurable: Dan will know how to determine a serving Measurable: Dan will demonstrate correct measurement of a one-serving portion

When preparing a teaching plan, the nurse differentiates between information the individual needs to know and information considered helpful to know to develop appropriate learning objectives. This process provides cues to the nurse for planning effective strategies for the necessary level of learning. As the level of learning to be achieved becomes complex, the educational strategies and methods selected involve the individuals in more active application and analysis of the content.

Designing Learning Strategies

Designing the learning strategies for an educational intervention involves selecting the methods and tools and structuring the sequence of activities. The teaching plan to this point provides the foundation on which to base the activity selection and sequence. The following questions guide the design of learning strategies:

- What are some basic considerations for selecting teaching methods for health education programs?
- How does the nurse, as instructor, establish and maintain a learning climate?
- What actions can the nurse perform to increase the effectiveness of the learning methods?
- What are the appropriate methods for each learning domain?
- What methods tend to promote behavior change?

Teaching Strategies

Numerous strategies for teaching are available (Table 10.3). A few of those most commonly used are listed and described here. Lecture is a well-known method in which the teacher verbally presents information and instructions to the person or audience. Lecture provides a way to present a large amount of information to a number of people in a nonthreatening way. This can be an effective method if active learning strategies such as questioning are integrated. Discussion involves interaction between the nurse educator and the individuals. The nurse prepares questions in advance to guide the discussion. This method gives the nurse an opportunity to gain a better perception of individuals' understanding of the topic and to clarify information.

Demonstration and practice are used in learning psychomotor skills such as performing exercises. The nurse demonstrates the expected behavior while the person observes. Then

TABLE 10.3 Domains of Learning, Teaching Strategies, and Examples of Desired Outcomes Related to a Behavior Change

Domain of Learning	Teaching Strategies	Examples of Desired Outcomes Related to a Behavior Change
Cognitive (thinking)	Lecture One-to-one instruction Discussion Discovery Audiovisual or printed materials Computer-assisted instruction	Describes and/or explains information relevant to the behavior change
Affective (feeling)	Role modeling Discussion Role-playing Simulation gaming	Expresses positive feeling, attitudes, values toward changing the behavior
Psychomotor (acting)	Demonstration or teach-back method Practice Mental imaging	Demonstrates performance of skills related to the behavior change

the nurse watches and provides feedback and encouragement while the person performs the behavior. Using the actual equipment the individual will use in their home facilitates successful performance. For complex tasks, teaching a few steps at a time, in sequence, aids skill development. The teach-back method previously described is an effective form of demonstration and practice.

Simulation gaming may involve computer learning, board games, or role-play. Obviously, computer learning games are dependent on the availability of hardware and software appropriate for the individual and the topic. Simple board games can be developed for cognitive learning. An example might be the development of a bingo game based on the food pyramid. Role-play involves acting out a potential scenario. This allows individuals to practice appropriate responses to challenging situations. For example, a person restricted to a low-fat diet can act out a response to being offered dessert by an insistent family member or friend played by the nurse (Fig. 10.2).

Considerations for Selecting Methods

The nurse's first consideration is to promote an environment and use methods that foster self-directed learning. An active participant usually learns more.

There will be many learning styles in a group audience; therefore, the nurse varies the teaching methods used in a given session. Taking into consideration the characteristics of the population (developmental stage, age, and knowledge of the topic), the nurse selects teaching methods that best support the goals and theme of the educational program. The order of content proceeds from simple ideas and skills to more complex concepts, from known material toward lesser-known data. The nurse is sensitive to the energy level and anxiety of the audience when presenting content that requires strong concentration or causes anxiety.

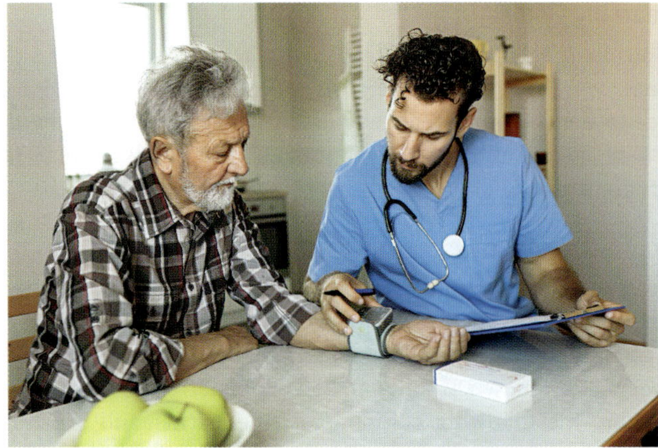

FIG. 10.2 Male nurse sitting at kitchen table with patient. (From iStock.com/ PixelsEffect).

Learning Climate

For group presentations, the nurse addresses several activities when seeking to establish an environment that is conducive to health behavior change. The first activity is creating a sense of preparedness and organization by providing physical facilities with adequate furnishings and suitable audiovisual materials and handouts. Even the instructor's appearance will lend credibility to or distraction from the presentation.

The second activity involves anticipating the needs of the group and communicating information about the schedule and the facilities. This action alleviates the group's apprehension and makes the group members more comfortable.

The third activity focuses on the nurse's assessment of the individual and group learning needs, possibly through questions and dialogue. Members of the group need to believe that the program will be beneficial and relevant to their situations. The instructor watches for and reinforces signs of motivation to participate in the experience.

Fourth, the nurse encourages, empowers, and engages students to continue to progress. As a reality check, the nurse might ask for periodic feedback from the group about the effectiveness of the program and its relevance to group needs. The nurse continues to assess the group throughout the learning experience.

Finally, the nurse works with the group to maintain the learning climate. This process involves observing group interactions, helping individuals participate, intervening to help the group deal with controlling its members, and remaining cognizant of dynamics in the group process that will facilitate or inhibit learning.

Teaching for Each Learning Domain

As mentioned, teaching is directed toward one or more of three learning domains: cognitive, psychomotor, and affective. Examples of appropriate teaching strategies for each domain and the expected outcomes in relation to behavior change are summarized in Table 10.3.

Evaluating the Teaching-Learning Process

The teacher can evaluate learning or measure achievement of learning objectives in all domains through the use of written or oral testing, demonstrations, observation, self-reports, and self-monitoring. Teaching methods for one domain may overlap with those for another domain.

The nurse can incorporate written, verbal, and nonverbal techniques for obtaining feedback about teaching performance into the teaching plan. End-of-program questionnaires are the usual method for obtaining written feedback. The nurse may ask for verbal feedback at various times from the group, from individual students, and from observers of the class. Nonverbal communication cues from participants may indicate their satisfaction, fatigue, or frustration with the educational intervention.

The overall process of the teaching-learning experience needs to be evaluated. The procedures used to organize and promote an educational program can affect its ultimate success. The nurse (or a program administration committee) records activities such as advertising, registration, fee collection, and availability and repair of equipment and materials. This evaluative information can then be used to improve subsequent programs. Surveys by telephone or by questionnaires help obtain the consumer's opinion about these implementation procedures. Word-of-mouth referrals to future programs and support from other community agencies and professionals may also indicate approval of the program format.

Occasionally the nurse is asked to justify a health education program in terms of its effect on the community's public health goals or social problems. Health promotion involves a combination of health-protection activities, preventive health services, and health education programs; therefore, drawing a direct correlation between an educational intervention and the statistical improvement of the health problem can be difficult.

Nurses can often describe the theoretical influence of an educational intervention on health behaviors, health problems, and social problems. Statistics such as the number of people served each year, the percentage of the target population reached, the number of service providers used, and the number and cost of programs are important and need to be preserved. As these statistics change over time, the data will provide cues to program successes and problems.

Referring Individuals to Other Resources

The end of a teaching plan includes resources for people to use for continuing education, counseling, peer support, and health services. Nurses encourage people to view health education as a lifelong learning process. Each person has different developmental needs and health concerns through their life cycle. Moreover, any one educational intervention may help a person move only from one phase of the behavior change process to the next. In addition, the Internet as a health education tool may influence a person's health practices.

TEACHING AND ORGANIZING SKILLS

To develop teaching and organizing skills in health education, the nurse often needs to learn new behaviors. A systematic guide can be used to learn these professional skills. To perform these steps, the nurse does the following:

- Seeks self-assessment opportunities
- Identifies, lists, and prioritizes learning needs
- Begins to identify the resources that are available for reading, instructor training, and practice teaching
- Drafts an initial set of learning goals
- Selects the target population and the general topic
- Works through the steps of the teaching-learning process, including the development of a teaching plan
- Identifies other people or a project team to help

After implementing the educational intervention, the nurse sets time aside to discuss what happened. Did the program go as planned? What changes were made in the teaching plan? What can be changed for the next program? The nurse reviews the self-developed learning goals and determines new ones.

In addition, health education research evaluates teaching interventions. This contributes to the evidence base from which nurses can implement new teaching strategies or question the effectiveness of traditional approaches. See Box 10.8: Evidence-Based Practice for an example of using technology to educate and promote behavior change.

As additional programs on either an individual or a group basis are provided, the nurse will be able to clarify specific instructor teaching and organizing skills that come naturally.

These skills tend to improve a program's effectiveness and enable the logistics to run smoothly. The teacher is first a learner; this is true in health education and any other form of education.

Ethical dilemmas must be considered as nurses create programs to provide health education and health promotion. See Box 10.9: Ethical Dilemmas, for information on a literature review that highlights ethical dilemmas in health promotion and offers recommendations on how to promote health in an equitable way.

BOX 10.8 EVIDENCE-BASED PRACTICE

Novel Interventions in Stroke Recovery

Stroke is one of the leading causes of death and disability around the world. Evidence shows that physical therapy and exercise poststroke provide tremendous positive health outcomes. Therapy is typically provided in the immediate period after a stroke, but patients often fail to continue exercise regimens as time goes on.

A study was conducted in the United Kingdom to examine whether a texting program titled Keeping Active with Texting After Stroke (KATS) made a difference in the activity level of patients poststroke. This program allowed patients to remain at home and create self-directed exercise plans. The program lasted for 12 weeks and began when patients were discharged from physical therapy.

Semistructured interviews were conducted via telephone halfway through the program at week 6 and again at the end of the intervention (the end of week 12). Twenty-four interviews were conducted on 12 patients in total. Results showed that patients not only felt encouraged to participate in physical activity but also expressed feeling less alone as they continued to recover. Unlike most stroke survivors, the participants mentioned not feeling abandoned at the point of discharge. Due to this finding, the researchers plan to add 2 extra weeks to the end of the 12-week program with text messages gradually declining. Overall, the participants found the program to be worthwhile and motivating (Farre et al., 2023).

BOX 10.9 ETHICS IN HEALTH PROMOTION

Ethical Dilemmas

A literature review was conducted to examine health professionals' ethical dilemmas in health promotion and education. The review was completed by examining publications from the last decade of the 20th century and the first 2 decades of the 21st century. The following keywords were used in the search: *ethics, health care workers, medical practice, health promotion,* and *public health.* Siljak et al. (2023) describe ethical dilemmas in health promotion as being related to the relationship between individual choice and health opportunities in the environment.

When health care professionals decide what is best for patients and populations, are we infringing on their rights? Is it considered paternalism when we decide wearing seat belts should be a law? Is this approach equitable when the result is the greatest good for the greatest number of people? These are all questions nurses consider as they work on health-promotion campaigns and with individuals to promote healthy behavior change.

Siljak et al. (2023) express the importance of patient education and empowerment and helping individuals see the benefits of healthy choices. Access to social conditions and community resources for health as part of the equation are also stressed. The hope is to educate the patient in a way that they are empowered to make the healthy choice even when it is not the easy choice.

CASE STUDY

Deshawn

Deshawn is a 40-year-old man who will be traveling to Dubai to give a business presentation in 3 months. Although he has traveled widely in the United States as a consultant, this is his first international trip. He requests information regarding immunizations needed before his trip. Deshawn states that because he will be in Dubai for only a few days, he is unlikely to contract a disease in such a short time and therefore believes that it is illogical to obtain immunizations. Deshawn states that he has heard that the side effects of the immunizations might be worse than the diseases they prevent. He is also concerned about leaving his wife at home alone because she is 6 months pregnant.

Reflective Questions

- How would you address Deshawn's beliefs?
- What learning would be needed in each domain?
- What learning theories would you consider?
- How might his family concerns be addressed?

SUMMARY

- Of all health professionals, nurses spend the most time in direct contact with individuals and often coordinate group programs.
- A comprehensive analysis of educational aspects of a health-promotion program is integral to program success.
- Assessment of the characteristics and learning needs of the target audience leads to greater influence on health behaviors.
- The principles of health education form a generic basis for implementing a variety of health topics.
- Planning to teach one person is different from planning to teach a group.
- One-to-one interventions tend to follow a counseling or problem-solving approach.
- Group interventions can range from guided discussions on concerns that evolve from the group to a more structured learning experience involving presentations, skill practice, and attitude-awareness exercises.
- The range of health education strategies provides nurses and all health care professionals with techniques and methods applicable in health service settings, schools, work sites, and other community facilities.

EVOLVE CHAPTER FEATURES

http://evolve.elsevier.com/Edelman/

- Study Questions

REFERENCES

Agency for Healthcare Research and Quality. (2020). *AHRQ health literacy universal precautions toolkit, 2nd edition.* http://www.ahrq.gov/professionals/quality-patient-safety/quality-resources/tools/literacy-toolkit/index.html

American Nurses Association. (2015). *Code of ethics for nurses with interpretive statements.* https://www.nursingworld.org/practice-policy/nursing-excellence/ethics/code-of-ethics-for-nurses/coe-view-only/

American Nurses Association. (2021). *Nursing: Scope and standards of practice* (4th ed.). American Nurses Association.

Bandura, A. (1997). *Self-efficacy: The exercise of control.* New York: W.H. Freeman.

Barton, A. J., Allen, P. E., Boyle, D. K., Loan, L. A., Stichler, J. F., & Parnell, T. A. (2018). Health literacy: Essential for a culture of health. *The Journal of Continuing Education in Nursing, 49*(2), 73–78.

Bastable, S. B., & Capacci, N. M. (2021). Behavioral objectives and teaching plans. In S. B. Bastable (Ed.), *Nurse as educator: Principles of teaching and learning for nursing practice* (6th ed.). Burlington, MA: Jones & Bartlett.

Bensley, R. J., & Brookins-Fisher, J. (2023). Laying the foundations for selecting community and public health education methods and strategies. In R. J. Bensley, & J. Brookins Fisher (Eds.), *Community and public health education methods: A practical guide* (5th ed.). Burlington, MA: Jones & Bartlett.

Botchwey, N. D., Park, E., & Kulbok, P. A. (2020). Building a culture of health to influence health equity within communities. In M. Stanhope, & J. Lancaster (Eds.), *Public health nursing: Population-centered health care in the community* (10th ed.). St. Louis: Elsevier.

Burkhardt, M. A., & Nathaniel, A. K. (2020). *Ethics and issues in contemporary nursing: Nursing Ethics for the 21st Century.* (1st ed.). Missouri: Elsevier.

Center for Disease Control and Prevention (CDC). (2022). *SMART Framework.* https://www.cdc.gov/youth-advisory-councils/action-plans/smart-framework.html?CDC_AAref_Val=https://www.cdc.gov/healthyyouth/yac/smart-framework.htm

Centers for Disease Control and Prevention (CDC), US Department of Health and Human Services. (2019). *The CDC clear communication index.* https://www.cdc.gov/ccindex/

Cottrell, R. R., Seabert, D. M., Spear, C. E., & McKenzie, J. J. (2023). *Principles of health education and promotion.* Burlington, MA: Jones and Bartlett Learning.

Farre, A., Morris, J. H., Irvine, L., Dombrowski, S. U., Breckenridge, J. P., Ozakinci, G., Lebedis, T., & Jones, C. (2023). Exploring the views and experiences of people recovering from a stroke about a new text message intervention to promote physical activity after rehabilitation. *Health Expectations: An international journal of public participation in health care and health policy, 26*(5), 2013-2022.

Fleming, L., & Van Riper, M. (2015). Genomics and family nursing across the life span. In M. D. Fowler (Ed.), *Guide to nursing's social policy statement.* American Nurses Association.

Gross, M., Knopp, A., & Brown, H. (2020). Major health issues and chronic disease management of adults across the lifespan. In M. Stanhope, & J. Lancaster (Eds.), *Public health nursing: Population-centered health care in the community* (10th ed.). St. Louis: Elsevier.

Kalevor, S., Kurts-Uveges, M., & Meyer, E. C. (2022). Using everyday ethics to address bias and racism in clinical care. *AACN Advanced Critical Care, 33*(1), 111–118.

Kutner, M., Greenburg, E., Jin, Y., & Paulsen, C. (2006). *The health literacy of America's adults: Results from the 2003 National Assessment of Adult Literacy. NCES 2006-483.* National Center for Education Statistics. https://nces.ed.gov/pubsearch/pubsinfo.asp?pubid=2006483

Massi, L., Hickey, S., Maidment, S. J., Roe, Y., Kildea, S., & Kruske, S. (2023). "This has changed me to be a better mum": A qualitative study exploring how the Australian Nurse-Family Partnership Program contributes to the development of First Nations women's self-efficacy. *Women and Birth, 36,* e613–e622.

National Academies of Sciences, Engineering, and Medicine. (2021). *The future of nursing 2020–2030: Charting a path to achieve health equity.* The National Academies Press. https://doi.org/10.17226/25982

National Council of State Boards of Nursing. (2019). *Clinical judgement measurement model: A framework to measure clinical judgment & decision making.* https://www.nclex.com/clinical-judgment-measurement-model.page

Ndugga, N., & Artiga, S. (2023). *Disparities in health and health care: 5 key questions and answers.* Kaiser Family Foundation. https://www.kff.org/racial-equity-and-health-policy/issue-brief/disparities-in-health-and-health-care-5-key-question-and-answers/

Niederhauser, V. P. (2020). Health education principles applied in communities, groups, families, and individuals for healthy change. In M. Stanhope, & J. Lancaster (Eds.), *Public health nursing: Population-centered health care in the community* (10th ed.). St. Louis: Elsevier.

Nurse-Family Partnership. (2023). *Nurse-Family Partnership Overview* [Fact sheet]. https://www.nursefamilypartnership.org/about/

Nurse-Family Partnership. (2024). *Public policy priorities.* https://www.nursefamilypartnership.org/public-policy-and-advocacy/2public-policy-priorities/

Prochaska, J. O., & DiClemente, C. C. (1984). *The transtheoretical approach: Crossing traditional boundaries of change.* Homewood, NJ: Dow Jones-Irwin.

Quality and Safety in Nursing Institute. (2022). *QSEN competencies.* Case Western Reserve University. https://www.qsen.org/competencies-pre-licensure-ksas

Riegelman, R. (2020). *Population health: A primer.* Burlington, MA: Jones & Bartlett.

Robert Wood Johnson Foundation. (2023). *Our vision.* https://www.rwjf.org/content/rwjf/en/cultureofhealth/taking-action.html

Rogers, E. M. (2003). *Diffusion of innovations* (5th ed.). New York: Free Press.

Siljak, S., Boricic, K., & Tosic, M. (2023). Ethical practice of health care professionals in health promotion. *Serbian Journal of the Medical Chamber, 4*(3), 303–310.

Simons-Morton, B., & Lodyga, M. G. (2023). *Behavior theory in public health practice and research.* Burlington, MA: Jones & Bartlett Learning.

Strickland, K., & Jones, M. (2021). ACHNE Innovative Teaching Strategies.
https://www.achne.org/aws/ACHNE/pt/sp/innovative-teaching-strategies

US Department of Health and Human Services (USDHHS). (2022). *Health literacy.* https://www.hrsa.gov/about/organization/bureaus/ohe/health-literacy

US Department of Health and Human Services (USDHHS). (n.d.). *Healthy People 2030.* https://health.gov/healthypeople

Videto, D. M., & Dennis, D. L. (2021). Report of the 2020 Joint Committee on Health Education and Promotion Terminology. *Health Educator, 53*(1), 4–21.

Webb, J. (2020). Working with families in the community for healthy outcomes. In M. Stanhope, & J. Lancaster (Eds.), *Public health nursing: Population-centered health care in the community* (10th ed.). St. Louis: Elsevier.

Weiss, D., Tilin, F. J., & Morgan, M. J. (2023). *The Interprofessional health care team: Leadership and development,* (3rd ed.). Jones & Bartlett Learning.

Woods A. (2022). Applying the principles of health promotion in nursing practice. *Nursing Standard.* https://doi.org/10.7748/ns.2022.e11774

Zschaebitz, E. J., Horn, J., & Lancaster, J. (2020). Genomics in public health nursing. In M. Stanhope, & J. Lancaster (Eds.), *Public health nursing: Population-centered health care in the community* (10th ed.). St. Louis: Elsevier.

11

Nutrition Counseling for Health Promotion

Pari Mokhtari

http://evolve.elsevier.com/Edelman/

OBJECTIVES

After completing this chapter, the reader will be able to:

- Interpret the nutrition and food safety objectives outlined in the United States' Healthy People initiative.
- Summarize and apply the recommendations within the Dietary Guidelines for Americans, the Dietary Reference Intake guidelines, and the MyPlate guidelines.
- Recognize appropriate uses of dietary supplements.
- Identify the food aid programs available for marginalized groups and older adults in the United States.
- Discuss the leading nutrition-related causes of morbidity and mortality in the United States and the corresponding nutrition interventions specific to each.

KEY TERMS

Body mass index
Botanicals
Cancer
Cardiovascular diseases
Cholesterol
Cirrhosis
Coronary heart disease
Diabetes mellitus
Dietary Approaches to Stop Hypertension (DASH)
Dietary Guidelines Advisory Committee
Dietary Guidelines for Americans
Dietary reference intakes
Dyslipidemia
Fiber
Food insecurity
Food security
Fortified foods
Heart disease
Hemolytic uremic syndrome
Hemorrhagic colitis
Herbals
High-density lipoprotein
Human immunodeficiency virus
Hyperglycemia
Hyperlipidemia
Hypertension
Incidence
Lacto-ovo-vegetarian
Low-density lipoprotein
Mediterranean diet
Metabolic syndrome; Microbiome
Micronutrients
MyPlate
Nutrigenomics
Nutrition screening
Nutritional genomics
Obese
Osteoporosis
Overweight
Prehypertension
Prevalence
Prohormone
Registered dietitian nutritionists
Salmonellosis
Serving sizes
Stroke
Sugar
Teratogenic
Trans fat
Triglyceride
Type 1 diabetes mellitus
Type 2 diabetes mellitus
Underweight
Vegan

THINK ABOUT IT

You can use this chart to evaluate your own nutrient intake or that of a client or patient. For further information access MyPlate at www.choosemyplate.gov.

1. Which food from each of the following food groups have you consumed in the last 24-hour period? Use a set of household measuring utensils (cups and spoons) to make accurate estimations where possible. If you are evaluating the diet of a client, start with this question: In the past 24 hours, how many foods did you eat from each of the following food groups?

Food Group (Recommended Servings for a 2000 Calorie Diet)	Grains (6 Ounces)	Vegetables (2½ Cups)	Fruits (2 Cups)	Dairy (3 Cups)	Proteins (5½ Ounces)	Oils, Added Sugars (Limit Use)
Examples of foods	Whole or refined grains, cereals, pasta, rice	Whole, canned, fresh, frozen, or juice	Whole fruits, fresh, canned, frozen, juices	Milk, skim or low-fat, cheese, yogurt; dairy substitutes (e.g., soy, rice, or almond milks)	Meat, poultry, fish, beans, lentils, nuts	Butter, margarine, cream cheese, sour cream, shortening; sugar, candy, syrup, jelly; sugar-sweetened beverages
Servings consumed in 24 hours:						

2. Use the measuring utensils to estimate amounts from each group and insert them in the previous corresponding boxes.
3. Create a person-specific MyPlate Plan by entering age, sex, weight, height, and physical activity at www.choosemyplate.gov/resources/MyPlatePlan.
4. Compare the 24-hour dietary intake obtained to the recommendations from the MyPlate Plan. Discuss actionable ways to improve the diet or make any other changes that may be of benefit.
5. A good starting point for dietary improvements is frequently curbing the intake of added sugar. Teach yourself and your clients how to convert grams of sugar into teaspoons. Use 5 g as equivalent to 1 teaspoon of sugar. This is close enough to provide a fair deal of accuracy. In one 12 oz. can of soda (or other sugar-sweetened beverage), you may get 37 g of sugar. This equals 7.4 teaspoons of added sugar. Use this same calculation to check the amount of sugar in candy, cereals, and baked goods. As many people do not use the metric system, this method will help visualize the added sugar in such foods.

NUTRITION IN THE UNITED STATES

Adequate and nutritious food is critical to health.

Classic Vitamin-Deficiency Diseases

Some nutrient-deficiency diseases, such as rickets, pellagra, scurvy, beriberi, xerophthalmia, and goiter, persist in some developing countries. However, they have virtually disappeared from developed areas of the world. The availability of an abundant food supply, the fortification of some foods with critical nutrients, and the implementation of better methods of assessing and increasing the nutrient contents of foods have contributed to the decline of nutrient-deficiency diseases.

The introduction of iodized salt in the 1920s, for example, contributed greatly to the elimination of iodine-deficiency goiter as a public health problem. Similarly, beriberi and pellagra disappeared after the discovery that inadequate thiamine and niacin levels, respectively, contribute to these diseases. Most grain and cereal products in the United States are enriched and fortified with the B vitamins (i.e., thiamin, riboflavin, niacin, folate) and iron. Likewise, food manufacturers fortify milk with vitamins A and D, greatly reducing the incidence of dietary inadequacies for those essential nutrients. Although undernutrition still occurs in some groups of people in the United States, diseases of dietary excess and imbalance (Table 11.1) have replaced these once-prevalent diseases of nutrient deficiency.

Nutrition-Related Health Status

A variety of diet-related factors exact a heavy toll on the population in the United States. The following statements give a broad-based view of some national health concerns:

- The vast majority of adults do not meet the daily recommendations for fruit and vegetable intake: only 10.0% of adults consume the recommended amount of vegetables, and only 12.3% consume the recommended amount of fruit (Lee et al., 2022).
- Very few high school-aged teenagers consume adequate fruits and vegetables: only 2.0% consume the recommended amount of vegetables daily, and only 7.1% meet the fruit intake recommendations (Lange et al., 2021).
- About half of adults (49.3%) and 63% of adolescents consume at least one sugar-sweetened beverage (e.g., soda, sport drinks, fruit drinks, punch, sweetened tea) each day (McElfish et al., 2022).
- Most American adults consume over twice the recommended average daily intake of sodium (USDA, 2021).
- 42.8% of the adult population was obese in 2017 and 2018, with a much higher prevalence meeting the overweight status (73.8%; Li et al., 2022).
- 19.7% of children between the ages of 2 and 19 years old were obese in 2017 through 2020 (Hu & Staiano, 2022).
- Only 24.2% of adults met the aerobic and muscle-strengthening guidelines on a regular basis (Elgaddal et al., 2022).
- Only 25.8% of infants are breastfed exclusively until 6 months of age (Meek et al., 2022).

TABLE 11.1 Health Problems Related to Poor Nutrition

Health Problem[a]	Contributing Lifestyle and Nutrition Practices[b]
Anemia	Inadequate intake or absorption of iron, folate, or vitamin B_{12} intake (depending on type of anemia); decreased ability to absorb nutrients
Cancer (breast, cervical, and colon)	Excessive calorie intake; abdominal obesity; high intake of dietary carcinogens; low intake of antioxidant-rich fruits and vegetables
Cirrhosis	Excessive alcohol intake
Constipation	Inadequate fiber or fluid intake; high fat intake; sedentary lifestyle
Dental caries	Excessive, frequent consumption of concentrated sweets or sugar-sweetened beverages; lack of fluoride; poor dental hygiene
Type 2 diabetes	Excessive calorie intake; abdominal obesity; sedentary lifestyle
Cardiovascular/heart disease	Excessive calorie intake; excessive simple sugar and fat intake (in particular saturated fat, trans fat); excessive sodium intake, inadequate fiber intake; sedentary lifestyle
Hypertension	Excessive sodium and insufficient potassium intake; excessive calorie intake; possible excess alcohol intake; sedentary lifestyle
Obesity	Excessive calorie intake; sedentary lifestyle
Osteoporosis	Low calcium intake; low vitamin D intake; excessive intake of animal protein, sodium, and caffeine; sedentary lifestyle
Underweight and growth failure	Inadequate calorie intake; poor diet; malabsorption

[a]A number of health problems are caused or exacerbated by poor nutrition. Health care professionals strive to prevent or delay these health problems.
[b]Not all causes apply in every case. Not an exhaustive list of contributing factors.

- In 2021, more than 13 million households (10.2%) were food insecure, meaning that they had limited access to adequate food subsequent to a lack of money or other resources (Coleman-Jensen et al., 2022). Individuals and families who experience food insecurity are more likely to experience being overweight or obesity, potentially because of the relatively lower cost of nutrient-poor calorie-dense foods (i.e., foods with a low nutrient density and high energy density).
- The Centers for Disease Control and Prevention (CDC) estimates that approximately one in six Americans (48 million people) becomes ill from food-borne diseases annually. Of those who are sick, 128,000 are hospitalized and 3000 die (CDC, 2023).
- Overcoming such health disparities to improve the well-being of the nation requires collaborative efforts in many aspects of health promotion and necessitates health care providers of many disciplines.

Dietary Inadequacy

Nutrient inadequacies can have devastating consequences for children in developing countries leading to wasting and stunting syndromes and a cycle of malnutrition that persists through generations. Although not to the same degree, impoverished areas in the United States show some degree of these imbalances.

Dietary inadequacy may originate from primary or secondary causes. A primary nutrient deficiency occurs when an individual does not consume adequate nutrition, regardless of the cause (e.g., socioeconomic, psychological, access). A secondary nutrient deficiency occurs when an individual cannot use the nutrients consumed or their condition requires more nutrients than what the diet is providing. For example, individuals with cystic fibrosis produce a thick sticky mucus that clogs the pancreatic ducts and inhibits the release of enzymes required to digest food and make the nutrients available for absorption and use by the body. Thus although their diet may contain adequate essential fatty acids, without proper treatment the nutrients pass in the feces undigested and unavailable for the cellular needs of the body, causing a secondary deficiency.

Although there are differences as to their causes, we classify eating disorders as calorie imbalances. Individuals of any sex and age group may experience eating disorders, with some starting early in childhood. For diagnostic purposes, there are four conditions: anorexia nervosa, bulimia nervosa, binge eating disorder, and other specified feeding or eating disorder. The latter diagnosis is appropriate for individuals that experience disordered eating behaviors but do not meet the diagnostic criteria for any other specified eating disorder.

Depending on the length of time and the age of the individual, the physiologic consequences, especially for anorexia nervosa, are life-threatening. Long-term complications may include alterations in the heart rate and blood pressure, depletion of lean mass, anemia, bone loss, amenorrhea, hypoglycemia, and psychological symptoms. Early diagnosis and treatment are critical to the success of recovery.

Dietary Excesses

Problems resulting from dietary imbalances (i.e., overconsumption of some foods groups and inadequate consumption of other food groups) are one of the leading causes of modifiable illness and death in the United States (English et al., 2021; Mokdad et al., 2018). Four leading causes of death directly associated with diet are coronary heart disease (CHD), some types of cancer, stroke, and type 2 diabetes mellitus. Four other major causes of death—accidents, cirrhosis, suicide, and homicide—are often associated with excessive alcohol intake. As stated in the Dietary Guidelines for Americans:

> [T]he US population, across almost every age and sex group, consumes eating patterns that are low in vegetables,

fruits, whole grains, dairy, seafood, and oil and high in refined grains, added sugars, saturated fats, sodium, and for some age-sex groups, high in the meats, poultry, and eggs subgroup (US Department of Agriculture & US Department of Health and Human Services, 2020).

Obesity serves as a risk factor for an extensive spectrum of medical conditions, encompassing type 2 diabetes, cardiovascular diseases, chronic kidney diseases, site-specific cancers, musculoskeletal complications, and infectious diseases (Kivimäki et al., 2022; Powell-Wiley et al., 2021). Statistics show that during 2017 and 2018, about 42.8% of American adults and 19.7% of children and adolescents aged 2 to 19 years were obese in 2017 through 2020 (Hu & Staiano, 2022; Li et al., 2022). These values do not include overweight individuals. Excess weight in children and adolescents is causing the same health problems that physicians previously only diagnosed in adults (e.g., hypertension, atherosclerosis, metabolic syndrome, type 2 diabetes mellitus; Kansra et al., 2021).

Reducing the incidence of obesity is beneficial to overall health and quality of life. Although people commonly view excess weight or obesity as an imbalance between energy intake and energy expenditure, health care professionals must consider other factors, such as the environment, race/ethnicity, and socioeconomic status. For example, genetics have a multifactorial effect on how the body processes and maintains energy balance that may predispose some individuals to overweight/obesity (Kleinendorst et al., 2019; Loos & Yeo, 2022; Verde et al., 2023). Additionally, recent investigations surrounding the human microbiome have explored the relationships between microbiota gut alterations and chronic diseases such as obesity, insulin resistance, diabetes, and cancer (de Vos et al., 2022; Hou et al., 2022; Sikalidis & Maykish, 2020). In both cases, the weight relationship goes beyond calories in and calories out.

FOOD AND NUTRITION RECOMMENDATIONS

This chapter introduces national nutrition guidelines, with the intent of motivating the reader to achieve three principal goals. The first goal is to encourage individual interest in the health-promoting power of balanced nutrition and to promote self-evaluation and comparison of one's own food habits and choices with respect to the evidence-based dietary recommendations presented. The second goal is to appreciate the many systemic factors contributing to the current nutrition-related health issues. These problems are so pervasive that a multisector approach, beyond traditional education about healthy food choices, is required. A final goal is to recognize the kinds and amounts of food that are essential for obtaining the necessary energy and nutrients required for health. The initiatives and guidelines covered in the following sections provide the foundation for national nutrition recommendations that experts have translated into law, policy, programs, and many consumer messages.

Healthy People Initiative: Nutrition Objectives

Every 10 years, the United States Department of Health and Human Services publishes a set of national objectives with the overarching goal of improving the health of all Americans. Encouraging healthy choices in diet, exercise, and weight control is one of the major themes of the Healthy People framework (US Department of Health and Human Services, 2023). It also includes objectives to address health disparities and health inequities, as well as focus on future measures to help healthy choices be the easy choice wherever people live, work, learn, and play (Fig. 11.1).

Poor dietary choices contribute substantially to the burden of preventable illness and premature death; thus, several objectives in the Healthy People framework aim at directing American dietary patterns toward current evidence-based nutrition recommendations. The nutrition and weight status objectives of the current Healthy People goals (Box 11.1: Healthy People 2030 Nutrition Objectives) reflect empirical evidence supporting the health benefits of consuming a nutritious diet and maintaining a healthy body weight. The objectives also emphasize that efforts to change diet and weight should address individual behaviors, as well as policies and environments that support these behaviors, in settings such as schools, worksites, health care organizations, and communities.

The Healthy People framework includes objectives involving all aspects of health and well-being. There is a smaller subset of topics deemed leading health indicators, as they are high-priority issues for the nation. Nutrition, physical activity, and obesity is one of these 23 urgent focuses. Although Chapter 12 covers the importance of physical activity separately from nutrition, the uniting of physical activity with nutrition and obesity as one topic in the leading health indicators illustrates how interconnected these lifestyle behaviors are to health. Box 11.1: Healthy People 2030 Nutrition Objectives details the leading nutrition health indicators.

Dietary Guidelines for Americans

The Dietary Guidelines for Americans acknowledge the importance of a coordinated, system-wide approach that engages all sectors of influence (e.g., home, school, work) to support healthy eating patterns for all. The guidelines in Fig. 11.2 demonstrate the

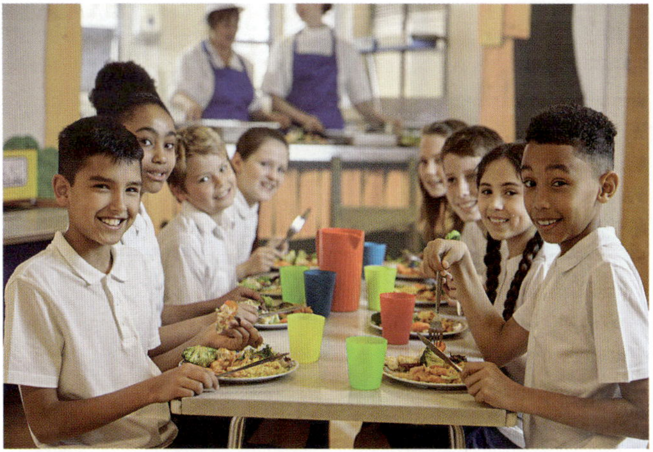

FIG. 11.1 Children who eat with each other in an appropriate environment often eat more nutritiously and try a wider variety of foods than when eating alone or at home. (From iStock photo 538486622, credit: monkeybusinessimages.)

BOX 11.1 HEALTHY PEOPLE 2030 NUTRITION OBJECTIVES

Objectives Related to Nutrition, Weight Status, and Food Safety

Weight Status

NWS–03	Reduce the proportion of adults with obesity.
NWS–04	Reduce the proportion of children and adolescents with obesity.
NWS–05	Increase the proportion of health care visits by adults with obesity that include counseling on weight loss, nutrition, or physical activity.

Food Insecurity

NWS-01	Reduce household food insecurity and hunger.

Food and Nutrient Consumption

NWS-06	Increase fruit consumption by people aged 2 years and over.
NWS-07	Increase vegetable consumption by people aged 2 years and older.
NWS-08	Increase consumption of dark green vegetables, red and orange vegetables, and beans and peas by people aged 2 years and over.
NWS-09	Increase whole grain consumption by people aged 2 years and over.
NWS-10	Reduce consumption of added sugars by people aged 2 years and over.
NWS-11	Reduce consumption of saturated fat by people aged 2 years and over.
NWS-12	Reduce consumption of sodium by people aged 2 years and over.
NWS-13	Increase calcium consumption by people aged 2 years and over.
NWS-14	Increase potassium consumption by people aged 2 years and over.
NWS-14	Increase vitamin D consumption by people aged 2 years and over.
NWS-16	Reduce iron deficiency in children aged 1–2 years.
NWS-17	Reduce iron deficiency in females aged 12–49 years.

Food Safety

FS-D01-D05	Reduce outbreaks of Shiga toxin-producing *Escherichia coli, Campylobacter, Listeria,* and *Salmonella* infections linked to beef, dairy, fruits and nuts, leafy greens, and poultry.
FS-07	Increase the proportion of people who wash their hands and surfaces often when preparing food.
FS-08	Increase the proportion of people who use separate cutting boards when preparing food.
FS-09	Increase the proportion of people who cook food to a safe temperature.

US Department of Health and Human Services (2023b).

complex layers of influence that shape a person's food and physical activity choices. Creating and supporting a healthy eating pattern means that nutrition-related community policies consider such influential factors and healthy food options are available and accessible to all people. In support of this guideline, the CDC has proposed strategies for both providing healthy food and preventing obesity in the United States (see Box 11.2: Best Practice).

Key recommendations from the Dietary Guidelines Advisory Committee include the following (US Department of Agriculture & US Department of Health and Human Services, 2020):

- Follow a healthy eating pattern across the life span. All food and beverage choices matter. Choose a healthy eating pattern at an appropriate calorie level to help achieve and maintain a healthy body weight, support nutrient adequacy, and reduce the risk of chronic disease.
- Focus on variety, nutrient density, and amount. To meet nutrient needs within calorie limits, choose a variety of nutrient-dense foods across and within all food groups in recommended amounts.
- Limit calories from added sugars and saturated fats and reduce sodium intake. Consume an eating pattern low in added sugars, saturated fats, and sodium. Cut back on foods and beverages higher in these components to amounts that fit within healthy eating patterns.
- Shift to healthier food and beverage choices. Choose nutrient-dense foods and beverages across and within all food groups in place of less healthy choices. Consider cultural and personal preferences to make these shifts easier to accomplish and maintain.
- Support healthy eating patterns for all. Everyone has a role in helping to create and support healthy eating patterns in multiple settings nationwide, from home to school to work to communities.

Other topics addressed in detail include guidance for specific population groups: children and adolescents, females of childbearing age, pregnant and breastfeeding females, and older adults, as well as individuals at high risk of chronic disease. A discussion of how to build healthy eating patterns embraces a variety of eating patterns with lacto-ovo-vegetarian, vegan, and dietary approaches to stop hypertension (DASH) variations provided at various calorie levels. (For details, see http://health.gov/dietaryguidelines.) Just like the Healthy People initiative, the report includes an emphasis on consumer aspects of food safety.

Representing the most current scientific evidence, the US Department of Health and Human Services intends these guidelines to reduce the nation's major diet-related health problems such as CHD, certain cancers, diabetes, high blood pressure, obesity, osteoporosis, and stroke. Nursing professionals play a key role in promoting the Dietary Guidelines of Americans as one component of healthful lifestyles. For more information about the articles and reports used to inform the development of the Dietary Guidelines for Americans, see the Report of the Dietary Guidelines Advisory Committee on the Dietary Guidelines for Americans and the related US Department of Agriculture's (USDA) Nutrition Evidence Library website at https://nesr.usda.gov.

MyPlate Guidelines

The USDA unveiled MyPlate to provide the public with easy to understand and useful advice regarding nutrient intake. MyPlate visually reminds consumers what a healthy plate looks like using a familiar place setting (Fig. 11.3). It is not a standalone teaching tool. Consumers and health professionals can

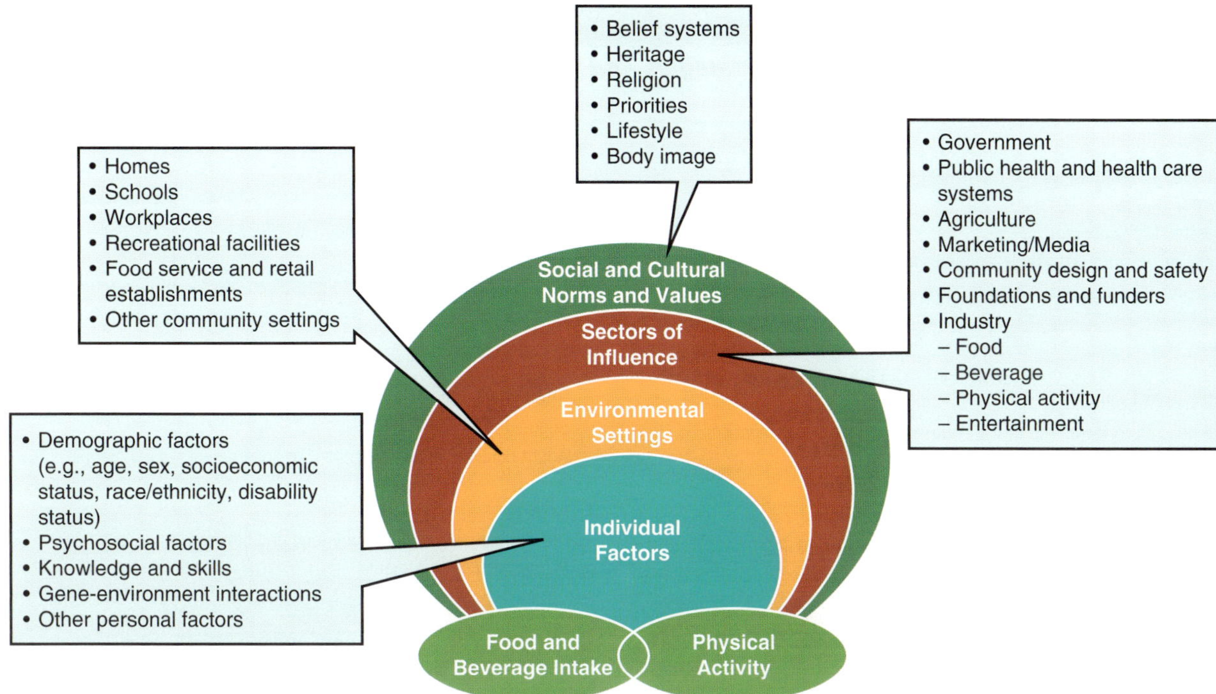

FIG. 11.2 Social-ecological framework for food and physical activity decisions. (From US Department of Health and Human Services, US Department of Agriculture, & Dietary Guidelines Advisory Committee, 2015.)

obtain person-specific details on the website (https://www.choosemyplate.gov). The food guidance system puts four of the food groups on the plate (grains, vegetables, fruits, and protein) with dairy (including milk and dairy substitutes) on the side.

Although the USDA's MyPlate food guidance system reflects general eating patterns of Americans, it has enough flexibility for different cultural traditions and eating patterns, including vegetarian (see Box 11.3: Health and Social Determinants/Health Equity).

Recognizing that food insecurity is a significant problem for millions of individuals in the United States, the MyPlate website includes an emphasis on resources for eating on a budget and tips to access nutrition assistance programs. The USDA also has resources available in Spanish. Experts update the website continuously, so it is worth checking periodically.

As noted, a considerable gap exists between public health recommendations and consumer practices. The overarching goal for nutrition is that food intake patterns change in the direction of the targeted goals recommended by the Healthy People initiative, the Dietary Guidelines for Americans, and the MyPlate food guidance system.

Dietary Reference Intakes

The Institute of Medicine of the National Academies of Sciences, Engineering, and Medicine developed the dietary reference intakes (DRIs) to reflect the latest understanding about nutrient requirements based on optimizing health in individuals and groups (US Department of Health and Human Services, 2023; Stallings et al., 2019). They are quantitative estimates of necessary nutrient intakes, which registered dietitian nutritionists (RDNs) can use to plan and assess the diets of healthy people in the United States. The recommended dietary allowances (RDAs) form the basis for the DRIs. We use the adequate intakes (AIs) whenever there is not enough scientific evidence to define the nutrient's RDA. See Box 11.4: Dietary Reference Intake Components and Definitions for details on these components and suggested uses.

It is important to note that in contrast to the routine 5-year review of the Dietary Guidelines for Americans, the DRI committees only update the DRIs when deemed necessary. In 2011, the United States and Canadian governments decided that there was enough new evidence and concern about vitamin D status to warrant the update of the DRIs for vitamin D and calcium (Institute of Medicine, 2011). The National Academy published the latest update in 2019 for sodium and potassium (Stallings et al., 2019). The revision of the vitamin D, calcium, sodium, and potassium DRIs demonstrates that scientists continue to research and revise the DRIs as evidence-based data become available.

The DRIs do have some shortcomings because of limited data relating to genetic diversity in the population or specific groups such as children, pregnant females, and elderly people. However, they are a good starting point based on best available data and probability of harm or benefit.

The expert panel intended for health care professionals to apply the DRIs to healthy people. It is possible that a provider will override the DRI for a specific nutrient based on clinical judgment and recommend more or less for a particular client. It is also helpful to remember that the DRIs apply over time. Thus if an individual does not meet the recommendation for a specific

BOX 11.2 BEST PRACTICE

Summary of Recommended Community Strategies and Measurements Related to Healthy Foods to Prevent Obesity in the United States[a]

Strategy 1
- Promote the availability of nutritious food and beverage options across public services.
- Suggested Measurement.
- Implement nutrition standards aligned with current Dietary Guidelines for Americans in local government and public-school food services.

Strategy 2
- Make healthy food and beverage choices more affordable in public venues.
- Suggested Measurement.
- Enact policies to lower the cost of nutritious options in comparison to less healthy alternatives in public service settings.

Strategy 3
- Expand access to supermarkets in underserved regions to improve geographical availability of healthy food options.
- Suggested Measurement.
- Increase the number of full-service grocery stores per capita in the most underserved areas.

Strategy 4
- Encourage food retailers to provide healthier options in underserved communities through incentives.
- Suggested Measurement.
- Offer incentives for retailers to enhance their selection of healthy food and beverage choices.

Strategy 5
- Foster mechanisms for direct farm-to-consumer food sales to increase the availability of fresh produce.
- Suggested Measurement.
- Boost the presence of farmers' markets and local farm produce in community food systems.

Strategy 6
- Encourage local farming through incentives.
- Suggested Measurement.
- Implement policies that promote local food production and distribution.
- Strategies to Support Healthy Food and Beverage Choices.

Strategy 7
- Restrict sales of unhealthy food and drinks in public venues.
- Suggested Measurement.
- Enforce policies against selling such items in government and school settings.

Strategy 8
- Offer smaller portion sizes in public venues.
- Suggested Measurement.
- Adopt policies for portion control in government facility menus.

Strategy 9
- Limit advertising of unhealthy food and beverages.
- Suggested Measurement.
- Establish policies to curb such advertisements in public and school areas.

Strategy 10
- Ban and limit sugary beverages in childcare settings.
- Suggested Measurement.
- Require facilities to exclude or limit sugar-added drinks.
- Strategy to Encourage Breastfeeding.

Strategy 11
- Enhance breastfeeding support in workplaces.
- Suggested Measurement.
- Mandate accommodations for breastfeeding in government facilities.
- **Introduction of New Weight Loss Medications[b].**

Strategy 12
- Explore and educate on new weight loss drug options.
- Suggested Measurement.
- Develop educational initiatives on medically supervised weight management options.
- Additional strategies can be found on the CDC website (https://www.cdc.gov/obesity/php/about/obesity-strategies-what-can-be-done.html).

[a]The entire report includes 24 strategies and measurements, including those related to physical activity. Because Chapter 12 covers physical activity, this excerpt includes nutrition advice only.

Institute of Medicine (US) Committee on Prevention of Obesity in Children and Youth (2005); Khan et al. (2009); Centers for Disease Control and Prevention (2023c).

[b]This strategy is informed by "an updated approach to antiobesity pharmacotherapy," advocating for broader goals in obesity treatment with new medications.

nutrient, such as vitamin C, on a certain day, that is not a cause for alarm. The trend matters with respect to food sources consumed throughout a week or month, as opposed to strictly daily intake.

Nutrition recommendations stated in terms of micrograms or milligrams of nutrients are of no use unless health care professionals advise people as to what types and quantities of foods they should consume to meet their recommendations. After all, people eat food, not nutrients. The intent of the Dietary Guidelines for Americans and the MyPlate guidelines is to translate the evidence-based DRI recommendations of nutrients into optimal dietary (i.e., food) guidelines so that the public can maximize healthy habits and minimize chronic disease. The DRIs also form the foundation for US nutrition policy, including nutrition-related programs such as the federal nutrition programs for families, children, and elderly people.

DIETARY SUPPLEMENTS AND HERBAL MEDICINES

Today's dietary supplements include vitamins, minerals, herbals and **botanicals**, amino acids, enzymes, probiotics, and fish oils, as well as powders, energy drinks, and energy bars. The

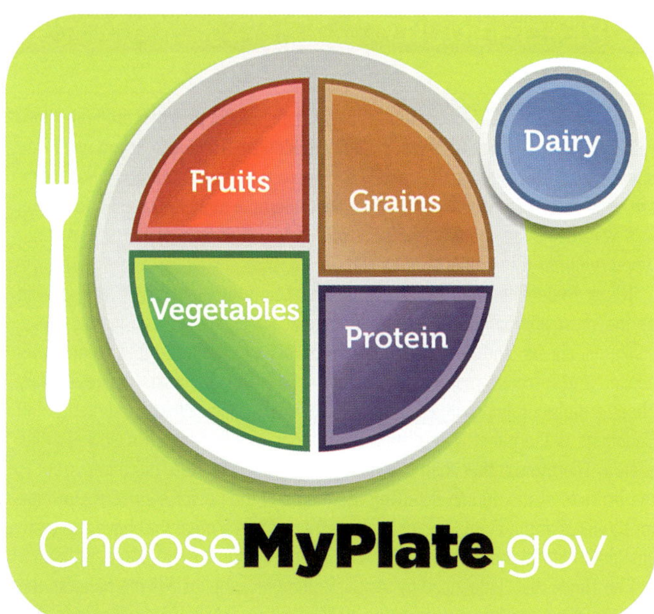

FIG. 11.3 Learn about healthy eating at www.choosemyplate.gov. (From US Department of Agriculture, Center for Nutrition Policy and Promotion. Choose MyPlate www.choosemyplate.gov.)

popularity of supplemental vitamins, minerals, proteins, fiber, and herbs has earned a high profile in the health field in recent decades. The explosive use of single-component dietary supplements in the 1980s instigated the change from the old RDAs (set to prevent nutrient deficiency) to the current DRIs (set to optimize health). With the availability of high-dose dietary supplements, individuals were consuming quantities of nutrients that were significantly higher than their needs. Adverse events of toxicity indicated that there was a point at which a nutrient could pose more of a risk than an advantage. As a result, experts established tolerable upper limit (UL) guidelines for specific life stages, ages, and sex.

It is the position of the Academy of Nutrition and Dietetics that micronutrient supplements are only warranted when individuals cannot meet their nutrient needs through diet alone (Marra & Bailey, 2018). Nevertheless, approximately more than half of the population in the United States regularly takes a dietary supplement (Mishra et al., 2021). The most frequently used supplement is the multivitamin or multimineral variety.

People sometimes use supplements as if they were medications. However, unlike the Food and Drug Administration (FDA)-approved medications, federal law does not require that dietary supplements be proven safe or effective before manufacturers market and sell them. To differentiate a dietary supplement from an over-the-counter (OTC) medication, the term "dietary supplement" must be clearly displayed on the product's labeling. Labels can include certain types of structure-function claims that address common conditions linked with aging, pregnancy, menopause, and adolescence, provided these do not refer to any disease. These claims can range from health-maintenance assertions (such as "supports a healthy circulatory system" or "promotes brain health") to nondisease claims (like "for muscle enhancement" or "aids in relaxation") and also cover claims for managing common, mild symptoms associated with different life stages (for instance, "eases typical premenstrual syndrome symptoms" or "alleviates hot flashes"). However, the FDA does not require that supplement manufacturers prove that the claim is accurate or truthful before using it on their products. Instead, the FDA requires that the following statement appear after any such claim: "This statement has not been evaluated by the Food and Drug Administration. This product is not intended to diagnose, treat, cure, or prevent any disease." The FDA provides a useful summary of facts regarding the regulation of dietary supplements on their website (http://www.fda.gov, search "FDA 101: Dietary Supplements"; US Food and Drug Administration, 2023).

Once a dietary supplement is on the market, the FDA monitors information on the product label and package insert to make sure that information about the supplement's content is not misleading. If the FDA finds a product to be unsafe or otherwise unfit for human consumption, it may take enforcement action to remove the product from the marketplace or it may work with the manufacturer to recall the product voluntarily. The FDA has recalled some supplements because of proven or potential harmful effects. The reasons for these recalls include microbiologic, pesticide, and heavy metal contamination; absence of a dietary ingredient claimed to be in the product; and the presence of ingredients causing illness and death.

The federal government can take legal action against companies and websites that sell dietary supplements when the companies make false or deceptive statements about their products, if they promote them as treatments or cures for diseases, or if their products are unsafe. Although laws exist to help protect the consumer, the reality is that it is a "buyer beware" environment because of historically low funding and resources for the FDA, along with political pressure and lack of scientific study on most supplements available in the United States.

Although the desirable way for the public to obtain recommended levels of nutrients is by eating a variety of foods, if people take dietary supplements, they should avoid taking them more than the UL for their age and sex group to preclude possible adverse effects. For other types of supplements, such as herbals or botanicals, note that "natural" does not necessarily mean that it is better or safer.

Micronutrient Toxicity

Excessive amounts of certain micronutrients can lead to various health issues, yet it's uncommon for such imbalances or toxicities to arise from consuming a balanced diet rich in whole foods. Most instances of nutrient toxicity stem from overuse of supplements, often compounded by consuming large amounts of fortified foods. It's particularly crucial to exercise caution with fat-soluble vitamins (A, D, E, and K) due to their ability to accumulate in the body, posing a risk of toxicity over time. Conversely, water-soluble vitamins, such as vitamin C and the B-complex vitamins, typically present a lower risk of toxicity because they are not stored in the body in significant amounts and are excreted in urine. However, it's important to acknowledge that extremely high intakes of these vitamins can still lead to health problems. Although not all micronutrients have

BOX 11.3 HEALTH AND SOCIAL DETERMINANTS/HEALTH EQUITY

Food and Culture

Numerous biologic and environmental factors guide individual food choices (Chen & Antonelli, 2020). Although it is true that without food people cannot survive, food is much more than a tool of survival. Studies have shown that food choices are shaped by a complex interplay of dietary, physiologic, cognitive-affective, familial, genetic, and cultural factors, as well as by the physical layout and offerings of food retail environments (Chen & Antonelli, 2020). Food transcends its basic role as a necessity for survival, serving multiple cultural and emotional purposes. It offers pleasure, as seen in invitations to dine out; comfort, reminiscent of cherished family recipes; and hospitality, through invitations for shared meals; and it can reflect personal choices or preferences without implying social status. Moreover, food is integral to various rituals and celebrations, such as toasting with champagne at significant milestones, the tradition of newlyweds saving their wedding cake's top layer, and the sharing of challah bread during the Jewish Sabbath meal, showcasing its deep-rooted significance in human connections and traditions.

The local environment significantly influences dietary preferences. In regions where wheat is abundant, such as the heartland of the United States, it becomes a primary food staple, leading to a variety of wheat-based foods like bread, cereal, crackers, pastries, and pasta. Similarly, in areas where rice is more readily available, it forms a central part of the diet, with numerous dishes centered around this grain.

Every culture has its particular food customs or activities interrelated to food (Kapelari et al., 2020). Food traditions include the activities that surround procuring, distributing, storing, preparing, consuming, and disposing of food, all of which define what is fit to eat, or what is edible (Jones-Garcia et al., 2022). When working with clients, it is important to consider factors that affect their food choices when making any dietary recommendations. It is also important to remember that just because a person is from a specific culture does not mean the person follows his or her traditional food patterns. These general guidelines are helpful as a starting point, but do not assume—ask questions to clarify specific eating habits with individuals and families. The following paragraphs provide a few examples of traditional and religious food values.

Chinese philosophies relate health and disease to the balance between the forces of yin and yang in the body (Cong & Chen, 2019). An individual may treat diseases that yang forces cause with yin forces to restore balance. Yin foods include low-calorie-density, low-protein foods, such as fresh fruits and vegetables. Yang foods are high in calories, cooked in oil, and irritating to the mouth, or are red, orange, or yellow. Examples include most meats, chili peppers, tomatoes, garlic, ginger, and alcoholic beverages. The hot-cold theory (Quinlan, 2022) in Puerto Rico follows the same basic principles as do yin and yang, but the food groupings differ somewhat.

Religious beliefs affect the food choices of millions of people worldwide (Imtiyaz et al., 2021). Many religions, including Buddhism, Hinduism, Islam, Judaism, and Seventh Day Adventism, specify the approved types and preparation methods of food that individuals may consume (Chouraqui et al., 2021). The following is a very basic summary of the principal dietary practices of these five major world religions (Chouraqui et al., 2021).

Many Buddhists practice vegetarianism. Foods of plant origin are viewed as the most appropriate for consumption, except pungent foods (garlic, leeks, scallions, chives, and onions), which are believed to generate lust when eaten cooked and to cause rage when eaten raw. For most Buddhists, however, they observe dietary rules such as these on a voluntary basis. What characterizes all Buddhists is the belief that all forms of life share a common link and are thus sacred. Therefore rather than the specific type of food eaten, more important is the attitude of the person receiving the food and the person's sincere gratitude for the lives of the plants and animals contained in the meal that have served to sustain and further enhance the life of the individual.

The Hindu diet, influenced by various traditions, emphasizes the belief in the equality of all life forms, leading many Hindus to adopt a lacto-vegetarian diet that excludes meat, fish, and eggs while allowing and encouraging dairy products. Cows are particularly revered and not consumed due to their sacred status and their symbolic representation of motherly provision and familial bond. Additionally, Hindu practices include fasting days and periods with dietary restrictions, such as consuming only plant-based foods.

Many Muslims follow Islamic food laws, which include foods that are halal (permitted), haram (prohibited), and questionable (mashbooh). Foods believed to be unclean, or haram, are animals that are improperly slaughtered or already-dead animals such as carrion, swine/pork and its by-products (bacon, lard, shortening), carnivorous animals with fangs (dogs, cats, and lions), birds of prey, and land animals without ears (frogs and snakes). Islamic food laws prohibit alcohol and intoxicants. Individuals may use halal-certified products.

Conservative Jews follow Judaic food laws, which prohibit the consumption of swine/pork, carrion, carrion eaters (scavengers), shellfish, animals with a cloven (split) hoof and that do not chew their cud (horses), and animals not slaughtered by the appropriate ritual method or kosher (fit). According to Jewish kosher dietary laws, meat (beef, lamb, veal, and poultry), fish, and meat products (eggs) cannot be served at the same meal or be cooked or eaten in the same vessels as dairy products. Individuals may consume kosher-certified products.

Many Seventh Day Adventists practice vegetarianism as the foundation of their dietary standard. They also abstain from alcohol, and many do not drink caffeine-containing beverages.

a determined upper intake level, for those that do, exceeding this limit can be harmful. Therefore individuals are advised to consult health care professionals before beginning any supplement regimen, especially with dosages approaching or exceeding these ULs, to avoid adverse health outcomes.

Large doses of vitamin A are teratogenic. Because of this risk, pregnant females should avoid supplementation with preformed vitamin A during pregnancy unless there is evidence of deficiency (see Box 11.5: Quality and Safety Scenario). Excess preformed vitamin A supplements during the first trimester of pregnancy have been linked to birth defects of the eyes, lungs, skull, and heart. Likewise, the FDA does not approve acne medications that contain large doses of vitamin A (e.g., isotretinoin) during pregnancy. Such a risk in early pregnancy raises the need for caution about general vitamin and mineral supplement use by females of childbearing age.

Besides problems with direct toxicity of some individual nutrients, high doses of a single nutrient may reflect interactions that result in a relative deficiency of another nutrient, or cause adverse interactions with prescribed medication (Marra & Bailey, 2018). The Office of Dietary Supplements provides detailed fact sheets on micronutrient supplements, including potential interactions and toxicity symptoms (https://ods.od.nih.gov/factsheets). Some examples follow:

- High doses of vitamin E and vitamin K can interfere with anticoagulation medications (e.g., warfarin). Examples such as this are one of the reasons that health care providers ask about

BOX 11.4 Dietary Definitions

Dietary Pattern

A dietary pattern comprises the full composition of foods and beverages that an individual consumes. It comprises the usual way of eating and may involve a listing of dietary intake.

Nutrient Dense

Nutrient dense foods and beverages provide the full range of vitamins, minerals and other health-promoting food choices. In general nutrient rich goods have less added sugar, saturated fat and sodium. Sugars should be less than 10% of calories, saturated fat less than 10%, and sodium less than 2,300 milligrams per day. Alcoholic beverages should be avoided. A healthy diet is not rigid but allows for variation in food and beverage choices.

Recommended Dietary Allowance

RDA is the average dietary intake level that is sufficient to meet the nutrient requirement of nearly all healthy individuals in a particular life stage and sex group. Scientists compute the RDA by moving the EAR two standard deviations to the right. In the past, the RDA of most nutrients represented the levels needed to prevent deficiency diseases. Now, the RDA includes the goal of preventing chronic diseases (e.g., heart disease or osteoporosis) and promoting health (as opposed to only preventing deficiency). Health care providers should not use the RDA to assess or plan nutrient intake for groups, but the RDAs may be useful in some individual applications.

Adequate Intake

An AI is set when there is not enough scientific evidence to determine the RDA. The AI is based on estimates of observed or experimentally determined mean nutrient intake of a group (or groups) of healthy people and assumes that the amount consumed is adequate to sustain health. The level is set to meet or exceed the needs of almost all people in a particular life stage and sex group. The RDAs include a range of appropriate intakes from the energy-yielding nutrients (i.e., carbohydrate, fat, and protein) that is associated with reduced risk of chronic disease while providing intakes of essential nutrients for a healthy person within an identified life stage and sex group.

Estimated Energy Requirement

This is the average dietary energy intake predicted to maintain energy balance in a healthy adult of a specific life stage and sex group calculated with a reference weight, height, and level of physical activity that is consistent with good health.

AI, Adequate intake; *RDA*, recommended dietary allowance; *UL*, upper intake level.

Data from US Department of Agriculture & US Department of Health and Human Services. (2020). *Dietary guidelines for Americans, 2020-2025. 9th edition.* https://www.dietaryguidelines.gov/sites/default/files/2021-03/Dietary_Guidelines_for_Americans-2020-2025.pdf

supplement use before surgery and recommend discontinuing the use of certain supplements for a period before and after surgery.

- Large amounts of calcium inhibit the absorption of iron and possibly other trace elements.
- Folic acid can mask hematologic signs of vitamin B_{12} deficiency, which, if untreated, can result in irreversible neurologic damage.
- High-dose zinc supplementation can reduce copper levels and high-dose iron supplements can reduce zinc absorption.

Nursing professionals can help people who suspect an adverse supplement effect by reporting the event to the FDA or by encouraging the individual to file a report. Report the event as soon as possible when there is a suspected problem.

BOX 11.5 QUALITY AND SAFETY SCENARIO

Supplements/Vitamin A

Adele is a 32-year-old female with no children and a history of two miscarriages. She and her husband have been trying to conceive for the past 4 years and have recently started talking about going to a fertility clinic. Always one to try the "natural way" first, she read that vitamin A is important for normal fetal development and decides to take a multivitamin supplement with 25,000 IU of preformed vitamin A. Adele knows that she can get vitamin A from food, but she also tries to read nutrition labels and choose fortified foods that have 20% or more of her daily value of vitamin A. She comes into the physician's office for a regular routine visit. Her health care team is aware that she and her husband are trying to have a baby.

Analyzing Cues and Reflective Questions

- Why is it important to discuss the use and type of supplements (and potentially fortified food use) during preconception/pregnancy?
- What is the vitamin A DRI recommendation for a female of her age?
- How can learning about simple changes in her eating habits and supplement use affect her risk of a spontaneous abortion or a birth defect in the event of pregnancy?
- What would your next step be in this situation?

Note: One retinol activity equivalent = 1 mcg of all-trans-retinol = 3.33 IU from retinol = 2 mcg of supplemental all-trans-β-carotene = 12 mcg of dietary all-trans-β-carotene = 24 mcg of other dietary provitamin A carotenoids.

DRI, Dietary reference intake.

Data from US Department of Agriculture & US Department of Health and Human Services. (2020). Dietary guidelines for Americans, 2020-2025. 9th edition. https://www.dietaryguidelines.gov/sites/default/files/2021-03/Dietary_Guidelines_for_Americans-2020-2025.pdf

Information on how to do this is available at http://www.fda.gov/food/dietary-supplements/how-report-problem-dietary-supplements. Another avenue is to alert the product's manufacturer or distributor to any serious side effects through the address or phone number listed on the supplement's label. By law, dietary supplement firms are required to forward reports they receive about serious adverse effects to the FDA within 15 days.

Circumstances When Nutrient Supplementation Is Indicated

Nutrient supplements or fortified foods, or sometimes a combination of both, are sometimes necessary for specific populations to obtain desirable amounts of particular nutrients. Some examples follow:

- The DRI committee recommends that pregnant females and females who are capable of becoming pregnant increase their intake of folic acid to 400 mcg/day from fortified foods and/or dietary supplements in addition to the folate that is already present in their diets to help prevent neural tube defects (Barry et al., 2023).
- The American Academy of Pediatrics recommends that all exclusively breastfed infants receive 400 IU of supplemental vitamin D daily to help prevent rickets. Infants who are not breastfed, children, and adolescents who do not consume at least 1 quart/day of vitamin D–fortified milk (or milk

substitute) or otherwise have an intake of less than 400 IU of vitamin D should also receive supplemental vitamin D daily (O'Callaghan et al., 2020).

- Numerous elderly individuals lack sufficient hydrochloric acid in their stomachs to effectively absorb vitamin B_{12} found in natural foods. Therefore it is recommended that people aged 50 and above primarily obtain their vitamin B_{12} from fortified foods or dietary supplements, as their bodies are generally more capable of absorbing the nutrient from these sources. For more information visit https://ods.od.nih.gov/factsheets/VitaminB12-Consumer/.

People can get their nutrition requirements from foods and, when necessary, from supplements. However, experts generalize the amounts needed to population groups (e.g., amounts for all females during pregnancy). These requirements do not account for individual genetic variations. In the future, it may be possible for physicians or registered dietician nutritionists (RDNs) to prescribe specific nutrients to individuals based on genomic maps. This new and exciting study of nutrigenomics explores the effects of nutrients on gene expression. However, when it comes to nutrients in foods and their effects on gene expression, the science is not yet available to create diets specific to an individual's genome makeup.

FOOD SAFETY

The combined efforts of the food industry and the regulatory agencies are often credited with making the food supply in the United States one of the safest in the world. Nonetheless, the CDC reports that each year an estimated one in six Americans—48 million people—become sick from food-borne illnesses caused by various microbial pathogen contaminations. Of these, an estimated 128,000 people require hospitalization and 3000 people die (USA Facts, 2023).

Attention to food-borne illnesses is becoming increasingly important with the globalization of the world's food supply. New disease-causing organisms have emerged, and food imports from countries without the same safety standards as the United States are on the rise. Furthermore, consumers are demanding fresh produce and seafood availability throughout the year as well as accessibility to less-processed foods, such as raw milk and fresh juices that are not cooked or pasteurized to kill bacteria. Consumers may also ignore warnings about unsafe food habits because of preferences for foods such as raw oysters, rare hamburgers, fresh juices, unpasteurized cheese, and runny egg yolks, which all carry higher risks of contamination.

To protect the public from numerous sources of food contamination (physical, chemical, biologic), private industry and numerous federal, state, and local agencies share responsibilities for regulating the safety of the food supply. On the food industry side, one example of initiatives is food processors that are working on programs to better trace products through the supply chain and monitor temperatures in trucks from remote locations. In late 2010, the US Congress passed sweeping food safety legislation called the "Food Safety Modernization Act" (FSMA), which gives the FDA new powers to police food safety and focus its efforts on preventing food contamination. Subject to adequate funding, the FSMA allows the FDA to increase its inspection of imported food, set safety standards for fresh produce, force companies to recall tainted products, and require companies to keep better production records.

When the safeguards built into this system fail, however, consumers themselves must serve as the final and sometimes most important guardian against unsafe food. Therefore, it is essential to inform and educate consumers about the potential dangers of food-borne illness and ways to avoid contaminated food products.

Food-Borne Illness

We classify a food-borne illness according to the source of its contamination (the unintended presence of harmful substances or microorganisms). Food contaminants may be biologic, chemical, or physical. Biologic contaminants include bacteria, viruses, parasites, and fungi (yeasts and molds). Chemical contamination refers to the presence of pesticides, kitchen-cleaning supplies, and leached toxic chemicals in food from worn metal cookware and equipment. Physical contamination includes dirt, glass chips, crockery, wood, splinters, stones, hair, jewelry, and metal shavings from dull can openers. Another physical contaminant may be an unintended allergen found in a food product that typically does not include that ingredient (such as peanuts) during food processing.

Common Food-Borne Pathogens

The safety of the US food supply is so important that there are specific objectives tied to the monitoring of common pathogens in the Healthy People initiative. These include outbreak-associated infections attributable to Shiga toxin–producing *Escherichia coli* O157, *Campylobacter, Listeria,* or *Salmonella* species associated with food commodity groups (e.g., beef, dairy, fruits and nuts, leafy vegetables, and poultry). We will cover two common types of food-borne pathogens next.

Salmonellosis

The most frequently reported cause of food-borne illness is from *Salmonella* bacteria. Each year in the United States, the CDC receives reports of approximately 1.35 million cases of salmonellosis infections, 26,500 hospitalizations, and 420 deaths from acute salmonellosis (US Food & Drug Administration, 2023). The actual number of infections may be closer to 1.2 million because milder cases frequently remain undiagnosed. Although the *Salmonella* family includes more than 2300 serotypes of the bacterium, the most common causes of illness are *Salmonella typhi* and *Salmonella paratyphi.*

The typical way humans are exposed to salmonellosis is by consuming foods contaminated with feces. Foods of animal origin such as beef, poultry, milk, and eggs are often the source of infection. However, all foods, including seafood from polluted water and vegetables, may become contaminated. Contamination may also occur from unsanitary handling of foods and utensils by infected food handlers and contact with the feces of some pets, especially those with diarrhea. Symptoms of salmonellosis include abdominal cramping, mild-to-severe diarrhea, nausea, vomiting, and fever. Symptoms may resolve within 4 to 7 days without treatment; however, infections can become life-threatening for people with weakened immune systems such as infants with an immature immune system, young children, pregnant females, older adults, and people with autoimmune disorders or those under cancer treatment. To prevent salmonellosis, avoid uncooked egg dishes, undercooked meat, shellfish, and unpasteurized milk and juice. Adherence to sanitary regulations, as well as proper food handling, is necessary to control salmonellosis outbreaks.

Escherichia coli Infection

The bacterium *Escherichia coli* was first identified by the German-Austrian pediatrician Theodor Escherich in 1885 within the intestinal flora of humans. Among the various strains of E. coli, those that produce Shiga toxin are particularly notorious for causing significant health issues in the United States each year. Infections by these strains can lead to severe symptoms, including intense abdominal cramps, diarrhea that may range from watery to bloody, dehydration, nausea, vomiting, and sometimes a low-grade fever. Typically, the condition, known as "hemorrhagic colitis," resolves itself within about 7 days.

Transmission of *E. coli* is most linked to fecal contamination, which can occur through the consumption of contaminated foods, inadequate hand washing after bathroom use or diaper changes, consumption of undercooked meats, and the intake of unpasteurized products like milk, apple cider, and soft cheeses. Furthermore, outbreaks can stem from person-to-person transmission in community settings such as homes, daycare centers, nursing homes, and hospitals, as well as through hand-to-mouth contact after touching animals or contaminated surfaces at petting zoos and agricultural fairs.

Although *E. coli* infections can affect individuals of any age, children and older adults are particularly at risk. In a small proportion of cases, ranging from 5% to 10%, the infection may escalate to hemolytic uremic syndrome (HUS), a serious condition that can cause permanent kidney damage among other complications (https://www.cdc.gov/ecoli/).

Food Safety Practices

The few examples provided demonstrate how serious food-borne illness can be. Individuals in their own homes can reduce contaminants and keep food safe to eat by following safe food handling practices. There are four basic food safety principles that work together to reduce the risk of food-borne illness. These four principles (detailed in the next section) are the cornerstones of Fight BAC!, a national food safety education campaign (https://www.fightbac.org). The Healthy People initiative includes a key food safety objective intended to increase the proportion of consumers following these guidelines:

- Clean: Wash hands, utensils, and cutting boards before and after contact with raw meat, poultry, seafood, and eggs.
- Wash all parts of the hands thoroughly with running warm water with soap and friction for approximately 20 to 30 seconds. Teach children to sing the "Happy Birthday" song twice to gauge the length of time they should continue washing their hands. If water is not available, use an alcohol-based (≥60%) hand sanitizer to clean hands.
- Clean all surfaces with warm, soapy water often (including all appliances, knobs, and handles) and clean spills immediately. Use a solution of one tablespoon of unscented, liquid chlorine bleach per gallon of water to sanitize surfaces.
- Discard refrigerated foods that are no longer safe to eat at least once a week. Discard cooked leftovers after 4 days; discard raw poultry and ground meats after 1 to 2 days.
- Separate: Do not cross-contaminate. While shopping, preparing, or storing foods, keep foods that you do not plan to cook separate from raw meat and poultry.
- Rinse unpackaged fresh fruits and vegetables thoroughly with running water before eating, cutting, or cooking them. Scrub firm surfaces (e.g., cantaloupes and cucumbers) with a produce brush. Commercial cleaners are unnecessary.
- Cook: Cook food to the proper temperatures and use a food thermometer. The appearance or smell of food does not indicate its safety.
- Cook seafood, meat, poultry, and egg dishes to the recommended safe minimum internal temperature to destroy harmful microbes. Cook eggs thoroughly. Do not allow children to consume raw batter of cake mixes containing raw eggs.
- Stir, rotate, and/or flip foods periodically to help them cook evenly when cooking food in a microwave oven.
- Chill: Refrigerate food promptly within 2 hours or in 1 hour for environments that are 90°F or hotter. This includes groceries, food being prepared, leftovers, and takeout foods. Keep the refrigerator at 40°F (4.4°C) or less and the freezer at 0°F (−17.7°C) or less and monitor temperatures with a thermometer.
- Keep hot food hot (140°F or hotter) and cold foods cold (32°F [0°C] to 40°F [4.4°C]). Between these temperatures is the danger zone in which harmful bacteria can grow rapidly.
- Thaw food properly to avoid bacteria growth: in the refrigerator; in cold water, such as in a leak-proof bag, changing the water for cold water every 30 minutes; or in the microwave oven, never on the countertop.

These guidelines also apply to carryout meals, restaurant leftovers, and home-packed meals to go. The Food Safety and Inspection Service website (https://www.fsis.usda.gov) provides safety publications for all types of foods and populations.

Making a food safe after improper handling may not be possible. For example, certain bacteria found in food that has been left at room temperature too long may produce a heat-resistant toxin that cannot be destroyed by cooking. Therefore the principal point is to be careful in preparing food, including cooking foods to the right temperatures, keeping track of the time food is exposed to certain temperatures, and being vigilant when eating out. If there is doubt about the safety of the food, it is better to dispose of it.

Without exception, everyone should exercise safe food handling practices when eating out, when handling their own food, or when handling the food of others. Prevention through education is the key to promoting healthy lives that are unscathed by the potentially severe and life-threatening effects of food-borne illness.

FOOD, NUTRITION, AND POVERTY

As already noted in the discussion of the Healthy People initiative, the current focus is on reducing health disparities and health inequities. Regarding nutrition, this goal manifests as promoting health, reducing chronic disease risk through the consumption of healthful diets, and achieving and maintaining healthy body weights. To accomplish this, we must make healthy food choices available wherever people live, work, learn, and play; eliminate very low **food security** for children; and reduce household food insecurity and hunger.

Poverty and Income Distribution

For most people in the United States, income has risen over time, providing more options for personal expenditures, including those on food. However, growth in income has not increased equally for all households. Hunger and malnutrition within the lowest socioeconomic status persist in the United States. More than 3 million households (10.2%) were food insecure, meaning that they do not have enough money and resources to obtain adequate food in socially acceptable ways (Coleman-Jensen et al., 2022). Households with the highest risk for food insecurity are those with young children (particularly those headed by a single adult), those with incomes below 185% of the poverty threshold, those headed by a Black non-Hispanic or Hispanic adult, and households in central city areas (Coleman-Jensen et al., 2022).

Additionally, the phenomenon of food deserts—areas with limited access to affordable and nutritious food—further exacerbates the challenge for households, particularly those in low-income and underserved communities, to maintain a nutritious diet. Living in a food desert can significantly restrict access to healthy food options, such as fresh fruits and vegetables, making it even more difficult for residents to achieve a balanced diet without substantial effort or assistance (Jin & Lu, 2021).

For households living at or below the national poverty line, obtaining a nutritious diet without assistance can be a challenge. Low-income families spend a significantly higher percentage of their annual income on food than other families, often with less access to healthier options such as fresh fruits and vegetables. Food assistance programs, as discussed next, are one mechanism to provide a limited safety net to help those in need of food, a necessity for life.

Food Assistance for Low-Income Individuals

A variety of federal, state, and local governments and private charitable organizations work to mitigate hunger in the United States. The primary responsibility at the federal level falls to the USDA, which administers 15 nutrition assistance programs through the Food and Nutrition Services (FNS) using a combination of federal funding and farm commodities. Programs target the diverse needs of different subgroups of low-income people by providing supplemental assistance through a variety of settings. Health care providers must be aware of the available food assistance programs (listed next) to make appropriate and timely referrals.

- Supplemental Nutrition Assistance Program (SNAP)
- Child Nutrition Program (includes the National School Breakfast Program [NSBP], the National School Lunch Program [NSLP], the Special Milk Program, the Child and Adult Care Food Program, and the Summer Food Service Program)
- Special Supplemental Nutrition Program for Women, Infants, and Children (WIC)
- Older Americans Act Nutrition Programs (Congregate Nutrition Services, Home-Delivered Nutrition Services, Nutrition Services Incentive Program)
- Food Distribution Program (includes the Food Distribution Program on Indian Reservations, the Commodity Supplemental Food Program, the Emergency Food Assistance Program, and USDA Foods in Schools)

One in four people in the United States receives federally funded food assistance at some point every year (Agriculture, 2022). The SNAP, NSLP, NSBP, WIC, and Older American Act programs are the main programs that provide food and nutrition assistance. With the tightening of federal and state budgets, these programs continually sustain funding cuts. Table 11.2 provides information on the various programs, along with their website addresses. Income eligibility requirements reflect household income and will change annually. Individuals may find instructions for applying to the programs directly on the respective websites.

Supplemental Nutrition Assistance Program

SNAP supplements the food-buying power of eligible low-income households and is the foundation of the nation's nutrition safety net. The program provides benefits through an electronic benefit transfer (EBT) card that participants use to purchase food at authorized stores. It helps low-income families and individuals purchase nutritionally adequate foods. Households can use their EBT card to purchase food or food products for home consumption, as well as seeds and plants for use in home gardens. Items that recipients cannot buy with EBT cards include alcoholic beverages, tobacco, nonfood items (e.g., cleaning supplies, paper products), hot ready-to-eat foods, lunch-counter items, dietary supplements, medicines, and pet foods.

Although there is no requirement that recipients use the EBT card to purchase nutrient-dense food, the goal of the SNAP nutrition education program is to increase the likelihood that recipients will make healthy food choices within a limited food budget. SNAP uses multiple strategies to facilitate healthy food choices and active lifestyles. These include providing nutrition education programs (SNAP-ed) aimed at guiding SNAP participants to make nutrient-dense food choices and encouraging more farmers' markets, small urban markets, and bodegas to participate in the program.

The FNS administers the program nationally, and local agencies administer the program in all 50 states, the District of Columbia, Guam, and the US Virgin Islands. Eligibility reflects financial factors such as income and expenses available to the household. SNAP requires most able-bodied adults aged between 16 and 59 years (with few exceptions) to register for work, to take part in employment/training programs referred by the SNAP office, and to accept or continue in suitable employment. Households may own certain limited resources.

TABLE 11.2 Federal Nutrition Assistance Programs

Program	Mission	To Find Out More
Child and Adult Care Food Program	Provide aid to child and adult care institutions and family or group day care homes for the provision of nutritious foods that contribute to the wellness, healthy growth, and development of young children, and to the health and wellness of older adults and chronically impaired disabled individuals	www.fns.usda.gov/cacfp
Child Nutrition Program	Provide healthy food to children from low-income families through a variety of programs, including the National School Lunch Program, the National School Breakfast Program, the Child and Adult Care Food Program, the Summer Food Service Program, and the Special Milk Program	www.fns.usda.gov/cn
SNAP	Offer nutrition assistance to low-income individuals and families and provide economic benefits to communities	www.fns.usda.gov/snap
WIC	Provide federal grants to states for supplemental foods, health care referrals, and nutrition education for low-income pregnant, breastfeeding, nonbreastfeeding postpartum females, and to infants and children up to age 5 years who are at nutritional risk	www.fns.usda.gov/wic
Food Distribution & Emergency Assistance Programs	To strengthen the nation's nutrition safety net by providing food and nutrition assistance to school-aged children and families and support American agriculture by distributing American-grown USDA foods. The programs include the Emergency Food Assistance Program, the USDA Food Disaster Assistance, and other programs	www.fns.usda.gov/usda-foods
Commodity Supplemental Food Program	Work to improve the health of low-income people over the age of 60 years by supplementing their diet with USDA food packages	www.fns.usda.gov/csfp
Food Distribution Program on Indian Reservations	Provide USDA foods to supplement the diet of low-income Native American households and households living on Indian reservations	www.fns.usda.gov/fdpir
Older Americans Act Nutrition Programs	Support nutrition services for older individuals. Programs include Congregate Nutrition Services, Home-Delivered Nutrition Services, and the Nutrition Services Incentive Program	https://acl.gov/programs/health-wellness/nutrition-services

SNAP, Supplemental Nutrition Assistance Program; *USDA,* US Department of Agriculture; *WIC,* Special Supplemental Nutrition Program for Women, Infants, and Children.

In addition to income, family size determines the EBT allotment. Approximately 40 million people participate in SNAP services in the United States monthly, at an annual cost of $65 billion. The average monthly benefit per person is $127 (Center on Budget and Policy Priorities, 2022).

Child Nutrition Program

Collectively called the "Child Nutrition Program," these programs provide cash reimbursement and commodity support for meals served to children in schools, childcare facilities, and summer settings. They include the NSLP, the NSBP, the Child and Adult Care Food Program, the Summer Food Service Program, and the Special Milk Program. The general purpose of these programs is to help ensure the health and well-being of children. We will describe the two biggest and most well-known programs next.

National school lunch program. The FNS administers the federally funded NSLP. On the state level, the US Department of Education usually administers the NSLP, which contracts with local public, nonprofit, private, and residential childcare centers and schools to provide balanced, low-cost, or free lunches. In 2019, before the onset of the coronavirus disease 2019 (COVID-19) pandemic, the NSLP distributed a total of 4.9 billion lunches to students (US Department of Agriculture, 2023a) including the following:

- Children from families with incomes at or below 130% of the federal poverty level were eligible for free school meals.
- Children from families with incomes between 130% and 185% of the poverty level were eligible for reduced-price school meals.

Schools that choose to take part in the lunch program must implement wellness policies that promote healthy eating, address obesity, and encourage physical activity. The USDA provides schools with cash subsidies and approved agricultural commodities. Current meal standards reflect the Institute of Medicine's recommendations to move subsidized meals into line with the Dietary Guidelines for Americans and the DRIs (US Department of Agriculture & US Department of Health and Human Services, 2020). The rules stipulate a doubling of previous amounts of fruits and vegetables served in schools, set limits on the levels of trans fats and salt, increase the amount of whole grains served, make 1% and fat-free milk the norm, and establish suitable ranges for daily calorie intake. They also require free drinkable water in food service areas.

National school breakfast program. The FNS designed the NSBP program to make it possible for all schoolchildren to receive a nutritious breakfast every day. Skipping breakfast can adversely affect children's performance potential. The NSBP aids states to initiate, maintain, or expand nonprofit breakfast programs in eligible schools and residential childcare institutions. Any child attending a participating school may receive a free, reduced-price, or full-price breakfast based on the same income criteria used by the NSLP. During the fiscal year 2019, which predates the COVID-19 pandemic, approximately 2.4 billion children received free breakfast annually at a cumulative expenditure of $4.5 billion (US Department of Agriculture, 2023b).

Special Supplemental Nutrition Program for Women, Infants, and Children

WIC supplies free nutritious supplemental food, nutrition counseling, breastfeeding support, and health and social service referrals to eligible low-income pregnant or postpartum females and to children younger than 5 years old who are at nutritional risk. Congress funds WIC every year as a federal grant program for FNS and 90 agencies (including 50 states, 34 Indian tribal organizations, the District of Columbia, and five US territories) to administer. WIC offers services in a wide variety of settings: county health departments, hospitals, mobile clinics, community centers, schools, public housing sites, Indian reservations, migrant health centers and camps, and Indian Health Service facilities.

The following factors determine eligibility: (1) income must be 185% or less of the US poverty income level (updated annually by the Department of Health and Human Services), and (2) participants must meet one of two major types of nutritional risk:

- Medically based risks, such as anemia, underweight, or a history of poor pregnancy outcome
- Diet-based risks, such as inadequate dietary pattern as determined by 24-hour recall, food frequency questionnaire, or diet history

Eligible participants in the program receive monthly vouchers for foods that supplement their diet with necessary nutrients. These items typically include iron-fortified cereals, vitamin C–rich juices, eggs, milk, cheese, and legumes. WIC emphasizes breastfeeding as the optimal nutrition source for infants, offering formula for those not breastfed and special formulas for medical conditions upon doctor's prescription. The program recently updated its food selection to include items like tofu, fruits and vegetables, and whole grains, aiming to cater to diverse dietary needs and align with current nutritional guidelines.

In 2022, WIC provided assistance to approximately 6.3 million participants every month, which accounted for an estimated 39% of all infants in the United States (US Department of Agriculture, 2023c). Financial constraints preclude WIC from serving all eligible people; therefore, the program has established a system of priorities for filling program openings. After a local WIC agency has reached its maximum caseload, they will fill vacancies with high-risk individuals in the order of medical priority.

The WIC Farmers' Market Nutrition Program provides additional coupons to WIC participants to purchase fresh fruits and vegetables at approved farmers' markets and roadside stands. The program has two goals: (1) to provide fresh, nutritious, unprepared, locally grown fruits and vegetables from farmers' markets to WIC participants, and (2) to expand consumers' awareness and use of farmers' markets.

The overall statistics on WIC demonstrate it is effective in improving the health of its participants. Females participating in WIC have a lower risk of preterm birth, low birth weight infants, and perinatal death compared with females that are eligible for WIC but do not participate (Venkataramani et al., 2022). Furthermore, WIC-eligible children who participate early in WIC services experience cognitive and academic benefits over their nonparticipating counterparts (Jackson, 2015).

Food and Nutrition Programs for Older Adults

A significant number of older people face obstacles that prevent their obtaining and consuming an optimal diet. Of particular concern are adults older than 75 years who are frail, alone, homebound, or restricted to a limited budget. Life changes such as the loss of a spouse/significant other, sensory changes in taste or smell, physical inability to obtain or consume food, and decreasing calorie needs can make acquisition of an adequate diet challenging.

Several nutrition assistance programs are available to this population. They include SNAP, the Senior Farmers' Market Nutrition Program, the Child and Adult Care Food Program, the Emergency Food Assistance Program, and the Commodity Supplemental Food Program. However, the programs that most people may be familiar with are some of those provided under the Older Americans Act, which are managed by the Administration on Aging (AoA) through the US Department of Health and Human Services. The Older Americans Act Nutrition Programs are designed to help older adults access nutritionally sound meals, obtain nutrition support services and other health-promotion services (including nutrition screening and counseling), and reduce the social isolation that may occur in old age. The AoA gives priority to older people with the greatest social and economic need, such as low income, minorities, those with limited English proficiency, those in a rural location, and frail seniors at risk of institutionalization.

The older adults nutrition services program. Services provided under the Older Americans Act include the Congregate Nutrition Services, the Home-Delivered Nutrition Services (i.e., "Meals on Wheels"), and the Nutrition Services Incentive Program (NSIP), which gives states, territories, and Indian tribal organizations the ability to purchase food or to cover the cost of commodities from the USDA for the meals provided through the Congregate Nutrition Services and the Home-Delivered Nutrition Services. The AoA provides funds to states, territories, and tribal organizations, and it awards money to Area Agencies on Aging for coordination with area food sites such as senior centers, faith-based sites, community centers, adult day care centers, and schools.

By law, age is the only factor used in determining eligibility. People aged 60 years or older and their spouse or caretaker, regardless of age, are eligible for benefits. Tribal organizations may select an age younger than 60 years for the definition of an older person for their tribes because of a shorter life expectancy and higher incidence of chronic illnesses. Additionally, disabled people who live in elder care housing facilities, people who accompany older participants to congregate feeding sites, and volunteers who assist in the meal service may also receive meals. For those receiving Home-Delivered Nutrition Services, spouses of any age and disabled persons may also participate if they live with the homebound elder.

There is no income requirement for meals. Each recipient may make a donation toward the cost of the meal, but meals are free to people who cannot contribute. Home-delivered meals provide more than a nutritional meal; they also help participants to stay in their own home for longer than they would otherwise be able to manage alone. In some cases, the person delivering the meal may be the only face-to-face contact or opportunity for conversation that the elderly individuals will have for the day or week.

NUTRITION SCREENING

Health care providers should assess the need for nutrition counseling by an RDN for any older person who has food-related problems that are affecting eating pleasure or quality of life. Malnutrition is a significant risk for patients as it contributes to morbidity, mortality, extended hospitalization, and significant additional medical costs (Fan et al., 2022; Inciong et al., 2022; Kabashneh et al., 2020). The diagnosis of malnutrition includes the following general characteristics: insufficient energy intake, weight loss, loss of muscle mass, loss of subcutaneous fat, localized or generalized fluid accumulation, and diminished functional status as measured by strength of handgrip (Serón-Arbeloa et al., 2022). A diagnosis requires that a patient meet two or more of these criteria. Table 11.3 provides the clinical diagnostic criteria for malnutrition.

Nutrition screening is the process of assessing risk factors that are associated with dietary problems and malnutrition. Its primary purpose is to identify individuals who are potentially at risk and initiate intervention. To serve this purpose, screening criteria must be simple, relatively straightforward, and easy to administer. Screening is also helpful in establishing priorities for the most efficient use of time and money. The single largest demographic group at risk of malnutrition is the elderly. The Mini Nutritional Assessment-Short Form (MNA-SF) is one of the standard assessment tools used to evaluate nutrition risk in elderly individuals (Fig. 11.4; Inoue, Misu, Tanaka, Kakehi, & Ono, 2019; Ozturk et al., 2022; Trampisch et al., 2022). The MNA-SF is a sensitive tool that can detect the risk of malnutrition early. Other assessment tools that health care providers may prefer to use in the geriatric population include the Mini Nutritional Assessment (standard form), the Nutritional Risk Screening 2002, the Malnutrition Universal Screening Tool, the Subjective Global Assessment, and the Geriatric Nutritional Risk Index. Using the nutrition screening results, the dietitian will assess the need for intervention using the least restrictive diet approach possible (Dorner & Friedrich, 2018).

NUTRITION-RELATED CHRONIC DISEASE

This section of the chapter examines the role of nutrition in the cause and prevention of the leading nutrition-related chronic diseases—heart disease, stroke, some forms of cancer, osteoporosis, obesity, and type 2 diabetes mellitus—and in the early treatment of people in whom human immunodeficiency virus (HIV) infection was recently diagnosed.

Cardiovascular Disease

Cardiovascular disease (CVD), principally CHD and stroke, is the leading killer of adults in the United States (Amini et al., 2021). As such, the Healthy People initiative has specific objectives to improve cardiovascular health and quality of life through prevention, detection, and treatment of risk factors for heart attack and stroke. Box 11.1: Healthy People 2030 Nutrition

TABLE 11.3 Clinical Diagnostic Criteria for Malnutrition

Characteristic	Acute Illness or Injury-Related Malnutrition	Chronic Disease-Related Malnutrition	Social or Environmental Related Malnutrition
Characteristics to Diagnose Severe Malnutrition			
Weight loss	>2%/1 week, >5%/1 month, >7.5%/3 months	>5%/1 month, >7.5%/3 months, >10%/6 months, >20%/1 year	>5%/1 month, >7.5%/3 months, >10%/6 months, >20%/1 year
Energy intake	≤50% for ≥5 days	≤75% for ≥1 month	≤50% for ≥1 month
Body fat	Moderate depletion	Severe depletion	Severe depletion
Muscle mass	Moderate depletion	Severe depletion	Severe depletion
Fluid accumulation	Moderate→severe	Severe	Severe
Grip strength	Not recommended in intensive care unit	Reduced for age/sex	Reduced for age/sex
Characteristics to Diagnose Moderate Malnutrition			
Weight loss	1%–2%/1 week, 5%/1 month, 7.5%/3 months	5%/1 month, 7.5%/3 months, 10%/6 months, 20%/1 year	5%/1 month, 7.5%/3 months, 10%/6 months, 20%/1 year
Energy intake	<75% for >7 days	<75% for ≥1 month	<75% for ≥3 months
Body fat	Mild depletion	Mild depletion	Mild depletion
Muscle mass	Mild depletion	Mild depletion	Mild depletion
Fluid accumulation	Mild	Mild	Mild
Grip strength	Not applicable	Not applicable	Not applicable

From Mogensen et al. (2019)

Mini Nutritional Assessment

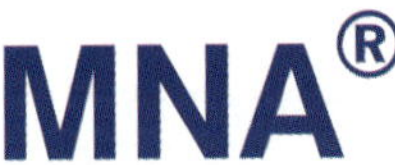

Nestlé NutritionInstitute

Last name: First name:

Sex: Age: Weight, kg: Height, cm: Date:

Complete the screen by filling in the boxes with the appropriate numbers. Total the numbers for the final screening score.

Screening

A Has food intake declined over the past 3 months due to loss of appetite, digestive problems, chewing or swallowing difficulties?
0 = severe decrease in food intake
1 = moderate decrease in food intake
2 = no decrease in food intake ☐

B Weight loss during the last 3 months
0 = weight loss greater than 3 kg (6.6 lbs)
1 = does not know
2 = weight loss between 1 and 3 kg (2.2 and 6.6 lbs)
3 = no weight loss ☐

C Mobility
0 = bed or chair bound
1 = able to get out of bed / chair but does not go out
2 = goes out ☐

D Has suffered psychological stress or acute disease in the past 3 months?
0 = yes 2 = no ☐

E Neuropsychological problems
0 = severe dementia or depression
1 = mild dementia
2 = no psychological problems ☐

F1 Body Mass Index (BMI) (weight in kg) / (height in m)^2
0 = BMI less than 19
1 = BMI 19 to less than 21
2 = BMI 21 to less than 23
3 = BMI 23 or greater ☐

IF BMI IS NOT AVAILABLE, REPLACE QUESTION F1 WITH QUESTION F2.
DO NOT ANSWER QUESTION F2 IF QUESTION F1 IS ALREADY COMPLETED.

F2 Calf circumference (CC) in cm
0 = CC less than 31
3 = CC 31 or greater ☐

Screening score
(max. 14 points) ☐☐

12-14 points: Normal nutritional status
8-11 points: At risk of malnutrition
0-7 points: Malnourished

Ref. Vellas B, Villars H, Abellan G, et al. *Overview of the MNA® - Its History and Challenges.* J Nutr Health Aging 2006;10:456-465.
Rubenstein LZ, Harker JO, Salva A, Guigoz Y, Vellas B. *Screening for Undernutrition in Geriatric Practice: Developing the Short-Form Mini Nutritional Assessment (MNA-SF).* J. Geront 2001;56A: M366-377.
Guigoz Y. *The Mini-Nutritional Assessment (MNA®) Review of the Literature - What does it tell us?* J Nutr Health Aging 2006; 10:466-487.
Kaiser MJ, Bauer JM, Ramsch C, et al. *Validation of the Mini Nutritional Assessment Short-Form (MNA®-SF): A practical tool for identification of nutritional status.* J Nutr Health Aging 2009; 13:782-788.

For more information: www.mna-elderly.com

FIG. 11.4 Mini Nutritional Assessment-Short Form. (From Nestle USA, Inc., Glendale, CA, 2009.)

Objectives lists specific nutrition-related objectives pertaining to CVD risks.

Atherosclerosis

The underlying disease process of CVD is the development of atherosclerotic plaques on the inside lining of the major blood vessels. The American College of Cardiology offers a 10-year atherosclerotic CVD Risk Estimator on their website (go to https://acc.org and search for "ASCVD Risk Estimator"). The current clinical practice guidelines recommend that health care providers regularly use this tool, along with blood lipid levels, as a means of evaluating a patient's risk level for CVD (Arnett et al., 2019). Major risk factors for atherosclerosis include age, family history, heredity, high total **cholesterol** levels, high low-density lipoprotein (LDL) levels, low high-density lipoprotein (HDL) levels, poor diet quality, physical inactivity, smoking, and comorbidities (e.g., hypertension, metabolic syndrome, type 2 diabetes; Bays et al., 2021; Björkegren & Lusis, 2022). Having an HDL cholesterol level greater than 60 mg/dL is protective against CVD.

In an attempt to reduce the incidence of CVD, the American College of Cardiology and the American Heart Association recommend that people adopt a healthy lifestyle throughout life (Arnett et al., 2019; Lichtenstein et al., 2021). Box 11.6: Evidence-Based Practice provides some modifiable lifestyle factors to achieve a healthy lifestyle. Many children, adolescents, and adults who already have unhealthy atherosclerotic lipid profiles should receive patient-centered nutrition counseling with a dietitian.

Nutrition Intervention for Atherosclerosis

Poor diet quality is one of the most significant risk factors for death and disability from CVD in the United States (Kris-Etherton et al., 2020; Mokdad et al., 2018). The primary focus of the current clinical practice guidelines for the prevention of CVD is a shift to a more balanced, well-rounded diet and lifestyle, as opposed to a focus on any specific nutrient (Arnett et al., 2019). Clients can adapt an eating pattern such as that described in Box 11.6: Evidence-Based Practice to meet their calorie requirements, personal and cultural food preferences, and nutrition therapy needs for other existing comorbidities (e.g., diabetes mellitus, obesity, kidney disease). The eating pattern should allow for the attainment and maintenance of a healthy weight. Clients may choose to achieve this pattern by following plans such as DASH (dietary approaches to stop hypertension) (discussed later in this chapter), the MyPlate guidelines, or the Mediterranean diet pattern. Dietary patterns such as these are beneficial for CVD risk reduction and are protective against other nutrition-related chronic diseases such as obesity and metabolic diseases.

In addition to the recommendations for a healthy eating pattern, the American College of Cardiology and the American Heart Association also recommend that adults participate in regular physical activity, minimize sedentary behaviors, abstain from tobacco, and avoid exposure to secondhand smoke as essential components of CVD risk reduction (Arnett et al., 2019). After the RDN and client have settled on an acceptable long-term healthy lifestyle plan, the client should schedule follow-up sessions with the health care team to monitor lipid levels and dietary adherence.

BOX 11.6 EVIDENCE-BASED PRACTICE

Nutrition Risk Factors and Heart Disease

Developing guidelines and recommendations for preventing heart disease is a topic that experts routinely reassess. You may ask, "Why do the recommendations change over time?" As with all things scientific, technology is ever growing and advancing. Such scientific progress brings new findings, which updated guidelines reflect. The gold standard in medicine is to base all medical intervention protocols on evidence-based practice. Evidence-based practice is the use of current evidence from available research coupled with clinical expertise to establish high-quality patient care.

CVD is the leading cause of death in the United States, and suboptimal diet quality is the single largest risk factor contributing to death and disability. A recent study notes that the poor dietary habits primarily contributing to CVD risk include a diet that is too high in sodium, processed meats, and sugar-sweetened beverages and too low in nuts/seeds, seafood, vegetables, and fruit (Kris-Etherton et al., 2020). Guidelines from the American College of Cardiology and the American Heart Association (Arnett et al., 2019) encourage Americans to aim for the following key components of a healthy lifestyle:

Foods to Focus On

- Eat a variety of nutritious foods from all food groups.
- Choose fresh vegetables and fruits, fiber-rich whole-grains, nuts, legumes, and fat-free or low-fat dairy products most often.
- Choose lean meats such as skinless poultry prepared without added saturated or trans fats.
- Eat a variety of fish, at least twice a week.
- Use monounsaturated and polyunsaturated fats instead of tropical oils and other forms of saturated fat.

Foods to Limit or Consume in Moderation

- Limit the intake of saturated fat. For those with elevated blood cholesterol levels, limit to a maximum of 5% to 6% of total daily calories.
- Avoid trans fat.
- Limit sodium intake. For those with elevated blood pressure, limit to a maximum of 2300 mg/day with a goal of reduction to 1500 mg/day.
- Limit red meat, processed meat, and refined carbohydrates.
- Consume less of the nutrient-poor foods, such as sugar-sweetened beverages.

Weight and Physical Activity

- Burn at least as many calories as consumed.
- Aim for at least 150 min of moderate physical activity or 75 min of vigorous physical activity (or an equal combination of both) weekly.
- To lose weight, increase the duration or intensity of physical activity to burn more calories than eaten every day.

General Recommendations

- Drink alcohol in moderation, if at all (e.g., one drink per day for females and two drinks per day for males).
- Do not smoke tobacco and avoid exposure to tobacco smoke.

CVD, Cardiovascular disease.

Barriers to Treatment Goals

The health care team should use behavioral theories to identify a person's level of readiness to change and focus on counseling strategies to match their level of readiness. The team must recognize that desire to change and ability to change are not synonymous terms. Social determinants of health contribute to a person's CVD risk, and such barriers (e.g., food access and socioeconomic factors) are not easily overcome. A successful long-term care plan will tailor the advice and treatment plan to the individual's financial status, education level, health literacy, and cultural, work, and home environments (Arnett et al., 2019). The health care team can address some treatment barriers and improve a person's adherence to dietary recommendations by developing protocols to encourage long-term follow-up, referring clients to food assistance resources as needed, reinforcing and celebrating compliance, and optimizing third-party reimbursement.

Hypertension

We record blood pressure, the force of blood against the walls of arteries, as the systolic blood pressure (SBP) over the diastolic blood pressure (DBP). Normal blood pressure is less than 120 mm Hg systolic and less than 80 mm Hg diastolic. The American College of Cardiology and the American Heart Association define prehypertension, or elevated blood pressure, as an SBP range of 120 to 129 mm Hg and a DBP less than 80 mm Hg to highlight the increased risk of progression to overt hypertension and CVD (Yano et al., 2018). Untreated hypertension can damage arteries and increase the risk of stroke and congestive heart failure. Hypertension is also responsible for many cases of kidney failure requiring dialysis and increases the risk of kidney failure in people with diabetes.

Epidemiology

Hypertension is a significant risk to the health of Americans. The most recent data estimate that 46% of adults with hypertension remain unaware of their condition. Moreover, only 42% of adults who have hypertension are diagnosed and are receiving treatment. Furthermore, high blood pressure is successfully managed in just about one-fifth of adults (21%; Farhadi et al., 2023). Of the adults with diagnosed hypertension, about half of them do not yet have their blood pressure under control. Based on this evidence, the Healthy People initiative includes objectives related to hypertension awareness and risk reduction strategies (see Box 11.1: Healthy People 2030 Nutrition Objectives). The incidence of hypertension is higher in Black or African Americans than in Whites, Hispanics, or Asian Americans (Abrahamowicz et al., 2023). Additional risk factors for hypertension include family history; obesity; smoking; excessive alcohol intake; high sodium intake; and a diet inadequate in potassium, magnesium, calcium, vegetable-derived protein, fiber, and unsaturated fat from fish (Ojangba et al., 2023).

Nutrition Intervention for Hypertension

The primary focus of nutrition intervention for hypertension is lifestyle modifications. The American College of Cardiology and the American Heart Association recommend the following lifestyle choices as a means to reduce the risk and severity of hypertension: (1) lose weight, if indicated; (2) adopt a heart-healthy diet such as the DASH diet; (3) reduce sodium intake (Box 11.7: Dietary Sources of Sodium); (4) increase potassium intake; (5) use alcohol moderately; (6) perform regular physical activity with a structured exercise program; and (7) stop smoking and prevent exposure to secondhand smoke, if indicated (Ojangba et al., 2023). Such lifestyle changes measurably improve blood pressure and reduce the risk of chronic disease. These recommendations apply to anyone with elevated blood pressure, whether they are using the modifications alone or in combination with drug therapy.

Dietary Approaches to Stop Hypertension

Using dietary changes only, the DASH landmark study was able to lower blood pressure significantly within a 2-week period (Appel et al., 1997). The DASH eating plan consists of four to five servings of fruits, four to five servings of vegetables, and two to three servings of low-fat dairy foods per day along with lean meats, nuts, seeds, dried beans, and high-fiber grains (for a 2000-kcal diet). In addition to a lowered blood pressure, individuals following the DASH eating plan experience the added benefits of an overall reduced occurrence of CVD, coronary heart disease, and stroke, and significantly lower total cholesterol, LDL-cholesterol, fasting blood insulin, HbA1c (a marker of blood glucose levels), and body weight (Appel et al., 1997; Onwuzo et al., 2023; Theodoridis et al., 2023). The DASH diet is not specifically a low-sodium diet; however, when combined with sodium-restriction, the blood-pressure–lowering effects are considerably greater than DASH alone (Filippou et al., 2022).

The American College of Cardiology and the American Heart Association recommend the DASH eating plan as an all-around healthy eating style. They specifically recommend it as a nutrition intervention strategy for individuals with high blood

BOX 11.7 Dietary Sources of Sodium

The following are the major sources of sodium in the typical American diet, in order of predominance:

- Salt added by food processing companies as an ingredient in almost all processed foods (including many foods that do not taste salty, such as baked goods); most processed foods have a high sodium content.
- Salt added by consumers to food during cooking or at the table.
- Salt from all animal products, which are a natural source of sodium.
- The following food tips help reduce salt and sodium intake:
    - Sodium occurs naturally in many foods and food manufacturers add salt to most processed foods; therefore, add salt only sparingly in home cooking and at the table.
    - Consume fewer foods that have high sodium levels, such as many cheeses; processed meats; most frozen dinners and entrees; packaged mixes; most canned soups and vegetables; salad dressings; and condiments such as soy sauce, pickles, olives, ketchup, and mustard.
    - Rinse canned vegetables before consuming them.
    - Eat salty, highly processed salty, salt-preserved, and salt-pickled foods only occasionally.
    - Check labels for sodium in foods and choose products lower in sodium (free, <5 mg per serving; low, <140 mg per serving; reduced or less, 25% less than standard-reference food; healthy, <480 mg per serving).

pressure, with blood pressure in the elevated range, for those with a family history of high blood pressure, and those who are using blood-pressure–lowering medications (Belanger et al., 2023). Clients following the DASH plan should continue other steps to control or prevent hypertension, including exercise, weight loss when necessary, not smoking, and limiting alcohol consumption. Clients and health care providers can freely obtain the complete DASH eating plan from https://www.nhlbi.nih.gov/education/dash-eating-plan.

Cancer

Cancer occurs because of mutations in DNA that alter the cellular control over normal cell reproduction. Several factors may contribute to the processes of (1) mutation, (2) promotion of mutated cellular growth, and (3) progression to malignancies capable of metastasizing. Some factors that initiate these changes include chemical carcinogens, radiation, dietary factors, oncogenic viruses, and epidemiologic components (e.g., race, age, heredity, occupation).

Epidemiology

The lifetime probability of being diagnosed with invasive cancer is 40.2% for males and 38.5% for females (Siegel et al., 2023). Cancer remains the second leading cause of death in the United States (Siegel et al., 2023). The most common cancers in males and females are breast, colorectal, lung, and prostate. Breast cancer alone accounts for 31% of newly diagnosed cases, and prostate cancer accounts for 29% of new cases (Siegel et al., 2023). Fig. 11.5 demonstrates recent trends in cancer prevalence for males and females.

Nutrition Intervention for Cancer Risk Reduction

Carcinogenic and anticarcinogenic compounds are both naturally found in many foods, which makes diet-related effects on cancer incidence difficult to discern. There are some well-documented connections between certain dietary patterns and specific forms of cancer (e.g., diets high in processed meat or meat cooked at high temperatures and the risk for colorectal and stomach cancer; Crowe et al., 2022; Veettil et al., 2021). However, many other questions about diet and cancer remain unanswered. Researchers agree that cancer prevalence increases along with obesity and poor dietary patterns, defined as a low intake of fruits, vegetables, whole grains, and dairy products, and high intake of processed meat, red meat, alcohol, and sugar-sweetened beverages (Key et al., 2020; McCullough et al., 2022; Pati et al., 2023; Zhao et al., 2023). As such, the American Cancer Society, the World Cancer Research Fund, and the American Institute for Cancer Research recommend a well-balanced diet combined with regular physical activity that maintains a healthy body weight for cancer prevention and all-around health promotion. The specific recommendations by the expert panel to reduce the risk of cancer include the following lifestyle factors (American Cancer Society, 2020):

1. Be as lean as possible within the normal range of body weight throughout life.
    - Balance caloric intake with physical activity.
    - Avoid excessive weight gain at all ages. For overweight or obese individuals, losing even a small amount of weight is helpful.
2. Adopt a physically active lifestyle.
    - Children and adolescents: participate in at least 60 minutes every day of moderate to vigorous physical activity,

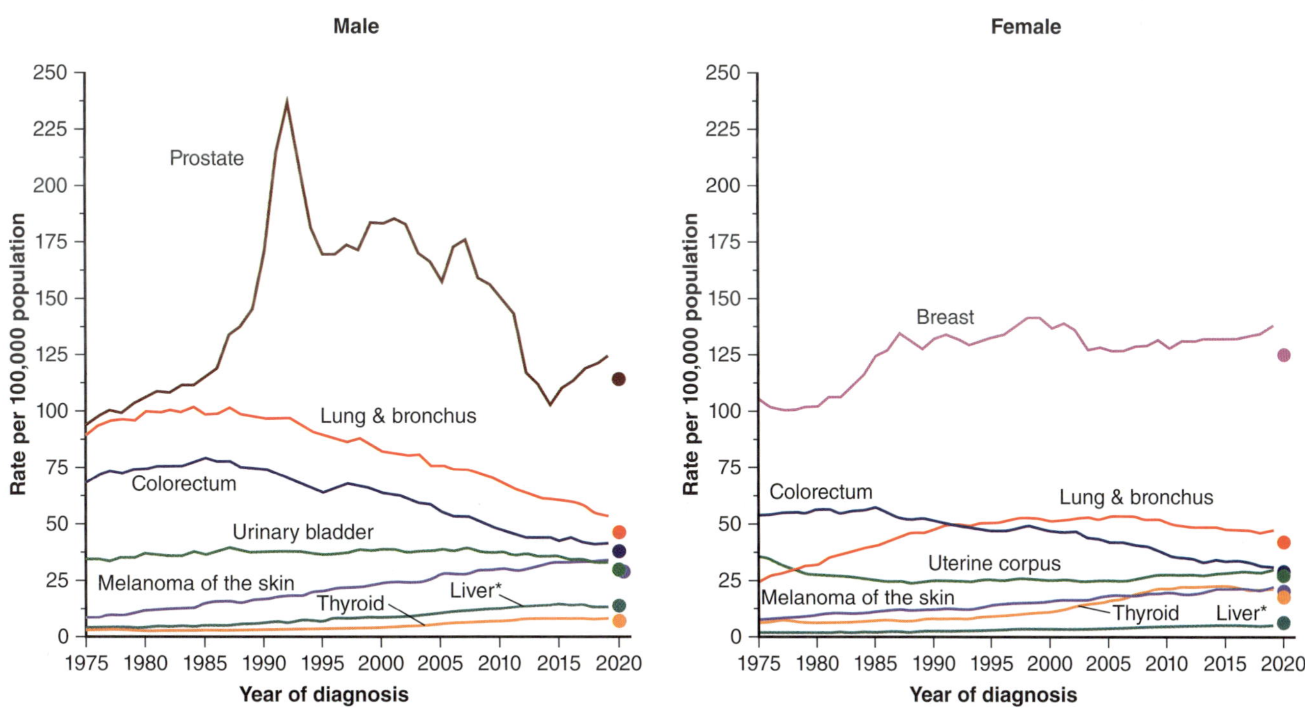

FIG. 11.5 Trends in incidence rates for selected cancers by sex, United States, 1975 through 2020. (From Siegel, Giaquinto, & Jemal, 2024).

with vigorous intensity activity included at least 3 days per week.
- Adults: engage in at least 150 minutes of moderate intensity or 75 minutes of vigorous physical activity each week, preferably spread throughout the week.
- Limit sedentary behaviors.

3. Consume a healthy diet that has an emphasis on plant-based food.
   - Become familiar with standard serving sizes and read food labels to become more aware of actual servings consumed. Choose foods that will help achieve and maintain a healthy body weight.
   - Limit the consumption of salty foods and salt-preserved foods.
   - Limit the consumption of energy-dense foods, particularly processed foods that are high in added sugar, low in fiber, or high in fat. Avoid sugar-sweetened beverages.
   - Choose a variety of different fruits and vegetables. Eat at least 2.5 cups of vegetables and fruits every day.
   - Choose whole grains instead of processed (refined) grains and sugars. Avoid moldy grains and legumes.
   - Choose fish, poultry, and beans as alternatives to red meat. Select lean cuts and small portions, and prepare the meat by baking, broiling, or poaching rather than frying. Avoid processed meats.
4. If consumed, limit alcohol intake. Limit alcohol intake to two drinks per day for males and one drink per day for females. One drink is defined as 12 oz of beer, 5 oz of wine, or 1.5 oz of 80-proof distilled spirits.
5. Meet nutrient needs through diet alone; do not rely on dietary supplements.
6. Aim to breastfeed infants exclusively for 6 months and continue to breastfeed while offering complementary food after 6 months.

The cancer-prevention recommendations are very consistent with the messages of the Dietary Guidelines for Americans, the MyPlate guidelines, and the dietary recommendations of other national agencies for general health promotion and prevention of other diet-related chronic conditions. Using either the Mediterranean dietary pattern or the MyPlate dietary pattern will provide a well-balanced diet that meets the cancer-prevention recommendations.

Nurses may find it is helpful to refer to the sections in the "Diet, Nutrition, Physical Activity and Cancer: A Global Perspective" expert report that refers to other aspects of food intake relating to prevention of cancer. The guidelines include specific suggestions for particular cancers, evidence specific to nutrient supplementation, and answers to other frequently asked questions. It is available free for download (subject to copyright if used) at http://www.wcrf.org/dietandcancer.

Osteoporosis

Osteoporosis is a skeletal disorder characterized by compromised bone strength and quality with increased risk of fracture, especially in the wrist, hip, and spinal area (Fig. 11.6). Bone strength reflects the integration of two main features: bone density and bone quality. Bone mineral density is expressed as grams of mineral per area or volume and, in any given individual, is determined by peak bone mass and the amount of bone loss. Bone quality refers to architecture, turnover, damage accumulation (microfractures), and mineralization.

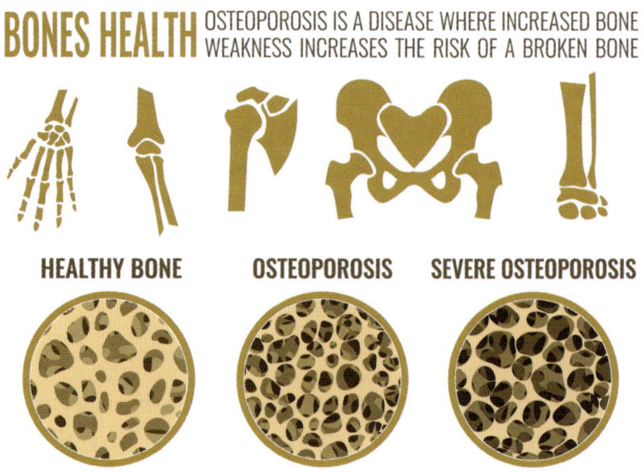

FIG. 11.6 Changes in bone from osteoporosis. (From iStock.com/Anna Bergbauer.)

Epidemiology

Osteoporosis is a substantial cause of morbidity in the United States: 30% of females and 16% of males over the age of 50 years meet the diagnostic criteria for osteoporosis. The prevalence of compromised bone strength and quality increases substantially with age. In adults over the age of 80 years, 77% of females and 46% of males are living with osteoporosis (Wright et al., 2017). An additional 47 million Americans have osteopenia (low bone mass), which is a significant risk factor for developing osteoporosis (Looker et al., 2017). Osteoporosis imposes a substantial global economic burden, primarily driven by fracture-related costs. Treating osteoporotic fractures alone costs an estimated annual total of 5000 to 6500 billion US dollars in Canada, Europe, and the United States. This figure does not include indirect costs like disability and productivity loss (Kemmak et al., 2020).

Nutrition Intervention for Osteoporosis

Maximizing bone mineral density early in life presents a vital opportunity to reduce the effect of age-related bone loss during the advanced years. Several nutrients are involved in healthy bone building, including protein; minerals such as calcium, phosphorus, copper, magnesium, manganese, potassium, and zinc; and vitamins such as C, D, and K. The bone mass attained early in life, the vast majority of which we accrue before the age of 30 years, is perhaps the most important determinant of lifelong skeletal health. Individuals with the highest peak bone mass have the greatest protective advantage when there is an unavoidable decline in bone density with increasing age.

Genetic, physiologic, environmental, and modifiable lifestyle factors exert a strong influence on peak bone mass acquisition. Certain medications that alter mineral bioavailability and bone turnover may influence bone mineral integrity as well. The Bone Health and Osteoporosis Foundation (2022) recognizes the following risk factors for osteoporosis:

Uncontrollable Risk Factors: older age, female sex, menopause, family history of osteoporosis, low body weight/being small or thin/excessive weight loss and experiencing broken bones or loss in stature as an adult

Controllable Risk Factors: a diet low in calcium and vitamin D; inadequate fruit and vegetable intake; excessive intake of protein, sodium, and caffeine; sedentary lifestyle, smoking, high alcohol intake

An overall healthy diet, adequate in calories and appropriate nutrients, is essential for normal growth and development of all tissues, including bone. For the purpose of this text, we will focus on two micronutrients required for bone development—calcium and vitamin D.

Calcium

A well-balanced diet includes foods that provide adequate calcium to meet the DRI throughout each life stage (Institute of Medicine, 2011). People of all ages should make sure they get adequate calcium intake by consuming calcium-rich foods (e.g., dairy products) and calcium-fortified foods (e.g., orange juice, dairy substitutes such as almond milk and rice milk), as they deliver the most bioavailable calcium of any food group. Other good sources of calcium include sardines, canned salmon (if the bones are eaten), and some dark green leafy vegetables, especially bok choy, collard greens, kale, and turnip greens. Many other vegetables contain oxalic acid and phytates, both of which inhibit the absorption of calcium, rendering them poor calcium sources. Examples include spinach, Swiss chard, beet greens, and wheat. Supplementation with calcium tablets may be appropriate for high-risk individuals with inadequate calcium intake. However, note that individuals should not exceed the tolerable upper intake levels.

Calcium from supplements comes in a variety of forms (e.g., calcium carbonate, citrate, phosphate, lactate, and gluconate). The bioavailability of calcium from these sources varies considerably. For those who do choose to take calcium supplements, calcium carbonate provides the most bioavailable form of calcium (Greupner et al., 2017). Calcium supplement absorption is most efficient for individuals with adequate gastric acid production at doses no greater than 500 mg at a time when taken with meals.

Health care providers should encourage anyone younger than 25 years old who does not ingest adequate calcium to develop strategies for increasing it. Females, particularly over the age of 50, are at the highest risk of inadequate calcium intake (Marshall et al., 2020). By modeling appropriate behaviors, health care professionals can help prevent or delay the onset of osteoporosis in themselves, their families, and the people in their care.

Vitamin D

Vitamin D is a prohormone found in two forms: vitamin D_2 (ergocalciferol) and vitamin D_3 (cholecalciferol). Both forms of vitamin D support bone health. The human body synthesizes cholecalciferol from a cholesterol-derived precursor when we expose the skin to the ultraviolet rays of the sun. Vigilant use of sunscreen and other situations that limit sun exposure may complicate this process. Similarly, some organisms such as invertebrates are capable of synthesizing ergocalciferol after they receive ultraviolet radiation. Vitamin D from foods, as well as that from sun exposure, must undergo two hydroxylation reactions in the liver and kidney to become an active functioning hormone in the body, known as 1,25-dehydroxyvitamin D_3, or calcitriol.

Food manufacturers commonly add vitamin D to milk and other commonly consumed foods (e.g., margarine, ready-to-eat cereals, milk substitutes). Natural sources of vitamin D include fatty fish (salmon and mackerel), butter, and eggs. During adolescence, when consumption of dairy products commonly decreases, vitamin D intake may be inadequate, which may affect calcium absorption adversely and ultimately affect bone health.

Obesity

Obesity is an excess of body fat. Obesity negatively affects health and longevity and is associated with the leading causes of death in the United States: CVD, type 2 diabetes, and some cancers (Pati et al., 2023; Powell-Wiley et al., 2021). Obesity is also associated with other chronic conditions that lower overall quality of life, such as the exacerbation of osteoarthritis in the weight-bearing joints.

Diagnostic Criteria for Adults

Health care providers diagnose obesity when a person's body weight is 20% or more above their desired weight for height or their body mass index (BMI) is 30 kg/m^2 or higher. We calculate a person's BMI by dividing their weight in kilograms by their height in meters squared. Table 11.4 provides the body weight classification by BMI. BMI classifications correlate to the effect that body weight has on the risk for morbidity and mortality. A BMI in the healthy range is associated with the lowest risk for weight-related chronic diseases.

We can use the BMI as an indicator of body weight status, but we cannot interpret it as a specific percentage of body fat. BMI is a marker of body weight to height, without consideration for other factors that influence the relationship of body fat. For example, females are more likely to have a higher percentage of body fat than males have for the same BMI. Furthermore, body weight in pounds does not allude to the proportion of lean body mass relative to fat body mass. For example, an elite athlete with a higher proportion of muscle to fat may have a higher body weight relative to height than a person of the same stature without exceptionally large skeletal muscles. Likewise, bone weight differs in people with smaller frames compared with those with

TABLE 11.4 BMI Classifications

Classification	BMI (kg/m2)
Underweight	<18.5
Healthy weight	18.5–24.9
Overweight	25–29.9
Obese	≥30

BMI, Body mass index.

larger frames and higher bone density. Nevertheless, BMI is an appropriate screening tool to identify health or nutrition-related disorders for much of the population.

On an individual basis, health care providers will combine BMI information with waist circumference to determine whether the client is at increased risk of chronic disease. The marker for elevated obesity-associated risk for males is a waist circumference ≥40 inches and for females it is a waist circumference ≥35 inches. Waist circumference is a helpful adjunct screening tool because the greater the amount of adipose tissue stored within the abdominal region, the higher the risk is for disease and all-cause mortality (Jayedi et al., 2020).

Diagnostic Criteria for Children

Pediatricians, nurses, and registered dietitians use growth charts to track growth and development in children and adolescents from birth to 20 years old. Growth charts consist of a series of percentile curves that illustrate the distribution in growth of healthy children across the United States. Fig. 11.7 illustrates a BMI-for-age growth chart for females aged 2 to 20 years. The CDC provides free online training for using and interpreting the growth charts at http://www.cdc.gov/nccdphp/dnpao/growthcharts.

Children at or above the 85th percentile are considered at risk for overweight. The growth chart provides a means of recognizing children who have the potential to become overweight as early as 2 years old. Early identification of obesity risk gives parents and care providers the opportunity to modify their family eating and activity patterns before their children develop a weight problem.

Epidemiology

The prevalence of overweight and obesity in the United States ranks high in comparison with that of other developed nations. Currently, 73.6% of adults are overweight, of which 41.9% are obese and 9.2% are extremely obese (defined as a BMI ≥ 40 kg/m^2; Stierman et al., 2023). Obesity is more common in females than in males (41% compared with 37%, respectively). There are significant differences in the prevalence of adult overweight/obesity among various races/ethnicities in the United States (Fig. 11.8). As mentioned before, 19.7% of children and adolescents between the ages of 2 and 19 years old are also obese (Stierman et al., 2023). Lifestyle, genetics, hormonal factors, and social-ecological factors are some of the many factors contributing to the problem.

Nutrition Intervention for Weight Management

The current exercise and weight-related recommendations in the Dietary Guidelines for Americans include the following (US Department of Agriculture & US Department of Health and Human Services, 2020):

- Choose a healthy eating pattern at an appropriate calorie level to help achieve and maintain a healthy body weight, support nutrient adequacy, and reduce the risk of chronic disease.
- Increase the amount of physical activity engagement each week.
- Limit screen time and decrease the amount of time spent in sedentary situations.

With the advances in nutrigenomics, it may be possible to individualize dietary recommendations based on a person's genotype at a point in the near future, thus having a greater affect on risk reduction in diet-related diseases such as obesity (Box 11.8: Genomics). A balanced diet to support weight reduction should include appropriate serving sizes to meet individual nutrient needs. Additionally, exercise is particularly important from the outset, because with exercise there is less needed to restrict food intake. Exercise also favors long-term maintenance of body weight (as described in Chapter 12). Health care providers make referrals to dietitians as appropriate for evidence-based patient-centered weight loss assistance.

There are many positive effects of even relatively small amounts of weight loss (5% to 10% of body weight) for obese individuals. Some noted benefits include improved blood glucose control, **triglyceride** levels, and HDL-cholesterol levels; decreased blood pressure; reduced sleep apnea; improved knee functionality in those with osteoarthritis; improved quality of life, mobility, and sexual function; and reduced health care cost and emergent depression (Horn et al., 2022; Tahrani & Morton, 2022).

Fad diets rarely provide a sustainable or effective way to lose weight. However, it is helpful for health care professionals to be able to discuss current fads intelligently and to guide clients as needed. The prevention-focused model of health care includes many facets needed to avoid and treat obesity in the United States. On an individual basis, for people who cannot or do not choose to maintain a BMI less than 30 kg/m^2 as a priority, Box 11.9 describes the paradigm Health at Any Size (Spark, 2001).

Diabetes Mellitus

For cells in the body to use glucose for energy, the glucose circulating in the blood must enter into the cell. For this to happen in most cells, insulin must be available and insulin receptors on the cell membrane must function properly. Diabetes mellitus (usually referred to as "diabetes") is a group of metabolic diseases causing defects in production, secretion, or action of insulin. The result is chronic hyperglycemia and a deficiency of available glucose to the cell. There are two main types of diabetes: type 1 and type 2. Type 1 diabetes mellitus results from an autoimmune destruction of the insulin-producing pancreatic β cells. Type 2 diabetes mellitus results from insulin resistance or insulin insufficiency and is frequently associated with obesity. Individuals with type 2 diabetes are either unable to use the insulin produced effectively or the pancreas does not produce adequate insulin.

Type 2 diabetes accounts for 90% to 95% of all diagnosed cases of diabetes. The risk factors include the following: age 45 years or older, family history of diabetes or a personal history of gestational diabetes or polycystic ovary syndrome, overweight (defined as BMI ≥ 25 kg/m^2), physical inactivity, hypertension, and dyslipidemia (e.g., high triglycerides, low HDL-cholesterol). Additionally, certain races or ethnic groups are at higher risk for diabetes, including African American, Hispanic/Latino, American Indian, Alaska Native, Asian American, Native

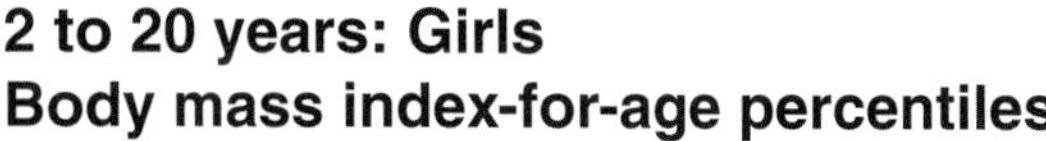

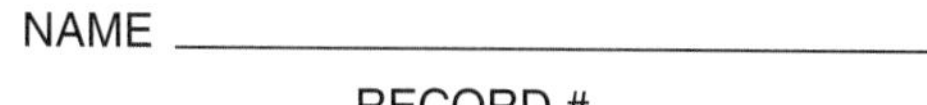

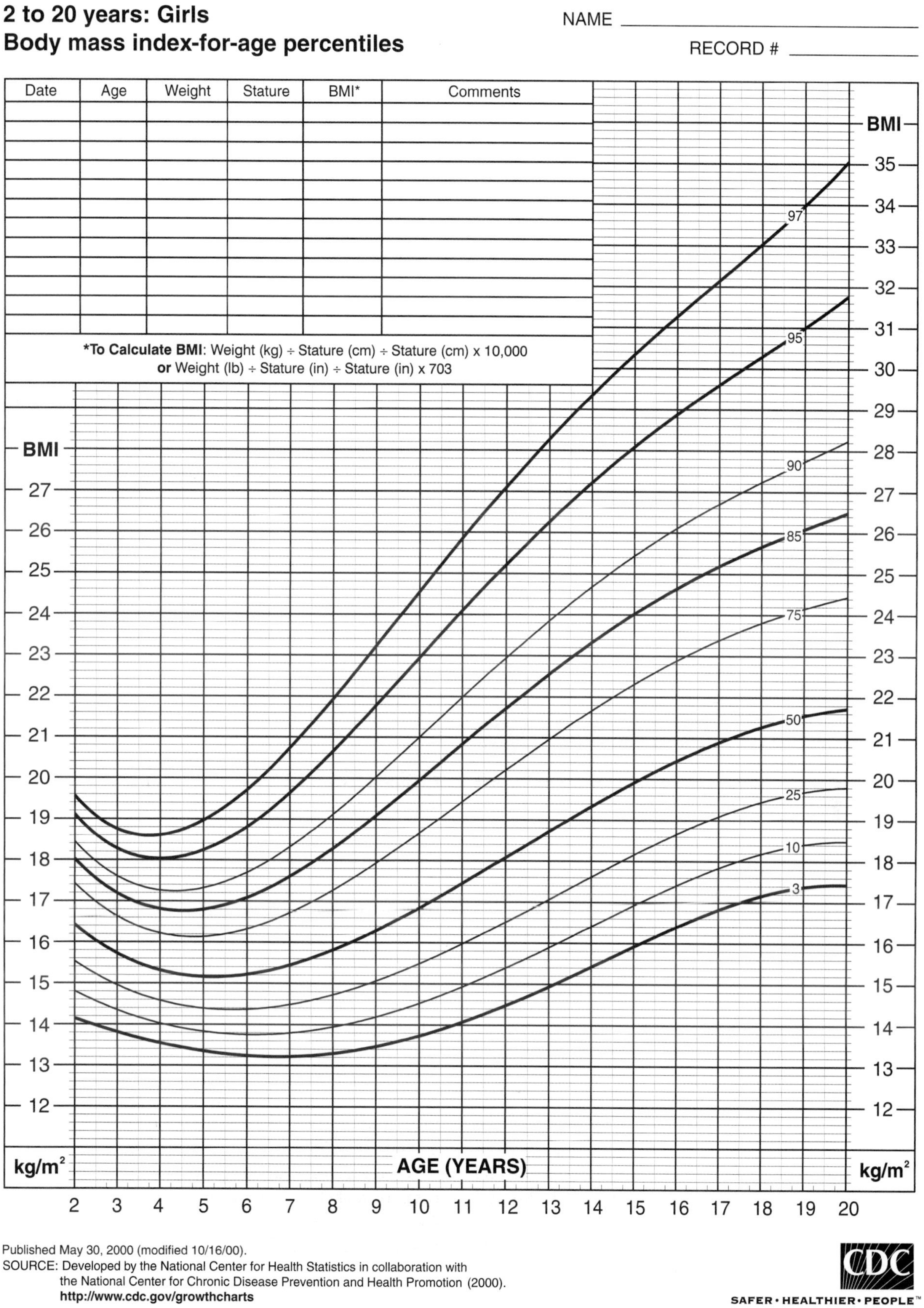
2 to 20 years: Girls
Body mass index-for-age percentiles
NAME
RECORD #
Date
Age
Weight
Stature
BMI*
Comments
*To Calculate BMI: Weight (kg) ÷ Stature (cm) ÷ Stature (cm) x 10,000
or Weight (lb) ÷ Stature (in) ÷ Stature (in) x 703
BMI
12
13
14
15
16
17
18
19
20
21
22
23
24
25
26
27
28
29
30
31
32
33
34
35
97
95
90
85
75
50
25
10
3
kg/m²
AGE (YEARS)
2
3
4
5
6
7
8
9
10
11
12
13
14
15
16
17
18
19
20
Published May 30, 2000 (modified 10/16/00).
SOURCE: Developed by the National Center for Health Statistics in collaboration with
the National Center for Chronic Disease Prevention and Health Promotion (2000).
http://www.cdc.gov/growthcharts
CDC
SAFER · HEALTHIER · PEOPLE™

FIG. 11.7 Example of a body mass index (BMI)-for-age growth chart for girls. (Courtesy National Center for Health Statistics, National Center for Chronic Disease Prevention and Health Promotion, Hyattsville, MD.)

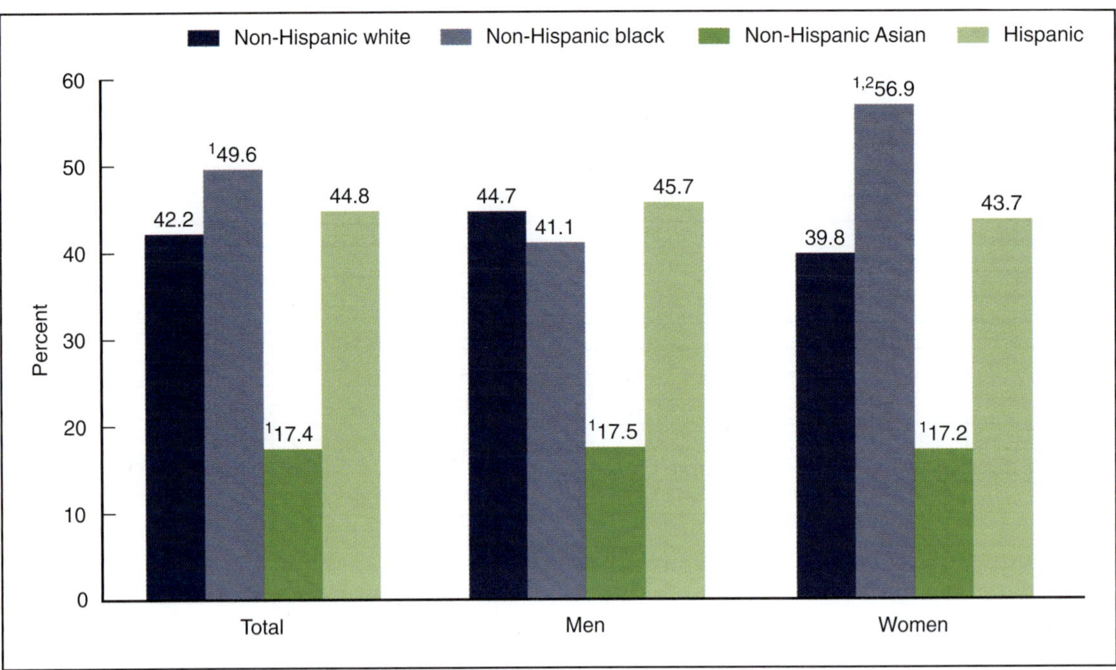

[1]Significantly different from all other race and Hispanic-origin groups.
[2]Significantly different from men for same race and Hispanic-origin group.
NOTES: Estimates were age adjusted by the direct method to the 2000 U.S. Census population using the age groups 20–39, 40–59, and 60 and over.
Access data table for Figure 2 at: https://www.cdc.gov/nchs/data/databriefs/db360_tables-508.pdf#2.
SOURCE: NCHS, National Health and Nutrition Examination Survey, 2017–2018.

FIG. 11.8 Age-adjusted prevalence of obesity in adults aged 20 and over, by sex and race and Hispanic origin: United States. (Hales et al., 2020)

BOX 11.8 GENOMICS

Nutrigenomics

The field of nutritional genomics is a multidisciplinary field of research that investigates the effects a person's diet has on that person's genes (i.e., nutrigenomics) and investigates how our genetic variations dictate our response to certain nutrients (i.e., nutrigenetics). We accept that slight variations in our genetic makeup account for the individuality of our physical appearances. Think about how you guess at what your height potential will be. We generally look to our biologic parents for answers regarding our physical appearance. Likewise, the study of nutrigenomics is attempting to predict how a specific genetic identity will influence a person's response to food and the nutrients within it.

There are many examples of how such individual genetic variants alter disease treatment in health care. For example, two people with hypertension may need different medications to treat the same condition because of their biologic response to certain medications. It makes sense then that the same two people may also benefit from different dietary interventions. Obesity is one of the primary health concerns in the United States and is a significant risk factor for all other major chronic diseases (Kivimäki et al., 2022). Nutrigenomics makes possible the use of a personalized diet prescription based on an individual's specific genetic profile. Researchers believe that the potential for personalized (i.e., precision) dietary intervention could change the prevalence of chronic disease such as obesity (Franzago et al., 2020; Horne et al., 2022). If such diet therapies are effective in managing or preventing disease, this will allow health care providers to focus more on health promotion instead of disease management. Such a shift in health care represents a significantly more sustainable and cost-effective strategy to enhance the health of the nation.

Hawaiian, and Pacific Islander (Centers for Disease Control and Prevention, 2022).

Epidemiology

The numbers of existing cases (prevalence) and new cases (incidence) of type 2 diabetes mirror the prevalence of obesity. Approximately 38.4 million people in the United States have diabetes, and the prevalence increases with age (Centers for Disease Control and Prevention, 2023b). Currently, over 29% of adults aged 65 years or older have diabetes (Centers for Disease Control and Prevention, 2023b).

Diabetes ranks as the eighth leading cause of death among Americans and is a primary reason for hospital admissions related to ischemic heart disease, stroke, amputations of lower extremities, and diabetic ketoacidosis (Centers for Disease Control and Prevention, 2023b). Early detection, improved delivery of care, and better education on disease self-management can prevent or delay much of the burden of diabetes.

Type 2 diabetes was previously known as "adult-onset diabetes" because it was primarily only identified in adults that were at least 40 years old. However, in recent decades, health care providers are increasingly diagnosing the disease in children and adolescents, and experts no longer classify it exclusively as an adult-onset disease. The epidemic of obesity in children and adolescents, the decrease in physical activity, the increase in calorie-dense foods, and the exposure to diabetes in utero are likely contributors to the increase in prevalence of type 2 diabetes in this younger population.

BOX 11.9 HEALTH AT EVERY SIZE (HAES)

The Size Acceptance Non-Diet Movement

The HAES paradigm has replaced the question "How can overweight people lose weight?" with the question "How can overweight people be healthy?" Recognizing that traditional weight loss interventions are often not successful and may even be damaging, the HAES philosophy advocates body acceptance and holistic approaches to health. The following principles are aligned with this movement (Association for Size Diversity and Health [ASDAH], 2020; Clarke et al., 2024):

- Weight loss should not be a main treatment goal. Instead of weight-centric approaches to health, a shift towards promoting healthy behaviors should occur, including a focus on intuitive eating and enjoyable physical activity.
- Human beings come in a variety of sizes and shapes; size diversity is a positive characteristic of humanity. Body acceptance should be encouraged.
- Access to health care is a human right, regardless of one's size. Health care providers should provide respectful, compassionate, and empathetic care and have the necessary skills and equipment (such as seating, exam tables, and patient gowns) available to treat individuals of all sizes.
- Antifat bias exists. Health care providers should carefully examine their own biases and advocate for nondiscriminatory health policies.

Numerous studies have examined HAES interventions' effect on a variety of outcomes, including general well-being, eating behaviors, quality of life, cardiometabolic indicators (blood pressure, blood lipids), physical activity, body perception, and anthropometric measures (weight, BMI, waist circumference). Although some of these studies showed improvement in outcomes, a recent meta-analysis (Clarke et al., 2024) addressed some of the limitations of these studies and found that there were no significant anthropometric, psychological, or cardiometabolic differences in outcomes compared with weight-focused interventions. There was, however, a significant reduction in susceptibility to hunger cues. Additional research is recommended.

BMI, Body mass index; *HAES,* health at every size.

Nutrition Intervention for Diabetes

The health care team for individuals with diabetes typically includes a physician, a registered nurse, an RDN, a pharmacist, and, in some practice settings, a mental health professional with expertise in diabetes management. The most critical and pivotal component of diabetes care is blood glucose management through medical nutrition therapy (MNT), for which the dietitian is responsible. MNT helps delay or prevent the development of complications (e.g., retinopathy, nephropathy, neuropathy, and CVD) for individuals with any form of diabetes (Evert et al., 2019).

No single "diet" for individuals with diabetes exists. Nutrition advice for people with diabetes is essentially the same as that for the general population: follow the Dietary Guidelines for Americans and consume a well-balanced healthy diet. Several established eating patterns meet the qualifications as a well-balanced diet, such as the Mediterranean and the DASH eating patterns. Dietitians will individualize the MNT for people with diabetes, with consideration given to usual eating habits, culture, food access, and other lifestyle factors. The client and RDN will work together to develop a nutrition care plan to meet treatment goals and improve outcomes using evidence-based recommendations (American Diabetes Association, 2019). Table 11.5 summarizes the MNT guidelines from the American Diabetes Association. Monitoring metabolic parameters, including blood glucose levels, glycosylated hemoglobin (HbA1C) levels, lipid values, blood pressure, body weight, renal function (when appropriate), and quality of life, helps guide continued care.

Regular exercise is also an important component of an overall healthy lifestyle that contributes to blood glucose management and reduces the risk for comorbidities (e.g., CVD, hyperlipidemia, hypertension). Individuals with diabetes should aim for 150 minutes per week or more of moderate-intensity aerobic physical activity (i.e., 50% to 70% of maximum heart rate) and two days per week of resistance training (also see Chapter 12; American Diabetes Association, 2019).

Human Immunodeficiency Virus and Acquired Immunodeficiency Syndrome

HIV is a virus that attacks the immune system. In advanced stages, the host's compromised immune system is unable to fight off even modest infections. Untreated HIV eventually leads to acquired immunodeficiency syndrome (AIDS) and death. HIV-infected individuals transmit the virus through sexual contact, shared needles or syringes, or mother-to-child transmission. Male-to-male sexual contact accounts for the majority of new HIV infections in the United States.

Epidemiology

Approximately 1.2 million people are infected with HIV in the United States, the majority of which are male (81%). An estimated 14% of them are unaware and undiagnosed, which increases the risk for transmission (Centers for Disease Control and Prevention, 2023a). AIDS is the ninth leading cause of death of American males between the ages of 25 and 54 years (Tian et al., 2023)

Nutrition Intervention for Human Immunodeficiency Virus

Attention to nutrition in early HIV intervention is essential for several reasons. People can now live for decades with HIV/AIDS, as long as their health care team diagnoses and treats them early. Nutritious diets can improve the sense of well-being, minimize disease symptoms and the side effects of medications, and reduce the risk of opportunistic infections. Implementation of good dietary habits early in the disease may have benefits for end-stage developments such as severe wasting.

Nutrition screening assessments help determine the extent to which the patient needs a referral for nutrition counseling. There are specific nutrition status screening tools available for use in individuals with HIV, such as the Subjective Global Assessment-HIV (Willig et al., 2018). Patients determined at nutrition risk will then see an RDN for a comprehensive nutrition assessment that establishes baseline information for evaluation of the progression of the disease. Because of a compromised immune system, exposure to food-borne organisms may cause severe illness in people with HIV/AIDS. Thus health care providers should address safe food handling practices with all HIV-affected patients. Involving the patient's significant others and caretakers in early discussions of optimal and safe nutrition is important.

TABLE 11.5 Medical Nutrition Therapy Recommendations from the American Diabetes Association

Topic	Recommendations
Eating patterns and macronutrient distribution	There is no single ideal dietary distribution of calories from carbohydrates, fats, and proteins for people with diabetes; therefore, meal plans should be individualized while keeping total calorie and metabolic goals in mind. A variety of eating patterns are acceptable for the management of type 2 diabetes and prediabetes.
Carbohydrates	Carbohydrate intake should emphasize nutrient-dense carbohydrate sources that are high in fiber, including vegetables, fruits, legumes, whole grains, and dairy products. People with diabetes and those at risk are advised to avoid sugar-sweetened beverages (including fruit juices) to control glycemia and weight and reduce their risk for cardiovascular disease and fatty liver and should minimize the consumption of foods with added sugar that have the capacity to displace healthier, more nutrient-dense food choices.
Protein	In individuals with type 2 diabetes, ingested protein appears to increase insulin response without increasing plasma glucose concentrations. Therefore carbohydrate sources high in protein should be avoided when trying to treat or prevent hypoglycemia.
Dietary fat	Data on the ideal total dietary fat content for people with diabetes are inconclusive, so an eating plan emphasizing elements of a Mediterranean-style diet rich in monounsaturated and polyunsaturated fats may be considered to improve glucose metabolism and lower cardiovascular disease risk and can be an effective alternative to a diet low in total fat but relatively high in carbohydrates. Eating foods rich in long-chain n-3 fatty acids, such as fatty fish (EPA and DHA) and nuts and seeds (ALA), is recommended to prevent or treat cardiovascular disease; however, evidence does not support a beneficial role for the routine use of n-3 dietary supplements.
Micronutrients and herbal supplements	There is no clear evidence that dietary supplementation with vitamins, minerals (such as chromium and vitamin D), herbs, or spices (such as cinnamon or aloe vera) can improve outcomes in people with diabetes who do not have underlying deficiencies, and they are not generally recommended for glycemic control.
Alcohol	Adults with diabetes who drink alcohol should do so in moderation (no more than one drink per day for adult females and no more than two drinks per day for adult males). Alcohol consumption may place people with diabetes at increased risk for hypoglycemia, especially if taking insulin or insulin secretagogues. Education and awareness regarding the recognition and management of delayed hypoglycemia are warranted.
Sodium	As for the general population, people with diabetes should limit sodium consumption to <2300 mg/day.
Nonnutritive sweeteners	The use of nonnutritive sweeteners may have the potential to reduce overall calorie and carbohydrate intake if substituted for caloric (sugar) sweeteners and without compensation by intake of additional calories from other food sources. For those who consume sugar-sweetened beverages regularly, a low-calorie or nonnutritive-sweetened beverage may serve as a short-term replacement strategy, but overall, people are encouraged to decrease both sweetened and nonnutritive-sweetened beverages and use other alternatives, with an emphasis on water intake.

ALA, Alpha-linolenic acid; *DHA,* docosahexaenoic acid, *EPA,* eicosapentaenoic acid.
American Diabetes Association (2018, 2019)

The aims of nutrition therapy and counseling for individuals with HIV/AIDS are personalized and focus on the following principles (Willig et al., 2018):

- Maintain adequate food intake to preserve appropriate body composition and nutrition status
- Review nutrition strategies and additional therapies available for symptom management to reduce the effects of disease progression, comorbidities, and medication intolerance
- Provide education and resources to address food safety and food security
- Review and address potential drug-nutrient interactions (with prescribed medications, supplements, alcohol, and other drugs)

The ultimate goal of nutrition intervention is to impose the least number of changes necessary in the person's normal food patterns to support optimal nutrition status while providing comfort and quality of life.

CASE STUDY

Obesity/Overweight: Estella

Estella is a 34-year-old single mother of three children sharing a small apartment with her 68-year-old mother in inner city Los Angeles. She is a full-time laborer in a local manufacturing facility and attends night classes to obtain her medical assistant's license. She is receiving some government assistance but is raising her children, aged 4, 7, and 10 years, on a meager income. Most days she arrives home too tired to prepare a well-balanced meal for her family and admits to eating a lot of fast food. Her mother, despite declining vision, works part-time evenings at a local fast-food restaurant to help with financial difficulties. Her mother is responsible for most of the meal preparation. Their diet consists mainly of inexpensive carbohydrates: flour tortillas, breads, pasta, cheese, and potatoes. The family budget does not allow for much fresh fruit or vegetables or expensive meats; therefore, she frequently serves bologna and hot dogs. There are few food stores accessible in her neighborhood.

The county hospital recently hired Estella as a nursing assistant. A required preemployment physical examination revealed several health risks. At 5 feet, 4 inches, she weighs 185 pounds. Her resting heart rate and blood pressure are also above normal levels. She has a family history of diabetes and heart disease:

her father died of a heart attack at age 55 years, and her mother has diabetes that requires daily insulin injections. The health care provider referred Estella to her primary care physician, who recommended immediate lifestyle changes, including walking 30 minutes per day, four to five days/week, as well as seeing an RDN for nutrition therapy.

Reflective Questions for Recognizing and Analyzing Cues

- What dietary habits would you address with Estella?
- What health-related risk factors does Estella exhibit that may be positively addressed through dietary changes?
- What resources may be helpful in increasing the access to fruits and vegetables for Estella and her family?

SUMMARY

- This chapter has introduced a wide range of subjects, including the Healthy People initiative and Dietary Guidelines for Americans nutrition objectives, the most current diet recommendations to reduce the risks of developing nutrition-related diseases, FDA regulations for food labeling, government nutrition assistance programs for disadvantaged and older Americans, and primary and secondary prevention strategies related to the most common nutrition-related chronic diseases.
- These topics form the basis of preventive nutrition, a requisite for the promotion of the nation's public health.
- Current, evidence-based nutrition education materials and continuing nutrition education literature for professionals are available at https://eatright.org from the Academy of Nutrition and Dietetics.

EVOLVE CHAPTER FEATURES

http://evolve.elsevier.com/Edelman/

- Study Questions

REFERENCES

Abrahamowicz, A. A., Ebinger, J., Whelton, S. P., Commodore-Mensah, Y., & Yang, E. (2023). Racial and ethnic disparities in hypertension: Barriers and opportunities to improve blood pressure control. *Current Cardiology Reports*, *25*(1), 17–27. https://doi.org/10.1007/s11886-022-01826-x

Agriculture, USDO. (2022). *National data sets useful in food and nutrition assistance research*. https://www.ers.usda.gov/topics/food-nutrition-assistance/food-assistance-data-collaborative-research-programs/national-data-sets/

American Cancer Society. (2020). *American Cancer Society guideline for diet and physical activity*. https://www.cancer.org/cancer/risk-prevention/diet-physical-activity/acs-guidelines-nutrition-physical-activity-cancer-prevention/guidelines.html

American Diabetes Association. (2018). Standards of medical care in diabetes—2019: introduction. *Diabetes Care*, *42*(Suppl. 1), S1–S2. https://doi.org/10.2337/dc19-Sint01

American Diabetes Association. (2019). Lifestyle management: Standards of medical care in diabetes-2019. *Diabetes Care*, *42*(Suppl. 1), S46–S60. https://doi.org/10.2337/dc19-S005

American Heart Association, Inc. (n.d.). *Diet and lifestyle recommendations*. https://www.heart.org/en/healthy-living/healthy-eating/eat-smart/nutrition-basics/aha-diet-and-lifestyle-recommendations. Accessed November 1, 2021.

Amini, M., Zayeri, F., & Salehi, M. (2021). Trend analysis of cardiovascular disease mortality, incidence, and mortality-to-incidence ratio: Results from global burden of disease study 2017. *BMC Public Health*, *21*(1), 401. https://doi.org/10.1186/s12889-021-10429-0

Appel, L. J., Moore, T. J., Obarzanek, E., Vollmer, W. M., Svetkey, L. P., Sacks, F. M. (1997). A clinical trial of the effects of dietary patterns on blood pressure. *New England Journal of Medicine*, *336*(16), 1117–1124. https://doi.org/10.1056/nejm199704173361601

Arnett, D. K., Blumenthal, R. S., Albert, M. A., Buroker, A. B., Goldberger, Z. D., Hahn, E. J. (2019). 2019 ACC/AHA guideline on the primary prevention of cardiovascular disease: a report of the American College of Cardiology/American Heart Association Task Force on Clinical Practice Guidelines. *Circulation*, *140*(11), e596–e646. https://doi.org/doi:10.1161/CIR.0000000000000678

Association for Size Diversity and Health. (2020). https://asdah.org/

Barry, M. J., Nicholson, W. K., Silverstein, M., Chelmow, D., Coker, T. R., Davis, E. M. (2023). Folic acid supplementation to prevent neural tube defects: US preventive services task force reaffirmation recommendation statement. *The Journal of the American Medical Association*, *330*(5), 454–459.

Bays, H. E., Taub, P. R., Epstein, E., Michos, E. D., Ferraro, R. A., Bailey, A. L., et al. (2021). Ten things to know about ten cardiovascular disease risk factors. *American Journal of Preventive Cardiology*, *5*, 100149. https://doi.org/10.1016/j.ajpc.2021.100149

Belanger, M. J., Kovell, L. C., Turkson-Ocran, R. A., Mukamal, K. J., Liu, X., Appel, L. J., et al. (2023). Effects of the dietary approaches to stop hypertension diet on change in cardiac biomarkers over time: results from the DASH-Sodium Trial. *Journal of the American Heart Association*, *12*(2), e026684.

Björkegren, J. L. M., & Lusis, A. J. (2022). Atherosclerosis: Recent developments. *Cell*, *185*(10), 1630–1645. https://doi.org/10.1016/j.cell.2022.04.004

Bone Health and Osteoporosis Foundation. (2022). *Are you at risk?* https://www.bonehealthandosteoporosis.org/preventing-fractures/general-facts/bone-basics/are-you-at-risk/

Center on Budget and Policy Priorities. (2022). *Policy basics: The Supplemental Nutrition Assistance Program (SNAP)*. https://www.cbpp.org/sites/default/files/policybasics-SNAP-6-9-22.pdf

Centers for Disease Control and Prevention. (2022). *Diabetes risk factors*. https://www.cdc.gov/diabetes/basics/risk-factors.html

Centers for Disease Control and Prevention. (2023a). *Estimated HIV incidence and prevalence in the United States, 2017–2021*. https://stacks.cdc.gov/view/cdc/149080

Centers for Disease Control and Prevention. (2023b). *National diabetes statistics report*. https://www.cdc.gov/diabetes/data/statistics-report/index.html

Centers for Disease Control and Prevention. (2023c). *Overweight and obesity: strategies to prevent obesity*. https://www.cdc.gov/obesity/resources/strategies-guidelines.html

Chen, P. J., & Antonelli, M. (2020). Conceptual models of food choice: Influential factors related to foods, individual differences, and society. *Foods*, *9*(12), 1898.

Chouraqui, J.-P., Turck, D., Briend, A., Darmaun, D., Bocquet, A., Feillet, F., et al. (2021). Religious dietary rules and their potential nutritional and health consequences. *International Journal of Epidemiology*, *50*(1), 12–26.

Clarke, E. D., Stanford, J., Gomes-Marin, M., & Collins, C. E. (2024). Revisiting the impact of health at every size interventions on health and cardiometabolic related outcomes: An updated systematic review with meta-analysis. *Nutrition and Dietetics*, *81*(3), 261–282. https://doi.org/10.1111/1747-0080.12869

Coleman-Jensen, A., Rabbitt, M. P., Gregory, C. A., & Singh, A. (2022). Household food security in the United States. *Economic Research Report*, *155*.

Cong, W., & Chen, K. (2019). Traditional Chinese medicine and aging: Integration and collaboration promotes healthy aging. *Aging Medicine (Milton)*, *2*(3), 139–141. https://doi.org/10.1002/agm2.12077

Crowe, W., Pan, X., Mackle, J., Harris, A., Hardiman, G., Elliott, C. T., et al. (2022). Dietary inclusion of nitrite-containing frankfurter exacerbates colorectal cancer pathology and alters metabolism in APCmin mice. *NPJ Science of Food*, *6*(1), 60. https://doi.org/10.1038/s41538-022-00174-y

de Vos, W. M., Tilg, H., Van Hul, M., & Cani, P. D. (2022). Gut microbiome and health: Mechanistic insights. *Gut*, *71*(5), 1020–1032.

Dietary Guidelines for Americans 2020-2025. https://www.dietaryguidelines.gov/sites/default/files/2021-03/Dietary_Guidelines_for_Americans-2020-2025.pdf.

Dorner, B., & Friedrich, E. K. (2018). Position of the Academy of Nutrition and Dietetics: Individualized nutrition approaches for older adults: Long-term care, post-acute care, and other settings. *Journal of the Academy of Nutrition and Dietetics*, *118*(4), 724–735. https://doi.org/10.1016/j.jand.2018.01.022

Elgaddal, N., Kramarow, E. A., & Reuben, C. A. (2022). *Physical activity among adults aged 18 and over: United States, 2020 (NCHS Data Brief, No. 443)*. https://www.cdc.gov/nchs/data/databriefs/db443.pdf

English, L. K., Ard, J. D., Bailey, R. L., Bates, M., Bazzano, L. A., Boushey, C. J., et al. (2021). Evaluation of dietary patterns and all-cause mortality: A systematic review. *The Journal of the American Medical Association Network Open*, *4*(8), e2122277.

Enright, C., Thomas, E., & Saxon, D. R. (2023). An updated approach to antiobesity pharmacotherapy: Moving beyond the 5% weight loss goal. *Journal of the Endocrine Society*, *7*(3), bvac195.

Evert, A. B., Dennison, M., Gardner, C. D., Garvey, W. T., Lau, K. H. K., MacLeod, J., et al. (2019). Nutrition therapy for adults with diabetes or prediabetes: A consensus report. *Diabetes Care*, *42*(5), 731–754.

Fan, Y., Yao, Q., Liu, Y., Jia, T., Zhang, J., & Jiang, E. (2022). Underlying causes and co- existence of malnutrition and infections: An exceedingly common death risk in cancer. *Frontiers in Nutrition*, *9*, 814095.

Farhadi, F., Aliyari, R., Ebrahimi, H., Hashemi, H., Emamian, M. H., & Fotouhi, A. (2023). Prevalence of uncontrolled hypertension and its associated factors in 50–74 years old Iranian adults: A population-based study. *BMC Cardiovascular Disorders*, *23*(1), 318. https://doi.org/10.1186/s12872-023-03357-x

Filippou, C., Tatakis, F., Polyzos, D., Manta, E., Thomopoulos, C., Nihoyannopoulos, P., et al. (2022). Overview of salt restriction in the Dietary Approaches to Stop Hypertension (DASH) and the Mediterranean diet for blood pressure reduction. *Reviews in Cardiovascular Medicine*, *23*(1), 36.

Franzago, M., Santurbano, D., Vitacolonna, E., & Stuppia, L. (2020). Genes and diet in the prevention of chronic diseases in future generations. *International Journal of Molecular Sciences*, *21*(7), 2633. https://doi.org/10.3390/ijms21072633

Greupner, T., Schneider, I., & Hahn, A. (2017). Calcium bioavailability from mineral waters with different mineralization in comparison to milk and a supplement. *Journal of the American College of Nutrition*, *36*(5), 386–390. https://doi.org/10.1080/07315724.2017.1299651

Hales, C. M., Carroll, M. D., Fryar, C. D., & Ogden, C. L. (2020). *Prevalence of obesity and severe obesity among adults: United States, 2017-2018. (NCHS Data Brief, No. 360)*. https://www.cdc.gov/nchs/data/databriefs/db360-h.pdf

Horn, D. B., Almandoz, J. P., & Look, M. (2022). What is clinically relevant weight loss for your patients and how can it be achieved? A narrative review. *Postgraduate Medicine*, *134*(4), 359–375. https://doi.org/10.1080/00325481.2022.2051366

Horne, J. R., Nielsen, D. E., Madill, J., Robitaille, J., Vohl, M. C., & Mutch, D. M. (2022). Guiding global best practice in personalized nutrition based on genetics: The development of a nutrigenomics care map. *Journal of the Academy of Nutrition and Dietetics*, *122*(2), 259–269. https://doi.org/10.1016/j.jand.2021.02.008

Hou, K., Wu, Z. X., Chen, X. Y., Wang, J.Q., Zhang, D., Xiao, C., et al. (2022). Microbiota in health and diseases. *Signal Transduction and Targeted Therapy*, *7*(1), 135.

Hu, K., & Staiano, A. E. (2022). Trends in obesity prevalence among children and adolescents aged 2 to 19 years in the US from 2011 to 2020. *The Journal of the American Medical Association Pediatrics*, *176*(10), 1037–1039.

Imtiyaz, H., Soni, P., & Yukongdi, V. (2021). Investigating the role of psychological, social, religious and ethical determinants on consumers' purchase intention and consumption of convenience food. *Foods*, *10*(2), 237. https://doi.org/10.3390/foods10020237

Inciong, J. F. B., Chaudhary, A., Hsu, H. S., Joshi, R., Seo, J. M., Trung, L. V., et al. (2022). Economic burden of hospital malnutrition: A cost-of-illness model. *European Society for Clinical Nutrition and Metabolism*, *48*, 342–350. https://doi.org/10.1016/j.clnesp.2022.01.020

Inoue, T., Misu, S., Tanaka, T., Kakehi, T., & Ono, R. (2019). Acute phase nutritional screening tool associated with functional outcomes of hip fracture patients: A longitudinal study to compare MNA-SF, MUST, NRS-2002 and GNRI. *Clinical Nutrition*, *38*(1), 220–226. https://doi.org/10.1016/j.clnu.2018.01.030

Institute of Medicine. (2011). *Dietary reference intakes for calcium and vitamin D*. Washington, DC: National Academies Press.

Institute of Medicine (US) Committee on Prevention of Obesity in Children and Youth. (2005). Preventing childhood obesity: Health in the balance. In J. P. Koplan, C. T. Liverman, & V. I. Kraak (Eds.), *The National Academies collection: reports funded by National Institutes of Health*. Washington, DC: National Academies Press.

Jackson, M. I. (2015). Early childhood WIC participation, cognitive development and academic achievement. *Social Science and Medicine*, *126*, 145–153. https://doi.org/10.1016/j.socscimed.2014.12.018

Jayedi, A., Soltani, S., Zargar, M. S., Khan, T. A., & Shab-Bidar, S. (2020). Central fatness and risk of all cause mortality: Systematic review and dose-response meta-analysis of 72 prospective cohort studies. *British Medical Journal*, *370*, m3324. https://doi.org/10.1136/bmj.m3324

Jin, H., & Lu, Y. (2021). Evaluating consumer nutrition environment in food deserts and food swamps. *International Journal of Environmental Research and Public Health*, *18*(5), 2675. https://doi.org/10.3390/ijerph18052675

Jones-Garcia, E., Bakalis, S., & Flintham, M. (2022). Consumer behaviour and food waste: Understanding and mitigating waste with a technology probe. *Foods, 11*(14), 2048. https://doi.org/10.3390/foods11142048

Kabashneh, S., Alkassis, S., Shanah, L., & Ali, H. (2020). A complete guide to identify and manage malnutrition in hospitalized patients. *Cureus, 12*(6), e8486. https://doi.org/10.7759/cureus.8486

Kansra, A. R., Lakkunarajah, S., & Jay, M. S. (2021). Childhood and adolescent obesity: A review. *Frontiers in Pediatrics, 8*, 866.

Kapelari, S., Alexopoulos, G., Moussouri, T., Sagmeister, K. J., & Stampfer, F. (2020). Food heritage makes a difference: The importance of cultural knowledge for improving education for sustainable food choices. *Sustainability, 12*(4), 1509.

Key, T. J., Bradbury, K. E., Perez-Cornago, A., Sinha, R., Tsilidis, K. K., & Tsugane, S. (2020). Diet, nutrition, and cancer risk: What do we know and what is the way forward? *British Medical Journal, 368*, m511. https://doi.org/10.1136/bmj.m511

Khan, L. K., Sobush, K., Keener, D., Goodman, K., Lowry, A., Kakietek, J., et al. (2009). Recommended community strategies and measurements to prevent obesity in the United States. *Morbidity and Mortality Weekly Report Recommendations and Report, 58*(RR-7), 1–26. https://www.cdc.gov/mmwr/preview/mmwrhtml/rr5807a1.htm

Kivimäki, M., Strandberg, T., Pentti, J., Nyberg, S. T., Frank, P., Jokela, M., et al. (2022). Body-mass index and risk of obesity-related complex multimorbidity: An observational multicohort study. *The Lancet Diabetes & Endocrinology, 10*(4), 253–263.

Kleinendorst, L., van Haelst, M. M., & van den Akker, E. L. (2019). Genetics of obesity. *Genetics of Endocrine Diseases and Syndromes*, 419–441.

Kris-Etherton, P. M., Petersen, K. S., Velarde, G., Barnard, N. D., Miller, M., Ros, E., et al. (2020). Barriers, opportunities, and challenges in addressing disparities in diet-related cardiovascular disease in the United States. *Journal of the American Heart Association, 9*(7), e014433. https://doi.org/10.1161/jaha.119.014433

Lange, S. J., Moore, L. V., Harris, D. M., Merlo, C. L., Lee, S. H., Demissie, Z., et al. (2021). Percentage of adolescents meeting federal fruit and vegetable intake recommendations—Youth Risk Behavior Surveillance System, United States, 2017. *Morbidity and Mortality Weekly Report, 70*(3), 69.

Lee, S. H., Moore, L. V., Park, S., Harris, D. M., & Blanck, H. M. (2022). Adults meeting fruit and vegetable intake recommendations—United States, 2019. *Morbidity and Mortality Weekly Report, 71*(1), 1.

Li, M., Gong, W., Wang, S., & Li, Z. (2022). Trends in body mass index, overweight and obesity among adults in the USA, the NHANES from 2003 to 2018: A repeat cross-sectional survey. *British Medical Journal Open, 12*(12), e065425.

Lichtenstein, A. H., Appel, L. J., Vadiveloo, M., Hu, F. B., Kris-Etherton, P. M., Rebholz, C. M., et al. (2021). 2021 dietary guidance to improve cardiovascular health: A scientific statement from the American Heart Association. *Circulation, 144*(23), e472–e487. https://doi.org/10.1161/cir.0000000000001031

Looker, A. C., Sarafrazi Isfahani, N., Fan, B., & Shepherd, J. A. (2017). Trends in osteoporosis and low bone mass in older US adults, 2005-2006 through 2013-2014. *Osteoporosis International, 28*(6), 1979–1988. https://doi.org/10.1007/s00198-017-3996-1

Loos, R. J., & Yeo, G. S. (2022). The genetics of obesity: From discovery to biology. *Nature Reviews Genetics, 23*(2), 120–133.

Marra, M. V., & Bailey, R. L. (2018). Position of the Academy of Nutrition and Dietetics: Micronutrient supplementation. *Journal of the Academy of Nutrition and Dietetics, 118*(11), 2162–2173.

Marshall, K., Teo, L., Shanahan, C., Legette, L., & Mitmesser, S. H. (2020). Inadequate calcium and vitamin D intake and osteoporosis risk in older Americans living in poverty with food insecurities. *Public Library of Science One, 15*(7), e0235042. https://doi.org/10.1371/journal.pone.0235042

McCullough, M. L., Hodge, R. A., Campbell, P. T., Guinter, M. A., & Patel, A. V. (2022). Sugar-and artificially-sweetened beverages and cancer mortality in a large US prospective cohort. *Cancer Epidemiology, Biomarkers & Prevention, 31*(10), 1907–1918.

McElfish, P. A., Rowland, B., Scott, A. J., Niemeier, J., Hoose, D. V., & Long, C. R. (2022). Sugar-sweetened beverage consumption is associated with higher body mass index among Marshallese adults in Arkansas. *Journal of Hunger & Environmental Nutrition, 17*(3), 333–346.

Meek, J. Y., Noble, L., & Section on Breastfeeding. (2022). Policy statement: Breastfeeding and the use of human milk. *Pediatrics, 150*(1), e2022057988.

Mishra, S., Stierman, B., Gahche, J. J., & Potischman, N. (2021). Dietary supplement use among adults: United States, 2017–2018. *National Center for Health Statistics Data Brief*, (399), 1–8.

Mogensen, K. M., Malone, A., Becker, P., Cutrell, S., Frank, L., Gonzales, K., et al. (2019). Academy of Nutrition and Dietetics/American Society for Parenteral and Enteral Nutrition consensus malnutrition characteristics: Usability and association with outcomes. *Nutrition in Clinical Practice, 34*(5), 657–665. https://doi.org/10.10002/ncp.10310.

Mokdad, A. H., Ballestros, K., Echko, M., Glenn, S., Olsen, H. E., Mullany, E., et al. (2018). The state of US health, 1990-2016: Burden of diseases, injuries, and risk factors among US states. *The Journal of the American Medical Association, 319*(14), 1444–1472.

National Academies of Sciences, Engineering, and Medicine. (2019). *Summary report of the dietary reference intakes*. https://www.nationalacademies.org/our-work/summary-report-of-the-dietary-reference-intakes

O'Callaghan, K. M., Taghivand, M., Zuchniak, A., Onoyovwi, A., Korsiak, J., Leung, M., et al. (2020). Vitamin D in breastfed infants: Systematic review of alternatives to daily supplementation. *Advances in Nutrition, 11*(1), 144–159.

Ojangba, T., Boamah, S., Miao, Y., Guo, X., Fen, Y., Agboyibor, C., et al. (2023). Comprehensive effects of lifestyle reform, adherence, and related factors on hypertension control: A review. *Journal of Clinical Hypertension (Greenwich), 25*(6), 509–520. https://doi.org/10.1111/jch.14653

Onwuzo, C., Olukorode, J. O., Omokore, O. A., Odunaike, O. S., Omiko, R., Osaghae, O. W., et al. (2023). DASH diet: A review of its scientifically proven hypertension reduction and health benefits. *Cureus, 15*(9), e44692.

Ozturk, Y., Sarikaya, D., Emin Kuyumcu, M., Yesil, Y., Koca, M., Guner Oytun, M., et al. (2022). Comparison of mini nutritional assessment-short and long form to predict all-cause mortality up to 7 years in geriatric outpatients. *Nutrition in Clinical Practice, 37*(6), 1418–1428. https://doi.org/10.1002/ncp.10878

Pati, S., Irfan, W., Jameel, A., Ahmed, S., & Shahid, R. K. (2023). Obesity and cancer: A current overview of epidemiology, pathogenesis, outcomes, and management. *Cancers (Basel), 15*(2), 485. https://doi.org/10.3390/cancers15020485

Powell-Wiley, T. M., Poirier, P., Burke, L. E., Després, J.-P., Gordon-Larsen, P., Lavie, C. J., et al. (2021). Obesity and cardiovascular disease: A scientific statement from the American Heart Association. *Circulation, 143*(21), e984–e1010.

Quinlan, M. B. (2022). Ethnomedicines: Traditions of medical knowledge. In M. Singer, P. Erickson, & C. Adadia-Barrero (Eds.), *A companion to medical anthropology* (2nd ed., pp. 315–341). Wiley & Sons.

Rashki Kemmak, A., Rezapour, A., Jahangiri, R., Nikjoo, S., Farabi, H., & Soleimanpour, S. (2020). Economic burden of osteoporosis in the world: A systematic review. *Medical Journal of the Islamic Republic of Iran, 34*, 154. PMCID: PMC7787041.

Serón-Arbeloa, C., Labarta-Monzón, L., Puzo-Foncillas, J., Mallor-Bonet, T., Lafita-López, A., Bueno-Vidales, N., et al. (2022). Malnutrition screening and assessment. *Nutrients, 14*(12), 2392.

Siegel, R. L., Giaquinto, A. N., & Jemal, A. (2024). Cancer statistics, 2024. *CA: A Cancer Journal for Clinicians, 74*(1), 12–49.

Siegel, R. L., Miller, K. D., Wagle, N. S., & Jemal, A. (2023). Cancer statistics, 2023. *CA: A Cancer Journal for Clinicians, 73*(1), 17–48.

Sikalidis, A. K., & Maykish, A. (2020). The gut microbiome and type 2 diabetes mellitus: Discussing a complex relationship. *Biomedicines, 8*(1), 8.

Spark, A. (2001). Health at any size: The size-acceptance nondiet movement. *Journal of the American Medical Women's Association (1972), 56*(2), 69–72.

Stallings, V. A., Harrison, M., & Oria, M. (2019). *Dietary reference intakes for sodium and potassium.* Washington, DC: National Academies Press.

Stierman, B., Afful, J., Carroll, M., Chen, T., Davy, O., Fink, S., et al. (2023). *National Health and Nutrition Examination Survey 2017–March 2020 Prepandemic data files development of files and prevalence estimates for selected health outcomes. National Health Statistics Reports No. 158. June 14, 2021.* National Center for Health Statistics. doi:10.15620/cdc:106273

Tahrani, A. A., & Morton, J. (2022). Benefits of weight loss of 10% or more in patients with overweight or obesity: A review. *Obesity (Silver Spring), 30*(4), 802–840. https://doi.org/10.1002/oby.23371

Theodoridis, X., Chourdakis, M., Chrysoula, L., Chroni, V., Tirodimos, I., Dipla, K., et al. (2023). Adherence to the DASH diet and risk of hypertension: A systematic review and meta-analysis. *Nutrients, 15*(14), 3261. https://doi.org/10.3390/nu15143261

Tian, X., Chen, J., Wang, X., Xie, Y., Zhang, X., Han, D., et al. (2023). Global, regional, and national HIV/AIDS disease burden levels and trends in 1990–2019: A systematic analysis for the global burden of disease 2019 study. *Frontiers in Public Health, 11*, 1068664.

Trampisch, U. S., Pourhassan, M., Daubert, D., Volkert, D., & Wirth, R. (2022). Interrater reliability of routine screening for risk of malnutrition with the Mini Nutritional Assessment Short-Form in hospital. *European Journal of Clinical Nutrition, 76*(8), 1111–1116. https://doi.org/10.1038/s41430-022-01080-y

US Department of Agriculture. (2023a). *Child nutrition programs, national school lunch program.* https://www.ers.usda.gov/topics/food-nutrition-assistance/child-nutrition-programs/national-school-lunch-program/

US Department of Agriculture. (2023b). *Child nutrition programs, school breakfast program.* https://www.ers.usda.gov/topics/food-nutrition-assistance/child-nutrition-programs/school-breakfast-program/#:~:text=In%20fiscal%20year%20(FY)%202019,the%20meals%20served%20to%20students

US Department of Agriculture. (2023c). *Food & nutrition assistance, WIC program.* https://www.ers.usda.gov/topics/food-nutrition-assistance/wic-program/

US Department of Agriculture & US Department of Health and Human Services. (2020). *Dietary guidelines for Americans, 2020-2025* (9th ed.). https://www.dietaryguidelines.gov/sites/default/files/2021-03/Dietary_Guidelines_for_Americans-2020-2025.pdf

US Department of Agriculture & US Department of Health and Human Services. (2020). *Dietary guidelines for Americans, 2020-2025. 9th edition.* https://www.dietaryguidelines.gov/sites/default/files/2021-03/Dietary_Guidelines_for_Americans-2020-2025.pdf

US Department of Health and Human Services. (2023a). *Dietary reference intakes development.* https://health.gov/our-work/nutrition-physical-activity/dietary-guidelines/dietary-reference-intakes/dietary-reference-intakes-development

US Department of Health and Human Services. (2023b). *Healthy People 2030 framework.* https://health.gov/healthypeople/about/healthy-people-2030-framework

US Department of Health and Human Services, US Department of Agriculture & Dietary Guidelines Advisory Committee. (2015). *Dietary guidelines for Americans, 2015–2020* (8th ed.). Washington, DC: US Department of Health and Human Services and US Department of Agriculture.

US Department of Agriculture, Agricultural Research Service. (2021). *Usual nutrient intake for food and bervarages, by gender and age, what we eat in America.* http://www.ars.usda/gov/ARSUserFiles/80400530/pdf/usual/Usual_Intake_gender_WWEIA-2015_2018.pdf

US Food and Drug Administration. (2023). *Dietary supplements guidance documents & regulatory information.* https://www.fda.gov/food/guidance-documents-regulatory-information-topic-food-and-dietary-supplements/dietary-supplements-guidance-documents-regulatory-information

US Food & Drug Administration. (2023). *Get the facts about salmonella.* https://www.fda.gov/animal-veterinary/animal-health-literacy/get-facts-about-salmonella

USA Facts. (2023). *How many people get sick from foodborne illnesses.* https://usafacts.org/articles/how-many-people-get-sick-from-foodborne-illnesses/

Veettil, S. K., Wong, T. Y., Loo, Y. S., Playdon, M. C., Lai, N. M., Giovannucci, E. L., et al. (2021). Role of diet in colorectal cancer incidence: Umbrella review of meta-analyses of prospective observational studies. *The Journal of the American Medical Association Network Open, 4*(2), e2037341. https://doi.org/10.1001/jamanetworkopen.2020.37341

Venkataramani, M., Ogunwole, S. M., Caulfield, L. E., Sharma, R., Zhang, A., Gross, S. M., et al. (2022). Maternal, infant, and child health outcomes associated with the special supplemental nutrition program for women, infants, and children: A systematic review. *Annals of Internal Medicine, 175*(10), 1411–1422.

Verde, L., Frias-Toral, E., & Cardenas, D. (2023). Environmental factors implicated in obesity. *Frontiers in Nutrition, 10*, 1171507.

Willig, A., Wright, L., & Galvin, T. A. (2018). Practice paper of the Academy of Nutrition and Dietetics: nutrition intervention and human immunodeficiency virus infection. *Journal of the Academy of Nutrition and Dietetics, 118*(3), 486–498. https://doi.org/10.1016/j.jand.2017.12.007

Wright, N. C., Saag, K. G., Dawson-Hughes, B., Khosla, S., & Siris, E. S. (2017). The impact of the new National Bone Health Alliance (NBHA) diagnostic criteria on the prevalence of osteoporosis in the USA. *Osteoporosis International, 28*(4), 1225–1232. https://doi.org/10.1007/s00198-016-3865-3

Yano, Y., Reis, J. P., Colangelo, L. A., Shimbo, D., Viera, A. J., Allen, N. B., et al. (2018). Association of blood pressure classification in young adults using the 2017 American College of Cardiology/American Heart Association blood pressure guideline with cardiovascular events later in life. *The Journal of the American Medical Association, 320*(17), 1774–1782. https://doi.org/10.1001/jama.2018.13551

Zhao, L., Zhang, X., Coday, M., Garcia, D. O., Li, X., Mossavar-Rahmani, Y., et al. (2023). Sugar-sweetened and artificially sweetened beverages and risk of liver cancer and chronic liver disease mortality. *The Journal of the American Medical Association, 330*(6), 537–546. https://doi.org/10.1001/jama.2023.12618

12

Physical Activity

Kevin K. Chui, Frank Tudini, Kent E. Irwin, Michele G. Criss and Mariana Wingood

http://evolve.elsevier.com/Edelman/

OBJECTIVES

After completing this chapter, the reader will be able to:

- Explain the physical activity and fitness goals of *Healthy People 2030* and the progress made toward these goals.
- Describe how physical activity positively influences physical and psychological health.
- Identify the benefits of physical activity throughout the aging process.
- Evaluate the prescriptions for and benefits of daily physical activity, aerobic exercise, and resistance training.
- Explain the interventions to promote exercise adherence and compliance.

KEY TERMS

Aerobic exercise
Anaerobic exercise
Arthritis
Cardiorespiratory fitness
Cool-down period
Cross-training
Exercise
Exercise prescription
Fat mass
Flexibility
Low back pain
Muscular fitness
Obesity
Osteoporosis
Physical activity
Physical fitness
Relaxation response
Resistance training
Rheumatoid arthritis
Tai Chi
Warm-up period
Yoga

 THINK ABOUT IT

Knowing versus Doing

Having knowledge of the benefits of exercise does not correlate well with long-term exercise compliance. Confidence in the ability to exercise and a sense of the meaning and purpose (core desire) of exercise in life ensure better success.

- What motivates an individual to put the effort into developing and maintaining an active lifestyle?
- Why is being active and physically fit important?

Regular physical activity and exercise enhance both physical and psychological health. Generally, people who exercise regularly, or those who naturally include physical activity in their daily routine, feel better mentally and physically, improve their health profiles, and safeguard their functional independence as they go through the aging process. A holistic approach to physical activity involves exercise for cardiorespiratory health (endurance), exercise for musculoskeletal health (strength, power, flexibility, and bone density), and body awareness. Body awareness and mindfulness during exercise facilitate self-inquiry and self-acceptance, helping to relieve psychological stress and preventing physical injury (Box 12.1: Health Effect of Physical Activity). Although an active lifestyle is an important component of primary prevention, regular physical activity is also an essential modality in the treatment of chronic disease, establishing the potential for benefit in all aspects of the biopsychosocial and spiritual model of health.

PHYSICAL ACTIVITY

Defining Physical Activity in Health

To ensure a full understanding of the *Healthy People 2030* core objectives regarding physical activity, this chapter will use the following definitions:

Physical activity: body movement that is produced by the contraction of skeletal muscles and that substantially increases energy expenditure; includes transportation and vocational and leisure-time activity, which can be further categorized into sports, recreational activities, and exercise training (Fig. 12.1)

Exercise (exercise training): planned, structured, and repetitive body movement performed to improve or maintain one or more components of physical fitness

Aerobic physical activity: activity that uses large muscle groups in a repetitive, rhythmical fashion over an extended period to increase the efficiency of the oxidative energy-producing system and increase cardiorespiratory endurance; uses stored adipose tissue as a major fuel source

BOX 12.1 Health Effect of Physical Activity

- Improves quality of life
- Improves mood and promotes a sense of well-being
- Increases flexibility
- Builds muscle strength
- Increases endurance
- Increases the efficiency of the heart
- Increases bone density
- Helps with weight reduction
- Decreases risk of stroke
- Decreases risk of heart disease
- Decreases risk of diabetes
- Decreases risk of several types of cancer

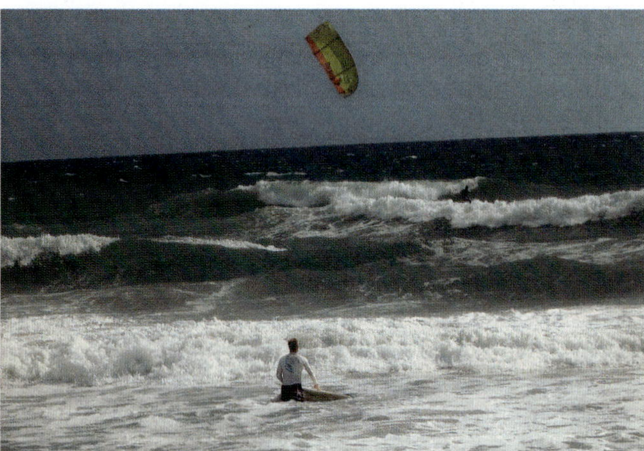

FIG. 12.1 Some people choose more vigorous types of exercise.

Anaerobic exercise: high-intensity, short-duration activity that increases the efficiency of the phosphocreatine and glycolytic energy-producing systems and increases muscle strength, power, and speed of reactivity; uses phosphagens and glucose-glycogen as major fuel sources

Physical fitness: a set of attributes (**cardiorespiratory fitness**, muscular fitness, and flexibility) that people have or achieve that relates to the ability to perform physical activity without undue fatigue or risk of injury

Physical inactivity: self-report of engaging in no leisure-time physical activity during the past month

Muscular fitness: the strength and endurance of muscles that allows participation in daily activities with low risk of musculoskeletal injury

Flexibility: adequate muscle length and joint mobility to allow free and painless movement through a wide range of motion (ROM)

Healthy People 2030 Objectives

Every decade, the *Healthy People* initiative, developed by the Department of Health and Human Services, generates 10-year national objectives with the goal of improving the health of all Americans. Unfortunately, of the 985 *Healthy People 2020* trackable objectives, only 33.9% met or exceeded goals, while 20.8% improved, 31% had no change, and 14.3% got worse. Furthermore, rates improved significantly more for those with higher incomes versus lower (64.8% vs. 38.4%), those with advanced degrees (69.6% vs. 38.6%), and those without disabilities compared with those with disabilities (47.2% vs. 32.5%). Only 24% of the adult population achieved the aerobic and muscle resistance training recommendations, and 25.4% of adults 18 years or older reported no leisure-time physical activity (US Department of Health and Human Services [USDHHS], 2018, 2023a). People were classified as being physically inactive if they responded "No" to the following question: "During the past month, other than your regular job, did you participate in any physical activities or exercises such as running, calisthenics, golf, gardening, or walking for exercise?" The percentage of adults who reported no leisure-time physical activity also differed by race and ethnicity, sex, educational level, geographical location, disability status, age group, and the presence or absence of **arthritis** symptoms. The tendency to be sedentary continues to increase with age and affects all the body's systems, such as the cutaneous, cardiovascular, respiratory, gastrointestinal, and urinary systems. As a result of a sedentary lifestyle, the risk of premature morbidity, death, impairment, functional limitation, and disability increases. The prevalence of physical inactivity decreased by a modest 0.7% from 2018 to 2020 (Van Dyke et al., 2023). The goal of the Physical Activity and Fitness Guidelines for Americans is to "improve health, fitness, and quality of life through regular physical activity" (USDHHS, 2023c). The guidelines recommend that preschool-aged children (aged 3–5 years) be physically active throughout the day to enhance growth and development. Children and adolescents (6–17 years) should perform at least 60 minutes of moderate to vigorous physical activity daily, and adults should perform at least: a) 150 minutes of moderate-intensity activity per week and muscle-strengthening activities 2 or more days per week, b) 75 minutes of vigorous activity per week and muscle-strengthening activities 2 or more days per week, or c) an equivalent mix of moderate- and vigorous-intensity aerobic activity 2 or more days per week and muscle-strengthening activities 2 or more days per week. In 2020, only 24.2% of adults met the guidelines for both aerobic and muscle-strengthening activities (Elgaddal et al., 2022).

Healthy People 2030 includes 359 core objectives, which are organized into topics including health conditions (e.g., cancer), health behaviors (e.g., physical activity), populations (e.g., children), settings and systems (e.g., environmental health), and social determinants of health (e.g., economic stability). A small subset of these objectives are considered leading health indicators, which cover the life span (i.e., infants, children and adolescents, and adults and older adults) and all ages. There are also developmental and research objectives, which may become core *Healthy People 2030* core objectives. The importance of physical activity for health is reflected in the *Healthy People 2030's* 13 core physical activity objectives (USDHHS, 2020b). Box 12.2 provides a summary of the updated physical activity objectives set for 2030. In addition to the *Healthy People* initiative, a National Physical Activity Plan complements the initiative and offers evidence-based strategies and tactics to attain these objectives. The plan considers the demonstrated relationship between physical

BOX 12.2 *HEALTHY PEOPLE 2030* PHYSICAL ACTIVITY OBJECTIVES

Symbol	*Healthy People 2030* Physical Activity Objectives
PA-01	Reduce the proportion of adults who do no physical activity in their free time
PA-02	Increase the proportion of adults who do enough aerobic physical activity for substantial health benefits
PA-03	Increase the proportion of adults who do enough aerobic physical activity for extensive health benefits
PA-04	Increase the proportion of adults who do enough muscle-strengthening activity
PA-05	Increase the proportion of adults who do enough aerobic and muscle-strengthening activity
PA-06	Increase the proportion of adolescents who do enough aerobic physical activity
PA-07	Increase the proportion of adolescents who do enough muscle-strengthening activity
PA-08	Increase the proportion of adolescents who do enough aerobic and muscle-strengthening activity
PA-09	Increase the proportion of children who do enough aerobic physical activity
PA-10	Increase the proportion of adults who walk or bike to get places
PA-11	Increase the proportion of adolescents who walk or bike to get places
PA-12	Increase the proportion of children and adolescents who play sports
PA-13	Increase the proportion of children aged 2 to 5 years who get no more than 1 hour of screen time a day

US Department of Health and Human Services. (n.d.). *Healthy People 2030: Browse objectives by topic.* https://health.gov/healthypeople/objectives-and-data/browse-objectives

activity and an improvement in the biologic markers associated with health, and it identifies the reasons for the trend toward a more sedentary lifestyle. The National Physical Activity Plan has a vision that all Americans be physically active in all aspects of their lives, including work and play (National Physical Activity Plan, 2022).

Physical Activity Objectives: Making Progress

The review of the physical activity data from *Healthy People 2020* (http://www.healthypeople.gov) provides evidence of the progress that has been made toward achieving the original objectives and the regress that has occurred.

Targets met or exceeded:

- Adults engaging in no leisure-time physical activity was 36.2% in 2008 and 25.4% in 2018.
- Adults engaging in regular physical activity—light or moderate for 150 minutes or more per week or vigorous for 75 minutes or more per week—was 43.5% in 2008 and 54.2% in 2018.
- Adults engaging in regular physical activity—light or moderate for 300 minutes or more per week or vigorous for 150 minutes or more per week—was 28.4% in 2008 and 37.4% in 2018.
- Adults performing muscle-strengthening activities 2 or more days per week was 21.9% in 2008 and 27.6% in 2018.
- Adults meeting aerobic physical activity and muscle-strengthening objectives was 18.2% in 2008 and 24.0% in 2018.

Worsening or little to no detectible changes:

- Adolescents meeting federal physical activity guidelines was 28.7% in 2011 and 26.1% in 2017.
- Adolescents meeting federal guidelines for muscle-strengthening activity was 55.6% in 2011 and 51.1% in 2017.
- Adolescents meeting federal guidelines for aerobic physical activity and muscle-strengthening activity was 21.9% in 2011 and 20.0% in 2017.
- Adolescents participating in daily school physical education was 33.3% in 2009 and 29.9% in 2017.
- Adolescents using a computer for nonschool work for 2 hours or less a day was 75.1% in 2009 and 57.0% in 2017.

Although adults are trending in a positive direction and have achieved some of the recommended physical activity goals set by *Healthy People 2020*, adolescents are trending in a negative direction. In 2019, only 23.2% of adolescents reported that they participated in at least 60 minutes of physical activity 7 days per week (compared with 26.1% in 2017), while 49.5% performed muscle-strengthening activity 3 days/week or more in 2019 (compared with 51.1% in 2017), and only 16.5% met both the aerobic and muscle-strengthening activity guidelines (compared with 20% in 2017).

The prevalence of obese children, adolescents, and adults has increased in the United States and is considered an epidemic. Children and adolescents (aged 2–19 years) are categorized as obese if their body mass index (BMI), expressed as weight in kilograms divided by height in meters squared, is equal to or greater than the 85th percentile in age- and sex-specific BMI growth charts (USDHHS, 2021). Results from the 2017–2018 National Health and Nutrition Examination Survey (NHANES) (2020) (https://www.cdc.gov/nchs/nhanes/index.htm) indicate that an estimated 19.3% of US children and adolescents aged 2 to 19 years have obesity, including 6.1% with severe obesity and another 16.1% who are overweight (Fryar et al., 2020).

Adults aged 20 years and older are considered overweight if their BMI is 25.0 to 29.9 kg/m^2, obese if their BMI is 30.0 kg/m^2 or higher, and extremely obese if their BMI is 40 kg/m^2 or higher. According to data from the NHANES for 2017 through 2018, the prevalence of obesity was 40.0% among adults aged 20 to 39, 44.8% among adults 40 to 59, and 42.8% among adults aged 60 and older. There were no significant differences in prevalence by age group (NHANES, 2020). The prevalence of obesity was lowest among non-Hispanic Asian adults (17.4%) compared with non-Hispanic White (42.2%), non-Hispanic Black (49.6%), and Hispanic (44.8%) adults. The prevalence of obesity was lowest among non-Hispanic Asian females (17.2%) compared with non-Hispanic White (39.8%), Hispanic (43.7%), and non-Hispanic Black (56.9%) females, and the prevalence among non-Hispanic Black females was higher than all other groups. Among males, the prevalence of obesity was lowest among non-Hispanic Asian males (17.5%) compared with non-Hispanic White (44.7%), non-Hispanic Black (41.1%), and Hispanic (45.7%) males. (NHANES, 2020). The prevalence of severe obesity increased from 7.7% to

9.2% during the same time frame. Females had a higher prevalence of severe obesity (11.5%) than males (6.9%). The prevalence was highest among adults aged 40 to 59 (11.5%) followed by adults aged 20 to 39 (9.1%) and adults aged 60 and over (5.8%). Non-Hispanic Black adults had the highest prevalence of severe obesity (13.8%), and non-Hispanic Asian adults had the lowest (2.0%).

The number of adults who combine good dietary practice with regular physical activity in an attempt to attain an appropriate body weight has decreased. This decidedly negative trend may be related to the decline in physical activity in and outside schools. According to Youth Risk Behavior Surveillance System (YRBSS) data, 29.9% of adolescents (9th to 12th graders) participated in daily school physical education in 2017, and that decreased to 25.9% in 2019 (USDHHS, 2020b). Youths attending physical education on 1 or more days per week also decreased from 56.4% in 2009 to 51.7% in 2017. Additionally, the proportion of elementary schools requiring daily physical education decreased from 4.4% in 2006 to 3.6% in 2014, while middle and junior high schools requiring daily physical education decreased from 10.5% to 3.4%. Compounding the problem is the significant increase in the percentage of 9th to 12th graders who report playing video or computer games or using a computer for 3 hours or more per day (31.1% in 2011, 41.3% in 2013, and 43% in 2017) and a decrease in the percentage who report playing on at least one sports team (58.4% in 2011, 54.0% in 2013, and 54.3% in 2017).

Physical activity during childhood and adolescence can affect later body composition through modifications in body fat induced during the early ages and prolonged into adulthood (Werneck et al., 2019). Maintaining normal BMI in youth is crucial to preventing obesity later in life. Early detection is key, as the majority of excess body weight in children who develop obesity is often gained before age 5 (Buscot et al., 2018). Thus if a standard is to be set for the importance of physical activity throughout the life span, it needs to start with children, who have the potential to develop lifelong healthy habits.

Due to the importance of preventing the consequences of inadequate physical activity, it is critical that health care providers empower their patients to become more physically active. Health care practitioners are in an ideal position to inquire about physical activity levels and utilize behavior change techniques. The importance of empowering patients to become more active is highlighted by the American Heart Association (AHA) and the US Preventive Taskforce (Lobelo et al., 2018). To assist with the integration of physical activity assessments and behavior change in clinical practice, the AHA has provided a list of recommendations for how to integrate assessment and promotion into clinical practice. For example, it is recommended that health care providers use simple assessment tools such as the Physical Activity Vital Sign (PAVS). Another recommendation is to use the transtheoretical model (stage of change model) to determine how to address a patient's inadequate activity levels (Lobelo et al., 2018). Although some progress has been made, particularly in physical activity for adults (CDC, 2018), obesity prevalence continues to rise in children, adolescents, and adults. Furthermore, there are still populations at greater risk of obesity based on race/ethnicity (such as non-Hispanic Black and Hispanic adults and youth), school type (public versus private) (Leal, 2018; Baniissa et al., 2020), and socioeconomic status (Hankonen, 2017; Anekwe, 2020). In a relevant systematic review, females of lower socioeconomic status had higher odds of obesity and a greater waist circumference compared with those in higher socioeconomic classes (Newton, et al., 2017). The same study called for improved public health strategies, reporting that at least 50% of noncommunicable disease–related deaths are preventable through modifiable risk factors such as obesity, physical activity, and nutrition (Newton et al., 2017) (Box 12.3: Populations with Low Rates of Physical Activity).

Aging

The biologic changes attributed to aging closely resemble the effects of physical inactivity. The changes seen with both aging and inactivity include an increase in body fat and decreases in all the following: aerobic capacity, muscle mass (sarcopenia), metabolic rate, strength and flexibility, bone mass, immune function, and sleep quality. Exercise is an effective, economical, nonpharmacologic strategy to mitigate the effects of aging and disease (CDC, 2023f). Among older adults, exercise can improve health, prevent disability and hospitalizations, improve blood lipid profiles, and reduce body fat. Older adults in particular need to be concerned about their nutritional status because the potential for malnutrition is associated with a decline in muscle strength and thus poorer outcomes, including decreased function and performance (Cheng et al., 2018; van Ancum, 2017).

According to the 2020 US census, the population aged 65 years and older has grown from 49.2 million people in 2016 to 55.9 million in 2020, or 16.8% of the population, and is projected to continue growing to 94.7 million by 2060. In 2030, for the first time in US history, older adults are projected to outnumber children (Vespa et al., 2020; US Census Bureau, 2018). Exercise is especially important for older individuals. Females in particular, who constitute the majority of the older population, benefit from the positive effects of exercise to improve bone health (Watson et al., 2018), reduce fall risk (Sherrington et al., 2019), and reduce fracture risk as part of a multidimensional approach (LaMonte et al., 2019).

By exercising, older people can improve levels of cardiovascular, cardiopulmonary, and metabolic functions, including muscle performance and aerobic capacity. Several researchers

BOX 12.3 Populations with Low Rates of Physical Activity

- Females are generally less active than males at all ages.
- People with lower incomes and less education are typically not as physically active as those with higher incomes and education.
- Black Americans and Hispanics are generally less physically active than Whites.
- Adults in northeastern and southern states tend to be less active than adults in north central and western states.
- People with disabilities are less physically active than people without disabilities.
- By age 75 years, one in three males and one in two females engage in no regular physical activity.

have reported significant increases or improvements in strength (Snijders et al., 2019), physical performance (Kidd et al., 2019), flexibility (Valenzuela et al., 2023), self-efficacy (Wada et al., 2019), quality of life (Chittrakul et al., 2020), continence (Kataria & Ilsley, 2021), bone density (Watson et al., 2018), balance (Thomas et al., 2019), safety (fewer falls and fall-related injuries) (Del Din et al., 2020), and ability to live independently (Olsen et al., 2022). Additional resources are available that discuss **exercise prescription** considerations and guidelines for the older adult; however, the weekly amount of moderate to vigorous physical activity for older adults is the same as for all adults (American College of Sports Medicine [ACSM], 2022a).

The health of the musculoskeletal system depends on movement and activity (Hart et al., 2020; Javaheri & Pitsillides, 2019). Bone is a dynamic tissue, constantly changing and adapting to the stresses to which it is subjected. Bone strength depends on stresses applied by muscular and weight-bearing activity (mechanical stress during active movement). Exercise may increase or maintain bone mineral density (BMD), but recent metaanalytic data suggest that the effects of exercises on BMD may depend on the mode of exercise, body part, combination of exercises (mixed loading), and other concurrent treatments such as pharmacologic intervention (Marin-Cascales et al., 2018). To stay healthy, joints also need to move and, in the lower extremities, bear weight. The health of the cartilage covering the joint surfaces is vital for maintaining proper joint function. The only way the cartilage can receive nourishment is through the cyclic loading and unloading of synovial fluid, which delivers nutrients, removes waste products, and lubricates joint surfaces. Movement is vital for the creation of this environment of blood and lymph in and out of joint structures and the adjacent soft tissues. Without the stress of weight-bearing activity, normal bone and cartilage metabolism and repair become dysfunctional, resulting in injury and disease.

In addition to the benefits of exercise on the musculoskeletal system, there are also positive relationships between fitness and cognitive performance. Physical training results in positive outcomes for brain structure, function, and cognition (Joubert & Chainay, 2018; Jia et al., 2019). There is evidence that moderate-intensity aerobic training, resistance training, and combination training are all associated with greater cognitive performance of executive functions (Northey et al., 2018). Furthermore, physical activity has been consistently found to be associated with reduced risk of developing dementia, Alzheimer disease, mild cognitive impairment, and cognitive decline (de Souto Barreto et al., 2018). In adults who already have mild cognitive impairment, physical exercise has been shown to have beneficial effects on global cognition (Song et al., 2018). However, the effects of specific exercise regimens (including frequency, type, intensity, and duration) have yet to be discovered (de Souto Barreto et al., 2018). Traditional Chinese exercise such as Tai Chi improved visuospatial function but had no effects on global cognitive functions (as measured with the minimental state examination), memory, executive function, verbal fluency, or depression in individuals with mild cognitive impairment (Zhang et al., 2019).

Effects of Exercise on the Aging Process

In 2020, 18% of adults ≥65 years had difficulty with at least one of the following functioning domains: hearing (29%), vision (21%), cognition (28%), ambulation (39%), self-care (8%) or communication (8%) (USDHHS, 2023b). Regular physical activity can help maintain functional independence and improve the quality of life throughout the aging process (Cunningham et al., 2020) (Fig. 12.2). Physical and psychological benefits of increased physical activity have been widely documented in healthy and in chronically ill older adults (Jourbert & Chainay, 2018). According to the CDC (2023c, 2023g), adults aged 65 and older need at least 150 minutes a week of moderate-intensity activity, such as brisk walking or 75 minutes a week of vigorous-intensity activity, such as hiking or running. The CDC also recommends 2 days a week of strengthening exercises. A recent study on community-dwelling older adults by Wingood et al. (2021) found that 91% of participants did not meet the full Physical Activity Guidelines for Americans. In addition, only 39% met the guidelines for moderate-vigorous physical activity, 26% for strength training, and 41% for balance activities. This is concerning, as low levels of physical activity are associated with higher risks of multimorbidity in older adults (Delpino et al., 2022). In combination with illness and injury, inadequate activity among older adults can accelerate multisystem decline and reduce quality of life, which can increase the risk of falls, frailty, and functional decline. The cumulative affect of illness, injury, and aging is illustrated by the Wellness Aging Model related to Inactivity, Illness, and Injury (WAMI-3) framework, a tool that promotes education on the critical importance of physical activity and encourages health care practitioners to look beyond current treatable impairments to envision the effect of prevention on future function (Billek-Sawhney et al., 2022).

Considerable research has investigated interventions to increase activity in populations of all ages, especially in older adults. Utilizing a personalized approach that aligns what matters to the older adult with exercise goals and action plans improves outcomes (Lachman et al., 2018; Wingood et al., 2023). This approach should also incorporate social support and

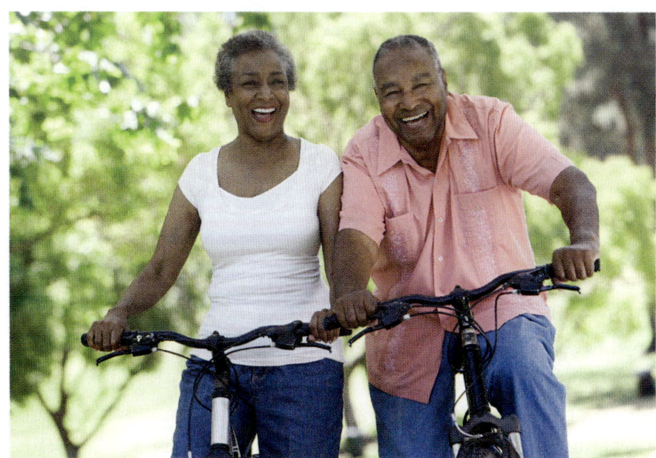

FIG. 12.2 Older adults can maintain functional independence while biking. From iStock.com/monkeybusinessimages

positive affect coupled with cognitive restructuring of negative and self-defeating attitudes and misconceptions. A few studies have even examined multicomponent cognitive-behavioral group interventions (Lachman et al., 2018). Lifestyle activity in older adults considers the accumulation of minutes of physical activity spread over the entire day. Some evidence suggests that lifestyle activity at any intensity combined with less sedentary time can substantially reduce the risk of premature mortality (Ekelund et al., 2019).

CARDIAC RISK FACTORS

The literature strongly demonstrates that the risk of cardiovascular disease (CVD) decreases as physical activity increases. A plausible relationship exists between decreased CVD risk and several exercise-induced physiologic and metabolic mechanisms such as (Liang et al., 2021):

- Increasing levels of high-density lipoprotein (HDL) cholesterol
- Decreasing levels of low-density lipoprotein (LDL) cholesterol
- Decreasing total cholesterol levels
- Decreasing serum triglyceride (TRG) levels
- Decreasing high blood pressure
- Improving glucose tolerance and insulin sensitivity
- Decreasing obesity; altering the distribution of body fat
- Reducing the sensitivity of the myocardium to the effects of catecholamines, thereby decreasing the risk of ventricular arrhythmias
- Enhancing fibrinolysis and altering platelet function

High-Density Lipoprotein and Serum Triglyceride Levels

For those with CVD, participation in exercise-based rehabilitation along with medical management reduces cardiovascular mortality, recurrent cardiac events, and hospitalizations while improving quality of life (Dibben et al., 2023). Exercise has a major influence on lipoprotein metabolism, primarily affecting plasma levels of HDL and serum triglyceride (TRG). There is a strong negative correlation between CVD and plasma HDL levels. Increases in HDL levels lower the total cholesterol-to-HDL ratio, thereby reducing CVD risk. Aerobic, resistance, and combined exercise helps control glucose and TRG levels (Liang et al., 2021). East Asian adults who performed moderate-intensity exercise in a volume of ≥150 minutes per week had significant improvements in HDL, LDL, total cholesterol, and TRG levels (Igarashi et al., 2019). Likewise, a metaanalysis of randomized controlled trials examining the effects of progressive resistance training on adults found significant reductions in total cholesterol levels; the ratio of total cholesterol to HDL; and the levels of non-HDL, LDL, and TRG (Ou et al., 2017; Costa et al., 2019). Other studies with school-aged and obese children found that physical activity training and exercise were associated with reductions in blood pressure, TRG levels, and overall cardiovascular risk profiles (Karaağaç, A., & Yıldırım, 2019; Lee, 2021; Seo et al., 2019).

Exercise intensity may explain changes in TRG levels, and volume may explain changes in HDL and LDL levels (Wood et al., 2021). At least moderate-intensity aerobic exercise training appears to have the greatest effect on HDL levels (Igarashi et al., 2019; Sarzynski et al., 2018). One systematic review found that high-intensity aerobic training promoted significant increases in HDL levels when performed in the range of 90 to 200 min/week. Additionally, resistance training resulted in a marked reduction in LDL levels, followed by a significant reduction in total cholesterol levels. Combining resistance and aerobic exercise led to remarkable reductions in LDL levels (Boeno et al., 2020), significant increases in HDL levels, and significant decreases in total cholesterol levels (Liang et al. 2021).

Hypertension

According to the CDC, nearly half of adults have hypertension (48.1%), defined as systolic blood pressure greater than 130 mmHg or diastolic blood pressure greater than 80 mmHg, or are taking medication for hypertension. Only 1 in 4 adults with hypertension have their hypertension under control. A greater percentage of males (50%) have high blood pressure compared with females (44%). High blood pressure is more common in non-Hispanic White adults (32%) than in non-Hispanic Black adults (25%), non-Hispanic Asian adults (19%), or Hispanic adults (25%) (CDC, 2023b).

The ACSM (2022b) and the AHA (2020) recommend **resistance training** in the prevention and treatment of hypertension (Box 12.4: Resistive Training Exercises). These recommendations are supported by study findings showing that in prehypertensive and hypertensive individuals, resistance training reduced both systolic and diastolic blood pressure (Nascimento et al., 2018). Evidence supporting the use of physical activity and exercise to improve and manage blood pressures is mixed. Part of this heterogeneity is the variability in the intervention (Saco-Ledo et al., 2020). Both low- to moderate-intensity aerobic exercise and high-intensity interval training result in comparable reductions in resting blood pressure in adults with pre- to established hypertension (Costa et al., 2018). Aquatic therapy has also been shown to reduce blood pressure in individuals 18 years and older, with decreases in systolic blood pressure similar to those performing land-based exercise (Reichert et al., 2018). In another metaanalysis of hypertensive populations, different types of exercise interventions appeared to be equally as effective as most antihypertensive medications (Naci et al., 2019). It seems that the blood pressure response to exercise is similar between sexes and different ethnicities. Although it is suggested that traditional Chinese exercise, including Tai Chi, Baduanjin Qigong, Wuqinxi, and YiJinjing, decreases blood pressure and blood lipids in individuals with hypertension, a recent systematic review and metaanalysis found no firm evidence to support the effectiveness and safety of this type of exercise due to the poor quality of the studies (Jin et al., 2019).

Hyperinsulinemia and Glucose Intolerance

Hyperinsulinemia and glucose intolerance account for the various types of diabetes. Diabetes mellitus encompasses a group of metabolic disorders that have in common an increase in blood glucose levels and associated metabolic dysfunction. According to the CDC (2023e), 38.4 million people

BOX 12.4 Resistive Training Exercises

Chest Press

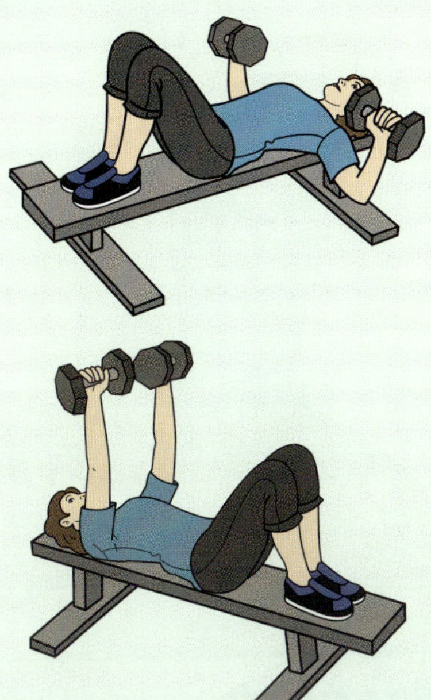

- Lie on a bench with feet flat on the bench, or lie on the floor with knees bent and feet flat, whichever is more comfortable.
- Hold weights near shoulders with elbows out and palms facing away from the body.
- Exhale while extending arms straight up, following an "A" pattern with the weights touching at the peak.
- Slowly lower the weights back to original position while inhaling.
- Repeat 8–12 times.

Chest Fly

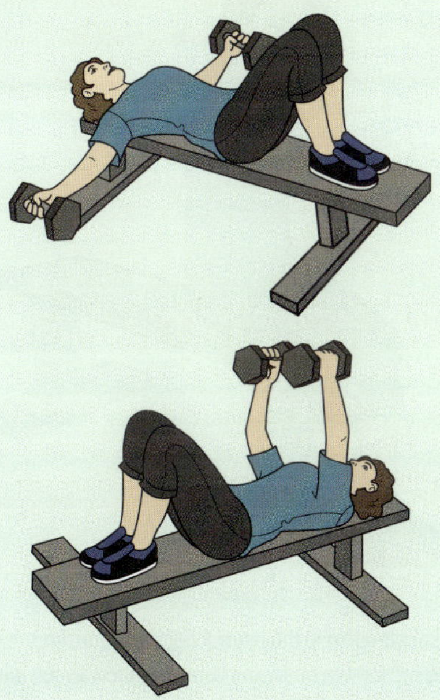

- Lie on a bench with feet flat on the bench, or lie on the floor with knees bent and feet flat, whichever is more comfortable.
- With palms facing each other, extend arms above chest, keeping elbows slightly bent at all times.
- Inhale and lower arms perpendicularly away from the body until arms are out of peripheral vision.
- Exhale while returning to starting position by visualizing arms hugging a barrel that is lying on the chest.
- Repeat 8–2 times.

Bent Over Row

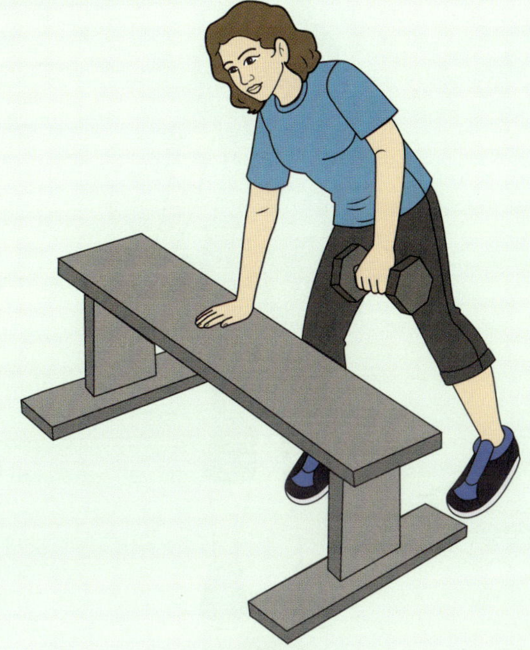

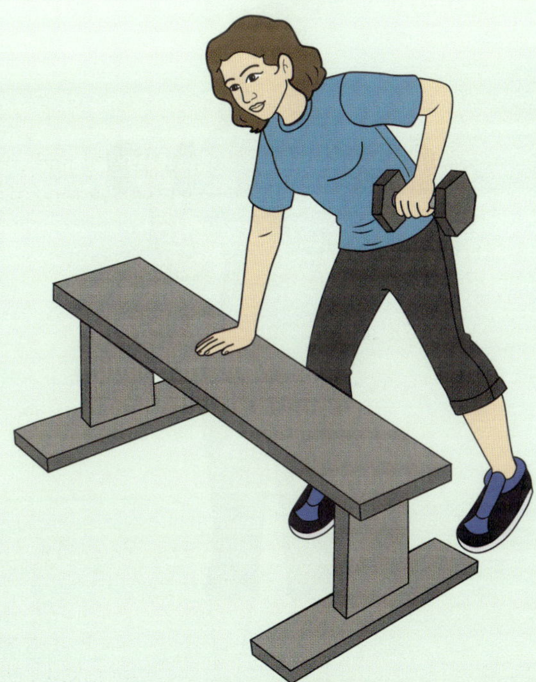

- Bend at waist while supporting the body with one hand (on table, bench, etc.) and holding a weight with the other hand in an overhand grip.
- Keep knees bent while the weight is hanging perpendicular to the torso.
- Slowly pull the weight up to the chest as if starting a lawn mower, exhaling and keeping the elbow away from the body.
- Slowly lower weight back to starting position while inhaling.
- Repeat 8–12 times on each side.

Continued

BOX 12.4 **Resistive Training Exercises—cont'd**

Dumbbell Curl

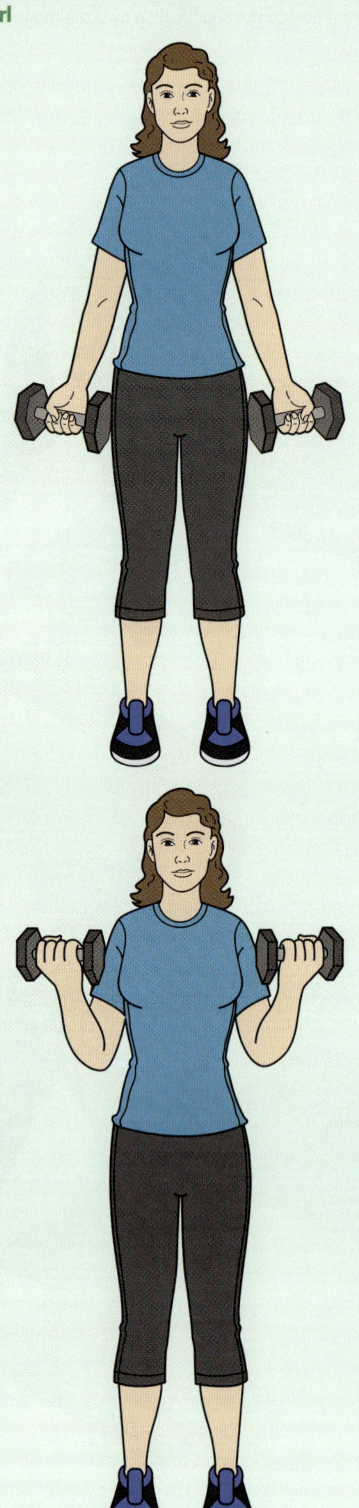

- Stand or sit with weights held at sides in an underhand grip, keeping elbows close to the body and upper arms stationary.
- Curl weights to the chin or upper chest while exhaling.
- Inhale while slowly lowering weights.
- Keep back straight throughout the duration of motion.
- Repeat 8–12 times.

Triceps Extension

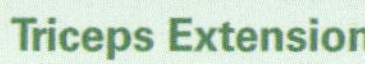

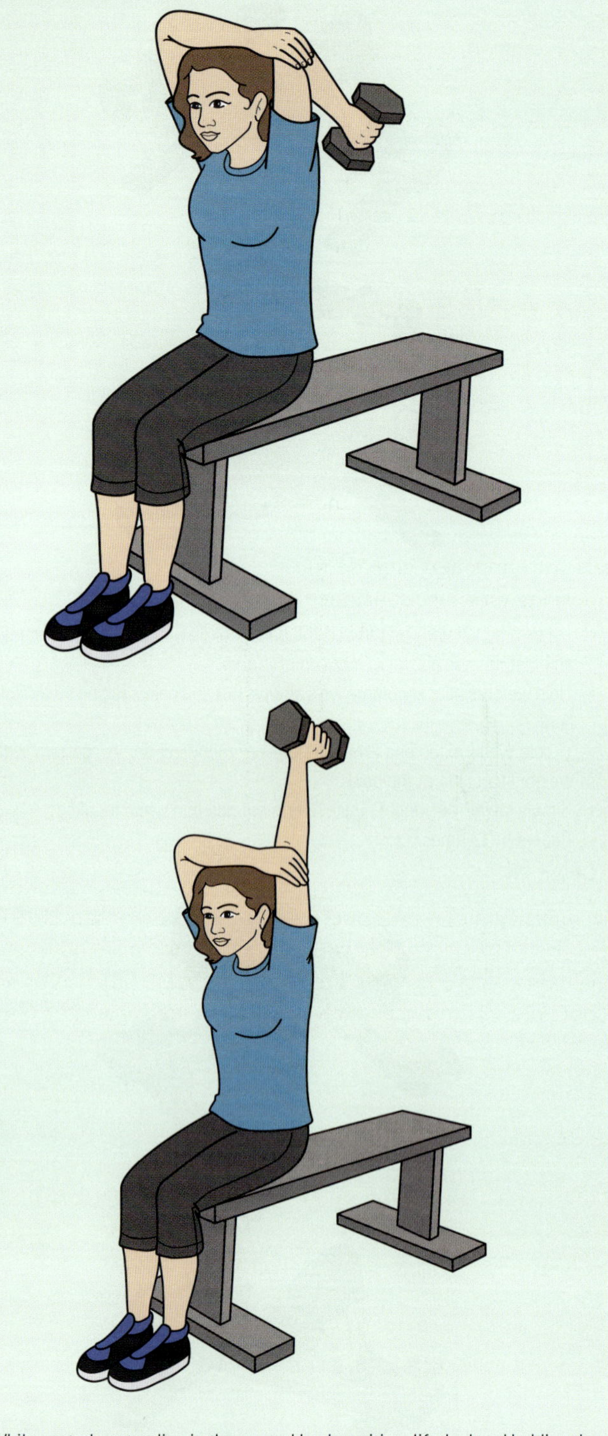

- While seated or standing in the neutral back position, lift the hand holding the weight straight above the head and in alignment with the ear.
- Keeping the upper arm tight, slowly bend the elbow to lower the weight between the shoulder blades.
- Use the free hand to support the elbow and to prevent movement in the upper arm.
- Raise the weight back to its original position by straightening the arm and exhaling.
- Repeat 8–12 times on each side.

have diabetes—almost 12% of the US population. Of those 38.4 million, 22.8%, or 8.7 million adults, are undiagnosed. Furthermore, 97.6 million adults are prediabetic. Diabetes was highest among Black and Hispanic/Latino adults, in both males and females (CDC, 2023e). In addition, adiposity and poor fitness are linked with insulin resistance. Complications of diabetes include heart disease (CDC, 2023d) and stroke, peripheral arterial disease, retinopathy, nephropathy, peripheral neuropathy, and lower-extremity amputation (Papatheodorou et al., 2018).

Exercise, in addition to diet, is a first-line intervention for diabetes. During physical activity, contracting skeletal muscles work with insulin to enhance glucose uptake into the cells (Nguyen et al., 2021). Exercise increases insulin sensitivity, improves the inherent effect of endogenous insulin, decreases obesity, and plays a role in lowering TRG levels and blood pressure (Sampath Kumar et al., 2019). In a metaanalysis of randomized controlled trials, both diet and lifestyle interventions including exercise and physical activity decreased 2-hour plasma glucose and fasting plasma glucose levels in individuals with impaired glucose tolerance (Gong et al., 2015). Other metaanalyses have concluded that lifestyle interventions including exercise and physical activity result in significant reductions in the level of hemoglobin A1c (HbA_{1c}), and cardiovascular risk parameters (Liang et al., 2021). Various modes of exercise, including aerobic interval type walking and both low- and high-intensity exercise, benefit people with type 2 diabetes; however, there is recent evidence that high-intensity resistance exercise may have a greater benefit in attenuation of HbA_{1c} and insulin than low- to moderate-intensity exercise (Liu et al., 2019). Although most of the previous studies focus on adults with type 2 diabetes, both resistance training (Reddy et al., 2019) and moderate to vigorous physical activity of at least 4 hours a week has also been found to be a promising treatment option for individuals with type 1 diabetes (Aljawarneh et al., 2019; Reddy et al., 2019; de Abreu de Lima et al., 2022).

With diet, weight control, and exercise, preventing or decreasing the need for oral antiglycolytic agents and insulin is possible while maintaining normal blood glucose levels. Physical activity may be most beneficial in preventing the progression of type 2 diabetes during the earlier stages of the disease process, before insulin therapy is required. Overall, physical activity has a significant positive effect on a chronic disease that is associated with a high risk of developing CVD (Box 12.5: Health and Social Determinants/Health Equity).

BOX 12.5 HEALTH AND SOCIAL DETERMINANTS/HEALTH EQUITY

Walk Away from Ethnic Glucose Intolerance

The Pima Indians of the Gila River Indian Community in Arizona have the highest documented incidence rates of type 2 diabetes in the world. On the island of Mauritius in the southwest Indian Ocean, all four ethnic groups (Hindu and Muslim Asian Indians, African Creoles, and Chinese) have unusually high rates of type 2 diabetes. In the United States, type 2 diabetes is 30% more prevalent in Blacks than in Whites. The presence of type 2 diabetes in each of these ethnic groups provides strong support for the existence of one or more modifiable risk factors in the cause of the disease.

Excessive weight gain is a strong independent predictor of type 2 diabetes. The development of type 2 diabetes (characterized by insulin resistance, hyperinsulinemia, and glucose intolerance) is related to weight gain in adults, particularly to fat accumulation around the waist, abdomen, and upper body (android or apple shape). This type of fat distribution is also associated with a higher risk of developing cardiovascular disease. Adipose tissue is a major site for insulin insensitivity, and most obese individuals have increased insulin resistance or some degree of glucose intolerance, or both.

Physical activity has an important role in the prevention and treatment of type 2 diabetes. By helping to maintain a proper lean-to-fat body mass, either by losing weight or by preventing weight gain, physical activity may indirectly protect against the development of type 2 diabetes. The modulating effect of physical activity on fat stores helps increase insulin sensitivity and glucose tolerance. Additionally, physical activity may directly affect glucose metabolism. The shorter-term effect of exercise can lower plasma glucose levels by enhancing the effect of insulin; long-term exercise improves insulin action and increases glucose tolerance.

Epidemiological studies of ethnic groups indicate that physical inactivity is also a risk factor for type 2 diabetes. In the United States, Blacks and Native Americans account for a disproportionate number of poor, unemployed, and disadvantaged individuals who lack access to the health care system. The least active individuals within these populations should be given the most attention because they have the most to gain. The methods and programs used to relay information to the public on the importance of physical activity need to vary depending on the socioeconomic and cultural factors specific to ethnic populations. Promotion of physical activity by schools, communities, and government and health agencies, with these factors in mind, will significantly help achieve the goal of improving lifestyles and decreasing the incidence of type 2 diabetes.

PHYSICAL ACTIVITY AND VARIOUS CHRONIC CONDITIONS

Obesity

Overweight and obesity are conditions of excess body fat (adipose tissue). Adults are considered overweight if their BMI is 25.0 to 29.9 kg/m^2 and obese if their BMI is 30.0 kg/m^2 or higher. More specifically, the ACSM (2022b) considers those with a BMI of 30.0 to 34.9 kg/m^2 as obese class I, 35.0 to 39.9 kg/m^2 as obese class II, and 40 kg/m^2 or more as obese class III. Obesity may also be defined as body weight that is equal to or greater than 120% to 125% of the ideal body weight. Fat mass (body fat percentage) is also important in determining the ideal body weight. The ACSM reports that body fat levels of 10% to 22% for males and 20% to 32% for females are considered satisfactory for health (Dumke, 2021). The average American male and female tend to exceed the recommended body fat level. An increase in fat mass and the development of obesity occurs when energy intake exceeds total daily energy expenditure for a prolonged period of time. Decreased physical activity may be both a cause and a consequence of weight gain over a lifetime.

The prevalence of obesity, as well as overweight and extreme obesity, is typically reported on the basis of BMI values, as is the case with NHANES. Nearly 1 in 3 adults (30.7%) are overweight, more than 2 in 5 adults (42.4%) have obesity, and about 1 in 11 adults (9.2%) have severe obesity (NIH, 2021). More than 2 in

5 non-Hispanic White adults (42.2%) have obesity. Nearly 1 in 2 non-Hispanic Black adults (49.6%) have obesity, more than 1 in 6 non-Hispanic Asian adults (17.4%) have obesity, and nearly 1 in 2 Hispanic adults (44.8%) have obesity (NIH, 2021). The CDC (2020) reports that 18.5% of children and adolescents (13.7 million) are affected by obesity. More specifically, obesity prevalence was 13.9% among 2- to 5-year-olds, 18.4% among 6- to 11-year-olds, and 20.6% among 12- to 19-year-olds. For children and by ethnicity, non-Hispanic Asians have an obesity prevalence of 11%, non-Hispanic Whites 14.1%, non-Hispanic Blacks 22%, and Hispanic 25.8% (CDC, 2020). A recent study indicated an apparent lack of parental awareness about the weight status of children, finding that only 5% to 6% of parents of children 2 to 12 years of age correctly classified their child as heavy or extremely heavy (Ruitere et al., 2020).

All states had more than 20% of adults with obesity. The number of states with an obesity prevalence of between 30% and 35% actually increased from 0 in 2000 to 19 in 2014, 20 in 2018, and 22 in 2023 (CDC, 2023a). Furthermore, the number of states with a prevalence of obesity between 35% and 40% increased from 8 in 2018 to 17 in 2023.

Increased fat mass and reduced physical activity increase the risk of CVD and overall mortality (CDC, 2023a). Both obesity and decreased activity are related to insulin resistance, elevated blood pressure, and elevated total and LDL cholesterol concentrations, all of which reduce with weight loss and fitness (Gong et al., 2015; Meng at al., 2022). Nevertheless, obesity should be considered an independent target for intervention in health promotion. On average, higher body weights are associated with higher death rates (Ward et al., 2022). Increases in physical activity may help with decreasing fat mass and counterbalance the risk associated with obesity and being overweight.

Maintaining fitness and health is closely related to controlling weight. The literature supports the positive influence that physical activity has on body weight and obesity. Research indicates that exercise results in weight loss for people across the life span who are overweight or obese (Barrow et al., 2019). For example, both high-intensity interval training with or without resistance training and moderate-intensity continuous training result in reduced weight and fat mass in postmenopausal females (Dupuit et al., 2020). Another recent study found that obese adolescents with diabetes, after a 12-week exercise intervention, made significant gains in overall fitness and body composition. Therefore, physical activity does the following:

- Promotes a negative energy balance (burns calories)
- Increases metabolic rate for an extended period after the activity
- Increases metabolic efficiency for burning calories by increasing lean body mass
- Helps counteract the decrease in metabolic rate associated with low-calorie diets by preserving lean body mass
- Is a good alternative to eating when eating is a response to stress rather than to hunger

Management of obesity involves a comprehensive program of nutrition management, behavior modification, and physical activity or exercise. The key to achieving a healthy body weight and optimizing body composition is long-term adherence and permanent lifestyle changes, not dieting or short-term exercise trials. Obesity treatments that demonstrate the best outcomes emphasize five components: behavioral techniques, cognitive strategies, social support, nutrition, and exercise. The effectiveness of physical activity is related to the frequency and duration of each activity session and the longevity of the activity program. Recommended ACSM-AHA guidelines for physical activity include the following (ACSM, 2022b):

- All healthy adults aged 18 to 65 years should participate in moderate-intensity aerobic physical activity for a minimum of 30 minutes 5 days per week or vigorous-intensity aerobic activity for a minimum of 20 minutes 3 days per week. (Combinations of moderate- and vigorous-intensity exercise can be performed to meet this recommendation.)
- Moderate-intensity aerobic activity can be accumulated to total the 30-minute minimum by performing bouts each lasting ≥10 minutes.
- Every adult should perform activities that maintain or increase muscular strength and endurance for a minimum of 2 days per week.
- Because of the dose-response relationship between physical activity and health, individuals who wish to further improve their fitness, reduce their risk for chronic diseases and disabilities, and/or prevent unhealthy weight gain may benefit by exceeding the minimum recommended amounts of physical activity.

As long as calorie expenditure is similar, moderate lifestyle activity may be as effective as structured exercise. Moderate intensity appears to be most effective for total and fat calorie consumption during the activity. Lean body mass is strongly correlated with resting metabolic rate (Flack et al., 2016). Females tend to have a 5% to 10% lower resting metabolic rate than males and a higher percentage of body fat than males of similar weight (McMurray et al., 2014). Consequently, females have a lower percentage of lean body mass and may not be as metabolically active as are males during exercise.

Osteoporosis

Osteoporosis, or porous bone, is the most common bone disease and a major health threat. It is characterized by low bone mass and structural weakness of bone tissue, leading to bone fragility and increased risk of fractures (National Institutes of Health Osteoporosis and Related Bone Diseases National Resource Center, 2020; Pouresmaeili et al., 2018). In the United States an estimated 10 million people have osteoporosis, and 44 million have low bone density and an increased risk of developing osteoporosis (Bone Health & Osteoporosis Foundation, 2020).

Bone mass increases during childhood and adolescence and usually peaks during the third decade of life (Burr, 2019). When a person reaches approximately 30 years old, age-related bone loss occurs throughout the skeletal system due to a reduction in glycosaminoglycans and bound water, both of which decrease bone toughness. However, there are significant differences in bone loss patterns between the sexes, with female sex being a risk factor for osteoporosis (Laurent et al., 2019). Females have less bone mass than males at all ages, and by their midthirties can expect age-related bone loss of approximately 1% annually. The rate of bone loss accelerates rapidly during the first 5 years after menopause, with annual losses of 3% to 5% being common. By the fifth decade, or during their forties, females can anticipate a 10% loss of vertebral bone mass. Cumulative bone loss can approach 40% of peak bone mass over a female's lifetime. Unfortunately, a loss of at least 30% of bone mass is required for detection on plain film radiographs (McKinnis, 2020). Therefore, it is important to detect females at risk early in the natural course of the disease and to target interventions toward lifestyle-oriented health promotion. Risk factors for osteoporosis include increased age, female sex, BMI less than 18.5 kg/m^2, history of smoking, and a history of major fractures (Xiao et al., 2022). Additional risk factors include White/Asian race, family history, low body weight for height, premature menopause, lack of physical activity, excessive alcohol consumption, living in poverty, and having food insecurities (Marshall et al., 2020).

Bone mass development is partially regulated by environmental factors such as nutrition. Inadequate calcium intake during early growth periods has implications for peak bone mass and bone health later in life. A recent systematic review of 74 countries found that people in many countries in Asia, Africa, and South America have low calcium intakes, between 400 and 700 mg/day. Only Northern European countries had national calcium intakes greater than 1000 mg/day (Balk et al., 2017). Although dietary sources are the preferred means of achieving adequate calcium intake, foods fortified with calcium are becoming more prevalent and are manufactured to provide approximately 300 mg of calcium in each serving (see Chapter 11).

In addition to the importance of optimizing the physiologic intake of calcium and vitamin D (Hill, 2017) and maintaining normal menstrual cycles for maximization of peak bone mass, physical activity plays a significant role in developing bone mass during childhood and adolescence and in maintaining skeletal mass into adulthood and old age (Zulfarina et al., 2016). Physical activities, those that involve weight-bearing in particular, increase BMD and provide support for a stronger skeletal foundation throughout aging. Thus activities such as walking, stair climbing, floor calisthenics, and aerobic dance have a positive effect on BMD and are an important component of reducing osteoporosis risk (Neuman, 2017). After the individual is diagnosed with osteoporosis, exercise continues to be important. The ACSM (2022b) recommends that people with osteoporosis engage in weight-bearing aerobic exercise in combination with some form of high-impact, high-velocity, high-intensity resistance training. Additionally, a systematic review and metaanalysis found that Tai Chi is effective in attenuating BMD loss at regions of the lumbar spine and proximal femur neck in older adults, perimenopausal and postmenopausal females, people with osteoarthritis, and cancer survivors (Zou et al., 2018) (Box 12.6: Evidence-Based Practice).

One of the most serious side effects of osteoporosis is increased fracture risk. Osteoporotic bone fractures are responsible for more hospitalizations for females than heart attacks, strokes, and breast cancer combined (Bone Health & Osteoporosis Foundation, 2020). It is estimated that 40% of White females and 13% of White males in the United States will have at least one fracture related to the fragility of their bones in their lifetime; however, 84% of older Americans who suffer fractures are not tested or treated for osteoporosis. It was also found that there is a 17% chance of hip, 16% chance of forearm, and 15% chance of vertebral fractures in White females at 50 years of age. The corresponding fracture rates for White males are 6%, 2.5%, and 5%, respectively (International Osteoporosis Foundation, 2024).

In older adults, fall prevention becomes equally important to maintaining and improving BMD. In addition to preserving BMD, an active lifestyle, exercise, and strength training may reduce fracture risk and improve functional performance in postmenopausal females with low bone mass and osteoporosis (Benedetti et al., 2018; Hong & Kim, 2018; Watson et al., 2018). Clinical practice guidelines for fall prevention and management strongly recommend risk stratification, gait and balance assessments, multifactorial interventions, medication reviews, physical exercise, vision and footwear intervention, physical therapy, environment modification, management of osteoporosis and fracture risk, and cardiovascular interventions (Montero-Odasso et al., 2021).

A recent Delphi study reported expert consensus findings on physical therapy interventions for the patient with suspected or confirmed osteoporosis including education on posture, body mechanics and activity modification to reduce fracture and fall risk, balance training, and resistance training (Avin et al., 2022). A new clinical practice guideline from the Academy

BOX 12.6 EVIDENCE-BASED PRACTICE

The purpose of the study was to investigate the effects of Tai Chi on fall prevention and balance in older adults. In this systematic review and meta-analysis, the authors used the PubMed, Embase, and Cochrane databases to search for randomized controlled trials (RCTs) from the time each database was established until 12/31/22. Study criteria included older adults aged ≥60 years, Tai Chi as an intervention, a control group receiving another form of low-level exercise, and an outcome assessment on falls and balance. After identifying and screening studies, 24 RCTs were included in the final review. Information was provided on publication year, country, risk of falls, mean age by group, description of Tai Chi and the control group participants, intensity, exposure time, and follow-up period. Six of the studies examined participants with a history of falls. Five studies examined participants with a history of a neurologic disease. Exercise frequency was typically one to three times per week and total exercise time was typically within 72 hours. The common follow-up period was 9 months (Chen et al., 2023).

Study results indicated that using Tai Chi exercise significantly reduced the number of fallers. Further analysis showed that Tai Chi was effective at reducing falls in any population at risk, regardless of the duration, follow-up time, or Tai Chi style. With respect to exercise frequency, exercising twice or ≥3 times a week showed greater benefits than exercising once a week.

Nurses and health care professionals may find that Tai Chi classes are offered in senior centers or as part of hospital community outreach initiatives. Tai Chi seems to be an effective exercise for preventing falls and improving balance in older adults. The effectiveness of Tai Chi increases with exercise time and frequency. Yang-style is more effective than Sun-style Tai Chi.

Chen, W., Li, M., Li, H., Lin, Y., & Feng, Z. (2023). Tai Chi for fall prevention and balance improvement in older adults: A systematic review and meta-analysis of randomized controlled trials. *Frontiers in Public Health, 11*, 1236050. https://doi.org/10.3389/fpubh.2023.1236050

of Geriatric Physical Therapy makes exercise recommendations for postmenopausal females to slow the decline of BMD of the a) hip and femoral neck, b) femoral neck, c) lumbar spine, and d) lumbar spine (Hartley et al., 2022).

Arthritis

Osteoarthritis (OA) is the most common disorder of the musculoskeletal system. The hip and knee are among the most common areas affected by OA, and its prevalence is expected to continue rising (Hunter & Bierma-Zeinstra, 2019). Although rheumatoid arthritis (RA) and OA have different causes and attack different parts of the joint, impaired joint function is the result in both conditions. Cartilage is destroyed, irregularities occur in the bone ends, and synovial inflammation occurs, leading to pain, stiffness, swelling, and loss of normal function (Kolasinski et al., 2020). As proper joint alignment changes, normal ROM is decreased, normal muscle balance and activity are altered, and disfigurement and dysfunction occur; ultimately, normal movement patterns are altered.

Although there is an ongoing controversy that arthritis cannot be reversed by exercise, a recent clinical practice guideline strongly recommend exercise for OA; exercise has a moderate effect on physical function, has limited side effects, and is cost-effective (van Doormaal et al., 2020). For the treatment of knee OA, the American Academy of Orthopaedic Surgeons strongly recommends supervised, unsupervised, and/or aquatic exercise to improve pain and function and moderately recommends neuromuscular training (e.g., balance, agility, coordination) with traditional exercises to improve function and walking speed (Brophy & Fillingham, 2022).

Physical activity helps restore health to synovium and cartilage, increase strength and flexibility, decrease joint vulnerability, and delay the onset of dysfunction. Exercise is also linked to improvements in patient outcomes regarding symptoms, mobility, quality of life, and psychological health (Wellsandt & Golightly, 2018). One common barrier to physical activity or exercise is a fear of exacerbating pain related to OA. However, this belief may be unfounded, as Wallis and colleagues (2015) demonstrated that individuals with moderate to severe knee OA were able to walk up to 70 minutes per week without exacerbating symptoms (ASCM, 2018).

Although researchers have concluded that regular exercise cannot cure arthritis, exercise has the following quality-of-life benefits for people with arthritis (Wellsandt & Golightly, 2018):

- Improved joint function and increased ROM
- Increased muscle strength and aerobic fitness that enhance activities of daily living
- Improvement in psychological state
- Decreased loss of bone mass and may promote increased BMD
- Decreased risk of chronic disease

The collective evidence strongly and consistently suggests that exercise is beneficial for individuals with OA. Although current evidence is insufficient to recommend the "best" and ideal prescribed amount (duration, intensity, and frequency) (Kolasinski et al., 2020) of exercise, "traditional" forms of exercise (strength, flexibility, and aerobic activities) have been shown to be beneficial for improvement in functional outcomes in individuals with hip or knee OA (Wellsandt & Golightly, 2018). The Osteoarthritis Research Society International has identified that therapeutic exercise is safe for patients with knee and hip OA (Bannuru et al., 2019; Holden et al., 2021). Numerous types of therapeutic exercise (including aerobic, strengthening, neuromuscular, and mind-body exercise) may be utilized at varying doses and in different settings to improve pain and function. Benefits from therapeutic exercise appear greater when dosage recommendations from general exercise guidelines for healthy adults are met. The ACSM (2022b) recommends aerobic exercise 3 to 5 days/week at a moderate to vigorous intensity that places low stress on arthritic joints (such as walking, cycling, or swimming); 2 to 3 days of resistance training at 60% to 80% with 1 repetition maximum; and daily flexibility. Based on the results of some smaller trials, higher intensity may result in greater benefit to people with OA, but only if tolerated (Maly et al., 2020). More research is needed to determine the optimal dosage parameters for exercise in individuals with OA.

In addition to traditional, land-based exercises, improvements have also been shown with other forms of exercise. The authors of an updated systematic review of aquatic exercise for patients with knee OA found that aquatic therapy programs had comparable results to land-based programs (Raposo et al., 2021; Xu et al., 2023). Tai Chi has also been found to be an excellent exercise for people with knee OA and has been found to improve gait and postural control (You et al., 2021; Yang et al., 2022a). Yoga may also be effective for improving pain, function, and stiffness in those with knee OA. However, at this time, only a weak recommendation can be made in favor of yoga due to the low quality of the studies and high risk of bias (Lauche et al., 2019; Zampogna et al., 2020).

Clinical practice guidelines suggest that education about physical activity and exercise should be included in the management of OA (Ariani et al., 2019; Kolasinski et al., 2020; The Royal Australian College of General Practitioners, 2018). Available evidence supports a small but positive benefit from education and self-management programs as complements to exercise (Kolasinski et al., 2020). In a much more robust study, the Better Management of Patients with Osteoarthritis Program delivered a consistent education- and exercise-based self-management message nationwide in Sweden (Jönsson et al., 2019). Individuals with knee and hip OA who participated in the self-management program reported significant improvements in pain, medication usage, desire for surgery, fear-avoidance behavior, and physical inactivity compared with those who did not participate.

Rheumatoid arthritis is a chronic, systemic autoimmune inflammatory disease that causes damage to both small and large joints. This damage can lead to physical deformities, functional disabilities, and significant adverse effects to quality of life. Additionally, people with RA are at increased risk for CVD as well as increased fat deposits and reduced muscle mass. Management of RA consists of both pharmacologic and nonpharmacologic treatments, of which physical activity and exercise should be considered an important component. Exercise has been shown to improve pain, function, and quality of life in people with RA (Sobue et al., 2022). In 2022 the American

College of Rheumatology published new guidelines for the treatment of RA (ACR, 2022). Strong recommendations were given for consistent engagement in exercise, aerobic exercise, aquatic exercise, resistance exercise, mind-body exercise, and occupational and physical therapy, among others. Exercise selection should be based on the presentation of symptoms. However, dosing (intensity, frequency, and volume) for the best results has not yet been determined (Hu et al., 2021).

Specific exercise recommendations also vary depending on the site and number of impaired joints, presence or absence of inflammation, joint stability, and any prior joint replacement. Increased physical activity and participation in different types of exercise, including high-intensity exercise, is safe for individuals with RA (Lange et al., 2019). Additionally, the physiologic benefits of exercise may have effects on both disease-related symptoms and systemic manifestations. In fact, evidence suggests that higher levels of physical activity correlate with a reduced risk of developing RA (Sun et al., 2021).

One of the manners in which physical activity has a positive effect is through antiinflammatory effects. Although a detailed discussion of the physiologic mechanisms through which this occurs is beyond the scope of this text, exercise is considered a major stimulus and can elicit beneficial reductions in acute and long-term inflammatory responses. There is also evidence that physical activity has an inverse relationship with disease activity in patients with RA (i.e., higher levels of physical activity correlate with lower disease activity), as assessed by the Disease Activity Score (DAS28) or the Simplified Disease Activity Index (SDAI) (Hernández-Hernández & Díaz-González, 2017).

Aerobic conditioning in people with stable RA is not only safe, but participants also report improvements in quality of life and functional ability (Hernández-Hernández & Díaz-González, 2017). The duration of both RA and aerobic exercise program participation appears to influence outcomes, with the quality of life benefiting more in those with earlier symptoms of RA who begin treatment sooner. Participating in a 20-week aerobic and resistance exercise program, 71% of patients rated their health as much or very much improved on the Patient Global Impression of Change Scale, had increased fitness, and had no serious adverse events (Lange et al., 2019).

Evidence regarding resistance exercise in patients with RA suggests that there are statistically significant improvements with regard to functional capacity, number of tender and swollen joints, and decrease in erythrocyte sedimentation rate (ESR) (a nonspecific measure of inflammation) (Hernández-Hernández & Díaz-González, 2017). A more recent metaanalysis supported these findings, revealing that participating in a resistance program resulted in a decreased Disease Activity Score (DAS28), ESR, and 50-foot walk time in patients with RA (Wen et al., 2021).

The barriers to participating in physical activity for those with RA are similar for those without the disease, such as cost and lack of time. In addition, those living with RA have cited disease-specific barriers such as pain, fatigue, and functional disabilities. Incidentally, each of these latter considerations can be improved once individuals begin exercising. Considering the benefits of managing disease-related symptoms and promoting improved physiologic function in response to exercise, physical activity is an important component to include with the management of RA.

In general, different exercises should be selected according to the symptoms, and any exercise is better than no exercise. However, the most effective intervention protocol has yet to be determined (Hu et al., 2021). During periods of high disease activity, resistance exercises should be avoided (Hernández-Hernández & Díaz-González, 2017). The inclusion of a multidisciplinary team of health care providers should be strongly considered for patients with RA. Adherence to long-term exercise programs can be challenging; support and encouragement from various providers can help patients adhere to physical activity and exercise programs, particularly during flare-ups, in a manner that continues to promote health and quality of life while adjusting to waxing and waning periods of RA symptoms.

Low Back Pain

Low back pain (LBP) is a common health and social problem worldwide. Nonspecific LBP (LBP not attributable to any known cause) comprises 90% to 95% of cases (Maher et al., 2017). Intermittent and chronic LBP may lead to loss of work and affect the overall economy. Of 154 conditions researched, low back and neck pain had the highest health care costs in 2016, with an estimated $134.5 billion in spending (Dieleman et al., 2020).

The spinal column is composed of 24 vertebrae stacked vertically, forming natural curves that allow the bony column to function with the resiliency of a spring. The intervertebral disks help with mobility and shock absorption. The health of the bony vertebrae and the cartilaginous disks depends on movement achieved through physical activity. The cartilage receives its nutrients from cyclical compression and decompression as a function of weight-bearing and non–weight-bearing movement. Similarly, repeated weight-bearing and non–weight-bearing activity stimulates vertebral bone integrity.

Muscles are intimately involved in the support and function of the spinal column. Maintaining the proper curves (anterior and posterior convexities) of lordosis in the cervical and lumbar vertebrae and kyphosis in the thoracic spine is vital for sustaining the spring and shock-absorption qualities of the spine. The lumbar curve is especially influenced by three sets of muscles that are attached to the pelvis and the lumbar vertebrae. By altering the tilt of the pelvis, these muscles can increase (iliopsoas muscle) or decrease (abdominal and hamstring muscles) the lumbar curve. In addition, the deep muscles of the back (paraspinal muscles) work in controlled synergistic and antagonistic fashions to control spinal planes of motion; they are also influential in supporting the spinal curves in posture. Weakness or shortening of any of these muscles can adversely affect posture and increase stress on the back. The result can be back pain from muscle strain, altered joint function (facet joints), and abnormal force on the intervertebral disks.

LBP is a multifactorial disorder, unlikely to be caused by any single factor. Many individual factors associated with LBP have been identified in the scientific literature, including genetics, sex, age, body build, strength, and flexibility. Obesity has been associated with an increased risk of LBP, as well as an increased likelihood of seeking care for subacute and chronic LBP in general (Zhang et al., 2018). Zhou et al. (2021) reported that BMI is significantly associated with increased risk for LBP. Other obesity-related traits such as hip circumference, body fat mass, fat-free mass, and fat percentage were also associated with LBP.

Additionally, psychosocial factors seem to play a more significant role in prognosis than physical factors (Delitto et al., 2012), particularly fear when pain has become persistent, and distress or depression are present in the earlier stages of LBP. Clinicians should therefore assess for fear, avoidance, depression, and physical distress using relevant screening tools, as they may be more important than physical performance factors in the successful management of LBP (Delitto et al., 2012). Furthermore, the authors of a metaanalysis concluded that individuals with symptoms of depression are at higher risk of developing new episodes of LBP compared with individuals without depressive symptoms; furthermore, more severe levels of depression correlate with higher risk (Pinheiro et al., 2015). In a similar study, Felício et al. (2022) found that depressive symptoms are a risk factor for LBP in older adults. However, the relationship between depressive symptoms and the intensity of LBP may depend on the duration of symptoms. In a metaanalysis by Wong et al. (2022), depressive symptoms were associated with pain intensity for chronic LBP but not for acute LBP.

Numerous studies have examined the relationship between sedentary behavior and risk for LBP. A recent metaanalysis of cross-sectional studies found that both nonoccupational and occupational sedentary behavior was associated with LBP (Dzakpasu et al., 2021). Interventions such as exercise programs (Fernandez-Rodrguez et al., 2022), including home exercise training (Quentin et al., 2021), physical activity (Geneen et al., 2017), and using sit-stand workstations (Agarwal et al., 2018), may reduce LBP.

For individuals experiencing LBP, exercise is advantageous, and its use is well-supported by scientific literature. In their Cochrane Review, Hayden and colleagues (2021a) concluded that in individuals with various levels of LBP, exercise was beneficial in terms of reducing pain and improving function. In a network metaanalysis, they found that specific types of exercise, such as Pilates, McKenzie therapy, and functional restoration, were more effective than other types of exercises at reducing pain and improving function in people with chronic LBP (Hayden et al., 2021b). The Academy of Orthopaedic Physical Therapy of the American Physical Therapy Association recommends exercise for acute and chronic LBP (George et al., 2021) (see the Acute and Chronic Low Back Pain: Clinical Practice Guideline for specific recommendations on exercise, education, and manual and other-directed therapies). A recent summary of recommendations for primary care management of nonspecific LBP emphasizes that encouragement to remain physically active and avoid bed rest is an important component of first-line care, before seeking pharmacologic or more invasive care (Almeida et al., 2018).

The goal of exercise programs for individuals with LBP is to prevent debilitation as a result of inactivity and to increase endurance, strength, and flexibility, allowing a return to usual functional activities. For this reason, ACSM currently recommends following similar guidelines to those used for the general population, which combine resistance, aerobic, and flexibility exercise that can be tailored to individuals on a case-by-case basis (ACSM, 2022b). The ACSM discourages patient education or counseling strategies that increase the threat or fear associated with LBP, the promotion of extended bed rest, and pathoanatomic explanations of LBP. The ACSM encourages patient education on the anatomic strength of the spine, pain neuroscience, the favorable prognosis of the condition, active pain coping strategies, and the importance of improving activity levels. The Acute and Chronic Low Back Pain: Clinical Practice Guideline makes recommendations for types of exercises, such as specific trunk muscular activation; trunk muscle strengthening and endurance; movement control; and aerobic, aquatic, and multimodal approaches, based on the duration of pain, symptoms of leg pain, impaired motor control, age, and postoperative status (George et al., 2021).

Various types of exercise have been examined and their effectiveness compared in persons with LBP. Walking appears to be effective in the management of chronic musculoskeletal pain. One group of authors found that walking could be as effective as other nonpharmacologic interventions, including exercise, education, and physiotherapy, in terms of pain and disability reduction (Sitthipornvorakul et al., 2018). A recent network metaanalysis concluded that the most beneficial interventions to reduce pain and disability in adults with chronic LBP were 1) Pilates or strengthening exercises, 2) core-based strength or mind-body exercises, and 3) Pilates and core-based exercises (Fernández-Rodríguez et al., 2022). It appears that the combination of stabilization and strengthening exercises is likely the most effective in the management of LBP but that a variety of forms of exercise (e.g., aerobic strengthening, stabilization, aquatic aerobic exercise, strengthening, and stretching) used individually or in combination appear to be more effective than usual care or no exercise (Tian & Zhao, 2018). Pocovi et al. (2022) found walking or running to be more effective than minimal or no intervention for reducing pain and disability when treating nonspecific LBP. Olaya-Contreras and colleagues (2015) examined the effects of advising a group of people with acute severe LBP to "stay active in spite of the pain," and they found no difference in pain intensity trajectory and a significantly higher level of physical activity when this group was compared with a group that was instructed to "adjust activity to the pain." Given the acknowledged detriments of bed rest, to stay active is good advice for individuals with LBP (Almeida et al., 2018).

In addition to physical benefits, exercise can have psychological benefits in the management of depression related to LBP. One study found that both low-dose (motor control plus manual therapy) and moderate-dose (general strength and conditioning training) exercises helped reduce depressive symptoms in adults with chronic LBP (Teychenne et al., 2019). In their Cochrane Review, Geneen and colleagues (2017) reported a variable effect of physical activity on psychological function and quality of life; they associated the inconsistency with the low quality of the studies or the mix of types of physical activity assessed. However, they did report few adverse events associated with physical activity and exercise.

Therefore, it appears that the inclusion of physical activity is an important component in the management of depressive symptoms to reduce the intensity and risk of new episodes of or contributing to existing episodes of LBP.

Advanced age, osteoporosis, arthritis, and LBP are not reasons to exclude exercise from anyone's lifestyle; in fact, the opposite is true. These conditions are reasons to remain as physically active as possible to facilitate the ability to function throughout the aging process. For individuals with multiple comorbidities, physical therapy may be beneficial. In fact, a referral to a physical therapist is warranted in most, if not all, cases of LBP pain to allow there to be proper comprehensive management, which may include exercise as well as other safe and effective interventions.

Immune Function

There is evidence suggesting that physical activity decreases the risk of developing many disease states, including osteoporosis (Tong et al., 2019), CVD (Tucker et al., 2022), and cancer (McTiernan et al., 2019). Part of this prevention is due to the effects of exercise on the immune system. Several studies demonstrate that people with impaired immune function can exercise safely without risk to their health status and can enhance their physiologic and psychological well-being as well as their quality of life with exercise (Gomes-Neto et al., 2021; Ibeneme et al., 2019a; Kalatzi et al., 2022).

A systematic review concluded that the combination of resistance and aerobic exercise produced the largest improvements in aerobic capacity and that of the physical function, general health, mental health, and energy/vitality domains of Health-Related Quality of Life (Gomes-Neto et al., 2021). Another metaanalysis suggests that aerobic exercise, either alone or in conjunction with progressive resistance exercise, can be safely performed by adults with HIV/acquired immunodeficiency syndrome (AIDS) and may increase fitness and improve body composition and well-being (Ibeneme et al., 2019a). Recommended parameters include moderate-intensity aerobic exercise (55% to 85% maximum heart rate) for 30 to 60 minutes, two to five times per week for 6 to 24 weeks (Ibeneme et al., 2019a). A recent metaanalysis added that exercise could have an antidepressant-like effect in adults with HIV/AIDS (Ibeneme et al., 2022).

In healthy young humans or animals, exercise seems to increase immune cell markers for HIV, which include CD4, CD8, and T-lymphocytes. However, the effects of exercise on immune-inflammatory system markers (e.g., CD4 levels, CD4/CD8 ratio, viral load, or other inflammatory modulators) in people with HIV/AIDS remains unclear. Similarly, metaanalytic data comparing the combination of aerobic and progressive resistance exercise with no exercise found no significant differences in CD4 count (Ibeneme et al., 2019b). Despite the fact that the CD4 count did not differ between exercising and nonexercising groups, there were significant beneficial changes in depressive symptoms, mean body weight, mean arm and thigh girth, and maximum heart rate for those in the exercising groups and one subdomain (role activity limitation due to physical health) of a quality-of-life assessment (Ibeneme et al., 2019b). In contrast, a recent metaanalysis compared the effects of resistance training versus no exercise on immune-inflammatory markers in people with HIV/AIDS and found a significant improvement in CD4 cell count but no difference in other immune-inflammatory markers (Zanetti et al., 2021). Other significant improvements in favor of resistance training were found in muscle strength (e.g., bench press and squat exercise) and body composition (lean body mass, fat body mass, and body fat percentage).

People with other diseases also benefit from physical activity and exercise. There is evidence supporting the health benefits of exercise in individuals with inflammatory bowel disease or functional gastrointestinal disorders (Costa et al., 2017). Physical activity and exercise may benefit gastric and pancreatic cancers (Parker et al., 2019), gastroesophageal reflux disease, peptic ulcer disease (Shephard, 2017), nonalcoholic fatty liver disease (van der Windt et al., 2018), cholelithiasis (Littlefield & Lenahan, 2019), diverticular disease (Rezapour, Ali, & Stollman, 2018), irritable bowel syndrome (Maleki et al., 2018), constipation (Gao et al., 2019), Parkinson disease, (Yang et al., 2023), and multiple sclerosis (Flores et al., 2023).

Physical activity also appears to lower the risk of developing pre- and postmenopausal breast cancers (Chan et al., 2019). Physical activity was also shown to reduce the risk of breast cancer recurrence and mortality due to recurrence (Zagalaz-Anula et al., 2022). Female with higher levels of recreational physical activity after a breast cancer diagnosis have a lower risk of all-cause mortality (Spei et al., 2019). For males, exercise may attenuate the risk of prostate cancer and also improve the side effects of cancer treatment (Campos et al., 2018). Additionally, a recent metaanalysis by Lavin-Perez et al. (2023) concluded that exercise should not be discouraged due to the known benefits of exercise and an absence of negative effects due to exercise in persons with breast cancer.

There are many potential mechanisms through which exercise may lower the incidence of cancer and improve cancer outcomes. These include reducing adiposity and systemic inflammatory markers, links to sex hormones, decreasing serum insulin levels, and promoting the immune system to increase the surveillance of tumor cells (Lee et al., 2018). Exercise has become so important in the treatment of cancer that the Clinical Oncology Society of Australia's 2018 Position Statement stated that exercise should be "embedded as part of standard practice in cancer care and as an adjunct therapy that helps counteract the adverse effects of cancer and its treatment." They further recommend that all members of the multidisciplinary cancer team promote physical activity and consider referral to an accredited exercise physiologist or physiotherapist with experience in cancer care (Cormie et al., 2018). Moreover, the American Cancer Society (ACS) established Guidelines on Diet and Physical Activity for Cancer Prevention with four recommendations: 1) achieve and maintain a healthy body weight, 2) be physically active, 3) follow a healthy eating pattern, and 4) limit alcohol consumption (Rock et al., 2020). With respect to physical activity for adults, the ACS recommends 150 to 300 minutes of moderate physical activity or 75 to 150 minutes of vigorous physical activity, or an equivalent combination, per week in addition to limiting sedentary behavior.

Mental Health

People who exercise regularly state that they feel better, have increased self-esteem, and have a more positive outlook on life. Not only do they feel better physically, but they also feel better mentally. The mental health benefits of physical activity include promoting mental health and well-being in healthy adults, preventing and treating mental disorders, and supporting psychosocial rehabilitation. In adults, exercise, yoga, and walking interventions have been shown to improve well-being across workplace settings (Abdin et al., 2018). Epidemiological research with both males and females suggests that physical activity may be associated with enhancements in positive affect and general sense of well-being. A cross-sectional study found that individuals who exercised had 43.2% fewer days of poor mental health in the past month compared with individuals who did not exercise but were otherwise matched in several other areas. Although the authors cautioned that more exercise was not always better, all exercise types were associated with lower mental health burden (Chekroud et al., 2018). A recent systematic review of longitudinal studies highlights sociodemographic, nutritional and lifestyle, and psychological determinants and indicators of successful aging (Rodrigues et al., 2023). Sustaining psychological well-being in adult life is a major determinant of successful aging.

Much of the work on mental health and exercise has focused specifically on depression (Heissel et al., 2023), anxiety (Piva et al., 2023), stress (Mariano et al., 2023), and schizophrenia (Gallardo-Gómez et al., 2023). Evidence from a review of the literature found that exercise protects against and is an intervention for mild to major depression (Gordon et al., 2018). Specifically, aerobic exercise and/or resistance training was effective in treating adults with major depressive disorder or with depressive symptoms (Heissel et al., 2023). Researchers examining major depressive disorder recommended an exercise prescription that is supervised, individually customized, lasts at least 30 minutes, and is performed at least three times per week (Gordon et al., 2018). A recent metaanalysis examined the effects of exercise on mental health during the COVID-19 pandemic, and there were significant improvements in anxiety, depression, stress and quality of life (Wang et al., 2023b). Subanalyses indicated that exercise sessions of 30 to 40 minutes three to five times per week is the most effective prescription for reducing anxiety and depression.

Investigations have also focused on populations across the life span, including children, young adults, and older adults. In children, replacing time spent playing sedentary video games with active video games or outdoor play is associated with more positive psychological outcomes (Grgic et al., 2018). Physical activity reduced depressive symptoms in children and adolescents when compared with the control condition (Recchia et al., 2023). Physical activity also improved the psychological health and cognitive function in children and adolescents with intellectual disabilities, with therapeutic and aerobic interventions more than120 minutes per week showing the best results (Yang et al., 2022b). A recent metaanalysis found that exercise improved different negative emotions, such as anxiety, depression, and stress, in children (Li et al., 2023a).

In older adults, depression is common, and many antidepressant medications may be contraindicated. According to 2019 data, in the past 2 weeks 18.4% of adults aged 65 years or older had experienced symptoms of depression, of which 12% were mild, 3.8% were moderate, and 2.6% were severe (Villarroel & Terlizzi, 2020). Fortunately, a recent systematic metaanalysis revealed that exercise is an effective treatment for older individuals with depression. In Thailand, there was an association of physical activity with self-reported general health in all age groups and with mental health in adults and older adults (Liangruenrom et al., 2019). Several recent metaanalyses have examined the effects of exercise on cognitive function and depression in older adults. Participating in a seated exercise program improved cognition function in older adults with and without cognitive impairment (Sexton & Taylor, 2019). Virtual reality–based exercise interventions improved depression, balance, and the quality of life in older adults (Vasodi et al., 2023). Resistance training improved depressions and circulating brain-derived neurotrophic factors, which are important for plastic changes related to learning and memory, in older adults (Setayesh et al., 2023).

The effects of exercise on individuals with various disorders or diseases, such as schizophrenia, cancer, or other chronic illnesses, has also been studied. Available evidence demonstrates that exercise improves cognitive functioning in people with schizophrenia, especially in the areas of social cognition, working memory, and attention (Firth et al., 2017). Another study suggested that exercise is effective in reducing anxiety and depression in previous methamphetamine users and level III-2 evidence that exercise is beneficial in improving the quality of life in this population (Morris et al., 2018).

Various types and modalities of exercise have been used in studies; an example of one such intervention is Tai Chi. A recent metaanalysis found that Tai Chi significantly improved depression in middle-aged and older adults (Zeng et al., 2023). This review found that a Tai Chi regimen lasting more than 24 weeks and for more than 2,400 minutes of total duration resulted in the best therapeutic effect. A recent metaanalysis examined the effects of Qigong on the mental and physical health of college students and found significant reductions in depression and anxiety symptoms as well as significant improvements in cardiorespiratory endurance and flexibility (Lin et al., 2022).

EXERCISE PRESCRIPTION

The literature certainly reflects both the physiologic and the psychological benefits that can be experienced with commitment to an active lifestyle. In short, regular physical activity or exercise can help people feel better, look better, and perform better. Unfortunately, as discussed, many Americans have failed to embrace the concept and health value of an active lifestyle. Some are overwhelmed by the misperception that to gain health benefits they must perform vigorous, continual exercise. The result has been discouragement in getting started and poor compliance in staying with it. "No pain, no gain" has been an unfortunate and common refrain. Although standardized exercise programs are the norm, one size does not fit all.

There is evidence that peer-led exercise groups (Burton et al., 2018) and integrated programs that turn daily routines into opportunities for exercise demonstrate increased adherence and improved motor performance (Weber et al., 2018). Replacing sedentary time with short periods of moderate to vigorous physical activity and frequent levels of light-intensity physical activity is also effective in increasing energy expenditure (Biswas et al., 2018). Sweden has developed a physical activity on prescription (PAP) model that consists of patient-centered dialogue, individually tailored physical activity recommendations with written prescription, and follow-up, which seems to increase physical activity levels (Onerup et al., 2019). It is the position of the ACSM (https://www.exerciseismedicine.org) and the Canadian Academy of Sport and Exercise Medicine (Thornton et al., 2016) that physicians and other health care providers should include physical activity assessment and prescription as part of routine health care (Box 12.7: Quality and Safety Scenario).

General physical fitness guidelines to promote optimal cardiorespiratory fitness and significantly increase muscle strength and endurance are presented in Fig. 12.3, the Physical Activity Pyramid. Major concepts incorporated into any general physical activity session should include frequency, intensity, time, and type as described in the following list (ACSM, 2022b).

BOX 12.7 QUALITY AND SAFETY SCENARIO

Less Pain, More Gain

In an attempt to encourage increased participation in physical activity, a panel of scientists from the CDC and the ACSM came together to review the evidence related to physical activity and to issue a public health message concerning the recommended types and amounts of physical activity. The evidence clearly indicates that the protective effects of exercise can be achieved at more moderate levels of intensity than had been recommended previously. The health and fitness benefits of exercise appear to be related more to the total amount of exercise performed (calories expended) rather than to the specific exercise intensity, frequency, and duration. The recommendations are as follows:

- Adults should perform 30 minutes or more of moderate-intensity (brisk) physical activity on most (or all) days of the week, for a weekly total of 3–4 hours.
- The activity need not be continuous; benefits can be realized with short bouts of activity (a minimum of 10 minutes) over the course of the day.
- This amount of activity will expend approximately 150–200 calories per day (the equivalent of walking 2 miles briskly) or 1000–1400 calories per week.
- All types of activity can be applied to the daily total (e.g., raking leaves, dancing, or gardening).
- Lower-intensity activities should be performed more often, or for longer periods, or both. More vigorous activities should be performed for shorter periods or less frequently.

Because most adults do not meet these standards, they have the most to gain by incorporating a few minutes of increased activity into their day, gradually building up to 30 minutes a day. People who are active on an irregular basis should strive to be more consistent. People who prefer more formal exercise can choose to participate in more vigorous, organized exercise regimens, sports, and recreational activities.

Sedentary individuals gain the most by increasing their activity to the recommended level. However, any person who already meets the standards can derive some additional benefit by becoming more active.

F (frequency) Aerobic exercise three to five times a week
Resistance training two to three times a week

I (intensity) Moderate to vigorous, by heart rate and perceived exertion
Able to complete each resistance exercise, 8 to 12 repetitions, without strain

T (time) 20–60 minutes, plus warm-up and cool-down periods
15–30 minutes to complete a series of 8–10 resistance exercises

T (type) Aerobic (walking, jogging, biking, swimming, rowing, cross-country skiing, elliptical trainer, NordicTrack, StairMaster, aerobics, dancing, skating, or rollerblading)
Multijoint resistance training, including free weights and machines (e.g., chest press, pull downs, push-ups, squats, etc.)

Aerobic Exercise

The benefits of aerobic exercise are cumulative; therefore, a frequency of three to five times a week is recommended. The benefits of exercising more than five times a week may be outweighed by the risk of injury, especially with higher-impact activities. If increased frequency or duration are a goal, using cross-training as an alternative to the more traditional aerobic activities (i.e., walking or jogging) may help prevent injury. **Cross-training** means performing different types of exercise on different days of the week or performing different types of exercise within one session. The benefits of cross-training include a decreased risk of musculoskeletal injury, an increased potential for total body conditioning, and improved long-term compliance because variety decreases boredom and eliminates the exercise barrier of limited choices (AAOS, 2020). Another potential method of decreasing the risk of injury is through the use of periodization. Periodization involves planned training variations relating to the volume, intensity, and frequency of exercise (Boggenpoel et al., 2018). Planned variations also help prevent the plateauing of physiologic gains that can occur during training that consistently stays the same.

The intensity of exercise that results in health and fitness benefits ranges from moderate to vigorous and is comfortable but challenging (brisk). Intensity is defined by the objective measure of heart rate (HR) and the subjective measure of perceived exertion. The increase in HR during exercise has a strong linear relationship with exercise intensity and aerobic capacity. Resting HR is the HR measured at rest. Maximum HR is the rate measured at the highest workload tolerated during exercise and decreases with age. A commonly used formula for determining maximum HR is 220 minus age. Due to the potential for an estimation error of 7 to 11 bpm (Visich 2003), many are now using the more accurate formula: $208 - (0.7 \times \text{Age})$ (Tanaka et al., 2001). These older formulas are still in use today. Most formulas for determining appropriate exercise HRs have been developed to take resting HR and maximum HR into consideration. Additional physical activity guidelines are provided by the USDHHS for preschool-aged children, children and adolescents, older adults, female during pregnancy, adults with chronic health conditions, and adults with disabilities.

For people who are unaccustomed to exercising or for those who are greatly deconditioned, short durations are recommended, gradually increasing to a beneficial, comfortable level

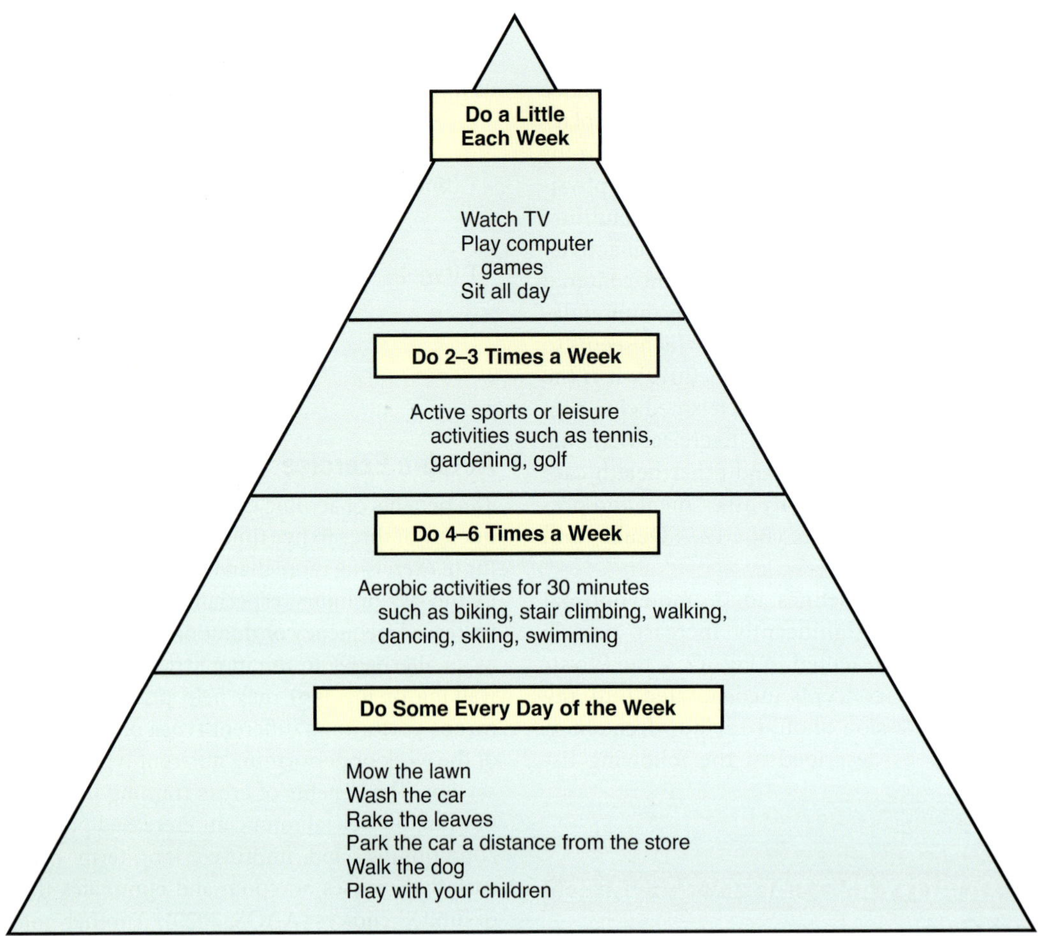

FIG. 12.3 Physical activity pyramid.

as tolerance and confidence increase. Everyone has to start somewhere, and doing a little is much better than doing nothing at all.

The benefit of sessions longer than 45 to 60 minutes may again be outweighed by the potential for injury. Exercising for more than 60 minutes on occasion is certainly not wrong, but a person who increases the duration should consider decreasing the intensity. Increases in cardiorespiratory fitness can also be accrued from intermittent bouts of moderate to vigorous exercise for a shorter duration on a workout day. As discussed, longer bouts of exercise are more beneficial for weight loss. The range of acceptable duration allows greater flexibility, giving reassurance of benefit to the individual who varies exercise choices daily based on capability, interests, and life demands.

As mentioned, many different choices for the mode of aerobic exercise are available. A question that is often asked is "What is the best type of aerobic exercise?" The answer is "The one that the individual is willing to do on a regular basis." Different aerobic exercises have different benefits; they all have their advantages and disadvantages. From a cardiovascular point of view, with relative intensity, frequency, and duration being equal, the benefit is about the same for all modes. Probably the best scenario for general fitness is cross-training, which results in the most optimal all-around benefits. However, the most important recommendation is that the person starts moving—choosing the person's favorite exercise will increase the likelihood of adhering to an exercise program.

Walking is probably the most accessible and popular form of aerobic exercise. Done briskly, walking provides a good cardiorespiratory challenge in 60% to 80% of the adult population. Walking at least twice daily for a total of 20 minutes is associated with less functional decline in older adults and also benefits individuals with lower functional status (Ley et al., 2019). Walking is also an activity that nearly everyone can do, requires little equipment or cost, can be done almost anywhere, and can be a social or a solitary activity, depending on individual needs. Walking is often the recommended exercise of choice for people who are greatly deconditioned or for those who have physical limitations. Considered a low-impact activity, walking can be easily regulated to accommodate a wide range of fitness levels and motor abilities. Cycling, rowing, and swimming (or water walking or other water aerobics) are non–weight-bearing to low–weight-bearing activities that may be good choices for individuals with physical limitations. Aquatic exercise is a good alternative for individuals with musculoskeletal limitations who need some weight relief with exercise, such as those with advanced OA. Although the buoyancy of the water provides this weight relief, the water also provides resistance to the limbs as they move, encouraging an increase in intensity and conditioning. Individuals should be encouraged to do the types of aerobic exercise that best fit their needs, interests, and lifestyles while providing reasonable benefits.

Warm-Up and Cool-Down Periods

In addition to the endurance phase of exercise, warm-up and cool-down periods should be a regular part of the exercise session. The **warm-up period** usually lasts 5 to 10 minutes, and may include light stretching, calisthenics, or performance of the chosen aerobic activity at a low intensity. This approach prepares both the musculoskeletal system and the cardiorespiratory system for the transition from rest to exercise by increasing blood flow, respiration, body temperature, and muscle flexibility. The warm-up period decreases the risks of injury and heart irregularities. Dynamic stretching exercises within a warm-up may enhance performance, including strength, jump, speed, and explosive movements (Hammami et al., 2018).

The **cool-down period** follows the endurance phase and usually lasts 5 to 10 minutes. This phase allows the body to readjust gradually from the demands of exercise back to the baseline. Stretching and slow, rhythmical movement help to increase muscle elasticity, prevent blood pooling and hypotension, and facilitate dissipation of body heat and removal of lactic acid. The result is the prevention of injury, light-headedness, fatigue, and muscle soreness.

Yoga is an excellent example of one form of exercise to use during warm-up and cool-down periods. The word *yoga* means union or "established in being," which implies a mind-body connection. Simply defined, yoga is mindful stretching. The mind is quiet, and awareness is focused on feeling the body as it moves. Movement into and out of yoga postures (called asanas) provides the necessary stimulation of weight-bearing activity to help keep bones strong, provides the movement to increase joint ROM, and stretches and tones muscles. The sun salute *(surya namaskar)*, a series of 12 flexion-extension yoga postures linked together as one fluid movement by the breath rhythm, is a wonderful practice to include in the warm-up and cool-down phases of exercise, providing both physiologic and mind-body benefits.

Yoga also helps develop an appreciation for the experience of the basic resting state, a mindfulness of how it feels to be relaxed physically and mentally during the activity. In this form, exercise becomes an inner experience: that is, quiet and settled on the inside, dynamic and lively on the outside. The yoga philosophy encourages an appreciation of body sensations, slow stretching, and maintenance of proper posture, all of which help to prevent injury and promote health. There is a growing body of evidence to support the use of yoga to improve ROM and flexibility, strength, balance, posture, function, mental health, blood pressure, glycemic control, quality of life, and sleep patterns; alleviate pain and cancer-related fatigue; and reduce disability in select populations (Ban et al., 2021; de Orleans Casagrande et al., 2023; Dhali et al., 2023; Dong et al., 2023; Ko et al., 2023; Martínez-Calderon et al., 2023; Shin, 2021; Zhou et al., 2023).

Flexibility

Flexibility is a basic component of physical fitness. Warm-up and cool-down periods provide the opportunity to work on stretching muscles and increasing joint ROM. ROM around a joint is improved immediately after flexibility exercise and shows chronic improvement after 3 to 4 weeks of regular stretching at a frequency of two to three times per week. There are various types of flexibility exercises, including static stretching, proprioceptive neuromuscular facilitation (PNF), and ballistic stretches (ACSM, 2022b). Static stretching is arguably the most common type of stretching, where a muscle or tendon is slowly stretched actively or passively and held usually for a duration of 10 to 30 seconds. PNF stretching involves an isometric contraction at 20% to 75% maximum voluntary isometric contraction (MVIC) of the targeted muscle for 3 to 6 seconds followed by a static stretch. Ballistic stretching uses the momentum of the moving body segment to produce a stretch. Stretching in older adults may be held for up to 60 seconds. A total of 60 seconds of flexibility exercise per joint is recommended by ACSM (2022b).

Resistance Training

Studies suggest that people who maintain or increase their flexibility and strength are better able to perform daily activities and avoid injury and disability (Martland et al., 2020). Resistance training increases muscle strength and endurance, increases muscle mass, increases metabolic efficiency, maintains or increases bone density, prevents limitations in performance of everyday tasks, decreases the effort required to perform these tasks, and decreases the potential for injury during physical activity. On average, after their early 20s people lose approximately half a pound of muscle every year through lack of use. This reduction in muscle mass is largely responsible for a decrease in resting metabolic rate, which may translate into weight gain. Resistance training is recommended for the older adult because it has a positive effect on many of the degenerative problems associated with the aging process.

Every individual should try to perform activities throughout the day that stimulate muscle strength and endurance. Activities that involve lifting, carrying, or performing repetitive movement against resistance (vacuuming, raking, shoveling, or baking bread) help preserve lean body mass. If these types of activities are not performed on a regular basis, then the guidelines for resistance training provided in Box 12.4 are suggested. These guidelines are not meant to represent workouts performed by bodybuilders or competitive weightlifters and are not meant to result in significant muscular hypertrophy. The purpose of weight training from a health perspective is to develop healthy muscles that provide the strength to do daily activities without risk of injury and to stimulate bone health.

The figures in Box 12.4 demonstrate several suggested resistance exercises for upper body strengthening. Resistance training for all major muscle groups is appropriate, but some individuals often choose to concentrate on the upper body because these muscles tend to be neglected in daily activity and other exercise regimens. The ACSM (2022b) recommends the incorporation of bilateral and unilateral as well as single and multijoint exercises, including total body exercises. Many people believe they need to spend a lot of time on strength training, but studies have found similar benefits to high- and low-frequency training (Thomas & Burns, 2016). In fact, one study found significant strength and endurance gains with just three 13-minute weekly sessions of resistance training (Schoenfeld et al., 2019). For muscle endurance training, the ACSM recommends three to five sets of 8 to 12 repetitions (ACSM, 2022b). The weight that is lifted should result in near muscle fatigue at the end of each set (this differs substantially depending on the muscle being trained, the amount of resistance, and the fitness level of the athlete) and should be performed without strain and while maintaining proper form. Once 12 to 15 repetitions can be completed without fatigue, the resistance can be increased (by 5% or less), or the same weight can be used to do an additional set to fatigue. The movements should be performed slowly, preferably coordinated with the breath, where exhalation occurs during exertion and inhalation occurs on return to the starting position. For strength and power development, ACSM recommends 2 to 4 sets of 8 to 12 repetitions with 2 to 3 minutes of rest between sets and a rest of ≥48 hours between sessions for any one muscle group (ACSM, 2022b). Slow, controlled movements result in greater benefits, lower risk of injury, and more appreciation of how the body feels as its muscles are challenged. Although these are general guidelines, the exercise variables that constitute the exercise prescription should always be chosen to meet the specific needs and limitations of each individual.

Exercise the Spirit: Relaxation Response

Exercise should not be considered merely a physical regimen with objective outcomes (calories burned and repetitions completed). Exercise is also a process of challenging the body and the mind to gain a sense of well-being and a feeling of accomplishment.

Most people understand the physical benefits of exercise, and some people enjoy the challenge of being physically active, but few realize the learning potential inherent in physical activity. Success in embracing a physically active lifestyle may involve a change in focus from the mechanics of exercise to an appreciation for how it feels and what it means to move. Physical activity can be time spent in meditation that fuels both the body and the spirit.

The **relaxation response** (RR) is an inborn set of physiologic changes that offset those of the fight-or-flight (stress) or sympathetic nervous system response. When elicited, the RR results in a "letting go" of physical, emotional, and mental tension. It is a physiologic response inborn in everyone and, although it can sometimes occur without the individual being aware of it, people generally need to develop techniques that help them let go on a more regular basis. Some techniques that are used commonly to elicit the RR include diaphragmatic breathing, meditation, imagery, mindfulness, yoga stretching, and repetitive exercise.

The RR can be combined with exercise to facilitate the release of tension and improve self-awareness and the feeling of well-being. However, a shift in attitude about exercise is also involved, with the focus becoming the process and awareness of movement. Successful elicitation of the RR involves two basic components: a repetitive focus (the breath, a mantra, and the cadence or rhythm of physical activity) and a nonjudgmental attitude (about everyday thoughts and the quality of performance) (Benson & Stuart, 1992). Berger and Owen (1988) have developed exercise characteristics that facilitate stress reduction and support an exercise environment that allows the successful elicitation of the RR. Activities should fulfill the following requirements:

- Be pleasant and enjoyable
- Be noncompetitive (competition implies judgment about the self and others)
- Be predictable (elicitation of the RR involves a shift in awareness from the external to the internal environment that will happen only with a sense of safety and reliability)
- Be repetitive and rhythmical (the cadence of activity provides a focus for awareness)
- Facilitate abdominal breathing (watching the breath serves to anchor thoughts in the moment; in combination with cadence, it provides a focused awareness)
    - Continue for 20 to 30 minutes at a comfortable intensity on most days of the week (continuity restores a sense of serenity)

All forms of exercise can be used to gain this experience. As discussed, yoga involves mindful stretching with a breathing focus, providing an environment for successful elicitation of the RR. **Tai Chi** is another exercise practice with roots in Eastern philosophy. Known as moving meditation, Tai Chi combines movement with focused awareness, involving a physical and cognitive focus for moving in choreographed forms that become a meditation. A recent systematic review found that Tai Chi and yoga may induce stress reduction through effects on the sympathetic and parasympathetic nervous system (Zou et al., 2018).

The quality of body awareness can also be brought into a more traditional exercise practice. Some types of aerobic exercise lend themselves well to changes in the RR because exercise is rhythmical and repetitive and facilitates abdominal breathing. The practitioner can focus on the breath rhythm, the step cadence of walking or jogging, the pedaling cadence of bicycling, or the stroke cadence of swimming. Mantras can be used to create a positive mindset and to focus the mind into the present moment as the experience unfolds. Resistance training takes on new meaning when coordinated with the breath. Focusing on the muscles and how it feels to move through the ROM enhances the knowledge of what feels good and what does not, providing feedback on accepting the physical challenge.

Exercise focus can and should vary daily depending on need, mood, and intent. Some days it feels right to focus on the more physical aspects of the activity, appreciating the challenge of working harder or longer. Other exercise sessions may be more contemplative, letting creativity run, working through the tension of a lingering stressor, quieting the mind for relaxation, listening to music, or appreciating nature. Focusing on the process rather than the outcomes brings meaning and purpose to the activity and helps achieve something more valuable than mere physical outcomes. There is a growing understanding of the effects exercise has on individuals with chronic pain and the potential benefits exercise offers when medical professionals, such as physical therapists, prescribe exercise to this population in the hopes of reducing the use of opioids and their potential for addiction (Capel-Alcaraz et al., 2023; Garland et al., 2019; Geneen et al., 2017; Gilanyi et al., 2023; Li et al., 2023b; Mueller et al., 2023; Rasmussen-Barr et al., 2023; Sun et al., 2018; Wang et al., 2023c). There is a growing body of evidence to support the use of Tai Chi to improve balance confidence, cognitive function, mental health, glucose and lipid metabolism, sleep quality, self-efficacy, quality of life, and functional mobility as well as to decrease pain, disability and fall risk in select populations (Chen et al., 2023; Huang et al., 2022; Liu et al., 2023; Park et al., 2023; Tajik et al., 2018; Wang et al., 2022; Xinzheng et al., 2022; Yin et al., 2023; Zhang et al., 2019, Zhang et al., 2023).

MONITORING THE INNER AND THE OUTER ENVIRONMENT

Activity Level and Physical Condition

The primary purpose of exercise is to enhance health. However, because exercise involves stress to the body, the potential to cause or exacerbate health problems is inherent. When a person is not feeling well, the exercise effort should be decreased or stopped until the individual is feeling better. With an infection or illness, the body is under stress, and overexertion will only increase that stress and possibly lengthen the healing time. The level of activity should be adjusted to accommodate how the individual feels, slowly progressing back to normal workout levels as strength and energy return. Exercise is a useful tool in coping with and managing chronic illness, including arthritis and HIV infection. During an acute exacerbation, activity should be limited to necessary activities of daily living; however, staying active on a regular basis is important, and individuals should adjust activity levels as tolerated. Some physical therapists advocate for having two different exercise programs: one regular program and a second "rescue" program to help during flare-ups (Bartholdy et al., 2016).

Missing an occasional workout will not affect the fitness level; choosing to stop or reduce the amount of exercise when not feeling well is the right choice. However, after missing workouts for 2 weeks, a decline in fitness is inevitable. When one starts again, resumption of the activity should be gradual, working back to the usual level of activity. Inactivity for 3 to 5 months results in the loss of all conditioning benefits gained, and resumption of exercise involves starting over (ACSM, 2022b). Being aware of the external exercise environment is also important. Extremes of heat and cold affect performance as the body adjusts to different temperatures and wind conditions. Changing the time of day for exercise (early morning and later evening are better choices for humid days), adjusting fluid intake, and varying the length of warm-up and cool-down periods will increase tolerance for environmental conditions and enhance exercise safety.

Hydration

Water is the most essential nutrient for the body. Water functions as a solvent, regulates cell volume, and plays a critical role in thermoregulatory and overall function (Lee et al., 2017). A hypohydrated state has been linked to decreases in exercise and sport performance, cognitive function, mood, and increases in risk of exertional heat illness or heatstroke for individuals exercising in hot and humid environments. Therefore, proper hydration before, during, and after exercise is an important component of a good fitness program. Extra fluid is needed to support physiologic homeostasis during exercise, especially in hot weather. The following hydration recommendations are from the ACSM (Dumke, 2021): Four hours before exercising, drink 5 to 7 mL/kg of fluid (12 to 17 oz for a 154-lb person). To achieve effective restoration of body water and retain ingested water, electrolytes lost in sweat should be replaced, so consuming beverages containing electrolytes and carbohydrates may be beneficial (Evans et al., 2017). According to the ACSM (2022b), a sports beverage should generally contain 20 to 30 mEq of sodium per liter, 2 to 5 mEq of potassium per liter, and 5% to 10% of carbohydrates. During exercise, weight changes should be monitored to estimate sweat loss. The amount and rate of fluid replacement depends on sweating rate, environment, and exercise duration. After exercise, consumption of normal meals and beverages will restore hydration. If a rapid recovery is needed, drinking 1.5 L/kg of body weight lost is beneficial. Table 12.1 provides a list of some sports drinks that hydrate and energize individuals.

SPECIAL CONSIDERATIONS

The ACSM (2022b) recommends preparticipation screening before participation with exercise. The ACSM (2023) has published two screening tools promoted by Exercise is Medicine (www.exerciseismedicine.org) to aid in exercise prescription and in identifying those who should receive medical clearance before exercising: the ACSM participation Screening Guidelines and ACSM Exercise Preparticipation Health Screen Recommendations. Most adults do not need medical clearance (i.e., clearance from a health care professional to exercise) before starting a light- to moderate-intensity physical activity program. However, individuals who do not participate in regular exercise (i.e., moderate-intensity physical activity for ≥30 minutes, more than three times per week, for the last ≥3 months) with a known cardiovascular, metabolic, or renal disease and who are asymptomatic should receive medical clearance before participation in an exercise program (ACSM, 2022b). Any individual who does not participate in regular exercise and has signs or symptoms suggestive of cardiovascular, metabolic, or renal disease

TABLE 12.1 Some Sports Drinks That Hydrate and Energize Individuals[a]

Brand (fl. oz)	Calories	Carbohydrate (g)
All Sport (12)	100	25
Cytomax (12)	90	23
Gatorade (12)	80	22
Powerade (12)	80	21
SoBe (12)	153	38
Muscle Milk (11)	170	9
BodyArmor (12)	90	21
Elecrolit (12)	70	18
Nutrilite (12)	91	21

[a]Exact calories and carbohydrates may depend on flavor.

BOX 12.8 Symptoms and Signs Suggestive of Cardiopulmonary Disease

- Pain, discomfort (or other anginal equivalent) in the chest, neck, jaw, arm, or other areas that may be ischemic in nature
- Shortness of breath at rest or with mild exertion
- Dizziness or syncope
- Orthopnea or paroxysmal nocturnal dyspnea
- Ankle edema
- Palpitations or tachycardia
- Intermittent claudication
- Known heart murmur
- Unusual fatigue or shortness of breath with usual activities

These symptoms should be interpreted in the clinical context in which they appear; they are not all specific to cardiopulmonary or metabolic disease.

(Box 12.8) should receive medical clearance before participation in an exercise program.

People with CVD or diabetes have special exercise needs. Limitations in the ability to exercise are related to the severity of the disease and the signs and symptoms of intolerance. For people with CVD and diabetes, safety starting a new exercise program requires supervision and guidance from knowledgeable health care providers. Before starting the program, these individuals should have a medical evaluation, including an exercise tolerance test, to determine functional capacity and the severity of disease.

Cardiovascular Disease

Exercise plays a major role in rehabilitation after a cardiac event such as myocardial infarction (MI), coronary artery bypass surgery, percutaneous transluminal coronary angioplasty or stent placement, and angina. Increased physical activity appears to benefit individuals from all these groups. Simple exercise methods can increase cardiac ejection fraction, exercise tolerance, physical status, and quality of living (Zhang et al., 2018). Other benefits include the following (Chair et al., 2021; He et al., 2022; Li et al., 2021; Prabhu et al., 2020; Wang et al., 2023a; Wu et al., 2022; Zheng et al., 2019):

- Reduction in blood pressure (systolic and diastolic)
- Reductions in HR
- Reduction in total and cardiovascular mortality
- Delay the progression of CVD
- Reduction in hospital admissions
- Reduction of symptoms
- Reduction in obesity and BMI
- Increase in exercise tolerance and fitness level
- Increase in physical and functional capacity
- Increase in the confidence and ability to carry out usual activities of daily living
- Increase in VO_2 max (maximum amount of oxygen that an individual can utilize during intense exercise)
- Decrease in anxiety and depression
- Improvement in psychological well-being

Despite the numerous benefits noted previously, cardiac rehabilitation and exercise training is underused by older adults. Generally, people with CVD demonstrate a reduction in VO_2 max and the ability to do submaximal levels of work. With exercise training, the increase in VO_2 max in persons with CVD averages approximately 20% after 3 months. This improvement in conditioning is the result of both central (cardiac) and peripheral (muscular) changes (ACSM, 2022b). Some of the most significant increases in exercise tolerance have been noted in individuals with angina. With a decrease in submaximal HR or a decrease in systolic blood pressure resulting from conditioning, myocardial oxygen demand is decreased, and individuals can do a greater amount of work before reaching the anginal threshold. An increase in functional capacity allows progression of exercise tolerance and improvement with daily, leisure, and vocational activities.

Appropriately prescribed and conducted exercise training programs increase exercise tolerance and physical fitness in individuals with CVD. Moderate and vigorous regimens are of value, but care should be taken to determine safe exercise parameters for each individual. Aerobic exercise increases cardiorespiratory fitness and functional capacity. Any of the aforementioned aerobic exercises are acceptable for this population, depending on level of fitness and musculoskeletal limitations. Traditionally, resistance training was not commonly recommended for individuals with CVD. The belief was that lifting weights resulted in a disproportionate rise in blood pressure, increased the myocardial oxygen demand, and increased the risk of angina and MI. However, data from several studies indicate that moderate, supervised weight training is feasible, tolerable, and beneficial for individuals with hypertension and CVD (Bjarnason-Wehrens et al., 2022; Fan et al., 2021). Strength training can keep the heart healthy by helping to control body weight, reduce cholesterol levels, and regulate blood glucose levels. Guidelines for determination of appropriate individual training include an aerobic capacity of at least four to five metabolic equivalents, an ejection fraction of greater than 30%, and the absence of severe, symptomatic aortic stenosis. However, clinical experience demonstrates that people with more serious disease can use small hand weights to increase muscle tone without risk of cardiovascular compromise.

Diabetes

As discussed, in addition to diet and weight loss, regular physical activity is an important modality in the prevention and treatment of type 2 diabetes. Regular physical activity reduces the risk of type 2 diabetes by 58% in high-risk individuals when combined with modest weight loss. Physical activity also positively affects lipid levels, blood pressure, cardiovascular health, mortality, and quality of life (de Sousa et al., 2019). Moderate muscular strength independent of cardiorespiratory fitness is also associated with a lower risk of developing type 2 diabetes (Lee et al., 2018). Numerous metaanalyses have demonstrated the benefits of physical activity for adults with type 2 diabetes, including improved glycemic control, vascular health, functional capacity, and quality of life as well as reduction in body fat, depressive symptoms, and inflammatory burden (Arrieta-Leandro et al., 2023; Arsh et al., 2023; Igarashi et al., 2023; Kang et al., 2023; Leonel et al., 2023; Papagianni et al., 2023; Sabag et al., 2023; Su et al., 2023; Zhao et al., 2023).

In a recently published consensus statement, the ACSM extends and updates their prior recommendations for individuals with type 2 diabetes, which includes engaging in physical activity regularly, reducing sedentary time, taking frequent activity breaks, and making accommodations for safe and effective participation when there are health complications (Kanaley et al., 2022). Recommendations for adults are provided for aerobic, resistance, flexibility, and balance exercises, including intensity, frequency, duration, and progression. Physical activity recommendations are also provided for adolescents and youths.

Exercise has long been regarded as part of the triad in the management of diabetes in conjunction with diet and medication (insulin or oral medication). In the early 1900s it was determined that exercise lowers the blood glucose concentration of people with diabetes. After the introduction of insulin, studies revealed that exercise can potentiate the hypoglycemic effect of injected insulin. More recently, findings suggest that in individuals who have poor control (i.e., excessive blood glucose levels), exercise may induce a further increase in blood glucose levels, resulting in ketosis. On average, people with diabetes have a lower maximum HR and higher blood pressure during exercise, resulting in lower maximal oxygen consumption. A recent metaanalysis reported that adults with type 2 diabetes have a lower level of cardiorespiratory fitness as measured by a lower VO_2 max and shorter-distance walk on the 6-Minute Walk Test (de Macedo et al., 2023). However, these individuals can increase their exercise capacity with training and can experience benefits related to overall fitness and cardiorespiratory training that are similar to those gained by people without diabetes.

People with type 2 diabetes should monitor their blood glucose levels and determine their responses to exercise. Although there are additional cautions for individuals with diabetes, such as elevated ketone levels and recent hypoglycemia, the health benefits of being physically active outweigh the risks of being sedentary (Riddell et al., 2017). For all adults living with diabetes, including those with type 1 diabetes, 150 minutes of accumulated physical activity is recommended each week, with no more than 2 consecutive days of no physical activity. Resistance training is also recommended two to three times per week. For children and young people with diabetes, at least 60 minutes of physical activity should be done per day (Riddell et al., 2017). Although the same exercise benefits can be achieved by people with type 1 diabetes, the inherent behavior and function of endogenous insulin makes exercising a more difficult proposition for these individuals. The major functions of insulin are to promote glucose uptake into the cells and to control metabolic homeostasis during exercise, working in synergy with the counter-regulatory hormones. With exercise, insulin secretion decreases slightly, and the concentrations of counter-regulatory hormones increase. This increase stimulates hepatic glucose production, which balances the increased use of glucose by the working muscles, maintaining normoglycemia. However, with injected insulin the plasma insulin concentration does not decrease with exercise, hepatic glucose is not produced as quickly as it is used, and a decrease in blood glucose concentration results. In contrast, people who have poorly controlled diabetes with decreased plasma insulin concentrations already have elevated blood glucose levels because there is insufficient insulin to assist glucose transport into cells. During exercise the liver is stimulated to produce more glucose, which causes a further elevation in blood glucose levels, worsening the hyperglycemic condition. Ketosis may also result from increased mobilization and incomplete combustion of free fatty acids in muscle cells and accelerated ketone body formation in the liver.

Although each person with diabetes should be evaluated and given individual exercise recommendations, the goals of an exercise program are universal:

- Maintain or increase cardiovascular fitness to prevent or minimize long-term cardiovascular complications
- Increase flexibility that is impaired as muscle collagen becomes glycosylated
- Increase muscle strength, which may deteriorate as a result of neuropathy
- Allow people with type 1 diabetes to safely participate in and enjoy physical activities or sports
- Assist with weight control for people with type 2 diabetes
- Allow people with diabetes to experience and gain the same benefits and enjoyment from regular exercise as do people without diabetes

Although blood glucose responses to various forms and intensities of exercise show high variability between and within individuals, Box 12.9 presents a list of general recommendations and precautions for people with diabetes who are interested in regular physical activity and exercise. Blood glucose levels should always be checked before exercise. The target range for blood glucose before exercise should ideally be between 90 and 250 mg/dL.

BUILDING A RHYTHM OF PHYSICAL ACTIVITY

Participation in regular physical activity increased gradually from the 1960s to the 1980s but seems to have plateaued in recent years. The progress made toward the *Healthy People 2020* physical activity goals indicates that most of the population has not embraced a physically active lifestyle (USDHHS, 2020a). Although the benefits of physical activity are common to all people, patterns of physical activity differ among population subgroups defined by sex, age, racial background, income, and body fat. The following generalities are true (Du et al., 2019):

- Males are more active than females.
- Physical activity declines with age.
- Ethnic minorities are less active than White Americans.
- Higher education and income are associated with more leisure-time activity.
- People who are obese are usually less active than their leaner counterparts.

Adherence and Compliance

In health care, adherence and compliance do not mean the same thing (Mir, 2023). Adherence is an active choice to follow through with a recommended treatment (e.g., physical activity) from a health care provider while taking responsibility for one's own health and wellness. Adherence ensures a person's autonomy while seeking behavior change. In contrast, compliance is

BOX 12.9 BEST PRACTICE

Recommendations and Precautions for People with Diabetes Who Are Interested in Regular Physical Activity and Exercise

- Notify primary care physician, ophthalmologist, and podiatrist of intent to exercise.
- Monitor blood glucose level before and 20–30 minutes after exercise to determine the response to exercise. Many individuals use continuous glucose monitors which show glucose levels during exercise.
- The target range for blood glucose is between 90 and 250 mg/dL.
- If possible, exercise approximately 1 hour after meals, when blood glucose level is highest. This plan helps with weight loss because extra food will not have to be eaten to ward off hypoglycemia. When exercising before meals, a snack may be necessary.
- Know the action and peak times of insulin dosage and avoid exercising at the peak.
- Consider adjusting oral medication or insulin dosage to prevent low blood glucose level during exercise. The adjustment will depend on the intensity of the exercise, the duration of the exercise session, and the type of insulin that is used during exercise.
- Be alert to the hypoglycemic lag effect that may occur 12–24 hours after vigorous exercise; an extra snack after exercise will help.
- Avoid injecting insulin into a muscle area that will be active during exercise; the pumping action of the muscle may accelerate absorption of the insulin and cause a rapid decrease of blood glucose level.
- Use proper footwear and frequently inspect the feet.
- Avoid high-impact activity when prone to neuropathy in the legs or feet or when there is a history of neuropathy.
- Keep systolic blood pressure below 180–200 mm Hg in the presence of eye or kidney disease.
- Exercising every day is best but should be done at least three to four times per week. Start with 10–20 minutes and gradually increase to 30–40 minutes at 50%–75% of maximum heart rate. Continuous aerobic activity helps maintain good blood glucose level control better than intermittent activities. Do not forget the 5–10-minute warm-up and cool-down periods.
- Avoid high-intensity anaerobic exercise, but low- to moderate-intensity resistance training is acceptable.
- Carry a concentrated form of carbohydrate (sugar packets, glucose tablets, or hard candy) when exercising.
- Wear some form of diabetes identification.
- People with type 2 diabetes need to test blood glucose levels with exercise and potentially adjust oral medications. Consider decreasing medication if blood glucose level is less than 80 mg/dL after exercise. For weight loss, plan the best time to exercise so that snacks can be avoided.

a passive behavior in which a person follows a recommendation from a health care provider. Compliance mandates treatment without seeking behavior change.

Physiologic, behavioral, and psychological variables influence the decision to adhere to diabetes treatment, including physical activity and medications. Each person is unique, and success with exercise over the long term comes from recognition of personal motivation or core desire and support from the social environment. Core desire defines the purpose behind putting the effort into developing and maintaining an active lifestyle; it is what motivates the individual to exercise. People should be encouraged to spend some quiet time meditating on why being adherent is important to them.

Physical activity is also influenced by multiple other factors, including social, economic, cultural, and environmental factors. Finding meaning and purpose in an active lifestyle can enhance behavior. Biopsychosocial and spiritual variables need to be considered in promoting physical activity. An individual's biopsychosocial factors and spiritual beliefs affect the behavioral and attitudinal factors that influence their motivation and ability to adhere to an active lifestyle. Generally, however, physical activity is more likely to be initiated and maintained if the individual does the following:

- Perceives a net benefit
- Chooses an enjoyable activity
- Feels competent doing the activity
- Feels confident in overcoming barriers that may interfere with the activity
- Feels safe doing the activity
- Can access the activity easily on a regular basis
- Perceives no significant negative financial or social cost
- Experiences minimal musculoskeletal discomfort
- Addresses competing time demands
- Is readily able to fit the activity into their daily schedule
- Balances the use of labor-saving devices with activities that involve physical exertion

Educating the public about physical activity helps provide guidelines for safe and effective exercise, reinforce potential benefits, and alleviate misperceptions that may interfere with the decision to change behavior. However, knowledge of exercise and the intent to exercise do not correlate well with long-term adherence. Confidence in the ability to be physically active—and the confidence that overcoming barriers produces positive benefits related to personal goals (self-efficacy)—is strongly related to participation and adherence (Fig. 12.4). Exercise self-efficacy is increased when people perform exercise successfully, receive positive feedback about success, view exercise role models, and learn more about the relationships among exercise, health, and body awareness (see the Case Study at the end of this chapter).

Creating a Climate That Supports Exercise

Clearly exercise and fitness need to be social norms. A climate that supports and encourages physical activity should be

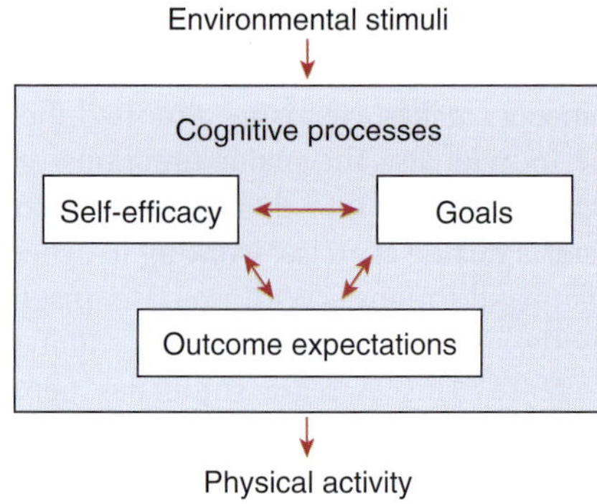

FIG. 12.4 Three interacting cognitive processes of Bandura's social-cognitive theory. (Modified from Beauchamp, M. R., Crawford, K. L., & Jackson, B. [2019]. Social cognitive theory and physical activity: Mechanisms of behavior change, critique, and legacy. *Psychology of Sports & Exercise, 42,* 110–117.)

fostered. Other people and organizations in the individual's social environment can influence the adoption and maintenance of physical activity.

Health Care Providers

People are more likely to increase their physical activity if counseled to do so by their health care providers. Health care providers should communicate the benefits of increased activity, assess a person's current level of activity and compare it with recommendations, identify the person's readiness to change behavior if their activity levels are not adequate, and then empower the person to increase or initiate physical activity (Wingood, 2023). Exploring perceived individual barriers to exercise and offering alternative viewpoints can help create new exercise paradigms. Teixeira and colleagues (2012) published an informative systematic review that summarizes the evidence for self-determination theory, which can be used to improve our understanding of exercise motivation and the importance of autonomous regulations in promoting physical activity. Health care providers also serve as role models by demonstrating enthusiasm regarding the health benefits of being physically active.

Recognizing the stages of behavioral change helps in meeting people at their stage of readiness to begin or increase exercise or physical activity. Providing information on physical activity designed for specific stages of readiness enables people to move from stages of contemplation and preparation into action. An individual in precontemplation is not ready to actively change behavior. This person may respond better to support and information about the benefits of changing behavior than to being placed in an action environment. The decision to change may come gradually. After an individual has made the commitment to change, the action phase lasts approximately 6 months. Leading clients in creating specific goals and an action plan to address their goals can improve their likelihood of success, and Wingood et al. (2023) developed step-by-step guidelines to assist health care providers in supporting physical activity behavior change. Readers are directed to their manuscript for step-by-step guidance.

Family and Friends

Social support can be a valuable resource for behavioral change. Significant others or friends can serve as buddies, providing a source of companionship and motivation. These people can offer to share daily responsibilities to make time for exercise (e.g., provide childcare). Parents can support their children's activity by having family outings and providing transportation and encouragement. Joining a fitness club or an exercise group at work provides various forms of stimulation and socialization, which increases the potential for new friendships grounded in an appreciation of the rewards of exercise.

Schools

Schools are one of the most important resources for increasing physical activity. Children are becoming less active (due to an increased use of electronic devices) and more obese while schools are providing fewer physical education opportunities. This has resulted in several new initiatives that assist schools in improving student health by incorporating physical activity into the classroom and as a regular part of a student's day. A few of these initiatives are Alliance for a Healthier Generation (https://www.healthiergeneration.org/), North Carolina Healthy Schools (https://www.dpi.nc.gov/districts-schools/classroom-resources/academic-standards/programs-and-initiatives/nc-healthy-schools), and Active Academics (https://www.activeacademics.org/). These programs help schools to choose physical activity opportunities that fulfill the following functions:

- Are appropriate and enjoyable for children of all skill levels and are not limited to competitive sports or physical education classes
- Appeal to young females and young males and to children from diverse backgrounds
- Are offered daily
- Can serve as a foundation for activities throughout life

Schools serve as a resource for the community. Research shows that children who participate in more physical activity each day have improved grades, concentration, memory, and classroom behavior. A recent network metaanalysis examined the effects of school-based exercise interventions on physical fitness (Wu et al., 2023). Researchers identified the outcome that each intervention was most effective at improving. High-intensity interval training improved BMI, VO_2 max, and sprint performance. Aerobic training reduced waist circumference. Active video games improved countermovement jump and shuttle run performance. Strength training improved standing long jump performance. Combined aerobic and strength training improved body fat percentage and push-up performance. Another metaanalysis found that physical education in school increased BMD and bone mineral content of the femoral neck and lumbar spine (Mello et al., 2022).

Communities

Participation in regular physical activity at the community level depends in large part on the availability and proximity of facilities and safe environments. Community government agencies, local health agencies, schools, and places of worship have the potential to provide activity resources to the population at large. Churches seem to be particularly successful in reaching ethnic minorities and older adults. Making neighborhoods safe for outdoor activities can have a major effect on improving activity habits, especially among low socioeconomic and disadvantaged populations, who report lower levels of daily physical activity. As more and more individuals use social media, a focus on posting material for others to see or following profiles such as CDC Community Health for more information may help facilitate further awareness in local communities (https://www.cdc.gov/makinghealtheasier/). Recognizing that many of the previous recommendations require a financial commitment, government agencies should respond to reports by health agencies and establish public policies that reinforce the importance of physical activity for the general population. Future genomic studies have the potential to refine exercise protocols and prescriptions (Box 12.10: Genomics). Individuals may make a personal commitment to be physically active, but that commitment needs to be supported by a social and political environment that values this lifestyle choice.

BOX 12.10 GENOMICS

Exercise and Genomics: Current Appraisal

Researchers have long tried to understand how genetic/genomic variations and the environment interrelate to facilitate exercise differences in healthy and diseased populations as well as elite athletes. It has been noted in various countries and globally that elite athletes often arise in the same families or within particular ethnic groups. So, there must be a heritable component that could be studied to gain a better understanding of how to better athletic performance and possibly decrease the likelihood of sports injuries (Hiam et al., 2023). A number of studies have examined genetic variants affecting exercise training and sport performance by looking at chromosome insertions/deletions and gene polymorphisms (same gene, different form). The coding of the human genome in the 2000s indicated that it might be possible to investigate exercise biologic variants, but it became clearer that the complex traits associated with exercise and training components are affected by thousands of genetic alterations. For example, one gene might have many inherited polymorphisms or forms, and exercise adaptation involves many genes. Newer approaches using bioinformation and advanced biostatistics allows for the combination of vast data sets connecting gene loci and gene expression types to discover molecular characteristics corresponding to various exercise habits, patterns, and prescriptions.

With the increase in the use and availability of metadata, there is a need for global collaboration to further exercise science. The COVID-19 pandemic showed the importance of using big data to enlarge scientific fields under the pressure of nearly day-to-day changes in information inputs. Further data analysis may support the utility of better genetic testing for more precise exercise prescriptions. Understandings about the human genome should not be siloed from understanding of exercise biology. Investigating important core questions about the identification of unrealized talent and genetic exercise biology is not only a public health measure but may also increase the potential of athletes, prevent athletic injuries, and speed recovery from all types of injuries (Hiam et al., 2023).

CASE STUDY

Exercise Self-Efficacy: Sharon G

Sharon G. is a 53-year-old account executive who is 2 years postmenopause, has insomnia, and has chronic LBP and left knee pain.

History: A motor vehicle accident 4 years ago resulted in Sharon receiving a bone graft to her left leg (her left leg is shorter than her right leg, and she uses a heel lift). As part of rehabilitation, Sharon started jogging, which was more comfortable than walking with chronic right-sided sacroiliac joint pain, located in the low back which would radiate into the groin and occasionally down the right leg. She started running marathons 2 years after the accident and continued to add more variety to her exercise routine by joining CrossFit and decreased her running. Sharon later had a fall that resulted in chronic LBP, and she was unable to continue aerobic exercise. She began to experience depression and insomnia, reporting difficulty falling and staying asleep 3 to 4 days/week. Exercise had been a significant coping mechanism in the past, and now her whole sense of well-being was affected. As Sharon attempted to rebuild her exercise practice, she would alternate between overexercising, exacerbating symptoms, and then having to stop and recuperate, reinforcing her negative self-image and battling fatigue. She decreased her attendance at CrossFit due to being unable to fully participate, which also removed a social support system from her life. Sharon continues to work, but her knees and back begin to stiffen, which limits her ability to sit for greater than 1 hour at a time. Stiffness and soreness are present in the morning for about 1 hour and then ease until midafternoon. Objectively, there are minimal- to moderate-strength deficits in the hips and trunk and difficulty performing squatting activities. There is also a slight decrease in knee flexion ROM bilaterally and moderate limitations to lumbar flexion, extension, and side bending. Standard X-rays of bilateral knees show osteoarthritis. T2 magnetic resonance imaging studies reveal lumbar spinal stenosis at L3–4.

Reflective Questions

- What are some of her barriers to exercise?
- How will a regular practice of mindfulness and the relaxation response benefit Sharon's exercise practice?
- How would she benefit from cross-training?
- What exercise is she doing that is beneficial for preventing osteoporosis?

SUMMARY

- Individuals need to incorporate deliberate physical activity into their lifestyles on a long-term basis, as exercise in the short term is of little overall benefit.
- Helping individuals gain knowledge (benefits of exercise and recommended parameters for exercise), skills (self-monitoring), and attitude (core desire) increases adherence.
- Individuals need to be motivated enough to start the activity, enjoy the activity enough to want to continue, and appreciate the value enough to start again if they lapse.
- Lapses should be anticipated to avoid the unrealistic sense of total success or total failure.
- Behavioral change is cyclical rather than linear; success often comes with repeated movement through stages of change, and it helps explore the reasons for the lapse and to view the lapse as a learning experience rather than a failure.
- The goal is to prevent a relapse that results in more permanent noncompliance.

EVOLVE CHAPTER FEATURES

http://evolve.elsevier.com/Edelman/smuck

REFERENCES

Abdin, S., Welch, R. K., Byron-Daniel, J., & Meyrick, J. (2018). The effectiveness of physical activity interventions in improving well-being across office-based workplace settings: A systematic review. *Public Health*, *160*, 70–76.

Agarwal, S., Steinmaus, C., & Harris-Adamson, C. (2018). Sit-stand workstations and impact on low back discomfort: A systematic review and meta-analysis. *Ergonomics*, *61*(4), 538–552. https://doi.org/10.1080/00140139.2017.1402960

Aljawarneh, Y. M., Wardell, D. W., Wood, G. L., & Rozmus, C. L. (2019). A systematic review of physical activity and exercise on physiological and biochemical outcomes in children and adolescents with type 1 diabetes. *Journal of Nursing Scholarship*, *51*(3), 337–345.

Almeida, M., Saragiotto, B., Richards, B., & Maher, C. G. (2018). Primary care management of non-specific low back pain: Key messages from recent clinical guidelines. *Medical Journal of Australia*, *208*(6), 272–275.

American Academy of Orthopaedic Surgeons (AAOS). (2020). *Staying healthy: Cross training*. https://orthoinfo.aaos.org/en/staying-healthy/cross-training/

American College of Rheumatology (ACR). (2022). *American College of Rheumatology (ACR) guideline for exercise, rehabilitation, diet, and additional integrative interventions for rheumatoid arthritis: Guideline summary*. https://assets.contentstack.io/v3/assets/bltee37abb6b278ab2c/bltb06bc74fd4810cce/integrative-ra-treatment-guideline-2022.pdf

American College of Sports Medicine (ACSM). (2022a). *Physical activity guidelines*. https://www.acsm.org/education-resources/trending-topics-resources/physical-activity-guidelines

American College of Sports Medicine (ACSM). (2022b). *ACSM's guidelines for exercise testing and prescription* (11th ed.). Philadelphia, PA: Wolters Kluwer.

American College of Sports Medicine (ACSM). (2023). *Exercise is medicine*. https://www.exerciseismedicine.org/

American Heart Association (AHA). (2020). *Getting active to control high blood pressure*. https://www.heart.org/en/health-topics/high-blood-pressure/changes-you-can-make-to-manage-high-blood-pressure/getting-active-to-control-high-blood-pressure

Anekwe, C. V., Jarrell, A. R., Townsend, M. J., Gaudier, G. I., Hiserodt, J. M., & Stanford, F. C. (2020). Socioeconomics of obesity. *Current Obesity Reports*, *9*(3), 272–279. https://doi.org/10.1007/s13679-020-00398-7

Ariani, A., Manara, M., Fioravanti, A., Iannone, F., Salaffi, F., Ughi, N., Prevete, I., Bortoluzzi, A., Parisi, S., & Scirè, C. A. (2019). The Italian Society for Rheumatology clinical practice guidelines for the diagnosis and management of knee, hip, and hand osteoarthritis. *Rheumatismo*, *71*(S1), 5–21.

Arrieta-Leandro, M. C., Moncada-Jiménez, J., Morales-Scholz, M. G., & Hernández-Elizondo, J. (2023). The effect of chronic high-intensity interval training programs on glycaemic control, aerobic resistance, and body composition in type 2 diabetic patients: A meta-analysis. *Journal of Endocrinological Investigation*, *46*(12), 2423–2443. https://doi.org/10.1007/s40618-023-02144-x

Arsh, A., Afaq, S., Carswell, C., Bhatti, M. M., Ullah, I., & Siddiqi, N. (2023). Effectiveness of physical activity in managing co-morbid depression in adults with type 2 diabetes mellitus: A systematic review and meta-analysis. *Journal of Affective Disorders*, *329*, 448–459. https://doi.org/10.1016/j.jad.2023.02.122

Avin, K. G., Nithman, R. W., Osborne, R., Betz, S. R., Lindsey, C., & Hartley, G. W. (2022). Essential components of physical therapist management of patients with osteoporosis: A Delphi study. *Journal of Geriatric Physical Therapy*, *45*(2), E120–E126. https://doi.org/10.1519/JPT.0000000000000347

Balk, E. M., Adam, G. P., Langberg, V. N., et al. (2017). Global dietary calcium intake among adults: A systematic review. *Osteoporosis International*, *28*(12), 3315–3324. https://doi.org/10.1007/s00198-017-4230-x

Ban, M., Yue, X., Dou, P., & Zhang, P. (2021). The effects of yoga on patients with Parkinson's disease: A meta-analysis of randomized controlled trials. *Behavioural Neurology*, *2021*, 5582488. https://doi.org/10.1155/2021/5582488

Baniissa, W., Radwan, H., Rossiter, R., Fakhry, R., Al-Yateem, N., Al-Shujairi, A., Hasan, S., Macridis, S., Farghaly, A. A., Naing, L., & Awad, M. A. (2020). Prevalence and determinants of overweight/obesity among school-aged adolescents in the United Arab Emirates: A cross-sectional study of private and public schools. *BMJ Open*, *10*(12), e038667. https://doi.org/10.1136/bmjopen-2020-038667

Bannuru, R. R., Osani, M. C., Vaysbrot, E. E., Arden, N. K., Bennell, K., Bierma-Zeinstra, S. M. A., Kraus, V. B., Lohmander, L. S., Abbott, J. H., Bhandari, M., Blanco, F. J., Espinosa, R., Haugen, I. K., Lin, J., Mandl, L. A., Moilanen, E., Nakamura, N., Snyder-Mackler, L., Trojian, T., Underwood, M., McAlindon, T. E. (2019). OARSI guidelines for the non-surgical management of knee, hip, and polyarticular osteoarthritis. *Osteoarthritis and Cartilage*, *27*(11), 1578–1589. https://doi.org/10.1016/j.joca.2019.06.011

Barrow, D. R., Abbate, L. M., Paquette, M. R., et al. (2019). Exercise prescription for weight management in obese adults at risk for osteoarthritis: Synthesis from a systematic review. *BMC Musculoskeletal Disorders*, *20*, 610. https://doi.org/10.1186/s12891-019-3004-3

Bartholdy, C., Klokker, L., Bandak, E., Bliddal, H., & Henriksen, M. (2016). A standardized "rescue" exercise program for symptomatic flare-up of knee osteoarthritis: Description and safety considerations. *Journal of Orthopaedic & Sports Physical Therapy*, *46*(11), 942–946.

Benedetti, M. G., Furlini, G., Zati, A., & Letizia Mauro, G. (2018). The effectiveness of physical exercise on bone density in osteoporotic patients. *BioMed Research International*, *2018*, 4840531. https://doi.org/10.1155/2018/4840531

Benson, H., & Stuart, E. (1992). *The wellness book: The comprehensive guide to maintaining health and treating stress-related illness*. New York, NY: Simon & Schuster.

Berger, B., & Owen, D. (1988). Stress reduction and mood enhancement in four exercise modes: Swimming, body conditioning, hatha yoga, and fencing. *Research Quarterly for Exercise and Sport*, *59*(2), 148–159.

Billek-Sawhney, B., Criss, M. G., Galantino, M. L., & Sawhney, R. (2022). Wellness aging model related to inactivity, illness, and injury (WAMI-3): A tool to encourage prevention in practice. *Journal of Geriatric Physical Therapy (2001)*, *45*(4), 168–177. https://doi.org/10.1519/JPT.0000000000000356

Biswas, A., Oh, P. I., Faulkner, G. E., Bonsignore, A., Pakosh, M. T., & Alter, D. A. (2018). The energy expenditure benefits of reallocating sedentary time with physical activity: A systematic review and meta-analysis. *Journal of Public Health (Oxford)*, *40*(2), 295–303.

Bjarnason-Wehrens, B., Schwaab, B., Reiss, N., & Schmidt, T. (2022). Resistance training in patients with coronary artery disease, heart failure, and valvular heart disease: A review with special emphasis on old age, frailty, and physical limitations. *Journal of Cardiopulmonary Rehabilitation and Prevention*, *42*(5), 304–315. https://doi.org/10.1097/HCR.0000000000000730

Boeno, F. P., Ramis, T. R., Munhoz, S. V., Farinha, J. B., Moritz, C. E. J., Leal-Menezes, R., Ribeiro, J. L., Christou, D. D., & Reischak-Oliveira, A. (2020). Effect of aerobic and resistance exercise training on inflammation, endothelial function and ambulatory blood pressure in middle-aged hypertensive patients. *Journal of Hypertension, 38*(12), 2501–2509. https://doi.org/10.1097/HJH.0000000000002581

Boggenpoel, B. Y., Nel, S., & Hanekom, S. (2018). The use of periodized exercise prescription in rehabilitation: A systematic scoping review of literature. *Clinical Rehabilitation, 32*(9), 1235–1248.

Bone Health & Osteoporosis Foundation. (2020). *Osteoporosis fast facts.* https://www.bonehealthandosteoporosis.org/wp-content/uploads/Osteoporosis-Fast-Facts-2.pdf

Brophy, R. H., & Fillingham, Y. A. (2022). AAOS clinical practice guideline summary: Management of osteoarthritis of the knee (nonarthroplasty), third edition. *Journal of the American Academy of Orthopaedic Surgeons, 30*(9), e721–e729. https://doi.org/10.5435/JAAOS-D-21-01233

Burr, D. B. (2019). Changes in bone matrix properties with aging. *Bone, 120*, 85–93. https://doi.org/10.1016/j.bone.2018.10.010

Burton, E., Farrier, K., Hill, K. D., Codde, J., Airey, P., & Hill, A. M. (2018). Effectiveness of peers in delivering programs or motivating older people to increase their participation in physical activity: Systematic review and meta-analysis. *Journal of Sports Sciences, 36*(6), 666–678.

Buscot, M. J., Thomson, R. J., Juonala, M., Sabin, M. A., Burgner, D. P., & Lehtimäki, T., et al. (2018). BMI trajectories associated with resolution of elevated youth BMI and incident adult obesity. *Pediatrics, 141*(1), e20172003. https://doi.org/10.1542/peds.2017-2003

Campos, C., Sotomayor, P., Jerez, D., et al. (2018). Exercise and prostate cancer: From basic science to clinical applications. *The Prostate, 78*, 639–645. https://doi.org/10.1002/pros.23502

Capel-Alcaraz, A. M., Castro-Sánchez, A. M., Matarán-Peñarrocha, G. A., Antequera-Soler, E., & Lara-Palomo, I. C. (2023). Effects of motor control exercises in patients with chronic nonspecific low back pain: A systematic review and meta-analysis. *Clinical Journal of Sport Medicine: Official Journal of the Canadian Academy of Sport Medicine, 33*(6), 579–597. https://doi.org/10.1097/JSM.0000000000001175

Centers for Disease Control and Prevention (CDC). (2023a). *Adult obesity prevalence maps.* Atlanta, GA: US Department of Health and Human Services. https://www.cdc.gov/obesity/data/prevalence-maps.html

Centers for Disease Control and Prevention (CDC). (2023b). *Hypertension cascade: Hypertension prevalence, treatment and control estimates among U.S. adults aged 18 years and older applying the criteria from the American College of Cardiology and American Heart Association's 2017 Hypertension Guideline—NHANES 2017–2020.* Atlanta, GA: May 12, 2023.

Centers for Disease Control and Prevention (CDC). (2023c). *How much physical activity do older adults need?* Atlanta, GA: US Department of Health and Human Services. https://www.cdc.gov/

Centers for Disease Control and Prevention (CDC). (2023d). *Know your risk for heart disease.* Atlanta, GA: US Department of Health and Human Services. https://www.cdc.gov/heartdisease/risk_factors.htm

Centers for Disease Control and Prevention (CDC). (2023e). *National Diabetes Statistics Report.* Atlanta, GA: US Department of Health and Human Services. https://www.cdc.gov/diabetes/data/statistics-report/index.html

Centers for Disease Control and Prevention (CDC). (2023f). *Physical activity among adults aged 18 and over: United States, 2020.* Atlanta, GA: US Department of Health and Human Services.

Centers for Disease Control and Prevention (CDC). (2023g). *Physical activity for everyone: Older adults.* Atlanta, GA: US Department of Health and Human Services.

Chair, S. Y., Zou, H., & Cao, X. (2021). Effects of exercise therapy for adults with coronary heart disease: A systematic review and meta-analysis of randomized controlled trials. *The Journal of Cardiovascular Nursing, 36*(1), 56–77. https://doi.org/10.1097/JCN.0000000000000713

Chan, D. S. M., Abar, L., Cariolou, M., et al. (2019). World Cancer Research Fund International: Continuous Update Project-systematic literature review and meta-analysis of observational cohort studies on physical activity, sedentary behavior, adiposity, and weight change and breast cancer risk. *Cancer Causes Control, 30*(11), 1183–1200.

Chekroud, S. R., Gueorguieva, R., Zheutlin, A. B., Paulus, M., Krumholz, H. M., Krystal, J. H., et al. (2018). Association between physical exercise and mental health in 1.2 million individuals in the USA between 2011 and 2015: A cross-sectional study. *The Lancet Psychiatry, 9*, 739–746. https://doi.org/10.1016/S2215-0366(18)30227-X

Chen, W., Li, M., Li, H., Lin, Y., & Feng, Z. (2023). Tai Chi for fall prevention and balance improvement in older adults: A systematic review and meta-analysis of randomized controlled trials. *Frontiers in Public Health, 11*, 1236050. https://doi.org/10.3389/fpubh.2023.1236050

Chen, S., Zhou, K., Shang, H., Du, M., Wu, L., & Chen, Y. (2023). Effects of concurrent aerobic and resistance training on vascular health in type 2 diabetes: A systematic review and meta-analysis. *Frontiers in Endocrinology, 14*, 1216962. https://doi.org/10.3389/fendo.2023.1216962

Cheng, H., Kong, J., Underwood, C., et al. (2018). Systematic review and meta-analysis of the effect of protein and amino acid supplements in older adults with acute or chronic conditions. *British Journal of Nutrition, 119*(5), 527–542.

Chittrakul, J., Siviroj, P., Sungkarat, S., & Sapbamrer, R. (2020). Multi-system physical exercise intervention for fall prevention and quality of life in pre-frail older adults: A randomized controlled trial. *International Journal of Environmental Research and Public Health, 17*(9), 3102. https://doi.org/10.3390/ijerph17093102

Cormie, P., Atkinson, M., Bucci, L., Cust, A., Eakin, E., Hayes, S., et al. (2018). Clinical Oncology Society of Australia position statement on exercise in cancer care. *Medical Journal of Australia, 209*, 184–187. https://doi.org/10.5694/mja18.00199

Costa, R. R., Buttelli, A. C. K., Vieira, A. F., Coconcelli, L., Magalhães, R. L., Delevatti, R. S., & Kruel, L. F. M. (2019). Effect of strength training on lipid and inflammatory outcomes: Systematic review with meta-analysis and meta-regression. *Journal of Physical Activity & Health, 16*(6), 477–491. https://doi.org/10.1123/jpah.2018-0317

Costa, E. C., Hay, J. L., Kehler, D. S., Boreskie, K. F., Arora, R. C., Umpierre, D., et al. (2018). Effects of high-intensity interval training versus moderate-intensity continuous training on blood pressure in adults with pre- to established hypertension: A systematic review and meta-analysis of randomized trials. *Sports Medicine, 48*(9), 2127–2142. https://doi.org/10.1007/s40279-018-0944-y

Costa, R. J. S., Snipe, R. M. J., Kitic, C. M., & Gibson, P. R. (2017). Systematic review: exercise-induced gastrointestinal syndrome-implications for health and intestinal disease. *Alimentary Pharmacology & Therapeutics, 46*(3), 246–265.

Cunningham, C., O' Sullivan, R., Caserotti, P., & Tully, M. A. (2020). Consequences of physical inactivity in older adults: A systematic review of reviews and meta-analyses. *Scandinavian Journal of Medicine & Science in Sports, 30*(5), 816–827. https://doi.org/10.1111/sms.13616

de Abreu de Lima, V., de Menezes, F. J., Júnior, da Rocha Celli, L., França, S. N., Cordeiro, G. R., Mascarenhas, L. P. G., & Leite, N. (2022). Effects of resistance training on the glycemic control of people with type 1 diabetes: A systematic review and meta-analysis. *Archives of Endocrinology and Metabolism, 66*(4), 533–540. https://doi.org/10.20945/2359-3997000000487

de Orleans Casagrande, P., Coimbra, D. R., de Souza, L. C., & Andrade, A. (2023). Effects of yoga on depressive symptoms, anxiety, sleep quality, and mood in patients with rheumatic diseases: Systematic review and meta-analysis. *PM & R: Journal of Injury, Function, and Rehabilitation, 15*(7), 899–915. https://doi.org/10.1002/pmrj.12867

de Macedo, A. C. P., Schaan, C. W., Bock, P. M., Pinto, M. B., Botton, C. E., Umpierre, D., & Schaan, B. D. (2023). Cardiorespiratory fitness in individuals with type 2 diabetes mellitus: A systematic review and meta-analysis. *Archives of Endocrinology and Metabolism, 67*(5), e230040. https://doi.org/10.20945/2359-4292-2023-0040

de Sousa, M. V., da Silva Soares, D. B., Caraca, E. R., & Cardoso, R. (2019). Highlight article: Dietary protein and exercise for preservation of lean mass and perspectives on type 2 diabetes prevention. *Experimental Biology and Medicine, 244*(12), 992–1004.

de Souto Barreto, P., Demougeot, L., Vellas, B., & Rolland, Y. (2018). Exercise training for preventing dementia, mild cognitive impairment, and clinically meaningful cognitive decline: A systematic review and meta-analysis. *The Journals of Gerontology Series A Biological Sciences and Medical Sciences, 73*(11), 1504–1511.

Del Din, S., Galna, B., Lord, S., Nieuwboer, A., Bekkers, E. M. J., Pelosin, E., Avanzino, L., Bloem, B. R., Olde Rikkert, M. G. M., Nieuwhof, F., Cereatti, A., Della Croce, U., Mirelman, A., Hausdorff, J. M., & Rochester, L. (2020). Falls risk in relation to activity exposure in high-risk older adults. *The Journals of Gerontology. Series A, Biological Sciences and Medical Sciences, 75*(6), 1198–1205. https://doi.org/10.1093/gerona/glaa007

Delitto, A., George, S. Z., Van Dillen, L., et al. (2012). Low back pain: Clinical practice guidelines linked to the International Classification of Functioning, Disability, and Health from the Orthopaedic Section of the American Physical Therapy Association. *Journal of Orthopaedic & Sports Physical Therapy, 42*(4), A1–A57.

Delpino, F. M., de Lima, A. P. M., da Silva, B. G. C., Nunes, B. P., Caputo, E. L., & Bielemann, R. M. (2022). Physical activity and multimorbidity among community-dwelling older adults: A systematic review with meta-analysis. *American Journal of Health Promotion, 36*(8), 1371–1385. https://doi.org/10.1177/08901171221104458

Dhali, B., Chatterjee, S., Sundar Das, S., & Cruz, M. D. (2023). Effect of yoga and walking on glycemic control for the management of type 2 diabetes: A systematic review and meta-analysis. *Journal of the ASEAN Federation of Endocrine Societies, 38*(2), 113–122. https://doi.org/10.15605/jafes.038.02.20

Dibben, G. O., Faulkner, J., Oldridge, N., Rees, K., Thompson, D. R., Zwisler, A. D., & Taylor, R. S. (2023). Exercise-based cardiac rehabilitation for coronary heart disease: A meta-analysis. *European Heart Journal, 44*(6), 452–469. https://doi.org/10.1093/eurheartj/ehac747

Dieleman, J. L., Cao, J., Chapin, A., Chen, C., Li, Z., Liu, A., Horst, C., Kaldjian, A., Matyasz, T., Scott, K. W., Bui, A. L., Campbell, M., Duber, H. C., Dunn, A. C., Flaxman, A. D., Fitzmaurice, C., Naghavi, M., Sadat, N., Shieh, P., Squires, E., Yeung, K., Murray, C. J. L. (2020). US health care spending by payer and health condition, 1996-2016. *JAMA, 323*(9), 863–884. https://doi.org/10.1001/jama.2020.0734

Du, Y., Liu, B., Sun, Y., Snetselaar, L. G., Wallace, R. B., & Bao, W. (2019). Trends in adherence to the physical activity guidelines for Americans for aerobic activity and time spent on sedentary behavior among US adults, 2007 to 2016. *The Journal of the American Medical Association Network Open, 2*(7), e197597. https://doi.org/10.1001/jamanetworkopen.2019.7597

Dumke, C. L. (2021). Chapter 4: Health Related Physical Fitness Testing and Interpretation. In G. Liguori (Ed.), *ACSM's Guidelines for exercise testing and prescription* (11th ed.). Philadelphia, PA: Wolters Kluwer.

Dupuit, M., Rance, M., Morel, C., et al. (2020). Moderate-intensity continuous training or high-intensity interval training with or without resistance training for altering body composition in postmenopausal women. *Medicine and Science in Sports and Exercise, 52*(3), 736–745. https://doi.org/10.1249/mss.0000000000002162

Ekelund, U., Tarp, J., Steene-Johannessen, J., et al. (2019). Dose-response associations between accelerometry measured physical activity and sedentary time and all cause mortality: systematic review and harmonised meta-analysis. *British Medical Journal, 366*, l4570.

Elgaddal, N., Kramarow, E. A., Reuben, C. (2022). *Physical activity among adults aged 18 and over: United States, 2020.* NCHS Data Brief, no 443. Hyattsville, MD: National Center for Health Statistics. https://dx.doi.org/10.15620/cdc:120213

Evans, G. H., James, L. J., Shirreffs, S. M., & Maughan, R. J. (2017). Optimizing the restoration and maintenance of fluid balance after exercise-induced dehydration. *Journal of Applied Physiology, 122*(4), 945–951.

Fan, Y., Yu, M., Li, J., Zhang, H., Liu, Q., Zhao, L., Wang, T., & Xu, H. (2021). Efficacy and safety of resistance training for coronary heart disease rehabilitation: A systematic review of randomized controlled trials. *Frontiers in Cardiovascular Medicine, 8*, 754794. https://doi.org/10.3389/fcvm.2021.754794

Felício, D. C., Filho, J. E., de Oliveira, T. M. D., Pereira, D. S., Rocha, V. T. M., Barbosa, J. M. M., Assis, M. G., Malaguti, C., & Pereira, L. S. M. (2022). Risk factors for non-specific low back pain in older people: A systematic review with meta-analysis. *Archives of Orthopaedic and Trauma Surgery, 142*(12), 3633–3642. https://doi.org/10.1007/s00402-021-03959-0

Fernández-Rodríguez, R., Álvarez-Bueno, C., Cavero-Redondo, I., Torres-Costoso, A., Pozuelo-Carrascosa, D. P., Reina-Gutiérrez, S., Pascual-Morena, C., & Martínez-Vizcaíno, V. (2022). Best exercise options for reducing pain and disability in adults with chronic low back pain: Pilates, strength, core-based, and mind-body. A network meta-analysis. *Journal of Orthopaedic and Sports Physical Therapy, 52*(8), 505–521. https://doi.org/10.2519/jospt.2022.10671

Firth, J., Stubbs, B., Rosenbaum, S., Vancampfort, D., Malchow, B., Schuch, F., et al. (2017). Aerobic exercise improves cognitive functioning in people with schizophrenia: A systematic review and meta-analysis. *Schizophrenia Bulletin, 43*(3), 546–556.

Flack, K. D., Siders, W. A., Johnson, L., & Roemmich, J. N. (2016). Cross-validation of resting metabolic rate prediction equations. *Journal of the Academy of Nutrition and Dietetics, 116*(9), 1413–1422. https://doi.org/10.1016/j.jand.2016.03.018

Flores, V. A., Šilić, P., DuBose, N. G., Zheng, P., Jeng, B., & Motl, R. W. (2023). Effects of aerobic, resistance, and combined exercise training on health-related quality of life in multiple sclerosis: Systematic review and meta-analysis. *Multiple Sclerosis and Related Disorders, 75*, 104746. https://doi.org/10.1016/j.msard.2023.104746

Fryar, C. D., Carroll, M. D., Afful, J. (2020). *Prevalence of overweight, obesity, and severe obesity among children and adolescents aged 2–19 years: United States, 1963–1965 through 2017–2018*. NCHS Health E-Stats. https://www.cdc.gov/nchs/data/hestat/obesity_child_15_16/obesity_child_15_16.pdf

Gallardo-Gómez, D., Noetel, M., Álvarez-Barbosa, F., Alfonso-Rosa, R. M., Ramos-Munell, J., Del Pozo Cruz, B., & Del Pozo-Cruz, J. (2023). Exercise to treat psychopathology and other clinical outcomes in schizophrenia: A systematic review and meta-analysis. *European Psychiatry: The Journal of the Association of European Psychiatrists*, *66*(1), e40. https://doi.org/10.1192/j.eurpsy.2023.24

Gao, R., Tao, Y., Zhou, C., Li, J., Wang, X., Chen, L., Li, F., & Guo, L. (2019). Exercise therapy in patients with constipation: A systematic review and meta-analysis of randomized controlled trials. *Scandinavian Journal of Gastroenterology*, *54*(2), 169–177. https://doi.org/10.1080/00365521.2019.1568544

Garland, E. L., Brintz, C. E., Hanley, A. W., et al. (2019). Mind-body therapies for opioid-treated pain: A systematic review and meta-analysis. *The Journal of the American Medical Association Internal Medicine*, *180*(1), 91–105. https://doi.org/10.1001/jamainternmed.2019.4917

Geneen, L. J., Moore, R. A., Clarke, C., Martin, D., Colvin, L. A., & Smith, B. H. (2017). Physical activity and exercise for chronic pain in adults: An overview of Cochrane Reviews. *The Cochrane Database of Systematic Reviews*, *4*(4), CD011279. https://doi.org/10.1002/14651858.CD011279.pub3

George, S. Z., Fritz, J. M., Silfies, S. P., Schneider, M. J., Beneciuk, J. M., Lentz, T. A., Gilliam, J. R., Hendren, S., & Norman, K. S. (2021). Interventions for the management of acute and chronic low back pain: Revision 2021. *Journal of Orthopaedic and Sports Physical Therapy*, *51*(11), CPG1–CPG60. https://doi.org/10.2519/jospt.2021.0304

Gilanyi, Y. L., Wewege, M. A., Shah, B., Cashin, A. G., Williams, C. M., Davidson, S. R. E., McAuley, J. H., & Jones, M. D. (2023). Exercise increases pain self-efficacy in adults with nonspecific chronic low back pain: A systematic review and meta-analysis. *Journal of Orthopaedic and Sports Physical Therapy*, *53*(6), 335–342. https://doi.org/10.2519/jospt.2023.11622

Gomes-Neto, M., Saquetto, M. B., Alves, I. G., Martinez, B. P., Vieira, J. P. B., & Brites, C. (2021). Effects of exercise interventions on aerobic capacity and health-related quality of life in people living with HIV/AIDS: Systematic review and network meta-analysis. *Physical Therapy*, *101*(7), pzab092. https://doi.org/10.1093/ptj/pzab092

Gong, Q.-H., Kang, J.-F., Ying, Y.-Y., Li, H., Zhang, X.-H., Wu, Y.-H., & Xu, G.-Z. (2015). Lifestyle interventions for adults with impaired glucose tolerance: A systematic review and meta-analysis of the effects on glycemic control. *Internal Medicine (Tokyo, Japan)*, *54*(3), 303–310.

Gordon, B. R., McDowell, C. P., Hallgren, M., Meyer, J. D., Lyons, M., & Herring, M. P. (2018). Association of efficacy of resistance exercise training with depressive symptoms: Meta-analysis and meta-regression analysis of randomized clinical trials. *The Journal of the American Medical Association Psychiatry*, *75*(6), 566–576.

Grgic, J., Dumuid, D., Bengoechea, E. G., Shrestha, N., Bauman, A., Olds, T., et al. (2018). Health outcomes associated with reallocations of time between sleep, sedentary behaviour, and physical activity: A systematic scoping review of isotemporal substitution studies. *International Journal of Behavioral Nutrition and Physical Activity*, *15*(1), 69.

Hammami, A., Zois, J., Slimani, M., Russel, M., & Bouhlel, E. (2018). The efficacy and characteristics of warm-up and re-warm-up practices in soccer players: A systematic review. *The Journal of Sports Medicine and Physical Fitness*, *58*(1-2), 135–149.

Hankonen, N., Heino, M. T. J., Kujala, E., et al. (2017). What explains the socioeconomic status gap in activity? Educational differences in determinants of physical activity and screentime. *BMC Public Health*, *17*, 144. https://doi.org/10.1186/s12889-016-3880-5

Hart, N. H., Newton, R. U., Tan, J., Rantalainen, T., Chivers, P., Siafarikas, A., & Nimphius, S. (2020). Biological basis of bone strength: Anatomy, physiology and measurement. *Journal of Musculoskeletal & Neuronal Interactions*, *20*(3), 347–371.

Hartley, G. W., Roach, K. E., Nithman, R. W., Betz, S. R., Lindsey, C., Fuchs, R. K., & Avin, K. G. (2022). Physical therapist management of patients with suspected or confirmed osteoporosis: A clinical practice guideline from the academy of geriatric physical therapy. *Journal of Geriatric Physical Therapy*, *44*(2), E106–E119. https://doi.org/10.1519/JPT.0000000000000346

Hayden, J. A., Ellis, J., Ogilvie, R., Malmivaara, A., & van Tulder, M. W. (2021a). Exercise therapy for chronic low back pain. *The Cochrane Database of Systematic Reviews*, *9*(9), CD009790. https://doi.org/10.1002/14651858.CD009790.pub2

Hayden, J. A., Ellis, J., Ogilvie, R., Stewart, S. A., Bagg, M. K., Stanojevic, S., Yamato, T. P., & Saragiotto, B. T. (2021b). Some types of exercise are more effective than others in people with chronic low back pain: A network meta-analysis. *Journal of Physiotherapy*, *67*(4), 252–262. https://doi.org/10.1016/j.jphys.2021.09.004

He, M., Wang, Q., & Zhang, W. (2022). Impact of exercise training in patients after CHD surgery: A systematic review and meta-analysis of randomised controlled trials. *Cardiology in the Young*, *32*(12), 1875–1880. https://doi.org/10.1017/S1047951122003201

Heissel, A., Heinen, D., Brokmeier, L. L., Skarabis, N., Kangas, M., Vancampfort, D., Stubbs, B., Firth, J., Ward, P. B., Rosenbaum, S., Hallgren, M., & Schuch, F. (2023). Exercise as medicine for depressive symptoms? A systematic review and meta-analysis with meta-regression. *British Journal of Sports Medicine*, *57*(16), 1049–1057. https://doi.org/10.1136/bjsports-2022-106282

Hernández-Hernández, M. V., & Díaz-González, F. (2017). Role of physical activity in the management and assessment of rheumatoid arthritis patients. *Reumatología Clínica*, *13*(4), 214–220.

Hiam, D., Jones, P., Pitsiladis, Y., & Eynon, N. (2023). Genomics and biology of exercise, where are we now? *Clinical Journal of Sport Medicine*, *33*(5), e112-e114. https://doi.org/10.1097/JSM.0000000000001012

Hong, A. R., & Kim, S. W. (2018). Effects of resistance exercise on bone health. *Endocrinology and Metabolism (Seoul)*, *33*(4), 435–444. https://doi.org/10.3803/EnM.2018.33.4.435.

Holden, M. A., Button, K., Collins, N. J., Henrotin, Y., Hinman, R. S., Larsen, J. B., Metcalf, B., Master, H., Skou, S. T., Thoma, L. M., Wellsandt, E., White, D. K., & Bennell, K. (2021). Guidance for implementing best practice therapeutic exercise for patients with knee and hip osteoarthritis: What does the current evidence base tell us? *Arthritis Care & Research*, *73*(12), 1746–1753. https://doi.org/10.1002/acr.24434

Hu, H., Xu, A., Gao, C., Wang, Z., & Wu, X. (2021). The effect of physical exercise on rheumatoid arthritis: An overview of systematic reviews and meta-analysis. *Journal of Advanced Nursing*, *77*(2), 506–522. https://doi.org/10.1111/jan.14574

Huang, C. Y., Mayer, P. K., Wu, M. Y., Liu, D. H., Wu, P. C., & Yen, H. R. (2022). The effect of Tai Chi in elderly individuals with sarcopenia and frailty: A systematic review and meta-analysis of randomized controlled trials. *Ageing Research Reviews*, *82*, 101747. https://doi.org/10.1016/j.arr.2022.101747

Hunter, D. J., & Bierma-Zeinstra, S. (2019). Osteoarthritis. *Lancet (London, England), 393*(10182), 1745–1759. https://doi.org/10.1016/S0140-6736(19)30417-9

Ibeneme, S. C., Irem, F. O., Iloanusi, N. I., Ezuma, A. D., Ezenwankwo, F. E., Okere, P. C., et al. (2019a). Impact of physical exercises on immune function, bone mineral density, and quality of life in people living with HIV/AIDS: A systematic review with meta-analysis. *BMC Infectious Diseases, 19*(1), 340.

Ibeneme, S. C., Omeje, C., Myezwa, H., et al. (2019b). Effects of physical exercises on inflammatory biomarkers and cardiopulmonary function in patients living with HIV: A systematic review with meta-analysis. *BMC Infectious Diseases, 19*(1), 359.

Ibeneme, S. C., Uwakwe, V. C., Myezwa, H., Irem, F. O., Ezenwankwo, F. E., Ajidahun, T. A., Ezuma, A. D., Okonkwo, U. P., & Fortwengel, G. (2022). Impact of exercise training on symptoms of depression, physical activity level and social participation in people living with HIV/AIDS: A systematic review and meta-analysis. *BMC Infectious Diseases, 22*(1), 469. https://doi.org/10.1186/s12879-022-07145-4

Igarashi, Y., Akazawa, N., & Maeda, S. (2019). Effects of aerobic exercise alone on lipids in healthy East Asians: A systematic review and meta-analysis. *Journal of Atherosclerosis and Thrombosis, 26*(5), 488–503.

Igarashi, Y., Akazawa, N., & Maeda, S. (2023). Effects of changes in body fat mass as a result of regular exercise on hemoglobin A1c in patients with type 2 diabetes mellitus: A meta-analysis. *International Journal of Sport Nutrition and Exercise Metabolism, 33*(4), 209–221. https://doi.org/10.1123/ijsnem.2022-0217

International Osteoporosis Foundation. (2024). *Osteoporosis facts and statistics*. https://www.iofbonehealth.org/facts-and-statistics/calcium-studies-map#category-299

Javaheri, B., & Pitsillides, A. A. (2019). Aging and mechanoadaptive responsiveness of bone. *Current Osteoporosis Reports, 17*(6), 560–569. https://doi.org/10.1007/s11914-019-00553-7

Jia, R. X., Liang, J. H., Xu, Y., & Wang, Y. Q. (2019). Effects of physical activity and exercise on the cognitive function of patients with Alzheimer disease: A meta-analysis. *BMC Geriatrics, 19*(1), 181. https://doi.org/10.1186/s12877-019-1175-2

Jin, X., Pan, B., Wu, H., & Xu, D. (2019). The effects of traditional Chinese exercise on hypertension: A systematic review and meta-analysis of randomized controlled trials. *Medicine (Baltimore), 98*(3), e14049.

Jönsson, T., Eek, F., Dell'Isola, A., Dahlberg, L. E., & Ekvall Hansson, E. (2019). The Better Management of Patients with Osteoarthritis Program: Outcomes after evidence-based education and exercise delivered nationwide in Sweden. *PLoS one, 14*(9), e0222657. https://doi.org/10.1371/journal.pone.0222657

Joubert, C., & Chainay, H. (2018). Aging brain: The effect of combined cognitive and physical training on cognition as compared to cognitive and physical training alone - a systematic review. *Clinical Interventions in Aging, 13*, 1267–1301.

Kalatzi, P., Dinas, P. C., Chryssanthopoulos, C., Karatzanos, E., Nanas, S., & Philippou, A. (2022). Impact of supervised aerobic exercise on clinical physiological and mental parameters of people living with HIV: A systematic review and meta-analyses of randomized controlled trials. *HIV Research & Clinical Practice, 23*(1), 107–119.

Kanaley, J. A., Colberg, S. R., Corcoran, M. H., Malin, S. K., Rodriguez, N. R., Crespo, C. J., Kirwan, J. P., & Zierath, J. R. (2022). Exercise/physical activity in individuals with type 2 diabetes: A consensus statement from the American College of Sports Medicine. *Medicine and Science in Sports and Exercise, 54*(2), 353–368. https://doi.org/10.1249/MSS.0000000000002800

Kang, J., Fardman, B. M., Ratamess, N. A., Faigenbaum, A. D., & Bush, J. A. (2023). Efficacy of postprandial exercise in mitigating glycemic responses in overweight individuals and individuals with obesity and type 2 diabetes-a systematic review and meta-analysis. *Nutrients, 15*(20), 4489. https://doi.org/10.3390/nu15204489

Karaağaç, A., & Yıldırım, A. (2019). How do diet and exercise programmes affect the cardiovascular risk profiles of obese children? *Cardiology in the Young, 29*(2), 200–205. https://doi.org/10.1017/S1047951118002093

Kataria, K., & Ilsley, A. (2021). Urinary incontinence in older adults: What you need to know. *British Journal of Hospital Medicine (London, England: 2005), 82*(4), 1–8. https://doi.org/10.12968/hmed.2020.0518

Kidd, T., Mold, F., Jones, C., et al. (2019). What are the most effective interventions to improve physical performance in pre-frail and frail adults? A systematic review of randomised control trials. *BMC Geriatrics, 19*, 184. https://doi.org/10.1186/s12877-019-1196-x

Ko, K. Y., Kwok, Z. C. M., & Chan, H. Y. (2023). Effects of yoga on physical and psychological health among community-dwelling older adults: A systematic review and meta-analysis. *International Journal of Older People Nursing, 18*(5), e12562. https://doi.org/10.1111/opn.12562

Kolasinski, S. L., Neogi, T., Hochberg, M. C., et al. (2020). 2019 American College of Rheumatology/Arthritis Foundation guideline for the management of osteoarthritis of the hand, hip, and knee. *Arthritis Care & Research, 72*(2), 149–162.

Lachman, M. E., Lipsitz, L., Lubben, J., Castaneda-Sceppa, C., & Jette, A. M. (2018). When adults don't exercise: Behavioral strategies to increase physical activity in sedentary middle-aged and older adults. *Innovation Aging, 2*(1), igy007. https://doi.org/10.1093/geroni/igy007

LaMonte, M. J., Wactawski-Wende, J., Larson, J. C., et al. (2019). Association of physical activity and fracture risk among postmenopausal women. *The Journal of the American Medical Association Netw Open, 2*(10), e1914084. https://doi.org/10.1001/jamanetworkopen.2019.14084

Lange, E., Kucharski, D., Svedlund, S., Svensson, K., Bertholds, G., Gjertsson, I., & Mannerkorpi, K. (2019). Effects of aerobic and resistance exercise in older adults with rheumatoid arthritis: A randomized controlled trial. *Arthritis Care & Research, 71*(1), 61–70. https://doi.org/10.1002/acr.23589

Lauche, R., Hunter, D. J., Adams, J., & Cramer, H. (2019). Yoga for osteoarthritis: A systematic review and meta-analysis. *Current Rheumatology Reports, 21*(9), 48. https://doi.org/10.1007/s11926-019-0846-5

Laurent, M. R., Dedeyne, L., Dupont, J., Mellaerts, B., Dejaeger, M., & Gielen, E. (2019). Age-related bone loss and sarcopenia in men. *Maturitas, 122*, 51–56. https://doi.org/10.1016/j.maturitas.2019.01.006

Leal, D. B., Assis, M. A. A., Conde, W. L., Lobo, A. S., Bellisle, F., & Andrade, D. F. (2018). Individual characteristics and public or private schools predict the body mass index of Brazilian children: A multilevel analysis. *Cadernos de Saúde Pública, 34*(5), e00053117.

Lee J. (2021). Influences of exercise interventions on overweight and obesity in children and adolescents. *Public Health Nursing, 38*(3), 502–516. https://doi.org/10.1111/phn.12862

Lee, D. C., Brellenthin, A., Sui, X., & Blair, S. (2018). Abstract MP32: Muscular strength and type 2 diabetes prevention. *Circulation, 137*(Supp 1), AMP32.

Lee, J., Wan, B. A., Malek, L., Lim, F., Lam, H., Silva, M. F., et al. (2018). Biological mechanisms linking exercise and cancer. *Journal of Pain Management, 11*(3), 207–215.

Lee, E. C., Fragala, M. S., Kavouras, S. A., Queen, R. M., Pryor, J. L., & Casa, D. J. (2017). Biomarkers in sports and exercise: Tracking health, performance, and recovery in athletes. *Journal of Strength & Conditioning Research, 31*(10), 2920–2937.

Leonel, L. D. S., Brum, G., Alberton, C. L., & Delevatti, R. S. (2023). Aquatic training improves HbA1c, blood pressure and functional outcomes of patients with type 2 diabetes: A systematic review with meta-analysis. *Diabetes Research and Clinical Practice, 197*, 110575. https://doi.org/10.1016/j.diabres.2023.110575

Ley, L., Khaw, D., Duke, M., & Botti, M. (2019). The dose of physical activity to minimise functional decline in older general medical patients receiving 24-hr acute care: A systematic scoping review. *Journal of Clinical Nursing, 28*(17-18), 3049–3064.

Li, J., Li, Y., Gong, F., Huang, R., Zhang, Q., Liu, Z., Lin, J., Li, A., Lv, Y., & Cheng, Y. (2021). Effect of cardiac rehabilitation training on patients with coronary heart disease: A systematic review and meta-analysis. *Annals of Palliative Medicine, 10*(11), 11901–11909. https://doi.org/10.21037/apm-21-3136

Li, J., Jiang, X., Huang, Z., & Shao, T. (2023a). Exercise intervention and improvement of negative emotions in children: A meta-analysis. *BMC Pediatrics, 23*(1), 411. https://doi.org/10.1186/s12887-023-04247-z

Li, Y., Yan, L., Hou, L., Zhang, X., Zhao, H., Yan, C., Li, X., Li, Y., Chen, X., & Ding, X. (2023b). Exercise intervention for patients with chronic low back pain: A systematic review and network meta-analysis. *Frontiers in Public Health, 11*, 1155225. https://doi.org/10.3389/fpubh.2023.1155225

Liang, M., Pan, Y., Zhong, T., Zeng, Y., & Cheng, A. S. K. (2021). Effects of aerobic, resistance, and combined exercise on metabolic syndrome parameters and cardiovascular risk factors: A systematic review and network meta-analysis. *Reviews in Cardiovascular Medicine, 22*(4), 1523–1533. https://doi.org/10.31083/j.rcm2204156

Liangruenrom, N., Craike, M., Biddle, S. J. H., Suttikasem, K., & Pedisic, Z. (2019). Correlates of physical activity and sedentary behaviour in the Thai population: A systematic review. *BMC Public Health, 19*(1), 414.

Lin, J., Gao, YF, Guo Y, Li M, Zhu Y, You R, Chen S, Wang, S. (2022). Effects of qigong exercise on the physical and mental health of college students: A systematic review and meta-analysis. *BMC Complement Med Ther, 8;22*(1), 287. https://doi.org/10.1186/s12906-022-03760-5. PMID: 36348349; PMCID: PMC9641907.

Littlefield, A., & Lenahan, C. (2019). Cholelithiasis: Presentation and management. *Journal of Midwifery & Women's Health, 64*, 289–297. https://doi.org/10.1111/jmwh.12959

Liu, H., Liu, S., Xiong, L., & Luo, B. (2023). Effects of traditional Chinese exercise on sleep quality: A systematic review and meta-analysis of randomized controlled trials. *Medicine, 102*(44), e35767. https://doi.org/10.1097/MD.0000000000035767

Liu, Y., Ye, W., Chen, Q., Zhang, Y., Kuo, C. H., & Korivi, M. (2019). Resistance exercise intensity is correlated with attenuation of HbA1c and insulin in patients with type 2 diabetes: A systematic review and meta-analysis. *International Journal of Environmental Research and Public Health, 16*(1), 140.

Lobelo, F., Rohm Young, D., Sallis, R., Garber, M. D., Billinger, S. A., Duperly, J., Hutber, A., Pate, R. R., Thomas, R. J., Widlansky, M. E., McConnell, M. V., Joy, E. A., & American Heart Association Physical Activity Committee of the Council on Lifestyle and Cardiometabolic Health; Council on Epidemiology and Prevention; Council on Clinical Cardiology; Council on Genomic and Precision Medicine; Council on Cardiovascular Surgery and Anesthesia; and Stroke Council. (2018). Routine assessment and promotion of physical activity in healthcare settings: A scientific statement from the American Heart Association. *Circulation, 137*(18), e495–e522. https://doi.org/10.1161/CIR.0000000000000559

Maleki, B. H., Tartibian, B., Mooren, F. C., FitzGerald, L. Z., Krüger, K., Chehrazi, M., et al. (2018). Low-to-moderate intensity aerobic exercise training modulates irritable bowel syndrome through antioxidative and inflammatory mechanisms in women: Results of a randomized controlled trial. *Cytokine, 102*, 18–25. https://doi.org/10.1016/j.cyto.2017.12.016

Maly, M. R., Marriott, K. A., & Chopp-Hurley, J. N. (2020). Osteoarthritis year in review 2019: Rehabilitation and outcomes. *Osteoarthritis and Cartilage, 28*, 249–266.

Mariano, I. M., Amaral, A. L., Ribeiro, P. A. B., & Puga, G. M. (2023). Exercise training improves blood pressure reactivity to stress: A systematic review and meta-analysis. *Scientific Reports, 13*(1), 10962. https://doi.org/10.1038/s41598-023-38041-9

Marin-Cascales, E., Alcaraz, P. E., Ramos-Campo, D. J., & Rubio-Arias, J. A. (2018). Effects of multicomponent training on lean and bone mass in postmenopausal and older women: A systematic review. *Menopause, 25*(3), 346–356.

Marshall, K., Teo, L., Shanahan, C., Legette, L., & Mitmesser, S. H. (2020). Inadequate calcium and vitamin D intake and osteoporosis risk in older Americans living in poverty with food insecurities. *PloS one, 15*(7), e0235042. https://doi.org/10.1371/journal.pone.0235042

Martínez-Calderon, J., Casuso-Holgado, M. J., Muñoz-Fernandez, M. J., Garcia-Muñoz, C., & Heredia-Rizo, A. M. (2023). Yoga-based interventions may reduce anxiety symptoms in anxiety disorders and depression symptoms in depressive disorders: A systematic review with meta-analysis and meta-regression. *British Journal of Sports Medicine, 57*(22), 1442–1449. https://doi.org/10.1136/bjsports-2022-106497

Martland, R., Mondelli, V., Gaughran, F., & Stubbs, B. (2020). Can high-intensity interval training improve physical and mental health outcomes? A meta-review of 33 systematic reviews across the lifespan. *Journal of Sports Sciences, 38*(4), 430–469.

McKinnis, L. N. (2020). *Fundamentals of orthopedic radiology* (5th ed.). Philadelphia, PA: F.A. Davis.

McMurray, R. G., Soares, J., Caspersen, C. J., & McCurdy, T. (2014). Examining variations of resting metabolic rate of adults: A public health perspective. *Medicine & Science in Sports & Exercise, 46*(7), 1352–1358. https://doi.org/10.1249/MSS.0000000000000232

McTiernan, A., Friedenreich, C. M., Katzmarzyk, P. T., et al. (2019). Physical activity in cancer prevention and survival: A systematic review. *Medicine & Science in Sports & Exercise, 51*(6), 1252–1261.

Mello, J. B., Pedretti, A., García-Hermoso, A., Martins, C. M. L., Gaya, A. R., Duncan, M. J., & Gaya, A. C. A. (2022). Exercise in school physical education increase bone mineral content and density: Systematic review and meta-analysis. *European Journal of Sport Science, 22*(10), 1618–1629. https://doi.org/10.1080/17461391.2021.1960426

Meng, C., Yucheng, T., Shu, L., & Yu, Z. (2022). Effects of school-based high-intensity interval training on body composition, cardiorespiratory fitness and cardiometabolic markers in adolescent boys with obesity: A randomized controlled trial. *BMC Pediatrics, 22*(1), 112. https://doi.org/10.1186/s12887-021-03079-z

Mir, T. H. (2023). Adherence versus compliance. *HCA Healthcare Journal of Medicine, 4*(2), 219–220. https://doi.org/10.36518/2689-0216.1513

Montero-Odasso, M. M., Kamkar, N., Pieruccini-Faria, F., Osman, A., Sarquis-Adamson, Y., Close, J., Hogan, D. B., Hunter, S. W., Kenny,

R. A., Lipsitz, L. A., Lord, S. R., Madden, K. M., Petrovic, M., Ryg, J., Speechley, M., Sultana, M., Tan, M. P., van der Velde, N., Verghese, J., Masud, T., Task Force on Global Guidelines for Falls in Older Adults. (2021). Evaluation of clinical practice guidelines on fall prevention and management for older adults: A systematic review. *JAMA Network Open*, *4*(12), e2138911. https://doi.org/10.1001/jamanetworkopen.2021.38911

Morris, L., Stander, J., Ebrahim, W., Eksteen, S., Meaden, O. A., Ras, A., et al. (2018). Effect of exercise versus cognitive behavioural therapy or no intervention on anxiety, depression, fitness and quality of life in adults with previous methamphetamine dependency: A systematic review. *Addiction Science & Clinical Practice*, *13*(1), 4.

Mueller, J., Weinig, J., Niederer, D., Tenberg, S., & Mueller, S. (2023). Resistance, motor control, and mindfulness-based exercises are effective for treating chronic nonspecific neck pain: A systematic review with meta-analysis and dose-response meta-regression. *The Journal of Orthopaedic and Sports Physical Therapy*, *53*(8), 420–459. https://doi.org/10.2519/jospt.2023.11820

Naci, H., Salcher-Konrad, M., Dias, S., Blum, M. R., Sahoo, S. A., Nunan, D., et al. (2019). How does exercise treatment compare with antihypertensive medications? A network meta-analysis of 391 randomised controlled trials assessing exercise and medication effects on systolic blood pressure. *British Journal of Sports Medicine*, *53*(14), 859–869.

Nascimento, D. D. C., da Silva, C. R., Valduga, R., et al. (2018). Blood pressure response to resistance training in hypertensive and normotensive older women. *Clinical Interventions in Aging*, *13*, 541–553. https://doi.org/10.2147/CIA.S157479

National Health and Nutrition Examination Survey. (2020). https://www.cdc.gov/nchs/nhanes/index.htm

National Health and Nutrition Examination Survey (NHNES). (2020). *NCHS fact sheet, July 2020.*

National Institutes of Health & Osteoporosis and Related Bone Diseases National Resource Center. (2020). *Osteoporosis*. http://www.niams.nih.gov/Health_Info/Bone/Osteoporosis

National Physical Activity Plan. (2022). *National physical activity plan.* https://paamovewithus.org/wp-content/uploads/2023/05/2022-National-PA-Plan-FINAL.pdf

Neuman, D. A. (2017). *Chapter 12: Hip. In Kinesiology of the musculoskeletal system* (3rd ed.). St. Louis, Missouri: Elsevier.

Newton, S., Braithwaite, D., & Akinyemiju, T. F. (2017). Socio-economic status over the life course and obesity: Systematic review and meta-analysis. *PLoS one*, *12*(5), e0177151.

Nguyen, T. P., Jacobs, P. G., Castle, J. R., Wilson, L. M., Kuehl, K., Branigan, D., Gabo, V., Guillot, F., Riddell, M. C., Haidar, A., & El Youssef, J. (2021). Separating insulin-mediated and non-insulin-mediated glucose uptake during and after aerobic exercise in type 1 diabetes. *American Journal of Physiology: Endocrinology and Metabolism*, *320*(3), E425–E437. https://doi.org/10.1152/ajpendo.00534.2020

Northey, J. M., Cherbuin, N., Pumpa, K. L., Smee, D. J., & Rattray, B. (2018). Exercise interventions for cognitive function in adults older than 50: A systematic review with meta-analysis. *British Journal of Sports Medicine*, *52*(3), 154–160.

Olaya-Contreras, P., Styf, J., Arvidsson, D., Frennered, K., & Hansson, T. (2015). The effect of the stay active advice on physical activity and on the course of acute severe low back pain. *BMC Sports Science, Medicine and Rehabilitation*, *7*, 19.

Olsen, P. Ø., Tully, M. A., Del Pozo Cruz, B., Wegner, M., & Caserotti, P. (2022). Community-based exercise enhanced by a self-management programme to promote independent living in older adults: A pragmatic randomized controlled trial. *Age and Ageing*, *51*(7), afac137. https://doi.org/10.1093/ageing/afac137

Onerup, A., Arvidsson, D., Blomqvist, Å., Daxberg, E. L., Jivegård, L., Jonsdottir, I. H., et al. (2019). Physical activity on prescription in accordance with the Swedish model increases physical activity: A systematic review. *British Journal of Sports Medicine*, *53*(6), 383–388.

Ou, S., Chen, Y., Shih, C., et al. (2017). Impact of physical activity on the association between lipid profiles and mortality among older people. *Scientific Reports*, *7*, 8399. https://doi.org/10.1038/s41598-017-07857-7

Papatheodorou, K., Banach, M., Bekiari, E., Rizzo, M., & Edmonds, M. (2018). Complications of Diabetes 2017. *Journal of Diabetes Research*, *2018*, 3086167.

Park, M., Song, R., Ju, K., Shin, J. C., Seo, J., Fan, X., Gao, X., Ryu, A., & Li, Y. (2023). Effects of Tai Chi and Qigong on cognitive and physical functions in older adults: Systematic review, meta-analysis, and meta-regression of randomized clinical trials. *BMC Geriatrics*, *23*(1), 352. https://doi.org/10.1186/s12877-023-04070-2

Parker, N. H., Ngo-Huang, A., Lee, R. E., et al. (2019). Physical activity and exercise during preoperative pancreatic cancer treatment. *Support Care Cancer*, *27*, 2275–2284. https://doi.org/10.1007/s00520-018-4493-6

Pinheiro, M. B., Ferreira, M. L., Refshauge, K., et al. (2015). Symptoms of depression and risk of new episodes of low back pain: A systematic review and meta-analysis. *Arthritis Care & Research*, *67*, 1591–1603.

Piva, T., Masotti, S., Raisi, A., Zerbini, V., Grazzi, G., Mazzoni, G., Belvederi Murri, M., & Mandini, S. (2023). Exercise program for the management of anxiety and depression in adults and elderly subjects: Is it applicable to patients with post-covid-19 condition? A systematic review and meta-analysis. *Journal of Affective Disorders*, *325*, 273–281. https://doi.org/10.1016/j.jad.2022.12.155

Pocovi, N. C., de Campos, T. F., Christine Lin, C. W., Merom, D., Tiedemann, A., & Hancock, M. J. (2022). Walking, cycling, and swimming for nonspecific low back pain: A systematic review with meta-analysis. *The Journal of Orthopaedic and Sports Physical Therapy*, *52*(2), 85–99. https://doi.org/10.2519/jospt.2022.10612

Pouresmaeili, F., Kamalidehghan, B., Kamarehei, M., & Goh, Y. M. (2018). A comprehensive overview on osteoporosis and its risk factors. *Therapeutics and Clinical Risk Management*, *14*, 2029–2049. https://doi.org/10.2147/TCRM.S138000

Prabhu, N. V., Maiya, A. G., & Prabhu, N. S. (2020). Impact of cardiac rehabilitation on functional capacity and physical activity after coronary revascularization: A scientific review. *Cardiology Research and Practice*, *2020*, 1236968. https://doi.org/10.1155/2020/1236968

Quentin, C., Bagheri, R., Ugbolue, U. C., Coudeyre, E., Pélissier, C., Descatha, A., Menini, T., Bouillon-Minois, J. B., & Dutheil, F. (2021). Effect of home exercise training in patients with nonspecific low-back pain: A systematic review and meta-analysis. *International Journal of Environmental Research and Public Health*, *18*(16), 8430. https://doi.org/10.3390/ijerph18168430

Raposo, F., Ramos, M., & Lúcia Cruz, A. (2021). Effects of exercise on knee osteoarthritis: A systematic review. *Musculoskeletal Care*, *19*(4), 399–435. https://doi.org/10.1002/msc.1538

Rasmussen-Barr, E., Halvorsen, M., Bohman, T., Boström, C., Dedering, Å., Kuster, R. P., Olsson, C. B., Rovner, G., Tseli, E., Nilsson-Wikmar, L., & Grooten, W. J. A. (2023). Summarizing the effects of different exercise types in chronic neck pain - a systematic review and meta-analysis of systematic reviews. *BMC Musculoskeletal Disorders*, *24*(1), 806. https://doi.org/10.1186/s12891-023-06930-9

Recchia, F., Bernal, J. D. K., Fong, D. Y., Wong, S. H. S., Chung, P. K., Chan, D. K. C., Capio, C. M., Yu, C. C. W., Wong, S. W. S., Sit, C. H. P., Chen, Y. J., Thompson, W. R., & Siu, P. M. (2023). Physical activity interventions to alleviate depressive symptoms in children and adolescents: A systematic review and meta-analysis. *JAMA Pediatrics*, *177*(2), 132–140. https://doi.org/10.1001/jamapediatrics.2022.5090

Reddy, R., Wittenberg, A., Castle, J. R., Youssef, J. E., Winters-Stone, K., Gillingham, M., et al. (2019). Effect of aerobic and resistance exercise on glycemic control in adults with type 1 diabetes. *Canadian Journal of Diabetes*, *43*(6), 406–414. https://doi.org/10.1016/j.jcjd.2018.08.193

Reichert, T., Costa, R. R., Barroso, B. M., da Rocha, V. M. B., Delevatti, R. S., & Kruel, L. F. M. (2018). Aquatic training in upright position as an alternative to improve blood pressure in adults and elderly: A systematic review and meta-analysis. *Sports Medicine*, *48*(7), 1727–1737.

Rezapour, M., Ali, S., & Stollman, N. (2018). Diverticular disease: An update on pathogenesis and management. *Gut Liver*, *12*(2), 125–132. https://doi.org/10.5009/gnl16552

Riddell, M. C., Gallen, I. W., Smart, C. E., et al. (2017). Exercise management in type 1 diabetes: A consensus statement. *Lancet Diabetes Endocrinol*, *5*(5), 377–390.

Rock, C. L., Thomson, C., Gansler, T., Gapstur, S. M., McCullough, M. L., Patel, A. V., Andrews, K. S., Bandera, E. V., Spees, C. K., Robien, K., Hartman, S., Sullivan, K., Grant, B. L., Hamilton, K. K., Kushi, L. H., Caan, B. J., Kibbe, D., Black, J. D., Wiedt, T. L., McMahon, C., Sloan, K., Doyle, C. (2020). American Cancer Society guideline for diet and physical activity for cancer prevention. *Cancer Journal for Clinicians*, *70*(4), 245–271. https://doi.org/10.3322/caac.21591

Rodrigues, C. E., Grandt, C. L., Alwafa, R. A., Badrasawi, M., & Aleksandrova, K. (2023). Determinants and indicators of successful aging as a multidimensional outcome: A systematic review of longitudinal studies. *Frontiers in Public Health*, *11*, 1258280. https://doi.org/10.3389/fpubh.2023.1258280

Royal Australian College of General Practitioners (RACGP). (2018). *Guideline for the management of knee and hip osteoarthritis* (2nd ed.). East Melbourne, Vic: RACGP.

Sabag, A., Chang, C. R., Francois, M. E., Keating, S. E., Coombes, J. S., Johnson, N. A., Pastor-Valero, M., & Rey Lopez, J. P. (2023). The effect of exercise on quality of life in type 2 diabetes: A systematic review and meta-analysis. *Medicine and Science in Sports and Exercise*, *55*(8), 1353–1365. https://doi.org/10.1249/MSS.0000000000003172

Saco-Ledo, G., Valenzuela, P. L., Ruiz-Hurtado, G., Ruilope, L. M., & Lucia, A. (2020). Exercise reduces ambulatory blood pressure in patients with hypertension: A systematic review and meta-analysis of randomized controlled trials. *Journal of the American Heart Association*, *9*(24), e018487. https://doi.org/10.1161/JAHA.120.018487

Sampath Kumar, A., Maiya, A. G., Shastry, B. A., Vaishali, K., Ravishankar, N., Hazari, A., Gundmi, S., & Jadhav, R. (2019). Exercise and insulin resistance in type 2 diabetes mellitus: A systematic review and meta-analysis. *Annals of Physical and Rehabilitation Medicine*, *62*(2), 98–103. https://doi.org/10.1016/j.rehab.2018.11.001

Sarzynski, M. A., Ruiz-Ramie, J. J., Barber, J. L., et al. (2018). Effects of increasing exercise intensity and dose on multiple measures of HDL (high-density lipoprotein) function. *Arteriosclerosis, Thrombosis, and Vascular Biology*, *38*(4), 943–952.

Schoenfeld, B. J., Contreras, B., Krieger, J., et al. (2019). Resistance training volume enhances muscle hypertrophy but not strength in trained men. *Medicine & Science in Sports & Exercise*, *51*(1), 94–103. https://doi.org/10.1249/MSS.0000000000001764

Seo, Y. G., Lim, H., Kim, Y., Ju, Y. S., Lee, H. J., Jang, H. B., Park, S. I., & Park, K. H. (2019). The effect of a multidisciplinary lifestyle intervention on obesity status, body composition, physical fitness, and cardiometabolic risk markers in children and adolescents with obesity. *Nutrients*, *11*(1), 137. https://doi.org/10.3390/nu11010137

Setayesh, S., & Mohammad Rahimi, G. R. (2023). The impact of resistance training on brain-derived neurotrophic factor and depression among older adults aged 60 years or older: A systematic review and meta-analysis of randomized controlled trials. *Geriatric Nursing (New York, N.Y.)*, *54*, 23–31. https://doi.org/10.1016/j.gerinurse.2023.08.022

Sexton, B. P., & Taylor, N. F. (2019). To sit or not to sit? A systematic review and meta-analysis of seated exercise for older adults. *Australasian Journal on Ageing*, *38*(1), 15–27.

Shephard, R. J. (2017). Peptic ulcer and exercise. *Sports Med*, *47*, 33–40. https://doi.org/10.1007/s40279-016-0563-4

Sherrington, C., Fairhall, N. J., Wallbank, G. K., Tiedemann, A., Michaleff, Z. A., Howard, K., Clemson, L., Hopewell, S., & Lamb, S. E. (2019). Exercise for preventing falls in older people living in the community. *The Cochrane Database of Systematic Reviews*, *1*(1), CD012424. https://doi.org/10.1002/14651858.CD012424.pub2

Shin, S. (2021). Meta-analysis of the effect of yoga practice on physical fitness in the elderly. *International Journal of Environmental Research and Public Health*, *18*(21), 11663. https://doi.org/10.3390/ijerph182111663

Sitthipornvorakul, E., Klinsophonb, T., Sihawongb, R., & Janwantanakulb, P. (2018). The effects of walking intervention in patients with chronic low back pain: A meta-analysis of randomized controlled trials. *Musculoskeletal Science and Practice*, *34*, 38–46.

Snijders, T., Leenders, M., de Groot, LCPGM., van Loon, L. J. C., & Verdijk, L. B. (2019). Muscle mass and strength gains following 6 months of resistance type exercise training are only partly preserved within one year with autonomous exercise continuation in older adults. *Experimental Gerontology*, *121*, 71–78. https://doi.org/10.1016/j.exger.2019.04.002

Sobue, Y., Kojima, T., Ito, H., Nishida, K., Matsushita, I., Kaneko, Y., Kishimoto, M., Kohno, M., Sugihara, T., Seto, Y., Tanaka, E., Nakayama, T., Hirata, S., Murashima, A., Morinobu, A., Mori, M., Kojima, M., Kawahito, Y., & Harigai, M. (2022). Does exercise therapy improve patient-reported outcomes in rheumatoid arthritis? A systematic review and meta-analysis for the update of the 2020 JCR guidelines for the management of rheumatoid arthritis. *Modern Rheumatology*, *32*(1), 96–104. https://doi.org/10.1080/14397595.2021.1886653

Song, D., Yu, D. S. F., Li, P. W. C., & Lei, Y. (2018). The effectiveness of physical exercise on cognitive and psychological outcomes in individuals with mild cognitive impairment: A systematic review and meta-analysis. *International Journal of Nursing Studies*, *79*, 155–164.

Spei, M. E., Samoli, E., Bravi, F., La Vecchia, C., Bamia, C., & Benetou, V. (2019). Physical activity in breast cancer survivors: A systematic review and meta-analysis on overall and breast cancer survival. *Breast*, *44*, 144–152. https://doi.org/10.1016/j.breast.2019.02.001.

Su, W., Tao, M., Ma, L., Tang, K., Xiong, F., Dai, X., & Qin, Y. (2023). Dose-response relationships of resistance training in Type 2 diabetes mellitus: A meta-analysis of randomized controlled trials. *Frontiers in Endocrinology*, *14*, 1224161. https://doi.org/10.3389/fendo.2023.1224161

Sun, E., Moshfegh, J., Rishel, C. A., Cook, C. E., Goode, A. P., & George, S. Z. (2018). Association of early physical therapy with long-term opioid use among opioid-naive patients with musculoskeletal pain. *The Journal of the American Medical Association Network Open*, *1*(8), e185909. https://doi.org/10.1001/jamanetworkopen.2018.5909

Sun, L., Zhu, J., Ling, Y., Mi, S., Li, Y., Wang, T., & Li, Y. (2021). Physical activity and the risk of rheumatoid arthritis: evidence from meta-analysis and Mendelian randomization. *International Journal of Epidemiology*, *50*(5), 1593–1603. https://doi.org/10.1093/ije/dyab052

Tajik, A., Rejeh, N., Heravi-Karimooi, M., Kia, P. S., Tadrisi, S. D., Watts, T. E., et al. (2018). The effect of Tai Chi on quality of life in male older people: A randomized controlled clinical trial. *Complementary Therapies in Clinical Practice*, *33*, 191–196. https://doi.org/10.1016/j.ctcp.2018.10.009

Tanaka, H., Monahan, K. D., & Seals, D. R. (2001). Age-predicted maximal heart rate revisited. *Journal of the American College of Cardiology*, *37*(1), 153–156.

Teixeira, P. J., Carraça, E. V., Markland, D., Silva, M. N., & Ryan, R. M. (2012). Exercise, physical activity, and self-determination theory: A systematic review. *International Journal of Behavioral Nutrition and Physical Activity*, *9*(78), 1–30.

Teychenne, M., Lamb, K. E., Main, L., Miller, C., Hahne, A., & Ford, J. (2019). General strength and conditioning versus motor control with manual therapy for improving depressive symptoms in chronic low back pain: A randomised feasibility trial. *PLoS one*, *14*(8), e0220442.

Thomas, M. H., & Burns, S. P. (2016). Increasing lean mass and strength: A comparison of high frequency strength training to lower frequency strength training. *International Journal of Exercise Science*, *9*(2), 159–167.

Thomas, E., Battaglia, G., Patti, A., Brusa, J., Leonardi, V., Palma, A., & Bellafiore, M. (2019). Physical activity programs for balance and fall prevention in elderly: A systematic review. *Medicine*, *98*(27), e16218. https://doi.org/10.1097/MD.0000000000016218

Thornton, J. S., Frémont, P., Khan, K., Poirier, P., Fowles, J., Wells, G. D., et al. (2016). Physical activity prescription: A critical opportunity to address a modifiable risk factor for the prevention and management of chronic disease: A position statement by the Canadian Academy of Sport and Exercise Medicine. *Clinical Journal of Sport Medicine*, *26*(4), 259–265.

Tian, S., & Zhao, D. (2018). Comparative effectiveness of exercise interventions for low back pain: A systematic review and network meta-analysis of 41 randomised controlled trials. *The Lancet*, *392*, S21.

Tong, X., Chen, X., Zhang, S., et al. (2019). The effect of exercise on the prevention of osteoporosis and bone angiogenesis. *BioMed Research International*, *2019*, 8171897.

Tucker, W. J., Fegers-Wustrow, I., Halle, M., Haykowsky, M. J., Chung, E. H., & Kovacic, J. C. (2022). Exercise for primary and secondary prevention of cardiovascular disease: JACC Focus Seminar 1/4. *Journal of the American College of Cardiology*, *80*(11), 1091–1106. https://doi.org/10.1016/j.jacc.2022.07.004

US Census Bureau. (2018). *Older people projected to outnumber children for first time in U.S. history*. Washington, DC: US Census Bureau. https://www.census.gov/newsroom/press-releases/2018/cb18-41-population-projections.html

US Department of Health and Human Services (USDHHS). (2018). *Physical activity guidelines for Americans* (2nd ed.). Washington, DC: US Department of Health and Human Services.

US Department of Health and Human Services (USDHHS). (2020a). *Healthy People 2020*. https://www.healthypeople.gov/

US Department of Health and Human Services (USDHHS). (2020b). *Healthy People 2030*. https://www.healthypeople.gov/

US Department of Health and Human Services (USDHHS). (2021). *Overweight & obesity statistics*. https://www.niddk.nih.gov/health-information/health-statistics/overweight-obesity

US Department of Health and Human Services (USDHHS). (2023a). *Healthy People 2020: An end of decade snapshot*. https://health.gov/sites/default/files/2020-12/HP2020EndofDecadeSnapshot.pdf

US Department of Health and Human Services (USDHHS). (2023b). *Healthy People 2030: Physical activity*. https://health.gov/healthypeople/objectives-and-data/browse-objectives/physical-activity#:~:text=Goal%3A%20Improve%20health%2C%20fitness%2C,life%20through%20regular%20physical%20activity

US Department of Health and Human Services (USDHHS). (2023c). *How has Healthy People changed?* https://health.gov/healthypeople/about/how-has-healthy-people-changed

Valenzuela, P. L., Saco-Ledo, G., Morales, J. S., Gallardo-Gómez, D., Morales-Palomo, F., López-Ortiz, S., Rivas-Baeza, B., Castillo-García, A., Jiménez-Pavón, D., Santos-Lozano, A., Del Pozo Cruz, B., & Lucia, A. (2023). Effects of physical exercise on physical function in older adults in residential care: A systematic review and network meta-analysis of randomised controlled trials. *The Lancet. Healthy Longevity*, *4*(6), e247–e256. https://doi.org/10.1016/S2666-7568(23)00057-0

van Ancum, J. M., Scheerman, K., Jonkman, N. H., et al. (2017). Change in muscle strength and muscle mass in older hospitalized patients: A systematic review and meta-analysis. *Experimental Gerontology*, *92*, 34–41.

van Doormaal, M. C. M., Meerhoff, G. A., Vliet Vlieland, T. P. M., & Peter, W. F. (2020). A clinical practice guideline for physical therapy in patients with hip or knee osteoarthritis. *Musculoskeletal Care*, *18*(4), 575–595. https://doi.org/10.1002/msc.1492

Van Dyke, M. E., Chen, T. J., Nakayama, J. Y., Moore, L. V., & Whitfield, G. P. (2023). Changes in physical inactivity among US adults overall and by sociodemographic characteristics, behavioral risk factor surveillance system, 2020 versus 2018. *Preventing Chronic Disease*, *20*, E65. https://doi.org/10.5888/pcd20.230012

van der Windt, D. J., Sud, V., Zhang, H., Tsung, A., & Huang, H. (2018). The effects of physical exercise on fatty liver disease. *Gene Expression*, *18*(2), 89–101. https://doi.org/10.3727/105221617X15124844266408

Vasodi, E., Saatchian, V., & Dehghan Ghahfarokhi, A. (2023). Virtual reality-based exercise interventions on quality of life, some balance factors and depression in older adults: A systematic review and meta-analysis of randomized controlled trials. *Geriatric Nursing (New York, N.Y.)*, *53*, 227–239. https://doi.org/10.1016/j.gerinurse.2023.07.019

Vespa, J., Medina, L., Armstrong, D. M. (2020). Demographic turning points for the United States: Population projections for 2020 to 2060. *Current Population Reports, P25-1144*. Washington, DC: U.S. Census Bureau.

Villarroel, M.A., & Terlizzi, E. P. (2020). *Symptoms of depression among adults: United States, 2019*. NCHS Data Brief, no 379. Hyattsville, MD: National Center for Health Statistics.

Visich, P. S. (2003). Graded exercise testing. In J. K. Ehrman, P. M. Gordon, P. S. Visich, & S. J. Keteyan (Eds.), *Clinical exercise physiology* (pp. 79–101). Champaign, IL: Human Kinetics.

Wada, T., Matsumoto, H., & Hagino, H. (2019). Customized exercise programs implemented by physical therapists improve exercise-related self-efficacy and promote behavioral changes in elderly individuals without regular exercise: A randomized controlled trial. *BMC Public Health, 19*, 917. https://doi.org/10.1186/s12889-019-7270-7

Wallis, J. A., Webster, K. E., Levinger, P., Singh, P. J., Fong, C., & Taylor, N. F. (2015). The maximum tolerated dose of walking for people with severe osteoarthritis of the knee: A phase I trial. *Osteoarthritis Cartilage OARS Osteoarthritis Res Soc, 23*(8), 1285–1293.

Wang, F., Cai, J., Liu, J., Duan, B., Yang, Y., & Yang, Q. (2023a). Effects of traditional Chinese exercise on physiological indicators and quality of life in patients with coronary heart disease: A systematic review and meta-analysis. *Medicine, 102*(26), e34233. https://doi.org/10.1097/MD.0000000000034233

Wang, C., Tian, Z., & Luo, Q. (2023b). The impact of exercise on mental health during the COVID-19 pandemic: A systematic review and meta-analysis. *Frontiers in Public Health, 11*, 1279599. https://doi.org/10.3389/fpubh.2023.1279599

Wang, T., Wang, J., Chen, Y., Ruan, Y., & Dai, S. (2023c). Efficacy of aquatic exercise in chronic musculoskeletal disorders: A systematic review and meta-analysis of randomized controlled trials. *Journal of Orthopaedic Surgery and Research, 18*(1), 942. https://doi.org/10.1186/s13018-023-04417-w

Wang, Y., Zhang, Q., Li, F., Li, Q., & Jin, Y. (2022). Effects of Tai Chi and qigong on cognition in neurological disorders: A systematic review and meta-analysis. *Geriatric Nursing (New York, N.Y.), 46*, 166–177. https://doi.org/10.1016/j.gerinurse.2022.05.014

Ward, Z. J., Willett, W. C., Hu, F. B., Pacheco, L. S., Long, M. W., & Gortmaker, S. L. (2022). Excess mortality associated with elevated body weight in the USA by state and demographic subgroup: A modelling study. *EClinicalMedicine, 48*, 101429. https://doi.org/10.1016/j.eclinm.2022.101429

Watson, S. L., Weeks, B. K., Weis, L. J., Harding, A. T., Horan, S. A., & Beck, B. R. (2018). High-intensity resistance and impact training improves bone mineral density and physical function in postmenopausal women with osteopenia and osteoporosis: The LIFTMOR randomized controlled trial. *Journal of Bone and Mineral Research, 33*, 211–220. https://doi.org/10.1002/jbmr.3284

Weber, M., Belala, N., Clemson, L., Boulton, E., Hawley-Hague, H., Becker, C., et al. (2018). Feasibility and effectiveness of intervention programmes integrating functional exercise into daily life of older adults: A systematic review. *Gerontology, 64*(2), 172–187.

Wellsandt, E., & Golightly, Y. (2018). Exercise in the management of knee and hip osteoarthritis. *Current Opinion in Rheumatology, 30*(2), 151–159.

Wen, Z., & Chai, Y. (2021). Effectiveness of resistance exercises in the treatment of rheumatoid arthritis: A meta-analysis. *Medicine, 100*(13), e25019. https://doi.org/10.1097/MD.0000000000025019

Werneck, A. O., Agostinete, R. R., Lima, M. C. S., Turi-Lynch, B. C., & Fernandes, R. A. (2019). The effects of physical activity during childhood, adolescence, and adulthood on cardiovascular risk factors among adults. *Revista da Associacao Medica Brasileira, 65*(11), 1337–1342.

Wingood, M., Bean, J. F., & Linsky, A. M. (2023). Incorporating physical activity assessments and behavior change techniques into geriatrics. *Archives of Rehabilitation Research and Clinical Translation, 5*(4), 100293. https://doi.org/10.1016/j.arrct.2023.100293

Wingood, M., Bonnell, L., LaCroix, A. Z., Rosenberg, D., Walker, R., Bellettiere, J., Greenwood-Hickman, M. A., Wing, D., & Gell, N. (2021). Community-dwelling older adults and physical activity recommendations: Patterns of aerobic, strengthening, and balance activities. *Journal of Aging and Physical Activity, 30*(4), 653–665. https://doi.org/10.1123/japa.2021-0194

Wong, J. J., Tricco, A. C., Côté, P., Liang, C. Y., Lewis, J. A., Bouck, Z., & Rosella, L. C. (2022). Association between depressive symptoms or depression and health outcomes for low back pain: A systematic review and meta-analysis. *Journal of General Internal Medicine, 37*(5), 1233–1246. https://doi.org/10.1007/s11606-021-07079-8

Wood, G., Taylor, E., Ng, V., Murrell, A., Patil, A., van der Touw, T., Sigal, R., Wolden, M., & Smart, N. (2021). Determining the effect size of aerobic exercise training on the standard lipid profile in sedentary adults with three or more metabolic syndrome factors: A systematic review and meta-analysis of randomised controlled trials. *British Journal of Sports Medicine*, bjsports-2021-103999. Advance online publication. https://doi.org/10.1136/bjsports-2021-103999

Wu, C., Bu, R., Wang, Y., Xu, C., Chen, Y., Che, L., & Wang, S. (2022). Rehabilitation effects of circuit resistance training in coronary heart disease patients: A systematic review and meta-analysis. *Clinical Cardiology, 45*(8), 821–830. https://doi.org/10.1002/clc.23855

Wu, J., Yang, Y., Yu, H., Li, L., Chen, Y., & Sun, Y. (2023). Comparative effectiveness of school-based exercise interventions on physical fitness in children and adolescents: A systematic review and network meta-analysis. *Frontiers in Public Health, 11*, 1194779. https://doi.org/10.3389/fpubh.2023.1194779

Xiao, P. L., Cui, A. Y., Hsu, C. J., Peng, R., Jiang, N., Xu, X. H., Ma, Y. G., Liu, D., & Lu, H. D. (2022). Global, regional prevalence, and risk factors of osteoporosis according to the World Health Organization diagnostic criteria: A systematic review and meta-analysis. *Osteoporosis International, 33*(10), 2137–2153. https://doi.org/10.1007/s00198-022-06454-3

Xinzheng, W., Fanyuan, J., & Xiaodong, W. (2022). The effects of Tai Chi on glucose and lipid metabolism in patients with diabetes mellitus: A meta-analysis. *Complementary Therapies in Medicine, 71*, 102871. https://doi.org/10.1016/j.ctim.2022.102871

Xu, Z., Wang, Y., Zhang, Y., Lu, Y., & Wen, Y. (2023). Efficacy and safety of aquatic exercise in knee osteoarthritis: A systematic review and meta-analysis of randomized controlled trials. *Clinical Rehabilitation, 37*(3), 330–347. https://doi.org/10.1177/02692155221134240

Yang, Y., Fu, X., Zhang, H., Ouyang, G., & Lin, S. C. (2023). The effect of home-based exercise on motor symptoms, quality of life and functional performance in Parkinson's disease: A systematic review and meta-analysis. *BMC Geriatrics, 23*(1), 873. https://doi.org/10.1186/s12877-023-04595-6

Yang, G. Y., Hunter, J., Bu, F. L., Hao, W. L., Zhang, H., Wayne, P. M., & Liu, J. P. (2022a). Determining the safety and effectiveness of Tai Chi: A critical overview of 210 systematic reviews of controlled clinical trials. *Systematic Reviews, 11*(1), 260. https://doi.org/10.1186/s13643-022-02100-5

Yang, W., Liang, X., & Sit, C. H. (2022b). Physical activity and mental health in children and adolescents with intellectual disabilities: A meta-analysis using the RE-AIM framework. *The International Journal of Behavioral Nutrition and Physical Activity, 19*(1), 80. https://doi.org/10.1186/s12966-022-01312-1

Yin, J., Yue, C., Song, Z., Sun, X., & Wen, X. (2023). The comparative effects of Tai Chi versus non-mindful exercise on measures of anxiety, depression and general mental health: A systematic review and meta-analysis. *Journal of Affective Disorders, 337*, 202–214. https://doi.org/10.1016/j.jad.2023.05.037

You, Y., Liu, J., Tang, M., Wang, D., & Ma, X. (2021). Effects of Tai Chi exercise on improving walking function and posture control in elderly patients with knee osteoarthritis: A systematic review and meta-analysis. *Medicine, 100*(16), e25655. https://doi.org/10.1097/MD.0000000000025655

Zagalaz-Anula, N., Mora-Rubio, M. J., Obrero-Gaitán, E., & Del-Pino-Casado, R. (2022). Recreational physical activity reduces breast cancer recurrence in female survivors of breast cancer: A meta-analysis. *European Journal of Oncology Nursing: The Official Journal of European Oncology Nursing Society*, *59*, 102162. https://doi.org/10.1016/j.ejon.2022.102162

Zampogna, B., Papalia, R., Papalia, G. F., Campi, S., Vasta, S., Vorini, F., Fossati, C., Torre, G., & Denaro, V. (2020). The role of physical activity as conservative treatment for hip and knee osteoarthritis in older people: A systematic review and meta-analysis. *Journal of Clinical Medicine*, *9*(4), 1167. https://doi.org/10.3390/jcm9041167

Zanetti, H. R., Lopes, L. T. P., Gonçalves, A., Soares, V. L., Soares, W. F., Hernandez, A. V., Tse, G., Liu, T., Biondi-Zoccai, G., Roever, L., & Mendes, E. L. (2021). Effects of resistance training on muscle strength, body composition and immune-inflammatory markers in people living with HIV: A systematic review and meta-analysis of randomized controlled trials. *HIV Research & Clinical Practice*, *22*(5), 119–127.

Zeng, L., Zhao, X., Yu, Y., Hu, T., Li, C., Wu, M., & Yang, F. (2023). Effects of Tai Chi on depression of middle-aged and older adults: An updated systematic review and meta-analysis. *BMC Complementary Medicine and Therapies*, *23*(1), 382. https://doi.org/10.1186/s12906-023-04207-1

Zhang, Q., Hu, J., Wei, L., Cao, R., Ma, R., Song, H., et al. (2019). Effects of traditional Chinese exercise on cognitive and psychological outcomes in older adults with mild cognitive impairment: A systematic review and meta-analysis. *Medicine (Baltimore)*, *98*(7), e14581.

Zhang, Y., Cao, H., Jiang, P., & Tang, H. (2018). Cardiac rehabilitation in acute myocardial infarction patients after percutaneous coronary intervention: A community-based study. *Medicine (Baltimore)*, *97*(8), e9785.

Zhang, W., Sun, J., Feng, X., Zhang, H., Zhang, Y., & Zhao, M. (2023). Effectiveness of Tai Chi exercise on fear of falling and balance in older adults: A meta-analysis. *Geriatric Nursing*, *51*, 194–201. https://doi.org/10.1016/j.gerinurse.2023.03.019

Zhao, H., Teng, J., Song, G., Fu, X., Pan, X., Shen, S., Yan, Y., & Liu, C. (2023). The optimal exercise parameters of Tai Chi on the effect of glucose and lipid metabolism in patients with type 2 diabetes mellitus: A meta-analysis. *Complementary Therapies in Medicine*, *79*, 102995. https://doi.org/10.1016/j.ctim.2023.102995

Zheng, X., Zheng, Y., Ma, J., et al. (2019). Effect of exercise-based cardiac rehabilitation on anxiety and depression in patients with myocardial infarction: A systematic review and meta-analysis. *Heart Lung*, *48*(1), 1–7.

Zhou, J., Mi, J., Peng, Y., Han, H., & Liu, Z. (2021). Causal associations of obesity with the intervertebral degeneration, low back pain, and sciatica: A two-sample Mendelian randomization study. *Frontiers in Endocrinology*, *12*, 740200. https://doi.org/10.3389/fendo.2021.740200

Zhou, W. S., Zheng, T. T., Mao, S. J., Xu, H., Wang, X. F., & Zhang, S. K. (2023). Comparing the effects of different exercises on blood pressure and arterial stiffness in postmenopausal women: A systematic review and meta-analysis. *Experimental Gerontology*, *171*, 111990. https://doi.org/10.1016/j.exger.2022.111990

Zou, L., Sasaki, J. E., Wei, G. X., Huang, T., Yeung, A. S., Neto, O. B., et al. (2018). Effects of mind–body exercises (tai chi/yoga) on heart rate variability parameters and perceived stress: A systematic review with meta-analysis of randomized controlled trials. *Journal of Clinical Medicine*, *7*, 404.

13

Stress Management

June Andrews Horowitz and Marni B. Kellogg

http://evolve.elsevier.com/Edelman/

OBJECTIVES

After completing this chapter, the reader will be able to:

- Analyze concepts of stress, stressor, eustress, and distress.
- Evaluate physical, psychological, social, spiritual, and behavioral stressors that are potential contributors to physical and mental health disorders.
- Analyze the pathophysiology of the stress response and effects on health and illness.
- Examine primary and secondary cognitive appraisals of stress.
- Develop evidence-based stress-management interventions that can be used in clinical practice.
- Explain the nurse's role in stress management and crisis intervention.

KEY TERMS

Active listening
Acupuncture
Affirmation
Allostatic load
Anxiety sensitivity
Aromatherapy
Assertive communication
Burnout
Caregiver stress/burden
Cognitive restructuring
Coping
Distress
Empathy
Eustress
Exercise
Expressive writing
Fight-or-flight response
Goal setting
Healthy diet
Healthy pleasures
Homeodynamics
Homeostasis
Humor
Hypnosis
Journal writing
Meridian
Mindfulness
Mini relaxations
Pet Therapy
Presence
Primary appraisal
Reflexology
Reiki
Relaxation response
Sandwich generation
Secondary appraisal
Self-awareness
Sleep hygiene
Social support
Sociophysiology
Spiritual practice
Stress
Stress management
Stressor
Stress response
Stress warning signs
Values clarification
Yoga

THINK ABOUT IT

Do We Live to Work or Work to Live?

When asked about yourself, what is your first response? Do you say what you do for work, or do you describe your characteristics? For most of us, our work roles, including being students, define us to a great extent. For most adults in industrialized countries and many other societies, employment is a primary source of income and social connection; working also contributes to a personal sense of accomplishment. However, how much work is too much? Americans take fewer yearly vacation days than their counterparts in other industrialized countries, and workplace pressures can increase the risk of various disorders. Work-related stress can be a significant problem.

- What aspects of work typically create stress? What aspects create meaning and satisfaction?
- How do people manage work-related stress? Which strategies are helpful, and which strategies increase health risks?
- How do people manage the work-life-home balance?
- What health-promotion strategies could you implement to reduce your work-related stress?
- What could you do to promote workplace health in your practice?

Stress is an expected physical or emotional reaction to challenges (National Center for Complementary and Integrative Health [NCCIH], 2022). Stress is an excellent paradigm for understanding the relationships among the determinants of health, the leading health indicators, and health outcomes. Chronic stress has been shown to cause or exacerbate many of the leading health problems in the United States today, including heart disease, diabetes, and mental health problems (American Psychological Association [APA], 2023a). Consequently, helping individuals, families, and communities find more effective ways to respond to stress is an essential health-promotion goal. The National Institutes of Health's NCCIH and the Centers for Disease Control and Prevention (CDC) provide excellent resources to help people of all ages learn to cope with stress in all areas of their lives (APA, 2023a; CDC, 2023; NCCIH, 2022).

Stress management has been an effective intervention framework for health promotion, disease prevention, and symptom management. Stress management strategies such as relaxation and imagery, self-monitoring, **goal setting, cognitive restructuring, mindfulness**, and problem-solving have long been staples of community health-promotion and online support programs, such as Alcoholics Anonymous, Smokenders, YMCA (Y-USA), Noom Weight, Calm.com, and WW International, Inc. (formerly Weight Watchers International, Inc.). These programs employ strategies to help people modify health-risk behaviors to improve their quality of life. A survey by the APA (2023b) found that the recent coronavirus (COVID-19) pandemic, international conflicts, social inequality, inflation, and climate-related disasters are all significant concerns on Americans' minds, and many are struggling to cope. Although the US health care system provides excellent, expensive, and often heroic care, it provides poor-quality, low-cost health promotion/preventive care, including stress management. Moreover, community-level health promotion is essential to ameliorate the many harmful effects of stress. Although shifting focus from providing acute care for individuals to enhancing the health of communities requires a revolution in our health care delivery systems and outlook, successful community health-promotion initiatives hold promise for the future (Fisher & Devlin, 2019).

Stress management aims to improve quality of life by increasing healthy, effective **coping**, thereby reducing unhealthy consequences of distress. This process produces a dynamic interaction of mind, body, and spirit, influencing physical health and well-being. Stress management is thus an essential tool for expert nursing practice, which recognizes the interface of knowledge on behavior change. Using critical reasoning to examine multiple factors contributing to symptom development provides a valuable contribution to meeting the goals of *Healthy People 2030*. Stress management can have a significant effect on leading health indicators and help in meeting many of the overarching goals of the *Healthy People* program, which strives to have all Americans achieve healthy lives free of preventable injury, illness, and disease (US Department of Health and Human Services, Office of Disease Prevention and Health Promotion [USDHHS ODPHP], 2021). This chapter outlines the multifaceted psychophysiological aspects of stress, examines strategies shown to mediate its harmful effects, reviews examples of clinical situations in which stress management has been effective, and explores the unique perspective nurses bring that helps individuals identify healthy stress-management strategies.

SOURCES OF STRESS

Key Concepts of Stress

A **stressor** is any psychological, social, environmental, physiologic, or spiritual stimulus that disrupts the tendency of a system, especially the physiologic system of higher animals, to maintain internal stability, resulting in the coordinated response of its parts to any situation or stimulus that would tend to disturb its normal condition or function. Although in use for more than 100 years, the term *homeostasis* has suggested balance and stability but has also denoted interchange and continuous regulated or balanced change (López-Otín & Kroemer, 2021). In other words, **homeostasis** has connoted a state of balance, thereby requiring change or adaptation—not a static state (Fig. 13.1). To reflect the continuously changing nature of an adaptive interaction among life processes in all of its manifestations, the term **homeodynamics** (López-Otín & Kroemer, 2021) is a better descriptor:

> *Homeodynamics extends homeostasis into a more inclusive term. There is no stasis in life; all of life is dynamic. Ninety-eight percent of a body's atoms are replaced each year. The Krebs cycle turns over 2.66 × 10^{21} times per minute. The half-life of an intestinal cell is measured in days. Stasis is nowhere to be found. Life is a verb rather than a noun.*

Stress is understood as a state of threatened homeostasis/homeodynamics that triggers an array of adaptive physiologic, behavioral, and even social responses in an effort to reestablish homeostasis or relative balance to avoid chaos. These descriptions

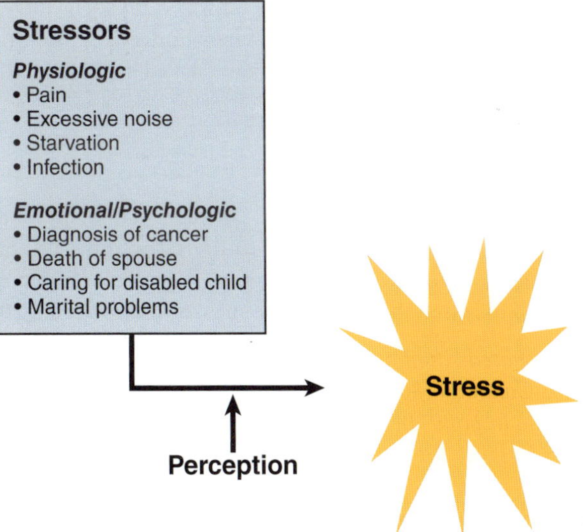

FIG. 13.1 Stressors can be physiologic or emotional/psychological. Perception of the stressors will determine whether they cause stress. (From Kwong, J., Roberts, D., Hagler, D., & Reinisch, C. [Eds.]. [2023]. *Lewis's medical-surgical nursing: Assessment and management of clinical problems* [12th ed.]. Elsevier.)

of stress underscore important ideas: even welcome events, such as a child's wedding, are stressors because they precipitate change. Nonetheless, stress is not intrinsically bad or unhealthy, and stress is experienced psychophysiologically and socially (i.e., as an interplay across all domains of individual and communal living). Stress is an essential component of being alive. Stress can be situational or maturational. One's coping strategies and resources will determine the outcomes of each stressful experience. Moreover, family and communal/social responses will affect many responses to shared stress. In this age of instant messaging and 24/7 news cycles, the collective shared nature of stress is intensified.

Individuals encounter a variety of physical, psychological, social, spiritual, and environmental stressors each day. These stressors are not simply additive but rather have an interactive effect within a homeodynamic human-ecological system. Stressors range from health and illness experiences, such as childbirth, physical illness, and trauma, to activities of daily living, such as caring for children, meeting work deadlines, and cleaning or repairing the house, to less frequent events, such as taking a critical examination, experiencing the death of a relative, losing possessions in a fire, losing a job, getting a divorce, or getting married. As a useful rubric, stressors can be organized into three categories: stressors over which people have no control (extrinsic factors), such as the weather, a traffic jam, or the death of a spouse; stressors that individuals can modify by changing their environment, social interactions, or behaviors; and stressors created or exacerbated (intrinsic factors) by poor time management, procrastination, poor communication, catastrophic negative thinking (expecting the worst), or struggling with self-defeating behaviors. However, stressors can never be neatly boxed into straightforward categories: Stress is a person-environment process. The person-environment fit model indicates that as a person appraises a situation as taxing or exceeding their resources, physical and emotional exhaustion often endangers one's well-being (Palmwood & McBride, 2019). Moreover, links between biologic pathways and social adversity to subsequent adverse health outcomes underscore the importance of stress as a health determinant (Javed et al., 2022; Lazarus & Folkman, 1984).

Stress Appraisal

Stress appraisal is an important concept that helps explain why two people react differently to the same situation. Stress appraisal involves considering coping resources and coping strategies to lessen the effect of the stressor (Landy et al., 2022).

The shared situation of Ms. Hernandez (86 years old) and Ms. Goldman (86 years old), both in good health, provides a case in point. Both individuals are about to become new residents at an assisted living retirement community in their hometown. Ms. Hernandez perceives this move as an opportunity to increase the ease of her socialization and activities of daily living. She looks forward to making new friends and participating in new recreational activities. In contrast, Ms. Goldman views this move as abandonment by her family and fears that the available resources will be inadequate. Although the event is virtually the same for Ms. Hernandez and Ms. Goldman, the homeodynamic consequences are personalized because each female perceives her situation differently. Even though the move to the new environment is the same, each female has different coping styles, expectations, and support systems, so the experience will differ in perception and, thereby, stress level.

Stress is the physical, psychological, social, or spiritual effect of life's pressures and events. Stress is an interactive homeodynamic process that involves appraisal and response to loss or the threat of loss of well-being at individual, family, and community levels (Lazarus & Folkman, 1984). Canadian physiologist Hans Selye (1950, 1974, 1982) first introduced the general adaptation syndrome, leading to a continual interest in stress and its effect on the body. Selye reported that, to a certain extent, stress can be challenging and valuable, which he identified as **eustress**. Selye also observed that when stress becomes chronic or excessive, the body cannot adapt and maintain homeostasis, and thus the process becomes **distress**. Therefore stress can be both beneficial and harmful. As stress increases, efficiency and performance also increase, but not endlessly. At a specific point, performance and productivity decrease significantly if the stress continues unabated. Understanding the many causes of stress and the negative physical, psychosocial, and spiritual consequences of distress is essential. Understanding the many-sided sources of stress provides the rationale for a multifaceted approach to its management. Notably, even in their early understanding, scientists and clinicians recognized the dynamic changing nature of the relationship between stress, epigenetics, and intrinsic human system responses (Box 13.1).

In nursing, we have operated within multiple frameworks to understand stress and its outcomes. Historically, nursing has been grounded in the biologic and medical sciences because of our long-standing roles in health promotion and caring for

BOX 13.1 GENOMICS

Relationship Between Stress and Development of Illness

Nurses and other clinicians have long appreciated that multiple factors operate in the development of various illnesses and have recognized the association of stressful life events with subsequent health. Researchers in epigenetics are exploring relationships between stress and vulnerability to a variety of health conditions. Mounting evidence has shown that childhood stress, or adverse childhood experiences/events (ACEs), produce a lifelong epigenetic effect and increased illness risk (Pelletier, 2019). Moreover, associations have been demonstrated between environmental stressors such as maternal prenatal psychological stress and altered DNA placental methylation patterns that affect fetal development (Argyraki et al., 2019). As epigenetic research continues, knowledge about the influences of stress on current and future health outcomes will mount. Given the evolving information about how stress can affect genes for individuals and how stress effects are transmitted generationally, nurses must be cognizant of current findings and integrate them into practice. Nurses are called to evaluate stress among all clients and to intervene to assist clients in recognizing stress triggers and employing stress-management skills. Moreover, community-level stressors require identification and management strategies, along with policy initiatives by nurses, to address disparity-related stressors and other community-based factors.

people experiencing illness. Yet, over many decades, nursing frameworks have also embraced concepts of continuous change and interaction in human-environmental fields. Most notably, Martha Rogers's science of unitary human beings (Phillips, 2015; Willis et al., 2015), Neuman's systems model, and Roy's adaptation model (Willis et al., 2015) have stressed the dynamic, interactive nature of human life. As a result, nurses have learned to balance and integrate traditional medical and bench science worldviews with the evolving and sometimes somewhat heretical nursing frameworks that focus more on continual change and interaction within and among human-environmental systems. Thus this chapter examines stress, its manifestations, and approaches to alleviating distress and associated health problems which involve weaving knowledge and understanding generated from diverse and sometimes conflicting perspectives.

The models for understanding human stress are multifaceted and complex. In the past, scientists and clinicians tended to examine and understand stress from their own disciplinary or scientific silos. In other words, understanding stress was typically split into neurobiologic and psychosocial camps. However, in recent decades, "**sociophysiology**" has emerged as a multidisciplinary perspective to integrate the "social" and "biologic." That is, individuals have physiologic responses associated with their social relationships and their emotions (Han et al., 2021).

Nursing science has long been interested in the dynamic interaction among human systems. Outstanding among nurses' voices calling for innovative perspectives to topple the traditional and accepted mechanistic medical worldview was Martha Rogers's theory of unitary human beings (Phillips, 2015). Phillips, a valued colleague of Rogers, described her as a heretic and a heroine because of her then-revolutionary views of nursing, health, and illness. Today, her ideas resonate well with contemporary understandings of the rapidly evolving interplay across all spheres of human life.

Thus understanding stress and its management involves attention to the interactions of social, environmental, and biologic life at individual and family/communal levels. It follows that stress-management strategies/interventions need to be multifaceted and could be aimed at neurophysiologic and interpersonal/social stressors and interactions and responses. Establishing empathy by the nurse in understanding stress is beneficial in designing interventions aimed at primary, secondary, and tertiary levels of prevention.

PHYSICAL, PSYCHOLOGICAL, SOCIOBEHAVIORAL, AND SPIRITUAL/ HOMEODYNAMIC CONSEQUENCES OF STRESS

First, it is necessary to set the groundwork for understanding stress and its multifaceted/interactive consequences. In the following discussion, facets of human responses are artificially categorized and discussed to assist the learner in discerning the many aspects of stress responses. This content should not be interpreted as meaning that stress responses are isolated to specific human systems or merely additive. Growing understanding of the homeodynamic interplay, including epigenetics, within individuals and across human and ecological systems forces us to examine the ever-changing nature of our knowledge of our world. As an example, in early 2020, health officials in China confirmed tens of thousands of cases of COVID-19 (Huang et al., 2023). The virus quickly spread worldwide as carriers traveled, resulting in rapid transmission of human infections and the declaration of a pandemic (Huang et al., 2023). Travel restrictions, social distancing, and quarantines ensued as the virus spread, and millions infected with COVID-19 died (WHO, 2023a). In addition to causing stress to many individuals, the virus had a substantial economic effect worldwide, as people were forced to stay in their homes for months (Kowal et al., 2020). Many lost their jobs, and most changed how they worked, played, learned, and interacted with others either temporarily or permanently (Kowal et al., 2020; Ng et al., 2021; Zhao & Watterston, 2021). We must remain mindful of the ongoing interplay within and among human, social, and ecological systems, even as we examine knowledge focused predominantly on specific response areas (i.e., human systems). Nevertheless, understanding stress effects at various micro to macro levels is needed to comprehend a holistic picture. The future challenges to do so are indeed exciting!

Physiologic Effects of Stress

An individual's homeodynamic response to stress provides a model to examine changes across biopsychosocial-spiritual domains. In response to a perceived threat (i.e., stressor), the body prepares to meet the challenge. Perception of threat stimulates a physiologic pattern of neuroendocrine activation and behavioral changes mediated by the central nervous system. Moreover, chronic stressful life circumstances likely exacerbate conditions favorable to adverse health outcomes (Fig. 13.2) (APA, 2023c). Nonetheless, in most cases, this reaction is an adaptive, short-term, acute response to a stressor. First termed the **fight-or-flight response** (Cannon, 1914) and later called the **stress response** (Selye, 1950, 1974, 1982), the individual's reaction to a real or imagined threat prepares the body for emergency reaction and fosters survival in circumstances of immediate, time-limited threat. The hypothalamus signals the sympathetic nervous system to release epinephrine, norepinephrine, and other related hormones. A resultant state of arousal is characterized by increased metabolism, pulse rate, blood pressure, respiration rate, and muscle tension. This physiologic arousal proceeds along three main pathways: the musculoskeletal system, the autonomic nervous system, and the psychoneuroendocrine system.

The musculoskeletal system responds by increasing tension and tone. At the same time, the autonomic nervous system, via the sympathetic branch, orchestrates a generalized arousal that includes increases in heart rate, blood pressure, and respiration rate. Additionally, a heightened awareness of the environment is triggered, and blood shifts from the visceral organs to the large muscle groups. Concurrently, the psychoneuroendocrine system stimulates the hypothalamic-pituitary-adrenal axis and the secretion of corticosteroids (primarily cortisol) and other neuroendocrine substances into the systemic circulation, increasing blood glucose levels, influencing sodium retention and, in the acute phase, increasing the antiinflammatory response.

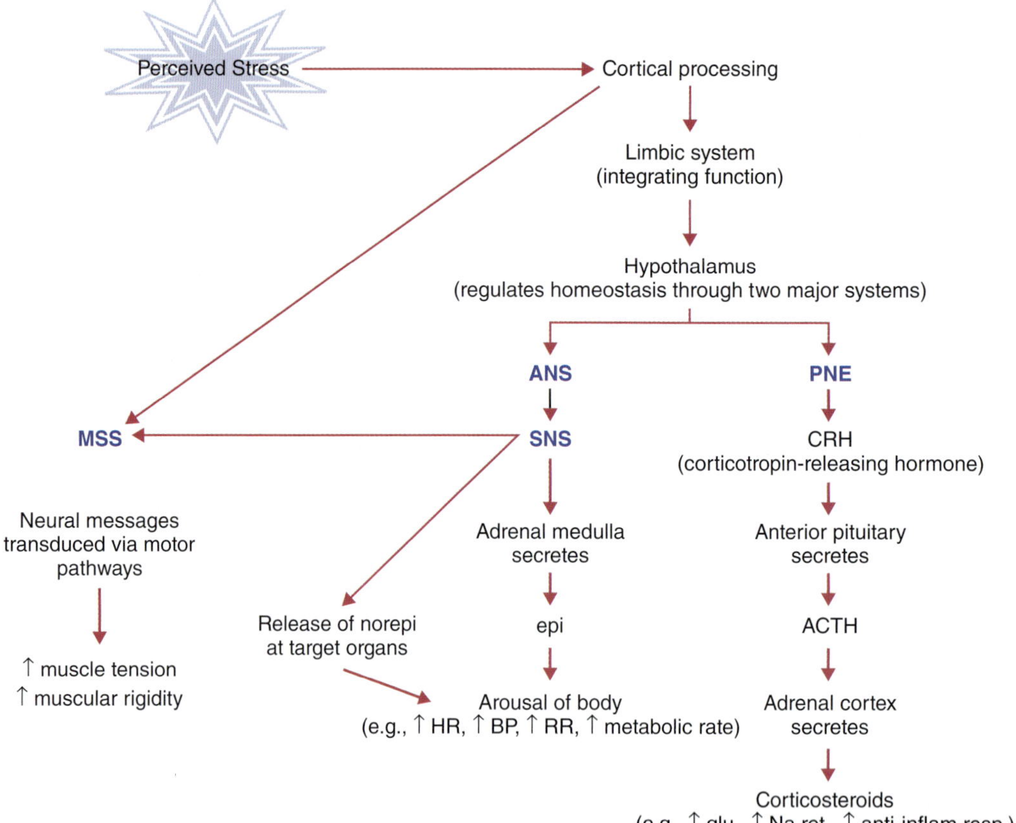

FIG. 13.2 The stress response. ACTH, Adrenocorticotropic hormone; ANS, autonomic nervous system; anti-inflam resp., antiinflammatory response; BP, blood pressure; CRH, corticotropin-releasing hormone; epi, epinephrine; glu., blood glucose level; HR, heart rate; MSS, musculoskeletal system; Na ret., sodium retention; norepi, norepinephrine; PNE, pituitary-neuroendocrine system; RR, respiration rate; SNS, sympathetic nervous system. (From Wells-Federman, C., Stuart-Shor, E., Deckro, J., Mandle, C. L., Baim, M., & Medich, C. (1995). The mind/body connection: The psychophysiology of many traditional nursing interventions. *Clinical Nurse Specialist, 9*, 60.)

Both stress and perceived stress can cause or exacerbate disease or symptoms of diseases and influence mental health (APA 2023c; Thorsén et al., 2022). Proinflammation associated with stress is emerging as a common pathway in a variety of diseases, such as asthma, angina, cardiac arrhythmias, pain, tension headaches, insomnia, depression, and gastrointestinal disorders. Additionally, stress can produce hyperreactivity or hyporeactivity of hormones regulated by the psychoneuroendocrine system (Parlindungan et al., 2023; Zänkert et al., 2019).

As mentioned previously, in most cases, the stress response is a beneficial adaptive pattern that increases the efficiency and quality of performance. Still, it can prove maladaptive when a stressor continues indefinitely. Maladaptive stress (distress) is an enduring and sometimes self-sustaining cascade of responses that degenerate physical, psychosocial, and spiritual well-being. Not surprisingly, stress and, specifically, depression have been associated with increased susceptibility to cardiovascular disease, as well as inadequate response to its treatment. Inflammation has been suggested as one of the processes underlying the association between cardiovascular disease and depression, two debilitating conditions (Halaris, 2016). Nonetheless, indirect influences of stress and depression on self-care health behaviors also help explain associations between these diseases.

Psychological Effects of Stress

The psychological effects of stress are best illustrated by its contributory role in negative mood states, including anxiety, depression, hostility, and anger. Exposure to stressful stimuli is associated with elevated cortisol levels and resultant effects on the immune system. The duration, intensity, and timing of a stressor have been shown to affect immune responses in animals. Although systematic studies to explain different patterns of immune response with humans are not yet adequate, the interactive nature of the mind and the immune system is an exciting area of investigation that may contribute to future evidence-based practice (Bennett & Molofsky, 2019).

A growing body of clinical research outcomes illustrates the interplay of stress and various health outcomes. For example, research on breast cancer patients suggested that a patient's subjective appraisal of stress influences depression, anxiety, and quality of life (Badana et al., 2019). The relationship between stress and cardiac symptoms is also well documented.

Wiesmaierova and colleagues (2019) found that social support minimized the adverse effects of stress on mental and physical well-being in patients hospitalized with acute coronary syndrome. Clinical implications include reducing perceived stress and encouraging reappraisal and support seeking. In conclusion, the evidence to date demonstrates a strong association between chronic stress and adverse health effects for individuals.

Sociobehavioral Effects of Stress

In response to stress, individuals often revert to or increase their reliance on less-healthy behaviors, such as overeating, excessive use of alcohol or drugs, and smoking. Recognizing that such behaviors are inconsistent with the healthy behaviors needed to cope with stress is easy; however, stopping these behaviors and using health-promoting strategies instead is not. Risky behaviors and traits, such as a sedentary lifestyle, obesity, overeating high-fat foods, smoking, and substance use disorder, have been linked to the development of chronic diseases and morbidity and mortality (National Center for Chronic Disease Prevention and Health Promotion [NCCDPHP], 2022). Conversely, **exercise**, a **healthy diet**, smoking cessation, healthy weight maintenance, and social interaction have been identified as leading health indicators in the United States (NCCDPHP, 2022). Encouraging these health behaviors supports the goals of *Healthy People 2030*. However, unless we understand how psychosocial factors affect health behaviors, the promotion of effective self-care is an unrealistic goal.

Spiritual Effects of Stress

Interest in the connection between spirituality and health is significant. Spirituality is defined in many ways, but critical components are typically that spirituality comprises feelings, thoughts, experiences, and behaviors that arise from a search for meaning and may include interconnectedness with self, others, nature, and a higher force called God, a lifeforce/higher power, nature, or the transcendent. Spirituality and religion intersect for many, yet they are not synonymous. Many individuals feel spiritual without a formal religious affiliation or practice. In response to stress, people often feel disconnected from life's meaning and purpose; harmful effects on their health and well-being can result. Stressful events can shatter individuals' spiritual center or, conversely, can move individuals to seek comfort in spirituality, religious practice, beliefs, or community. Encouraging involvement with one's religious/spiritual practices is recommended to improve resilience to stress-related problems (Manning et al., 2019; McClintock et al., 2019).

As an example, spirituality and religious support were found to be the most common protective factors in a study of African American adults providing kinship care for children who have experienced abuse, substance misuse, neglect, or whose parents are incarcerated (Wu et al., 2024). African American children are overrepresented in the child welfare system and placed disproportionately to be cared for by close friends or relatives who may not be equipped to do so (Wu et al., 2024). Results of this research reveal that African Americans most often relied on spirituality/religion as a protective factor while caring for a child in need (Wu et al., 2024). This result provides a foundation for future interventions to improve kinship care. Engaging a pastoral counselor of the individual's choice may prove effective in promoting parenting skills in African Americans providing temporary care to children, thus resulting in better health outcomes for the child.

The previous section discussed how stress could adversely affect biologic, cognitive, emotional, behavioral, and spiritual well-being. Understanding the psychophysiology of the mind-body-spirit connection is fundamental to applying stress management in nursing and provides an obvious rationale for a multifaceted approach. Further support is provided by research endorsing the health-promoting effects of managing stress (USDHHS ODPHP, 2022).

Health Benefits of Managing Stress

Evidence underscores the importance of managing stress to reduce allostatic load and promote health and quality of life for people with various health problems (Guan et al., 2023; Guidi et al., 2021). **Allostatic load** is the cumulative effect of life events and ongoing stress, involves the interaction of several physiologic systems operating at various intensities, and may be a key factor for understanding the physiologic effects of long-term exposure to chronic stressors on chronic diseases, including cancer, cardiovascular disease, and diabetes (Guan et al., 2023; Guidi et al., 2021). Promoting lifestyle modifications and the pursuit of psychological well-being may provide positive outcomes. Psychotherapeutic approaches, such as cognitive-behavioral psychotherapies that focus on the perception and management of life stressors, are effective treatments for depression and related mental health disorders (Gautam et al., 2020). These psychotherapies have been incorporated into various treatment and secondary prevention programs, such as cardiac rehabilitation, with great potential for wider adapted use (Li et al., 2021; Wurst et al., 2019). Targeting primary prevention programs is the aim of nurses in assisting individuals with stress reduction before becoming symptomatic.

Promoting a positive attitude and development of skills to cope with stress is foundational to many stress-management interventions. As early as 1982, Kobasa and colleagues (1982) made a groundbreaking contribution to our understanding of the stress-illness relationship when they identified characteristics of hardiness. They described individuals with stress-hardy characteristics who were less vulnerable to stress-related symptoms and diseases when exercising and accessing **social support**. The characteristics of stress hardiness are control, challenge, and commitment. For stress-hardy individuals, stress is viewed as a challenge rather than a threat; they feel in control of situations in their lives and are committed to, rather than alienated from, work, home, and family. Hardiness continues to be assessed (recognized) by nurses in assisting individuals and families dealing with a crisis and promoting the strengths of survivorship in coping with new stressors. Another term that is often used is *resilience*.

Stress management is critical in situations such as caregiving, which extends over long periods. **Caregiver stress/burden** can be described as a multifaceted strain as a result of psychological distress, impaired social relationships, physical symptoms, spiritual distress, and financial troubles in the caregiver resulting from long-term caregiving tasks (Choi & Seo, 2019; Liu et al., 2020). As the setting for care increasingly becomes the home, and family members take on mounting responsibility for caring for loved ones (i.e., children, spouses, or aging parents with chronic conditions), the importance of caring for the caregiver to prevent significant burnout grows. As a result of current trends of delayed parenting and increased lifespan, the "**sandwich generation**" of middle-aged adults who have concurrent responsibility for their children and aging parents are at particular risk of severe caregiver burden. Research evidence supports the usefulness of interventions aimed at helping family caregivers to find meaning in their activities and role in buffering caregiver stress (Fernández Sánchez et al., 2020; Graham et al., 2019). Moreover, the quality of the caregiver–care recipient relationship can reduce caregiver burden (Graham et al., 2019).

In summary, the evidence proves that thoughts, feelings, behaviors, beliefs, and biologic activity are interrelated. Perceptions, or the way individuals view situations, can lead to stress and, in turn, adversely affect biologic activity, emotions, behavior, and the connection with life's meaning and purpose. This interaction among perceptions, stress, and multifaceted effects, in turn, can increase stress and foster a negative stress cycle. The remainder of this chapter presents an assessment of stress relating to the homeodynamic framework, including the facets of physical, psychosocial, and spiritual health and well-being of individuals, and describes the application of a variety of strategies shown to help break the negative stress cycle and mitigate its harmful effects across the biologic, psychosocial, and spiritual domains (see Box 13.1).

ASSESSMENT OF STRESS

Methods for Assessing and Appraising Stress

Assessment of the stress-coping abilities of an individual, family, or community is part of a comprehensive health assessment that includes past and present subjective and objective data. Collecting these data enables the individual and the nurse to determine the status of the person's stress-coping pattern and actual and potential strengths and weaknesses.

The nurse thoroughly collects data during the history, physical examination, and health patterns assessment (see Chapters 6 to 8). Identifying the stress-coping pattern is especially important. Asking for specific examples of events with probes to elicit the person's thoughts, feelings, and actions leads to a discussion of appraisal and ideas for alternative actions in the future (see Chapter 4). Each individual is the primary data source; no other person can explain accurately the individual's perceptions of the stressors, stress responses, and resources to prevent or alleviate stress.

Stress is experienced across biologic, psychosocial, and spiritual domains; therefore, all perceptions are essential for the assessment. Throughout the assessment process, individuals may become aware of information of which they were previously unaware, or they may identify information related to their perceived problems. For example, a male may be mindful of the stress of his job but may be unaware that his high blood pressure was caused, at least in part, by this stress.

Lazarus and Folkman (1984) proposed the transactional model of stress and coping comprising primary and secondary appraisals of stressful events, situations, or demands and the effectiveness of an individual's coping skills. **Primary appraisal** of coping includes descriptions of perceived actual and potential positive and negative outcomes. Negative outcomes refer to harm, whereas positive outcomes refer to the challenges resulting from stressors that an individual perceives can be overcome. Examples of negative outcomes include physical injury; disease; loss of a cherished relationship, position, or possession; and death. Positive outcomes include graduation, promotion, and developing essential relationships (see the Case Study at the end of this chapter).

Secondary appraisal follows primary appraisal. Secondary appraisal consists of the individual's identification of choices to cope with the actual or potential harm, threat, or challenge. The choices may be internal or external resources and responses. For example, a social resource in coping with the needs of a toddler might be learning strategies in a parent-effectiveness training course. A coping response to the challenges of parenting a toddler might be restructuring the toddler's and parent's schedules to allow for more frequent cycles of activities and rest.

The individual's primary and secondary stress appraisals provide opportunities to consider the stress experiences differently. Resources that had been forgotten may be remembered, or a threat may be newly viewed as a challenge and an opportunity for enhanced development and status. The appraisal process mediates stress responses. This understanding supports using cognitive-behavioral therapy (CBT) as a practical intervention for stress-related problems (Cole, 2022). Nurses appropriately may refer individuals for CBT and are encouraged to obtain advanced training in CBT to integrate this evidence-based intervention into their practice. Using good-quality texts for the general population is also a practical psychoeducational approach. For example, Brewer's *Unwinding Anxiety* (2021) and Gillihan's *Mindful Cognitive Behavioral Therapy: A Simple Path to Healing, Hope, and Peace* (2021) are examples of materials that can serve as springboards for discussion of ways to adjust the meaning of life stressors, responses, and ways to cope.

Instruments for Measuring Stress

Measuring stress and related symptoms/responses is essential to assessing and evaluating treatment outcomes. Using measurement instruments with established reliability and validity, nurses can improve the assessment of an individual's stress and coping. Tools can help nurses distinguish between diagnoses that have many signs and symptoms in common. For example, disturbances in thinking and feeling processes can be challenging to distinguish and may have confounding clinical pictures. These disturbances can occur separately or simultaneously in the same person. An example of this complexity is the overlapping symptoms of depression and dementia. To develop an effective care plan, the nurse determines whether one health problem is the cause of the other (see the Case Study at the end of this chapter).

Various instruments are available to help nurses assess orientation, attention, cognitive skills and patterns, traits and states of emotions, symptoms of mental health distress and disorders, and overall quality of life. For example, the Schedule of Recent Experiences (Holmes, 1981) and the Impact of Event Scale (Horowitz et al., 1979; Weiss & Marmar, 1997) are well-established instruments used widely in clinical assessment and research to measure stress associated with life changes and events. **Burnout**, work-related or personal, is understood as emotional exhaustion, depersonalization, and a sense of reduced personal accomplishment. The Maslach Burnout Inventory (Maslach & Jackson, 1986) is a psychometrically robust instrument to assess perceptions about work-life balance. (Box 13.2; Evidence-Based Practice, which investigates the quality of life of critical care nurses and its correlation with anxiety, depression, stress, burnout, and sleep quality.)

Before using any instrument, clinicians and researchers need to check information about its reliability and validity, updates/revisions, training requirements, and copyright restrictions (e.g., purchase requirements) that can affect access to its use. Older instruments typically have an established record of demonstrated reliability and validity; however, phenomena may evolve with time, and revised versions may have been developed and tested for specific populations. Therefore exploring the literature to seek updated information to inform users is always wise. Additionally, seeking consultation from clinical experts/researchers regarding appropriate instrument selection for the population is recommended.

Using standardized instruments promotes accuracy in developing diagnoses and care plans and assists in evaluating the effectiveness of care. For example, a nurse may compare an individual's self-evaluation and symptom preintervention scores with postintervention scores and revise the care plan accordingly. Additionally, nurses may analyze population baseline scores for relevant characteristics and develop programs of research and quality-improvement efforts aimed at enhancing outcomes.

Assessment at the family and community levels is also recommended. Family assessment consists of three major categories: structural, developmental, and functional components (Shajani & Snell, 2019). Environmental factors also contribute to the determinants of health and thus stress, so a thorough nursing assessment requires consideration of the community. For example, examination of community-level data for unemployment, population density, housing, school quality, crime, suicide incidence, and disease occurrence patterns (i.e., health profiles of the community), as well as the availability of various amenities such as green space and access to transportation and healthy foods, provides a more complete stress assessment than individual assessment alone (DeMarco & Healey-Walsh, 2020). Moreover, family and community assessment can point to possible stress-reduction interventions, such as marshaling available social support or engaging in outdoor activities and exercise.

BOX 13.2 EVIDENCE-BASED PRACTICE

Quality of Life of Critical Care Nurses and Effect on Anxiety, Depression, Stress, Burnout and Sleep Quality

This cross-sectional study aims to understand the effect of anxiety, depression, stress, burnout, and sleep quality on the quality of life (QoL) of critical care nurses (N = 140). Data collection utilized well-established scales such as the Depression Anxiety Stress Scale (DASS), Maslach Burnout Inventory, Pittsburgh Sleep Quality Index, and Nursing Quality of Life Scale. Findings suggest that critical care nurses face a high risk of experiencing anxiety, depression, burnout, stress, and suboptimal sleep quality. Specifically, the study reveals a significant effect on emotional and work-life quality of life, with emotional exhaustion and high DASS scores associated with poor QoL in the emotional and work-life dimensions. This study emphasizes the importance of recognizing and addressing the QoL of critical care nurses and the need for health care professionals to prioritize their mental health and adopt positive health behaviors. Creating conducive work conditions is essential for the critical care nurse's well-being and maintenance of a high standard of care for critically ill patients. This research highlights the intricate relationship between mental health, burnout, and the overall QoL of critical care nurses, urging health care systems to implement strategies that promote the well-being of these essential frontline workers (From Cecere et al., 2023).

STRESS-MANAGEMENT INTERVENTIONS

Stress-management strategies benefit people across a broad spectrum of chronologic, sex, cultural, and ethnic characteristics. Male and female, young and old, from divergent socioeconomic, cultural, and ethnic backgrounds can benefit from stress-management interventions. Sensitivity to the needs and values of individuals and communities, particularly for high-risk groups (i.e., vulnerable populations), guides assessment and intervention techniques. The language, belief system, and cultural distinctions of individuals and families in the community guide the choice and adoption of stress-management strategies. Understanding stress and its management involves paying attention to the interactions of social and biologic life at the individual and family/communal levels; therefore, interventions may need to encompass a variety and combination of psychosocial and biologic approaches at the primary, secondary, and tertiary levels of prevention. Population-based interventions may be expanded from the individual to the community and a system- or population-focused practice (Demarco & Healey-Walsh, 2020).

Stress intersects all areas of health, wellness, and illness. Many of the proposed *Healthy People 2030* objectives involve stress management; however, Box 13.3 highlights a few of the most relevant objectives for consideration. These objectives can guide nurses' intervention plans for health promotion and disease/symptom management.

Developing Self-Awareness

Self-awareness is one of the most effective stress-management tools. Self-awareness helps people learn about mind, body, and spirit interactions; increases a sense of control; and counters self-defeating perceptions. Interventions that promote self-awareness help people make sense of life events and circumstances that may be bewildering or discomforting. Many

BOX 13.3 *HEALTHY PEOPLE 2030* OBJECTIVES

Stress relates to many proposed objectives for *Healthy People 2030* due to its multifaceted influences on health and illness. The following proposed objectives are of particular interest to stress management.

Access to Health Services

- Increase the capacity of the primary care and behavioral health workforce to deliver high-quality, timely, and accessible patient-centered care
- Increase the use of telehealth to improve access to health services

Disabilities and Health

- Reduce the proportion of adults with disabilities aged 18 years and older who experience serious psychological distress

Mental Health and Mental Disorders

- Increase the proportion of primary care physician office visits where adolescents and adults are screened for depression

Nutrition and Weight Status

- Increase consumption of dark green vegetables, red and orange vegetables, and beans and peas in the population aged 2 years and older

Source: US Department of Health and Human Services, Office of Disease Prevention and Health Promotion. (2021). *Healthy People 2030 framework.* https://health.gov/healthypeople/about/healthy-people-2030-framework

experiences in life lead to feelings of emptiness and disharmony because people cannot connect the experience with thoughts, feelings, actions, and physiologic responses. Self-awareness helps individuals recognize the stress they create through negative, exaggerated, unrealistic thinking. This recognition allows for changes to these negative thought patterns, thereby decreasing stress and increasing control. Strategies that increase self-awareness can empower individuals to make new connections and reframe and reinterpret their experiences in light of their inner strengths and wisdom.

A closely related concept is mindfulness, which is nonjudgmental self-awareness characterized by intentional acceptance of the unfolding of experience in the moment. Mindfulness requires dedicated practice to achieve and reduce adverse stress effects (Yue et al., 2023). A variety of mindfulness approaches have been proposed and tested. Mindfulness interventions can be combined with other efficacious treatments or serve as primary stress-management interventions. Mindfulness as both a state and an intervention is not simple, although it may appear so initially. Therefore nurses are urged to obtain specialized training in mindfulness approaches to use them in their practice. Mindfulness interventions have shown promise in improving the quality of life in coping with various health conditions (Feldman & Kuyken, 2019; Presciutti et al., 2023). For example, Fan and colleagues (2023) demonstrated that mindfulness-based interventions could be a viable and acceptable supplementary treatment for cancer patients, helping to control symptoms associated with the disease. The neuroscience basis of mindfulness remains a fruitful field of investigation. Evidence suggests mindfulness meditation may precipitate neuroplastic changes (Yue et al., 2023). The horizons are vast and exciting for future nurse scientists to engage in team science to explore the underpinnings of interventions such as mindfulness.

Techniques for Developing Self-Awareness

Monitoring Stress Warning Signs. The negative stress cycle can be challenging to interrupt. Recognizing warning signs of stress is a necessary first step. Often, individuals have long ignored physical, emotional, or behavioral cues or reactions to a stressor, which are **stress warning signs**. A male who has chronic, intermittent backaches and ignores the daily muscle tension caused by the poor posture that precedes the backaches provides an example. If he had attended to his early stress warning signs of poor posture and muscle tension, he might have avoided the backache that kept him from exercising and socializing. Becoming aware of these stress warning signs is the first step. Attending to these cues is the next step. After this connection has been made, the development of skills to reduce negative mood states, unhealthy behaviors, and physical symptoms becomes much more accessible. Furthermore, some people misinterpret physiologic signs of anxiety (e.g., shortness of breath, racing heartbeat) as indicative of severe physical danger (e.g., suffocation, myocardial infarction). This tendency to misinterpret physical anxiety cues is referred to as **anxiety sensitivity**, a belief that body sensations associated with anxiety indicate imminent and dangerous outcomes, and is associated with various anxiety disorders and health anxiety. By helping individuals who are prone to anxiety sensitivity to interpret body sensations accurately or to distract from the sensation, nurses can help reduce individuals' misinterpretations, as well as the likelihood of escalation of anxiety symptoms and possibly even the development of anxiety disorders.

Nurses teach people to identify their warning signals of stress, stop, take a few breaths, and break the cycle. Fig. 13.3 shows a sample form for identifying and recording this information. These signals or cues differ among individuals and can be physical, emotional, behavioral, cognitive, relational, or spiritual. Individuals become more consciously aware of these cues when asked to monitor their responses to a particular event. Although this heightened awareness initially may increase an individual's consciousness of physical pain or emotional discomfort, awareness is a necessary first step in recognizing the adverse effects of stress and the relationship between thoughts, feelings, behavior, and biologic processes. In addition, nurses and other clinicians are responsible for screening individuals for emotional distress to help them recognize and monitor their own physical and mood states. For individuals with health conditions such as coronary artery disease, which is known to have high comorbidity with emotional distress and specifically depression, routine screening should be the standard of care (Henry et al., 2019).

Try this: Ask an individual to identify a stressful experience and the physical or emotional reactions (stress warning signals) to that particular experience. For example, after being instructed to stop, take a breath, and notice the physical and emotional response to a stressful situation, one female related the following:

> *I sat in a massive traffic jam on my way to work yesterday. I noticed that my heart was racing, my breathing had*

Physical Symptoms

___	Headaches	___	Back pain
___	Indigestion	___	Tight neck and shoulders
___	Stomachaches	___	Racing heart
___	Sweaty palms	___	Restlessness
___	Sleep difficulties	___	Tiredness
___	Dizziness	___	Ringing in ears

Behavioral Symptoms

___	Excess smoking	___	Grinding of teeth at night
___	Bossiness	___	Overuse of alcohol
___	Compulsive gum chewing	___	Compulsive eating
___	Attitude critical of others	___	Inability to get things done

Emotional Symptoms

___	Crying	___	Overwhelming sense of pressure
___	Nervousness and anxiety	___	Anger
___	Boredom (no meaning to things)	___	Loneliness
___	Edginess (ready to explode)	___	Unhappiness for no reason
___	Feeling powerless to change things	___	Easily upset

Cognitive Symptoms

___	Trouble thinking clearly	___	Inability to make decisions
___	Lack of creativity	___	Thoughts of running away
___	Memory loss	___	Constant worry
___	Forgetfulness	___	Loss of sense of humor

	Spiritual Symptoms		Relational Symptoms
___	Emptiness	___	Isolation
___	Loss of meaning	___	Intolerance
___	Doubt	___	Resentment
___	Unforgiving	___	Loneliness
___	Martyrdom	___	Lashing out
___	Looking for magic	___	Hiding
___	Loss of direction	___	Clamming up
___	Cynicism	___	Lowered sex drive
___	Apathy	___	Nagging
___	Needing to "prove" self	___	Distrust
		___	Lack of intimacy
		___	Using people

FIG. 13.3 Stress warning signals. (From Medical Symptom Reduction Clinic Patient Notebook. [n.d.]. Boston: The Benson-Henry Institute for Mind Body Medicine of Massachusetts General Hospital, Harvard Medical School.)

changed, and my hands gripped the steering wheel. I felt angry and frustrated because I would be late for work.

Although these responses seem quite obvious, most people are unaware of the effects of stress on their minds and bodies. In the preceding example, the building of the female's stress may continue to escalate at work, influencing her interactions with coworkers. Once individuals become aware of these effects, they may be able to release tension more easily, countering the adverse effects of stress and increasing a sense of control. Techniques that help reduce the negative effects of stress include distraction by purposefully shifting focus to pleasant thoughts or engaging in a diversion activity and using a **relaxation response** technique, as described in the following section.

Learning and Practicing a Relaxation Response Technique. Eliciting the relaxation response is another technique that helps people develop awareness and counter the adverse effects of stress. Relaxation response techniques oppose the stress response by reducing sympathetic arousal (Benson, 1975). The immediate physiologic effects of relaxation are decreases in heart rate, blood pressure, respiration rate, and muscle tension. The long-term physiologic effect is decreased central nervous system arousal with a concomitant reduction of the musculoskeletal, autonomic, and psychoneuroendocrine system arousal. To the extent that stress causes or exacerbates a symptom, elicitation of the relaxation response can break this stress-symptom cycle. In addition to these physiologic changes, psychological changes, such as improved mood and behavioral changes, can occur. The relaxation response has demonstrated the ability to improve glucose control and quality of life in patients with type 1 diabetes (Stahl et al., 2022).

The relaxation response is an innate physiologic response (Benson, 1975); therefore, several techniques that involve mental focusing can be used. Details on relaxation response techniques such as meditation and yoga and guidelines for clinical applications can be found in Chapter 14. All these techniques have two primary components:

- The repetition of a word, sound, phrase, prayer, image, or physical activity
- The passive disregard of everyday thoughts when they occur

Electronic applications (i.e., apps), easily accessible via mobile devices, can help guide this process of focusing, especially during the initial learning phase. Many health apps are available to support the use of relaxation techniques.

Nurses can often introduce individuals to the immediate calming effects of the relaxation response in less than 5 minutes. One effective way is to have the person make a fist and notice what happens to the breathing pattern. Most people tend to hold their breath while tensing a body part. Now ask the person to take a few deep diaphragmatic breaths while making a fist. Most people will notice that the tension is much harder to maintain while taking a deep breath. This awareness helps recognize the relationship between breath and tension. Lamaze techniques for assisting females in managing pain during labor and delivery are based on this connection between breathing and relaxation. Most people hold their breath when they perceive a threat (stress), feel anxious, or become angry. By stopping and taking a few deep breaths when they become aware of physical changes (holding their breath or clenching the jaw) or emotional changes (feeling anxious or angry), individuals can elicit a relaxation response, reduce sympathetic arousal, calm negative mood states, and gain a sense of control. **Yoga** and deep breathing can assist with **mindfulness** (i.e., awareness of perception) and promote relaxation (Komariah et al., 2022; La Torre et al., 2020). Notably, evidence supports the benefits of yoga on stress reduction. A systematic review demonstrated that practicing yoga regularly was associated with improved antioxidants and reduced oxidative stress (Pai & Gupta, 2019).

Using Mini Relaxations. **Mini relaxations** can be taught quickly and used throughout the day to help develop awareness and counter the adverse effects of stress on the mind, body, and spirit. Individuals can be taught to monitor minor stress warning signs (jaw and shoulder tension) and to use a mini relaxation exercise to keep these initial symptoms of stress from developing into an incapacitating tension headache. A mini relaxation exercise can be anything from a few conscious, deep diaphragmatic breaths to several minutes of sitting quietly (Box 13.4: Quality and Safety Scenario). Practice is needed to elicit the response quickly when stress, pain, or tension is recognized. The power of using relaxation, including visualization and breathing techniques, is illustrated by the personal experience of a nurse who had coached pregnant females and partners in Lamaze preparation for childbirth for 10 years before having her third baby. During Pitocin induction, due to a postdate determination, the female was experiencing significant contractions. Her experienced labor nurse commented that she was an advertisement for childbirth preparation. The female managed a smile in response. The female later reflected: *The contractions were tough. I think that the Pitocin escalated the process so that contractions increased quickly from mild to intense. Did my Lamaze relaxation techniques help? Oh yes. Was it still painful? Oh yes. However, I was able to make it through this and two previous labors and deliveries without an epidural by using relaxation techniques that I had been taught and practiced. I cannot emphasize enough that relaxation techniques are powerful tools, including breathing, visualization, distraction, and partner/nurse*

BOX 13.4 QUALITY AND SAFETY SCENARIO

A Stress-Management Strategy for Nurses

Develop the skill of personal presence. Presence is the gift of self through availability and attention to needs. Presence means "being there" for another person. To be available to others in this way, first practice the skill of being present with yourself. One effective way of developing this skill is through mindfulness, which is the ability to focus attention on what you are experiencing from moment to moment. Mindfulness encompasses the ability to slow down and bring your full attention (thoughts, feelings, and body sensations) to the action you are engaged in. The practice can be beneficial in allowing yourself to extend the benefits of eliciting the relaxation response in more areas of your daily life (Miller, 2019).

The following are some ideas for practicing personal presence (mindfulness):

- When you awaken each morning, bring your full attention to your breathing. Allow your awareness to expand gradually into the room, and then slowly begin to listen to the sounds of the outdoors.
- On your way to work, focus on how you walk, drive, or ride the transit. Take some deep diaphragmatic breaths and relax your body as you travel.
- Take a moment to attend to your breath, relax your body, and focus your mind before entering a care recipient's room.
- As you eat a meal, carefully examine it through all your senses—the sight, smell, touch, taste, and the sound of each bite. Mindfully enjoy this new experience.
- Recurring events of the day can become cues for a mini relaxation (the ringing telephone; auscultating a heartbeat; answering a call light; before, during, and after rounds or report).
- Make the transition home from work mindful. Leave thoughts and worries about work at work, and be conscious of your home environment daily.

Once again, focus on your breathing and become completely aware of your surroundings as you go to sleep. Practice mindfully letting go of today and tomorrow as you allow your mind and body to rest.

coaching support. These techniques require practice to be called upon in an instant of pain or stress. Medication and/or anesthesia remain helpful tools in situations of acute pain, such as labor, surgery, injury, or ongoing stress. Still, our capacities to harness our abilities are powerful and should not be overlooked. Let's empower ourselves so that pharmacotherapeutics is a tool but not the immediate or sole go-to solution for stress and pain!

Alternative and Complementary Therapies. A variety of alternative and complementary therapies and techniques can prevent and reduce harmful effects of stress (Lindquist et al., 2022). These therapies include **acupuncture**, **hypnosis**, **aromatherapy**, **reflexology**, **reiki**, and chiropractic and herbal therapies. These approaches have developed outside the mainstream of traditional Western medicine; however, developing evidence of efficacy has promoted growing acceptance of some of these approaches. People are increasingly using alternative and complementary practices as self-help measures, and research to study their effects has exploded in recent years. Nurses can help individuals evaluate the safety and efficacy of various alternative and complementary therapies. In particular, herbal remedies require cautious use because they can have harmful as well as beneficial effects, and they sometimes interfere with other treatments and medications. Among the alternative therapies available, there is strong evidence of effectiveness of acupuncture and hypnosis, and they are becoming widely accepted within mainstream health care.

Acupuncture is an ancient Chinese technique used to reduce pain and to prevent and manage various disorders by placement of fine needles at specific **meridian** points on the body. Acupuncture is not a self-help approach, so seeking treatment from an experienced acupuncturist is required. The Western scientific community cannot explain why acupuncture works but acknowledges its effectiveness. Even the World Health Organization has listed illnesses that can be managed with acupuncture (WHO, 2023b), and some health insurance plans provide reimbursement for acupuncture treatments. Additionally, acupressure is a related intervention that involves use of pressure at specific points but does not involve needles (Lindquist et al., 2022).

Hypnosis comes from a Greek word meaning "sleep." Hypnosis narrows consciousness and elicits relaxation, inertia, and passivity, like sleep, yet awareness is never lost completely, and the hypnotized person can respond (Lynn et al., 2019). The exact mechanisms through which hypnosis works are not known, although its ability to induce deep relaxation and its possible action in shifting brain activity from the "analytical" left side to the "nonanalytical" right side might be explanatory. Nevertheless, its effectiveness in managing a variety of conditions, notably smoking and anxiety-related problems, and managing pain is well-recognized. Trained therapists provide hypnotherapy to manage stress and various mental health problems, including phobias, addictions, and posttraumatic stress disorder. Self-hypnosis, a form of deep relaxation similar to the relaxation techniques described in this chapter, can be a useful stress-reduction tool. Self-help guides provide safe and easy-to-follow guidelines. One note of caution is warranted: hypnosis is not recommended for people with organic brain disorders, psychotic disorders, or other severe mental disorders. For individuals with trauma histories, practice with an expert clinician is recommended.

Reiki (pronounced ray-kee) is made up of two Japanese words: *rei*, or "universal spirit" (sometimes thought of as a supreme being), and *ki*. Thus the word *reiki* means "universal life energy." Reiki is a therapy that uses energy fields with the intent to affect health. To transmit ki, believed to be a lifeforce energy, the reiki practitioner places hands on or near the person receiving treatment. In the United States, reiki is designated as a form of complementary and alternative medicine (Lindquist et al., 2022).

Expressive Writing. Transforming thoughts and emotions related to stressful experiences into written language has demonstrated positive effects on health (Demarco & Healey-Walsh, 2020; Lindquist et al., 2022). In its therapeutic meaning, **expressive writing** involves telling a "story" about traumatic, emotionally charged, or stressful events and personal reactions. **Journal writing**—more specifically, self-confessional writing—is a form of expressive writing that is typically done via entries in a journal over time that describe unfolding personal responses to life events. Expressive writing is useful in disclosing and processing emotions and in measurably improving physical and mental health.

Expressive writing, including journaling, can help people reflect on stressful events and their reactions to these events. Such reflection is an opportunity to reform perceptions and to consider alternative ways to manage stress. Individuals may find resolutions to conflicts that work uniquely for them. These resolutions may then increase a sense of control and mediate negative consequences of stress. This self-reflective process shares elements of cognitive-behavioral therapy (CBT)—an intervention effective in reducing harmful effects of stress (see Chapter 4).

Nurses can advise people to get a special notebook or a journal (or to use an electronic tablet or computer) to write about a stressful event for 15 minutes a day in a setting in which they will not be interrupted. From a health perspective, journaling will be more effective when they make themselves the only audience. The nurse should warn the individual that they may feel sad or depressed immediately after the writing session, but these feelings usually dissipate within an hour. Nonetheless, exploring deep thoughts and feelings on paper is not a panacea. When an individual is coping with death, divorce, or some other major stressor, feeling better instantly after writing cannot be expected. A person can, however, develop a clearer understanding of feelings and of the situation through journal writing. In other words, journal writing helps people objectify experiences, identify the influence of stress on symptoms, and develop insights into more effective problem-solving. Some individuals may recognize the need for psychotherapeutic support through journal writing, and an appropriate referral can then be made. Nurses can use the same approaches to examine their own stressful work-related situations to reflect, analyze their responses/reactions, and generate effective responses to similar experiences in the future.

Nutrition: Healthy Diet

Countering negative effects of stress requires caring for physical health and well-being. The mind and body are connected; therefore, paying attention to one while ignoring the other does not promote overall health. The body requires rest, a **healthy diet** of balanced food choices, and exercise. In the last few decades, nutrition has moved to the forefront as a major component of health promotion, disease prevention, and symptom management. Food is now viewed as a positive influence on health, physical performance, and state of mind rather than simply a fuel needed to prevent disease and sustain life. Adaptive eating is characterized by balanced eating patterns and calorie intake, as well as appropriate body weight for height. Nutrition is an important component of early intervention strategies to improve physical, cognitive, emotional, social, and spiritual functioning.

However, the American lifestyle has made practicing healthy eating habits increasingly difficult. Americans frequently replace nutritionally balanced meals with readily available high-fat, high-calorie food (US Department of Agriculture, 2020). One of the frustrations that nurses experience is trying to help children and adults develop healthy eating habits. This effort requires planning and correctly choosing a variety of foods and eating a diet low in fat, saturated fat, and cholesterol, with plenty of vegetables, fruits, and grain products. The current US dietary guidelines (US Department of Agriculture, 2020) are based on the following two overarching concepts: focus on calorie balance over time to achieve and maintain a healthy weight and focus on consuming nutrient-dense foods and beverages. Daily food choices should be made from the five food groups. Key recommendations also highlight the importance of calorie control and physical activity. Guidelines continue to undergo evaluation and revision; for example, guidelines about "healthy foods" are under ongoing review, so nurses are urged to check for updated guidelines. A detailed discussion of the health benefits of balanced nutrition and guidelines throughout the lifespan can be found in Chapter 11.

Encouraging healthier dietary choices helps people recognize that control over their health and well-being is possible. This knowledge, in turn, helps counter the negative effects of stress and lower the stress-disinhibition effect that can influence poor dietary choices. Nurses encourage people to monitor their daily dietary patterns to gain awareness of how they use food in times of stress. Tools such as food diaries (24-hour recall) help people to monitor the amount and quality of what they eat and drink and to set realistic goals. An example of a free online program is MyFitnessPal (2023), which combines nutrition tips and a way to monitor exercise in a journal format. Notably, numerous health apps that vary in cost are available to help individuals lose and manage weight. Such programs boast convenience and fingertip access. Although convenience is a clear advantage over traditional face-to-face programs, maintaining ongoing engagement with mobile app programs remains a challenge.

Physical Activity

Combining a healthy diet with a regular exercise routine has many health benefits and can positively affect quality of life. For example, one of the most effective ways to lose weight and improve self-esteem is to combine exercise with nutritious eating. Exercise (physical activity that increases strength and flexibility and improves conditioning) and balanced nutrition serve as protective factors against several major chronic diseases. Regular physical activity decreases the risk of death from heart disease, lowers the risk of developing diabetes, and is associated with a decreased risk of colon cancer (CDC, 2020). Exercise helps prevent high blood pressure and helps lower blood pressure in people with elevated levels. Regular physical activity, even at moderate levels, is associated with lower death rates for adults of any age. Psychological well-being is enhanced, and the risk of developing depression can be reduced; regular physical activity appears to reduce symptoms of depression and anxiety and to improve mood.

Additionally, children and adolescents need weight-bearing exercise for normal skeletal development, and young adults need this type of exercise to achieve and maintain peak bone mass (CDC, 2023). Regular physical activity also increases the ability of older people, and people with certain chronic, disabling conditions, to perform activities of daily living. Nevertheless, high stress can increase injury risk for athletes, and injured athletes may experience greater stress than noninjured peers when they are sidelined from competition. Chapter 12 provides a comprehensive discussion of the benefits of exercise and its clinical application throughout the lifespan.

Regular physical activity helps people adopt a more active lifestyle as they begin to feel better physically and emotionally, thereby breaking the negative stress cycle (Fig. 13.4). Positive effects can be obtained with exercise of only moderate intensity. For example, a brisk walk of 30 to 60 minutes, three to five times a week, promotes fitness and decreases the risk of disease. Being physically active on a daily basis is extremely important; therefore, nurses can help individuals increase their physical activity by suggesting a variety of activities in which they might engage each day (Box 13.5: Helping Individuals Increase Physical Activity). An exercise diary can generate a baseline for usual activity to set realistic goals and monitor progress. By simply changing a few daily routines, individuals can gain enormous physical, psychosocial, and spiritual rewards that promote health and break the negative stress cycle.

Sleep Hygiene

Health and the ability to meet life's many demands and manage stress effectively require proper rest. Many people experience sleep deprivation and sleep disorders (e.g., sleep apnea) that can cause or exacerbate conditions such as depression and fatigue and contribute to poor concentration and ineffective problem-solving. Poor sleep quality has been linked to a variety of serious chronic health problems (Gaffney & Foster, 2023; National Heart, Lung, and Blood Institute, 2024). Insomnia can be induced by stress or other cognitive-behavioral factors, such as unrealistic expectations, inappropriate scheduling of sleep, trying too hard to sleep, consuming caffeine, getting inadequate exercise, and a number of other factors, including illness, alcohol use, or drug use, Determining the extent to which sleep disturbance is the result of behavior or stress-related issues is a necessary assessment. Overcoming sleep disturbances cannot be done quickly. Changing these behaviors requires patience and persistence. Once the factors associated with sleep disturbance have been identified, nurses can help individuals improve their sleep patterns by counseling them to follow several **sleep hygiene** or behavior guidelines (keeping a sleep diary, having a

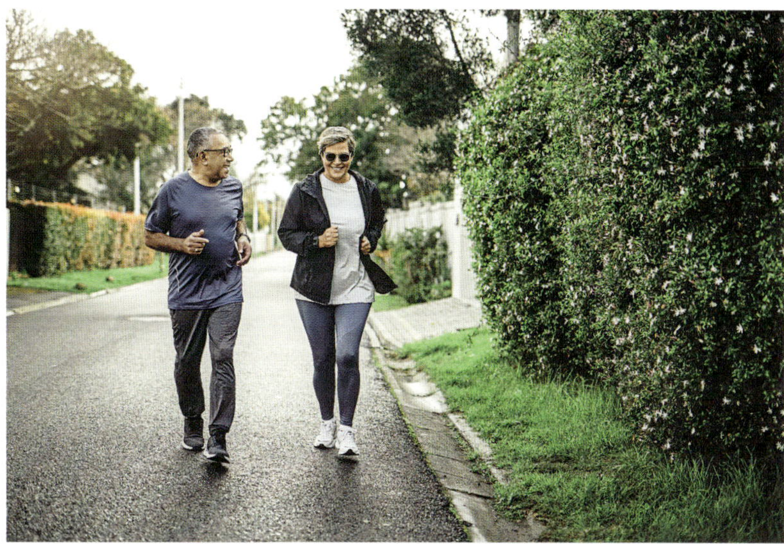

FIG. 13.4 Regular physical activity helps individuals adopt a more active lifestyle. (From iStock.com/Charday Penn.)

BOX 13.5 Helping Individuals Increase Physical Activity

Nurses can suggest ways for individuals to increase physical activity throughout the day based on their interests and activity ability, including the following:

- Have fun and play active games with children.
- Engage in a sport.
- Find a friend with whom to walk or jog.
- Take a class in yoga or Tai Chi.
- Get and walk a dog.
- Garden on the weekends.
- Walk or bicycle to school or work.
- Take the stairs, never the elevator.
- Park the car at the farthest point in the parking lot at work, school, or the store.

By simply changing a few daily routines, a person can gain enormous physical, psychosocial, and spiritual rewards that promote health and break the negative stress cycle.

regular sleep-wake cycle, and making prudent dietary changes). Referral for appropriate evaluation of possible disorders such as sleep apnea is also a necessary nursing intervention. Assisting people in making healthy behavior changes in their sleep habits provides another opportunity for people to increase self-regulation, confidence, and control, thereby reducing stress and improving quality of life. Box 13.6 presents several sleep hygiene strategies.

Cognitive-Behavioral Restructuring

Many stressful situations can be created or exacerbated by negative, exaggerated, catastrophic thinking. CBT is a conceptually based short-term intervention to modify this thinking and related behaviors, thereby reducing stress. In the context of therapy, cognitive-behavioral restructuring is a technique or a series of strategies that help people evaluate their thoughts, challenge them,

BOX 13.6 Sleep Hygiene Strategies

Nurses find the following suggestions to be helpful for individuals with sleep disturbance resulting from behavioral or stress-related issues:

- Keep a sleep diary, which helps determine sleep patterns more accurately and assess progress; it reinforces behavior change.
- Have a regular sleep-wake schedule whenever work schedules allow.
- Avoid consuming caffeine in the afternoon or evening.
- Avoid consuming alcohol before going to bed.
- Limit your fluid intake before going to bed.
- Turn off electronic devices at least 30 minutes before bed.
- Limit exposure to bright light.
- Avoid the use of sleeping pills.
- If you cannot fall asleep within 20 minutes, or if you wake up and cannot fall back to sleep within that time, get out of bed and do something until you are tired again. During that time, avoid bright lights or electronics.
- Focus on relaxation, not sleep. Use a relaxation tape, and practice diaphragmatic breathing. Limit naps during the day to less than 45 minutes. Longer naps reset the biologic clock and disturb nighttime sleep.
- Exercise within 3–6 hours of bedtime. Exercise improves sleep by significantly increasing body temperature, which is followed by a compensatory drop a few hours later, making it easier to fall and stay asleep. Furthermore, because exercise is a physical stressor, the brain compensates for this by increasing the amount of deep sleep.
- Take a hot bath 2 hours before bedtime. The temperature drop after the bath helps induce sleep.
- Sleep in a cool room. Individuals become sleepier and less active when their body temperature falls.
- Try a sleep application, such as calm.com, to quiet brain activity.

Adapted from American Academy of Sleep Medicine Foundation (AASM). (2020). *Healthy sleep habits.* https://sleepeducation.org/healthy-sleep/healthy-sleep-habits/; Gaffney, D. A., & Foster, N. C. (2023). *Courageous well-being for nurses: Strategies for renewal.* Johns Hopkins University Press, Baltimore, MD.

and replace them with more rational cognitive and behavioral responses (Beck, 1976, 1979; Gaffney & Foster, 2023; Najavits, 2019). Although advanced training is needed to provide CBT and nurses are encouraged to do so, nurses can safely and effectively use basic strategies. A helpful resource for nurses is the Beck Institute for Cognitive Behavior Therapy (2024).

Appraisal, or the way in which a situation is viewed, can be a major cause of stress, making CBT especially suited for stress management. When situations are viewed in a negative, distorted, or illogical manner, such perceptions can adversely affect emotions, behaviors, beliefs, and physiologic parameters. Cognitive-behavioral restructuring teaches people to recognize that negative thinking often causes emotional distress and associated behaviors. This recognition, in turn, alters problematic thinking and behavior, reduces the negative consequences of stress, and enhances health (Stuart, 2013). Mindfulness is a complementary approach that focuses on awareness that emerges from attending to one's purpose in the present moment nonjudgmentally. A strong evidence base supports its use as a practiced approach to manage stress effectively (Gaffney & Foster, 2023).

Cognitive-behavioral restructuring does not gloss over or deny misfortune, suffering, or negative feelings. Many circumstances exist in peoples' lives for which it is appropriate to feel sad, anxious, angry, or depressed. More accurately, cognitive-behavioral restructuring is a technique that helps some people become unstuck from these moods so that they can experience a broader range of feelings and try out new behaviors (Stuart, 2013). In this structured method, individuals are asked to consider their cognitive appraisal of a situation and how this assessment affects feelings, behaviors, and physiologic processes. Reframing, or cognitive reappraisal, educates individuals in monitoring thoughts and replacing those that are negative and irrational with those that are more realistic and helpful. Adding behaviors that are consistent with reframed thinking follows.

For example, a female may have plans to meet a friend for lunch on a day she wakes up with a migraine headache. She might begin to think such thoughts as "This always happens to me when I have plans," "This headache will never go away," "I shouldn't have to deal with this," or "My day is ruined." The result of this negative, irrational self-talk is disappointment, frustration, and anger. This emotional arousal will, in turn, increase muscle tension and a variety of other stress-related symptoms, which may exacerbate the headache. To help individuals develop the skill of cognitive-behavioral restructuring, nurses can teach them to examine a stressful situation using the four-step innovative practice CBT approach highlighted in Box 13.7: Best Practice.

In the previous example, the female may reflect that "I am having a migraine headache, and I hate that it is on a day that I had made plans, but I will take my medication, listen to my relaxation recordings, and rest. I'll call my friend and see if we can change our plans. Perhaps she can come over to visit me for tea this afternoon if I feel better." Although it is understandable that anyone would be disappointed and upset over this situation, application of the four-step cognitive restructuring technique can help individuals identify healthy choices and gain a sense of control.

BOX 13.7 BEST PRACTICE

The Four-Step Approach to Cognitive Restructuring Enhanced With Technology

To help individuals develop the skill of cognitive restructuring, nurses can teach them to examine a stressful situation using the following four-step approach:

- Stop (break the cycle of escalating, negative thoughts).
- Breathe deeply (elicit the relaxation response and release tension).
- Reflect (Ask, "What is going on here? What am I thinking? Is the thought true? Is the thought helpful? Am I jumping to conclusions or magnifying the situation?").
- Choose a more realistic, rational response. Try out the alternative response in a future situation.

Alternative Approach

Teaching/coaching can be done face-to-face or via technology (e.g., a website and/or smartphone application that shows the previous steps with a feedback interface) (Adams et al., 2019). Via technology, feedback can be given via text or email to correct negative thoughts and provide suggestions and positive reinforcement for steps 2–4 when success is reported. Phone and face-to-face interaction can augment contact via technology when possible. Tracking successful cognitive restructuring via online entry can provide valid outcome data. As Internet and smartphone penetration increase and costs decrease, such technologic interventions will increasingly be a cost-effective way to reach more individuals and can be applied across various technologic platforms (e.g., computers, smartphones, and tablets). Generic affirmations can also be added via text messaging at a very low cost to encourage the practice of the steps (Adams et al., 2019).

Based on the work of pioneers such as Aaron Beck (1976, 1979) and Albert Ellis (Ellis, 1962; Ellis & Dryden, 1987), cognitive therapy has emerged during the past several decades as a treatment designed to alter dysfunctional beliefs and thoughts associated with depression, anxiety disorders, and other emotional problems (Najavits, 2019). Over time, theorists, clinical researchers, and clinicians recognized the effectiveness of this approach for many people, as well as the value of linking helpful alterations in thinking to complementary behavioral changes. As a result, CBT emerged. CBT and mindfulness, a related method, are evidence-based approaches for many stress-related and mental health disorders (Gillihan, 2021; Gaffney & Foster, 2023).

Research provides strong support for use of cognitive-behavioral restructuring and mindfulness as stress-management approaches. For example, evidence from a robust systematic review of 44 meta-analyses involving over 30,000 participants across 336 randomized clinical trials supported the efficacy of mindfulness in improving a variety of mental health conditions, including depression (Goldberg et al., 2021).

Thought, perception, and stress appraisals are also situated within a person's culture and experience. Cultural sensitivity to such influences is critical to providing quality care. Box 13.8 presents relevant information related to the effects of racial/ethnic discrimination on cognitive appraisals of interactions as threatening and harmful, resulting in increased overall stress burden.

BOX 13.8 HEALTH AND SOCIAL DETERMINANTS/HEALTH EQUITY

Social Stressors and Depression Can Lead to Unfavorable Outcomes for Vulnerable Populations

Health is perceived through one's spiritual beliefs, holistic practice, and biomedical perspectives. Nurses understand the importance of cultural sensitivity when providing care and of clear communication when providing multicultural care. Greater concern for health literacy and improved coordination with support organizations are needed. Social determinants of health, including racial differences, may affect the ability to cope with frustration and may influence health care outcomes. *Healthy People 2030* identifies the need to increase the proportion of adults that are screened for depression. For example, a recent study found that pregnant Black females might be more susceptible to social stressors and depression symptoms, causing chronic inflammation (Saadat et al., 2022). This is concerning, as increased inflammation during pregnancy has been linked to a greater likelihood of unfavorable perinatal outcomes (Saadat et al., 2022). Thus to enhance overall maternal well-being and lower the risk associated with racial disparities, adequate screening for social stressors and depressive symptoms during pregnancy is essential.

Affirmations

Affirmations can be an effective stress-management and cognitive-behavioral restructuring skill because they are a method of countering self-defeating negative thoughts and attitudes in addition to being helpful in addressing spiritual needs. An affirmation is a positive thought, in the form of a short phrase or saying, which has meaning for the individual. By reinforcing new ways of thinking or behaving in the present moment, affirmations are statements that people can use to reaffirm new intentions and to clarify goals.

Nurses coach individuals to create an affirmation as a way of developing a more helpful, realistic belief system. For example, thoughts such as "I can't handle this" and "My day is ruined" can be countered with "I can handle this" and "I know ways to increase my comfort." Repeating an affirmation often throughout the day, perhaps after elicitation of the relaxation response or as part of a breathing exercise, can become second nature and can help to enhance self-esteem and reduce stress.

Social Support

Having supportive family, friends, and coworkers is, for many individuals, an important contributor to effective coping and stress hardiness (Rink et al., 2022). Many people believe that confiding in others and talking out problems can be a helpful way to get good advice or uncritical support. Social support comprises a network of close family, friends, coworkers, and professionals. The social support literature notes that both the number of supports and the quality of the relationships are important (McNamara et al., 2021). Furthermore, the context of social support and personal history can also affect health outcomes. Karatekim and Ahluwalia (2020) examined the effects of adverse childhood experiences (ACEs), stress, and social support on the health of college students. Results showed that those with higher levels of ACEs had higher stress and lower social support. Stress made the greatest contribution to negative health outcomes. Findings indicated that social support interacts with contextual factors such as history and current stress to affect health.

Nursing interventions are aimed at facilitating social support to promote effective coping and reduce stress. Using information available in their local communities or through national organizations, nurses suggest support groups (see Chapter 8), website chat rooms, social networking sites, educational classes, and exercise facilities. Individuals and their families are often referred to volunteer organizations such as the American Lung Association, the American Heart Association, the American Cancer Society, and the Arthritis Foundation for resources related to specific health-promotion/maintenance needs that also may provide social support opportunities.

Use of PET Therapy. Pet therapy can augment the benefits of social support by providing unconditional affective or emotional responsiveness. Pet therapy is the therapeutic use of an animal to offer comfort to individuals experiencing stress or illness. It can be used in a variety of settings, including hospitals, long-term-care settings, hospice centers, and schools. The most frequently used animals in pet therapy programs include cats, dogs, birds, guinea pigs, fish, rabbits, horses, and dolphins, although many other animals can be used in a therapeutic way (Perkins, 2020). Pets can provide unconditional regard and a comforting physical presence that often evokes touch as a human stress-reducing response. Nevertheless, animals in pet therapy programs require screening and training so their behaviors are predictable, safe, and "friendly." Also, allergies to specific animals, notably cats, dogs, and horses, need assessment for individuals before implementing pet therapy. Moreover, individuals' perceptions of animals and related meanings from life experience also require assessment for pet therapy to be effective.

Assertive Communication

Effective communication is an important stress-management skill. An important coping and problem-solving skill, communication can be adversely affected by exaggerated negative thoughts and deeply held negative beliefs and assumptions (Stuart, 2013). (See Chapter 4 for additional discussion of communication.) People who have difficulty with communication usually have one or all of the following problems:

- Disparity between what they say (statement) and what they want (intent)
- Confusion about or resistance to stating clearly how they feel, what they want, or what they need (lack of assertiveness), with either a tendency to deny their own feelings (passiveness) or indifference toward the feelings of others (aggressiveness)
- Difficulty listening to others

The importance of matching the statement with intention is illustrated by the following example:

As Timothy is leaving for his basketball game on a Saturday afternoon, his mother tells him, "Remember to be home early tonight." When Timothy arrives home at 9:00 p.m., his mother, who is waiting at the front door, yells, "Where were you? Is this your idea of early? You know your father and I had plans tonight. We were counting on you. You think only of yourself. This always happens. You'll never change. You'll always be irresponsible and selfish."

The first guideline for effective communication is that people need to be clear about what they want and what they need (intent) in statements to others. Although it would be wonderful if a son or daughter, spouse, friend, or others were great mind readers, assuming that people automatically know what is meant does little to help with communication. Nurses help individuals match statements with intentions. This process requires that individuals recognize distorted, exaggerated thoughts and emotions and take responsibility for their part of the conversation. Communicating effectively is a learned art and skill.

In reviewing the previous example, it is helpful to note that if the mother's intention was to have her son home before 8:00 p.m., then her statement needed to indicate this. She could have said, "I hope you enjoy the game, but remember your father and I are going out tonight. We need to have you home before 8:00 p.m. to take care of your sister." It is important that the person understands that the other person in the conversation is not obligated to respond as one would wish. However, a request can be much clearer when the statement reflects the intent.

The next guideline for effective communication is to be assertive. **Assertive communication**, in most cases, is the most effective way to communicate. An assertive statement is nonjudgmental, expresses feelings and opinions, and reaffirms perceived rights. The general format of an assertive statement is "I feel [emotion] when you [the behavior] because [explanation]."

The formula requires that all three elements be included. **Cognitive restructuring**, as described earlier, facilitates assertive communication because it requires individuals to identify their thoughts and feelings. In the previous example, Timothy's mother could:

- Stop (breaking the cycle of escalating, negative thoughts)
- Breathe deeply (releasing physical tension; promoting relaxation)
- Reflect:
  - How do I feel emotionally? (e.g., frustrated)
  - What are my automatic thoughts? ("If he cared about us, then he would have been home on time. He's always selfish and irresponsible. He's never going to change.")
- *Choose*:
  - A more realistic, helpful way of thinking ("He's not always selfish and irresponsible. Even though it feels like he doesn't care about us when he does this, I know he cares.")

Becoming aware of her automatic thoughts and feelings and tone of voice would help Timothy's mother plan an assertive statement when Timothy comes home. She could then say, "I feel frustrated [emotion] when you are late [behavior] because I expected you would be home in time to care for your sister while your father and I went out or that you would have called if you were going to be late [explanation]." This statement both makes her feelings clear and explains why she feels this way, which in turn provides a better opportunity to work on problem-solving. When people cannot verbalize both their feelings and their needs, in the appropriate tone, others are forced to figure out what they are. When others fail to do so correctly, individuals may feel victimized and blame the others for not understanding. Nurses help people recognize that they have a right and a responsibility to speak up and to do so in an assertive manner. The nurse helps individuals match their emotions with the explanation (frustration equals unmet expectation). It is important to remind individuals that this way of communicating may feel awkward and uncomfortable at first. Practicing this technique many times will be required before communication improves. Role play can be a useful technique to practice. Other people need time to become accustomed to the changes. Effective communication takes both practice and patience for everyone involved.

Health Education and Communication. Effective communication by the nurse is also a critical ingredient in providing health education. Health education is more than providing people with materials and resources. Applying the strategies described here will clarify expectations and elicit the other person's feelings, thoughts, and goals. Alignment of feelings, thoughts, and goals will enhance effectiveness of health education. Moreover, adjusting communication used in health education to match the individual's health literacy is essential. Techniques such as teach-back, when the nurse asks the person to explain or show what was communicated or taught, is a brief, user-friendly, and effective strategy. Moreover, it provides immediate feedback about what was or was not effectively communicated so the nurse can reinforce the health education.

Empathy

Empathy is an effective stress-management intervention because it assists with communication. It is the ability to consider another person's perspective and to communicate this understanding back to that person. Empathy guides individuals to become better listeners.

Empathy can be facilitated through the technique of active listening. **Active listening** requires conscious, empathic, nonjudgmental awareness. Listening also helps clarify the issues involved and can deescalate many emotional exchanges. The use of focus groups can assist the nurse in understanding concerns, such as those of a parent group concerned about nutrition choices in the lunchroom. For example, during a situation in which a parent announces, "I'm fed up with the food selection in the cafeteria," the response may be important to resolving the issues without promoting further miscommunications and increasing problems. Rather than being caught by a defensive, emotional reaction, individuals can learn to communicate empathetically by using the four-step approach:

- Stop (breaking the cycle of escalating, negative thoughts)
- Breathe deeply (releasing physical tension; promoting relaxation)
- Reflect:
  - How do I feel emotionally? (Hurt, angry)
  - What are my automatic thoughts? ("How could [person] say that? It's not my fault. I have things to do. [Person] always accuses me. This is never going to change.")
  - What are the thoughts and emotions being expressed by the other person?

- *Choose*:
  - "My feelings are hurt, but I don't have to react defensively."
  - "I'm going to try to understand [person's] perspective by using the phrase 'You sound ____ about____' and listening to [person's] response."

By using this phrase (you sound ____ about____), an individual can gain awareness of another person's perspective (Rogers, 1951). If we continue with the scenario, the response might be "You sound upset about the choice of food available." Possible responses to this empathetic statement might include "It's not just about that. Everything went wrong today, and this was just one more thing when my child complains about lunch," or "You're right. I hate having to pay for food that my child will not eat."

When one uses active listening, the other person often feels heard. An opportunity to clarify any misunderstanding becomes available. This exercise may help reduce emotional arousal, defensive behavior, and conflict. Active listening allows the individual to buy time and to get a better perspective on what the other person is thinking and feeling. Individuals can then make a choice as to how they want to respond. They may choose to use assertive communication or to step away from the interaction. Active listening promotes empathic, objective, and nonjudgmental communication. Nurses recommend the use of stress-management skills that include active listening techniques to facilitate effective communication, which, in turn, reduces conflict and stress.

Healthy Pleasures

Engaging in **healthy pleasures** (activities that bring feelings of peace, joy, and happiness) is, for most individuals, an important part of life. However, for individuals who are feeling overwhelmed with daily hassles of work-life balance, illness, or loss, this practice may have been lost. Individuals may feel that they do not deserve to have pleasure or that they are waiting for happiness until they feel better, until the stressors are resolved, or until the stressors go away. This belief makes breaking the stress cycle even more challenging; however, rewards motivate behavior. By asking people to pursue a healthy and pleasurable activity every week, motivating them to become more involved in their lives and break this cycle is often easier. The activity can be simple, and it need not cost money. For example, people often find pleasure in enjoying nature, spending time with a friend, reading a book, or watching a movie. Hobbies are purposeful leisure-time activities that can balance hectic, stressful lives. A hobby should be chosen from interest and/or talent. Many hobbies or pleasurable interests have added benefits of increasing activity (e.g., gardening) or promoting social engagement (e.g., a book club or chorus). Nurses advise individuals to make leisure-time activities a regular part of the week as a purposeful and conscious plan to break the stress cycle. Evidence supports the efficacy of well-being activities to detoxify stress (McNamara et al., 2021).

Spiritual Practice

In response to stress, people can feel disconnected from life's meaning and purpose, which in turn affects spiritual health and well-being. Meeting spiritual needs may be facilitated by **spiritual practice** or activities that help people find meaning, purpose, and connection. For example, individuals may choose to elicit the relaxation response through prayer. This focused, relaxed state of mind might help them develop a spiritual perspective that can engender a shift in values and beliefs to help them cope with a stressor they cannot change, such as chronic illness or loss of a loved one. Expression of anger or confusion in the face of difficulties, trauma, or tragedy also can provide a therapeutic outlet but conversely may engender spiritual or religious doubt or a sense of alienation from one's beliefs. Nurses suggest a referral to a chaplain or clergy member, provide spiritual music or art work, recommend spiritual reading material, and provide personal **presence** (see Box 13.4: Quality and Safety Scenario). Willis and colleagues (2015) have explicated how spiritual healing manifested itself in the aftermath of childhood maltreatment and pointed out the potential helpfulness of "constructing caring-healing interventions aimed at both cultivating spiritual consciousness and facilitating loving-kindness and acts of letting go in the healing process."

Nurses propose activities that provide a sense of meaning and purpose. Keeping a journal can be an important strategy to help individuals focus on aspects of life that are more positive and that become clouded from view when a person is feeling overwhelmed by stress. Even listing worries on paper or in a phone's notes feature can reduce rumination fueled by anxiety. Finding ways of helping others (e.g., tutoring children, reading to persons with sight impairment, or visiting an older adult) can have a positive influence on spiritual health and well-being. Altruism, generosity, kindness, and service to others are more than moral virtues. These attributes not only help to make the world a better place but also help people find meaning and purpose in life. Religious and existential well-being has provided some defense against depression for people with chronic and life-threatening conditions. Older, chronically ill, and homebound people can be encouraged to produce written or oral histories that can be a legacy or, when able, to contact others needing care or to make telephone calls or send mailers to raise funds for a favorite charity. In addition, nurses and other health care professionals can assist individuals and families in describing and clarifying their personal religious and spiritual perspectives, especially in light of evolving practices/meaning structures and high rates of interfaith marriages/partnerships. Spirituality and religious affiliation cannot be equated. Many experience a sense of spirituality or "awe" from nature, art, or music. Nonetheless, being part of a "faith community" can provide an important source of social support for many people. Within faith communities, nurses (also known as "parish" nurses) act as facilitators, educators, and referrers to individuals and families in promoting holistic care. Nurses can encourage individuals to search for a community that is comfortable, accepting, and supportive.

Clarifying Values and Beliefs

To manage stress and develop a balanced lifestyle, people must recognize the things and values that are important to them, reflect on where they are in life, evaluate what needs to be changed, and generate an action plan for that change (see Chapter 4). This process is known as **values clarification**. The first step is to identify what is important, meaningful, and valuable to assess whether actions are consistent with beliefs. What people believe and value guides their actions by endorsing certain behaviors and changing others. When people assess their values and beliefs, they use the ability to make their own choices rather than relying on beliefs and values dictated by others.

One method nurses use to help people identify what they value and, ultimately, to clarify the relationship between their beliefs and actions is to ask them to identify what is important or meaningful to them. The form in Fig. 13.5 is an example of questions used in the Medical Symptom Reduction Program at the Benson-Henry Institute for Mind Body Medicine of Massachusetts General Hospital (2021) in Boston. Individuals are asked to identify what is important and meaningful to them. Nurses need to know the values and beliefs of the individuals they are counseling. After reviewing the results, individuals may find that they have not been doing certain things that are important to them (becoming more physically active, eating a healthier diet,

"What Is Important and Meaningful to You in Life?"

In each of the following areas, what do you want for yourself, today, next week, a year from now?

Under each of the following categories, please ask yourself these important questions.

Professional, educational, and intellectual
Today ______
Next week ______
A year from now ______

Relationships
Today ______
Next week ______
A year from now ______

Creative things
Today ______
Next week ______
A year from now ______

Spiritual
Today ______
Next week ______
A year from now ______

Volunteer and altruistic
Today ______
Next week ______
A year from now ______

Health
Today ______
Next week ______
A year from now ______

Fun and play
Today ______
Next week ______
A year from now ______

Material objects
Today ______
Next week ______
A year from now ______

FIG. 13.5 What is important and meaningful to you in life? (From Medical Symptom Reduction Program Patient Notebook. [n.d.]. Boston: The Benson-Henry Institute for Mind Body Medicine of Massachusetts General Hospital, Harvard Medical School.)

volunteering, or spending time with their children). When people detect inconsistencies between their values and their actual living habits, they can begin to develop a working plan for correcting these inconsistencies. This process enables them to make conscious choices and to have more control (see Fig. 13.5).

Setting Realistic Goals

Developing an action plan for change to work toward a more balanced health-promoting lifestyle that is consistent with a person's values and beliefs is an important stress-management strategy. Setting realistic, attainable goals facilitates this exercise. Goal setting is a dynamic process that involves both the individual and the nurse. Goals should be specific, concrete, measurable, and achievable. Nurses facilitate this process by respecting the individual's input and using a values clarification exercise (such as the one mentioned) to facilitate a more complete database to guide individuals to identify and prioritize problems to be addressed and set mutually agreed upon long-term and short-term goals. Nurses encourage individuals to challenge themselves when their behaviors are not consistent with what they identified as important and meaningful to them. For example, when an overweight male with hypertension and high cholesterol levels continues to smoke and eat high-fat foods, nurses help him to look at these behaviors relative to what is meaningful to him, such as his family. The costs and benefits are usually clear, and the responsibility for the change is with the individual, not the nurse. Nurses ask the following questions to help individuals clarify long-term goals:

- What is important to you?
- What would you like to change about your life?
- What can you do to start that change?
- When will you take that action?
- How will you measure success?
- How will you maintain the desired change?
- How can I help you to reach your goal?

Setting realistic, attainable goals helps create a sense of confidence and achievement and to build enthusiasm to set future goals. This process, in turn, increases a sense of control and mitigates the negative effects of stress.

Humor

Humor is an enjoyable and effective antidote to stress for many people. Humor can have health-promoting properties (Lindquist et al., 2022; Stuart, 2013; Gaffney & Foster, 2023). When acting as a stress reducer, humor produces laughter. Laughter creates predictable physiologic changes in the body. Similarly to how it behaves with other forms of exercise, the body responds in two stages: an arousal phase with an increase in physiologic parameters and a resolution phase during which these parameters return to resting values or lower values.

Humor can open different perspectives on problems and facilitate objectivity, which increases a sense of self-protection and control. Finding humor in a stressful situation can help people reframe perceptions of the event. Some hospital staffs are using laughter libraries, humor rooms, comedy carts that can be wheeled into an individual's hospital room, and clowns to bring laughter and joy to the bedside. Humor has potential as an accessible, enjoyable, and inexpensive stress-reduction strategy that can offer people new perspectives on their world and themselves. Nevertheless, recognizing that humor can mask conflict or be hurtful is critically important in judging when and how to use it in clinical and work-setting encounters (Box 13.9: Humor Strategies for Stress Reduction).

> **BOX 13.9 Humor Strategies for Stress Reduction**
>
> Nurses can help individuals use humor for health promotion and stress reduction in a variety of ways, including:
>
> - Smiling
> - Counting humorous experiences and blessings in a journal
> - Seeking out laughter—when you hear laughing, move to it
> - Spending more time with fun, lighthearted, and humorous people
>
> For more information about using humor to reduce stress, see Box 6.4.

From HelpGuide.org (n.d.). *Laughter is the best medicine.* https://www.helpguide.org/articles/mental-health/laughter-is-the-best-medicine.htm

Engaging in Pleasurable Activities

A variety of pleasurable activities can mitigate harmful effects of stress (McNamara et al., 2021). Finding activities that are enjoyable to the person can be a key strategy to reduce stress, promote healthy behaviors, and encourage positivity (Gaffney & Foster, 2023). Asking individuals what they do for enjoyment and exploring how to incorporate pleasurable activities, even in small ways, can help manage stress. Encouraging "bite-size" realistic steps will likely result in positive outcomes that can grow with time and practice.

EFFECTIVE COPING

When people believe they can cope effectively, the harmful effects of stress can be minimized. The stressful situation is perceived as a challenge rather than a threat. This often-elusive difference has vital mind, body, and spirit effects. When people believe that their lives are more balanced and under control, they are productive, but not driven; aroused, but not anxious; and perhaps even physically or mentally tired, but not exhausted.

Effective coping helps people face great adversity (such as illness) and recognize the opportunity that the situation often presents. First and foremost, individuals must recognize that coping is the ability to find a balance between acceptance and action, between letting go and taking control. Many stress-management strategies help individuals distinguish these differences by providing a format for observing or objectifying their experiences. Other strategies such as exercise and balanced nutrition help individuals promote physical health and well-being to counter the harmful effects of stress. In addition, epigenetics (i.e., how environmental factors such as stress trigger or mute the expression of genetic traits) is a vast canvas for the exploration of causes and intervention across a variety of physical and mental health disorders for individuals and populations (Pelletier, 2019) (Box 13.1: Genomics).

Nurses help individuals improve effective coping by guiding them in the art of choosing the right strategy at the right time. In doing so, people gain a sense of control that minimizes or buffers harmful effects of stress. Nurses use the interventions described in this chapter to assist individuals to manage extrinsic and intrinsic stressors.

When individuals cannot control or influence the situation (extrinsic stressors), nurses advise the following:

- Take care of physical health and well-being: exercise; eat healthy, balanced meals; and practice sleep hygiene.
- Accept: learn to accept that some situations or people cannot be changed or avoided. Forgiveness and letting go of resentment are often a part of acceptance.
- Use distraction: distraction involves putting a worry aside, when necessary, until the situation can be dealt with directly. Prioritizing is quite different from procrastinating or denial, because it is a necessary delay rather than avoidance.
- Reduce emotional arousal: practice mini relaxations, listen to a relaxation recording, use the four-step cognitive-behavioral restructuring technique, exercise, seek social support, pray, meditate, use humor and affirmations, write in a journal, or engage in a healthy pleasure.

When individuals can alter or influence the situation, or when they are contributing to or creating the stress (intrinsic stressors), nurses advise them to do the following:

- Take care of physical health and well-being: exercise; eat healthy, balanced meals; and practice sleep hygiene.
- Reduce emotional arousal: practice mini relaxations, listen to music or a relaxation podcast, engage in exercise, seek social support, pray, meditate, use humor and affirmations, write in a journal, engage in a healthy pleasure, and/or use the four-step cognitive-behavioral restructuring strategy:
- Stop (breaking the cycle of escalating, negative thoughts)
  - Breathe deeply (eliciting the relaxation response and releasing tension)
  - Reflect (Ask, "What is going on here? What am I thinking? Is the thought true? Is the thought helpful? Am I jumping to conclusions or magnifying the situation?")
  - Choose a more realistic, rational response and related behavioral reaction.
- Problem-solve:
  - Clarify values, beliefs, and expectations.
  - Gather information.
  - Seek advice, support, assistance, or information.
  - Use assertive communication and empathy.
  - Set realistic goals, design action strategies, and determine the best steps to handle the problem.
  - Take action.

See the Case Study for John DeBruno as an example.

CASE STUDY

Health Assessment: John DeBruno

John DeBruno, a 29-year-old male separated from his wife, walked into the health maintenance organization stating he had a severe sore throat, could not eat, had not worked for 2 days, and was feeling "awful." He wanted to see the physician or nurse practitioner and get a prescription for an antibiotic. The medical record revealed two episodes within the last 9 months of reports of a sore throat, the culture of the organism, and antibiotic treatment. The separation from his wife occurred 1 year ago. He had not had a routine physical examination in 2 years. During the assessment interview, the nurse gathered the following information: John DeBruno appeared tired; he presented his problem in short, terse statements; he was irritable about the clinic's slow service; and he expressed a need to get back to work. Within the last 3 weeks, he had been required to work overtime because he faced deadline penalties, and his boss said that Mr. DeBruno's upcoming promotion depended on his performance now. The company Mr. DeBruno worked for was struggling, with possible layoffs pending. Mr. DeBruno said that, in general, things were "fine." His wife was apparently happy without him, and he was too busy to care or to think about the loss of that relationship. He made one remark about his boss: "What do you do when you have a nervous boss?" He described his diet as fast food "taken on the run." He said he gets about 6 hours of sleep per night and awakens one to two times during the night. He had infrequent contact with family members who live in the area. In accordance with the clinical protocol for the health center, the nurse collected a throat culture.

Analyzing Cues and Reflective Questions

- As Mr. DeBruno's nurse, how would you comprehensively assess his health?
- What cues regarding Mr. DeBruno's health would the nurse recognize?
- What coping strategies might the nurse recommend for Mr. DeBruno?
- What stressors might be modifiable for Mr. DeBruno?
- Identify two SMART goals (i.e., specific, measurable, achievable, relevant, and time-bound goals) or outcomes for Mr. DeBruno related to his current state.

SUMMARY

- Health requires the ability to cope effectively with the many demands of work-life balance and effective management of stress.
- Nurses play a crucial role in helping people cope with actual or potential stressors through careful assessment and implementation of effective interventions along with thoughtful and honest feedback and continued support.
- Research to discern the interplay of homeodynamic physiologic, psychological, social, and spiritual responses to stress has yielded essential knowledge for practice.
- Stress-management strategies allow individuals to acquire the necessary skills to cope more successfully and to become confident in self-management.
- Self-management empowers individuals to challenge and change perceptions, decrease stress reactivity, improve self-management skills, and minimize the harmful consequences of stress, positively influencing health promotion, disease prevention, and symptom management.
- Understanding the influences of stress on health and illness is essential to all nursing practice.

EVOLVE FEATURES

http://evolve.elsevier.com/Edelman/

- Study Questions

REFERENCES

Adams, S. M., Rice, M. J., Jones, S. L., Herzog, E., Mackenzie, L. J., & Oleck, L. G. (2019). Telemental health: Standards, reimbursement, and interstate practice. *Journal of the American Psychiatric Nurses Association*, *24*(4), 295–305. https://doi.org/10.1177/1078390318763963

American Psychological Association (APA). (2023a). *Stress*. https://www.apa.org/topics/stress

American Psychological Association (APA). (2023b). *Stress in America 2023*. https://www.apa.org/news/press/releases/stress/2023/collective-trauma-recovery

American Psychological Association (APA). (2023c). *How stress affects your health*. https://www.apa.org/topics/stress/health

Argyraki, M., Damdimopoulou, P., Chatzimeletiou, K., Grimbizis, G. F., Tarlatzis, B. C., Syrrou, M., & Lambropoulos, A. (2019). In-utero stress and mode of conception: Impact on regulation of imprinted genes, fetal development and future health. *Human Reproduction Update*, *25*(6), 777–801. https://doi.org/10.1093/humupd/dmz025

Badana, A. N. S., Marino, V. R., Templeman, M. E., McMillan, S. C., Tofthagen, C. S., Small, B. J., & Haley, W. E. (2019). Understanding the roles of patient symptoms and subjective appraisals in well-being among breast cancer patients. *Supportive Care in Cancer*, *27*(11), 4245–4252. https://doi.org/10.1007/s00520-019-04707-2

Beck, A. T. (1976). *Cognitive therapy and the emotional disorders*. New York: International Universities Press.

Beck, A. T. (1979). *Cognitive therapy of depression*. New York: Guilford Press.

Beck Institute for Cognitive Behavior Therapy. (2024). *Beck Institute for Cognitive Behavior Therapy*. https://www.beckinstitute.org/get-informed/tools-and-resources/

Bennett, F. C., & Molofsky, A. V. (2019). The immune system and psychiatric disease: A basic science perspective. *Clinical and Experimental Immunology*, *197*(3), 294–307. https://doi.org/10.1111/cei.13334

Benson, H. (1975). *The relaxation response*. New York: William Morrow & Co.

Benson-Henry. (2021). Institute for Mind Body Medicine of Massachusetts General Hospital. *Stress*. https://www.bensonhenryinstitute.org

Brewer, J. (2021). *Unwinding anxiety: new science shows how to break the cycles of worry and fear to heal your mind*. Avery.

Cannon, W. (1914). The emergency function of the adrenal medulla in pain and the major emotions. *American Journal of Physiology*, *33*, 356–372.

Cecere, L., de Novellis, S., Gravante, A., Petrillo, G., Pisani, L., Terrenato, I., Ivziku, D., Latina, R., & Gravante, F. (2023). Quality of life of critical care nurses and impact on anxiety, depression, stress, burnout and sleep quality: A cross-sectional study. *Intensive & Critical Care Nursing*, *79*, 103494. https://doi.org/10.1016/j.iccn.2023.103494

Centers for Disease Control and Prevention (CDC). (2023). *Stress*. https://www.cdc.gov/howrightnow/emotion/stress/index.html

Choi, S., & Seo, J. (2019). Analysis of caregiver burden in palliative care: An integrated review. *Nursing Forum*, *54*(2), 280–290. https://doi.org/10.1111/nuf.12328

Cole, G. (2022). The trans-theoretical model for mindful cognitive behavioral therapy a paradigm for systematically advancing evidence-based practice and research. *Cogent Psychology*, *9*(1). https://doi.org/10.1080/23311908.2022.2080320

DeMarco, R., & Healey-Walsh, J. (2020). *Community and public health nursing: Evidence for Practice* (3rd ed.). Philadelphia: Wolters Kluwer.

Ellis, A. (1962). *Reason and emotion in psychotherapy*. New York: L. Stuart.

Ellis, A., & Dryden, W. (1987). *The practice of rational emotive therapy (RET)*. New York: Springer.

Fan, M., Wang, Y., Zheng, L., Cui, M., Zhou, X., & Liu, Z. (2023). Effectiveness of online mindfulness-based interventions for cancer patients: A systematic review and meta-analysis. *Japanese Journal of Clinical Oncology*, *53*(11), 1068–1076. https://doi.org/10.1093/jjco/hyad101

Feldman, C., & Kuyken, W. (2019). *Mindfulness: Ancient wisdom meets modern psychology*. NY, NY: Guilford Press.

Fernández Sánchez, H., Hernández, E., C. B., Sidani, S., Osorio, C. H., Contreras, E. C., & Mendoza, J. S. (2020). Dance intervention for Mexican family caregivers of children with developmental disability: A pilot study. *Journal of Transcultural Nursing*, *31*(1), 38–44. https://doi.org/10.1177/1043659619838027

Fisher, S. G., & Devlin, A. (2019). Development of an urban community-based cohort to promote health disparities research. *International Journal of Public Health*, *64*(7), 1107–1115. https://doi.org/10.1007/s00038-019-01267-4

Gaffney, D. A., & Foster, N. C. (2023). *Courageous well-being for nurses: Strategies for renewal*. Baltimore, MD: Johns Hopkins University Press.

Gautam, M., Tripathi, A., Deshmukh, D., & Gaur, M. (2020). Cognitive behavioral therapy for depression. *Indian Journal of Psychiatry*, *62*(Suppl 2), S223–S229. https://doi.org/10.4103/psychiatry.IndianJPsychiatry_772_19

Gillihan, S. J. (2021). *Mindful cognitive behavioral therapy: A simple path to healing, hope, and peace*. HarperOne.

Goldberg, S. B., Riordan, K. M., Sun, S., & Davidson, R. J. (2021). The empirical status of mindfulnesss-based interventions: A systematic review of 44 meta-analyses of randomized controlled trials. *Perspectives on Psychological Science*, *17*(10):108–130. https://doi./10.1177/1745691620968771

Graham, K. M., Kreutzer, J. S., Marwitz, J. H., Sima, A. P., & Hsu, N. H. (2020). Can a couples' intervention reduce unmet needs and caregiver burden after brain injury? *Rehabilitation Psychology*, *65*(4), 409–417. https://doi.org/10.1037/rep0000300

Guan, Y., Shen, J., Lu, J., Fuemmeler, B. F., Shock, L. S., & Zhao, H. (2023). Association between allostatic load and breast cancer risk: A cohort study. *Breast Cancer Research: BCR*, *25*(1), 1–12. https://doi.org/10.1186/s13058-023-01754-w

Guidi, J., Lucente, M., Sonino, N., & Fava, G. A. (2021). Allostatic load and its impact on health: A systematic review. *Psychotherapy and Psychosomatics*, *90*(1), 11–27. https://doi.org/10.1159/000510696

Halaris, A. (2017). Inflammation-associated co-morbidity between depression and cardiovascular disease. *Current Topics in Behavioral Neurosciences*, *31* 45–70. https://doi.org/10.1007/7854_2016_28

Han, S. C., Schacter, H. L., Timmons, A. C., Kim, Y., Sichko, S., Pettit, C., Chaspari, T., Narayanan, S., & Margolin, G. (2021). Romantic partner presence and physiological responses in daily life: Attachment style as a moderator. *Biological Psychology*, *161*, 108082. https://doi.org/10.1016/j.biopsycho.2021.108082

Henry, T. L., Schmidt, S., Lund, M. B., Haynes, T., Ford, D., Egwuogu H., Schmitz, S., McGregor, B., Toomer, L., & Bussey-Jones, J. (2019). Improving depression screening in underserved populations in a large urban academic primary care center: A provider-centered analysis and approach. *American Journal of Medical Quality*, *35*, 315–322. https://doi.org/10.1177/1062860619884639

Holmes, T. H. (1981). *The schedule of recent experiences*. Seattle: University of Washington Press.

Horowitz, M., Wilner, N., & Alvarez, W. (1979). Impact of event scale: A measure of subjective stress. *Psychosomatic Medicine, 41*(3), 209–218.

Huang, J., Tian, W., & Döring, O. (2023). January 23: A date for COVID-19 research and reflection. *Journal of Global Health, 13*, 03056. https://doi.org/10.7189/jogh.13.03056

Javed, Z., Haisum Maqsood, M., Yahya, T., Amin, Z., Acquah, I., Valero-Elizondo, J., Andrieni, J., Dubey, P., Jackson, R. K., Daffin, M. A., Cainzos-Achirica, M., Hyder, A. A., & Nasir, K. (2022). Race, racism, and cardiovascular health: Applying a social determinants of health framework to racial/ethnic disparities in cardiovascular disease. *Circulation. Cardiovascular Quality and Outcomes, 15*(1), e007917. https://doi.org/10.1161/CIRCOUTCOMES.121.007917

Karatekim, C., & Ahluwalia, R. (2020). Effects of adverse childhood experiences, stress, and social support on the health of college students. *Journal of Interpersonal Violence, 35*(1/2), 15–172.

Kobasa, S. C., Maddi, S. R., & Kahn, S. (1982). Hardiness and health: A prospective study. *Journal of Personality and Social Psychology, 42*, 391–404.

Komariah, M., Ibrahim, K., Pahria, T., Rahayuwati, L., & Somantri, I. (2022). Effect of mindfulness breathing meditation on depression, anxiety, and stress: A randomized controlled trial among university students. *Healthcare, 11*(1), 26. https://doi.org/10.3390/healthcare11010026

Kowal, M., Coll-Martín, T., Ikizer, G., Rasmussen, J., Eichel, K., Studzi´nska, A., Koszałkowska, K., Karwowski, M., Najmussaqib, A., Pankowski, D., Lieberoth, A., Ahmed, O. (2020). Who is the most stressed during the COVID-19 pandemic? Data from 26 countries and areas. *Applied Psychology: Health and Well-Being, 12*, 946–966. https://doi.org/10.1111/aphw.12234

Kwong, J., Roberts, D., Hagler, D., & Reinisch, C. (Eds.). (2023). *Lewis's medical-surgical nursing: Assessment and management of clinical problems* (12th ed.). Elsevier.

Landy, J. F., Shigeto, A., Laxman, D. J., & Scheier, L. M. (2022). Typologies of stress appraisal and problem-focused coping: Associations with compliance with public health recommendations during the COVID-19 pandemic. *BMC Public Health, 22*(1), 784. https://doi.org/10.1186/s12889-022-13161-5

La Torre, G., Raffone, A., Peruzzo, M., Calabrese, L., Cocchiara, R. A., D'Egidio, V., Leggieri, P. F., Dorelli, B., Zaffina, S., Mannocci, A., & Yomin Collaborative Group. (2020). Yoga and mindfulness as a tool for influencing affectivity, anxiety, mental health, and stress among healthcare workers: Results of a single-arm clinical trial. *Journal of Clinical Medicine, 9*(4), 1037. https://doi.org/10.3390/jcm9041037

Lazarus, R., & Folkman, S. (1984). *Stress, appraisal, and coping*. New York: Springer.

Li, Y. N., Buys, N., Ferguson, S., Li, Z. J., & Sun, J. (2021). Effectiveness of cognitive behavioral therapy-based interventions on health outcomes in patients with coronary heart disease: A meta-analysis. *World Journal of Psychiatry, 11*(11), 1147–1166. https://doi.org/10.5498/wjp.v11.i11.1147

Lindquist, R., Tracy, M. F., & Snyder, M. (2022). *Complementary/alternative therapies in nursing: promoting integrative care* (9th ed.). New York: Springer.

Liu, Z., Heffernan, C., & Tan, J. (2020). Caregiver burden: A concept analysis. *International Journal of Nursing Sciences, 7*(4), 438–445. https://doi.org/10.1016/j.ijnss.2020.07.012

López-Otín, C., & Kroemer, G. (2021). Hallmarks of health. *Cell, 184*(1), 33–63. https://doi.org/10.1016/j.cell.2020.11.034

Lynn, S. J., Green, J. P., Craig, P., Ellenberg, S., Gautem, A., & Asken, D. (2019). Hypnosis, hypnotic phenomena, and hypnotic responsiveness: Clinical and research foundations—a 40-year perspective. *International Journal of Clinical & Experimental Hypnosis, 67*, 475–511. http://doi.org/10.1080/00207144.2019.1649541

Manning, L., Ferris, M., Rosario, C. N., Prues, M., & Bouchard, L. (2019). Spiritual resilience: Understanding the protection and promotion of well-being in the later life. *Journal of Religion, Spirituality & Aging, 31*(2), 168–186. https://doi.org/10.1080/15528030.2018.1532859

Maslach, C., & Jackson, S. E. (1986). *Burnout inventory (manual research ed.)* (2nd ed.). Palo Alto, CA: Consulting Psychologists Press.

McClintock, C. H., Worhunsky, P. D., Balodis, I. M., Sinha, R., Miller, L., & Potenza, M. N. (2019). How spirituality may mitigate against stress and related mental disorders: A review and preliminary neurobiological evidence. *Current Behavioral Neuroscience Reports, 6*, 253–262.

McNamara, N., Stevenson, C., Costa, S., Bowe, M., Wakefield, J., Kellezi, B., Wilson, I. Halder, M., & Mair, E. (2021). Community identification, social support, and loneliness: The benefits of social identification for personal well-being. *The British Journal of Social Psychology, 60*(4) 1379–402. https://doi.org/10.1111/bjso.12456

Miller, J. J. (2019). Mindfulness. *Psychiatric Times, 36*(12), 6–7.

MyFitnessPal. (2023). *Free calorie counter*. http://www.myfitnesspal.com/

Najavits, L. M. (2019). *Finding your best self: Recovery from addiction, trauma, or both*. NY, NY: Guilford Press.

National Center for Chronic Disease Prevention and Health Promotion (NCCDPHP). (2022). *About chronic diseases*. https://www.cdc.gov/chronic-disease/about/?CDC_AAref_Val=https://www.cdc.gov/chronicdisease/about/index.htm

National Center for Complementary and Integrative Health (NCCIH). (2022). *Stress*. https://www.nccih.nih.gov/health/stress

Ng, M. A., Naranjo, A., Schlotzhauer, A. E., Shoss, M. K., Kartvelishvili, N., Bartek, M., Ingraham, K., Rodriguez, A., Schneider, S. K., Silverlieb-Seltzer, L., & Silva, C. (2021). Has the COVID-19 pandemic accelerated the future of work or changed its course? Implications for research and practice. *International Journal of Environmental Research and Public Health, 18*(19), 10199. https://doi.org/10.3390/ijerph181910199

National Heart, Lung and Blood Institute. (2024). *Sleep disorder treatments*. https://www.nhlbi.nih.gov/health/sleep-disorder-treatments

National Heart, Lung, and Blood Institute. (2024). *Sleep health*. https://www.nhlbi.nih.gov/health-topics/education-and-awareness/sleep-health

Pai, R., & Gupta, N. (2019). Yogic practices on oxidative stress and of antioxidant level: A systematic review of randomized controlled trials. *Journal of Complementary and Integrative Medicine, 16*(40). https://doi.org/10.1515/jcim-2017-0079

Palmwood, E. N., & McBride, C. A. (2019). Challenge vs. threat: The effect of appraisal type on resource depletion. *Current Psychology, 38*(6), 1522–1529. https://doi.org/10.1007/s12144-017-9713-6

Parlindungan, F., Hidayat, R., Ariane, A., & Shatri, H. (2023). Association between proinflammatory cytokines and anxiety and depression symptoms in rheumatoid arthritis patients: A cross-sectional study. *Clinical Practice and Epidemiology in Mental Health, 19*(1), e174501792304261. https://doi.org/10.2174/17450179-v19-e230510-2022-34

Pelletier, K. R. (2019). Mind matters: Turn off genetic vulnerabilities by reducing stress. *Alternative and Complementary Therapies, 25*(3), 155–159. https://www.libproxy.umassd.edu/

Perkins, A. (2020). The benefits of pet therapy. *Nursing Made Incredibly Easy!, 18*(1), 5–8. https://doi.org/10.1097/01.NME.0000613652.69241.d7

Phillips, J. R. (2015). Martha E. Rogers: Heretic and heroine. *Nursing Science Quarterly*, *28*, 42–48.

Presciutti, A. M., Bannon, S. M., Yamin, J. B., Newman, M. M., Parker, R. A., Elmer, J., Wu, O., Donnino, M. W., Perman, S. M., & Vranceanu, A.-M. (2023). The relationship between mindfulness and enduring somatic threat severity in long-term cardiac arrest survivors. *Journal of Behavioral Medicine*, *46*(5), 890–896. https://doi-org.libproxy.umassd.edu/10.1007/s10865-023-00405-x

Rink, L. C., Silva, S. G., & Sexton. B. (2022). The association between well-being behaviors and resilience in health care workers. *Western Journal of Nursing Research*, *44* (No. 8), 743–754. https://doi.org/10.1177/01939459211017515

Rogers, C. (1951). *Client-centered therapy*. Boston, MA: Houghton Mifflin.

Saadat, N., Zhang, L., Hyer, S., Padmanabhan, V., Woo, J., Engeland, C. G., Misra, D. P., & Giurgescu, C. (2022). Psychosocial and behavioral factors affecting inflammation among pregnant African American women. *Brain, Behavior, & Immunity - Health*, *22*, 100452. https://doi.org/10.1016/j.bbih.2022.100452

Selye, H. (1950). *Stress*. Montreal: Acta.

Selye, H. (1974). *Stress without distress*. Philadelphia: J. B. Lippincott & Co.

Selye, H. (1982). History and present status of the stress concept. In L. Goldberger & S. Breznitz (Eds.), *Handbook of stress: Theoretical and clinical aspects* (pp. 7–17). New York: Free Press.

Shajani, Z., & Snell, D. (2019). *Wright & Leahey's Nurses and families: A guide to family assessment and intervention* (7th ed.). Philadelphia: F.A. Davis.

Stahl, J. E., Ammana, H. R., Kwak, L., & Comi, R. J. (2022). SMART-ly managing type 1 diabetes - modifying glucose metabolism with an online mind-body intervention: A feasibility and pilot study. *Frontiers in Clinical Diabetes and Healthcare*, *3*, 802461. https://doi.org/10.3389/fcdhc.2022.802461

Stuart, G. W. (2013). *Principles and practice of psychiatric nursing* (10th ed.). St. Louis: Mosby.

Thorsén, F., Antonson, C., Palmér, K., Berg, R., Sundquist, J., & Sundquist, K. (2022). Associations between perceived stress and health outcomes in adolescents. *Child and Adolescent Psychiatry and Mental Health*, *16*(1), 75. https://doi.org/10.1186/s13034-022-00510-w

US Department of Agriculture. (2020). *Food and nutrition*. https://www.usda.gov/topics/food-and-nutrition

US Department of Health and Human Services Office of Disease Prevention and Health Promotion (USDHHS ODPHP). (2021). *Healthy People 2030 framework*. https://health.gov/healthypeople/about/healthy-people-2030-framework

US Department of Health & Human Services Office of Disease Prevention and Health Promotion (USDHHS ODPHP). (2022). *Manage stress*. https://healthfinder.gov/healthtopics/category/health-conditions-and-diseases/heart-health/manage-stress#take-action_1

Weiss, D. S., & Marmar, C. R. (1997). Impact of Event Scale-revised. In S. Wilson & T.M. Keane (Eds.), *Assessing psychological trauma and PTSD: A practitioner's handbook* (pp. 399-411). New York: Guilford Press.

Wells-Federman, C., Stuart-Shor, E., Deckro, J., Mandle, C. L., Baim, M., & Medich, C. (1995). The mind/body connection: The psychophysiology of many traditional nursing interventions. *Clinical Nurse Specialist*, *9*, 60.

Willis, D. G., DeSanto-Madeya, S. Ross, R., Sheehan, D.L., Fawcett, J. (2015). Spiritual healing in the aftermath of childhood maltreatment: Translating men's lived experiences utilizing conceptual models and theory. *Advances in Nursing Science*, *38*, 162–174. https://doi.org/10.1097/ANS.0000000000000075

Wiesmaierova, S., Catena, A., Petrova, D., Garcia-Retamero, R., Hernández, Ramírez, A., J., & Arrebola Moreno, A. (2019). Social support buffers the negative effects of stress in cardiac patients: A cross-sectional study with acute coronary syndrome patients. *Journal of Behavioral Medicine*, *42*(3), 469–479. https://doi.org/10.1007/s10865-018-9998-4

World Health Organization (WHO). (2023a). *WHO COVID-19 dashboard*. https://data.who.int/dashboards/covid19/cases?n=c

World Health Organization (WHO). (2023b). *Traditional, complementary and integrative medicine*. https://www.who.int/health-topics/traditional-complementary-and-integrative-medicine#tab=tab_1

Wu, Q., Zhu, Y., Brevard, K., Wu, S., & Krysik, J. (2024). Risk and protective factors for African American kinship caregiving: A scoping review. *Children & Youth Services Review*, *156*, 107279. https://doi.org/10.1016/j.childyouth.2023.107279

Wurst, R., Kinkel, S., Lin, J., Goehner, W., & Fuchs, R. (2019). Promoting physical activity through a psychological group intervention in cardiac rehabilitation: A randomized controlled trial. *Journal of Behavioral Medicine*, *42*(6), 1104–1116. https://doi.org/10.1007/s10865-019-00047-y

Yue, W. L., Ng, K. K., Koh, A. J., Perini, F., Doshi, K., Zhou, J. H., & Lim, J. (2023). Mindfulness-based therapy improves brain functional network reconfiguration efficiency. *Translational Psychiatry*, *13*(1), 345. https://doi.org/10.1038/s41398-023-02642-9

Zänkert, S., Bellingrath, S., Wüst, S., & Kudielka, B. M. (2019). HPA axis responses to psychological challenge linking stress and disease: What do we know on sources of intra- and interindividual variability? *Psychoneuroendocrinology*, *105*, 86–97. https://doi.org/10.1016/j.psyneuen.2018.10.027

Zhao, Y., Watterston, J. (2021). The changes we need: Education post COVID-19. *Journal of Educational Change 22*, 3–12. https://doi.org/10.1007/s10833-021-09417-3

14

Complementary, Integrative, and Alternative Strategies

Donna M. Dello Iacono

OBJECTIVES

After completing this chapter, the reader will be able to:

- Compare and contrast holistic, allopathic, complementary, integrative, and alternative health modalities.
- Describe the nursing role in complementary health therapies.
- Explain the origin and practice of selected holistic health strategies.
- Identify and evaluate complementary and alternative therapy resources.
- Discuss complementary, integrative, and alternative medicine safety and effectiveness.
- Provide client education regarding complementary health therapies, resources, and possible safety concerns.
- Develop awareness of cultural aspects of holistic health practices.
- Identify the rationale for including the use of herbal and other supplements in medication reconciliation.

KEY TERMS

Acupressure
Acupuncture
Affordable Care Act
Allopathic medicine
Allopathy
Alternative therapy
American Holistic Nurses Association
Aromatherapy
Attunement
Ayurvedic medicine
Biofeedback
Centering
Chi
Chiropractic medicine
Complementary and alternative medicine
Complementary therapy
Cranial and craniosacral therapies
Dance therapy
Distant healing
Energy healing or therapy
Energy therapy
Energy work
Genetics
Healing touch
Health
Herbal therapy
Holism
Holistic health
Homeopathy
Hydrotherapy
Hypnotherapy
Imagery
Integrative therapy
Jin Shin Jyutsu
Massage
Meditation
Meridians
Moxibustion
Music therapy
National Center for Complementary and Integrative Health
National Prevention Strategy
Naturopathy
Nursing presence
Nutritional counseling
Pet therapy
Physical therapy
Polarity therapy
Prayer
Presence
Probiotics
Qi
Qigong
Reflexology
Reiki
Shiatsu
Spinal or bone manipulation
Tai chi
Therapeutic presence
Therapeutic touch
Touch therapies
Traditional Chinese medicine
Visual or guided imagery
Wellness
Whole medical systems
Yoga

THINK ABOUT IT

Ms. Sarinda Choi, a normally healthy 55-year-old scientist, sees her primary care provider for shortness of breath and fatigue. She is diagnosed with mitral valve prolapse that requires surgery. A cardiac catheterization test reveals two-vessel obstructive coronary artery disease. She has never smoked; she doesn't exercise. For lunch she mostly eats take-out fried foods; she has a strong family history of heart disease. Her family and work friends are very concerned and have provided her with various complementary and alternative medicine modalities to treat her symptoms. They have provided their reasoning for these agents. She is taking 650 mg aspirin, as it is "good for the heart," she has been taking fish oil, omega 3, and garlic, which are supposed to lower her cholesterol, turmeric for her immune system, and lemon balm for her "frazzled nerves." She has recently begun yoga classes. She and her life partner go to the multidisciplinary clinic to discuss optimization and a plan for surgery. She is frightened, and she believes that she feels more in control since starting these therapies. She has never taken prescription medications and is afraid of addiction if she takes prescribed pain medication. She understands that these complementary therapies may help to relieve some of her symptoms, but she believes they may also treat her heart disease and maybe she will not need surgery. After researching internet sites, including the National Institutes of Health Office of Dietary Supplements (n.d.) and the National Center for Complementary and Integrative Health (NCCIH, n.d.), she feels overwhelmed and confused as to what is best for her, as there is not a great deal of science to support what she has been told by her friends.

Other questions that you or your clients may have:

- Are these therapies evidence-based?What is the best understanding of the physiologic mechanisms for these therapies?
- What is the best understanding of the safety of these therapies?
- Which therapies are covered by her insurance?

For Ms. Choi:

- Would Ms. Choi's therapies be considered complementary, alternative, or integrative?
- What is known about the safety and efficacy about the supplements she is taking to lower cholesterol, improve her immune system, and help her anxiety?
- What does the evidence report about yoga?

BACKGROUND

Key Definitions and Terminology

Although many complementary and alternative therapies date back more than 5000 years to the Han Dynasty, Hippocrates, and Indian cultures with Ayurveda practices, only a few have been evaluated with well-conducted research (NCCIH, n.d.). "**Complementary and alternative medicine**" (CAM) is the term for medical products and practices that are not part of standard medical care. In the United States, the CAM movement, which includes herbal agents used by Native Americans, chiropractic, meditative, and a variety of therapies, began in the 19th century. The first center for alternative medicine, the Office of Alternative Medicine, was commissioned by Congress in 1991 (NCCIH, 2024). The working definition of CAM at that time was "a group of medical, health care, and healing systems other than those included in mainstream health care in the United States" (NCCIH, 2024b).

The field is broad and constantly changing, but an authoritative governmental source, the National Institutes of Health's NCCIH (2024), now describes CAM as a set of medical and health care systems, practices, and products that are not used in conventional medicine, also known as "Western allopathic medicine" (NCCIH, 2024). NCCIH has separate definitions of complementary, alternative, and integrative therapy. Interested participants and practitioners can search for research and the latest-known science for a variety of therapies and supplements, with easy-to-use search bars or alphabetically by topic or agent.

NCCIH defines **complementary therapy** as a nonmainstream practice that is used together with conventional medicine, thus considered "complementary." One example is the use of acupuncture to treat pain. **Alternative therapy** is a nonmainstream practice that is used in place of conventional medicine practices. One example is the use of a special diet or herbs to treat abnormalities instead of drugs prescribed by providers. **Integrative therapy** is a total approach to medical care that combines standard medical and surgical interventions with the complementary approaches in a coordinated way, thus treating the whole person. Integrative approaches to health and wellness have increased in care settings, with multidisciplinary providers collaborating on a clients' care. They treat the individual's mind, body, and spirit (NCCIH, 2024). Complementary and alternative therapies are more holistic than traditional medicine practices have been in the past. The most common of these practices (psychological, physical, and nutritional) can be seen in Fig. 14.1.

Although heterogeneous, the major complementary, alternative, and integrative approaches have many common characteristics, including a focus on individualizing treatments, treating the whole person, promoting self-care and self-healing, and recognizing the multiple interconnected domains of health: biologic, behavioral, social, and environmental. A large gap exists between our current level of scientific evidence and the knowledge needed to provide evidence-based advice. More rigorous scientific research is being conducted in many countries, including the United States, to enrich our knowledge base.

Some Known Facts

- In the World Health Organization's January 2023 newsletter (*Integrating Traditional Medicine in Health Care*), it is estimated that more than 80% of the world's population currently use some form of alternative medicine, such as herbal medicine, yoga, Ayurveda, acupuncture, or acupressure (who.int)
- A scientific statement from the American Heart Association (Chow et al., 2023) notes that health care professionals rarely inquire or document use of CAM as part of the medical record, and patients do not often disclose their use.
- The percentage of patients undergoing surgery who use herbal products has been reported to range from 32% to 51%. Some agents have been associated with positive effects on postoperative pain, anxiety, and postoperative nausea and vomiting. However, they have also been associated with adverse effects that include:
  - Prolonging the effects of anesthesia
  - Increasing the risks of bleeding
  - Raising blood pressure

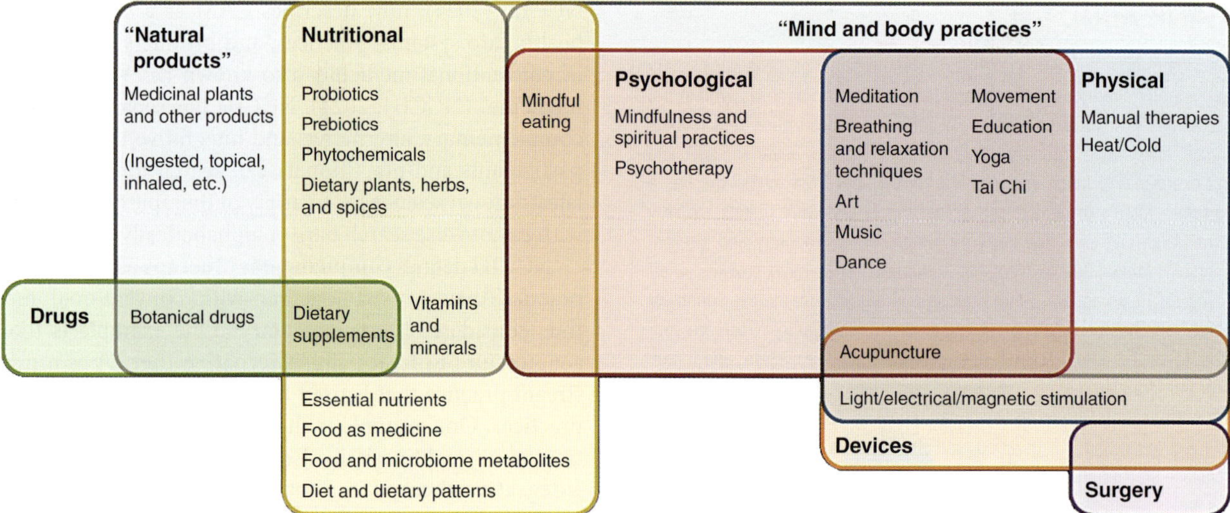

FIG. 14.1 Examples of complementary health approaches that fall within the categories: psychological, physical, and nutritional.

- Interfering with other medications
- Causing heart, respiratory, or digestive problems (Arruda et al., 2019)

Accurate risk assessments are unknown as there is/are:

- No regulation of these agents by the US Food and Drug Administration (FDA), unlike prescription and over-the-counter medications. This means the companies that make them don't have to prove that they are safe or even that they are effective. It also means the ingredient levels or preparations of each product can vary, and some levels might not be safe.
- No standard manufacturing process; the place of origin of the product is not always known; the label may state "distributed by" a company the United States, but that may not be where the product was created.
- No method to determine ingredients, dosage, or bioavailability.
- No quality controls or standardization.
- No protection against contamination.
- No reporting of adverse reactions. Unlike postmarket surveillance and reporting for prescription medications, over-the-counter medications, vaccines, and other agents, the US FDA does not require reporting of adverse reactions of alternative therapies.

There is no evidence for most of the claims made, and the American public assumes:

- That the FDA reviews the safety and effectiveness of dietary supplements before they are marketed
- That supplements have to list potential side effects on their labels
- That herbal-pharmaceutical interactions occur (US Food and Drug Administration, n.d.)

WHAT IS THE DIFFERENCE BETWEEN HOLISM AND ALLOPATHY?

Holism Versus Allopathy

Health care in the United States is most often **allopathic medicine**, a system in which providers, such as physicians, nurses, advanced practice professionals, pharmacists, and therapists, treat symptoms and diseases using medications, radiation, lasers, or surgical interventions. **Allopathy** is also called "biomedicine," "conventional medicine," "mainstream medicine," "orthodox medicine," and "Western medicine" (NCCIH, 2024).

Holistic health considers the whole person: their biology, genetics, behaviors, and how they interact with their social environment. It emphasizes the connection of mind, body, and spirit. **Holistic health** is a system of preventive care that considers the whole individual, one's own responsibility for one's well-being, and the total influences—social, psychosocial, spiritual, environmental—that affect health, including nutrition, exercise, and mental relaxation. **Holism** entails a focus on proactive, healthy living and considers not only prevention of illness but also the root cause of the illness. When disease occurs, holistic practitioners seek to support the person's natural healing systems, to consider the whole person, and to consider the environment, both physical and mental, surrounding the person. This movement in the healing arts reflects the theory of holism and recognizes that all aspects of the person must be considered when care is being planned and delivered (NCCIH, 2024).

Person-Centered Care

There are a variety of reasons why people seeking care desire a more holistic approach to care and use CAM. Those receiving traditional medicine therapies are often disappointed in the lack of effective treatments or cures for many disorders, are afraid of the safety and long-term effects of drugs or treatments, believe herbal products are safe because they are derived from "nature," and have a desire to have control of their own health, so they choose alternative and/or complementary methods. One study found that the prevalence of CAM use was greater than 66% in cancer-care recipients, with a higher percentage in females, as available therapies did not treat all the symptoms or complications associated with cancer (Wu et al., 2023). There is a great deal of advertising, media, and peer or family influence that affects the range of holistic choices.

Many people are seeking alternative styles of health care that focus on seeing care recipients as whole people, increasing well-being, and giving them greater control over self-care. According to the most recent National Health Interview Survey, as reported in Missenda et al. (2023), people in the United States spent $33.9 billion out of pocket for CAM therapies, $14.8 billion on nonvitamin, nonmineral natural products, and $11.9 billion on CAM practitioner visits, for a total of $60.6 billion in 2019.

Many traditional medical centers now include a holistic viewpoint and integrative therapies, including Harvard, Stanford, Duke, and the Mayo Clinic. Most of them offer acupuncture, massage, healing gardens, essential oils, energy-based therapies, imagery, music, acupressure, and nutrition counseling along with the traditional allopathic approach. The Van Elslander Cancer Center at St. John Hospital and Medical Center in Detroit, Michigan, has a clinic that also offers qigong, tai chi, yoga classes, hypnotherapy, and guided imagery (www.healthcare.ascension.org). The Birchtree Center in western Massachusetts offers professional holistic development classes for nurses that can help them to prepare for holistic nursing certification (Birch Tree Center for Healthcare Transformation, n.d.). At the Dana Farber Cancer Institute in Boston, Massachusetts (Dana Farber Patient and Family Resource Centers, n.d.), the Eleanor and Maxwell Blum Patient and Family Resource Center provides individuals undergoing cancer therapies and their family members with a comfortable environment to learn more about disease treatment and management, including nutrition, palliative care, spirituality, stress management, and emotional health (https://www.dana-farber.org/patient-family/support-services/patient-family-resource-centers). In addition, the Institute has the Leonard P. Zakim Center for Integrative Therapies and Healthy Living, which seeks to enhance the quality of life of patients with cancer through integrative therapies such as acupuncture, massage, and healthy living programs such as exercise and nutrition counseling (https://www.dana-farber.org/patient-family/support-services/integrative-therapies). In an integrative review of the use of CAM by those living with cancer, the reasons for use include (Balneaves et al., 2022):

- Managing cancer and treatment-related symptoms and side effects
- Improving overall quality of life
- Providing a sense of control
- Boosting the immune system
- Fighting the disease
- Preventing a recurrence
- As a "last resort"

This integration of holistic practices with standard allopathic medicine (Box 14.1: Genomics) serves to introduce more people to complementary and integrative therapies and may give these practices more credibility, especially with those who currently question their value. Complementary/integrative therapies are used as an adjunct to conventional medical care, and many are now covered by insurers, meet consumer demand, and thus satisfy the definition of care recipient- or person-centered care.

BOX 14.1 GENOMICS

Genetics contributes to scientific knowledge of a person's risk of developing many common diseases. Diet, lifestyle, and environmental exposures are factors in many conditions and risk factors for many types of cancer. Genetics is one factor that contributes to health and illness. Genetics has a role in targeted therapies. A better understanding of the interface of CAM practices with genetics may identify measures to mitigate health risks. Mapping the genetic components of cells, explaining how all the various elements work together to affect the human body in both health and disease, and developing targeted therapies will help providers to better educate and advise those in their care.

CAM, Complementary and alternative medicine.

HEALTH AND WELLNESS

The World Health Organization's timeless definition of **health** is "a state of complete physical, mental and social well-being and not merely the absence of disease or infirmity" (World Health Organization, n.d.-a). The Wellness Initiative of Healthy People 2030 defines wellness as "overall well-being." It includes the mental, emotional, physical, occupational, intellectual, and spiritual aspects of a person's life (https://health.gov/healthypeople). Working toward health and wellness is an ongoing process that includes self-knowledge and self-care and is viewed as essential to a thriving and equitable society. The wellness-related reasons that people use a variety of nontraditional therapies include:

- To treat a specific health condition
- To promote general wellness or disease prevention
- To improve immune function
- To improve energy
- To focus on the whole person—mind, body, and spirit
- To improve memory or concentration

Use of holistic modalities can also help to meet the goals of Healthy People 2030. This includes increasing quality and number of years of life, improving nutrition, increasing physical activity, and eliminating health disparities (Box 14.2: Healthy People 2030). The Affordable Care Act of 2010 includes provisions that allow CAM providers to participate in health care delivery teams.

Health Policy

Clinical Practice Guidelines

Clinical practice guidelines for CAM modalities exist to identify and describe evidence-based recommended courses of intervention in general (NCCIH, 2024) and for specific disorders (Tables 14.1 and 14.2). See Box 14.3: Quality and Safety Scenario for guidelines on quality and safety and Box 14.4 for a sample list of NCCIH practice guidelines to provide best evidence-based practice support (Balneaves et al., 2022).

Healthy People 2030

Holistic interventions are used to promote wellness and are used to meet the Healthy People 2030 vision of improving the

BOX 14.2 HEALTHY PEOPLE 2030 OBJECTIVES

Symbol	Healthy People 2030 Objective
AOCBC-D01	Increase self-management of high-impact chronic pain
C-R01	Increase the mental and physical health-related quality of life of cancer survivors
ECBP-D02	Increase the proportion of work sites that offer employee health promotion program(s) to their employees
ECBP-DO6	Increase the number of community-based organizations providing population-based primary prevention services
ECBP-DO9	Increase the inclusion of core clinical prevention and population health content in undergraduate nursing and graduate nurse practitioner training programs
D-DO1	Increase the proportion of eligible individuals completing CDC-recognized lifestyle change programs
PA-01	Reduce the proportion of adults who engage in no leisure-time physical activity
HRQOL/WB-1	Increase the proportion of adults who self-report good or better physical health

CDC, Centers for Disease Control and Prevention.
US Department of Health and Human Services (n.d.)

TABLE 14.1 Herbs as Medicine

Drug Name	Plant/Tree
Digitalis (heart drug)	Foxglove plant
Paclitaxel (cancer drug)	Pacific yew tree
Aspirin	Willow tree
Quinine (malaria drug)	Cinchona tree
Morphine	Opium poppy
Galantamine (Alzheimer disease drug)	Daffodil bulb
Vincristine (cancer drug)	Rosy periwinkle
Reserpine (blood pressure drug)	Indian snakeroot plant

What are herbs? An herb (also called a "botanical") is a plant or plant part used for its scent, flavor, and/or therapeutic properties. An herbal supplement is a type of dietary supplement that contains herbs, either alone or in mixtures.
NCCIH (2024)

health of Americans and helping them live long and healthy lives. This includes increasing quality and number of years of life; improving nutrition; increasing physical activity and flexibility in all age groups; decreasing pain, including chronic pain; and reducing health disparities (https://health.gov/healthypeople). Examples of some of the holistic modalities include integrative and complementary measures to address chronic pain and smoking cessation (Agency for Healthcare Research and Quality [AHRQ], 2021; see Box 14.2: Healthy People 2030).

Affordable Care Act and National Prevention Strategy

The Affordable Care Act (https://www.healthcare.gov) mandates that insurers do not discriminate against licensed health care providers, including those who practice alternative medicine, such as naturopaths, massage therapists, and acupuncturists. CAM practitioners and integrative practices are mentioned in several areas of the law, including workforce planning; care recipient–centered medical homes; wellness, prevention, and health-promotion services; comparative effectiveness research; and birthing services. The **National Prevention Strategy**, originating in 2011 as a result of the Affordable Care Act, updated in June 2020, has the following four strategic directions:

- Healthy and safe community environments: Create, sustain, and recognize communities that promote health and wellness through prevention.
- Clinical and community preventive services: Ensure that prevention-focused health care and community prevention efforts are available, integrated, and mutually reinforced.
- Empowered people: Support people in making healthy choices.
- Elimination of health disparities: Eliminate disparities, improving the quality of life for all Americans (DeCosta, 2023).

The National Prevention Strategy lists the following priorities:

- Tobacco-free living
- Prevention of drug abuse and excessive alcohol use
- Healthy eating
- Active living
- Injury and violence-free living
- Reproductive and sexual health
- Mental and emotional well-being

One year after the start of the coronavirus disease 2019 (COVID-19) pandemic, the use of supplements to boost the immune system had doubled according to the *National Business Journal* (Crawford et al., 2022). The *Journal of the American Medical Society (JAMA),* analyzed selected supplements and found the majority had inaccurate labeling (Crawford, et al., 2022). Legislative efforts to improve the oversight of supplements have not been successful to date. The proposed Dietary Supplement Listing Act of 2022 (GovTrack.us, n.d.) would have required companies to provide the FDA with information about their products, a list of all ingredients, claims on the label, allergen statements, and more; it was not voted on in the last Congress.

Nursing and Nursing Education

As a variety of holistic, complementary, and alternative practices are now very prevalent and part of mainstream health care practice, nurses must understand the nature of these interventions to provide safe, effective care and to discuss these practices with individuals who are using them to facilitate integrative care. Nurses who understand holistic practices will be able to make appropriate referrals to alternative/complementary and integrative practitioners. Nurses also find that holistic interventions such as **energy work**, bodywork, aromatherapy, prayer, meditation, massage, guided imagery, music therapy, and the movement arts of yoga, tai chi, and qigong provide a useful adjunct to current nursing theory and practice.

The **American Holistic Nurses Association** (AHNA, 2024) defines holistic nursing as nursing practice that heals the whole person. It is a "specialty practice that draws on nursing

TABLE 14.2 **Commonly Used Herbs: Safety Profiles**

Herb	Uses	Side Effects	Interactions	Evidence
St. John's wort	Depression	Dizziness, restlessness, sensitivity to sunlight, sleep disturbances, constipation	Seizure medications, alcohol, warfarin, calcium channel blockers, digoxin, oral contraceptives, statins	No statistically significant effect other than placebo effect on depression scores
Ginseng	Depression, anxiety, energy, concentration, immunity	Chest pain, headache, hypertension, impotence, palpitations	Diabetic agents, including insulin	Some evidence for concentration, no benefit for energy, mood, or immune modulation
Milk thistle	Liver ailments	Laxative effects	Flagyl	Cirrhosis; individuals may have longer survival; may be protective against hepatotoxic agents
Black cohosh	Menopausal symptoms	Low blood pressure, dizziness	Iron, antihypertensive drugs, warfarin, aspirin	No better than placebo
Echinacea	Immune system booster	Well-tolerated	Immunosuppressants	Decreases time to resolution of symptoms; no preventative effect
Saw palmetto	Benign prostate hyperplasia	Abdominal issues, headache, urinary retention	Hormones: leuprolide, birth control agents	As effective as many prescribed medications for benign prostate hyperplasia
Gingko biloba	Memory, asthma, vision	Gastrointestinal upset, seizures, bleeding or bruising	Anticoagulants, warfarin, aspirin, acetaminophen, seizure medications, antidepressants	No measurable long-term benefit
Garlic	Asthma, diabetes, high cholesterol level, cancer	Dizziness, rash, diaphoresis, bleeding	Antiplatelet drugs, warfarin, aspirin, HIV medications	No long-term benefits
Cranberry	Urinary tract infection, cancer	Diarrhea	None	Reduces risk of infection; no effect on treatment
Soy	Menopause, cancer, heart disease	Bloating, constipation, diarrhea, and nausea	Antibiotics, estrogens, warfarin, tamoxifen, losartan, carvedilol, levothyroxine	No effect on blood pressure; inconclusive results for hot flashes to date
Fish oil	Cholesterol, blood pressure, heart disease	Prolonged bleeding, negative impact on immunity	Anticoagulants, birth control agents	May worsen depression
Glucosamine	Joint health	Gastrointestinal upset	Blood thinners, insulin, heart medications	Those with a shellfish allergy should avoid it
Coenzyme Q_{10}	Heart, fatigue, immunity	Rash, gastrointestinal upset	Chemotherapy, blood pressure medications, coumadin	Inconclusive for all diseases already studied
Ephedra	Weight loss	Heart attack, respiratory depression, death	Theophylline, digoxin, caffeine	Banned by the US Food and Drug Administration in 2003 but available on the internet

From NCCIH (2024)

BOX 14.3 **QUALITY AND SAFETY SCENARIO**

- What government oversight of CAM practices should be more closely regulated?
- What standards of evidence should the nurse require before adopting an alternative/complementary therapy in clinical practice?
- Have all (or even some) of the alternative/complementary therapies commonly used by nurses nowadays been subjected to these standards?
- Have all (or even most) of the standard therapies commonly used by nurses and medicine today been subjected to these standards?

CAM, Complementary and alternative medicine.

knowledge, theories, expertise, and intuition to guide nurses in becoming therapeutic partners with people in their care. This practice recognizes the totality of the human being—the interconnectedness of body, mind, emotion, spirit, social/cultural, relationship, context, and environment" by integrating CAM modalities into clinical practice to broaden and enrich nursing treatment of physiologic, psychological, and spiritual needs. Florence Nightingale is thought to be one of the first holistic nurses because she believed in care of the person, focusing on unity, wellness, and the interrelationship of human beings with their environment. Holistic therapy is considered an "attitude, a philosophy, a way of being," although some holistic nurses specialize in one or more modalities.

The AHNA "advances the profession of holistic nursing by providing continuing education in holistic nursing, helping to improve the health care workplace through the incorporation of the concepts of holistic nursing, educating professionals and the public about holistic nursing and integrative health care, and promoting research and scholarship in the field of holistic nursing" (AHNA, 2024). The AHNA website offers a variety of resources, including a directory of holistic

BOX 14.4 Complementary and Alternative Medicine Clinical Practice Guidelines

***Samples of Featured Guidelines*[a]**

Allergy and Immunology

- Diagnosis and Management of Food Allergy (*Journal of Allergy and Clinical Immunology*)
- Guidelines for the Diagnosis and Management of Asthma (*National Heart, Lung, and Blood Institute*)

Cardiology

- Soy, Isoflavones, and Cardiovascular Health *(Circulation)*

Family Medicine

- Vitamin D and Calcium Supplementation to Prevent Fractures in Adults *(US Preventive Services Task Force)*
- Evaluation and Management of Chronic Insomnia in Adults *(Journal of Clinical Sleep Medicine)*
- Practice Parameters for the Psychological and Behavioral Treatment of Insomnia *(Sleep)*
  - NSAIDS and Other Complementary Treatments for Episodic Migraine Prevention in Adults *(Neurology)*
- American Cancer Society Guidelines on Nutrition and Physical Activity for Cancer Prevention *(CA: A Cancer Journal for Clinicians)*
- Guidance for the Prevention and Control of Influenza in the Peri- and Postpartum Settings *(CDC)*

Gastroenterology

- Probiotics and Children (*Journal of Pediatric Gastroenterology and Nutrition*)

Neurology

- Practice Parameter: Neuroprotective Strategies and Alternative Therapies for Parkinson Disease *(Neurology)*
- Complementary and Alternative Medicine in Multiple Sclerosis *(American Academy of Neurology)*

Oncology

- Exercise Guidelines for Cancer Survivors *(Medicine & Science in Sports & Exercise)*
- Use of Integrative Therapies as Supportive Care in Breast Cancer Patients *(Journal of the National Cancer Institute)*

Pain Management

- Practice Guidelines for Chronic Pain Management *(Anesthesiology)*
- Diagnosis and Treatment of Low-Back Pain *(Annals of Internal Medicine)*

Pediatrics

- Management of Children with Autism Spectrum Disorders *(Pediatrics)*
- Pediatric Integrative Medicine *(American Academy of Pediatrics)*

Psychiatry and Mental Health

- Nonpharmacologic Versus Pharmacologic Treatment of Adults With Major Depressive Disorder *(American College of Physicians)*

Rheumatology/Orthopedics

- Guidelines for the Nonsurgical Management of Knee Osteoarthritis *(OA Research Society International)*
- Nonpharmacologic and Pharmacologic Therapies for Osteoarthritis of the Hand, Hip, and Knee *(American College of Rheumatology)*

Women's Health

- Use of Botanicals for Management of Menopausal Symptoms *(Obstetrics and Gynecology)*

CDC, Centers for Disease Control; *NSAIDS,* nonsteroidal antiinflammatory drugs; *OA,* osteoarthritis.

[a]Complete list at National Center for Complementary and Integrative Health. *Clinical practice guidelines.* https://nccih.nih.gov/

practitioners based on modality and location, descriptions of healing modalities, and guidance on starting a holistic private practice (AHNA, 2024). The AHNA has created a Pain Tool Kit (AHNA Tool Kit, 2024) that includes the nonpharmacologic interventions of aromatherapy, physical/healing touch, energy and thermal applications, progressive muscle relaxation (PMR), meditation, mindfulness-based stress reduction, visualization, yoga, and tai chi. The association provides laminated instructions of some of the methods in a variety of languages.

INTERVENTIONS

NCCIH divides CAM modalities into several loose domains and an additional whole medical system category that incorporates all domains. The domains are not formally defined but include biologically based practices, mind and body techniques, manipulative body-based practices, energy therapies, and ancient medical systems. See Table 14.3 for examples of these categories. These domains are neither mutually exclusive nor mutually inclusive because many modalities could belong to several categories. Because each modality has its own identified guidance for purpose, efficacy, and safety, this section will not be specific but will briefly define many of the modalities and highlight a few of the more common ones with current known evidence.

TABLE 14.3 Categories and Examples of Complementary and Alternative Therapies

Whole medical systems	Chinese, ayurvedic, traditional/folk healers, naturopathy, homeopathy
Biologically based practices	Herbal remedies, vitamins, dietary supplements, diets, probiotics, chelation therapy, hydrotherapy, aromatherapy
Manipulative and body-based practices	Massage, reflexology, chiropractic, craniosacral therapies, physical therapy
Mind-body techniques	Meditation, guided imagery, hypnosis, music, biofeedback, yoga, tai chi, qigong, acupuncture, dance
Energy therapies	Magnetic field therapy, reiki, therapeutic touch, prayer

Whole Medical Systems

Whole medical systems are complete systems of theories and practices that have evolved culturally over time, and because they are different from Western allopathic medicine, they are considered CAM. Examples include traditional healers or folk healers.

Ayurvedic Medicine

Ayurvedic medicine has evolved over thousands of years, originating in India. This treatment uses herbs in their natural state, as prepared herbal drugs; massage; and special individualized diets, based on the seasons of one's life and one's constitutional type. There are 10 types. Ayurvedic supplements can be made either of herbs only or a combination of herbs, metals, and minerals. Some of these products may be harmful if used improperly or without the direction of a trained practitioner (NCCIH, 2024).

The goals of Ayurvedic medicine are treatment of disease, prevention of disease, and improving a person's quality of life, by balancing the body, mind, and spirit. Basic premises include the beliefs that all living and nonliving things in the universe are joined together, and good health is achieved when one's mind and body are in harmony with all the elements (NCCIH, 2024). Two ancient books, more than 2000 years old and written in Sanskrit, are considered the heart of the practice and identify eight branches of ayurvedic medicine: internal medicine, surgery, treatment of head and neck disease, gynecology/obstetrics, pediatrics, toxicology, care of the elderly, and rejuvenation and sexual vitality. Treatment practices include eliminating impurities, decreasing symptoms, increasing resistance to disease, and reducing worry and increasing harmony. Nearly 80% of the Indian population continues to use ayurvedic medicine. No states in the United States currently license ayurvedic practitioners (NCCIH, 2024).

Traditional Chinese Medicine

Traditional Chinese medicine (TCM) has evolved over thousands of years in China and includes herbs, acupuncture, and other CAM treatments. The theoretical framework includes the complementary yet opposing yin and yang life forces, and the balance and harmony of the vital energy, or life force (**qi**), circulating through the body's pathways. TCM describes the organs and tissues in the body through corresponding elements of fire, earth, metal, water, and wood. It also uses eight principles to analyze symptoms and categorize conditions, including cold/heat, interior/exterior, excess/deficiency, and yin/yang (NCCIH, 2024).

Naturopathy

Naturopathy, also called "naturopathic medicine," evolved from a combination of traditional and other modalities in 19th-century Europe guided by the healing power of nature (NCCIH, 2024). The underlying principles are first do no harm, illness is seen as a purposeful process of the organism, and symptoms are viewed as life forces attempting to heal the organism. Practitioners do not use prescription drugs, injections, x-rays, or surgery but instead implement a variety of CAM modalities, emphasizing the adoption of a healthy lifestyle, strengthening and cleansing the body, special diets, therapies, and use of manipulation and exercise (NCCIH, 2024).

Homeopathy

Homeopathy principles have been documented since at least the time of Hippocrates, but not until early in the 19th century were they brought into modern use. Samuel Hahnemann, a German physician and chemist, is credited with founding homeopathy (www.homeopathycenter.org). When Hahnemann first named the discipline in 1807, mainstream medicine involved ineffective practices such as bloodletting and purging. Homeopathy treats the whole person and believes that symptoms are a body's effort to rid itself of disease. It is based on four principles: (1) the law of similar, or like cures; (2) the minimum dose, determining the least amount of medicine needed to treat a disease; (3) totality of symptoms, matching the complete symptom profile of the person to the symptom profile of the remedy; and (4) single remedy, administration of one remedy at a time (Substance Abuse and Mental health Services Administration, n.d.; National Center for Homeopathy, n.d.; https://www.homeopathycenter.org/).

Homeopathy is based on the whole person rather than on the symptoms. Treatment stimulates the body's healing ability through the administration of small amounts of dilute substances that are believed to cause illness or symptoms. There is a wider acceptance of homeopathy in other countries, including France, Germany, Mexico, Argentina, India, and Great Britain, than there is in the United States. The World Health Organization estimates that homeopathy is currently practiced by more than 500 million people worldwide. The FDA does not regulate homeopathic products or herbal supplements; thus, there is no regulation, no safety reporting, or efficacy data. The lack of scientific evidence, lack of consumer understanding and health literacy, the lack of regulation, and the lack of safety monitoring are areas for further analysis and research.

Biologically Based Practices/Natural Products

Biologic or natural products are the oldest form of CAM. Medicinal herbs were found in the personal effects of a mummified prehistoric male in the Italian Alps (NCCIH, 2024). Botanical remedies were inventoried in detail in the Middle Ages. This area of CAM includes nutritional counseling, herbs, vitamins, minerals, probiotics, and aromatherapy. According to NCCIH, daily multivitamin and calcium supplements are not thought of as CAMs.

According to the US National Nutritional Research Roadmap (www.nal.usda.gov, 2016), nutritional **counseling** uses education, dietary guidance, and supplementation therapeutically as the primary or adjunctive measure to prevent or treat illness. Multiple studies have demonstrated the efficacy of nutritional interventions, vitamins, therapeutic diets, and individual instruction. Diet teaching for those receiving hemodialysis showed efficacy in stabilization of laboratory values. The National Kidney Foundation (NKD) has an eat right program (NKFS, n.d.) that details the quality improvements in handgrip strength, energy, and laboratory values. Nutritional interventions for those undergoing chemotherapy help manage nausea, maintain weight and muscle mass, and improve laboratory values. Nutritional guidelines are available for several diseases including diabetes, kidney disease, heart disease, and anemia.

Herbal therapy is the use of herbs or their chemical properties to treat specific conditions or to enhance the function of various body systems, such as boosting the immune system, treating allergies, or preventing a cold. Herbal medicines may act on the body in a similar way as prescription drugs and may interact with prescription medications (Prieto-Garcia et al., 2023);

thus, it is important to elicit a full profile of what care recipients are taking and in what doses as part of medication reconciliation. A table of common agents, their common uses, side effects, interactions, and the current evidence has been compiled from NCCIH data (NCCIH, 2024); also see Table 14.2.

Probiotics are live microorganisms ("friendly bacteria") found in the human digestive tract. They are taken to enhance the digestive system either as a supplement or in natural forms, such as yogurt or other fermented foods. The human intestinal tract is colonized by a variety of microbes and is influenced by a variety of factors. Ferraris and colleagues (2020) note that exogenous factors, such as diet, drugs, supplements, and environment, and endogenous factors, such as age, sex, and genetic features, influence the composition of the gut microbes, and thus the health of the individual. The authors suggest that a Mediterranean diet or diets with high fiber content may improve the number of beneficial microbes; they caution that more research is needed (Ferraris et al., 2020)

Hydrotherapy, or water therapy, is the use of water at various temperatures or as ice or steam to relieve discomfort and promote physical well-being. Treatments include full-body immersion, hydrotherapy, steam baths, saunas, spas, and the application of hot and/or cold compresses.

Aromatherapy, also referred to as "essential oil therapy," is defined by the National Association for Holistic Aromatherapy (n.d.) as the art and science of using naturally extracted oils from plants, flowers, or trees to balance, harmonize, and promote the health of body, mind, and/or spirit. The most common reasons for the use of aromatherapy are for pain, nausea, stress, anxiety, and depression. The therapeutic use of the oils may be via inhalation, external application, or ingestion. The use of aromatherapy, like that of many CAMs, without professional clinical training is strongly discouraged. Individuals must be trained to know the specific warnings and contraindications for each oil, as well as to understand how to handle the oils.

Manipulative and Body-Based Practices

Manipulative and body-based practices focus on the manipulation of bones and joints, soft tissues, and the circulatory and lymphatic systems.

Spinal or Bone Manipulation

Spinal or bone manipulation is the application of controlled force on a bone or joint and is performed by chiropractors, physical therapists, osteopathic physicians, and some conventional physicians. Spinal manipulation was recorded in ancient Greece and became foundational to chiropractic and osteopathic medicine in the late 19th century.

Chiropractic medicine focuses on manipulation of the spine and joints, focusing on spinal alignment for optimal functioning. Chiropractors often integrate other CAMs such as massage, nutrition, and specialized kinesiology into their practice.

Cranial and craniosacral therapies also focus on a natural configuration of the skeletal system, focusing on the skull and flow of cerebrospinal fluid for the treatment of body imbalances. Craniosacral therapy originated in osteopathy and focuses on the bones of the cranium, spine, and sacrum, using gentle pressure to restore free movement of cerebrospinal fluid, allowing normal functioning.

Physical therapy integrates a variety of modalities, including massage, manipulation, heat and cold, movement, and electrical impulses, to treat the body after damage or injury, reduce swelling, relieve pain, and restore function and range of motion to the body.

Massage

Massage incorporates different techniques in the manipulation of muscles and soft tissues of the body, such as rubbing or kneading, to increase circulation, facilitate healing, and reduce stress and increase relaxation. It is one of the oldest therapies and is referred to in writing in ancient China, Japan, India, Egypt, Greece, and Rome. Even Hippocrates mentions it in his writings. Different types of therapies have different techniques and purposes, such as lymphatic therapy, neuromuscular therapy, and trigger point therapy.

Reflexology is a mixed method of CAM because it involves a type of manipulation and the concept of energy fields. A reflexologist applies pressure with the thumbs to mapped points on the feet or hands, or both, by pressing deeply into the point to release tension and stimulate circulation of blood, lymph, and energy. Reflexology is more than massage because practitioners believe that the points correspond to the organs of the body and that stimulating the points will stimulate the organs to heal (Reflexology Association of America, n.d.). Reflexology along with aromatherapy and acupuncture was found to be useful for pregnancy symptoms, including low back and pelvic girdle pain (Hughes et al., 2018).

Mind-Body Medicine

Mind and body practices focus on the interactions between the brain, the body, and behavior, using the mind to affect the body and the body to affect the mind. Categories include meditation, imagery, and various methods of body movement. This concept dates back 2000 years to TCM and ayurvedic medicine practices (NCCIH, 2024). Hippocrates noted that treatment relied on attitude, environmental influences, and natural remedies. Deep breathing, meditation, yoga, guided imagery, and progressive relaxation are common CAM therapies. **Visual or guided imagery** encourages individuals to relax by focusing on calming thoughts or experiences.

Meditation

Meditation is a method of focused attention to increase relaxation, quiet the mind, and reduce stress. Although it is often a part of many religious cultures, it is not necessarily a religious activity and can be practiced while one is still or while one is active, such as during walking. Like massage, different types have a variety of purposes and techniques. Breath meditation is the simplest because it can be done anywhere and can evoke the relaxation response (Box 14.5). It can be taught easily and is useful for anyone. Centering focuses on a chosen word. Mindfulness meditation is a way of paying attention to or being mindful of a variety of topics, such as thoughts, actions, or the environment. Walking meditation is a form of mindfulness because the

BOX 14.5 Teaching the Technique of Breath Meditation

- You may stand, sit, or lie quietly as you begin to focus on your breath.
- Inhale, and feel the air come into your nostrils, move down your throat, and into your lungs. Do not try to control the breath. Just observe it.
- Exhale, and feel the air move up from your lungs and into your throat. Feel the warmth of the exhaled air in your nostrils.
- Breathe. Feel the air move in and out. Concentrate on the breath. Do not try to control the breath. Just observe it.
- Continue watching the breath for 5 to 10 min. As other thoughts come into focus, notice them and let them go. Focus again on the breath.
- As you become comfortable with breath meditation, you may easily add simple imagery to this technique.
- As you inhale, imagine breathing in peace, love, or wellness.
- As you exhale, imagine breathing out pain, sorrow, or grief.
- As you inhale, breathe in whatever it is that you need.
- As you exhale, breathe out whatever you wish to be free of in your life.

individual is mindful of the interaction of the inner body, the external body, and the environment with each step.

Hypnotherapy is a form of guided relaxation and focused attention of the unconscious mind. It is used with differing success for memory recall of suppressed events and for behavior changes such as discontinuation of the use of tobacco products. **Biofeedback** is a relaxation technique concentrating on vital functions such heart rate, breathing rate, and blood pressure. This visualization identifies which actions can change the rates and is used for stress and an irregular heart rate. Neurolinguistic programming changes behavior by changing patterns of thinking and speaking (NCCIH, 2024).

Movement Therapy

Movement therapies use movement and bodywork to promote physical, mental, emotional, and spiritual well-being. The movement arts such as qigong, tai chi, and yoga are helpful for body, mind, and spirit, and, although technically not energy work, do manipulate life energies. **Qigong** (pronounced "chee gung") is part of TCM, combining relaxed movements with a meditative aspect and controlled breathing to move qi energy through the energy channels and increase vital energy. **Tai chi** (pronounced "tie chee") began as a Chinese martial art and combines physical movement, breath control, and meditation in a dancelike sequence of poses based on the movements of animals. One pose flows into the next in a slow, relaxed, gentle, unbroken rhythm, bringing an awareness of the moment-to-moment state of the body and producing a meditative state.

Yoga is a meditative movement practice that originated in India as a form of spiritual practice and aids in flexibility, agility, balance, and relaxation. The postures have names such as "proud warrior," "waterfall," "runner's pose," "downward-facing dog," "mountain pose," and "eagle pose." There are many types and branches of yoga. Hatha yoga, a combination of many styles, is one of the most popular forms of yoga. It is a more physical type of yoga rather than a still, meditative form. The goal during yoga practice is to challenge yourself physically but not to feel overwhelmed. Several studies of individuals with a variety of diagnoses and in a variety of health states have documented health-related benefits from the practice of yoga, including reducing stress and anxiety, improving pain management, increasing flexibility, and increasing strength (Oka & Lkhagvasuren, 2021). Yoga has been shown to relieve tension and anxiety but also has been shown to increase strength and balance and improve immune function and heart health (https://www.yogaalliance.org/). Given the increase in this practice in traditional medicine centers and during the COVID-19 pandemic on virtual platforms, the prevalence of yoga will likely continue to rise.

Dance therapy is another movement-based mind-body modality, using dance to allow the body and mind to move freely in response to music.

Energy Therapies

Energy healing or therapy is practiced in many cultures and involves the use of assumed energy fields to heal and maintain wellness (Box 14.6). Believers in energy therapy describe disruptions in the energy field as a cause for illness and teach that balancing energy can aid in healing when this is done by an energy practitioner. Certain types of body energy are well-known. Electrical energy in the body is reflected in diagnostic studies, including electrocardiographic, electromyographic, and electroencephalographic tracings. Nerves and cells have electromagnetic action potential. Magnetic resonance imaging uses powerful magnets to measure the array of charged particles in the human body and produce diagnostic images. People can be affected by the energy of their environments, including the energy of other people. For example, anxiety is contagious and moves readily and quickly from person to person.

There are medical uses for energy that come from the environment. The energy of radiation is used to shrink tumors; sound energy, in the form of ultrasound waves, is used to break up kidney stones. Lasers, focused light energy, are used in many

BOX 14.6 Feel Your Own Energy

This exercise will help you feel your own energy, or chi.

- Sit quietly, back straight, feet touching the floor.
- Place your hands in your lap.
- Take a few deep breaths. Become quiet and still.
- Breathe slowly in and out for a few minutes.
- Slowly raise your hands in front of you, palms facing you, hands approximately 15 inches apart. Cup your fingers as though you are holding a basketball between your hands.
- Concentrate on the space between your hands. What is there? Can you feel anything?
- Slowly bring your palms closer together, focusing on the space between your hands.
- Can you feel warmth? Does it feel spongy? Can you move your hands around a shape?
- What you are feeling is the energy coming from the energy centers in your hands. Focus on the energy. Try to increase the sensation of fullness in the space between your hands.
- If you do not feel anything immediately, bring your hands back out to 15 inches apart and slowly move your hands together again. Try this no more than three times each time you attempt the exercise.

types of surgery to seal a scar, remove superficial abnormalities, and to treat disorders such as psoriasis. Light energy is useful in treating seasonal affective disorder. Color, another form of light energy, has been shown to influence emotions and behaviors.

Energy fields may be characterized as measurable or as yet unmeasured. Practices based on measurable forms of energy include those involving electromagnetic fields such as magnet therapy and light therapy. Practices based on other energy fields, also called "biofields," generally reflect the concept that human beings are infused with subtle forms of energy, and various CAM therapies aim to treat these biofields (NCCIH, 2024).

Any illness, stress, emotional upset, or spiritual distress can affect the flow of life energy. These disruptions in the flow of life energy can cause or exacerbate illness in the physical body and can increase emotional and spiritual distress (Box 14.7: Diversity Awareness). The basic goal behind the various modalities of **energy therapy** is to release blockages of energy flow, stimulate deficient life energy, and rebalance life energy.

Acupuncture

Acupuncture manipulates life energy, referred to as "**chi**" or "qi" in some cultures, by stimulating precisely mapped points on the skin surface (Box 14.8: Evidence-Based Practice). The points overlie the channels, called "**meridians**," through which chi travels. The channels are named for the organs they affect, such as the "lung meridian," "heart meridian," and "kidney meridian." Acupuncture may be used to diagnose disharmony; the points become tender to palpation in the **presence** of a disturbance in energy flow. The acupuncture points act as valves in the meridian system. When the points are stimulated, acupuncture acts as a treatment modality to correct disturbances in flow. When stimulated, the valve may open to release blocked or excess chi or close to allow chi to collect if chi is deficient. Stimulation of the points may be accomplished in several ways: by inserting fine needles into the points, by electrostimulation, by laser, by light stimulation, and by burning herbs on or over the points to increase point stimulation, a technique called "**moxibustion**." Acupuncture is one of the oldest healing practices in the world; according to the World Health Organization, acupuncture is used in 103 of 129 countries that have reported data (NCCIH, 2024). Some evidence exists for the efficacy of acupuncture in a variety of treatments. The NCCIH (2024) site reports that research has shown that acupuncture may be helpful for several pain conditions, including back or neck pain, knee pain associated with osteoarthritis, postoperative pain, and joint pain associated with the use of aromatase inhibitors, which are drugs used in people with breast cancer. An analysis of data from over 20 studies with 6376 participants with painful conditions showed that the beneficial effects of acupuncture continued for a year after the end of treatment for all conditions except neck pain (NCCIH, 2024).

Acupressure is a form of acupuncture, where the meridian points are stimulated with pressing, rubbing, squeezing, and stretching movements. The stimulation of the sites moves, enhances, or modulates the individual's energy to achieve balance and well-being. The technique is taught in some massage schools because it is often used along with massage to move and balance the body's energies. Evidence suggests that self-acupressure is effective in reducing perceived stress and fatigue among nurses (Srivali Teal, 2024). **Shiatsu** uses a sequence of rhythmic pressure on acupressure meridians. A systematic review revealed that auricular point acupressure, the application of acupuncture-like stimulation to specific points on the ear, is a promising treatment for anxiety for inpatients and perioperative patients (Chen et al., 2022).

BOX 14-7 Diversity Awareness

The WHO held the first of its kind Traditional Medicine Global Summit in 2023 to seek collaboration for evidence-based TCIM. They established goals aimed at research, safety, effectiveness, and sharing of knowledge. This initiative will provide evidence and resources for practitioners. The site information is available in several languages. The WHO indicates that 88% of the world's population primarily uses complimentary or "nontraditional" practices.

Their chief aims include:

- Harnessing the potential contribution of TCIM to health, wellness, and people-centered health care
- Promoting safe and effective use of Traditional and Complementary Medicine (T&CM) through the regulation, research, and integration of TCIM products, practices, and practitioners into the health system
- Reviewing and assessing the existing models of integration in member states to record and recommend best practice
- Creating a clinical evidence database and knowledge platform
- Developing global guidelines on quality and safety of herbal medicines
- Identifying any technical issues for the safe use of herbal medicines with reference to interaction with other medicines
- Developing benchmarks for training and practice in acupuncture, ayurveda, naturopathy, osteopathy, traditional Chinese medicine, yoga, and others
- Conducting regular global surveys for building a database of member states and assessing the global trends of the use of TCIM

TCIM, Traditional, complementary, and integrative medicine; *WHO,* World Health Organization.
World Health Organization (n.d.-b)

BOX 14.8 EVIDENCE-BASED PRACTICE

A systematic review of randomized control trials revealed a positive, sustainable effect of mindfulness therapy on stress, anxiety, and depression experienced by university students. Surveys by the WHO indicate that anxiety, mental stress, and emotional distress among university students ranged from 20.3% to 45%, with higher rates during the COVID-19 pandemic. These negative emotions led to insomnia and poor self-image and negatively affected their physical health. Mindfulness therapy is a standardized psychological intervention of meditation, breathing exercises, guided imagery, and other practices. These activities are designed to reduce stress, encourage positive thinking habits, and provide tools to manage difficult emotions. The principle of mindfulness is to suspend judgment, ideas, and opinions and accept things as they are while focusing on one's breathing and body reactions. Results of the systematic review showed that mindfulness therapy had statistically significant effects in reducing anxiety, perceived stress, and depression and improving self-kindness and physical health. No significant differences between control groups and the therapy groups was found for sleep quality, social functioning, or self-perception of well-being (Pan et al., 2024).

COVID-19, Coronavirus disease 2019; *WHO,* World Health Organization.

Touch Therapies

In **touch therapies**, such as therapeutic touch, healing touch, and reiki, practitioners use their hands to direct life energies drawn from the environment to the individual to restore balance and harmony within the human energy system (Fig. 14.2). **Reiki** comes from Japanese tradition and requires training by a reiki master. In addition to teaching the hand placements and symbolic gestures used in reiki, the master attunes the student (Box 14.9: Best Practice). **Attunement** opens the energy channel, enabling the student to bring universal energy through the body and to the recipient. During these therapies, the hands can be placed directly on the person's body or at a distance from the body. The NCCIH notes that reiki has not been shown to be effective in well-controlled studies.

Therapeutic touch was conceptualized by nursing theorist Martha Rogers. According to her theory, humans are energy fields that interact with the environment, an energy field that consists of everything external to the individual, encompassing the whole universe (Hedlund, 2023). Therapeutic touch practice comprises three essential elements. The first element is centering by the practitioner. **Centering** is a process of becoming calm, present in the moment, and connected with the individual being treated, allowing the practitioner to give the person undivided attention. The centered practitioner is able to let go of personal feelings and emotions and is more open to inner perceptions. During assessment, the second element, the practitioner's hands move over the individual's body at a height of approximately 3 inches above the skin to sense disturbances or imbalances in the person's energy field. The final element is a series of techniques to change the patterns in the human energy field, unruffling, to direct energy to the person to replenish depleted energy, modulation, and to balance or redistribute the individual's energies. **Healing touch** is like therapeutic touch but adds full-body techniques for moving energy and disorder-specific energetic interventions to the modulation phase of therapeutic touch.

Jin Shin Jyutsu uses fingertips pressed on specific healing point combinations to balance energy along specific pathways. **Polarity therapy** is a combination of energy work, caring intention, movement exercises, and dietary regimens and is aimed at clearing energy blockages and building health (American Polarity Therapy Association, 2024). Many practitioners use magnets or magnet therapy to control magnetic fields around many body systems to aid in healing and in the functioning of the systems.

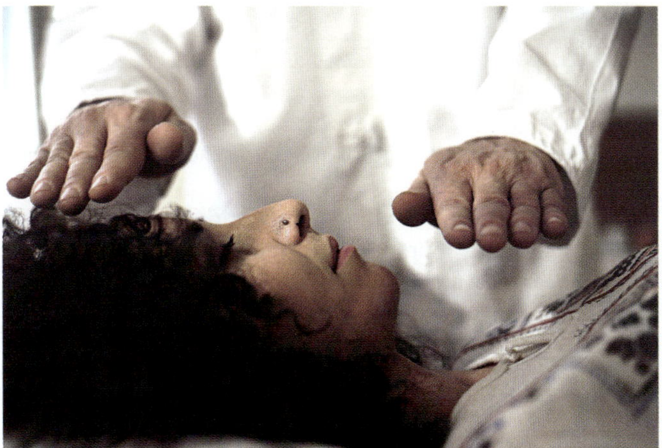

FIG. 14.2 The assessment phase of therapeutic touch. The practitioner is attempting to sense disturbances or imbalances in the person's energy field. (From iStock.com/gevende)

> **BOX 14.9 BEST PRACTICE**
>
> Inclusion of alternative and complementary practices is a challenge in an acute care hospital. At BWH in Boston, Massachusetts, an integrative care program, including a reiki volunteer program, has helped to provide a means for integrating healing practices for both nurses and patients. BWH has the largest reiki volunteer program in the country, with 60 volunteers who have provided more than 35,000 treatments in the past 5 years. They noted that "many times, patients become so relaxed they fall asleep. Nurses also request reiki for themselves and staff on their unit." The team also offers music therapy, **pet therapy**, and meditation. To increase the availability of these therapies, educational offerings are available on the internal television program channel. Staff reiki sessions were used to help caregivers deal with the stress of caring for seriously ill patients or after traumatic events. Sessions can be requested by a group or unit.
>
> *BWH,* Brigham and Women's Hospital.

Other Energy Modalities

The basis for many religious faiths, **prayer** focuses on the subtle energy life force known by different names. Prayer has different meanings to different people. A prayer may be a request for divine intervention, a type of meditation, or a form of intentionality that is useful in healing. Praying for others may be a form of **distant healing**. One method of participating in distance healing is the healing circle. The members of the healing circle join hands. Each member sends healing energy to his or her neighbor on the right until the energy is flowing around the circle. When the energy is flowing readily, each member of the group focuses the energy on one group member, who acts to send the energy to someone that person knows who needs healing. Each member of the circle may, in turn, receive energy from the group and send it to an individual in need of healing.

Music therapy uses a variety of methods in a therapeutic relationship to address physical, emotional, cognitive, and social needs of individuals. Music influences the limbic system, the area of the brain involved with emotions and feelings. Music is a form of sound energy, and this energy can be relaxing or stimulating and has been used to decrease pain, depression, and disability. Dependent on the person and the mood desired, all forms of music can be used. Music therapy is used as a treatment for the improvement of cognitive function and to reduce distress in people with dementia. An integrative review and meta-analysis found that:

- The intervention based on listening to music presents the greatest effect on patients with dementia, followed by singing.
- Music therapy improved the quality of life of people with dementia.
- Music has a long-term effect on depression symptoms associated with dementia (Moreno-Morales et al., 2020).

Pets. Two-thirds of US households have at least one pet; nearly half of all older Americans own a pet, but research on the therapeutic benefit of pets has been limited or not well-designed. Dogs have been studied the most, and the benefits of reducing anxiety, assisting with posttraumatic stress disorder (PTSD), and improving physical dexterity have been supported by research (Gee et al., 2021).

NURSING PRESENCE

Nurses have the potential to alleviate suffering and improve health care outcomes through their **therapeutic presence**. By connecting deeply with individuals and their families, nurses are in a unique position to facilitate their journey toward recovery or a peaceful death. When using **nursing presence** as a holistic intervention and establishing a therapeutic relationship, nurses are fulfilling the definition of nursing as an art and a science.

Holistic health involves knowing the physical self, the emotional self, the mental self, and the spiritual self, seeking a comfortable balance among these aspects of being (Table 14.4), and knowing what changes need to be made to achieve this balance (AHNA, 2024). This knowledge is vital to both the nurse attempting holistic practice and the individual interested in pursuing holistic health.

The Wellness Quiz can assist both nurses and individuals in the exploration of self that begins the process of self-care (Box 14.10). When self-knowledge is gained, one or more of the holistic health strategies mentioned in this chapter, as well as emerging therapies, can be useful in helping people achieve optimal wellness. Every person is a whole, unique being; therefore, each person needs to explore the possible strategies and individually decide which modalities are the best methods to achieve an improved state of wellness. People beginning this self-exploration and the practice of holistic health strategies may find that the practice changes their lives. Using presence and giving the gift of self enhances personal growth in the caregiver.

Safety and Effectiveness

Most CAM therapies lack a strong scientific evidence base because many have not been studied with rigorous, well-designed clinical trials. The National Institutes of Health is sponsoring research to fill the knowledge gap and build this foundation for safety, efficacy, and suitability for specific conditions. The FDA regulates dietary supplements, but the regulations are less strict than those for prescription or over-the-counter medications. For example, safety and efficacy do not have to be proven before a product is marketed, although once the product is on the market, the FDA does monitor label claims and inserts.

An aptly titled patient education brochure, *Made for This Moment, the American Society of Anesthesiologists, ASA©* provides some guidance on herbal and dietary supplements and anesthesia (American Society of Anesthesiologists, 2020). It includes the following information regarding the potential risks of common herbs and supplements:

Ephedra (Ma-Huang): An appetite suppressor, it can interact with some blood pressure medication to cause dangerous increases in blood pressure or heart rate.

Garlic: Some people take it to lower their cholesterol and blood pressure, but it can increase bleeding.

Ginkgo: Used to improve memory, it can increase the risk of bleeding.

Ginseng: Taken to improve concentration, ginseng can increase your heart rate and the risk of bleeding.

Kava: Used to ease anxiety, kava can increase the effect of anesthesia.

St. John's Wort: Used to ease anxiety and help with sleep problems, but it may prolong the effects of anesthesia.

Valerian: A sleep aid, it can prolong the effects of some types of anesthesia.

Vitamin E: Some people take it to slow the aging process, but it can increase bleeding and cause blood pressure problems.

TABLE 14.4 Being There Versus Being With

The Nurse Who Is There	The Nurse Who Is "With"
Is attentive	Is available with whole self
Is task oriented	Enters the person's world
Does the right thing	Becomes vulnerable
Fulfills a role	Is present as a whole person
Assists with coping	Alleviates suffering
Provides security	Enables growth

BOX 14.10 Wellness Assessment and Management

In the last decades, the medical establishment has been rightly criticized for focusing on elimination of disease rather than on wellness. During the same period, a number of wellness-assessment measurements have been proposed. Some of these measurement tools ask questions such as:

- Do you wake up with enthusiasm for the day ahead?
- Do you have the high energy you need to do what you want?
- Do you laugh easily and often, especially at yourself?
- Do you confidently find solutions for the challenges in your life?
- Do you feel valued and appreciated?
- Do you appreciate others and let them know it?
- Do you have a circle of warm, caring friends?
- Do the choices you make every day get you what you want? (Caton, 2003).

A current systematic review attempted to answer questions about what wellness assessments have been evaluated in clinical settings and the reliability and validity of the instruments used (Bart et al., 2018). There is no doubt that during the last two decades wellness/well-being choices have been more guided by individual preferences and knowledge that there is a wider multidimensional scope to wellness. Bart and colleagues (2018) reviewed 23 wellness assessments identified with search-preferred reporting guidelines. Key words used were "assessment, evaluation, measurement, wellness, and well-being." The study identified five tools that had the best reliability profiles; however, it was not possible to identify one single tool that would be the best for clinical settings. Part of this difficulty in identifying the most appropriate instruments was the lack of consensus on a definition of wellness. It appears that the understanding of wellness is open and evolving toward achieving a person's full potential. As the definition is general, holistic, and abstract, it may encompass lifestyle, spiritual, and environmental domains. There is need for future studies to describe further the best working definition of wellness, whether it can be measured, and how to use information from some proprietary assessment instruments in clinical practice (Bart et al., 2018).

Most CAM providers are not credentialed in a standardized national system, so credentialing regulations and standards differ nationally (NCCIH, 2024). Some require training, testing, and continuing education, but most do not. Many practitioners belong to professional organizations that establish the requirements for their profession. It is imperative that nurses and other health care professionals have knowledge of CAM practices, safety, and guidelines for use to inform and protect users. Many medical and nursing schools now include alternative/complementary therapies in their curricula. To help ensure care-recipient safety, practitioners and users should review the following principles:

- Carefully select CAM practitioners with appropriate training and experience. The US National Library of Medicine (2024), a division of the National Institutes of Health, provides a directory of providers, services, and facilities.
- Take time to research and understand the treatment and its effectiveness.
- Be aware of scams and fraudulent claims.
- Know the costs and if the treatment is covered by insurance.
- Be aware that quality is not always regulated for dietary supplements, and they may have side effects or react dangerously with other medications and supplements. In addition, they may not have been tested on children or pregnant females, so check labels with care.
- Be aware that some energy treatments may have side effects and cause inflammation that can affect other conditions and may not have been tested on children or pregnant females.
- Always inform the care providers and both traditional and holistic practitioners about the use of CAM therapies.

The American Nurses Association recognizes holistic nursing as an official nursing specialty with its own defined scope and standards of practice. The AHNA defines holistic nursing as "all nursing that has healing the whole person as its goal and integrates **complementary and alternative medicine** approaches into clinical practice." According to the AHNA, a holistic nurse:

- Is a legally licensed nurse who takes a mind-body-spirit-emotion approach to the practice of nursing
- Serves as a bridge between conventional healing and complementary and alternative healing practices and is trained in both health care models
- Works in a variety of settings—from hospitals to universities to private practice
- May specialize in one or more modalities (or methods of healing), such as acupuncture, chiropractic, or energetic healing (AHNA, 2024)

Care of Ms. Choi

Let us return to Ms. Choi and review what is known about her CAM options and their safety and efficacy for her. To review, Ms. Choi has been diagnosed with heart disease, coronary artery blockages, and mitral valve disease that requires surgery. Her family and friends have offered their opinions, and she has heeded their advice and is taking various CAM modalities as well as aspirin, albeit at too high a dose for heart health. She has been taking fish oil, omega 3, and garlic, which are supposed to lower her cholesterol; turmeric for her immune system; and lemon balm for her "frazzled nerves." She has also begun yoga classes. She has been advised to have surgery, take traditional cholesterol-lowering agents, and begin a β-blocker to lower her heart rate and blood pressure.

Teaching Points for Ms. Choi

- Aspirin prolongs bleeding, and 81 mg is the recommended dose to prevent platelet aggregation. She should stop the 650 mg dose.
- Fish oil or omega 3 is claimed to have three main possible benefits: lower cholesterol levels, improve vision, and improve cognition or prevent cognitive decline. The NCCIH (2024) reports the health benefits of eating fish, a rich source of omega 3. Evidence to support fish oil supplements is lacking; those who took fish oil did no better in vision and cholesterol testing than those who took a placebo. Omega-3 dietary supplements may interact with medications, and they may cause bleeding when taken with warfarin or other anticoagulants.
- Garlic, one of the most studied of the herbal supplements, may reduce low-density lipoprotein (LDL) cholesterol levels by a small amount. Taking garlic supplements may increase the risk of bleeding and cause stomach upset. Garlic supplements may interfere with the effectiveness of some drugs, including saquinavir, a drug used to treat HIV infection.
- Although turmeric is promoted for a variety of health conditions, it has low bioavailability (not much of it reaches the bloodstream) when it's taken orally, and the NCCIH reports that turmeric's health effects remain uncertain. Safety concerns include increased bleeding and bile duct and liver effects.
- Lemon balm seems to have a sedative and calming effect, but side effects include increased appetite, nausea, dizziness, and wheezing. It may interact with sedatives and thyroid medications.
- Yoga, reiki, and acupuncture have demonstrated positive outcomes, and she should be referred to licensed practitioners.
- A careful assessment of her dietary supplements is necessary because many interact with other agents and may interfere with anesthesia if she does opt for surgery.

Now see if you can answer these questions:

- Are these therapies evidence-based?
- What is the best understanding of the biologic and physiologic mechanisms for these therapies?
- What is the best understanding of the safety of these therapies?
- Which therapies are covered by her insurance?
- Would Ms. Choi's therapies be considered complementary, alternative, or integrative?

Every person is a unique individual; therefore, some exploration of self, the various strategies, and the practitioner will be necessary before it is determined which strategy is the right fit for each individual. Nurses must understand holistic health strategies (Box 14.11: More Website Information) because individuals are using them in increasing numbers, and they are evolving and expanding into new methods, such as hot yoga, where the therapy is conducted in a heated room at a temperature greater than 90°F. Nurses who begin to practice holistic interventions may find them a useful and exciting adjunct to their nursing practice and their personal lives.

BOX 14.11 More Website Information

- The NCCIH webpages at https://nccih.nih.gov provide further guidance on how to be an informed consumer, how to obtain information for the health care professional, and how to find and select a CAM practitioner.
- The Office of Dietary Supplements (https://ods.od.nih.gov) seeks to strengthen knowledge and understanding of dietary supplements by evaluating scientific information, supporting research, sharing research results, and educating the public. Its resources include publications (e.g., *Dietary Supplements: What You Need to Know*), fact sheets on a variety of specific supplement ingredients (e.g., vitamin D and black cohosh), and the *PubMed Dietary Supplement Subset.*

CAM, Complementary and alternative medicine; *NCCIH,* National Center for Complementary and Integrative Health.
PubMed (http://www.ncbi.nlm.nih.gov/sites/entrez) is a service of the US National Library of Medicine and contains publication information and (in most cases) brief summaries of articles from scientific and medical journals.

CASE STUDY

Use of Therapeutic Touch: David P.

David P., an 82-year-old male, came to the clinic reporting neck pain and stiffness of approximately 4 months' duration. He was previously treated with ibuprofen (Motrin), acetaminophen, and oxycodone as well as with physical therapy. At the time of the initial clinic visit, David P. was still taking ibuprofen but had stopped taking oxycodone because the pain "isn't bad enough to take drugs [narcotics]." He rated his neck pain as 5 on a scale of 1 to 10. Neck range of motion had increased, but he had problems when driving. David P. lives next to a very busy street and did not feel that he could turn his neck well enough to see the traffic coming. He was afraid to pull out into the street. His daughter had driven him to the clinic. She said, "Pop is still in pain. He has little interest in doing anything. He walks like an old man, and he can't work in his garden because of the pain." The goal of treatment for David P. is pain relief and increased range of motion.

Reflective Questions

- What holistic health strategies might be used to relieve David's pain and to help him increase his range of motion?
- After the treatment goals have been reached, what holistic health strategies would you recommend to assist David P. in maintaining and improving his health?

Therapeutic touch was offered to David P. Although he was skeptical that this treatment would be effective, he agreed to the treatment to please his daughter. Increased heat was noted in the neck and shoulder areas. A 30-minute therapeutic touch treatment was performed, with special attention given to the neck and shoulder area. Immediately following the therapeutic touch, David P. rated his pain as 0 on a scale of 1 to 10 and reported that he "couldn't remember when he'd been so relaxed," and the excess heat had dissipated. David P. was also given some simple yoga exercises for the neck and advised to perform the exercises twice a day, five gentle repetitions each time. David P. was seen in the clinic a total of eight times for therapeutic touch and was given increasingly difficult yoga stretches for the neck and shoulders. His pain rating at the end of treatment remained at 0 on the 1 to 10 scale. He had stopped taking ibuprofen, saying, "I don't need it anymore." His neck range of motion had increased, and he was driving and working in his garden again. He continues his yoga stretches and has started performing daily qigong exercises.

SUMMARY

- Holistic health strategies are designed to view the individual as a biopsychosocial-spiritual whole being.
- Many holistic health strategies have been practiced in other cultures for thousands of years; some began as religious practices.
- Many of these strategies can be used to help nurses and those they serve to reach the Healthy People 2030 goals. However, high-quality, evidence-based research is lacking, although there is an increased awareness of the practices and more research is being done.
- Holistic health practitioners and many consumers are convinced that these practices help to promote and maintain health or cure a variety of health conditions. Believing is sometimes therapy. The placebo effect is not well-understood but has a strong influence on the results of any research study, whether in conventional or complementary medicine.

EVOLVE CHAPTER FEATURES

http://evolve.elsevier.com/Edelman/

- Study Questions

REFERENCES

Agency for Healthcare Research and Quality (AHRQ). (2021). *Integrated and comprehensive pain management programs: effectiveness and harm*. https://effectivehealthcare.ahrq.gov/products/integrated-pain-management/research

American Holistic Nurses Association (AHNA). (2024). https://www.ahna.org/

American Holistic Nurses Association Tool Kit for Pain. (2024). *AHNA tool kit*. https://www.ahna.org/American-Holistic-Nurses-Association/Resources/Holistic-Pain-Tools

American Polarity Therapy Association. (2024). *About polarity therapy*. http://www.polaritytherapy.org/

American Society of Anesthesiologists. (2020). *Made for this moment*. https://www.asahq.org/madeforthismoment/wp-content/uploads/2020/10/ASA_Supplements-Anesthesia_Updated.pdf

Arruda, A. P., Zhang, Y., Gomaa, H., de Cassia Bergamaschi, C., Guimaraes, C. C., Righesso, L. A., et al. (2019). Herbal medications for anxiety, depression, pain, nausea and vomiting related to preoperative surgical patients: A systematic review and meta-analysis of randomised controlled trials. *BMJ Open*, *9*(5), e023729. https://doi.org/10.1136/bmjopen-2018-023729

Balneaves, L. G., Watling, C. Z., Hayward, E. N., Ross, B., Taylor-Brown, J., Porcino, A., et al. (2022). Addressing complementary and alternative medicine use among individuals with cancer: An integrative review and clinical practice guideline. *JNCI: Journal of the National Cancer Institute*, *114*(1), 25–37. https://doi.org/10.1093/jnci/djab048

Bart, R., Ishak, W. W., Ganjian, S., Jaffer, K. Y., Abdelmesseh, M., Hanna, S., et al. (2018). The assessent and measurement of wellness in the clinical medical setting: A systematic review. *Innovations in Clinical Neuroscience*, *15*(09-10), 14.

BirchTree Center for Healthcare Transformation. (n.d.). *Holistic nursing certification and re-certification.* https://birchtreecenter.com/p/4/Holistic-Nursing-Certification-and-Re-Certification

Caton, S. (Ed.). (2003). *Wellness from within: The first step*. Anaheim, CA: American Holistic Health Association.

Chen, S.-R., Hou, W.-H., Lai, J.-N., Kwong, J. S. W., & Lin, P.-C. (2022). Effects of acupressure on anxiety: A systematic review and meta-analysis. *Journal of Integrative and Complementary Medicine*, *28*(1), 25–35. https://doi.org/10.1089/jicm.2020.0256

Chow, S. L., Bozkurt, B., Baker, W. L., Bleske, B. E., Breathett, K., Fonarow, G. C., et al. (2023). Complementary and alternative medicines in the management of heart failure: A scientific statement from the American Heart Association. *Circulation*, *147*(2). https://doi.org/10.1161/cir.0000000000001110

Crawford, C., Avula, B., Lindsey, A. T., Walter, A., Katragunta, K., Khan, I. A., et al. (2022). Analysis of select dietary supplement products marketed to support or boost the immune system. *JAMA Network Open*, *5*(8), e2226040. https://doi.org/10.1001/jamanetworkopen.2022.26040

Da Costa, M. (2023). How culture impacts health: The Hispanic narrative. *Creative Nursing*, *29*(3), 273–280. https://doi.org/10.1177/10784535231211695

Dana Farber Patient and Family Resource Centers. (n.d.). https://www.dana-farber.org/for-patients-and-families/care-and-treatment/support-services-and-amenities/patient-and-family-resource-centers/

GovTrack.us. (n.d.). *Dietary supplement listing act of 2022 (2022 - S. 4090).* https://www.govtrack.us/congress/bills/117/s4090

Ferraris, C., Elli, M., & Tagliabue, A. (2020). Gut microbiota for health: How can diet maintain a healthy gut microbiota? *Nutrients*, *12*(11), 3596. https://doi.org/10.3390/nu12113596

Gee, N. R., Rodriguez, K. E., Fine, A. H., & Trammell, J. P. (2021). Dogs supporting human health and well-being: A biopsychosocial approach. *Frontiers in Veterinary Science*, *8*, 630465.

HealthCare.gov. (2024). *Affordable Care Act*. healthcare.gov.

Hedlund, A. (2023). Martha Rogers' science of unitary human beings in relation to workers health and well-being: A scoping review. *Work*, *76*(3), 953–968. https://doi.org/10.3233/wor-220681

Hughes, C. M., Liddle, S. D., Sinclair, M., & McCullough, J. E. M. (2018). The use of complementary and alternative medicine (CAM) for pregnancy related low back and/ or pelvic girdle pain: An online survey. *Complementary Therapies in Clinical Practice*, *31*, 379–383. https://doi.org/10.1016/j.ctcp.2018.01.015

Interagency Committee on Human Nutrition Research. (2024). *National Nutritional Research National Agricultural Library*. http://www.nal.usda.gov/

Missenda, M., Morris, D., & Nault, D. (2023). Herbal supplement use for evidence-based indications in US adults: An analysis of national survey data. *Journal of Integrative and Complementary Medicine*, *29*(9), 584–591. https://doi.org/10.1089/jicm.2022.0722

Moreno-Morales, C., Calero, R., Moreno-Morales, P., & Pintado, C. (2020). Music therapy in the treatment of dementia: A systematic review and meta-analysis. *Frontiers in Medicine*, *7*, 160. https://doi.org/10.3389/fmed.2020.00160

National Agricultural Library. (2016). *National Nutritional Road Map*. www.nal.usda.gov.

National Association for Holistic Aromatherapy. (n.d.). https://naha.org/

National Center for Complementary and Integrative Health. (n.d.). https://www.nccih.nih.gov

National Center for Complementary and Integrative Health. (2021). https://www.nccih.nih.gov/health/complementary-alternative-or-integrative-health-whats-in-a-name

National Center for Complementary and Integrative Health (NCCIH). (2024a). *Clinical practice guidelines.* https://nccih.nih.gov

National Center for Complementary and Integrative Health (NCCIH). (2024b). *Complementary, alternative, or integrative health: What's in a name?* https://www.nccih.nih.gov/

National Center for Homeopathy. (n.d.). http://www.nationalcenterforhomeopathy.org

National Institutes of Health Office of Dietary Supplements (ODS). (n.d.). https://ods.od.nih.gov

National Kidney Foundation. (n.d.). *Eating right for CKD patients (NKFS).* https://nkfs.org/kidney-failure/eating-right-for-ckd-patients/

Office of Disease Prevention and Health Promotion. (2024). *Wellness initiative of Healthy People 2030.* Healthy People 2030. odphp.health.gov.

Oka, T., & Lkhagvasuren, B. (2021). Health-related benefits and adverse events associated with yoga classes among participants that are healthy, in poor health, or with chronic diseases. *BioPsychoSocial Medicine*, *15*(1), 17. https://doi.org/10.1186/s13030-021-00216-z

Pan, Y., Li, F., Liang, H., Shen, X., Bing, Z., Cheng, L., et al. (2024). Effectiveness of mindfulness-based stress reduction on mental health and psychological quality of life among university students: a grade-assessed systematic review. *Evidence-Based Complementary and Alternative Medicine*, *2024*, 8872685.

Prieto-Garcia, J. M., Graham, L., Alkhabbaz, O., & Mazzari, A. L. (2023). Potential pharmacokinetic interactions of common cardiovascular drugs and selected European and Latin American herbal medicines: a scoping review. *Plants*, *12*(3), 623. https://doi.org/10.3390/plants12030623

Reflexology Association of America. (n.d.). http://reflexology-usa.org/

Srivali Teal, J. (2024). Self-acupressure to reduce stress and fatigue. *American Nurse Journal*, *19*(1), 62–66. https://doi.org/10.51256/anj012462

Substance Abuse and Mental Health Services Administration. (n.d.). *Wellness initiative.* http://www.samhsa.gov

US Department of Health and Human Services. (n.d.). *Healthy People 2030.* https://www.healthypeople.gov/

US Food and Drug Administration. (n.d.). *Homeopathic product regulation.* https://www.fda.gov/drugs/information-drug-class/homeopathic-products

US National Library of Medicine. (2024). *Directories: MedlinePlus.* http://www.nlm.nih.gov/medlineplus/directories.html

World Health Organization. (n.d.-a). *Constitution of the World Health Organization.* https://www.who.int/

World Health Organization. (n.d.-b). *WHO global traditional medicine centre.* https://www.who.int/initiatives/who-global-centre-for-traditional-medicine

World Health Organization (WHO). (2023). *Integrating traditional medicine in health care.* www.who.int.

Wu, A., Wu, Y., Natarajan, V., Singh, P., Cheema, W., Hossain, R., et al. (2023). Complementary and alternative medicine use in patients with cancer and immigration background. *JCO Global Oncology*, *9*, e2200303. https://doi.org/10.1200/go.22.00303

Yoga Alliance. (2024). *Scientific research on yoga.* https://www.yogaalliance.org

15 Overview of Growth and Development Framework

Elizabeth Connelly Kudzma

OBJECTIVES

After completing this chapter, the reader will be able to:

- Define the terms *growth*, *development*, and *maturation*.
- Describe factors that influence growth in an individual.
- Explain the importance of growth and development theory as a framework for assessing and promoting health.
- Outline Erikson's theory of psychosocial development.
- Differentiate Piaget's and Vygotsky's theories of cognitive development.
- Compare Kohlberg's and Gilligan's theories of cognitive moral development.
- Analyze examples of individual growth and development, distinguishing normal and abnormal processes.

KEY TERMS

Cephalocaudal
Development
Developmental patterns
Differentiation
Erikson's Theory of Psychosocial Development
Gilligan's Theory of Moral Development
Growth
Growth charts
Growth patterns
Lawrence Kohlberg's Theory of Moral Development
Learning
Maturation
Piaget's Theory of Cognitive Development
Proximodistal
Scaffolding
Vygotsky's Theory of Cognitive Development
Zone of proximal development

THINK ABOUT IT

Vaccine Controversies and Misinfodemics

A 4.5-year-old child begins to scream as the nurse approaches with her "kindergarten shots." The mother tries to comfort her child as she turns anxiously to the nurse and states, "I've read and seen online postings that vaccinations can be dangerous. No wonder she's frightened. Are they really necessary?"

- What influence might the mother's anxiety have on the child's behavior?
- What approach can the nurse use and what information can the nurse have for the mother?
- What approaches can the nurse take to gain the child's cooperation?
- What resources might the mother use to review recommendations for childhood vaccinations?
- What types of online sources can be trusted?
- What can nurses do to promote vaccination programs and minimize pockets of unvaccinated populations?
- How does population vaccination coverage and vaccination policy contribute to herd immunity?

Online misinformation about vaccines and treatments can provoke epidemics (misinfodemics). Recent outbreaks of measles and measles vaccination hesitancy can be traced to the rapid spread of online postings. Public health misinformation can be spread quickly through social media (Rittle, 2019). For measles and other vaccination-preventable infections, some postings on social media sites can quickly link to information sites which are not science-based. The misinformation about vaccines and treatments spread during the coronavirus disease 2019 (COVID-19) epidemic caused excessive loss of life. Social media use for education is essential within comprehensive public health education and practice. Nurses should recommend vaccinations and associated education and reduce treatment barriers for hard-to-reach patients and families (Gyenes, 2019; Rittle, 2019; Thomas & Senkpeni, 2020).

Unit 4 introduces growth and development as a framework for health assessment and promotion throughout the life span. Understanding human growth and development facilitates nursing assessment and collection of cues about health and behavior. Furthermore, health education is more effective when the nurse acknowledges and incorporates growth and developmental needs, as well as the individual's prior understanding of and beliefs about health and health-related concepts.

Growth and development theory is incorporated throughout Healthy People 2030. Throughout Unit 4, specific topics and objectives from Healthy People 2030 will be examined in chapters appropriate to the age and individual developmental level in the life span under discussion. Although these objectives will serve as guides for the promotion of health care at each level, Healthy People 2030 emphasizes social determinants of health, which include economic stability, education access and quality, health care access, neighborhood and environment, and the social and community context (US Department of Health and Human Services, 2023). Without access to health services, health promotion cannot occur, and a person has difficulty achieving and maintaining health. This chapter focuses on the study of health promotion at individual developmental levels by exploring basic concepts foundational to growth and development, as well as providing an overview of representative theories of development. Healthy People 2030 has an embedded life stages perspective, as the Healthy People 2030 leading health indicators (LHIs) vary across the life span. Interventions at specific points in the life cycle can reduce risks and protect health. In the last decade, as a result of the Affordable Care Act (2010), more adults have gained health insurance; however, many still lack coverage and there are significant differences in access to care, stratified by age, sex, ethnicity, family income, and education. Many of these access problems are related to geography; there is a critical need to develop the primary care workforce in rural areas (US Department of Health and Human Services, 2023).

Each of the following nine chapters provides health-assessment and health-promotion strategies appropriate for selected age groups across the life span. The age groups described are the childbearing/prenatal period, infant, toddler, preschool child, school-aged child, adolescent, young adult, middle-aged adult, and older adult (Table 15.1).

TABLE 15.1 GROWTH AND DEVELOPMENT

Developmental Periods Condensed and at a Glance

Period	Age	Characteristics
Infant	Birth to 12 months	Fully dependent on others for basic needs Ends as infant begins to explore environment, walks alone, and develops basic communication skills
Toddler	12 months to 3 years	Motor development progresses significantly Child achieves a degree of physical and emotional autonomy while maintaining a close identity with the primary family unit
Preschool child	3–5 years	Child has increased interest in and involvement with peers and may have social interactions with many people
School-aged child	5–12 years	Marked by entry to elementary school; interests turn away from family toward peers
Adolescent	12–18 years	Period of transition, adjustment, and personal exploration; ends when adolescent demonstrates readiness to assume full adult responsibilities of financial, emotional, and social independence
Young adult	18–35 years	Establishing an occupation or career, finding and learning how to live with a partner, and starting and rearing a family
Middle-aged adult	35–65 years	Being established in a marriage, an occupation or career, and a community; may continue to be a time of transition; adjusts to physiologic changes of middle age
Older adult	>65 years	May be a time of continued involvement in work and active socializing; adjusts to decreased physical strength and health; retirement; reduced income; decreasing independence; deaths of spouses, friends, and self

OVERVIEW OF GROWTH AND DEVELOPMENT

Fuller understanding of growth and development has continued to expand with advances in science. Currently, the genomic era is intersecting with the digital age, and nursing educators are striving to integrate genomic content (Aiello & Calzone, 2018; Barbato et al., 2019; Calzone et al., 2018). The contribution of genomic knowledge to growth and development is huge, and there has been an explosion of findings on genetics and on the long-term effects of early development on later health and health-related behaviors.

Individuals continue to evolve throughout the life span, and developmental transitions occur beyond childhood and adolescence, extending into the early, middle, and later adult years. Aging adults are receiving increased attention as the average life expectancy increases, and the adult population older than 85 years has become the fastest growing age group, providing new challenges for health protection and promotion.

Growth

Growth refers to a quantifiable change in structure size. In the body this change increases the number and/or size of the cells, resulting in an increase in the size and weight of the whole or any of its parts. During childhood, physical changes in height, weight, and head circumference, or growth parameters, are measured and recorded regularly. Growth refers to both the obvious changes in the whole individual and to the increases (and as we age, decreases) in the size of specific organs and systems. The health history and physical assessment of an individual should include all body systems and should emphasize systems undergoing the most change. The growth of some systems, such as the skeletal and muscular systems, is more influenced by sex, whereas the growth of other systems, such as the nervous and respiratory systems, is less dependent on sex. Growth changes that occur in young, middle-aged, and older adults should be noted. Thinking of growth only as it applies to infants, children, and adolescents misses important changes that occur from conception and throughout all the stages of life.

Influences on an individual's potential for growth include genetic factors, prenatal and postnatal exposures, nutrition, and environmental factors (see the Case Study at the end of this chapter). Other influences include emotional health and traditional cultural practices that influence childrearing, lifestyle, and health care practices (Box 15.1: Social Determinants). Although much of the potential for growth is primarily determined by individual genetics, health and environmental exposures influence the attainment of that potential. The timing of contact with environmental hazards and stressors may determine to a great extent the amount and kind of effects of these influences. If a pregnant mother is exposed to a virus in utero (e.g., cytomegalovirus or Zika virus), the developing fetus is more vulnerable than either the mother or an older child, especially during the first trimester, when all organ systems are in a stage of rapid growth and development. Teens who fracture a limb at the bone's growth plate also have more difficulty healing than older teens and young adults who have completed their growth spurt. Older adults may be more susceptible to severe complications of COVID-19.

Growth Patterns

Expected **growth patterns** exist for all people. Growth is not steady or uniform throughout life. The periods of extremely rapid growth—childbearing period, infancy, and adolescence—are contrasted with slower rates of growth during the toddler, preschool, and school-age periods. Infants typically double their birth weight by 6 months of age and triple their birth weight by 1 year of age. The well-known early adult "growth spurt" in height typically occurs early in adolescence for girls and later in adolescence for males.

Different parts of the body increase in size at different rates. For example, during early life the head is the fastest-growing section, followed by the trunk, and then the arms and legs. Newborns' heads account for one-quarter of their overall length, as opposed to adults' heads, which account for one-ninth of their overall height. The growth changes in proportions of body parts from infancy to adulthood are demonstrated in Fig. 15.1.

Growth Charts

Growth is one of the most important indications of a child's overall health and well-being. Accurate growth assessment depends on precise measurement of growth parameters with proper equipment, correct and consistent techniques, careful plotting of measurements, and thoughtful interpretation of the data.

On the basis of input from an expert panel, the Centers for Disease Control and Prevention (CDC) recommended that health practitioners in the United States use the 2006 World Health Organization (WHO) international **growth charts** for children from birth to 24 months and continue to use the revised CDC growth charts (including the body mass index [BMI] and the 3rd and 97th percentiles) for children aged 2 to 20 years (Box 15.2). The exceptional strength of the WHO growth charts is that they are globally representative. The CDC and the WHO growth charts both describe weight for age, length (or stature) for age, weight for length, and BMI for age, and include the 5th and 95th and the 3rd and 97th percentiles (CDC, 2022). The WHO and the CDC growth charts for each sex with percentile curves can be viewed at the CDC website. These charts with revisions have been used by pediatricians, nurses, and parents to compare infant, child, and adolescent growth since 1977 and are still current.

When one is assessing growth data for use in the growth charts, it is important to remember that a single measurement taken at one point in time, although helpful in providing a baseline, does not allow the best assessment of a child's growth. Serial measurements plotted over time on a growth chart best reflect a child's pattern of growth. Slowed growth, plateaus, or decreases in height, weight, and head circumference, as well as rapid increases, raise questions for health care providers about the adequacy of a child's nutritional intake, disease states, neglect, or emotional problems. See Box 15.2: Evidence-Based Practice on the use of growth charts and application to health of young children.

Concept of Development

Development refers to change and expansion of ability and advancement in skill from a lower to a more advanced capability. In contrast to growth, which is a quantitative or precisely measurable change, development is a qualitative change. Qualitative changes are more challenging to describe because they are more gradual and may not be easily measured in precise units. Development has

BOX 15.1 HEALTH AND SOCIAL DETERMINANTS

Childhood Lead Poisoning and Latino Families

Whereas the United States has made tremendous progress in eliminating some of the more significant sources of lead (lead paint was banned in 1978; leaded gasoline was phased out in the early 1990s), lead poisoning remains a significant threat to today's children. Lead exposure results in behavior and learning problems, decreased intelligence, attention deficits, lower academic achievement, impaired growth, poor eye-hand coordination, and hearing loss. The CDC (2021) has lowered the reference level to 5 mcg/dL to identify children with lead exposure. As a consequence, more children will likely be identified as having lead exposure. During the past 2 decades, public health and provider efforts have resulted in a 90% decline in the overall number of children affected in the United States. There is substantial evidence that children living in disadvantaged neighborhoods are at greater risk (CDC, 2021).

There are also specific risks for Latino and migrant families. One-third of the Latino population resides in Western states and is exposed to pesticides, fertilizers, and chemical residues contaminating the water. Food and culturally defined health practices pose additional risks of lead exposure to this population (CDC, 2021). Immigrant and refugee children from underdeveloped countries are at higher risk of being exposed to lead due to lower standards for protection of children from lead exposure in their country of origin. Foods packaged or canned outside the United States (especially in Mexico or South America); foods cooked in, stored in, eaten from, or drunk from ceramic containers or pottery made outside the United States (especially in Mexico or South America); Mexican or South American raisins; and wrapped Mexican candies may all contain lead.

When screening for lead poisoning in children, the nurse remembers to ask about the use of folk remedies, pottery, imported foods, and candies, as well as the use of boiled or hot tap water. In addition, the nurse encourages a diet with less fat, because lead is retained in fat, and a greater vitamin C, calcium, and iron intake, which reduces the amount of lead in the body.

CDC, Centers for Disease Control.

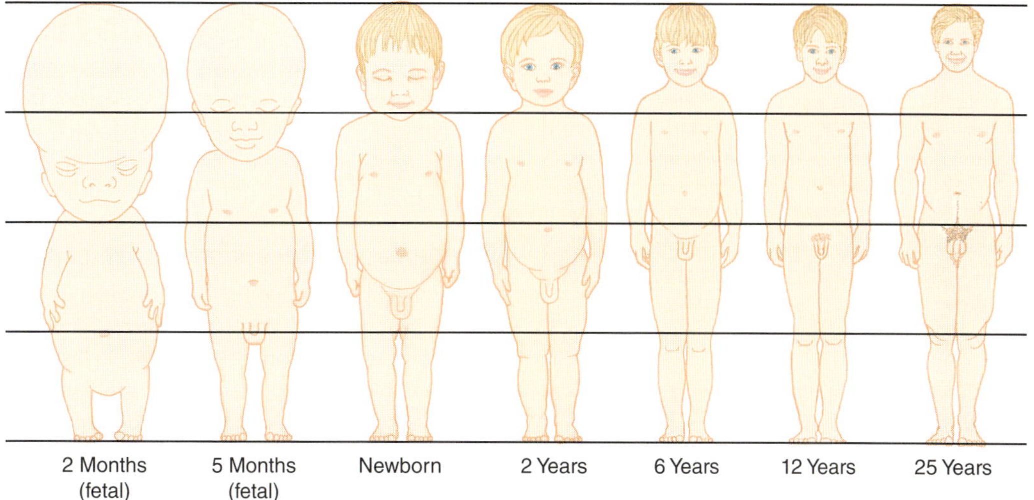

FIG. 15.1 Changes in body proportions from birth to adulthood. (From McKinney et al., 2022)

BOX 15.2 EVIDENCE-BASED PRACTICE

Growth Charts: Did You Know?

Growth charts are constructed percentile graphs illustrating the variance in selected body measurements of children. As such, they are used by health professionals to monitor the growth of infants and children through adolescence. Other forms of growth charts are also used to monitor intrauterine growth. The CDC (2022) recommends that health care professionals use WHO growth standards for infants and children ages 0 to 2 years. For children ages 2 and older, CDC (2022) recommends CDC Growth Charts. Health care professionals should know that use of WHO standards is recommended for younger children because WHO standards are based on breastfeeding as a norm for growth. The WHO standard weights and measurements reflect measurements of babies who are predominantly breastfed during at least the first 4 months of life, if not during the first year. The CDC young children charts reflect measurements of typical children in the United States who may be formula fed. Slower growth of breastfed infants is normal during the first 6 months. CDC charts are also used for older children as the WHO charts only provide measurements on children up to 5 years of age. WHO charts also reflect measurement statistics from six countries including the United States. These are optimal growth rates and may not reflect actual growth rates in many countries where mothers may not have access to nutritious foods for either themselves or their children (CDC, 2022).

CDC, Centers for Disease Control; *WHO,* World Health Organization.

best been conceptualized as a process that can be assessed because it follows certain sequencing or patterns, although the timing of milestones and this advancement is individual.

Developmental Patterns

All individuals follow similar **developmental patterns**, with one stage of development building on and leading to the next. Early development proceeds as follows:

- **Cephalocaudal**, from head to toe
- **Proximodistal**, from midline to periphery
- **Differentiation** follows a pattern: simple to complex and general to specific

The following are examples of patterns of development:

- Cephalocaudal: Infants advance in neck and head control before controlling the movements of the extremities.
- Proximodistal: Infants' central nervous systems develop before peripheral nervous systems.
- Differentiation: Infants use a whole-hand grasp before learning the finer control of the pincer grasp, and they coo or babble before they speak.

Although the sequence of development is predictable, the exact timing of the sequencing depends on the individual. Individuals develop at their own rate on their own schedule. For example, infants creep and crawl before they walk and their primary teeth erupt in a predictable sequence, but each will walk and develop primary teeth on an individual schedule. However, there are guidelines or parameters that assist parents and health care providers in assessing whether children are progressing in an acceptable developmental sequence within a reasonable time frame. Areas of assessment usually focus on personal and social skills, gross and fine motor skills, and language development. Combining developmental screening tests improves the predictive detection value. A single developmental test may be insufficient, indicating that less than 50% of those who are referred have an actual developmental delay, subjecting some children to further screening that may not be warranted (Camp & Bonnell, 2020).

Social expectations can influence developmental tasks with expectations that an individual achieve certain landmarks during each period of development. However, the age at which a child is expected to master certain developmental tasks is determined partly by cultural expectations. Some cultures are comfortable with breastfeeding their children well into childhood, whereas others expect the transition to self-feeding with a cup much earlier. When assessing a child's abilities, nurses are aware that a child who has never been given the opportunity to learn or master a skill may be developmentally capable but fails when tested. For example, a child who is capable of learning colors or numbers can do so only if taught, just as the child who was

BOX 15.3 QUALITY AND SAFETY SCENARIO

Anticipatory Guidance

The nurse is often in a position to provide anticipatory guidance to parents, which involves teaching parents ways to handle a situation before it becomes an issue or problem. Knowledge of normal growth and development provides a foundation for this teaching. For example, the toddler period is one of intense exploration of the environment, when locomotion is the major gross motor skill acquired. The nurse, knowing the number one cause of death in toddlers is accidents, provides the following teaching to the parents of a child who is entering the toddler period:

- Use a federally approved car restraint/car seat and check for proper installation and placement.
- Supervise a child closely near any source of water, including buckets, bathtubs, toilets, and especially swimming pools.
- Move pot handles toward the back of the stove and use the back burners whenever possible.
- Place toxic substances in a locked cabinet and have the poison control contact number easily accessible. Avoid the use of syrup of ipecac unless advised by a poison control representative to use it.
- Move the toddler from the crib to a bed.
- Provide barriers on open windows.
- Decrease water temperature to avoid scald burns from tap water.
- Avoid foods that pose a choking hazard such as nuts, hard candies, raisins, fresh carrots, whole grapes, chewing gum, hot dogs, and fish with bones.
- Guard against the toddler running into the street when walking and playing outside.

breastfed well into childhood, never having been offered a cup, may well be developmentally capable of drinking from a cup but probably will fail in early attempts.

Development is closely interrelated with the concepts of both learning and maturation. **Learning** is the process of gaining specific knowledge or skills that result from exposure, experience, education, and evaluation. **Maturation** is an increase in competence and adaptability that reflects understandings in the complexity of a structure that makes it possible for that structure to begin to function or to function at a higher level. Maturation of a structure, system, or individual refers to the emergence of the genetic potential of that structure, system, or individual. Learning cannot occur unless the individual is mature enough to understand and control behavior. Children can be toilet trained only when their bodies have matured to the point of developing internal and external sphincter control. Earlier attempts will be frustrating for both the child and the parent.

Growth and development are complex, interrelated processes that are influenced by and, in turn, influence the health of an individual. The nurse who understands this relationship is aware of the need for age-specific health-assessment, health-protection, and health-promotion strategies (Box 15.3: Quality and Safety Scenario).

THEORIES OF LIFE SPAN DEVELOPMENT

Specific aspects of development of the person have been studied for centuries. Many theories of development are used in the study of individuals throughout the life span; the nurse may wish to refer to a text on developmental psychology to become familiar with some of these theories. In this unit, five theories are discussed to gain a holistic view of the progression of individual development throughout the life span. These theories were originally advanced by Erikson, Piaget, Vygotsky, Kohlberg, and Gilligan. Whereas these theories can assist in understanding developmental tasks, they are not definitive, and individuals may exhibit variations and stage activities may overlap.

Psychosocial Development: Erikson's Theory

Erik Erikson described the development of identity of the individual self through successive stages that unfold throughout the life span (Erikson, 1968, 1995; Erikson & Erikson, 1998; McLeod, 2008/2013). Although he studied with Freud and supported the psychosexual theory of development, **Erikson's Theory of Psychosocial Development** is based on the need of each person to develop a sense of trust in self and others and a sense of personal worth. Erikson described a healthy personality in positive terms, not merely through the absence of disease.

According to Erikson, psychosocial development is composed of critical stages, each requiring resolution of a conflict between two opposing forces (e.g., intimacy versus isolation). Each stage depends on the preceding stage, which must be accomplished successfully for the person to proceed to the next stage. Erikson's use of a psychosocial framework acknowledges the influence of socialization and the environment but maintains that it is ultimately the individual who must master each of the conflicts. Although each of the conflicts is predominant at a certain stage in life, it is important to recognize that all the conflicts exist in each person, to some extent, at all times and that a conflict, once resolved, may emerge again in appropriate situations. For example, the renunciation and wisdom of old age is accomplished by a person reflecting on the crises of early development and coping with the physical and mental changes of aging. Erikson wrote volumes and there is much for a current researcher to investigate. Changes in current society such as modern technology, the internet, globalization, migration, prolonged education, and delay in transition to adulthood may be viewed through Erikson's theory (Schachter & Galliher, 2018). Erikson's theory has gaps; it does not discuss the causes of development, for instance, or the experiences that a person must have to move to the next stage. Erikson acknowledged that his schema of stages was more a description of human social and emotional development rather than an explanation of how maturing through a stage affects personality at a later time (McLeod, 2008/2013). These stages are summarized in Table 15.2 and are discussed more fully in the chapters on each developmental age group. The Case Study at the end of this chapter is about a potentially disabled infant girl and how hospitalization could affect her stage of psychosocial development.

Cognitive Individual Development

Cognitive development is another aspect. Jean Piaget, a Swiss psychologist, also trained in biology and philosophy, is well known for his theory of cognitive development. He viewed children as biologic organisms interacting with their environment, and his theory contends that cognitive development reflects children's attempts to make sense of their worlds. Piaget developed

TABLE 15.2 GROWTH AND DEVELOPMENT

Erikson's Eight Stages of Human Development

Age Group	Psychosocial Stage	Lasting Outcomes
1. Infancy	Basic trust versus basic mistrust	Faith and hope
2. Toddler stage	Autonomy versus shame and doubt	Self-control and willpower
3. Preschool stage	Initiative versus guilt	Direction and purpose
4. School age	Industry versus inferiority	Method and competence
5. Adolescence	Identity versus role confusion	Devotion and fidelity
6. Young adulthood	Intimacy versus isolation	Affiliation and love
7. Middle adulthood	Generativity versus stagnation	Production and care
8. Older adulthood	Ego integrity versus despair	Renunciation and wisdom

Erikson (1995); Erikson & Erikson (1998); McLeod (2008/2013)

his cognitive theory by observing his own children (Piaget, 1950). Hence, one major criticism of his work is that he underestimated children's capabilities and gave little or no consideration to cultural differences. Lev Vygotsky, a Russian contemporary, was also trained in both the physical sciences and psychology. His theory of cognitive development maintains that a child's development cannot be separated from the social and cultural context in which it occurs. He also credited children with more innate ability to learn and emphasized the importance of language (Vygotsky, 1986). The theories of Piaget and Vygotsky are presented in more detail in the following sections.

Cognitive Development: Piaget's Theory

Jean Piaget's theory of cognitive development is concerned primarily with structure rather than content, with how the individual mind works rather than what it works with. Piaget uses the word "scheme" to describe a pattern of action or thought. A scheme is used to take in or assimilate new experiences or may be modified or accommodated by new experiences. Each person is striving to maintain a balance, or equilibrium, between assimilation and accommodation (Phillips, 1975; Piaget, 1950).

Piaget described the stages of cognitive development throughout the developmental years. Through a natural unfolding of ability, the child acquires sequentially predictable cognitive abilities. Given adequate environmental stimuli and an intact neurologic system, the child gradually matures toward full conceptualized reasoning. Piaget's Theory of Cognitive Development encompasses the time from birth to approximately 15 years of age. Each of the four distinct stages is summarized in Table 15.3, and they are discussed more fully in the specific chapters on each developmental age. Piaget suggests that quantitative, but no further qualitative, changes in cognitive function occur after approximately age 15 years. Although some developmental theorists may dispute a portion of Piaget's findings, this scheme of cognitive development assists the nurse in assessing growth and development in children and adolescents. A search

TABLE 15.3 GROWTH AND DEVELOPMENT

Piaget's Stages of Cognitive Development

Stage	Age	Characteristics
Sensorimotor	Birth to 2 years	Begins with a predominance and reliance on reflexes that permit the body to learn Reflexes decrease and voluntary acts develop Imitation predominates Thought is dominated by physical manipulation of objects and events Develops the concept of object permanence and the ability to form mental representations
Preoperational	2–7 years	Advancing use of language and movement Development of egocentric, animistic, and magical thinking Uses representational thought to interpret and learn, not in terms of general properties but in terms of the relationship or use to themselves No cause-and-effect reasoning Thought is dominated by the senses—what is seen, heard, or experienced
Concrete operations	7–11 years	Mental reasoning processes assume logical approaches to solving concrete problems, including cause and effect Collecting; mastering facts Can consider other points of view Thought influenced by social contacts Language is perfected
Formal operations	11–15 years	True logical thought and manipulation of abstract concepts emerge Morality established

Piaget (1959); Piaget & Inhelder (2000); Leifer & Fleck (2022)

of current literature on nursing and health indicates that many studies use this as a basis for their investigations (Rapanta, 2023; Rapanta & Felton, 2021).

Cognitive Development: Vygotsky's Theory

One of the significant differences between the cognitive theories of Piaget and Vygotsky is that Piaget believed that development precedes learning. Piaget proposed that a certain level of cognitive development must be reached before learning can occur. Vygotsky thought that by viewing development and learning in this way, adults would teach to the lowest ability, aiming instruction at those mental functions or intellectual operations that had already matured in the child. In contrast, Vygotsky proposed that learning precedes development. He states that learning pulls development, which is in stark contrast to Piaget, who felt children are not capable of learning something until they are developmentally ready. Vygotsky's theory has substantial influence upon current thinking about cognitive development (Zhang & Wang, 2018).

Vygotsky argued that, while learning may be similar among children at certain times or phases of development, it is not identical in all children because of their differing social and cultural experiences (Vygotsky, 1978). He felt Piaget overemphasized the intellectual and biologic universality of developmental stages. Vygotsky was more interested in the cultural and social influences on learning and development, as well as how individual children actively internalize what they learn from others. For Vygotsky, development begins as an interpersonal process of "meaning making," which then becomes an individualized process of "making sense." There are no predetermined levels of development; rather, experience is in the front—leading and expanding development in unlimited ways. Where Piaget believed that children learn through doing, Vygotsky emphasized that children may be more adaptable and can learn by observing a task.

Although **Vygotsky's Theory of Cognitive Development** is less known to health care professionals, educators have embraced his theory, especially what he refers to as the "zone of proximal development." The **zone of proximal development** is the distance between the actual developmental level and a potential developmental level. In this proximal zone, children are pulled toward new learning through their interaction with others and the environment. The guidance given by others in this zone is referred to as "**scaffolding**." Expert guidance is important, as is the availability of repeated practice (Sadideen et al., 2018). According to Vygotsky, all people need to understand not only the way in which an individual learns and develops but also the social, cultural, and political context in which learning and development occur. This difference can profoundly affect how the nurse approaches teaching and learning (Box 15.4: Best Practice).

BOX 15.4 BEST PRACTICE

Managing the Use of Electronic Devices

It is almost impossible to restrict the use of electronic devices for young children. These devices may include a wide range of promoted aids, including video games, television, mobile phones, internet and phone applications, computers, tablets (of all sizes), and smaller simpler gaming devices for even younger children. Many parents may also use these devices to keep children occupied or in one place for a period of time. It is not difficult to find children in strollers using tablets to allay impatience while waiting in queue lines for restaurants and movies. Electronic devices can benefit children by stimulating imagination, promoting language, encouraging learning, and improving manual dexterity and engineering skills. However, they can also miss out on learning essential practical skills and time spent indoors on electronic devices limits the time spent outdoors. Less time outdoors involved in walking and sports can lead to unhealthy eating habits and obesity (Yapbeelee, 2023). Some video game use may be beneficial if the type of video game stresses beneficial social functioning and well-being. However, violent video games have been shown to be related to more social bullying and dissatisfaction (Shoshani et al., 2021).

- How can nurses talk to parents about young children using electronic devices?
- How can nurses teach parents that face-to-face interaction and two-way conversations with their children promote cognitive development more than watching television, videos, or other virtual media?
- Nurses should emphasize that role modeling is important and young children will observe the parent's online politeness and use of media.
- How can nurses reinforce a focus that content matters and content quality is more influential than the electronic device or media platform?

Moral Development: Kohlberg's Theory

Another aspect of cognitive development is the development of moral thinking and judgment. **Lawrence Kohlberg's Theory of Moral Development** is based on interviews that focused on hypothetical moral dilemmas, such as: Should a man steal an expensive drug that would save his dying wife? This question forms the basis of Kolhberg's classic Heinz pilfered drug dilemma/scenario. From interviews with young males, Kohlberg developed his cognitive development ethical theory, which is outlined in Table 15.4 (Kohlberg, 1969, 1981). The three stages of moral development—preconventional, conventional, and postconventional—were based on Piaget's theory of cognitive development and emphasize the ethics of rights and justice. Progression through the successive stages of moral development generally occurs during the school-aged, adolescent, and young-adult years. Beyond the young-adult years, stabilization or increased consistency of thought and perhaps an increased correlation between moral judgment and moral action occur (Kohlberg, 1981).

TABLE 15.4 GROWTH AND DEVELOPMENT

Kohlberg's Stages of Moral Development

Stage	Goal
Preconventional	Avoiding punishment
	Gaining reward
Conventional	Gaining approval
	Avoiding disapproval
Postconventional	Agreeing upon rights
	Establishing personal moral standards
	Achieving justice

Kolhberg (1981)

Moral Development: Gilligan's Theory

Carol Gilligan's Theory of Moral Development (Gilligan, 1982; Gilligan & Snider, 2018; Gilligan et al., 1988) suggests that the process of moral development differs in females. While a doctoral student, Gilligan conducted research with Lawrence Kohlberg at Harvard University. She discovered that Kohlberg's original research was conducted with only males and that females often scored lower in Kohlberg's scaling of moral levels. She asserted that females were not inferior in their moral development, just different. In developing her own research with females, she proposed an alternative theory of moral development, which, like Kohlberg's, has three stages (Table 15.5). Gilligan concluded that the transitions between stages are based on changes in one's sense of self rather than on changes in cognitive development, as Kohlberg proposed. Gilligan more clearly differentiated the "voice of care" from the "voice of justice." She also reported that females think and act more from a base of caring and relationships than do males, who are more inclined to think in terms of justice, rights, and rules. The voice of justice promotes

TABLE 15.5 **GROWTH AND DEVELOPMENT**

Gilligan's Stages of Moral Development (for Women)

Stage	Characteristics	Goal
Preconventional	What is practical to others and best for self, realizing connection to others	Individual survival
Conventional	Sacrifices wants and needs to fulfill others' wants and needs	Self-sacrifice is goodness
Postconventional	Moral equal of self and others	Principle of nonviolence, do not hurt self or others

Gilligan (1982); Gilligan et al. (1988); Gilligan & Snider (2018)

legislative policies (e.g., concerning immigration) and development of codes of ethics; the voice of caring speaks to the importance of social relationships. Care ethics and Gilligan's work reside within pluralist feminist theory informed by historically important philosophical methods and schools (Gary, 2022). Gilligan's writings reflect that male patrimony and female sense of self emanate from reaction to psychological trauma. Females tend to back off into caregiving when managing loss; males tend to recede into not caring, social isolation, and desire for greater achievement (Gilligan & Snider, 2018).

BEHAVIORAL BIOLOGICAL DEVELOPMENT

All the preceding theories discuss the importance of experience and environmental exposure on behavior and learning. One of the fundamental questions in the nature versus nurture debate is understanding how environmental stress (physical and behavioral) alters biologic development (epigenetics). Evidence in animals and from human epidemiologic studies indicates that experiences and the environment change the functioning of genes and thus provide a basis for a model of gene-environment interaction. Early life experiences and social exposures may alter the way in which genes direct cell activities (Box 15.5: Genomics); early life adversity, including living in poverty, appears to result in DNA changes in the brain and other body tissues, which can, for instance, increase the risk of obesity (Schafte & Bruna, 2023). Recent studies suggest that even past parental experiences can affect the behavior of children; brain plasticity theory describes brain cell development that can potentially modify ways individuals learn and experience their outside environment. This has implications for physical disease as well as attention, behavioral, and mental disorders and even the transmission of behavioral traits to the next generation (see Box 15.5: Genomics).

BOX 15.5 **GENOMICS**

Epigenetics

- What is epigenetics?
- What are the associations between environmental stressors and physical and behavioral disorders?
- How can environmental exposures, including malnutrition, stress, and poverty, affect more than one generation?

Epigenetics is the scientific investigation of the capacity of cells to react differently or regulate to variations in environmental stimuli that are not related to the DNA code itself. The term "epigenetics" means "top of genetics" (McIntosh, 2019; US National Institutes of Medicine, US National Library of Medicine, 2021; Sprouse, 2024). Variations in cell response were historically attributed to changes in DNA gene sequences and the manufacture of cellular proteins with RNA transcription. However, this description does not fully explain why cells sharing identical DNA sequences can have differing appearances and effects. Some of this was attributed to cell mutations or alternative forms of genes (alleles). Again, this did not fully explain the full variety of appearances seen. Further scientific investigations showed that in two cells having identical DNA, the genes may be expressed differently. In summary, DNA sequence is not destiny. Cells can regulate gene expression via the presence of regulatory proteins that wrap around DNA and RNA and can change cell function negatively or positively. Some of these regulatory proteins may turn off or silence cell function. Epigenetics may have implications for cellular memory and plasticity and for why events occurring during gestation or development may affect later health problems (Cavilli & Heard, 2019; McIntosh, 2019, Sprouse, 2024). Epigenetic investigations demonstrate that regulatory changes can be long-lasting. Stressors, trauma, and/or maltreatment affecting one generation may have lasting behavior effects on subsequent generations. This is sometimes termed as "intergenerational trauma," as traumatic events (war, economic depressions, family dysfunction) in one generation may have behavioral and mental effects on the next, including risk of obesity (Schafte & Bruna, 2023). There are also associations with attention-deficit disorders, learning problems, and acquisition of language and numeral skills. Epigenetic age may be accelerated by high body mass index and decreased by high levels of education and physical activity, low body mass index, and consumption of fish, poultry, fruits, and vegetables (Cavilli & Heard, 2019). Whereas this science is in its infancy and it is difficult to study human intergenerational effects, there is no question that various stressors and physical and learning disorders affecting parents and children may be a problem for the next generation, even when the original precipitating stressors are removed.

CASE STUDY

Birth of a Disabled/Chronically Ill Child: Avery

Avery is a 36-year-old female pregnant with her third child; her other two children are aged 5 and 10 years. At 26 weeks of gestation, Avery is hospitalized for contractions and premature labor. Despite pharmacologic attempts to stop labor, Avery's labor continues to the active phase. Avery and her partner just learned that a baby born this prematurely may have many problems, including cerebral palsy. As the perinatologist leaves the room, Avery turns to the nurse and starts to cry.

Reflective Questions

- What is the nurse's role when the parents learn a child may have a chronic disease and/or disability?
- What can the nurse anticipate for these new parents during the labor? At the birth of the baby?
- If the infant is born with cerebral palsy, what can the nurse anticipate in the first 2 weeks after birth? Over the baby's first year of life? Over the first 5 years?

Continued

CASE STUDY—cont'd

Birth of a Disabled/Chronically Ill Child: Avery

- How will this child's growth, development, and goals for health promotion be affected? What about those of the parents? What about the child's siblings?
- What factors might contribute to Avery's development of chronic sorrow? If Avery becomes depressed, how might this affect the growth and development of the new baby? What effect might this have on her relationship with her partner? What effect might her depression have on her other children?
- What will be the effect of this child's disabilities on the siblings?
- How might the nurse intervene to lessen the effects of chronic sorrow?

The birth of a disabled and chronically ill child exemplifies the theory on chronic sorrow (Batchelor & Duke, 2019; Carroll, 2019). Chronic sorrow is the cyclical, recurring, and potentially progressive pattern of pervasive sadness experienced by the caregiver in response to continual loss.

There are numerous potential theoretical and actual potential nursing actions (Pereira et al., 2018). Nursing interventions may include grief work facilitation—for example, the nurse listens to expressions of grief, encourages identification of fears, and assists in identifying needed modifications in lifestyle. Another intervention might entail hope/inspiration—for example, the nurse helps identify areas of hope, demonstrates hope by recognizing the disability as only one facet of the child, and provides parents with opportunities to be involved with support groups. Coping enhancement might involve assisting caregivers to adapt to perceived stressors and changes to meet life demands and roles. For example, the nurse provides an atmosphere of acceptance, seeks to understand each parent's perspective on the situation, and assists the parents to identify positive strategies. Resiliency promotion might be used to strengthen protective factors; for example, the nurse encourages positive health-seeking behavior and facilitates development and use of neighborhood resources.

SUMMARY

- Individuals make many choices that affect their health each day, and a number of factors influence how these choices are made.
- The stage of growth and development, as well as the context in which learning occurs, influences how individuals experience different situations and realize the choices available.
- Understanding the most widely used theories of human growth and development assists nurses to have a clear understanding of the challenges an individual is likely to encounter as well as the skills the individual is likely to need for successful growth, development, and maturation throughout the life span.
- Theories provide nurses with frameworks, resources, and comparisons for health assessment, promotion, and intervention.

EVOLVE CHAPTER FEATURES

http://evolve.elsevier.com/Edelman/

- Study Questions

REFERENCES

Aiello, L., & Calzone, K. (2018). Precision medicine: Preparing nurses in genomics for today's healthcare. *Dean's Notes: National Student Nurses' Association*, *40*(2), 1–2.

Barbato, E. S., Daly, B. J., & Darrah, R. J. (2019). Educating nursing scientists: Integrating genetics and genomics into PhD curricula. *Journal of Professional Nursing*, *35*(2), 89–92.

Batchelor, L. L., & Duke, G. (2019). Chronic sorrow in parents with chronically ill children. *Pediatric Nursing*, *45*(4), 163–173, 183.

Calzone, K. A., Kirk, M., Tonkin, E., Badzek, L., Benjamin, C., & Middleton, A. (2018). Increasing nursing capacity in genomics: Overview of existing global genomics resources. *Nursing Education Today*, *69*, 53–59.

Camp, B. W., & Bonnell, L. N. (2020). Combining two developmental screening tests to improve predictive accuracy. *Academy Pediatrics*, *20*(3), 413–420. https://doi.org/10.1016/j.acap.2019.06.010

Carroll, K. (2019). Bringing joy-sorrow to light: Informing practice utilizing theoretical and research perspectives. *Nursing Science Quarterly*, *32*(10), 29–32.

Cavilli, G., & Heard, E. (2019). Advances in epigenetics link genetics to the environment and disease. *Nature*, *571*, 489–499.

Centers for Disease Control and Prevention (CDC). (2021). *Lead poisoning prevention*. https://www.cdc.gov/nceh/lead/prevention/populations.htm

Centers for Disease Control and Prevention (CDC). (2022). *Growth charts*. https://www.cdc.gov/growthcharts/

Erikson, E. H. (1968). *Identity, youth, and crisis*. New York: Norton.

Erikson, E. H. (1995). *Childhood and society* (35th anniversary ed.). New York: Norton.

Erikson, E. H., & Erikson, J. M. (1998). *The life cycle completed*. New York: Norton.

Gary, M. E. (2022). From care ethics to pluralist care theory: the state of the field. *Philosophy Compass*, *17*(4), e12819. https://doi.org/10.1111/phc3.12819

Gilligan, C. (1982). *In a different voice: Psychological theory and women's development*. Cambridge, MA: Harvard University Press.

Gilligan, C., & Snider, N. (2018). *Why does patrimony persist?* Cambridge: Polity Press.

Gilligan, C., Ward, J. V., & Taylor, J. M. (Eds.). (1988). *Mapping the moral domain: A contribution of women's thinking to psychology theory and education*. Cambridge, MA: Harvard University Press.

Gyenes, N. (2019). Fighting misinfordemics. *Harvard Public Health*, Spring, 7.

Kohlberg, L. (1969). Continuities and discontinuities in childhood and adult moral development. *Human Development*, *12*, 93–120.

Kohlberg, L. (1981). *The philosophy of moral development* (Vol. 1). San Francisco: Harper & Row.

Leifer, G., & Fleck, E. (2022). *Growth and development across the lifespan* (3rd ed.). St. Louis: Elsevier.

McIntosh, B. (2019). The science of sex. *Harvard Magazine*, Nov-Dec, 34–38.

McKinney, E. S., Smith Murray, S., Mau, K., James, S. R., Nelson, K., Aswill, J. W., et al. (2022). *Maternal child nursing* (6th ed.). St Louis: Saunders.

McLeod, S. A. (2008/2013). *Erik Erikson/psychological stages-simply psychology*. http://www.simplypsychology.org/Erik-Erikson.html

Pereira, A., Ferreira, J. M., & Barbieri-Figueiredo, C. (2018). Nursing theories in palliative care investigation: A review. *Hospice & Palliative Medicine International Journal*, *2*(4), 231–234.

Phillips, J. L. (1975). *The origins of intellect: Piaget's theory* (2nd ed.). San Francisco: W. H. Freeman.

Piaget, J. (1950). *The psychology of intelligence*. London: Routledge and Kegan Paul.

Piaget, J. (1959). *Language and thought of the child*. New York: Routledge.

Piaget, J., & Inhelder, B. (2000). *The psychology of the child*. New York: Basic Books.

Rapanta, C. (2023). Piaget, Vygotsky and young people's argumentation: Sociocognitive aspects and challenges of reasoning "together" and "alone." *Learning, Culture and Social Interaction*, *39*, 100698. https://doi.org/10.1016/j.lcsi.2023.100698

Rapanta, C., & Felton, M. K. (2021). Learning to argue through dialogue: A review of instructional approaches. *Educational Psychology Review*, *34*, 477–509. https://doi.org/10.1007/s10648-021-09637-2

Rittle, C. (2019). What's new about measles? *American Nurse Today*, *14*(9), 81.

Sadideen, H., Plonczak, A., Saadeddin, M., & Kneebone, R. (2018). How educational theory can inform the training and practice of plastic surgeons. *Plastic and Reconstructive Surgery Global Open*, *6*(12), e2042.

Schachter, E. P., & Galliher, R. V. (2018). Fifty years since "Identity: Youth and Crisis": A renewed look at Erikson's writings on identity. *Identity, International Journal of Theory and Design*, *18*(4), 247–250. https://doi.org/10.1080/15283488.2018.1529267

Schafte, K., & Bruna, S. (2023). The influence of intergenerational trauma on epigenetics and obesity in indigenous populations - a scoping review. *Epigenetics*, *18*(1), 22601218. https://doi.org/10.1080/15592294.2023.2260218

Shoshani, A., Braverman, S., & Meirow, G. (2021). Video games and close relations: Attachment and empathy as predictors of children's and adolescents' video game social play and socio-emotional functioning. *Computers in Human Behavior*, *114*, 106578.

Sprouse, E. (2024). *How are genes turned on and off?* https://science.howstuffworks.com/life/genetic/genes-turned-off-on.htm

Thomas, K., & Senkpeni, A. D. (2020). What should health science journalists do in epidemic responses? *AMA Journal of Ethics*, *22*(1), E55–E60.

U.S. Department of Health and Human Services. (2023). *Healthy People 2030 topics and objectives*. http://www.healthypeople.gov

U.S. National Institutes of Medicine, National Library of Medicine. (2021). *What is epigenetics?* https://medlineplus.gov/genetics/understanding/howgeneswork/epigenome/

Vygotsky, L. S. (1978). *Mind in society: The development of higher psychological processes*. Cambridge, MA: Harvard University Press.

Vygotsky, L. S. (1986). *Thought and language*. Cambridge, MA: MIT Press.

Yapbeelee. (2023). *WeHaveKids: Positive and negative impacts of electronic devices on children*. https://wehavekids.com/parenting/dlectronic-devices-and-gadgets-to-Children

Zhang, X., & Wang, H. (2018). Embodied cognition from the perspective of Vygotsky's socio-cultural theory. *Philosophy Study*, *8*(8), 362–367.

16

The Childbearing Period

Courtney Coffey

http://evolve.elsevier.com/Edelman/

OBJECTIVES

After completing this chapter, the reader will be able to:

- Differentiate fetal development and the newborn transition to extrauterine life.
- Analyze changes in the maternal system during pregnancy on the basis of their influences on pregnancy adaptation.
- Interpret the role of the nurse in promoting the physical, mental, and spiritual health of the childbearing family.
- Compare and contrast fetal problems caused by maternal drinking, smoking, drug use, and viral exposure during pregnancy.
- Outline the nursing role during labor and birth with a focus on the physical, emotional, spiritual, and educational needs.
- Evaluate the influence of factors such as ethnicity, legislative priorities, and the sociopolitical context of the health care delivery system on prenatal and childbirth care and the needs of families.

KEY TERMS

Acquired immunodeficiency syndrome
Amniocentesis
Amniotic membranes
Anemia
Apgar scoring system
Bacterial vaginosis
Bradycardia
Candida albicans
Cervical effacement
Chlamydia
Chloasma
Chorionic membranes
Chorionic villi
Colostrum
Conception
Congenital defect
Cytomegalovirus
Dilation
Diversity
Down syndrome
Embryo
Endometrium
Estrogen
Fertilization
Fetal alcohol spectrum disorder
Fetal alcohol syndrome
Fetal heart monitor
Fetus
First stage of labor
Fourth stage of labor
Fundus
Gestation
Gestational hypertension
Gonococcus
Group B streptococcus
Health outcomes
Hepatitis B
Hepatitis B virus (HBV)
Herpes simplex
Human chorionic gonadotropin (hCG)
Human immunodeficiency virus
Hydramnios
Infant mortality rate
Infertility
Labor
Lamaze
Linea nigra
Meconium
Miscarriage
Neonatal abstinence syndrome
Obesity
Pica
Placenta
Positive signs of pregnancy
Prejudices
Presumptive signs of pregnancy
Preterm birth
Probable signs of pregnancy
Progesterone
Quickening
Rh blood group incompatibility
Risk factors
Rubella
Second stage of labor
Sexually transmitted infections
Spontaneous abortion
Stages of labor
Station
Stillbirth
Striae gravidarum
Syphilis
Tachycardia
Teratogen
Third stage of labor
Toxoplasmosis
Trimesters
Ultrasound
Zika virus
Zygotic cells

THINK ABOUT IT

First Pregnancy Labor

Tia is a 40 y/o gravida 1 para 0 and is currently 41 weeks pregnant. Tia is married to their partner S.J. This is an vitro fertilization (IVF) pregnancy. They both identify as nonbinary and prefer they/them pronouns. Tia is admitted at 2:00 a.m. to Memorial Medical Center with uterine contractions occurring every 8 minutes since midnight. Their cervix is dilated to 2 cm and is 80% effaced, station is −3. S.J. is out of town on a business trip, and Tia's family friend has accompanied them to the hospital. Although Tia attended Lamaze classes with S.J., they are anxious about the labor. Tia says to the nurse, "My back is about to break, I have so much bottom pressure, and I wanted to go natural, without medication and all this high-technology stuff, including the monitor."

- On the basis of your knowledge of ethical and legal principles of care, how would you as a caregiver appropriately respond to Tia's desire to labor and give birth without fetal heart rate monitoring?
- What factors in Tia's history would support the use of the fetal heart monitor? What factors would not support use of the monitor?
- What political, legal, ethical, and other factors might be relevant to the widespread use of monitors in American maternity units nowadays?
- How does the use of fetal heart rate monitoring fit into a health-promotion approach to labor and birth?
- What considerations are important when caring for Tia and their partner S.J. as a family unit? How can you as a health care provider provide care that is inclusive?

The process of conception, pregnancy, and birth involves a complex interaction of many factors, including the physiologic and psychological changes in the birthing parent and family and the development of a fetus into a viable newborn. The nurse's role during the pregnancy cycle should encompass evidence-based practice recommendations for effective health-promotion interventions in the antepartum, intrapartum, and postpartum periods to improve maternal and newborn health outcomes. The focus of this chapter is on the birthing parent, their family, and the developing fetus; discussing one without the others is impossible. The nurse must consider all three entities when seeking to promote a healthy pregnancy and healthy family system after birth.

Note: The language in this chapter is intended to be inclusive. It is essential to acknowledge that individuals with varied gender identities and sexual orientations may become pregnant. The term "birthing parent/individual" is used to reflect the diversity of those who conceive and carry a pregnancy. Nurses must aim to provide care that is inclusive to all with the aim of providing evidence-based and patient-centered care. Part of the nurse's role in providing inclusive care is through the use of inclusive language, which is reflected in this chapter.

BIOLOGY AND GENETICS

Cells are the basic units of life. Pregnancy begins with fertilization, the fusion of a sperm from a male and an egg from a female. Each one contains half of the genetic material to form a new individual. Their combination forms a diploid cell, which contains all of the genetic material needed to form a human. Fertilization is the first embryonic event in a series that culminates in the birth of an infant. The physical changes during pregnancy include natural processes involving fertilization of the egg by the sperm, implantation of the fertilized egg into the uterus, embryonic or fetal growth and development, placental development and function, and maternal changes related to the pregnancy process.

Duration of Pregnancy

Pregnancy begins with the union of a sperm and an egg, a process called "fertilization." Under normal healthy circumstances, a full-term pregnancy lasts approximately 10 lunar months, or 40 weeks. An accurate estimated date of delivery is determined by use of the Nägele rule. One does this by adding 7 days to the date of the first day of the last normal menstrual period and subtracting 3 months, plus 1 full year. A usual pregnancy is divided into three equal periods called "trimesters." Often, these trimesters form the basis for discussion of expected fetal and maternal changes during pregnancy (American College of Obstetricians and Gynecologists [ACOG], 2024).

Fertilization

The union of a sperm and an egg requires several crucial factors, many of which are not fully understood. When a sperm cell penetrates an egg in the ampulla of the fallopian tube, the beginning of a human being (called a "zygote") results. Early cell divisions occur while the zygote is slowly being transported through the fallopian tube toward the uterus. Additional division of zygotic cells results in more differentiated structures that eventually produce an embryo and subsequently a fetus.

An absence of one or more critical factors may cause infertility (inability to become pregnant despite usual sexual activity in a period of 1 year for those 35 years old and younger and in a period of 6 months for those 35 years old and older). For example, both a sperm cell and an egg cell must be mature and in the fallopian tube for approximately 5 hours for union of the sperm and egg to occur (the process of conception). The sperm must be of uniform size, be normally formed, possess high motility, and have an ability to secrete enzymes that dissolve the membrane surrounding the egg. Cellular changes within the egg prevent other sperm from entering the ovum after the sperm penetrates it (Webster et al., 2018). The birthing parent attempting pregnancy must have a certain basal body temperature and fallopian tubes free of adhesions or obstructions. Pregnancy is likely conceived within 24 hours after ovulation.

Implantation

The process of attachment and placental formation is called *implantation*. A pregnancy has not occurred until successful implantation has happened, which usually begins by day 8 postfertilization. Up to this point, the cells have relied upon the energy stored within the cells and nutrients within the uterine fluid. For the zygote to grow, it needs to get nutrients from the maternal blood, which it does by developing the placenta. The placenta is an organ that serves to prevent the direct exchange between the blood and nutrients to the fetus. It also functions as an endocrine gland, manufacturing and secreting hormones that play a vital role in maintaining the pregnancy. Transplantation of the fertilized egg in the uterine cavity after its trip through the fallopian tube requires approximately 6 days (Jordan et al., 2019). Once the zygote reaches the uterus, it stays there for up to 5 days, receiving nutrition from the **endometrium**, the inner lining of the uterus (Blackburn, 2018). The process of fertilization and implantation triggers the production of large amounts of the hormone **progesterone**, which stimulates the formation of endometrial cells known as the *decidua*, meaning "to shed." The decidua provides nutrition for the "**embryo**," a term that defines the growing conceptus up to 8 weeks of age.

Fetal Growth and Development

Much is known about the stages of physical development in each structural system of the embryo. However, metabolic functions, particularly those relevant to the endocrine and neurologic systems, are less well-defined. Appropriate fetal development depends on these events occurring in a specified period and order during each trimester of pregnancy. If this does not occur, an abnormality in structure or function (a **congenital defect**) may result. This defect may be noted at birth and did not occur at conception (called a "genetic defect"), but most likely resulted from some disruption that occurred after conception and during fetal development.

Placental Development and Function

After implantation of the zygote, the **placenta** develops through an integration of embryonic and decidual cells. The **chorionic membranes** and **amniotic membranes**, which surround the fetus throughout **gestation**, also begin to form. The amniotic fluid, manufactured by the amniotic membrane, supports the developing fetus and protects it from injury.

The basic structure of the placenta allows maternal-fetal blood exchange to nourish the fetus and allow excretion of fetal waste products. Throughout most of gestation, increasing placental development allows maternal blood to flow through the intervillous spaces and fetal blood to flow through the **chorionic villi** (Cunningham et al., 2022). The unique structure of the placenta permits the exchange of certain molecules but prevents fetal and maternal blood supplies from mixing for most of the pregnancy. Substances with larger and heavier molecules (e.g., heparin or insulin) normally do not pass through the placenta to the fetus, but lighter molecules (e.g., anesthetic gases, oxygen, carbon dioxide, and electrolytes) readily cross the placenta. Because of the difficulty involved in predicting exactly which substances will cross the placenta, a shared decision-making process should be utilized when discussing an intake of substances by the birthing parent and those contemplating pregnancy to avoid harm to the fetus. Some substances or medications such as antidepressants have been shown to be beneficial to continue despite a small risk to the fetus, because the benefit of stable mental health in the birthing parent outweighs the risk of fetal harm (Mayo Foundation for Medical Education and Research, 2023b)

The placenta has four major functions: metabolic, endocrine, immunologic, and transport. The placenta manufactures and secretes four hormones throughout pregnancy. The primary hormones produced by the placenta include **estrogen**, progesterone, **human chorionic gonadotropin (hCG)**, and human placental lactogen (hPL). Estrogen's role is to increase uterine blood flow and increase uterine and breast growth. Progesterone maintains the uterus in a quiet state throughout the pregnancy to prevent labor contractions occurring too early. hCG's main role is to sustain estrogen and progesterone production in early pregnancy, and it is also the hormone detected in pregnancy tests. hPL ensures adequate fetal nutrition, increases insulin resistance, and stimulates production of growth hormones (King et al., 2019).

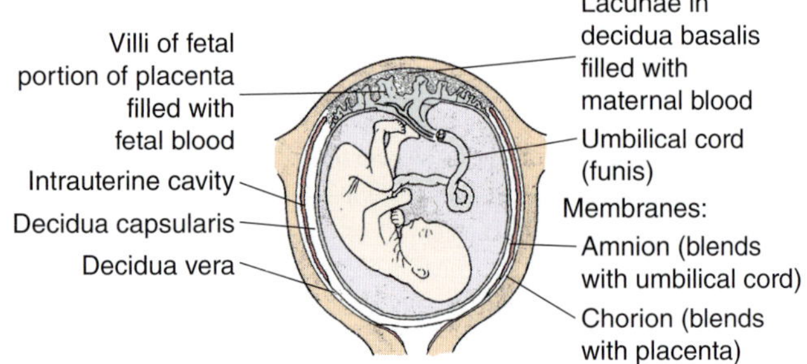

FIG. 16.1 Relationship of fetus, placenta, membranes, and uterus during gestation. (From Lowdermilk et al. [2024].)

The fetus, which continues to gain strength and maturity during the later weeks of gestation, generally rests its head in the lower maternal pelvis by the end of pregnancy (Fig. 16.1). The membranes protect the fetus from infection and act as a container for the amniotic fluid. As birth begins, the membranes may rupture, causing the loss of amniotic fluid and stronger uterine contractions, reflective of the **labor** process. If the membranes rupture more than 24 hours before birth, uterine infection and potential fetal harm may result.

As gestation nears completion, placental function gradually decreases, which may serve as a stimulus for the onset of labor. When pregnancy continues beyond 42 weeks, or 2 weeks beyond the calculated due date, placental function decreases even more, posing concerns about the well-being of the fetus (Blackburn, 2018).

The discussion of fetal development provides only a brief glimpse of the prenatal period. It is also important to address maternal changes and culmination of the prenatal period, labor, and birth.

Physiologic Changes

The birthing parent experiences various physiologic effects based on a combination of hormonal and mechanical changes during pregnancy. Hormonal influences tend to increase as the pregnancy progresses. The mechanical (hemodynamic) changes reach a peak in the seventh or eighth month and then gradually decline as the pregnancy nears completion (Cunningham et al., 2022). Clinical symptoms will manifest themselves during this peak stress time.

Signs of Pregnancy

Virtually every body system is affected by dynamic hormonal, anatomic, physiologic, and biochemical changes that occur with conception. Pregnancy may be suspected if there is a missed menstrual period or experiences of nausea and vomiting, changes in breast sensations and size, or increased urinary frequency (presumptive signs of pregnancy). **Presumptive signs of pregnancy** are the least-reliable indicators of pregnancy because any one of them can be caused by conditions other than pregnancy. If pregnancy is suspected, a home urine pregnancy test can be used. If it is performed too early, a home pregnancy test may produce a false-negative result attributable to a low level of hCG. This hormone, produced by the placenta and found in urine and blood, triggers a positive pregnancy result. These home pregnancy tests have a high degree of accuracy (97%) if the instructions are followed exactly. If the pregnancy test is positive, a prenatal visit should be scheduled to confirm gestational age and for the birthing parent to receive appropriate pregnancy counseling, which should include taking folic acid supplementation to prevent neural tube defects (NTDs). It is recommended that those who are sexually active and could become pregnant should supplement their diet before conception with 0.4 to 1.0 mg of folic acid daily as part of their multivitamins. The incidence of NTDs (approximately 1 in 3000 live births in the United States annually) has fallen since the inclusion of folic acid supplementation, but recent research suggests folic acid supplementation is underused because of low adherence (March of Dimes, 2022). As the pregnancy progresses, **presumptive signs of pregnancy** are subjectively experienced, **probable signs of pregnancy** are objectively observed by the health care provider, and **positive signs of pregnancy** are positive signs that verify that a pregnancy exists (Box 16.1). During the first trimester of pregnancy, using sophisticated testing with **ultrasound**, health care providers can determine fetal presence and placental adequacy early in pregnancy. This technology, which uses high-frequency sound waves that bounce off the fetus and are interpreted by a computer, allows visualization of the fetus and gestational structures throughout pregnancy (Norwitz et al., 2019).

Nausea and vomiting occurs in up to 80% of pregnancies, and there is a tendency for many health care providers to minimize it. The US Food and Drug Administration has approved Diclegis to treat nausea and vomiting in those whose symptoms have not abated with a change in diet or other nonmedical treatments. It is a delayed-release medication containing a combination of doxylamine (antihistamine) and pyridoxine (vitamin B_6). The major side effect is drowsiness (King et al., 2019).

Adaptive Changes of Other Systems

In addition to pregnancy-related changes in the reproductive system, adaptive changes in other body systems occur. The urinary system undergoes dramatic changes during gestation as follows:

- A 50% increase in glomerular filtration rate occurs related to the influences of **estrogen** and progesterone.
- Ureters increase in diameter by 25% secondary to progesterone influence.
- Urinary output increases by approximately 80% related to the total body water increase.
- Bladder capacity increases to approximately 1500 mL to accommodate extra fluids.

BOX 16.1 Signs of Pregnancy and Time of Occurrence

Presumptive

- Breast changes (e.g., tenderness) (3–4 weeks)
- Fatigue (12 weeks)
- Urinary frequency (6–12 weeks)
- Nausea and vomiting (4–14 weeks)
- Amenorrhea (4th week)
- Quickening (16–20 weeks)

Probable

- Enlargement of the uterus (12–14 weeks)
- Softening of the uterine isthmus (Hegar sign) (6th–12th weeks)
- Bluish or cyanotic color of cervix and upper vagina (Chadwick sign) (6th–8th weeks)
- Softening of the cervix (Goodell sign) (5th week)
- Ballottement of the fetus (16th–28th weeks)
- Positive test result for human chorionic gonadotropin in the maternal urine or blood serum (4th–12th weeks)
- Changes in skin pigmentation (chloasma and linea nigra) (2nd half of pregnancy)

Positive

- Detection of fetal heart tones by auscultation, ultrasonography, or a Doppler scan (8–17 weeks)
- Palpation of fetal body parts with Leopold maneuvers (19–22 weeks)
- Fetal movements visible and detected by examiner (late pregnancy)
- Radiologic or ultrasonographic demonstration of fetal parts (6–16 weeks)

The cardiovascular system changes also begin early in pregnancy as follows:

- Cardiac output increases by up to 50% to meet the demands of pregnancy.
- Total blood volume increases by up to 45% during pregnancy. Physiologic **anemia** of pregnancy may result because of a greater increase in the volume of plasma compared with the volume of red blood cells.
- Heart rate increases by 10 beats/minute to compensate for the increase in blood volume.

Respiratory system changes include the following:

- Tidal volume (volume of air inspired) increases by 30% to 40% to increase the effectiveness of air exchange. Total oxygen consumption increases by approximately 20%.
- The diaphragm is displaced upward secondary to the enlarging uterus and causes shortness of breath during the last trimester.

Increased elasticity and softening of connective tissue of the musculoskeletal system cause the following changes during pregnancy:

- The joints relax, especially the pelvic joints that support the pregnancy and create pliability at the time of birth. This occurs due to the increase in the hormone relaxin. Separation of the symphysis pubis also occurs secondary to this hormonal increase.
- Lumbar and dorsal curves of the spine increase late in pregnancy and contribute to low back pain and the waddle of pregnancy.

Changes in the integumentary system occur, which may include the following:

- Hormonal changes and stretching of the connective tissue of the abdomen, attributable to an enlarging uterus, lead to stretch marks (**striae gravidarum**).
- A narrow, brownish line (**linea nigra**) divides the abdomen, running from the umbilicus to the symphysis pubis. The linea nigra fades after the pregnancy ends.
- An increase in pigmentation caused by melanocyte-stimulating hormone causes darkened areas on the face termed the "mask of pregnancy" (**chloasma**).

The gastrointestinal system undergoes dramatic changes during pregnancy, such as the following:

- The enlarging and space-occupying uterus cramps the intestinal region, causing a slowing of peristalsis and an increase in the emptying time of the stomach.
- Relaxin causes a decrease in gastric motility leading to constipation.
- Frequent "heartburn" results from reflux of stomach contents into the esophagus secondary to upward displacement of the stomach and a relaxed gastroesophageal sphincter (Dutton et al., 2020; King et al., 2019).

Reproductive System

The effects on the reproductive system include changes in the uterus, breasts, vagina, vulva, and ovaries. The prepregnant uterus is approximately the size of a closed fist. The uterus at term has the capacity to contain an approximately 3.2- to 4.5-kg (7- to 10-pound) infant and the placenta. As the uterus enlarges, the **fundus** (the upper uterine segment) moves higher in the abdomen (Fig. 16.2). The breasts begin enlarging early in the pregnancy, and in late pregnancy they may secrete small amounts of **colostrum**, a precursor of mature breast/chest milk. The vagina and vulva receive a greater blood supply and appear darker (cyanotic) as a result. Mucous glands in the cervix become enlarged with increased blood supply, making it more prone to bleeding from superficial injury. Some will notice an increase in vaginal secretions and experience a whitish discharge (Webster et al., 2018).

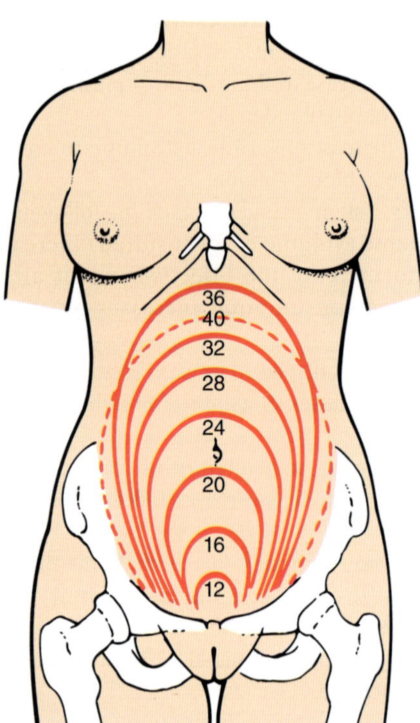

FIG. 16.2 Upper level of enlarging uterus by weeks of normal gestation with a single fetus. (From Seidel et al. [2019].)

Hormones such as hCG and estrogen, secreted by the placenta and the fetus, create an optimal intrauterine environment for the fetus and stimulate many changes in the pregnant person's body. The developing fetus contributes to the provision of an adequate environment for its own growth and nourishment, despite the possibility of creating discomforts for the pregnant individual.

Preconception Care

During the prenatal period, health promotion, risk assessment, and targeted interventions are paramount. Preconception health promotion is a primary intervention that benefits people of reproductive age and their potential children. Prenatal care has been used as secondary prevention to improve the health of the birthing parent during their pregnancy, but by the time prenatal care has generally started at weeks 8 to 12, a considerable amount of fetal development has already occurred. The fetus is most sensitive to maternal health and environmental exposures from weeks 4 to 10 of pregnancy, and many people may not know they are even pregnant then. The rates of adverse birth outcomes (preterm and low birth weight, infant deaths, and birth defects) and maternal pregnancy complications in the United States are all higher than the goals in Healthy People 2030. Given the adverse trends seen in **preterm birth** rates and related maternal and infant death rates, a global summit was convened by the US Department of Health and Human Services (USDHHS; Douthard et al., 2021). The summit put forth the following key suggestions:

- Improve access to individual-centered, comprehensive care before, during, and after pregnancy, especially in rural and underserved areas.
- Improve quality of maternity services through efforts such as utilization of safety protocols in all birthing facilities.
- Provide continuity of care before, during, and after pregnancies by increasing the types and distribution (access to and utilization of a variety of) of health care providers.
- Provide continuous team-based support and use a life course model of care before, during, and after pregnancies.
- Improve the quality and availability of national surveillance and survey data, research, and common terminology and definitions.
- Improve quality and consistency of maternal mortality review committees through collaborations and technical assistance with US states.
- Engage in opportunities for productive collaborations with multiple summit participants.

The key points introduced focus on improving maternal health outcomes and addressing health disparities through access to quality health services, a skilled workforce, and applying evidence-based interventions (Health Resources & Services Administration [HRSA], 2019).

Not all couples who seek preconception care are able to conceive on their own. Conception requires ovulation of a mature ovum, normal fallopian tubes, the presence of progressively motile sperm in the female reproductive tract, and an endometrium favorable for implantation. For many couples, the experience of fertility problems and aspects of the care with uncertain outcomes can be stressful and distressing. Infertility affects more than 6 million American couples (Office on Women's Health [OWH], 2021). Frequently, couples will seek treatment for their infertility issues and undergo testing that may include a semen analysis, assessment of ovulation, evaluation of tubal patency, and tests for ovarian reserve (Lockwood et al., 2023). The nurse's role is that of support and education of the couple. The nurse can assist in educating the couple about the various methods to treat infertility and allow them to make their own decision as to which method is best for them. Infants conceived through IVF technologies have a higher risk of genetic abnormalities, a higher risk of being part of a multiple pregnancy, and a higher risk of being born prematurely (American Pregnancy Association, n.d.). The nurse must be knowledgeable to be able to respond to questions that will come up throughout the treatment experience. One of the greatest risks of assisted reproduction is the risk of obtaining a multifetal pregnancy after intrauterine insemination with more than one embryo. Compared with a single pregnancy, the risks of a multifetal pregnancy include iron- and folate-deficiency anemia, placenta previa, dysfunctional labor, gestational hypertension, preeclampsia, hydramnios, gestational diabetes, and a high surgical birth rate (Jordan et al., 2019). Most couples need a great deal of emotional support, and it is important for the nurse to be able to act as an advocate for them, particularly those using gestational surrogacy as a means of achieving parenthood.

Surrogacy is an arrangement in which someone carries and gives birth to a child for another couple. The fundamental nature of families has changed over the years, whereby gestational surrogacy as an option for infertile couples is widely accepted. Gestational surrogacy, where the surrogate is not genetically related to the embryo, has become the norm. The legal aspects of surrogacy are very complex and differ among countries (Phillips et al., 2019).

Preconception care before a pregnancy implies health-promotion activities that are conducted before a pregnancy occurs to address risk factors across the life span—including during adolescence. Although most pregnancies during adolescence are unintended, health behaviors initiated during this period can have a great effect, not only on future reproductive outcomes but also on present and future health.

Preconception care offers an effective and efficient means to reduce complications of pregnancy for both the birthing parent and their newborn. The components of preconceptual care can be grouped into three broad areas: risk assessment and screening (health history, physical exam, and diagnostic tests); health promotion and counseling (reproductive life plan, nutritional status, optimal body mass index [BMI], physical activity, supplements, and vaccinations); and appropriate interventions based on risk factors identified (Box 16.2; Jordan et al., 2019). The following interventions may be included in preconception care:

- Folic acid supplementation to reduce the risk of NTDs
- Screening for medical and social risk factors
- Rubella vaccination to reduce the risk of severe congenital defects
- Diabetes management to reduce the risk of birth defects threefold
- Hypothyroidism management to promote healthy fetal neurologic development
- Hepatitis B vaccination to prevent chronic liver disease
- Human immunodeficiency virus (HIV)/acquired immunodeficiency syndrome (AIDS) screening and treatment to prevent transmission to the fetus
- Healthy diet instruction throughout pregnancy
- Physical activity needs throughout pregnancy
- Substance misuse and medication safety
- Intimate partner violence screening (Case Study)
- Counseling individuals about immunizations for themselves and their infants
- Assessment of chronic health conditions such as diabetes, hypertension, and thyroid disease
- Screening and treatment for sexually transmitted infections (STIs) to reduce the risk of ectopic pregnancy and/or fetal anomalies
- Oral antiepileptic medication management to minimize birth defect potential
- Cessation of acne treatment with isotretinoin (Accutane) to prevent defects

BOX 16.2 QUALITY AND SAFETY SCENARIO

Intimate Partner Violence and Birth Outcomes in Abused Pregnant Individuals

Intimate partner violence is a significant public health problem with negative physical and psychological outcomes. According to the CDC (2021), approximately 34% of females experience physical violence from their partner. It has been associated with increased levels of STIs, suicide attempts, low self-esteem, preterm labor, low birth-weight infants, anxiety, substance abuse behaviors, and postpartum depression or psychosis (AWHONN, 2019).

Overall, nurses need to screen for high-risk factors prenatally, to be aware of the health risks secondary to violence, and to tailor nursing interventions supportive of those facing abuse. Nurses need to be aware of the issues surrounding pregnancy violence and should provide patients with the resources and information necessary to ensure their safety.

Questions

- How do the current health care system and the sociopolitical context of care in the United States contribute to the high numbers of pregnant individuals facing abuse from their intimate partners?
- What kind of interventions do you believe would be effective for those who are abused?
- How should US health care policy ethically and legislatively address the problem of intimate partner abuse during pregnancy?

AWHONN, Association of Women's Health, Obstetric and Neonatal Nurses; *CDC*, Centers for Disease Control; *STI*, sexually transmitted infections.

- Smoking cessation counseling to reduce negative perinatal outcomes
- Screening and treating of depression to reduce the risk of postpartum depression
- Elimination of alcohol use to prevent **fetal alcohol spectrum disorders (FASDs)**
- **Obesity** control to reduce the risk of cerebrovascular disease, diabetes, or surgical births (Centers for Disease Control and Prevention [CDC], 2023a; Norwitz et al., 2019)

Normal Discomforts of Pregnancy

Although pregnancy is a physiologic event, it poses a burden and stress. Although health professionals regard these pregnancy changes as minor and not in need of treatment, they can be perceived as problematic by the patient. Therefore it is important that the well-being of the pregnant patient be assessed and maintained throughout the gestation (Yikar & Nazik, 2019). There may be a sense of relief that other pregnant people have these concerns and that interventions exist to increase their comfort at various points during gestation. Particularly for those experiencing a first pregnancy, the nurse serves as a valuable support person to help expectant couples adjust to the challenges and discomforts of pregnancy.

Teaching About Changes to Expect in the Body During Pregnancy

In addition to serving as a caregiver, advocate, and support person, the nurse serves as a teacher throughout the pregnancy care process. Active teaching responsive to an individual's concerns about pregnancy may occur in the clinic, physician's office, or other health care environments. Nursing interventions should address recommended professional practice guidelines for education during the prenatal period, to prevent complications for the family. For example, the nurse may offer textbooks, pamphlets, videos, and referrals to websites and other media to increase a couple's knowledge of fetal, maternal, and family changes during gestation and then encourage and answer any questions based on the material. Going beyond one-to-one teaching, the nurse may also refer couples to early pregnancy and **Lamaze** childbirth preparation classes to enlarge their social support network and increase knowledge of labor and birth. Throughout the care process the nurse is sensitive to the cultural and ethnic beliefs and behaviors of the individual and family.

A summary of perinatal care guidelines is provided in Table 16.1. Prenatally, pregnant people experience a wide variety of physiologic adaptations. Nurses must possess a broad and deep understanding of these changes combined with accurate and early risk assessment to identify deviations. This knowledge base is vital for nurses caring for patients during the childbearing cycle.

Total Weight Gain

Total weight gain during pregnancy reflects not only the growth of the baby and placenta, but also the growth of the uterus and breasts, the storage of maternal fat, and the increased amounts of blood and other body fluids. It has been nearly two decades since guidelines for how much weight should be gained during pregnancy were issued by the Institute of Medicine (IOM), since renamed the "National Academy of Medicine" (NAM). More research has been conducted on the effects of weight gain in pregnancy on the health of both the birthing parent and their baby. Excessive weight gain is one of the most important potentially modifiable factors associated with adverse pregnancy outcomes. The then IOM released new weight gain guidelines in 2009 that were based on revised BMI categories and now have a recommendation for obese individuals. However, the IOM did not differentiate by age, race/ethnicity, or subclasses of obesity. As a result, the weight gain guidelines span a wide range, and nurses are challenged to individualize their dietary counseling for the obese individual. To meet the recommendations of the report, weight gain should fall within the weight gain ranges for their BMI category. Achieving the recommended weight gain will require individualized guidance from health care providers. Nurses are uniquely positioned to educate about the NAM guidelines for weight gain in pregnancy and the importance of a healthy diet and adequate physical exercise. In addition, the internet, social media, and eHealth technologies provide unprecedented opportunities to efficiently reach and educate influential family members, friends, and the media (Cunningham et al., 2022).

The NAM guidelines reflect changing US demographics, particularly the surge in the number of those who are overweight or obese. The guidelines advise that those at a normal weight for their height (BMI of 18.5–24.9 kg/m^2) should gain 25 to 35 pounds during pregnancy. Those who are underweight (BMI less than 18.5 kg/m^2) should gain more, 28 to 40 pounds, and overweight (BMI of 25–29.9 kg/m^2) should gain less, 15 to 25 pounds. Patients with obesity (BMI greater than 30 kg/m^2) should limit their gain to 11 to 20 pounds (NAM, 2009).

Obesity is a public health concern worldwide and has reached alarming proportions. It is arising from multifaceted and complex causes that relate to individual choices and lifestyles and the influences of wider society. In addition to a long-standing focus on both childhood and adult obesity, there has been more recent concern relating to maternal obesity. Obese pregnant patients are at increased risk for an array of maternal and perinatal complications. The risks are amplified with the more weight that is gained. Obesity in pregnancy can lead to infants being more likely to be born prematurely, to be stillborn, or to die in the first 28 days of life. Obesity increases the risk of obstetric complications during the prenatal, intrapartum, and postnatal periods, as well as contributing to technical difficulties with fetal assessment. In addition, infants of obese individuals are more likely to be born with a congenital abnormality (Ramsey & Schenken, 2023). Overweight and obese individuals are at increased risk of several pregnancy complications that include abortion, preterm birth, gestational diabetes, hypertension, preeclampsia, thromboembolism, surgical birth, and postpartum weight retention. Despite the serious health implications of obesity in pregnancy, the current level of awareness of such risks among childbearing patients is limited. In addition, many health care providers do not address this health issue with the patient (Jordan et al., 2019).

TABLE 16.1 **Perinatal Care Guidelines**

First Trimester	Second Trimester	Third Trimester	Labor Stages	Postpartum
Complete assessment to identify risk factors	Assess adaptation to pregnancy and fetal well-being	Review physiologic changes	Admission to birthing facility	Complete a head-to-toe physical assessment: breasts, uterus, bladder, bowels, lochia; emotional status; circulatory status; episiotomy
Awareness of subtle or overt physical, sexual, or emotional abuse	Update heath history	Monitor changes related to pregnancy	First stage: Complete maternal/fetal assessments Determine labor progress Assist with comfort measures Monitor fetal heart rate Support family in their efforts Praise efforts	Assess for postpartum blues/ depression
Assess physical and psychosocial progress in adaptation to pregnancy	Continue to recognize cultural influences	Assess expectant family's readiness for labor, birth, and parenting role	Second stage: Offer encouragement Assist with pushing efforts Document activities	Encourage bonding and attachment
Inquire about physical changes and discomforts; explain causes and identify appropriate relief measures	Encourage informed decision-making and positive health care practices	Review finalized birth plan	Third stage: Provide care as needed Document time of placental delivery Administer medications as ordered	Demonstrate breast/chestfeeding techniques
Provide anticipatory guidance appropriate for individual needs	Review potential risk factors and when to report them	Identify community resources available to the family	Fourth stage: Monitor vital signs; fundus, assess bladder status Encourage parental-infant interaction Monitor newborn's well-being Provide perineal care, food, fluids Provide family support	Provide anticipatory guidance needed for the family
Educational needs: hazards during pregnancy Use of drugs, alcohol, and smoking	Ensure community referrals/resources as needed. Educational needs: Oral hygiene Nutritional needs	Explain any diagnostic tests ordered. Meet educational needs: needs for newborn care		Educational needs: Nutrition Fatigue Child care
Seat belts, high-risk behaviors Warning/danger signs to report Nutrition and weight management Sexuality	Safety issues in workplace Discomforts of pregnancy Relief of common discomforts of pregnancy Prepared childbirth classes	Monitor fetal movements Strategies to cope with discomforts Promote family safety Include partner in process Childbirth preparation		Immunizations Sexuality Family planning Breast engorgement Family adaptation Follow-up care needed Danger signs to report Sibling readiness for new member Self-care activities

Ideally, those with a BMI greater than 30 kg/m^2 should be provided at a preconception visit with accurate and accessible information about the risks associated with obesity in pregnancy. Weight-loss interventions would be most appropriately used before pregnancy, but if that is not possible, nurses need to recognize the need for opportunistic health promotion aimed at disseminating information about the risks of obesity in pregnancy to overweight and obese patients of childbearing age. Most birthing parents are highly motivated to have healthy infants, and this could be a key factor in health-promotion discussions that inform of the risks of obesity in pregnancy and promote healthy lifestyle choices and weight-loss strategies preconceptually and between pregnancies.

Labor and Birth

Pregnancy culminates with labor and giving birth. Giving birth is a life-changing event, and the care that an individual receives during labor has the potential to affect her both physically and emotionally for a long period. The process of giving birth elicits a significant emotional response from the delivering family.

Several theories offer explanations for the cause of labor. Many factors likely interact, including uterine distention, mechanical irritation, progesterone deprivation, placental aging and hormones, and posterior pituitary activity. Labor usually begins at approximately 40 weeks of gestation, suggesting that hormonal control similar to that regulating the menstrual cycle also contributes to its onset (Cunningham et al., 2022).

Labor may be divided conveniently into the following four distinct stages:

- **Dilation** stage—lasts from the onset of true labor contractions to complete dilation of the cervix. It is divided into three phases: latent (0 to 3 cm dilation), active (4 to 7 cm dilation), and transition (8 to 10 cm dilation)
- Pushing stage—lasts from complete dilation (10 cm) of the cervix to birth
- Placental stage—lasts from the time of birth of the newborn to delivery of the placenta and membranes, which can range from 2 to 15 minutes
- Recovery stage—defined as the first 4 hours after childbirth, where physiologic and psychological adjustments begin to occur

The **first stage of labor** starts with regular timing of uterine contractions and ends with complete **dilation** (opening) and **cervical effacement** (thinning of the cervix). The signs of beginning labor include those listed in Box 16.3. The cervix, the lower portion of the uterus, must dilate from a closed position (0 cm) to a totally open position (10 cm or 4 inches in diameter). During the first stage, the cervix must also completely efface or shorten from a length of 1 to 2 inches to a barely palpable (paper-thin) thickness. For most, painless Braxton Hicks contractions throughout pregnancy cause some cervical dilation and thinning, or at least cervical softening, before the onset of active labor.

During the first stage of labor, the presenting part of the fetus begins to press on the cervix, lower uterine segment, and nerve endings around the cervix and vagina. The birthing parent's responses to this process differ; pain thresholds and cultural perceptions of and responses to pain differ among laboring individuals. The fundus, the active contractile part of the uterus, becomes thicker as labor progresses, retracts the lower uterine segment and cervix, and helps push the fetus toward the cervix and eventually through the vagina for birth (Blackburn, 2018). The first stage lasts an average of 8 to 12 hours for those experiencing a first birth and somewhat less for those having a second or additional child. Based on a laboring patient's needs, various pain medications, nonpharmacologic measures, Lamaze breathing, and other distractive techniques may alleviate the discomfort associated with first-stage labor. Periodic vaginal examinations by the nurse or other health care provider can indicate a laboring patient's cervical dilation, effacement, and descent of the fetus into the birth canal (a concept called "**station**"). It is important to note that vaginal exams should be reserved for instances in which the information is necessary for the plan of care and should only be performed with a patient's consent. In a full-term pregnancy, loss of the amniotic membrane usually increases pressure of the fetal head against the cervix, making dilation and effacement more efficient, and tends to augment the labor process.

During the **second stage of labor**, the fetus descends through the lower birth canal toward the perineum. It is the time elapsing from the full cervical dilation to the birth of the newborn. The upper uterine segment greatly thickens, and the abdominal muscles assist in the descent and expulsion of the fetus. Birthing parents who have attended childbirth classes are often better prepared to actively push the baby through the pelvis and perineum during contractions. Cultural practices may support pushing from a squatting or upright position and not in a supine one. Nurses must acknowledge that the maternity health care system has a unique culture that may clash with the cultures of many of our care recipients. For many, an overwhelming urge to bear down during uterine contractions occurs at this time. The fetal head accommodates to the pelvis and vaginal structure and, finally, the head becomes flush with the vaginal opening on the perineum. At this point, the birthing parent actively pushes to expel the newborn.

The **third stage of labor** begins after the birth of the newborn and lasts until placental expulsion. Placental separation usually occurs within 2 to 30 minutes after completion of the second stage. After delivery of the placenta, the health care provider examines the placenta to determine that all placental tissue is intact and to detect any abnormalities that could affect the infant's condition and adaptation to extrauterine life.

The **fourth stage of labor** generally consists of the first 2 hours after childbirth, during which the birthing parent faces the greatest risk of postpartum hemorrhage. An expected blood loss of 250 to 500 mL may cause the birthing parent to experience a moderate decline in blood pressure, but nurses should not wait or rely on this change to intervene. A postpartum hemorrhage is defined as blood loss greater than 500 mL with signs and symptoms of hypovolemia within 24 hours of giving birth (Vogel et al., 2019). The birthing parent may also experience an increase in pulse rate (**tachycardia**) to compensate for blood loss during the early postpartum period. The care plan at the end of this chapter addresses the nurse's role in managing the **stages of labor**.

BOX 16.3 Signs of Beginning Labor

- Bloody show or loss of the mucous plug that seals cervical canal during pregnancy
- Regular uterine contractions
- Contractions increasing in intensity, duration, and frequency
- Palpable hardening of the uterus during contractions
- Pain in the lower back radiating to the front of the abdomen

Overview of Care

Professional members of the health care team (nurses, midwives, physicians) play an important role in labor and birth, but a birthing parent's family, partner, or significant other also inherently contributes to her care during labor and birth, particularly in certain cultures. Many practitioners suggest that the expectations and beliefs of a birthing couple have a great effect on how the parents fulfill their roles. Therefore the nurse needs to collaborate with the people who care for the birthing parent to meet that family's needs during pregnancy, labor, and childbearing.

With increases in reproductive technology, alternative methods of conception are now widely available. Those who identify with the lesbian, gay, bisexual, transgender, queer, and other groups (LGBTQ+) population may opt to utilize reproductive technology for their family planning. Nurses need to have a clear understanding of the needs of the LGBTQ+ patients and identify ways to improve the disparities that exist for this population. Many challenges that LGBTQ+ couples face include making complex childbearing decisions, navigating a health care system designed for heterosexual couples, and confronting barriers such as health insurance issues and uncertain legal rights. Changes in health care settings to address the needs of this population might include the need to display equality signs, use of gender-neutral language on medical records, in-service education for all health care personnel to confront any heterosexist bias, and discussion of privacy issues throughout the perinatal period (Landry & Kensler, 2019).

The importance of the nurse's knowledge, caregiving, and support cannot be underestimated during the first stage of labor. Active emotional and physical nursing support decreases the length of many birthing parents' labors, use of analgesics and anesthetics, and number of operative deliveries and may help in reaching their birthing goals (King et al., 2019). Provided that they are accepted by the birthing parent's culture, independent nursing interventions to increase comfort (e.g., giving backrubs or massages, offering ice or warm fluids by mouth, assisting with ambulation and position changes, and providing a clean and dry environment) may help the laboring patient to cope with the challenges of labor. Many laboring patients will request medication to diminish the pain of labor and birth, and the nurse may need to review the options for medication. A laboring patient may depend on the nurse to model breathing techniques to relieve labor discomfort. The nurse may need to explain usual interventions during this stage of labor, including the use of a **fetal heart monitor** (a machine that detects and records fetal heart rate and activity during labor), intravenous fluids, a digital blood pressure machine, and a urinary catheter. Open and clear communication among the health care providers and laboring patient and their significant others, particularly during frequent and difficult uterine contractions, will improve coping before the pushing stage begins.

Contemporary childbearing has benefited from many medical and technical advances, but the current high rate of maternity care interventions may bring about many disadvantages for the healthy majority. Current understanding suggests that safely avoiding unneeded interventions would improve outcomes. Promoting and supporting physiologic births, which are low-technology health and wellness approaches to childbearing, yields better outcomes. Currently, physiologic childbearing refers to childbearing conforming to healthy biologic processes. Evidence-based research reveals that physiologic childbearing facilitates better outcomes by promoting fetal readiness for birth and safety during labor, enhancing labor effectiveness, providing physiologic help with labor stress and pain, providing maternal satisfaction, promoting maternal and newborn transitions, and optimizing breast/chestfeeding and maternal-infant attachment (Calik et al., 2018). Selected physiologic principles include limiting use of maternity care interventions, providing prenatal care that reduces stress and anxiety, fostering the physiologic onset of labor and not artificial intervention, encouraging hospital admission in active labor, providing privacy and reducing anxiety in labor by continuous support, making nonpharmacologic pain measures available, using pharmacologic measures sparingly, fostering spontaneously vaginal births, and supporting continuous skin-to-skin contact between the parents and the newborn and early breast/chestfeeding after birth (USDHHS, 2020).

During the second stage of labor the patient needs reassurance and support for their pushing efforts. Constant reinforcement and education by the nurse about labor progress, fetal heart monitor tracings, and other interventions will give the birthing parent and their support system the guidance needed to give birth to the infant. Throughout labor, the nurse considers the specific cultural and ethnic needs to support nursing assessment and positive responses to labor by the childbearing family.

Active nursing support during the third and fourth stages of labor includes observing the patient for excessive vaginal bleeding after the placenta has been expelled, assisting in breast/chestfeeding their new baby, monitoring vital signs, and implementing uterine massage if the uterus becomes boggy or fails to contract over the placental site. Emotional support during assessments and delivery of information to explain the rationale for assessments are also important nursing roles supported by professional practice standards.

Current hospital guidelines call for birthing parent-baby dyad care on postpartum units. Nurses must therefore be competent in caring for both populations and be able to share a large amount of information in a short time (typically 1 to 3 days) to prepare for discharge. Although teaching and support related to breast/chestfeeding take priority, other topics nurses must address before discharge include bathing, car seat safety, jaundice, safe sleep, vaccinations, follow-up care for both, postpartum mood disorders, and nutrition for both the birthing parent and the baby. Having a standard discharge checklist and pamphlets to give the parents to read will help nurses to ensure a successful transition from the hospital to the home.

Throughout the entire labor and birth process, the nurse carefully observes the laboring patient and fetus so that they can detect early any difficulties with the progress of labor or with maternal or fetal health. Problems may include unusual fetal or uterine activity, the presence of **meconium** (fetal stool) in the amniotic fluid, fetal tachycardia (heart rate greater than 160 beats/min) or fetal **bradycardia** (heart rate less than 110 beats/min) in a full-term infant, and a fetal heart rate that decreases with uterine activity during labor (Coleman, 2019). These events must be reported immediately to the health care provider, with a complete oral and electronic description of the event. The nurse must be aware that abnormal fetal and maternal signs and patterns may be related to factors such as maternal diabetes or hypertension; the type, timing, or dosage of labor medications; uterine contraction pattern; maternal or fetal infections; maternal anemia; preeclampsia; the presence and character of amniotic fluid; bleeding in the pregnant patient or fetus; or early gestational age of the infant (Lockwood et al., 2023).

Our major role as nurses is to provide safe and evidence-based care to promote optimal birth outcomes for all birthing parents. Nurses need to remember there is more than one way to provide this care. Nurses are educated to assess every patient as an individual and to plan care with mutual goal setting for the best outcomes. By assisting all people seeking care from diverse cultures and by adopting our practices as much as possible to embrace the cultural traditions of others, we will enhance the childbearing experience and promote the health of the birthing parent, newborns, and families.

CHANGES DURING TRANSITION FROM FETUS TO NEWBORN

Birth is a relatively hypoxic experience, as newborns undergo a transition from the placenta as the organ of gas exchange to the newborn's lungs. Most newborns experience a smooth transition from intrauterine to extrauterine life. The fetus-to-newborn transition is complex and depends on several factors, including maternal health and chronic medical conditions, the status of the placenta, gestational duration, the presence of fetal anomalies, and birthing room care. When difficulty occurs, however, the newborn's viability depends on the nurse's understanding of the fine balance of chemical, physiologic, and anatomic changes that occur as it makes the transition to postnatal life (Blackburn, 2018).

Nursing Interventions

Nursing activities during this adaptation process include assessment and interventions aimed at specific protection of the infant and prevention of complications. Cold stress should be avoided by the newborn being kept dry and warmly wrapped and by avoidance of environments that cause heat loss. Overall, the nurse should minimally disturb but maximally observe and document the newborn's behavior during reactive periods.

Apgar Score

Assessment of the newborn after the first few hours of life is essentially the same as assessment of the young infant (see Chapter 17). One technique, specific to timing after birth, is the **Apgar scoring system**. It is used as an assessment of overall newborn well-being and stands for "appearance, pulse, grimace, activity, and respiration." This scoring system has historically been used to provide a simple clinical measure to evaluate the newborn's general condition at birth. The Apgar score, obtained at 1 and 5 minutes of age, may be obtained again at 10 minutes of age until the infant's condition has stabilized. A total score is calculated by addition of the values allotted to the categories noted in Table 16.2. The highest possible score is 10. A score of 8 to 10 indicates that the baby is adapting well. The Apgar score does not predict the neurologic development of an infant but may relate to the infant's risk of illness or death during the first year of life, which is important information for parents of an infant with a low Apgar score (Hammond, 2019).

Sex

Sex differences occur in fetal growth. In general, boys grow faster than girls in the third trimester, and at birth boys are slightly heavier, are longer, and have a larger head circumference than girls (Martin et al., 2019). Although more boys are conceived, they tend to be aborted spontaneously more often than girl embryos; the two X chromosomes possessed by female embryos may protect them from the early hazards of pregnancy. After birth, boys continue to have a lower survival rate than do girls (Kliegman et al., 2020).

Race and Culture

Race may affect the health of the fetus in several ways. For example, in the United States, non-Whites (mainly Blacks) have more fraternal twin pregnancies than Whites (Cunningham et al., 2022). Twin fetuses face an increased risk of **preterm birth** because of gestational factors in the birthing parent. Currently, the United States ranks 174th out of 227 countries for **infant mortality rate (IMR)**, with a rate of 5.1 per 1000 live births (Central Intelligence Agency, 2023). This rate reflects the number of infants who die before the end of their first year of life and is the leading indicator of a nation's health. It reveals the higher IMRs and low birth-weight outcomes of Blacks, American Indians, and other ethnic minority populations in the United States. This rate illustrates the complex sociopolitical issues that produce birth outcomes in the United States and those needing attention to reduce the IMR (CDC, 2023b).

Race is also a factor in the frequency of certain genetic and congenital malformations (Box 16.4: Genomics). For example, more babies of Native American, Latino, and Asian descent

TABLE 16.2 Apgar Scoring

	SCORE		
SIGN	0	1	2
Heart rate	Absent	Slow (<100)	>100
Respiratory effort	Absent	Weak cry, hypoventilation	Good strong cry
Muscle tone	Flaccid, limp	Some flexion of extremities	Active motion, extremities well-flexed
Reflex irritability	No response	Grimace	Cry
Color	Blue, pale	Body pink, extremities blue	Completely pink

From Kliegman et al. (2020)

BOX 16.4 GENOMICS

Genetic Testing May Lead to Ethical Dilemmas

Prenatal genetic testing provides important opportunities for assessment of genetic risk and diagnosis. However, some genetic tests do not identify all the possible gene mutations that can cause a particular condition, or they have limited predictive value. Because some genetic tests may not provide all the information that families may want, the test may subsequently require difficult decisions without providing full information. As an example, a cystic fibrosis carrier test can identify couples who are both carriers. When the cystic fibrosis mutations are identified in the parents, prenatal diagnosis can be performed to determine whether a fetus has inherited a cystic fibrosis gene mutation from each parent. However, knowing that a fetus has inherited two cystic fibrosis mutations does not, at this time, predict the severity of the disease in the infant. For couples in this situation, the ethical dilemma involves the decision to continue or to end a pregnancy without having knowledge of the severity of the disorder.

Should the Information Be Obtained if No Treatment or Intervention Exists?

Genetic testing can lead to specific treatments or interventions for some conditions but not for others. This is the case with some disorders that can be detected in expanded newborn screening. When phenylketonuria is identified, dietary intervention allows individuals with this condition to lead healthy and productive lives. Currently, however, not all conditions can be adequately treated. Genetic testing for some conditions for which there are no treatments might have the potential to cause psychological harm, stigmatization, and discrimination. Genetic testing for Huntington disease, a progressive motor and cognitive disorder with onset in midlife, is one example. There are no effective treatments or preventive measures currently available. Thus choosing to have genetic testing for Huntington disease is highly personal, and it is recommended that individuals consider extensive pretest counseling. These tests may lead to decisions that cannot be reversed and are based on a best guess as to what would be the best course of action for the patient and their family. The dilemma that occurs then is whether a newborn should be tested for disorders that we cannot treat.

Ethical decision-making models/frameworks are valuable tools that can assist nurses in addressing ethical dilemmas. Principles of autonomy, informed consent, privacy/confidentiality, beneficence, nonmaleficence, and justice are applicable to use in the ethics involved in genetic testing. These principles should be sensitive to human needs, should be responsive to contextual considerations, and should emphasize the uniqueness of each situation.

- What might be the nurse's role in assisting the family in the decision-making process?
- What assurances can be made regarding privacy and confidentiality of the genetic information to prevent future employment or health insurance discrimination?
- What resources are available to nurses to keep current on prenatal genetic testing?

have cleft palates (an opening in the oral palate) than do Black babies (Wu et al., 2019). Black babies have higher rates of sickle cell anemia (abnormally shaped red blood cells) than do White babies. The total proportion of malformations tends to be approximately the same in all races that have been studied (Whites, Blacks, Hispanics, and Asians; March of Dimes, 2019).

A patient's ethnic background may also influence the health of her fetus on the basis of a link to socioeconomic status. For increasing numbers of homeless and immigrant pregnant individuals, income may support family survival needs but not prenatal care. Minority group pregnant individuals may have fewer economic resources to obtain a nutritious diet or early and consistent high-quality prenatal care. These outcomes may relate to access to health care factors or cultural beliefs that do not support recommended foods or prenatal care (Box 16.5: Healthy People 2030).

BOX 16.5 *HEALTHY PEOPLE 2030*

Selected National Health Promotion and Disease Prevention Objectives for the Prenatal Period

- MICH-01: Reduce the rate of fetal deaths at 20 or more weeks of gestation.
- MICH-02: Reduce the rate of all infant deaths.
- MICH-04: Reduce the rate of maternal deaths.
- MICH-05: Reduce severe maternal complications of pregnancy identified during labor and delivery hospitalizations.
- MICH-06: Reduce cesarean births among low-risk females with no prior births.
- MICH-07: Reduce preterm births.
- MICH-08: Increase the proportion of pregnant females who receive early and adequate prenatal care.
- MICH-09: Increase abstinence from alcohol among pregnant females.
- MICH-10: Increase abstinence from cigarette smoking among pregnant females.
- MICH-11: Increase abstinence from illicit drugs among pregnant females.
- MICH-12: Increase the proportion of females of childbearing age who have optimal red blood cell folate concentrations.
- MICH-13: Increase the proportion of females delivering a live birth who had a healthy weight before pregnancy.
- MICH-14: Increase the proportion of infants who are put to sleep on their backs.
- MICH-15: Increase the proportion of infants who are breast/chestfed exclusively through 6 months.

MICH, Maternal, Infant, and Child Health.

Genetics

The science of genetics has expanded recently to genomics (the science that studies genes that make up the human genome). The completion of the mapping and sequencing of the human genome led to the expansion of research technologies that are currently used to identify genetic and genomic factors that have an influence on people's health. "Genomics" is a fancy word for all of a person's DNA that guides body growth, maintenance, organ development, and repair and is unique to every individual. In humans, a copy of the entire genome—more than 3 billion DNA base pairs—is contained in all cells that have a nucleus. Genetic influences affect the survival and later well-being of the child through several known mechanisms. Extra chromosomes, deleted chromosomes, or translocations usually cause multiple malformations incompatible with life, causing early loss of the fetus via **spontaneous abortion**. Single malformations in an otherwise normal fetus (e.g., clubfoot, cleft palate, or NTD) probably result from a combined effect of many genes (National Human Genome Research Institute, 2019). These defects, found at birth, may be surgically corrected or managed during the child's life. Invasive techniques of **amniocentesis**, chorionic villus sampling, and chromosome analysis have expanded genetic counseling options and interventions when facing possible fetal genetic defects. Nurses now will have to deal with the challenges of the explosion of genomic information to provide personalized health care based on genomics. The nurse, as a vital member of the health care team, needs to assist in informing of genetic and high-risk screening resources when family history or other factors indicate that a fetal genetic defect may be likely.

GORDON'S FUNCTIONAL HEALTH PATTERNS

Box 16.6 provides an example of a pregnancy assessment using Gordon's (2016) functional health patterns.

Health Perception–Health Management Pattern

On the basis of their culture and life experience, a patient may view pregnancy as an illness, as a completely natural and healthy state, or as a combination of the two. This perception will influence their view of their changing body, their attitude toward the usual discomforts of pregnancy such as fatigue or backache, their choice of health-oriented or illness-oriented care, and their decision to seek prenatal care. The patient who sees themselves as healthy and pregnancy as a normal part of her life most likely will seek a health care provider with a similar outlook. Another patient with the same perception may seek help from a socially approved group, as defined by her culture, and avoid standard Western medicine during pregnancy (e.g., Roma [gypsies]). In general, patients with a positive view of pregnancy will continue with active participation in their respective social circles and careers. However, the patient who sees their pregnancy as a time of illness may use this as a reason to withdraw from their work and social obligations.

One's acceptance of their pregnancy influences their health-management practices and choices. The patient who denies or has strong negative feelings about their pregnancy may fail to eat properly, get enough rest and exercise, breast/chestfeed, or seek prenatal care. Some may deny a pregnancy because they never intended to become pregnant despite having sexual intercourse without using birth control. Approximately 50% of American pregnancies are unintended, particularly among vulnerable aggregates such as females aged 18 to 24; those who cohabitate; females with low income; females of color; females who lack health care access, cultural acceptance, and education; those who experience sexual violence; and those who lack financial resources to purchase or use contraceptives. A decrease in the unintended pregnancy rate by 30% was promoted as one of the first Healthy People goals in 2000 but has been changed in Healthy People 2030 (Guttmacher Institute, 2024; USDHHS, 2023b).

BOX 16.6 Assessment for Pregnancy According to Gordon's Functional Health Patterns

Health perception–health management pattern: Aware of or participates in management of pregnancy, or both; expects an uncomplicated pregnancy on the basis of the individual's or significant other's active involvement in their own care; able to state complications of pregnancy that mandate physician notification; engages in health-promotion behaviors specific to pregnancy.

Nutritional-metabolic pattern: Follows diet changes of pregnancy as recommended by nurse; has appropriate weight for height and has gained adequate weight for gestational age of pregnancy; eats three meals a day and two snacks (afternoon and evening), focusing on increased amounts of vegetables and fruits; drinks healthy fluids, including at least eight glasses of water per day; has elastic skin turgor.

Elimination pattern: Experiences occasional constipation from progesterone influence of gastrointestinal peristalsis relaxation, usually corrected by increased fluids, nightly walking, and more diet roughage; voids 7–10 times a day, depending on amount of fluids consumed; no known hemorrhoids or difficulty in elimination; voiding without excess frequency, urgency, or burning; understands signs of urinary tract infection.

Activity-exercise pattern: Walks three times a week for 20 minutes without reports of unusual fatigue or soreness; active at home with housework and at work teaching in a primary school; swam two times a week before pregnancy and moved to current residence.

Sleep-rest pattern: Generally, sleeps 7–8 hours a night; has increased total daily sleep somewhat with fatigue of pregnancy—naps for 1 hour on weekends and 30 minutes after work; sleeps on side and with two pillows for comfort; uses no sleep aids; generally able to relax and initiate sleep without difficulty; occasionally has headache at end of workday and takes acetaminophen (Tylenol) for relief or listens to soft music after work to enhance relaxation.

Cognitive-perceptual pattern: Realizes the need to decrease work activity and increase rest periods as she nears end of pregnancy; answers questions in appropriate tone and words during pregnancy visits; has intact memory (alert and remote); reads about pregnancy and early parenthood to prepare for the birth.

Self-perception–self-concept pattern: States she is excited about pregnancy after 1 year of trying to conceive; well groomed.

Roles-relationships pattern: Lives with husband of 3 years; visits extended family, 60 miles away, every month; shares family roles with husband, accepts this balance; has many friends who support her pregnancy; perceives extensive employee and employer support with pregnancy and time off after delivery.

Sexuality-reproductive pattern: States, "I have a satisfying love life and enjoy my husband"; before pregnancy, engaged in sexual intercourse four to five times a week with desire to become pregnant; with pregnancy and fatigue, has intercourse generally two to three times a week, with pattern acceptable to both partners; no known sexually transmitted infections in past or present.

Coping–stress tolerance pattern: Concerned about fatigue affecting performance as primary school teacher; walks three times a week for 20 minutes to "center myself and feel good"; smiles often, good sense of humor; supportive family excited about her pregnancy.

Values-beliefs pattern: Protestant religion; prays daily and gains strength from religion.

Other data:

- Medication history:
  Prenatal vitamin, one tablet each morning
  Ferrous sulfate, one tablet each morning
  Acetaminophen (Tylenol) 650 mg for occasional headaches
- Physical examination:
  5 feet, 4 inches tall
  Weight 140 pounds (at 14 weeks of pregnancy; weight gain of 5 pounds with pregnancy)
  29 years of age
  Pupils equally round and reactive to light and accommodation
  Temperature 98.2°F; pulse 76 beats/min; respiration 16 breaths/min
  Blood pressure 114/78 mm Hg right arm (sitting, left arm)
  Peripheral pulses equal, strong bilaterally
  Skin warm, dry, elastic turgor; mucous membranes intact, moist; alert, oriented

Modified from Gordon (2016); Potter et al. (2020)

Individuals who are faced with an unplanned or a closely spaced pregnancy may be more likely to have exposures to alcohol, tobacco, and **sexually transmitted infections** or may fail to obtain follow-up care for a high-risk child (i.e., one who experienced complications from childbirth; USDHHS, 2023b; US Preventive Services Task Force [USPTF], 2020a).

Nurses encounter patients with reproductive health needs and concerns in all practice settings and play an important role in caring for them as an integral member of the health care team. The nurse who works with a pregnant population must be sensitive to a wide range of views expressed and work with each to effectively manage their pregnancies. For example, Hispanic individuals are less likely to receive early prenatal care because of a belief that pregnancy is not an illness. The nurse targets interventions that focus on this group's needs and beliefs while adhering to professional practice standards that will improve their outcomes.

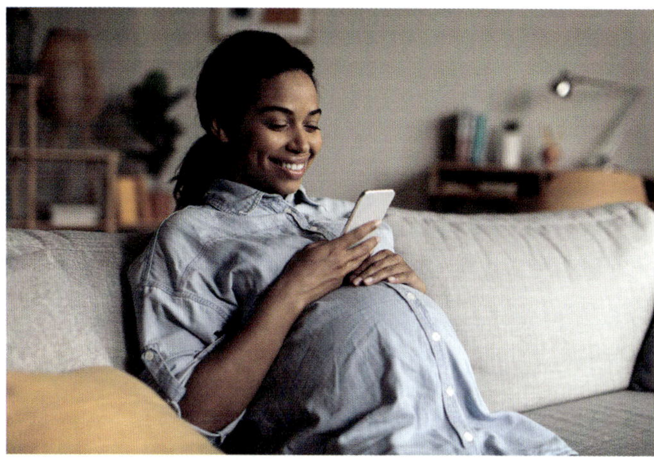

FIG. 16.3 A pregnant female uses technology to connect with her provider virtually. (From iStock.com/ Prostock-Studio.)

Nutritional-Metabolic Pattern

A pregnant person's nutritional status should be assessed preconceptually with the goal of optimizing maternal and fetal health. Pregnancy-related dietary changes should begin before conception, with needed modifications during pregnancy and lactation. Most nutritional requirements of pregnant and lactating patients can be met by their consuming a variety of foods according to government-endorsed guidelines. Massive amounts of literature support the importance of optimal nutrition during pregnancy for maternal and fetal well-being. The key components of nutritional management during pregnancy include consumption of a variety of foods; appropriate weight gain; appropriate micronutrient supplementation; physical activity; and avoidance of alcohol, tobacco, and other harmful substances. Maternal malnutrition before and during pregnancy may exert a teratogenic effect on the fetus. A **teratogen** is an agent or factor that causes developmental malformation. Teratogens principally affect the central nervous system of the fetus, leading to impaired intelligence and performance later in life. They are discussed more in the Environmental Processes section later in the chapter.

Various factors influence the quality of nutrition needed for positive fetal development and birth outcome. Fetal development suffers in cases of adolescent pregnancy or in pregnancies of older individuals who experience poor nutrition between and during several pregnancies. Maternal nutritional deficiencies during an individual's own fetal, infant, and childhood periods also contribute to the development of structural and physiologic disadvantages to supporting a growing fetus. For example, people who are severely underweight before pregnancy often experience higher rates of low birth-weight infants and preterm labor than do people of appropriate prepregnant weight (Cunningham et al., 2022). Inherited maternal stature and pelvic development may influence pregnancy and efficiency of labor and delivery. A lack of income to buy healthy food may also exist, and sometimes cultural values related to food intake influence the quality of nutrition during pregnancy.

To meet increased metabolic, energy, and structural needs for pregnancy, most nutritionists recommend that a pregnant patient increase her intake by approximately 300 calories each day (USDHHS, 2021). This results in a total weight gain of approximately 25 to 35 pounds. It is suggested that 1 to 4 pounds be gained during the first 3 months and 2 to 4 pounds per month during the fourth to ninth months (Fig. 16.3). If at the end of 20 weeks of gestation the patient has not gained at least 10 pounds, they risk delivering an ill infant with fetal growth restriction. This risk also exists when a patient continues to gain insufficient weight throughout the pregnancy or in a patient who was underweight or overweight before pregnancy. Although the rate of gain and the total gain during pregnancy differ among patients, a correlation exists between an erratic pattern of weight gain or a too-rapid weight gain and a lack of fetal well-being (Seymour et al., 2019). The nurse advises the pregnant patient to eat a well-balanced diet. Educating and supporting birthing parents during pregnancy to make healthy food choices to fulfill their needs and the needs of their growing fetus will help promote a healthy start to life.

A well-balanced diet for a pregnant patient parallels that needed by all human beings, with increases in the amounts of certain components as recommended by ACOG (2023a). The nurse recommends that the entire family eat a healthy diet. The nurse encourages the pregnant patient to drink 8 to 10 glasses of water per day to develop amniotic fluid and prevent urinary tract infections (UTIs) often seen with pregnancy. The nurse may also need to encourage the patient to modify her diet to include more fiber and roughage to avoid constipation during pregnancy (Table 16.3).

Protein requirements during pregnancy increase to approximately 70 g/day during the second and third trimesters, or a daily increase of 25 g greater than normal (Sizer & Whitney, 2019). This ensures an adequate supply of amino acids for fetal growth and development, blood volume expansion, and maternal tissue growth. Other protein sources, such as cheese, cream soups, puddings, tofu, and yogurt, may be better tolerated by some and by those from cultures (Hispanic) that do not drink milk. Animal protein and less-expensive legume sources provide protein and, if combined with other healthy food sources, provide high-quality meals (e.g., tuna and rice, peanut butter, and

TABLE 16.3 **Nutritional Needs for Pregnant and Lactating Individuals**

Nutrient	Pregnancy	Lactation	Sources	Comments
Calories	+300	+500	Eat a variety from all food groups	Begin to increase calories in second and third trimesters
Protein	70 g	70 g	Lean meat, fish, eggs, poultry, milk, and dairy products	Supports fetal growth and development; formation of placenta and amniotic fluid; and expanded blood volume
Calcium	1000 mg/day	1000 mg/day	Milk, cheese, dark green leafy vegetables, nuts, and dried fruit	Low calcium intake requires calcium supplements with vitamin D
Iron	27 mg/day	9 mg/day	Lean meats, dark green leafy vegetables, eggs, whole grains, dried fruit, and shellfish	Provides iron for fetal liver storage, which sustains infant for first 4–6 months of life
Folic acid	600 mcg	500 mcg	Fresh green leafy vegetables, liver, peanuts, whole-grain breads, and cereals	All those of childbearing age should take 400 mcg of folic acid daily to prevent neural tube defects in first trimester
Fats	30% of daily calories	30% of daily calories	Low-fat dairy products and lean cuts of meat	Provide a valuable source of energy for the body during pregnancy
Carbohydrates	7–11 servings daily	7–11 servings daily	Dairy products, fruits, vegetables, whole-grain cereals, and breads	Provide fiber necessary for proper bowel functioning. Carbohydrate intake needs to be sufficient to prevent ketoacidosis from protein use for energy

From Sizer, F. S., & Whitney, E. N. (2019). *Nutrition: Concepts and controversies* (15th ed.). Boston, MA: Cengage Learning Inc. Reproduced by permission. www.cengage.com/permissions

whole wheat bread). Protein foods cost more than other foods; therefore, the nurse may need to teach pregnant couples about economical ways to meet protein needs for fetal development.

Mineral intake must also increase during pregnancy. Increased protein intake usually provides the extra needed essential minerals, particularly phosphorus and calcium. The rapid deposit of calcium in fetal bones and teeth during the third trimester of pregnancy requires adequate maternal calcium stores from early pregnancy and continued calcium intake to prevent maternal bone demineralization. Other calcium sources include green, leafy vegetables and calcium-fortified foods, sources more acceptable to cultures with a history of lactose intolerance (African, Mexican, and some European groups).

Sufficient iodine intake by pregnant and lactating individuals is crucial for thyroid hormone production, which contributes to the offspring's neurocognitive development. Approximately one-third of pregnant patients are marginally deficient in iodine. The American Academy of Pediatrics calls for those who are pregnant and lactating to use iodized salt and take a supplement of 150 mcg of iodine daily, which typically is not contained in prenatal vitamins. Because processed and convenient foods make up a large portion of American diets nowadays, patients need to be informed that the salt used in them is not iodized (American Academy of Pediatrics, 2021).

A patient who eats a well-balanced diet should gain sufficient vitamins and minerals for maternal and fetal needs during pregnancy. However, most health care providers recommend that pregnant patients include 27 mg of elemental iron daily to benefit both herself and the fetus, particularly during the last trimester (ACOG, 2023a). Anemia of pregnancy is a global health problem affecting nearly half of all pregnant patients worldwide. High fetal demands for iron, increased erythrocyte mass, and in the third trimester, expanded maternal blood volume render iron deficiency the most common cause of anemia of pregnancy. In certain geographic populations, human pathogens such as hookworms, malarial parasites, and HIV are important factors contributing to anemia of pregnancy. The hemoglobinopathies—sickle cell disease and thalassemia—represent diverse causes of anemia of pregnancy, requiring specialized care. Iron deficiency anemia is common among pregnant patients, and anemia contributes to hemorrhage, postpartum infection, and preterm birth. Anemia occurs more often among pregnant adolescent, Black, and older White patients. The World Health Organization (WHO) defines anemia in pregnancy as a hemoglobin concentration of less than 11 g/dL at any stage of pregnancy (International Federation of Gynecology and Obstetrics (FIGO) Working Group, 2019).

There are almost universal recommendations for periconceptual folic acid supplementation to prevent NTDs. NTDs are congenital malformations that include anencephaly, encephalocele, and spina bifida caused by the failure of fusion of the neural tube, which normally closes between the 22nd and 28th days after conception (at an average of 40 to 42 days after the first day of the last menstrual period). The occurrence of NTDs differs among the population. In the United States, 3000 pregnancies are affected by NTDs annually, and it is estimated that more than 300,000 pregnancies are affected every year worldwide. Increased consumption of folic acid among those of childbearing age can help to prevent approximately 150,000 to 210,000 NTDs that occur globally (CDC, 2023c). However, research has shown that only a small percentage of individuals of childbearing age consume the recommended amount of folic acid, which is critical for early fetal development (USDHHS, 2023b).

Fats and carbohydrates must supply the caloric requirements during pregnancy. Although increased protein intake provides more calories, the body-building requirements of pregnancy and fetal growth demand most of the added protein. Fats and carbohydrates remain the most important sources of energy and essential vitamins and minerals. Supplemental vitamins and minerals, although not known to cause maternal or fetal harm if taken in reasonable doses, probably cost more to meet the nutritional needs of pregnancy than does a well-balanced diet.

Pica is an eating disorder characterized by the ingestion of nonfood substances such as dirt, clay, laundry starch, ashes, plaster, raw rice, paint chips, coffee grounds, and ice. No one knows what causes these cravings, but a combination of biochemical, psychological, and cultural factors may be at work (Young & Cox, 2023). Pica is a symptom of iron deficiency anemia and malnutrition. This practice may contribute to iron deficiency anemia and interfere with nutrient absorption, particularly among those of lower economic status. The first-line treatment for pica involves testing for mineral or nutrient deficiencies and correcting those (National Eating Disorders Association [NEDA], 2019).

The best time to teach a patient about prenatal nutrition is before they become pregnant. Most people do not seek prenatal care until they suspect pregnancy. Therefore the nurse often delivers information about optimal nutrition to the pregnant patient after critical fetal development has already begun. Nutrition is typically monitored during pregnancy through laboratory testing of iron levels, assessment of the patient's feelings of well-being, determination of the actual intake of essential nutrients, and assessment of their pattern and total weight gain during the pregnancy.

In June 2011, the US Department of Agriculture (USDA) unveiled a new food icon, ChooseMyPlate, which replaces MyPyramid as the government's primary food group symbol. ChooseMyPlate is meant to serve as a simple guide to help consumers choose healthful foods. To build a "healthy plate," ChooseMyPlate suggests that consumers choose fruits, vegetables, whole grains, low-fat dairy products, and lean protein foods to get essential nutrients without excess calories. The strategies for creating such a plate include filling half your plate with fruits and vegetables, using whole grains for at least half of your daily grains consumed (e.g., 100% whole-grain cereals, breads, and pasta), switching from whole milk to skim or 1% milk, and choosing a variety of protein sources (e.g., seafood, small portions of lean meat and poultry, and beans). It also recommends that patients should avoid shark, swordfish, king mackerel, or tilefish when they are pregnant or breast/chestfeeding. These fish contain high levels of mercury and should be avoided. In summary, the pregnant patient needs to follow the USDA Daily Food Plans for Moms as follows:

- Fruits and vegetables—seven or more servings daily (three servings of fruit and four of vegetables)
- Whole-grain or enriched breads/cereals—six to nine servings daily
- Dairy products—three to four servings of low-fat or nonfat milk, yogurt, or cheese daily
- Meat and beans—three servings daily (one serving is equivalent to 2 ounces; USDA, 2019)

See Chapter 11 for more specific information on nutrition.

Elimination Pattern

Fetus

The fetus accomplishes all essential elimination functions through the placenta. Carbon dioxide, water, urea, and other waste products pass through the placenta to be eliminated. By the end of the first trimester, the fetus swallows, makes respiratory movements, and urinates. However, these abilities become truly functional only after birth.

Pregnant Patient

The pregnant patient experiences changes in their elimination pattern because of the enlarging uterus and hormonal influences. These changes (urinary frequency during the first and third trimesters, constipation, and hemorrhoids) cause normal, minor discomforts. Anticipatory guidance by the nurse helps the patient to cope with these changes and prevent complications of pregnancy. For example, teaching commonsense measures (Box 16.7: Best Practice) may prevent UTIs, typically a problem that is more common during pregnancy. With a known correlation between UTIs and preterm labor, a focus on preventing and managing these infections must occur during pregnancy.

Activity-Exercise Pattern

Fetus

Early spontaneous movements of the fetus may be reflexive, stimulated by passive uterine movement. Ultrasonographic observation of fetal movement shows repetitive movements early in pregnancy; at approximately 16 weeks, the pregnant individual feels these movements, termed "quickening." By the end of the second trimester, fetal movement occurs less frequently because of lack of space in the uterus. The birthing parent and their partner look forward to the regular daily cycle of movements, indicators of fetal well-being. An absence of or a dramatic increase in fetal movements for more than 8 hours may indicate fetal distress. The nurse routinely teaches the birthing parent to count the number of fetal movements each day typically starting at 28 weeks of gestation and report any decrease in fetal activity to the health care provider.

Pregnant Patient

The physical changes during pregnancy and the rigors of labor and delivery require that a pregnant person be in the best physical condition of their life. Fortunately, many pregnant patients view pregnancy as a normal, natural state, and they often participate actively in physical activities or sports enjoyed before pregnancy. In general, a pregnant person should avoid high-risk sports, such as sky diving and high-altitude climbing, because these could cause trauma to the fetus from low oxygen pressure or a maternal fall. Nurses encourage each patient to choose activities on the basis of their interests, comfort, and good judgment. When a sport or activity causes exhaustion or pain, it should be modified or discontinued. Later in pregnancy, the patient should be encouraged to choose safe

BOX 16.7 **BEST PRACTICE**

Evidence-Based Practice for Preventing UTIs and Promoting Genitourinary Health

Pregnancy can increase susceptibility to UTIs because of physiologic changes. Current management of UTIs in pregnancy is with a short course of antibiotics. Excessive and unnecessary use of antibiotics is associated with a rise in antimicrobial resistance, which may lead to life-threatening infections that resist therapy. It is essential that primary prevention of UTIs be used to address this growing antimicrobial resistance.

- Increase fluid intake to approximately 8–10 glasses per day; plain water is best to flush the body's systems of potential toxins; drink a glass of water before sexual intercourse to allow urinary output afterward to prevent UTIs.
- Avoid bladder irritants such as caffeine products, alcohol, artificial sweeteners, spicy foods, and carbonated beverages.
- Make urination a regular habit; avoid waiting to urinate until bladder is full.
- Wash the genitals after sexual intercourse.
- Avoid taking tub baths.
- Use liquid soap to prevent colonization from bar soap.
- Be aware that vigorous or frequent intercourse may contribute to increased risk of UTIs.
- Maintain consistently good perineal hygiene, including wiping from front to back after urination and defecation.
- Take all prescription medications given for UTIs, even when the symptoms of the infection have been alleviated.
- Drink cranberry juice to acidify the urine or take cranberry pills; these products may relieve some of the symptoms of a UTI. Cranberry (*Vaccinium macrocarpon*) has demonstrated antiinflammatory, antiadhesive, and antioxidant properties.
- Seek health care advice for a vaginal infection, which may contribute to development of a UTI.
- Nurses need to be aware that most UTIs are caused by *Escherichia coli*, and most are asymptomatic. Obtaining a urine specimen and culture is needed with any degree of suspicion of a UTI.
- Approximately half of UTIs in pregnancy occur in those with preexisting asymptomatic bacteriuria, and these UTIs have poor outcomes, including preterm rupture of membranes, preterm birth, neonatal infection, preeclampsia, maternal anemia, amnionitis, and maternal septic shock.
- The nurse should assess for increased risk of developing a UTI: congenital or structural abnormalities of the genitourinary system, previous surgery to the genitourinary system; pregnancy; previous UTIs; high intake of carbonated beverages; and poor intake of water.

UTI, Urinary tract infections.
From Ghouri et al. (2019)

physical activities because of changes in their center of gravity attributable to the enlarging uterus and changes in the musculoskeletal system.

The patient with a sedentary lifestyle before pregnancy should slowly increase their activity level during pregnancy. A daily swim or 30-minute walk provides a good introduction to a regular exercise program. Regular exercise contributes to joint flexibility, increased cardiovascular and gastrointestinal fitness, decreased uterine tone for an efficient labor, fewer pregnancy discomforts, weight control and a lower risk of diabetes by maintaining glycemic control, and overall feelings of well-being in the pregnant patient (USDHHS, 2023b). For most, group exercise with other pregnant people is more enjoyable than exercising alone. The benefits of physical activity in the general population are established and include strengthening and toning muscles, boosting energy level, promoting better sleep, relieving stress, and helping weight loss. Research finds that regular physical activity following childbirth is linked to improved health outcomes. However, many do not resume prepregnancy exercise levels (ACOG, 2022).

In an uncomplicated pregnancy, a couple may continue their usual sexual activity, as the fetus is protected by strong uterine muscles, amniotic fluid, and a mucous plug that develops around the cervix. However, threatened abortion or a history of abortion in the first trimester, early rupture of membranes, and other complications may call for restrictions on sexual intercourse or orgasm.

Sleep-Rest Pattern

Fetus

Electroencephalographic studies have shown four cyclical states of activity in the fetus: complete wakefulness, drowsy wakefulness, rapid eye movement sleep, and quiet sleep. Evidence suggests that a diurnal (day-night) pattern exists during the fetal period. Sleep is required for somatic and brain growth and development. Sleep-wake patterns change with central nervous system maturation. In one research study, the median relative percentage of time spent in a quiet state was 26%. The median duration of time spent in a quiet state can be up to 60 minutes. Both quiet states and active states were established in 84% of the fetuses studied (Umana & Siccardi, 2023). Infant development entails increasing amounts of quiet sleep as well as increasing periods of quiet alertness. Both states require remarkable neural organization; thus sleep-wake patterns are an excellent window into the infant's neurologic status.

Pregnant Patient

Fatigue reflects the significant physical and emotional changes occurring during the pregnancy. The nurse counsels that fatigue usually subsides by the fourth month but may return later in pregnancy. Rest breaks during the day and 8 hours of sleep each night help prevent fatigue and increase comfort. The nurse encourages rest based on when the body signals it is tired because of the rapidly growing fetus and the patient's needs for physical renewal. This encouragement must be directed particularly toward working pregnant people, who may need a physician's note for their employer that validates the need for rest during the workday.

Many people experience significant sleep disruption and inadequate sleep throughout pregnancy. This is due to the need to urinate several times a night during the first and third trimesters. In addition, some experience positional discomfort in late pregnancy that prevents effective sleep and therefore increases their fatigue. The nurse helps the patient to express their thoughts and feelings and find ways to support better sleep and rest patterns (e.g., sleeping upright in a chair at night for easier breathing).

Cognitive-Perceptual Pattern

Fetus

During the prenatal period, although motor functions lag behind, all fetal sensory systems function or nearly function.

BOX 16.8 Topics for Prenatal Care Teaching

- Rationale for and interpretation of physical findings and laboratory results
- Value of keeping appointments
- Danger signs that should be reported
- Breast care to prepare for lactation
- Breast/chestfeeding versus bottle feeding
- Exercise and rest
- Fetal growth and development
- Physical and psychological changes during pregnancy and relief measures
- Effects of smoking, drinking, and drugs on the fetus
- Nutrition
- Work and play
- Body mechanics
- Personal hygiene
- Sex during pregnancy
- Preparation for labor and birth
- Superstitions and old wives' tales
- Signs of impending labor
- Supplies and preparations for the baby
- Partner and sibling responses

These systems include vision, hearing, taste, smell, touch, and proprioceptive and vestibular senses (Blackburn, 2018). The fetus with all senses intact experiences the discomfort of pregnancy and the pain of labor contractions. The visual system matures relatively late in gestation, especially compared with the tactile, olfactory, and auditory systems. Although capable of seeing by 30 weeks of age, the fetus has little opportunity to use this ability in utero because of the absence of light (Blackburn, 2018). After approximately 25 weeks, babies respond to a loud, sudden noise. Some pregnant people and their partners offer sensory stimulation to the fetus by singing or rubbing the abdomen. This parental behavior may assist in the bonding process between the parent and the baby. Thus the nurse may wish to include this kind of information in prenatal teaching sessions (Box 16.8: Topics for Prenatal Care Teaching).

Pregnant Patient

Physical and psychological processes remain closely intertwined as pregnancy progresses. Psychological stresses and normal emotional growth affect the physical status of the pregnancy, interactions of the family members, and the eventual relationship between the parents and the infant. When considering the emotional aspects of pregnancy, the nurse recognizes that the patient's personality, environment, physical state, family, and sociocultural and spiritual background affect the ways in which she handles the psychological changes (Fig. 16.4).

Two major categories of psychological influences are normal psychological growth required of parents to emotionally and physically prepare them for parenthood and internal or external stressors on the pregnant patient that decrease their ability to provide the best environment for the developing fetus. The pregnant patient undergoes many cognitive changes that ultimately result in their psychological readiness for parenthood. Nurses can plan strategies and instruct on ways to promote resilience to cope with all the changes experienced throughout pregnancy.

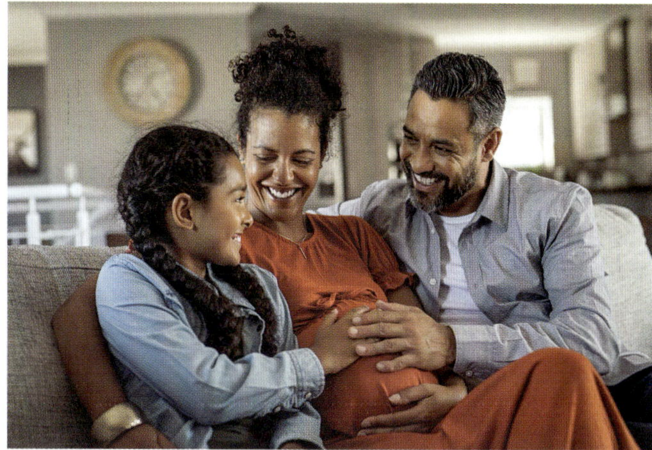

FIG. 16.4 A pregnant female enjoys time with her family. (From iStock.com/ Ridofranz.)

Emotional Changes. Biologic and psychosocial changes during pregnancy affect emotional well-being and the ability to cope with stress. Hormonal and other physical changes assist in the psychological work of pregnancy. Progesterone level increases affect the general mood, causing more introverted behavior. These mood changes help to focus energy on the growing child and the birthing parent's own growth and development. In addition to hormonal changes, the presence, growth, and movements of the fetus become more a part of the birthing parent's experiential self. According to Rubin (1984), the classic researcher on maternal-infant bonding, the pregnant person receives immediate sensations of touch, motion, and weight from the fetus that they can share only partially with others. These support a maternal feeling of separateness and uniqueness that causes the pregnant person to turn inward. They frequently worry that the shift in energy away from the world toward themselves and their child may cause them to lose contact, drift away from valued relationships, and lose feelings of competence in areas of achievement. They spend time analyzing their experiences and their possible influence on their effectiveness as a future parent. They constantly study the qualities of human relationships and show increased sensitivity and perceptiveness to many people. To others, the pregnant person may seem overly sensitive and analytical during pregnancy (Jordan et al., 2019).

Although mood varies on the basis of a variety of factors and at different times during the pregnancy, many people experience wide mood swings, emotional lability, irritability, and changes in sexual desire. Physical discomforts, hormonal changes, feelings about altered body image, cultural considerations, work and relationship adjustments, and demanding cognitive maturational processes may also cause these emotional changes.

Rubin's classic work stimulated nurses to look beyond the physiologic and pathologic aspects of childbearing to the intricate process of becoming a parent and to identify areas for providing help. The parental role is developed over time as the parent learns to love, respond to, and care for their newborn. Current research identifies two simultaneous processes in the transition to parenthood: engagement and growth and transformation. Engagement is making a commitment and being engrossed in parenting through active involvement in the child's care. At the same time, the engagement leads to growth and transition as they become a parent. The bond between a parent and their newborn is one of strength, power, and potential (Denbow, 2019).

Current descriptions for the stages in the process of becoming a parent include the following:

- Commitment, attachment, and preparation for the pregnancy
- Acquaintance, learning, and physical restoration during the first 6 weeks after birth
- Movement toward a new normal from 2 weeks to 4 months

Nurses can promote the parental-newborn bond through encouraging skin-to-skin contact, breast/chestfeeding, eye contact, and newborn massage during the first hour after childbirth.

Perinatal Mental Health. Family planning, trying to conceive, pregnancy, the transition to parenthood, pregnancy loss, and the postpartum period are all vulnerable times in which a birthing parent or their support person can develop a perinatal mental health disorder. Although stress and times of transition can be difficult, when symptoms begin to affect one's ability to function in their day-to-day life is when there is cause for concern. Postpartum depression has become an overarching diagnosis category for any mental health disorder occurring in the perinatal period; however, many individual mental health disorders can occur in the perinatal period. The Mental Health Technology Transfer Center (MHTTC) Network (2023) states that the following mental health disorders are included in the category of perinatal mental health disorders:

- Perinatal depression
- Perinatal anxiety and panic disorders
- Obsessive compulsive disorder (OCD)
- Posttraumatic stress disorder (PTSD)
- Perinatal bipolar disorder and postpartum mania
- Postpartum psychosis
- Perinatal substance use
- Parental suicide
- Complicated grief after perinatal loss

It is estimated that one in seven females experience postpartum depression. In addition, and importantly, is that approximately 7% to 9% of new fathers experience postpartum depression (Healthy Children.org, 2023). Although the majority of available research focuses on male partners or fathers, partners of all genders are susceptible to perinatal depression. The nurse's role in educating patients on perinatal mental health warning signs is an essential first step to early identification and intervention for those in need. Patients should be screened for perinatal mental health disorders preconceptually, at the first prenatal visit, in each trimester thereafter, before discharge postpartum, and at any postpartum or infant visit for the first 6 months postpartum. According to Healthy Children.org (2023), signs and symptoms to report include:

- Excessive feelings of sadness, worry, and/or anxiety
- Obsessive fears or anxiety regarding infant's health and well-being
- Low energy, even after rest
- Mood swings
- Frequent crying
- Feelings of anger or irritability
- Brain fog that affects basic decision-making
- Inability to take care of oneself and complete activities of daily living
- Difficulty falling or staying asleep
- Difficulty eating or loss of appetite
- Not bonding with the infant
- Thoughts of harming oneself or their infant

Due to the colossal hormonal shifts that occur during the postpartum period, it is common to have what is referred to as "baby blues" during the first 1 to 2 weeks in the postpartum period. The baby blues may include feeling tearful, mood changes, and some mild anxiety. Symptoms extending beyond 2 weeks or severe symptoms such as the ones noted previously, should be reported to the health care provider.

Unfortunately, due to the stigma that exists, it is estimated that as many as 50% of patients with diagnosable perinatal mental health disorders are often not willing to disclose symptoms (Mughal et al., 2022). This can be due to a multitude of reasons including personal shame and even fear that their infants could be taken away. Perinatal mental health disorders extend beyond the individual. Children of parents who have untreated depression can develop behavioral and emotional problems. These can include delays in language development, sleeping problems, eating difficulties, excessive crying, and attention-deficit hyperactivity disorder (ADHD; Mughal et al., 2022).

Stressors Influencing Development. Age, fears related to a previous fetal loss, feelings about the pregnancy, life situation and culture, degree of stress, loss of control at times, unintended pregnancy, the presence of other children, and the influence of loved ones may serve as stressors that influence the ways in which the parents complete the developmental tasks of parenthood. People with unwanted pregnancies have multiple risk factors and would benefit from targeted interventions that will promote emotional well-being (Guttmacher Institute, 2024). A young pregnant person facing the additional developmental task of adolescence may have difficulty incorporating the pregnant body or the role of being a parent into their still undefined self-image. Cognitively, they may still be unable to make plans for the baby or even accept the pregnancy until they feel the baby move. Anticipatory guidance is critical when an adolescent faces overlapping developmental challenges of age and pregnancy.

A pregnant person with other children moves through the developmental tasks differently from a person who is pregnant for the first time. Even with a desired pregnancy, they may worry about incorporating the new infant into their relationships and managing the time needed for a new baby. They may have fears and anxieties about labor and delivery because of a previous negative experience. They may be much more aware of the problems involved with caring for a new infant and may not be excited about another pregnancy experience that demands a redefinition of parenthood or additional childrearing expenses.

Developmental Tasks

Rubin (1984) describes four major developmental tasks that a pregnant person seeks to accomplish as they learn to become a parent. These include ensuring safe passage through pregnancy and childbirth, ensuring acceptance of the child by significant people in their family, binding to their unknown child, and learning to give of self. According to Rubin, all four tasks must be confronted simultaneously, but each task assumes greater priority at certain times than do other tasks. Each person works through these tasks on the basis of their unique style, cultural values, and life priorities. However, at the end of pregnancy, all tasks must be integrated to create a presentation, similar to a tapestry (Rubin, 1984).

Ensuring Safe Passage. The pregnant person engages in a variety of prenatal care options appropriate to their culture and life experience (Rubin, 1984).

Ensuring Acceptance of the Child. The pregnant person must believe that their child will be accepted into her family based on her definition of family (Rubin, 1984).

Binding to Their Unknown Child. This task is the most complex cognitive process for the pregnant person. To accomplish this task, they must integrate the fetus as an integral part of themself but also as a separate being. Completion of this task occurs with birth of the baby (Rubin, 1984).

Learning to Give of Themselves. Although the actual parenting activity occurs after birth, the learning process to become a parent often begins during pregnancy (Rubin, 1984).

ENVIRONMENTAL PROCESSES

Physical Agents

A healthy infant is the desired outcome of most pregnancies. However, genetic abnormalities and environmental hazards may cause fetal harm, spontaneous abortion (natural loss of conceptive products), or minor or serious congenital defects. The WHO (2023a) estimates that congenital defects affect 3% to 4% of all live births and contribute to IMRs by causing structural or functional disability incompatible with life. Every year, an estimated 303,000 infants worldwide die of congenital anomalies within 1 month after their birth. Real-time ultrasonography identifies approximately 85% of fetal anomalies by 36 weeks of gestation. The best time for a fetal scan is at 18 to 20 weeks of gestation (Cunningham et al., 2022). This knowledge, gained before giving birth, permits expectant couples and the health care delivery team to access resources for improving the baby's life or to support a grieving family if the baby is not expected to live. With progress made in diagnostic tools and the Human Genome Project, some couples may be able to prevent fetal defects or manage them during pregnancy to improve the quality of their baby's life after birth (see the Case Study at the end of this chapter). Unfortunately, even when no genetic or congenital defects exist, the fetus may still be injured during the process of labor and delivery and face a lesser quality of life.

Teratogens are environmental agents that cause spontaneous abortions or congenital defects. Examples would include mercury, potassium iodide, radiation, alcohol, tobacco, lead, and certain infections. Unlike genetic abnormalities, which occur only at conception, environmental agents may affect the developing infant at any point during gestation. Fetal organs have critical periods of development, and if affected at that time by a teratogen, the infant may have a defect in that organ system. Teratogens normally do not cause a congenital defect during the first 14 days after conception. However, the embryo may be lost later during early gestation (a spontaneous abortion). Therefore as a primary prevention strategy, anyone contemplating or attempting pregnancy should be counseled to avoid teratogens that might cause fetal loss or damage.

Physical Factors and Diagnostic Tools

Modern diagnostic tools, such as ultrasonography, amniocentesis, chorionic villus sampling, and alpha fetoprotein screening, have been used to identify a number of fetal problems. Certain risk factors, some of which may be found in the family history, or maternal and paternal age, maternal illness, or previous fetal abnormalities, may indicate the need for these diagnostic tools during a person's pregnancy. These tools commonly identify problems related to abnormal size or rate of fetal growth, chromosomal abnormalities, NTDs, and fetal lung immaturity. The nurse, in consultation with the health care team, must participate in providing informed consent to the patient before these diagnostic tools are used.

Biologic Agents

Biologic processes in the fetal environment, which include infections and other health problems, may affect fetal growth and development. A pregnant person who acquires an asymptomatic viral infection may not seek health care because she believes that the fetus will not be harmed. However, viral agents may cause fetal damage early in pregnancy. The patient with a chronic health problem, such as diabetes, may also cause fetal damage if she fails to adhere to her health care provider's directives to keep her blood glucose under control.

When the nurse discusses with pregnant couples the effects of biologic processes on the fetus, they must emphasize that the timing of the maternal infection or illness is critical to predicting fetal defects. Maternal infections during the first trimester of pregnancy may cause severe fetal defects or death, depending on the organism. Infections later in pregnancy may also seriously affect the fetus, but this does not happen as often. Unfortunately, pregnancy renders many susceptible to viral illness, supporting an argument for all people of childbearing age to be fully immunized. Many vaccines (measles, mumps, rubella, and polio) cannot be given during pregnancy because of potential risk to the fetus, but others present no risk (tetanus and diphtheria). A TORCH (**toxoplasmosis**, other agents, rubella, **cytomegalovirus** [CMV], **herpes simplex**; other infections include *Treponema pallidum*, hepatitis viruses, HIV, varicella, parvovirus B19, and enteroviruses) screen may be done to detect the presence of teratogenic perinatal infections: toxoplasmosis, hepatitis B, rubella, CMV infection, and herpes simplex (Table 16.4). TORCH infections are major contributors to prenatal, perinatal, and postnatal morbidity and death. Evidence of infection may be seen at birth, in infancy, or years later. For many of these pathogens, treatment or prevention strategies are available, but early recognition, including prenatal screening, is essential.

TABLE 16.4 Perinatal Infections

Infection	Agent	Source	Fetal-Neonatal Risks	Comments
Toxoplasmosis	Protozoan *Toxoplasma gondii*	Raw or undercooked meat; unpasteurized goat's milk; feces of infected cats	Fetal growth restriction, hydrocephaly, seizures, neurologic and cognitive effects, chorioretinitis, intracranial calcifications	Instruct to not eat undercooked or raw meat; avoid exposure to cat litter
Other/hepatitis B	Hepadnavirus	Blood or blood products; sexually transmitted via body fluids	Generally asymptomatic, but majority become chronically infected	Newborn should receive HBIG within 12 h after birth and hepatitis B vaccine postpartum
Rubella	Rubella virus	Direct or indirect contact with droplets of infected person	CNS defects, developmental delay, deafness, cataracts, IUGR, microcephaly, cardiac defects, glaucoma	Screen all pregnant patients with rubella antibody titers
Cytomegalovirus	Herpes virus	Transmitted by droplet infection from person to person	Microcephaly, fetal growth restriction, CNS abnormalities, deafness, blindness, jaundice, gastrointestinal defects, seizures	Prevention of maternal primary infection in early pregnancy; stress good personal hygiene
Herpes simplex	HSV-1 and HSV-2	Sexually transmitted infection; fetus contracts it during birth from genital lesions	Intense herpetic lesions on eyes, mouth, and skin; keratitis; conjunctivitis	Practice safer sex; careful handwashing; surgical birth if active lesions

CNS, Central nervous system; *HBIG,* hepatitis B immune globulin; *HSV-1,* herpes simplex virus type 1; *HSV-2,* herpes simplex virus type 2; *IUGR,* intrauterine growth restriction.
From Norwitz et al. (2019); Cunningham et al. (2022); Phillippi & Kantrowitz-Gordon (2023).

Toxoplasmosis

Toxoplasmosis is caused by a protozoan that infects people through consumption of undercooked meat, handling of feces of cats that become infected by eating infected rodents and birds, and exposure to contaminated soil, in countries outside the United States (CDC, 2022a). An infected pregnant person is usually asymptomatic but may have flulike symptoms or mild-to-severe upper respiratory tract symptoms believed to be unrelated to an infection. Vertical transmission from an infected pregnant person to the fetus predominantly occurs when infection is acquired for the first time during pregnancy. Overall, approximately one-third of infected pregnant people give birth to an infant with toxoplasmosis, and the risk of vertical transmission rises sharply with gestational age at maternal infection. However, fetuses infected during an early pregnancy period are much more likely to show clinical signs of infection, such as chorioretinitis, hydrocephalus, or intracranial calcification (King et al., 2019). Approximately 60% of maternal infections acquired during the third trimester will result in fetal infection, which might manifest itself as rashes, enlarged lymph nodes and liver, blindness, inflammation of the heart, pneumonia, jaundice, or severe central nervous system damage after birth or years later (CDC, 2022a). Nurses can offer some simple hygiene suggestions that reduce the risk of infection. For example, humans can acquire toxoplasmosis from eating undercooked or raw meat (especially lamb and pork), from being exposed to contaminated soil or water, or from consuming uncooked vegetables. Clearly, nurses should advise pregnant patients to cook meat thoroughly and wash and scrub vegetables well, especially those eaten raw. Good handwashing hygiene should be encouraged, eating raw meat should be avoided, food should be cooked to safe temperatures, gloves should be worn when gardening, handling cats and cleaning cat litter boxes should be avoided, cats should be kept indoors, and outdoor sandboxes should be kept covered to avoid exposure to toxoplasma.

Syphilis

Syphilis is an STI that can be transmitted through oral, anal, or vaginal contact. The WHO (2023b) estimates approximately 1.5 million females are diagnosed with syphilis infections each year, whereas 520,000 present with complications in pregnancy. An infected patient transfers syphilis, caused by a bacterium, to her fetus. The causative organism, *Treponema pallidum*, can be transferred across the placenta and can infect the developing fetus as early as 9 weeks of gestation. The risk of vertical transmission and infection in the newborn is directly related to the stage of syphilis during pregnancy; transmission occurs more frequently during primary or secondary syphilis in the patient than during latent stages of the disease. Although syphilis is preventable and treatable, the number of congenital and neonatal syphilis cases has increased in the past several years (CDC, 2023d). Maternal risk factors for acquiring syphilis include homelessness, **HIV**-positive status, single marital status, and a history of STIs. Maternal syphilis has been associated with complications such as **hydramnios**, spontaneous abortion, fetal death, and preterm birth. Fetal complications such as fetal syphilis, fetal hydrops, prematurity, fetal distress, and **stillbirth** also occur. Neonatal complications can include congenital syphilis, seizures, neonatal death, and late sequelae (Kliegman et al., 2020). The infant may be born with localized mucocutaneous lesions, nasal congestion, anemia, and generalized septicemia but may appear healthy at birth only to have symptoms appear later. Routine testing for syphilis at the first prenatal visit and during the third trimester and antibiotic treatment (benzathine penicillin G intramuscularly) for affected patients and their partners have reduced the number of infants with congenital syphilis (Lockwood et al., 2023).

Rubella

Rubella is a viral illness that can lead to complications and death. Despite the broad use of the measles, mumps, and rubella (MMR) vaccine and the resulting immunity to rubella, approximately 20% of females reach their childbearing period without immunity to this disease. Rubella was declared eliminated from the United States in 2004 but has reemerged recently due to a decrease in vaccination rates. Because rubella continues to circulate throughout the world, an estimated 100,000 infants are born with congenital rubella syndrome annually worldwide (CDC, 2020a). The risk of vertical transmission from a nonimmune individual with primary rubella infection in the first trimester of pregnancy is considerably high at up to 90%. Beyond the first 12 weeks of gestation, fetal organogenesis is nearly complete, and deafness may be the only consequence in the infected infant. Deafness, cataracts, psychomotor delays, and cardiac defects are the classic congenital anomalies associated with a rubella infection (Kliegman et al., 2020). The symptoms of rubella may cause the individual to think they have a minor viral infection, but rubella during the first trimester may cause improper fetal development of the ears, eyes, and heart. No treatment exists for an infected fetus; however, a pregnant person may receive the vaccine to protect future pregnancies if she has no history of rubella infection. After giving birth, individuals often receive the vaccine before being discharged with a recommendation to avoid pregnancy for at least 3 months to prevent fetal harm from the vaccine.

Cytomegalovirus

CMV is a virus in the herpes virus family and is a leading cause of congenital infections and long-term neurodevelopmental disabilities among children. Contact with young children has been identified as the main source of virus transmission. It is the most common infection that can cause serious fetal complications. More than half of adults by age 40 have been infected with CMV. It infects an estimated 1 out of every 200 newborns, and approximately 1 in 5 of those infants with congenital CMV will experience long-term health problems (CDC, 2020b). Most people infected with CMV have mild, often nonspecific symptoms, but their infants may experience hearing loss, blindness, enlarged liver and spleen, seizures, intracranial calcifications, and neurodevelopmental disabilities (Kliegman et al., 2020). Unfortunately, no means exist to prevent or manage this viral infection. Perhaps an immunization similar to that for rubella will be developed in the future. Until vaccines and nontoxic antiviral agents are available, hygienic measures are important as prophylaxis and should be emphasized by all nurses to their prenatal care recipients.

Herpes Simplex Virus

Herpes simplex virus infections remain extremely common nowadays, with up to 90% of people unaware that they have the disease. It is estimated that 16% of adults in the United Sates are infected with herpes simplex virus. Herpes is a lifelong infection that has the potential for transmission throughout the life span (King et al., 2019). Neonatal herpes is one of the most serious complications of genital herpes and can be fatal for newborns. The estimated rate of neonatal herpes ranges from 1 in 3000 and 1 in 20,000 live births (Fernandes et al., 2024)). Herpes simplex may cause spontaneous abortion or fetal neurologic damage. Infants infected at birth may show localized or generalized disease with symptoms of vesicular skin lesions, microcephaly, hydrocephalus, chorioretinitis, conjunctivitis, seizures, respiratory distress, or gastrointestinal bleeding. These symptoms may cause newborn death. An infant delivered vaginally by someone with active genital herpes has a 50% chance of being infected (CDC, 2023e), supporting a decision for a cesarean delivery for any individual with active vaginal or perineal herpes lesions. Risk factors for the transmission of herpes from the birthing parent to the newborn have been detailed. The pregnant person who acquires genital herpes as a primary infection in the latter half of pregnancy rather than before pregnancy is at greatest risk of transmitting this virus to her newborn. This is true for both herpes simplex virus type 1 and herpes simplex virus type 2 (Kenner et al., 2019). In general, an antiviral agent is recommended during pregnancy for treatment of viral lesions. The nurse educates the infected patient about comfort measures at this time, including ways to keep the lesions dry and application of comfort measures to reduce the pain of the lesions. In addition, meticulous hand hygiene is essential to prevent transmission of the virus (Jordan et al., 2019).

Zika Virus Disease

Zika virus is transmitted to humans primarily through the bite of an infected *Aedes* species mosquito during the daytime. The most common symptoms of Zika virus disease are fever, rash, headaches, bone pains, joint tenderness, and conjunctivitis. The illness is typically mild, with symptoms lasting for several days to a week after the person has been bitten. In the United States, approximately 15% of pregnant people with confirmed Zika virus infection in the first trimester will have infants with Zika-associated birth defects—microcephaly, brain damage, eye anomalies, seizures, developmental delays, and hypotonia (CDC, 2022b). The virus has been reported to be spread through blood transfusions, organ transplants, and sexual contact, but can also be passed from a pregnant person to her fetus. The CDC recommends abstaining from oral, anal, or vaginal sexual contact with anyone who has traveled to areas with active infections.

Chlamydia, Gonococcus, Group B Streptococcus, Bacterial Vaginosis, and Candida albicans

Infections caused by chlamydia, gonococcus (GC), group B streptococcus, and yeast (*Candida albicans*) may occur in the vagina or cervix, infecting the infant during a vaginal birth. Chlamydia, the most common bacterial STI, appears most often among poor individuals, with almost two-thirds of new infections occurring among youth aged 15 to 24 years. It is estimated that 1 in 20 sexually active females aged 14 to 24 years has chlamydia (CDC, 2023f). Although few symptoms are seen, infection may cause preterm labor, premature rupture of membranes, low birth-weight infants, newborn conjunctivitis, or pneumonia. Routine treatment of the newborn's eyes after birth with erythromycin or other effective antibiotic ointment destroys the organisms. Gonococcus infection can be transmitted to the newborn from the birthing parent's genital tract at the time of birth and can cause ophthalmia neonatorum, a systemic neonatal infection, maternal endometritis, or pelvic infection. The risk of transmission from an infected patient to their infant is nearly 30% (Kliegman et al., 2020). Newborn infants often receive an antibiotic ointment in the eyes to prevent GC infection. Group B streptococcus is found in the vagina and/or rectum in approximately 25% of all healthy females. Screening at 36 to 37 weeks of pregnancy for group B streptococcus infection has been recommended because this infection causes preterm rupture of the amniotic membranes, preterm labor, fetal respiratory distress syndrome, fetal septicemia, and meningitis (ACOG, 2023b). **Bacterial vaginosis** is caused by an imbalance in the normal vaginal bacteria and is linked to preterm labor and birth (Shimaoka et al., 2019). *Candida albicans*, the cause of a common vaginal fungal infection, may also cause an oral infection called "thrush" in the mouth of the newborn. Routine assessment of pregnant patients and occasionally their sexual partners (GC) for these bacterial and yeast infections must occur during pregnancy so that treatment can occur and prevent fetal infection at the time of birth.

Human Immunodeficiency Virus and Acquired immunodeficiency syndrome

The US Public Health Service and the USPTF recommend that all pregnant individuals in the United States be tested for HIV infection, ideally at the first prenatal visit. HIV infection should be identified before pregnancy to provide the best opportunity to improve maternal health and pregnancy outcomes and prevent infant acquisition of HIV and so that therapy can be started as soon as possible (USDHHS, 2023a). Anyone in a high-risk group (e.g., intravenous drug users, those who have bisexual partners or multiple sexual contacts, those with a history of STIs, or those who engage in sex for money or drugs) should be tested for antibodies to HIV. For the HIV-positive individual or one who engages in high-risk sexual practices, counseling must occur before conception. Counseling should include both the direct effect of the virus on pregnancy and the effect of pregnancy on HIV disease progression. Although unclear, it appears that HIV infection becomes worse during pregnancy because of a patient's altered immune status. Some early pregnancy discomforts, such as fatigue, anorexia, and weight loss, may mask the early symptoms of HIV infection and thus postpone a definitive diagnosis.

Infants born to HIV-positive birthing parents who have taken antiretroviral medications during their pregnancy, in whom the virus is undetectable, and who have avoided breast/chestfeeding have a less than 1% perinatal transmission rate (CDC, 2023g). Affected infants may not be seropositive for HIV for many months after birth and then later develop the disease. The use of antiretroviral medications throughout pregnancy has improved the prognosis of an HIV-positive patient and has decreased viral transmission to the fetus, although the drugs remain expensive and may be inaccessible for those who do not receive prenatal care.

The pregnant person who has **AIDS** or who is HIV positive should be carefully monitored by a health care team for opportunistic infections that occur frequently. The nurse can be instrumental in helping coordinate their contacts with care providers, answering their questions, and working as a member of the team to provide optimal care for the patient and their child. Frequently, the pregnant person with AIDS does not seek care because of fears of being reported for her disease. Involving the patient in continuous prenatal care decreases their risk of preterm rupture of membranes, problems with fetal growth, postpartum infection, drug and alcohol abuse, and difficulty in addressing sociocultural barriers to a better life (Peterson, 2022).

Although important in decreasing the transmission of any disease, astute preventive measures are mandatory for nurses who are exposed to HIV-infected body fluids, such as blood, amniotic fluid, and vaginal secretions (standard precautions should be followed). All health care providers must follow hospital and birth center policies regarding the use of gloves and gowns and the disposal of needles and other potentially contaminated equipment to prevent the transmission of this disease in particular.

Hepatitis B

Hepatitis B virus (HBV) is a serious global public health problem, with more than 2 billion people infected and more than 1 million deaths occurring annually because of cirrhosis and liver carcinoma (Lee & Lok, 2023). HBV infection remains a significant concern during pregnancy because it affects the maternal liver and has a high fetal transmission rate (40%) if present during the third trimester. Approximately 90% of infected infants become chronically infected, which can lead to cirrhosis and liver cancer. High-risk groups for HBV infection include individuals from Asia, Pacific Islands, and sub-Saharan Africa, as well as health care workers, intravenous drug users, and those with multiple sexual partners (CDC, 2022c). On the basis of the large number of infected individuals who fail to show symptoms until liver damage has occurred, the USPTF (2020a) recommends that all pregnant individuals and those at risk should be screened routinely for HBV on their first prenatal visit (Jin, 2019). HBV immunization (three injections over a period of 6 months) may be given before or during pregnancy to an individual who is seronegative (CDC, 2022c). According to the American Academy of Family Physicians (AAFP, 2019), most people harboring HBV transmit it vertically through the placenta to the fetus or through contaminated urine, feces, saliva, or vaginal fluids during birth. Many individuals carrying HBV experience preterm births, and some infants may have acute hepatitis or later develop liver cancer.

Hepatitis C

Globally, there has been an increase in both acute and chronic **hepatitis C virus** (HCV) infections among individuals ages 20 to 39 years old. With this increased occurrence rate occurring in those who are of childbearing age, there are more pregnancies being affected by HCV. The CDC recommends screening all pregnant patients for HCV (CDC, 2024). The risk of transmission from the pregnant individual to the infant is approximately 6%. Although this rate of transmission is lower than that of HBV, it is important to note that there are no available treatments for HCV in pregnancy. Individuals with HCV in pregnancy should be referred for treatment in the postpartum period. Infants exposed to HCV during pregnancy should be tested at 2 to 6 months of life. Curative treatment is approved for children over 3 years old (CDC, 2024).

Other Health Concerns

Pregnant people may also develop any of the infections of non-pregnant persons. For example, pregnant people frequently experience upper respiratory tract and gastrointestinal tract infections, adding to the discomforts of pregnancy. However, there is no evidence the viruses causing these infections have a teratogenic effect on the fetus.

Fever frequently occurs with illness and may have a teratogenic effect in a pregnancy. A high temperature for a prolonged time (hyperthermia) in a pregnant person may harm the fetus, especially during the first trimester. Some literature indicates that fever is associated with miscarriages, low birth weight, stillbirths, preterm births, and neonatal neurodevelopmental disorders (Gustavson et al., 2019). Whether the fever or an underlying illness causing the fever has created the problem must be determined. Some reports have also correlated prolonged use of a sauna or hot tub, causing hyperthermia, with birth defects such as microcephaly, anencephaly, NTDs, and hypotonia (Sahni & Ohri, 2023). Until health care providers understand this issue better, the nurse should advise pregnant patients to avoid prolonged sauna or hot tub use and spending time with people who are ill or carrying disease. When a pregnant person develops a fever, she should be advised to contact her health care provider immediately.

COVID-19 in Pregnancy. Coronavirus disease 2019 (COVID-19) continues to infect millions of people worldwide. Despite available vaccines, there remains an overall low vaccination rate in the US. Although the risk of severe illness in pregnancy from COVID-19 is low, severe implications such as preterm birth and stillbirth are associated with the virus. The risks of severe illness increase with comorbidities such as diabetes or hypertension (Mayo Foundation for Medical Education and Research, 2023a). In addition, there are higher rates of intensive care unit (ICU) admission, need for ventilator-assisted breathing, blood clots, preeclampsia, and eclampsia associated with COVID-19 in pregnancy. It is important to consider the racial inequities that exist related to COVID-19 in pregnancy. Black and Hispanic pregnant individuals are more likely to have severe illness or die from complications of COVID-19. The increased rate of morbidity and mortality are not related to a biologic cause but rather due to the social, economic, and health care inequities that are present for people of color (Emeruwa et al., 2021). It is recommended that pregnant individuals stay up to date on COVID-19 vaccinations.

Diabetes. Diabetes mellitus is approaching epidemic proportions worldwide, which parallels the rise in obesity. Diabetes may exist before pregnancy (preexisting diabetes) or start during pregnancy (gestational diabetes), affecting both the birthing parent and the fetus. Pregnancy increases the need for maternal insulin to balance the blood glucose level. Currently, the ACOG recommends that all pregnant patients complete a glucose tolerance test at 28 weeks of gestation to identify abnormal blood glucose use and the need for additional monitoring. Complications from diabetes during pregnancy include hydramnios (excessive amniotic fluid volume), spontaneous abortion, acidosis, increased rate of infection, preeclampsia, vascular complications, and increased risk of a surgical birth. Because of an increased incidence of intrauterine death after 36 weeks of gestation attributable to an aging placenta, close monitoring in the last month is essential to prevent stillbirth. Neonatal complications from diabetes include hypoglycemia, respiratory distress syndrome, hyperbilirubinemia, fetal anomalies, fetal demise, macrosomia, and hypocalcemia. Infants of parents with diabetes also have a higher incidence of congenital anomalies, such as a heart lesion or meningocele (American Diabetes Association, 2022). The diabetic pregnant patient needs close health care team supervision and ongoing health teaching, including diet and exercise management, to control her disease effectively for an optimal pregnancy outcome.

Heart Disease and Hypertension. The physiologic changes that occur in pregnancy can place extra demands on cardiac function. Cardiac disease complicates approximately 4% of all pregnancies in the United States (Iftikhar & Biswas, 2023). Heart disease and hypertension are two serious maternal cardiovascular problems during pregnancy. Rheumatic heart disease, a common problem that affects globally more than 33 million people annually, contributes to congestive heart failure, threatening the lives of both the birthing parent and the fetus. The greatest tragedy of all is that it is eminently preventable (Elkayam, 2020). The fetus may require preterm birth to prevent complications. Chronic hypertension, seen more frequently in first-time birthing parents older than 35 years, increases the chances of stillbirths, pulmonary embolus, preterm births, preeclampsia, chronic hypertension, and development of gestational hypertension, which increase both maternal and IMRs. Hypertension complicates up to 10% of pregnancies and is a significant cause of maternal and perinatal morbidity and mortality. Pregnant people with cardiac problems must be monitored closely throughout pregnancy to prevent complications (Braunthal & Brateanu, 2019).

Rh Blood Group Incompatibility. **Rh blood group incompatibility**, which is a rare occurrence nowadays because of implementation of anti–D immune globulin prophylaxis given to the patient prenatally and postnatally, sometimes affects fetal development. This problem usually occurs when the patient has Rh-negative red blood cells and the fetus has Rh-positive red blood cells, inherited from a father who has Rh-positive blood. In this disorder, maternal antibodies develop, cross the placental membranes, and destroy the Rh-positive red blood cells of the fetus. Depending on the severity of the response, the infant may develop various levels of hyperbilirubinemia after birth or may die in utero from the anemia of erythroblastosis fetalis (hemolytic disease of the newborn).

All patients should be assessed for blood type, Rh factor, and development of antibody to Rh-positive cells at their first prenatal care visit and again at 24 to 28 weeks of pregnancy unless the father of the baby is Rh negative (Cunningham et al., 2022). Rh incompatibility between a patient and a future fetus may be prevented by administration of Rho(D) immune globulin

(RhoGAM) to a Rh-negative patient at 28 weeks of gestation and within hours after childbirth. The immunization prevents the patient's sensitization to fetal Rh-positive cells by inactivating fetal red blood cells in the patient before they can develop an antibody response. The ideal injection time is after the patient's first birth of an Rh-positive infant, miscarriage, or therapeutic abortion. Incompatibility generally does not occur during the first pregnancy, and the immunization prevents problems with later pregnancies.

Chemical Agents

Substance abuse in pregnancy remains a major public health problem worldwide. The misuse and abuse of alcohol and other mind-altering drugs have political, legal, socioeconomic, health, mental health, and familial effects felt widely around the world (Box 16.9: Evidence-Based Practice). Drugs ingested by the birthing parent may be teratogenic to the fetus. The tragic experience with the tranquilizer drug thalidomide, which caused limb deformities during the early 1960s, led to a recommendation that medications should be avoided during pregnancy unless necessary. However, the fact remains that during the most critical early weeks of fetal development and growth, when many do not know they are pregnant, ingested drugs may seriously affect the fetus. Depending on fetal gestational age and drug metabolism, drugs may alter the placenta itself or directly affect development and growth of the fetus. The drugs that most commonly cause congenital defects are prescription medications, over-the-counter (OTC) drugs, street drugs, nicotine (cigarettes), caffeine, and alcohol.

BOX 16.9 EVIDENCE-BASED PRACTICE

Substance Use in Pregnancy

It is well known that tobacco, alcohol, and marijuana use during pregnancy are linked to poor birth outcomes. With limited research on predictors of substance abuse during pregnancy, the primary objective of this study was to assess the relative effects of socioeconomic, demographic, and mental health risk factors associated with drug use during pregnancy. A retrospective cohort study (Brown et al., 2019) consisted of 25,734 pregnant females whose mean maternal age was 29 years. Data were prospectively acquired from perinatal and neonatal databases at tertiary hospitals. Neighborhood-level socioeconomic variables were labeled by recording maternal postal codes. Separate logistic regressions were computed for all outcome variables. In this study, the rates of alcohol (1.9%), tobacco (16.2%), and marijuana (2.3%) use continued throughout pregnancy. Maternal age was inversely associated with alcohol, tobacco, and marijuana use, and single-parent households were associated with depression and anxiety, which increased the risk of substance use. Depression was the highest risk factor contribution to the use of all three drug substances. Compared with females not depressed during pregnancy, females who were depressed were more likely to use these substances (Brown et al., 2019). Based on the findings of this study, it is evident that maternal depression is a primary risk factor of drug use during pregnancy. Early prenatal identification of depression and targeted interventions aimed at these at-risk individuals are important considerations to improve maternal mental health and ultimate birth outcomes. Nurses need to reach out to these high-risk patients on their first prenatal visit to secure appropriate resources to optimize their outcomes.

Prescription Medications

People frequently become pregnant while taking medications for illnesses diagnosed before pregnancy, such as hypertension, or they may receive medication to treat an illness acquired during pregnancy, such as a UTI. Some of the more common drugs that have been studied for fetal effects include antibiotics and anticonvulsants.

Most short-term and usual-dose antibiotics do not cause fetal harm. The tetracyclines are harmful to baby teeth formation because they combine with calcium ions and are deposited in deciduous teeth (causing discoloration) and bones (inhibiting bone growth and causing deformities) (King et al., 2019). Primary teeth seem most affected, but when the antibiotic is given near the time of delivery, the permanent teeth may also be damaged.

On the basis of our current state of knowledge, the vast majority of antibiotics do not cause serious harm to the unborn child if used properly and at the appropriate doses during pregnancy. In a recent large population-wide cohort study, it was found that there was no increase in risk of congenital fetal anomalies following first-trimester exposure to 10 commonly prescribed systemic antibiotics. However, ultimately no medicine, including antibiotics, can be described as absolutely 100% safe (Damkier et al., 2019).

The prevalence of antiepileptic drug use in pregnancy is currently very low. Although their main indication is for management of epilepsy, antiepileptic drugs are increasingly being used in the treatment of bipolar mood disorders, migraine, and neuropathic pain syndrome, which means their prevalence will increase (Arshida et al., 2019). The effects of anticonvulsants on the fetus have been documented thoroughly. Those with seizure disorders have carried infants to term while being treated with hydantoin, barbiturates, and other antiseizure medications. Infants born to those taking hydantoin (Dilantin) may have fetal hydantoin syndrome, reflected in microcephaly, retardation, cleft lip and palate, and congenital heart disease. Barbiturates, such as phenobarbital, may cause newborn addiction. Valproic acid, carbamazepine, phenytoin, phenobarbital, lamotrigine, and oxcarbazepine are some of the common antiepileptics prescribed during pregnancy, and more studies need to be done to identify their potential teratogenic effect (Kallen, 2019; Tomson et al., 2019). Patients with seizure disorders should discuss their medication requirements with their physicians before becoming pregnant and have close health care team monitoring throughout pregnancy.

Over-the-Counter Drugs

Pregnant people frequently choose to treat minor illnesses with OTC drugs. Research on acetylsalicylic acid (aspirin) and acetaminophen (Tylenol) indicates that both medications are safe in the recommended dosages. However, aspirin alters platelet function and may cause maternal and newborn bleeding if taken close to delivery. Acetaminophen can be toxic to the liver. Certain ingredients in common cold remedies have been associated with fetal irritability (Stanley et al., 2019). Ibuprofen has been known to prolong labor on the basis of its antiprostaglandin effect. Many OTC medications have documented safety for use during pregnancy, but research is limited based on ethical concerns of exposing the fetus to potential risks. Any drug may harm a fetus, so all drugs should be avoided during pregnancy unless prescribed by the health care provider.

The nurse includes information on the known and probable effects of medications on the fetus in prenatal teaching of couples. Discussion of herbal treatments is included, because little research exists on their effects and interactions with OTC and prescribed medications. The nurse recognizes that many cultural groups use these nontraditional agents because they believe that they will effectively manage pregnancy-related concerns. The nurse may need to encourage an individual to reconsider the use of herbs when evidence exists that these may harm the fetus or individual.

Drug Abuse

Given the prevalence of drug use and abuse in our society, it is imperative that nurses be able to recognize, manage, and refer as appropriate substance abuse problems for their care recipients. Substance abuse during pregnancy poses a significant risk because all substances consumed by the birthing parent pass freely through the placenta, and thus the fetus as well as the birthing parent experiences substance use, abuse, and addiction. All pregnant people and individuals of childbearing age should be screened periodically for alcohol, tobacco, and prescription and illicit drug use.

Use of narcotics, tranquilizers, marijuana, cocaine, vaping, amphetamines, and other drugs may cause serious health problems to both the birthing parent and the unborn child. These drugs represent an enormous cost to society by causing increased risks of low birth-weight and preterm infants, as well as deficits in child development, if the birthing parent ingests them during pregnancy. Frequent marijuana use is associated with changes in the fetal brain involved in attention, memory, decision-making, and motivation and increasing risk of addiction. Severe acute and chronic respiratory illness and potential death are linked to vaping (American Psychiatric Association, 2023). Treatment resources are scarce for this vulnerable population in terms of addressing their complex needs of drug misuse.

To optimize the care of patients with substance use disorder (SUD), it is essential for nurses to understand it is a disease process independent of pregnancy. It is a primary, chronic disease of brain reward, motivation, memory, and related circuitry. Just like any other chronic diseases, without treatment, substance misuse is progressive and can result in disability or death (Prasad & Metz, 2019).

Narcotics. Long-term narcotic use during pregnancy is increasing in prevalence. Signs of narcotic withdrawal in the newborn include tremors, irritability, hyperactivity, vomiting, diarrhea, sweating, poor feeding, and possibly convulsions. There is an increased risk of preterm births, neonatal irritability, placental abruption, fetal seizures, fetal demise, premature rupture of membranes, and fetal distress (ACOG, 2020). Frequent maternal marijuana use during pregnancy may cause fetal immunologic problems, but there is conflicting evidence about the effect. Current research has shown that some infants born to individuals who used marijuana during their pregnancies display altered responses to visual stimuli, increased tremulousness, and a high-pitched cry, which could indicate problems with neurologic development (National Institute on Drug Abuse [NIDA], 2019). To avoid these problems, nurses must recognize patients who abuse drugs and assist them in seeking appropriate help. This task may be difficult because individuals with SUD may try to hide their addiction and may be unable to change their lifestyle without extensive intervention.

Drug and substance misuse is a serious public health issue in the United States, especially among people of childbearing age. The problem of drug abuse during pregnancy has affected those in all communities, those of all races and cultures, and those of all ages and socioeconomic levels. As a result, many infants are born exposed to illicit substances in utero, are addicted, and develop the complex disorder known as **"neonatal abstinence syndrome" (NAS)**. This is a drug withdrawal syndrome that most commonly occurs after an exposure to addictive prescriptive or illicit drugs, such as opioids, which has been increasing in prevalence during the past decade. Current treatment interventions to address NAS focus on nonpharmacologic measures and rooming-in to reduce the length of hospital stay and medication use (Grossman & Berkwitt, 2019).

For early identification of newborns needing interventions, the nurse should observe newborns with a history of maternal drug abuse for the following: hyperactivity, shrill cry, muscle tension, tremors, seizures, sneezing, yawning, restless sleep, disorganized suck, vomiting, diarrhea, poor feeding, tachypnea, scratches on face, flushing, and sweating. Supportive care for these infants with NAS includes placing them in a quiet area with dim lights; using a tight swaddling position on the side or back; using calming techniques and rocking; clustering infant-care activities with gentle handling; encouraging nonnutritive sucking; providing small, frequent feedings; and administering pharmacologic agents to control withdrawal symptoms if warranted.

Alcohol. Alcohol is the most widely used recreational substance worldwide. Many today drink alcohol regularly. Researchers found that approximately one in nine pregnant females report drinking alcohol when surveyed (Denny et al., 2019). Research has demonstrated that alcohol is a teratogen, a substance that can cause abnormal development in a growing fetus, as it crosses the placenta readily. Recognition of the effects that even low levels of prenatal alcohol exposure can have on the physical and cognitive development of a child led to the coining of the umbrella term "fetal alcohol spectrum disorder" (FASD). FASD is a serious, lifelong, disabling condition that affects individuals from all racial, ethnic, and socioeconomic backgrounds. Fetal exposure to alcohol throughout pregnancy may cause **fetal alcohol syndrome** (FAS) or FASD, a collection of symptoms including intrauterine growth restriction, increased risk of facial anomalies, structural brain abnormalities, mental health problems, ADHD, and retardation. It is clinically proven that alcohol consumption during all stages of pregnancy puts the fetus at risk of being born with lifelong alcohol-related brain damage (Nowak & Michno, 2019). Recent studies have reported symptoms of fetal alcohol disorder in those who may have consumed just a couple of drinks a day at certain stages of pregnancy. Another study confirmed that FAS is not the only problem connected with drinking during pregnancy: it is also a risk factor for early alcohol abuse and dependence in the child (Reid & Moritz, 2019). Numerous studies have shown that no safe level of alcohol use exists during pregnancy; therefore alcohol consumption should be avoided during this time and when conception is being attempted. The consequences of prenatal alcohol exposure are often grave, inhibiting both physical and intellectual development, societal acceptance, and adult success. The evidence is clear—alcohol can be more damaging to the developing fetus than heroin, cocaine, or any other drug, producing by far the most serious neurobehavioral effects in the fetus. Prenatal alcohol exposure is the leading preventable cause of intellectual disability in the United States. As many as 1 in 13 infants born are affected by prenatal exposure to alcohol (Popova et al., 2019). Nurses are an important partner in addressing at-risk alcohol consumption. Nurses need to stress this risk to make all aware of avoiding alcohol consumption during their pregnancy. Nurses can help to deliver the message that alcohol poses grave risks during pregnancy. Eliminating alcohol consumption during pregnancy is an important measure to take to provide future generations with a healthy start in life so that they can reach their full potential in life.

Nicotine. Tobacco use is the leading cause of preventable death in the United States. Smoking during pregnancy is a leading cause of negative pregnancy and perinatal outcomes. In the United States, it is estimated that approximately 16% of those who are pregnant smoke. Carbon monoxide, tar, and nicotine from tobacco smoke may interfere with the oxygen supply to the fetus. Nicotine also readily crosses the placenta, and concentrations in the fetus can be as much as 15% higher than maternal levels. Nicotine concentrates in fetal blood, amniotic fluid, and breast/chest milk. Combined, these factors can have severe consequences for the fetuses and infants of those who smoke (NIDA, 2022). The USPTF (2020b) recommends that clinicians ask all pregnant patients about tobacco use and provide an augmented, pregnancy-tailored counseling framework for engaging in smoking cessation discussions:

- Ask about tobacco use.
- Advise to quit through clear, personalized messages.
- Assess willingness to quit.
- Assist to quit.
- Arrange follow-up and support.

Evidence indicates that maternal smoking causes increased rates of spontaneous abortion and ectopic pregnancy, decreased fertility, fetal growth restriction, increased numbers of low birth-weight or preterm infants, placental abnormalities, vaginal bleeding, congenital anomalies, perinatal death, sudden infant death syndrome (SIDS), neonatal morbidity and mortality, and premature rupture of the membranes. The best advice for pregnant individuals or those considering pregnancy is to cease all use of tobacco products, decreasing smoking and avoiding places where smoking occurs. The nurse needs to understand the context of smoking in a patient's life and the complexity of their choice to quit smoking to propose solutions to decrease fetal exposure to nicotine (see Box 16.9: Evidence-Based Practice).

Caffeine. Caffeine is a widely consumed psychoactive substance that may affect the normal course of pregnancy, so its intake should be limited. It is a stimulant found in tea, coffee, cola, chocolate, and some OTC medications. Caffeine is an addictive substance. Gene mutations have been found in laboratory animals exposed to moderate amounts of caffeine; however, these defects have not been found in human beings. One study found an association between excess caffeine intake (>200 mg daily) and a higher risk of low birth-weight infants (Wierzejska et al., 2019). Until additional research clarifies the relationship between caffeine intake and fetal effects, nurses should teach pregnant individuals to avoid excess caffeine intake.

Chemical Substances

The influence of chemicals on human development remains unclear. Some natural substances found to be teratogenic in animals, but not necessarily in human beings, include insect and bacterial toxins, insecticides, herbicides, and fungicides, including dichlorodiphenyltrichloroethane (DDT). Fish are a source of several nutrients that are important during pregnancy for healthy fetal development, including iodine; selenium; zinc; omega-3 polyunsaturated fatty acids; and vitamins A, D, and B_{12}. Studies involving pregnant people who eat large amounts of fish with high mercury levels (shark, swordfish, king mackerel, marlin, orange roughy, canned tuna, or tilefish) support evidence that mercury negatively affects fetal development, particularly brain development, and may be associated with preterm labor (US Food & Drug Administration [FDA] & Environmental Protection Agency, 2022). Pregnant people can safely eat up to 12 ounces of cooked fish weekly. Some studies report stillbirths, abortions, preterm births, and intellectual disabilities in fetuses exposed to lead. This area needs more study, particularly with more females working in traditional male workplaces where there are environmental contaminants. Nurses assess and provide individuals in their first trimester with information on environmental agents that are potentially damaging throughout gestation and counsel them on ways to avoid exposure.

Medications Given During Childbirth

The final time that the fetus encounters drugs through the birthing parent is during the birthing process. Many desire medications for labor discomforts, and usually only medications deemed safe and monitored closely during labor and birth have been used (e.g., epidural anesthetics, opiate agonists in small doses). Some analgesic drugs administered during labor can cause neonatal sedation and respiratory depression and can influence the rate and quality of the infant's adaptation to extrauterine life. Studies of visual attentiveness and sucking behavior, as well as neurologic tests and electroencephalography, suggest that fetal depressant effects may last as long as days after birth (Grant, 2022).

Mechanical Forces

The amniotic fluid reservoir protects the fetus during pregnancy and during mild-to-moderate trauma to the abdomen. However, major trauma to the abdomen, such as that sustained in a severe car accident, may cause maternal bleeding, preterm labor, and other concerns. The nurse instructs the proper way to wear both a lap belt and a shoulder harness to protect the fetus while driving. All those in the second and third trimesters should be encouraged to seek medical care following an accident believed to influence the health of the birthing parent or fetus.

The uterus, another mechanical force, also influences the fetus. Near the end of pregnancy, the fetus outgrows the uterus and becomes molded by it, particularly in cases of multiple pregnancy. Some children have congenitally dislocated hips from uterine pressure and fetal position in utero. Most deformities resolve either naturally or with repositioning after birth. Fetal malposition cannot be prevented; therefore the neonate is assessed for problems, and support is provided to the parents about the newborn's appearance.

The actual labor and birth process represent the final mechanical force. Few newborns experience injury during this process, and those who do usually recover with limited effect. It is difficult to predict and prevent birth traumas, such as when delivery of an infant who is larger than expected requires vacuum extraction, which may injure the child. In these cases, based on health care team assessment, the patient may undergo cesarean section to protect herself and the baby.

Radiation

Radiation exposure during pregnancy has been debated for years, but various experiences are continuing to show that there are increasingly negative effects on the growing fetus, as well as effects later in life. Scientific evidence indicates that exposure to x-rays, especially early in pregnancy during organogenesis, may cause chromosomal changes, spontaneous abortion, growth restriction, microcephaly, fetal loss, or malignancy later in life. The fetus is most sensitive to radiation effects between 8 and 15 weeks of pregnancy and thus should be spared any radiation exposure during that period (CDC, 2020c). The literature supports a greater incidence of leukemia in those exposed to x-rays during pregnancy compared with children who were not exposed. Unless the benefits of radiographic information clearly outweigh the risks of exposing the fetus to x-rays, these examinations should not be performed during gestation. If radiography is deemed necessary, the wearing of a lead apron, use of as low a radiation dose as possible, and application of other recommendations made by the National Council on Radiation Protection and Measurements should be used to protect the developing fetus.

DETERMINANTS OF HEALTH

Social Factors and Environment

Community and Work

As each individual considers or experiences pregnancy, they will need to ask themselves questions that will optimize their pregnancy outcome. These questions include the following: Is my work strenuous or possibly dangerous to my baby because of exposure to toxic substances? Do I need to work for long periods, influencing my need for rest? Will workplace stressors influence my coping with pregnancy and my family needs?

A safe workplace environment (one that does not involve exposure to hazardous substances or organisms and provides adequate breaks for worker rest and body movement) will allow a pregnant person to work until their baby is due, unless their health becomes impaired. The nurse helps each patient to assess the safety of their workplace and suggests ways to decrease hazards in that setting. These hazards include exposure to viruses, fungi, industrial products (hydrocarbons or pesticides), second-hand smoke, radiation emitted by medical diagnostic equipment, air pollutants, and asbestos and the possibility of workplace violence, mental and physical stress, and even noise pollution. The nurse encourages the pregnant worker to consider workplace ergonomics, addressing how the current work space will meet their changing physical needs.

Some employers in the United States have been designated creators of "family friendly" work environments because they have willingly made accommodations to support breast/chestfeeding and pregnant workers and their families. However, as a rule, too few employers support flexible work schedules for prenatal care visits, rest periods for pregnant workers, or removal of vending machines to support optimal nutrition for pregnant working-class individuals. Some individuals, regardless of workplace status, believe that once they announce their pregnancy, they will face workplace pressure to stop working or change positions in the company to suit their gestational needs.

Secondly, health advice on pregnancy might also be difficult to implement within some workplaces because of underlying assumptions, reflected in health advice, that pregnancy care is most appropriately performed in the home (Covert, 2019).

Culture and Ethnicity

With the increasing **diversity** and globalization in the US populations, nurses are challenged to develop culturally competent skills that meet the social, cultural, and linguistic needs of those for whom they care. Cultural competence is not static and requires frequent relearning and unlearning about diversity. Nurses must acknowledge the implications of their own "cultural lens" and continuously reflect on their own assumptions, biases, and stereotypes. Cultural groups have unique ideas and beliefs related to pregnancy, childbirth, and childbearing that must be understood by the nurse to render individualized care to each pregnant person. The goal of providing culturally sensitive care is to provide consistent quality of care to every individual, regardless of their culture, ethnic, racial, or religious background (Box 16.10: Nursing Roles in Providing Culturally Competent Care).

Nonconscious stereotyping and **prejudice** contribute to racial and ethnic disparities in health care. Contemporary training in cultural competence is insufficient to reduce these problems because even educated, culturally sensitive nurses can activate and use their biases without being aware they are doing so. This implies that, when activated, implicit negative attitudes and stereotypes shape how nurses evaluate and interact with minority groups. These negative attitudes and stereotypes can contribute to minority group-care recipients feeling uncomfortable and potentially discourage them from seeking care or adhering to treatment (Swihart & Martin, 2023). Nurses need an awareness of how culture, tradition, and acculturation may affect the patients for whom they provide care, because this is the first step toward understanding diverse cultural behavior.

BOX 16.10 Nursing Roles in Providing Culturally Competent Care

Nursing is considered a caring profession that provides holistic care to all diverse individuals. Nurses need to research, understand, and respect diverse cultures so as to provide appropriate measures in caring for individuals from diverse cultural backgrounds. In recent years, greater emphasis has been placed on nurses recognizing and appreciating **diversity** so as to acquire cultural competency. Cultural knowledge is the most important construct of cultural competence for nurses, being crucial for the accurate appreciation of a care recipient's worldview. Delivery of culturally competent care implies that a nurse acknowledges and acts on the unique history that a pregnant patient and their family bring to a health care interaction. The essence of both the individual centeredness and competence for the nurse is the importance of seeing the patient as a unique individual. The nurse supports culturally competent care by:

- Recognizing that cultural diversity exists and affects the process and outcome of health care
- Respecting people as unique individuals who, by their differences from the majority, bring a broadened definition of appropriate health care
- Using data gained from a cultural assessment for completion of a care plan
- Encouraging cultural behavior that protects the biopsychosocial, spiritual, and safety needs of the individual
- Gaining insight into the nurse's own beliefs and values about people who may be different from or have needs different from those of the majority or those of the nurse's own culture; understanding how these beliefs and values influence the outcomes of health care delivery with childbearing families
- Recognizing the values of the health care system reflected in the customs and practices of birthing facilities
- Providing interpreters to improve communication between the individual and health care providers
- Becoming literate in languages, customs, and cultural practices of people commonly seen in the health care environment
- Developing cultural humility by maintaining an interpersonal stance as it relates to the other person from a different culture
- Recognizing and valuing the diversity of those seeking care and entering all therapeutic relationships acknowledging that nurses are always in the process of learning and growing

From Lin et al. (2019); Sheperd et al. (2019); Purnell & Fenkl (2019)

Racial Inequities and Disparities in Pregnancy. As discussed previously, Black individuals experience twice the rate of hypertension and diabetes mellitus as White individuals in pregnancy. These higher rates may account for the three to four times higher mortality rate seen among pregnant Black individuals as compared with White individuals. Approximately 800 people in the United States die each year during pregnancy and within 42 days after childbirth. All other developed nations ranked better (Slomski, 2019). The maternal mortality rate in the United States has been increasing, whereas in other nations this rate has been decreasing. Greater than 80% of pregnancy-related deaths in the United States are preventable (The White House, 2022). It is essential to recognize that the higher mortality rate for people of color is not solely caused by increased occurrence rates of hypertension and other comorbidities. The inequities and disparities present in health care are caused by racism, bias, and economic injustices. Health care providers are less likely to listen to and address the concerns of Black pregnant individuals. In addition, and equally as concerning is that Black, Indigenous, and Hispanic pregnant individuals report substantially higher levels of mistreatment from providers including yelling at and patronizing patients. Increased action is needed on a political and social level to reduce inequities within obstetrical care. The Blueprint for Addressing the Maternal Health Crisis was released in 2022 by the Biden Administration. The goal of the Blueprint is to improve access to care and coverage for care for marginalized individuals. Another goal of the Blueprint is increased diversity within the perinatal labor force, as studies have demonstrated improved outcomes when patients are cared for by providers of the same racial background (The White House, 2022).

Levels of Policy Making and Health

Legislative actions and social movements can influence individual and family childbearing decisions. The Family and Medical Leave Act (FMLA) is a federal regulation that requires employers with more than 50 employees to provide 12 weeks of unpaid parental leave. The United States is one of only five countries in the world to provide no federal benefit to new parents. Thirteen states have passed family leave laws as of January 2024 (Center for American Progress, 2024). For the promotion of health throughout society, it is essential for governments to prioritize the wellbeing of families by giving new parents time off from work during the early months of parenthood and providing safe and equitable health care.

Historically, states have used federal aid from Medicaid and Title V maternal and child health block programs to provide services for pregnant patients and children. Many countries provide universal access to prenatal care, but in the United States, low-income patients rely on Medicaid, a joint federal-state program, to cover most of the cost of prenatal care. With constraints on state and federal budgets, many of which fund community prenatal clinics, concerns have been expressed about whether there will be sufficient money to fund obstetrical and children's care programs. Local health departments may offer free or low-cost prenatal care for those who are pregnant, but again the extent of services depends on state government or local allocation of funds. Despite this free or low-cost care and Affordable Care Act health insurance with subsidies, more than 25 million Americans still lack health insurance and therefore face barriers that affect their easy access to prenatal care (Kaiser Family Foundation, 2023; USDHHS, 2023b). In addition, the closing of thousands of birthing units across the county has limited pregnant individual's access to care and has disproportionally affected communities of color. This lack of access to care further contributes to the disparities that people of color face within their obstetrical care (Harvard School of Public Health, 2023). Many ethnically diverse populations lack insurance and a level of education that could increase their understanding of health-related information (low health literacy) for family health promotion. Education during the childbearing cycle is particularly important to increase the chances of families obtaining and understanding health-promotion information (USDHHS, 2023b).

With the nurse's help in data collection, consumers should be encouraged to express their views and opinions on pregnancy and parenting topics to their elected governmental representatives. This expression indeed works; many states legislated hospital stays of at least 48 hours for patients with vaginal deliveries and even longer stays for those with cesarean deliveries. These laws evolved from public concern over premature discharges of birthing parents as part of managed care insurance directives. Longer stays help health care providers to identify potential problems in the birthing parent or the baby before discharge. Continued legislative work on insurance reform may improve family planning services so that individuals can plan pregnancies to better meet their sociocultural and financial goals and needs (USDHHS, 2023b). The Patient Protection and Affordable Care Act of 2010 was the most sweeping health care legislation in a generation and affected reproductive health tremendously. Insurance reform, driven by legislative change, may also improve health care coverage for underinsured individuals who lack a consistent source of prenatal care or report difficulties in receiving care because of communication, structural, or personal barriers within their insurance system.

Economics

When the pregnant person begins prenatal care, personal financial resources influence the kind of care they receive, the need to remain employed during or after a pregnancy, the acceptance of their pregnancy, their nutritional status, and other choices. The expenses of planning and experiencing a pregnancy may determine whether the pregnant person or their family faces a financial crisis. The nurse needs to understand the financial history and priorities of the pregnant individual because this information will affect access to and use of prenatal care.

The nurse can make appropriate referral to resources for care (e.g., Title V or Medicaid programs). Until recently, Medicaid provided no adolescent family planning services, a situation that may have influenced high rates of pregnancy in some sectors of this country (USDHHS, 2023b). Many low-income individuals qualify for the USDA's Special Supplemental Nutrition Program for Women, Infants, and Children. This program provides essential foods such as milk, cheese, and eggs to pregnant and lactating individuals. During prenatal visits, the nurse may help a patient or family to plan a budget for food and other essential requirements based on individual family needs, cultural values, the need for a healthy diet during pregnancy, and income level. Occasionally, patients may access free transportation and childcare at the prenatal clinic if the nurse provides information about this program.

Health Services/Delivery System

Options for care during pregnancy range from medical-based care by a health care professional to more health promotion–focused care by a nurse practitioner or midwife. Globally, 80% of people alive today were born with the assistance of midwives (Midwives Alliance of North America, 2023). Midwives have a long tradition that includes watchful waiting; sharing empirical knowledge; protecting the normal, nonmedicalized birth process; and engaging in research to incorporate the findings into evidence-based practice. Midwifery is distinguished by characteristics that define a partnership with females by listening; being sensitive to cultural, sexual, and generational needs; encouraging shared decision-making; and practicing patience to be "with women" during their most vulnerable periods (King et al., 2019). Geographic availability of options, finances, previous experience, partner's preference, cultural or social acceptability of certain options, and preexisting or newly recognized risk factors will influence choice of care. Because of some cultural beliefs that pregnancy is not an illness, some may not seek Western medical prenatal care but rather may rely on individuals from their community to provide care until the actual labor, when they will go to a hospital.

A doula is another health care professional who can support pregnant individuals before, during, and following pregnancy. Compared with other obstetrical health care providers, it has been estimated that doulas spend up to 11 times more time with their patients. Per ACOG, a doula is one of the single most effective interventions for reducing pregnancy- and delivery-related complications. Doulas have also been shown to have a significantly positive effect on reducing racial disparities in pregnancy, particularly disparities faced by Black individuals. A community-based doula is a doula who resides within the community in which they provide care. This provides a unique opportunity for the doula to intimately relate to the community members and their needs (National Health Law Program, 2022).

Unless complications arise, the birthing parent generally chooses where they will labor and give birth. The movement toward home birth that began during the early 1970s continues to meet some people's needs for a more family-oriented, natural, health-focused experience. However, most Americans choose a hospital birth setting because of the availability of emergency equipment and personnel in case of complications. Some insurance companies will reimburse births that occur only in hospitals and in birth centers or birthing rooms attached to a hospital. The nurse helps pregnant patients to become aware of the care and birthing alternatives to make an informed choice for a positive labor and birth experience. People who lack resources to access the health care delivery system and teaching by the nurse during regular prenatal visits are generally less able to make informed decisions that affect their childbearing experiences.

Many expectant couples also make an informed choice about the actual process of labor and birth by developing a birth plan—those components of care and intervention that the couple desires for the birth experience. A pregnant person may choose natural childbirth or a method of analgesia or anesthesia. The nurse helps the pregnant patient choose the most appropriate method by providing information about options and encouraging questions about each option.

Pregnant individuals or couples are advised to attend prenatal classes. These provide valuable information and preparation for birth for many couples. The International Childbirth Education Association, the American Society for Psychoprophylaxis in Obstetrics (ASPO), and many local groups offer a variety of classes for the expectant couple. These classes may include information on early pregnancy, Lamaze-ASPO or Bradley methods, cesarean birth, breast/chestfeeding, infant cardiopulmonary resuscitation, and parenting. Sibling classes for the newborn and involvement of children in the birth experience

BOX 16.11 Nursing Strategies to Help Parents Prepare Siblings for the Neonate

- Explain the pregnancy and birth appropriate to the child's age.
- Answer all the child's questions.
- Involve the older sibling in planning for the new family member by fixing up the baby's room, picking out clothes, and buying diapers.
- Use relevant literature to educate the child about the coming baby.
- Encourage discussion and questions by talking about the new baby during relaxed family times rather than during busy, rushed times.
- Have the child participate in decisions, such as choosing a name, clothes, and toys for baby.
- When sibling classes are available as part of the childbirth education process, encourage parents and the child to attend.
- Suggest that the child go with the parent during clinic or office visits.
- Allow and discuss negative comments about the pregnancy or baby.
- Encourage the child to make drawings or give small gifts to the baby when it is born.

also promotes sibling bonding. See Box 16.11 for nursing strategies to help parents prepare siblings for the neonate.

NURSING APPLICATION AND ACTION

Teaching the pregnant patient and their partner during the prenatal period is the most important role of the nurse. Even the patient who has previously given birth or who has a high degree of education may need or want information from the health care team that will assist their family to adapt effectively to changes of pregnancy to support a healthy birth outcome.

To provide appropriate teaching, the nurse performs a comprehensive assessment that involves the entire family. Assessment, the first step in the nursing process, allows the nurse to determine maternal and fetal physical and psychological risks, the parents' knowledge base for pregnancy and birth, and cultural and family needs. Assessment should also include physical, spiritual, emotional, and sociocultural inspection and recognition of abuse. Pregnant patients at high risk of abuse include adolescents, those with low incomes, low self-esteem, limited education, or limited support system, and those with a history of alcohol or drug abuse, as well as those with a partner with a similar history, poor impulse control, or aggressive behaviors (Gosselin, 2019). In cases of suspected abuse, the nurse, in consultation with other members of the health care team, provides support and resources for the patient to make an informed decision about protecting themselves and their fetus during pregnancy. The nurse may also want to refer the patient to a professional counselor for a brief counseling outreach intervention or abuse shelter for personal safety (Hrelic, 2019).

As discussed in this chapter, assessment may also be made by use of Gordon's (2016) Functional Health Patterns, a common conceptual framework for clinical assessment (see Box 16.6). Data used in the assessment process will likely be collected during the prenatal visit and may change depending on life occurrences. A patient may be defined as high risk during their pregnancy if they experience heavy bleeding, preterm labor, elevated blood pressure, or extreme anxiety; if there is fetal distress; or if the patient shows unexpected behavior or symptoms. After noting these high-risk conditions, the nurse should refer the pregnant patient to an obstetric specialist or other resources for pregnant patients and their families (see the Case Study at the end of this chapter).

After a complete assessment during each prenatal visit, the nurse develops a teaching plan for the individual. Throughout the prenatal course, the nurse collaborates with the patient and their partner to assess their learning and support needs. For example, literature on bottle feeding or breast/chestfeeding may be provided to help a birthing parent to decide on a method, and books, videos, and websites may help couples understand more about birth and therefore feel that they have more control during labor and in meeting their birthing goals. If the birthing parent plans to attend group prenatal classes, the nurse should coordinate their teaching content and process with those expected in the classes, thereby preventing undue repetition. The nurse teaching prenatal classes should provide a list of topics to participants in the class to share with their health care providers. Box 16.8 covers relevant topics to be covered by the nurse during prenatal care interactions with pregnant patients. These topical areas relate to nursing interventions discussed earlier in this chapter. Basic handouts detailing danger signs of pregnancy can be posted in the home to consult if there are unexpected complications of pregnancy.

CASE STUDY

Active Labor: Melissa Martinez

Melissa Martinez, a gravida 1 para 0, is admitted to the birthing suite in early labor after spontaneous rupture of membranes at home. She is at 38 weeks of gestation with a history of abnormal alpha-fetoprotein levels at 16 weeks of pregnancy. She was scheduled for ultrasonography to visualize the fetus to rule out an open spinal defect or Down syndrome but never followed through. Melissa and her husband disagreed about what to do (keep or terminate the pregnancy) if the ultrasonography indicated a spinal problem, so they felt they did not want this information.

Reflective Questions

- As the nurse, what priority data would you collect from this couple to help define relevant interventions to meet their needs?
- How can you help this couple if they experience a negative outcome in the birthing suite?
- How can you process your own beliefs and preconceptions on a topic such as pregnancy termination while simultaneously providing evidence-based high-standard care to your patients?
- Based on the influence of the Human Genome Project and the possibility of predicting open spinal defects earlier in pregnancy, how will maternity care change in the future?

More About Identifying Prenatal Defects

Presently, every newborn in the United States is tested at birth for 30 to 50 severe, inherited, treatable genetic diseases through newborn state-wide public health metabolic screening programs. Using genome sequencing, a much larger number of diseases and conditions can be identified. Early identification and interventions would improve the quality of life for most.

SUMMARY

- Dramatic changes occur during pregnancy: a new life forms and develops and the expectant family members experience major changes in their roles and relationships with each other.
- Although all fetal development processes, changes in pregnant individual's bodies, and role transitions among family members share common elements, each family uniquely experiences pregnancy because of life experience and personal values.
- The focus is the entire family, although the nurse most often deals directly with the pregnant patient.
- The nurse provides valuable resources and information that the family may use to meet its specific needs.
- The overall nursing goal involves assisting each family to have a healthy pregnancy and birth outcome, to lay the foundation for satisfactory parenting and family life.

EVOLVE CHAPTER FEATURES

http://evolve.elsevier.com/Edelman/

- Study Questions

REFERENCES

American Academy of Family Physicians [AAFP]. (2019). *Screen pregnant women for HBV at first prenatal visit*. https://www.aafp.org/news/health-of-the-public/20190114hepbscreen.html

American Academy of Pediatrics [AAP]. (2021). *Nutrition and exercise during pregnancy*. https://www.healthychildren.org/English/ages-stages/prenatal/Pages/Nutrition-and-Exercise-During-Pregnancy.aspx

American College of Obstetricians and Gynecologists [ACOG]. (2020). *Tobacco, alcohol, drugs, and pregnancy*. https://www.acog.org/womens-health/faqs/tobacco-alcohol-drugs-and-pregnancy

American College of Obstetricians and Gynecologists [ACOG]. (2022). *Exercise after pregnancy*. https://www.acog.org/Patients/FAQs/Exercise-After-Pregnancy?IsMobileSet=false

American College of Obstetricians and Gynecologists [ACOG]. (2023a). *Nutrition during pregnancy*. https://www.acog.org/Patients/FAQs/Nutrition-During-Pregnancy?IsMobileSet=false#does

American College of Obstetricians and Gynecologists [ACOG]. (2023b). *Group B strep and pregnancy*. https://www.acog.org/Patients/FAQs/Group-B-Strep-and-Pregnancy?IsMobileSet=false#why

American College of Obstetricians and Gynecologists [ACOG]. (2024). How your fetus grows during pregnancy. https://www.acog.org/womens-health/faqs/how-your-fetus-grows-during-pregnancy

American Diabetes Association [ADA]. (2022). Management of diabetes in pregnancy: Standards of medical care in diabetes-2022. *Diabetes Care* ;*45*(Suppl 1):S232–S243. https://doi.org/10.2337/dc22-S015

American Pregnancy Association. (n.d.). *In vitro fertilization: IVF*. https://americanpregnancy.org/infertility/in-vitro-fertilization/

American Psychiatric Association. (2023). *Perinatal mental and substance use disorder*. https://www.psychiatry.org/getmedia/344c26e2-cdf5-47df-a5d7-a2d444fc1923/APA-CDC-Perinatal-Mental-and-Substance-Use-Disorders-Whitepaper.pdf

Arshida, P., Sreejith, K., Thehsin, K. S., Nadiya Banu, M., Sulaikha, S., & Midhun, K. (2019). Antiepileptics use in pregnant women. *Journal of Drug Delivery and Therapeutics*, *9*(4-s), 705–708. https://doi.org/10.22270/jddt.v9i4-s.3287

Association of Women's Health, Obstetric and Neonatal Nurses [AWHONN]. (2019). Intimate partner violence. *Journal of Obstetric, Gynecologic and Neonatal Nursing*, *48*(1), 112–116.

Blackburn, S. T. (2018). *Maternal, fetal, neonatal physiology: A clinical perspective*. St Louis, MO: Elsevier.

Braunthal, S., & Brateanu, A. (2019). Hypertension in pregnancy: Pathophysiology and treatment. *SAGE Open Medicine*, *7*, 2050312119843700. https://doi.org/10.1177/2050312119843700

Brown, R. A., Dakkak, H., Gilliland, J., & Seabrook, J. A. (2019). Predictors of drug use during pregnancy: The relative effects of socioeconomic, demographic, and mental health risk factors. *Journal of Neonatal-Perinatal Medicine*, *12*(2), 179–187. https://doi.org/10.3233/NPM-1814

Calik, K. Y., Karabulutlu, O., & Yavuz, C. (2018). First do no harm – interventions during labor and maternal satisfaction: A descriptive cross-sectional study. *BMC Pregnancy and Childbirth*, *18*(1), 415. https://www.ncbi.nlm.nih.gov/pmc/articles/PMC6201531/

Center for American Progress. (2024). *Paid leave*. https://www.americanprogress.org/topic/paid-leave/

Centers for Disease Control and Prevention [CDC]. (2020a). *Rubella: clinical overview*. https://www.cdc.gov/rubella/hcp.html

Centers for Disease Control and Prevention [CDC]. (2020b). *Cytomegalovirus (CMV) and congenital CMV infection*. https://www.cdc.gov/cmv/

Centers for Disease Control and Prevention [CDC]. (2020c). *Radiation and pregnancy: a fact sheet for clinicians*. https://www.cdc.gov/nceh/radiation/emergencies/prenatalphysician.htm

Centers for Disease Control and Prevention [CDC]. (2021). *Intimate partner violence*. https://www.cdc.gov/violenceprevention/intimatepartnerviolence/index.html

Centers for Disease Control and Prevention [CDC]. (2022a). *Toxoplasmosis: pregnant women*. https://www.cdc.gov/parasites/toxoplasmosis/gen_info/pregnant.html

Centers for Disease Control and Prevention [CDC]. (2022b). *Fact sheets on Zika and pregnancy*. https://www.cdc.gov/pregnancy/zika/materials/pregnancy-resources.html

Centers for Disease Control and Prevention [CDC]. (2022c). *Hepatitis B: perinatal transmission*. https://www.cdc.gov

Centers for Disease Control and Prevention [CDC]. (2023a). *Planning for pregnancy*. https://www.cdc.gov

Centers for Disease Control and Prevention [CDC]. (2023b). *Infant mortality rates by race and ethnicity*. https://www.cdc.gov/reproductivehealth/maternalinfanthealth/infantmortality.htm

Centers for Disease Control and Prevention. (2023c). *Folic acid recommendations*. https://www.cdc.gov

Centers for Disease Control and Prevention [CDC]. (2023d). *Congenital syphilis – CDC fact sheet*. https://www.cdc.gov/std/syphilis/stdfact-congenital-syphilis.htm

Centers for Disease Control and Prevention [CDC]. (2023e). *STDs during pregnancy*. https://www.cdc.gov/std/pregnancy/stdfact-pregnancy-detailed.htm

Centers for Disease Control and Prevention [CDC]. (2023f). *Chlamydia*. https://www.cdc.gov/std/chlamydia/stdfact-chlamydia-detailed.htm

Centers for Disease Control and Prevention [CDC]. (2023g). *HIV and pregnant women, infants, and children*. https://www.cdc.gov

Centers for Disease Control and Prevention [CDC]. (2024). *HCV infection challenges*. https://www.cdc.gov/nchhstp/pregnancy/challenges/hcv.html

Central Intelligence Agency [CIA]. (2023). *World Factbook: infant mortality rate*. https://www.cia.gov

Coleman, A. (2019). *Obstetrics and gynecology: A case-based approach*. New Delhi, India: ML Books International.

Covert, B. (2019). *The American workplace still won't accommodate pregnant workers*. The Nation. https://www.thenation.com/article/archive/pregnant-workers-discrimination-workplace-low-wage/

Cunningham, F. G., Leveno, K. J., Dashe, J. S., Hoffman, B. L., Spong, C. Y., & Casey, B. M. (2022). *William's obstetrics* (26th ed.). New York, NY: McGraw-Hill Education.

Damkier, P., Bronniche, L. M. S., Korch-Frandsen, J. F. B., & Broe, A. (2019). In utero exposure to antibiotics and risk of congenital malformations: A population-based study. *American Journal of Obstetrics and Gynecology, 221*(6), 648.e1–648.e15. https://doi.org/10.1016/j.ajog.2019.06.050

Denbow, J. (2019). Good mothering before birth: Measuring attachment and ultrasound as an affective technology. *Engaging Science, Technology, and Society, 5*. https://doi.org/10.17351/ests2019.238

Denny, C. H., Acero, C. S., Naimi, T. S., & Kim, S. Y. (2019). Consumption of alcohol beverages and binge drinking among pregnant women aged 18-44 years – United States, 2015-2017. *Morbidity and Mortality Weekly Report, 68*(16), 365–368.

Douthard, R. A., Martin, I. K., Chapple-McGruder, T., Langer, A., & Chang, S. (2021). U.S. maternal mortality within a global context: Historical trends, current state, and future directions. *Journal of Women's Health, 30*(2), 168–177. https://doi.org/10.1089/jwh.2020.8863

Dutton, L. A., Densmore, J. E., & Turner, M. B. (2020). *A pocket guide to clinical midwifery: The efficient midwife* (2nd ed.). Burlington, MA: Jones & Bartlett Learning.

Elkayam, U. (2020). *Cardiac problems in pregnancy* (4th ed.). Hoboken, NJ: John Wiley & Sons.

Emeruwa, U. N., Gyamfi-Bannerman, C., & Miller, R. S. (2022). Health care disparities in the COVID-19 pandemic in the United States: A focus on obstetrics. *Clinical Obstetrics and Gynecology, 65*(1), 123–133. doi:10.1097/GRF.0000000000000665

Fernandes, N. D., Arya, K., Syed, H. A., & Ward, R. (2024). Congenital herpes simplex. *StatPearls*. https://www.ncbi.nlm.nih.gov/books/NBK507897/

FIGO Working Group on Good Clinical Practice in Maternal-Fetal Medicine. (2019). Good clinical practice advice: Iron deficiency anemia in pregnancy. *International Journal of Gynecology & Obstetrics, 144*(3), 322–324.

Ghouri, F., Hollywood, A., & Ryan, K. (2019). Urinary tract infections and antibiotic use in pregnancy- Qualitative analysis of online forum content. *BMC Pregnancy and Childbirth, 19*(1), 289. https://doi.org/10.1186/s12884-019-2451-z

Gordon, M. (2016). *Manual of nursing diagnosis* (13th ed.). Sudbury, MA: Jones & Bartlett Learning.

Gosselin, D. K. (2019). *Family & intimate partner violence: Heavy hands*. New York, NY: Pearson.

Grant, G. J. (2022). *Pharmacologic management of pain during labor and delivery*. UpToDate. https://www.uptodate.com/contents/pharmacologic-management-of-pain-during-labor-and-delivery

Grossman, M., & Berkwitt, A. (2019). Neonatal abstinence syndrome. *Seminars in Perinatology, 43*(3), 173–186.

Gustavson, K., Ask, H., Ystrom, E., Stoltenberg, C., Lipkin, W. I., & Reichborn-Kjennerud, T. (2019). Maternal fever during pregnancy and offspring attention deficit hyperactivity disorder. *Scientific Reports, 9*(1), 9519. https://www.nature.com/articles/s41598-019-45920-7

Guttmacher Institute. (2024). *Guttmacher*. https://www.guttmacher.org/

Hammond, A. C. R. (2019). *Heroes of progress: Virginia Apgar*. https://www.humanprogress.org/article.php?p=2019

Harvard School of Public Health. (2023). *Maternity ward closures exacerbating health disparities*. https://www.hsph.harvard.edu/news/features/maternity-obstetric-closure-health-disparities/#:~:text=The%20reasons%20cited%20for%20the,effect%20of%20new%20antiabortion%20laws

Health Resources & Services Administration [HRSA]. (2019). *About HRSA*. https://www.hrsa.gov/about/index.html

HealthyChildren.org. (2023). *Perinatal depression in partners: can both parents get the baby blues?* https://www.healthychildren.org/English/ages-stages/prenatal/delivery-beyond/Pages/dads-can-get-postpartum-depression-too.aspx#:~:text=Any%20parent%20may%20become%20depressed,or%209%2D1%2D1

Hrelic, D. A. (2019). *Intimate partner violence in pregnancy*. American Nurse Today. https://www.americannursetoday.com/intimate-partner-violence-in-pregnancy/

Iftikhar, S. F., & Biswas, M. (2023). *Cardiac disease in pregnancy*. StatPearls. https://www.ncbi.nlm.nih.gov/books/NBK537261/

Jin, J. (2019). Screening for hepatitis B in pregnant women. *The Journal of the American Medical Association, 322*(4), 376. https://doi.org/10.1001/jama.2019.9229

Jordan, R. G., Farley, C. L., & Grace, K. T. (2019). *Prenatal and postnatal care: A woman-centered approach* (2nd ed.). Hoboken, NJ: Wiley Blackwell.

Kaiser Family Foundation. (2023). *Key facts about the uninsured population*. https://www.kff.org/uninsured/issue-brief/key-facts-about-the-uninsured-population/

Kallen, B. (2019). *Maternal drug use and infant congenital malformations*. Cham, Sweden: Springer Publishers.

Kenner, C., Altimier, L. B., & Boykova, M. V. (2019). *Comprehensive neonatal nursing care* (6th ed.). New York, NY: Springer Publishing Company.

King, T. L., Brucker, M. C., Jevitt, C., & Osborne, K. (2019). *Varney's midwifery* (ed.). Burlington, MA: Jones & Bartlett Learning.

Kliegman, R. M., St. Geme, J. W., Blum, N. J., Shah, S. S., Tasker, R. C., & Wilson, K. M. (2020). *Nelson textbook of pediatrics* (21st ed.). Philadelphia, PA: Elsevier.

Landry, J., & Kensler, P. (2019). Providing culturally sensitive care to women who are the sexually minority or are gender nonconforming. *Nursing for Women's Health, 23*(2), 163–171.

Lee, H., & Lok, A. S. F. (2023). *Hepatitis B and pregnancy*. UpToDate. https://www.uptodate.com/contents/hepatitis-b-and-pregnancy/print

Lin, M. H., Wu, C. Y., & Hsu, H. C. (2019). Exploring the experiences of cultural competence among clinical nurses in Taiwan. *Applied Nursing Research, 45*, 6–11. https://doi.org/10.1016/j.apnr.2018.11.001

Lockwood, C. J., Moore, T. R., Copel, J. A., Silver, R. M., Resnik, R., Dugoff, L., et al. (2023). *Creasy & Resnik's maternal-fetal medicine: principles and practice*. Philadelphia, PA: Elsevier.

Lowdermilk, D., Perry, S., Cashion, K., & Alden, K. R. (2024). *Maternity and women's health care* (13th ed.). St. Louis: Mosby

March of Dimes. (2019). *Birth defects and other health conditions.* https://www.marchofdimes.org/complications/birth-defects-and-health-conditions.aspx

March of Dimes. (2022). *Neural tube defects.* https://www.marchofdimes.org/complications/neural-tube-defects.aspx

Martin, R., Fanaroff, A., & Walsh, M. (2019). *Fanaroff and Martin's neonatal-perinatal medicine* (11th ed.). Philadelphia, PA: Elsevier.

Mayo Foundation for Medical Education and Research. (2023a). *Understand how Covid-19 might affect your pregnancy.* Mayo Clinic. https://www.mayoclinic.org/diseases-conditions/coronavirus/in-depth/pregnancy-and-covid-19/art-20482639#:~:text=Pregnant%20women%20with%20COVID%2D19,as%20stillbirth%20and%20pregnancy%20loss

Mayo Foundation for Medical Education and Research. (2023b). *Antidepressants: safe during pregnancy?* Mayo Clinic. https://www.mayoclinic.org/healthy-lifestyle/pregnancy-weekby-week/in-depth/antidepressants/art-20046420#:~:text=SSRIs%20are%20generally%20considered%20an,t%20associated%20with%20birth%20defects

Mental Health Technology Transfer Center (MHTTC) Network. (2023). *Perinatal mental health.* https://mhttcnetwork.org/

Midwives Alliance of North America [MANA]. (2023). *About midwives.* https://mana.org/about-midwives

Mughal, S., Azhar, Y., & Siddiqui, W. (2022). *Postpartum depression.* National Library of Medicine [NIH]. https://www.ncbi.nlm.nih.gov/books/NBK519070/

National Academy of Medicine [NAM]. (2009). *Reexamination of IOM pregnancy weight guidelines.* http://www.nationalacademies.org/hmd/Reports/2009/Weight-Gain-During-Pregnancy-Reexamining-the-Guidelines.aspx

National Eating Disorders Association [NEDA]. (2019). *Pica.* https://www.nationaleatingdisorders.org/learn/by-eating-disorder/other/pica

National Health Law Program. (2022). *Doula care improves health outcomes, reduces racial disparities and cuts cost.* https://healthlaw.org/doula-care-improves-health-outcomes-reduces-racial-disparities-and-cuts-cost/

National Human Genome Research Institute. (2019). *About genomics.* https://www.genome.gov/About-Genomics/Introduction-to-Genomics#three

National Institute on Drug Abuse. (2024). *Cannabis (Marijuana).* https://nida.nih.gov/research-topics/cannabis-marijuana

National Institute on Drug Abuse. (2022). *Cigarettes and other tobacco products.* https://www.drugabuse.gov/publications/drugfacts/cigarettes-other-tobacco-products

Norwitz, E. R., Zelop, C. M., Miller, D. A., & Keefe, D. L. (2019). *Evidence-based obstetrics and gynecology.* Hoboken, NJ: Wiley Blackwell.

Nowak, A., & Michno, A. (2019). FADS – Fetal alcohol syndrome disorder. *World Scientific News, 129,* 242–254.

Office on Women's Health [OWH]. (2021). *Infertility.* https://www.womenshealth.gov/a-z-topics/infertility

Peterson, A. T. (2022). *HIV in pregnancy.* eMedicine. https://emedicine.medscape.com/article/1385488-overview

Phillippi, J., & Kantrowitz-Gordon, I. (2023). *Varney's midwifery* (7th ed.). Burlington, MA: Jones & Bartlett Learning.

Phillips, A. M., Magann, E. F., Whittington, J. R., Whitcombe, D. D., & Sandlin, A. T. (2019). Surrogacy and pregnancy. *Obstetrical & Gynecological Survey, 74*(9), 539–545.

Popova, S., Lange, S., Shield, K., Burd, L., & Rehm, J. (2019). Prevalence of fetal alcohol spectrum disorder among special sub-populations: A systematic review and meta-analysis. *Addiction, 114*(7), 1150–1172.

Potter, P. A., Perry, A. G., Stockert, P., & Hall, A. (2020). *Clinical companion for fundamentals of nursing* (10th ed.). St. Louis, MO: Elsevier.

Prasad, M. R., & Metz, T. D. (2019). *Substance abuse in pregnancy. Clinical Obstetrics and Gynecology, 62*(1), 110–111.

Purnell, L. D., & Fenkl, E. A. (2019). *Handbook for culturally competent care.* Cham, Switzerland: Springer Publishers.

Ramsey, P. S., & Schenken, R. S. (2023). *Obesity in pregnancy: Complications and maternal management.* UpToDate. https://www.uptodate.com/contents/obesity-in-pregnancy-complications-and-maternal-management/print

Reid, N., & Moritz, K. M. (2019). Caregiver and family quality of life for children with fetal alcohol spectrum disorder. *Research in Developmental Disabilities, 94,* 103478. https://doi.org/10.1016/j.ridd.2019.103478

Rubin, R. (1984). *Maternal identity and the maternal experience.* New York: Springer.

Sahni, M., & Ohri, A. (2023). *Meningomyelocele.* StatPearls. https://www.ncbi.nlm.nih.gov/books/NBK536959/

Seidel, H. M., Ball, J. W., Dains, J. E., Flynn, J. A., Solomon, B. S., & Stewart, R. W. (2019). *Seidel's guide to physical examination: An interprofessional approach (Mosby's guide to physical examination): an interprofessional approach* (9th ed.). St Louis: Mosby.

Seymour, J. V., Beck, K. L., & Conlon, C. A. (2019). Nutrition in pregnancy. *Obstetrics, Gynecology, & Reproductive Medicine, 29*(8), 219–224.

Sheperd, S. M., Willis-Esqueda, C., Newton, D., Sivasubramaniam, D., & Paradies, Y. (2019). The challenge of cultural competence in the workplace: perspectives of healthcare providers. *BMC Health Services Research, 19*(1), 135–145. https://doi.org/10.1186/s12913-019-3959-7

Shimaoka, M., Yo, Y., Doh, K., Suzuki, A., Tsuji, I., Mandai, M., et al. (2019). Association between preterm delivery and bacterial vaginosis with or without treatment. *Scientific Reports, 9*(1), 509. https://doi.org/10.1038/s41598-018-36964-2

Sizer, F. S., & Whitney, E. N. (2019). *Nutrition: Concepts and controversies* (15th ed.). Boston, MA: Cengage Learning.

Slomski, A. (2019). Why do hundreds of US women die annually in childbirth? *The Journal of the American Medical Association, 321*(13), 1239–1241. https://doi.org/10.1001/jama.2019.0714

Stanley, A. Y., Durham, C. O., Sterrett, J. J., & Wallace, J. B. (2019). Safety of over-the-counter medications in pregnancy. *MCN: The American Journal of Maternal/Child Nursing, 44*(4), 196–205.

Swihart, D. L., & Martin, R. L. (2023). *Cultural religious competence in clinical practice.* StatPearls. https://www.ncbi.nlm.nih.gov/books/NBK493216/

Tomson, T., Battino, D., & Perucca, E. (2019). Teratogenicity of antiepileptic drugs. *Current Opinion in Neurology, 32*(2), 246–252.

Umana, O. D., & Siccardi, M. A. (2023). *Prenatal non-stress test.* https://www.ncbi.nlm.nih.gov/books/NBK537123/

US Department of Agriculture [USDA]. (2019). *ChooseMyPlate: Professionals.* https://www.choosemyplate.gov/browse-by-audience/view-all-audiences/professionals; https://www.myplate.gov/professionals

US Department of Health and Human Services [USDHHS]. (2020). *Healthy women, healthy pregnancies, healthy futures: action plan to improve maternal health in America.* https://aspe.hhs.gov/system/files/aspe-files/264076/healthy-women-healthy-pregnancies-healthy-future-action-plan_0.pdf

US Department of Health and Human Services [USDHHS]. (2021). *Pregnancy: calorie needs.* https://www.womenshealth.gov/pregnancy/youre-pregnant-now-what/staying-healthy-and-safe#a

US Department of Health and Human Services [USDHHS]. (2023a). *Maternal HIV testing and identification of perinatal HIV exposure.* https://clinicalinfo.hiv.gov/en/guidelines/perinatal/maternal-hiv-testing-identification-exposure

US Department of Health and Human Services [USDHHS]. (2023b). *Healthy People 2030*. https://health.gov/healthypeople

US Food & Drug Administration [FDA] & Environmental Protection Agency [EPA]. (2022). *Advice about eating fish*. https://www.fda.gov/food/consumers/advice-about-eating-fish

US Preventive Services Task Force [USPTF]. (2020a). *Sexually transmitted infections: behavioral counseling*. https://www.uspreventiveservicestaskforce.org/uspstf/recommendation/sexually-transmitted-infections-behavioral-counseling

US Preventive Services Task Force [USPTF]. (2020b). *Prevention and cessation of tobacco use in children and adolescents: primary care interventions*. https://www.uspreventiveservicestaskforce.org/Page/Document/draft-recommendation-statement/tobacco-and-nicotine-use-prevention-in-children-and-adolescents-primary-care-interventions

Vogel, J. P., Williams, M., Gallos, I., Althabe, F., & Oladapo, O. T. (2019). WHO recommendations on uterotonics for postpartum haemorrhage prevention: what works, and which one? *BMJ Global Health*, *4*(2), e001466. https://doi.org/10.1136/bmjgh-2019-001466

Webster, S., Morris, G., & Kevelighan, E. (2018). *Essential human development*. West Sussex, UK: Wiley Blackwell.

White House. (2022). *The Blueprint for Addressing the Maternal Health Crisis*. https://nmppcares.org/sites/default/files/2022-08/White%20House%20Maternal-Health-Blueprint.pdf

Wierzejska, R., Jarosz, M., & Wojda, B. (2019). Caffeine intake during pregnancy and neonatal anthropometric parameters. *Nutrients*, *11*(4), 806–816. https://doi.org/10.3390/nu11040806

World Health Organization [WHO]. (2023a). *Congenital anomalies*. https://www.who.int/en/news-room/fact-sheets/detail/congenital-anomalies

World Health Organization [WHO]. (2023b). *Syphilis screening and treatment for pregnant women*. https://apps.who.int/iris/bitstream/handle/10665/259003/9789241550093-eng.pdf?sequence=1

Wu, R. T., Peck, C. J., Shultz, B. N., Travieso, R., & Steinbacher, D. M. (2019). Racial disparities in cleft palate repair. *Plastic and Reconstructive Surgery*, *143*(6), 1738–1745.

Yikar, S. K., & Nazik, E. (2019). Effects of prenatal education on complaints during pregnancy and on quality of life. *Patient Education and Counseling*, *102*(1), 119–125.

Young, S., & Cox, J. T. (2023). *Pica in pregnancy*. UpToDate. https://www.uptodate.com/contents/pica-in-pregnancy

17

Infant

Courtney Coffey

http://evolve.elsevier.com/Edelman/

OBJECTIVES

After completing this chapter, the reader will be able to:

- Evaluate the infant's health status and give examples of basic growth and developmental principles.
- Analyze the developmental tasks for the infant and the behavior indicating that these tasks are being accomplished.
- Explain the immunization schedule and other safety and health-promotion measures to a parent.
- Detect common parental concerns about infants and describe a model for parent education to allay these concerns.
- Examine accidents that occur during infancy and recommend appropriate counseling for accident prevention and safety.
- Differentiate ways in which nurses can be active in promoting major policies and influencing legislation concerning health.
- Outline governmental strategies to meet the goals of improving infant health.

KEY TERMS

Active immunization
Birth defect
Body mass index
Growth
Growth index
Infant/child abuse
Oral stage of development
Passive immunization
Poor growth
Reflexes
Sensorimotor period
Sickle cell anemia
Sudden infant death syndrome (SIDS)
Trust versus mistrust
Weaning

THINK ABOUT IT

Car Safety Seats

Infants are at particular risk in automobile accidents. The proper use of occupant protection systems (infant car safety seats with seat belts) can reduce the risk of death and injury significantly. Although many public service campaigns encourage parents to restrain their infants while riding in automobiles (and all states have laws requiring some type of passenger safety restraint for infants), some parents neglect this or remain unaware of the importance of providing safety for their vulnerable infants.

Another time that it is recommended that infants are restrained in their car seat is while riding on an airplane. While it is rare for airplanes to crash, sudden onset of turbulence and runway accidents place the infant at risk of injury. While the Federal Aviation Administration does not require car seats, a car seat is the best way to keep an infant safe while travelling by air (University of Vermont Health Network, 2022)

Nurses must have up-to-date knowledge of car-occupant protection systems and their proper use to help parents find new products and obtain the most current information available. Parents often rely on the person selling the infant car seat for their information about protection systems and the proper use of car seats. However, informational brochures and media campaigns fall short because they usually fail to provide explanations or demonstrations. As a result, parents may misinterpret the information that they receive. *Car seats should always be purchased new and never used second-hand. Car seats should never be used after an accident. Insurance companies will often reimburse for a new car seat following an automobile accident. Many states require that the infant is discharged from the hospital in an approved car seat. If parents do not have an approved car seat, hospitals sometimes have new, never-used ones available to give to a family in need.*

- What type of program might you develop to reach and inform parents about the importance of car seat safety?
- In what settings might such a program be implemented? Childbirth classes, birthing centers?
- How would you modify your teaching plan to meet the learning needs of parents with lower reading levels or different learning types?
- How would you modify your program to ensure that parents who come from cultural backgrounds different from your own would respond well to the information?

Infants are born requiring the care and support of adult caregivers for survival. They are unique individuals who are unable to communicate with language and must rely on their caretakers for prompt, safe, and effective interpretation of their behaviors so that correct care can be provided. Infants are recognized as the most vulnerable and dependent members of society, and their well-being is often used to measure the overall health of society. Health is shaped by a broad set of determinants, including socioeconomic status, physical and social environments, genetics and biologic influences, and access to health care. Providing a safe and sound source of attachment and interaction is paramount to healthy infant development. Caregiving and parenting activities are the primary ingredients of an infant's preparation for life and ultimate independence. Nurses play a vital role in influencing this positive interaction through health promotion and education. An understanding of infant growth and development patterns and concepts is essential for parents and caregivers to create a nurturing and caring environment that will stimulate an infant's learning.

This chapter focuses on the infant and the infant's family during the infant's developmental period of 1 to 18 months. Because the infant is completely dependent on others, this chapter addresses the infant's parents and significant others as sources of health-promotion activities. The relationship initiated at birth between parents and the infant is the basis for the interdependence that is required for proper psychological and physical infant development. Health care professionals must focus on parent education as a means of fostering healthy, satisfying relationships within the family unit and promoting the development of healthy future generations.

The principles of normal growth and development are used as a structural framework for this chapter. Understanding these principles helps the nurse identify deviations from the norm and institute appropriate health-promoting interventions.

To promote and maintain health during infancy, a balance between the infant's internal and external environmental forces must be established; any disruption places the infant at risk. Several processes that greatly influence this balance are identified, and appropriate interventions are outlined to assist the nurse in promoting a healthy infant population (American Academy of Pediatrics [AAP], 2023a). Box 17.1 outlines some of the Healthy People 2030 population health goals for the infant population in the United States.

Of note: the term(s) *breast/chest feeding* are used interchangeably in this chapter. It is important that the terminology used in health care is inclusive for all. It is essential to acknowledge that not only those who identify as female breastfeed, and some may feel more comfortable referring to it as "chestfeeding" for a multitude of reasons. When inclusive care is provided, patients are more likely to have a safe and trusting relationship with their providers, which will promote health for both parents and their infants.

BOX 17.1 *HEALTHY PEOPLE 2030*

Selected National Health-Promotion and Disease-Prevention Objectives for Infants

Symbol	*Healthy People 2030* Objective
MICH-02	Reduce the rate of infant deaths
MICH-16	Increase the proportion of infants who are breastfed at 1 year
IID-05	Reduce cases of pertussis among infants
MICH-07	Reduce preterm births
IID-06	Increase the coverage level of four doses of the DTaP vaccine in children by age 2 years

DTaP, diphtheria-tetanus-pertussis.

BIOLOGY AND GENETICS

Human development begins when a single sperm penetrates a mature ovum. The changes that follow are undeniable and wondrous. During this early period of growth and development the infant depends completely on others, primarily the parents, to meet all personal needs (Table 17.1). To assist the parents in their understanding of their infant's needs and progress, the nurse must know what behaviors to expect at certain ages. These developmental landmarks serve as a basis for anticipatory guidance (Table 17.2). Parents are aware of age-appropriate behavior to anticipate and facilitate these developmental landmarks. This knowledge, along with the nurse's anticipatory guidance, can also promote closer family relationships. In addition to the growth landmarks, the infant must accomplish developmental tasks to form a healthy personality.

Developmental Tasks

Infant development begins before birth. A healthy pregnancy and a positive early childhood environment are essential to normal infant physical and mental health. Every infant faces developmental tasks and must accomplish them individually. Developmental change is a basic fact of human existence, and each infant is developmentally unique. Different practices in various societies affect the perception and resolution of the tasks, but all must be faced (Ruffin, 2019).

The infant's first and most basic task is survival, which includes the physical tasks of breathing, sucking, eating, digesting, eliminating, and sleeping. Because many of these tasks involve the infant's mouth, this stage of life often is referred to as the **oral stage of development**, reflecting the primary importance of the mouth as the center of pleasure. Piaget outlines five stages within the sensorimotor period that describe the infant's development, from the early reflexive behavior to differentiation between self and the environment (Table 17.3). In the first year, infants learn to focus their vision, reach out, explore, and seek out things around them. During this time, infants also develop bonds of love and trust with their caregivers and others as part of their social and emotional development. Nurses can provide the infant's caregivers with guidance to encourage their infant's development through:

- Talking to their infant, especially in a calming fashion
- Repeating sounds that their infant makes to help the infant learn to use language
- Reading to their infant to help develop and understand language and sounds
- Singing and playing music to help the infant develop a love for music and to help with brain development
- Giving their infant a great deal of loving attention to make the infant feel secure
- Praising their infant when something has been accomplished or learned (Centers for Disease Control and Prevention [CDC], 2021a).

To assist the infant's parents in encouraging achievement of these tasks, the nurse discusses the importance of stimulation and environmental interactions. Many neurologic structures are far from completely developed at birth. In parallel to growing

TABLE 17.1 Examples of Growth and Development Milestones During Infancy

1 Month
- Follows and fixes on bright object with eyes when it moves within field of vision
- Still has head lag when pulled to sitting position
- Displays tonic neck, grasp, and Moro reflexes
- Turns head when prone, but unable to support it
- Displays sucking and rooting reflexes
- Holds hands in fists
- Looks intently at caregiver when talked to
- Lifts head momentarily when prone

2 Months
- Has closed posterior fontanel
- Lifts head almost 45 degrees off table when prone
- Follows moving object with eyes
- Grasp reflex decreases
- Recognizes familiar faces
- Pays attention to speaking voice
- Begins to have social smile

3 Months
- Visually inspects object and stares at own hand with apparent fascination when either appears in field of vision
- Has longer periods of wakefulness without crying
- Laughs aloud and shows pleasure in vocalization
- Holds head erect and steady; raises chest, usually supported on forearms
- Smiles in response to mother's face
- Recognizes faces, voices, and familiar objects
- Opens and closes hands, shakes toys
- Begins prelanguage vocalizations (coos, babbles, and chuckles)

4 Months
- Begins drooling
- Holds head steady when in sitting position
- Recognizes familiar objects
- Shows almost no head lag when pulled to sitting position
- Rolls from back to side and from abdomen to back
- Inspects and plays with hands; pulls clothing or blanket over face in play
- Begins eye-hand coordination
- Chews and bites

5 Months
- Reaches persistently, grasps with entire hand
- Begins to discover parts of their body
- Smiles at mirror image
- Shows signs of tooth eruption
- Weighs twice the birth weight
- Sits with slight support
- Vocalizes displeasure when desired object is taken away
- Rolls from back to stomach or vice versa

6 Months
- Gains approximately 3–5 ounces weekly during the second 6 months
- Grows approximately 1 inch monthly for 6 months
- Is able to lift cup by handle
- Sits in highchair with straight back
- Begins to imitate sounds
- Vocalizes to toys and mirror image
- Recognizes caregivers
- Babbles with one-syllable sounds: "ma, ma, da, da"
- Chewing and biting occur

7 Months
- Bears weight when held in standing position
- Sits, leaning forward on both hands
- Fixates on one very small object
- Produces vowel sounds: "ba-ba" and "da-da"
- Shows fear of strangers
- Displays emotional instability by easy and quick changes from crying to laughing
- Repeats activities that are enjoyed

8 Months
- Feeds self with finger foods
- Sits well alone
- Stretches out arms to be picked up
- Greets strangers with bashful behavior
- Releases object at will
- Shows nervousness with strangers
- Pulls toy toward self

9 Months
- Creeps and crawls
- Shows good coordination and sits alone
- Responds to adult anger; cries when scolded
- Explores object by sucking, chewing, and biting it
- Responds to simple verbal requests
- Pulls self to standing position
- Imitates waving "bye-bye"
- Uses thumb and index finger in pincer grasp

10 Months
- Sits by falling down
- Says "da-da" and "ma-ma" with meaning
- Understands "bye-bye"
- Looks at and follows pictures in book
- Object permanence begins to develop
- Plays interactive games such as pat-a-cake
- Crawls and cruises about well
- Pays attention to own name

11 Months
- Is able to push toys and place several objects in container
- Attempts to walk without assistance
- Begins to hold spoon
- Explores objects more thoroughly
- Stands erect with help of person's hand
- Imitates definite speech sounds
- Reacts to restrictions with frustration

12 Months
- Loses Babinski sign
- Understands simple verbal commands
- Develops evident hand dominance
- Weighs triple the birth weight

Continued

TABLE 17.1 Examples of Growth and Development Milestones During Infancy—cont'd

- **Knows own name**
- **Turns pages in book**
- **Has slow vocabulary growth because of increased interest in walking**
- **Drops object deliberately for it to be picked up**
- **Shakes head for "no"**
- **Recovers balance when falling over**

15 Months

- **Creeps up stairs**
- **Uses "da-da" and "ma-ma" labels for correct parents**
- **Tolerates some separation**
- **Drinks from cup**
- **Asks for object by pointing**
- **Plays interactive games such as peek-a-boo and pat-a-cake**
- **Expresses emotions; may have temper tantrums**
- **Walks without help**

18 Months

- **Has closed anterior fontanel**
- **Has long trunk, short and bowed legs, and protruding abdomen**
- **Walks upstairs with help**
- **Turns pages of book**
- **Has short attention span**
- **Is extremely curious**
- **Places object in a hole or slot**
- **Imitates behavior of parents, such as mimicking household chores (Ruffin, 2019)**

TABLE 17.2 GROWTH AND DEVELOPMENT

Developmental Tasks Accomplished in Infancy

- **Achieves physiologic equilibrium after birth**
- **Establishes self as a dependent person but separate from others**
- **Becomes aware of animate versus inanimate objects and familiar versus unfamiliar objects and develops rudimentary social interaction**
- **Develops a feeling of affection for others and the desire for affection from others**
- **Manages the changing body and learns new motor skills, develops equilibrium, begins eye-hand coordination, and establishes rest-activity rhythm**
- **Learns to understand and control the physical world through exploration**
- **Develops a beginning symbol system, conceptual abilities, and preverbal communication**
- **Directs emotional expression to indicate needs and wishes**

Centers for Disease Control and Prevention (CDC) (2023d); Center for Parenting Education (2023)

TABLE 17.3 GROWTH AND DEVELOPMENT

Piaget's Five Stages of Infant Development

Stage	Description
1: Birth to 1 month	Modification of reflexes Practices and perfects reflexes present at birth Sucking reflex becomes more refined and voluntary
2: 1–4 months	Primary circular reactions Repeats behavior that previously led to an interesting event Only the infant's own body involved in activities
3: 4–10 months	Secondary circular reactions begin Repetitions involve events or objects in the external world Appears to perform actions with a purpose Hand-eye coordination
4: 10–12 months	Coordination of secondary reactions Combines two or more previously acquired strategies to obtain a goal
5: 12–18 months	Tertiary circular reactions Uses active experimentation to achieve previously unattainable goals Purposely varies movements to observe results

Malik & Marwaha (2023); Ruffin (2019)

in size, infants will acquire new skills and abilities as their brain develops. This process involves a complex interaction of genes and the environment. The genes determine the basic "wiring plan" by forming neuronal connections between different brain regions, while the environment influences the extent to which the infant achieves that potential through interaction (Webster, Morris, & Kevelighan, 2018). To continue growing, the brain depends not only on internal, embryologic, and maturational forces, but also on external stimulation. This external stimulation appears to influence the internal, anatomical, and maturational processes by different mechanisms. Age-appropriate stimulation, through play, is the chief way that infants learn how to move, communicate, socialize, and understand their surroundings (Kliegman et al., 2020):

- Stimulation favors progressive complex branching of dendrites (the connection between nerve cells).
- Stimulation increases the degree of vascularization of certain anatomical structures of the brain, such as the centers associated with vision.
- Stimulation through social experiences is the portal to linguistic, cognitive, and emotional development in infants.
- Stimulated infants tend to have higher intelligence quotients (IQs) and better memory as they grow older.

- Stimulation increases the process of myelination, which is closely related to the rate of development of a variety of functions. Myelin coats the brain and nerve tissue, which then becomes activated.

When counseling parents, the nurse stresses the importance of a variety of stimuli within the infant's environment. A variety of auditory and visual stimuli should be available, such as colorful mobiles, radio, blocks, puzzles, coloring books, balls, push-and-pull toys, and spoken voice, to assist the infant in achieving developmental tasks. The sense of touch is an extremely important stimulus, bringing the infant in tune with caregivers in different environments, making the environment a reality. Ensuring that appropriate sensory stimuli are available is vital to the infant's growth and developmental progression (AAP, 2021a).

Concepts of Infant Development

As infants develop, they go through a series of developmental stages that are important for all aspects of their personhood, including physical, intellectual, emotional, and social aspects. Experience plays an essential role in building brain architecture after birth. The role of their caretakers is to provide encouragement, support, and access to activities that enable them to master key developmental tasks. The study of how a helpless infant grows and develops into a fully functioning, independent adult has fascinated many researchers. Their theories describe the development of human behavior as overlapping stages that occur in somewhat predictable patterns in an individual's life (Academies of Sciences, Engineering, and Medicine, 2019). Because these developmental theories are presented in Chapter 15, only their specific application to the infant is discussed here.

Psychosocial Development

Erikson's Psychosocial Developmental Theory is concerned primarily with a series of tasks or crises that each individual must resolve; each must be resolved before the next one can be mastered. The central task during infancy is the development of a sense of **trust versus mistrust**. This occurs when adults meet an infant's basic needs for survival. The establishment of this basic trust or mistrust determines the way the infant approaches all future stages of growth. The infant develops a sense of trust first in their parents and then in other significant people. Trust influences the infant's future relationships, allowing deeper commitment and intimacy. To develop trust, the infant requires maximal gratification and minimal frustration to experience a healthy balance between inner needs and outer satisfaction. If the parent is consistently responsive to the infant, meeting physical and psychological needs, the infant will likely learn to trust their caretaker, view the world as a safe place, and grow up to be secure, self-reliant, trusting, cooperative, and helpful toward others.

A prompt, skillful, and consistent response to the infant's needs helps foster security and trust because it enables the infant to predict what will happen within the environment. When unpredictability and disorganized routines exist, the infant will develop fear, anger, anxiety, and insecurity, which eventually lead to mistrust. The infant can demonstrate desire by crying but depends on the sensitivity and willingness of others to provide relief. If the most important people fail to do this, the infant has little foundation on which to build faith in others or self in adulthood. If the infant's needs are not met appropriately, the infant will grow up with a sense of mistrust and may view the world as unpredictable.

Cognitive Development

Piaget's cognitive developmental theory focuses on intellectual changes that occur in a sequential manner because of continual interaction between the infant and the environment. The theory is based on the idea that infants actively construct knowledge as they explore and manipulate the world around them (Babakr, Mohamedamin, & Kakamad, 2019). Piaget's sensorimotor period (up to age 18 months) describes the time during which infants develop the coordination to master activities that allow them to interact with the environment. During this period, the infant solves problems using sensory systems and motor activity rather than symbolic processes, which develop later.

Fetuses can distinguish light from dark, and sight is present at birth. Rod cells in the retina of the eyes, which are responsible for light perception, are functional at birth, although the retina (the organ of visual perception) is not fully developed until approximately 4 months of age. However, the infant can perceive color and shape. Infants are startled by loud noises and are soothed by soft voices, indicating that their sense of hearing is functioning. Their hearing can also be tested with audio equipment at birth. Babies cry when pricked with a diaper pin and fuss when too hot or too cold; therefore, the senses of pain and temperature are also operative. Touching, stroking, and rocking typically comfort a fussing infant. Infants will also react to odors and tastes.

In addition to perceiving stimulation, the newborn is capable of reflexive behavior. **Reflexes** are responses that are normally exhibited after particular types of new stimulation (Malik & Marwaha, 2023). Because the response occurs after the stimulus, reflexes are unlearned. Some infant reflexes, such as rooting and sucking, have survival value. The rooting reflex, activated by the angle of the lips or cheek being lightly stroked, helps the infant locate the food source. The infant will turn toward the side that is being stroked and will open the lips to suck. The sucking reflex is initiated when an object is placed in the infant's mouth. Together these reflexes ensure that the infant can obtain food. Infants also have reflexes that result in grasping, yawning, hiccoughing, coughing, and sneezing.

Armed with these reflexes and sensory capabilities, the infant is ready to begin interacting with the environment (seeing, hearing, touching, tasting, and smelling) to acquire valuable information.

The infant in the sensorimotor period uses behavioral strategies to manipulate objects, to learn some of their properties, and to reach goals by combining several behaviors. The infant's behavior is tied to the concrete and the immediate; schemes can be applied only to objects that can be perceived directly.

Knowledge of child developmental theories is extremely valuable to the nurse during interactions with infants. Understanding the infant's level of cognitive thought and emotional and social development helps the nurse to decipher a child's communications more meaningfully and to interpret behaviors and processes that motivate the child more accurately. This knowledge can be incorporated in the anticipatory guidance offered to the parents. The nurse stresses that a variety of sensory and motor stimuli foster learning within the infant's environment.

The Infant Development Inventory is a 60-question infant assessment tool parents can complete that screens children from birth to 18 months. It tracks developmental skills in five areas: social, self-help, gross motor, fine motor, and language. Monthly developmental milestones on the development chart help parents obtain a more comprehensive picture of how infants develop. Parents can also report any questions or concerns about their infant's health, development, or behavior. Health care providers may also further assess the infant's development by observing behaviors and recording them on the chart, in which case the baby's progress will be scored "typical," "borderline," or "delayed" in each developmental area.

The infant's **growth index**—height and weight measurements plotted on a standard growth chart to assess the infant for normal progression—is also important. Physical growth (height and weight) is a valid health status indicator that should be measured during each routine office or clinic visit. During the first year of life, growth is rapid (CDC, 2019).

The nurse plots the infant's length and weight measurements against exact chronologic age on growth grids. The World Health Organization (WHO) releases international growth charts for children aged 0 to 59 months. The growth charts are international standards that show how healthy children should grow. It is recommended by the AAP and CDC that the WHO international growth charts be used for children younger than 24 months and that the CDC growth charts be used for children older than 24 months (CDC, 2019). **Body mass index** (BMI) is a feature of the new pediatric growth charts that have been released by the CDC. BMI is the individual's weight in kilograms divided by the square of height in meters. In infants and children, a high amount of body fat can lead to weight-related diseases and other health issues. A BMI calculator for children and teens can be found on the CDC's website: https://www.cdc.gov/healthyweight/bmi/calculator.html. Growth charts are not intended to be used as sole diagnostic instruments. Instead, growth charts are tools that contribute to the formation of an overall clinical impression of the child being measured (CDC, 2019).

An infant's **growth index**, as determined by length and weight, is only one factor used in the assessment of health status. Differences in **growth** curves can influence the diagnosis of undernutrition and overnutrition and the interpretation of adequate growth following nutritional intervention. The nurse has an overall understanding of growth and developmental principles to counsel parents regarding their infant's progress.

Sex

Sex is a biologic concept, while gender is a social concept and refers to the social and cultural differences a society assigns to people based on their sex. The infant's sex is determined at the moment of fertilization. An embryo with two X chromosomes will become a female, while an embryo with a X-Y combination results in a male.

There are many biologic and behavioral differences between male and female infants. Males are, on average, larger and have proportionately more muscle mass at birth. Females are generally smaller but physiologically more mature at birth and are less vulnerable to stress. Males show more motor activity, whereas females display a greater response to tactile stimulation and pain. As the infant develops, further differences are noted. By 6 months, females respond to visual stimulation with longer attention spans and are more socially responsive than are males; females also tend to sit up, walk, and crawl earlier than do males. Females also tend to learn to communicate with language at an earlier age, whereas male infants use their whole bodies in communicating.

Health intervention focuses on the identification of high-risk families and the promotion of positive relationships between infants and parents. The nurse promotes the good health, appearance, and developmental potential of the infant. Increasing the parents' feelings of adequacy and self-esteem will promote their acceptance and care of the infant. Most importantly, follow-up care for these families is a high priority to ensure that adequate support and help are available (Ruffin, 2019).

Assessing Diverse Populations

A range of normal anatomic and physical variation exists among different populations regarding growth rate, dentition, body structure, blood groups, and susceptibility to certain diseases. In assessing an infant, the nurse not only collects data, but also compares the data with established norms, such as a standardized growth chart. The nurse who works with families from a variety of populations understands each background and how it relates to health and health care. To facilitate nursing care for a family from a cultural group different from that of the health care provider, effective communication must be established. This communication will help foster an understanding of the other's point of view and frame of reference. Each family member is viewed as an individual, as well as a family unit. Despite common language, skin color, or historical background, not all members of a particular group are alike. Universal norms by which to measure one's growth and skill capacity do not exist. Education surrounding health maintenance and disease prevention is basic to future health practices. This concept is the focus of all health care.

Genetics

In the past several decades, remarkable progress has been made in our understanding of the structure and function of genes and chromosomes. These advances have been aided by the complete sequencing of human DNA—our genome. This knowledge can now be applied to medical care. The desired and expected outcome of any pregnancy is the birth of a healthy, perfect baby. Parents experience disappointment when they discover that their baby has been born with a defect. A **birth defect** is an abnormality of structure, function, or metabolism as a result of a genetic or environmental influence on the fetus, often a combination of both. Couples may refrain from having another child because they have had one with a serious birth defect and do not want to risk another. In these situations, genetic counseling provides information that is needed to understand a hereditary disorder and its associated risks. The main goal of counseling is to explain birth defects to affected families and to allow prospective parents to make informed decisions about childbearing.

Using the basic laws governing heredity and knowing the frequency of specific birth defects in the population, the genetic counselor often predicts the probability of recurrence of a given abnormality in the same family. An important aspect of primary prevention is identifying families at increased risk and referring them for genetic counseling (Clarke, 2020). The aspects to be reviewed in the initial interview include the following:

- Maternal age. The risk of having a child with Down syndrome increases significantly for the female older than 35 years. In Down syndrome, there are three chromosomes in the 21-chromosome group (trisomy 21). Characteristic features of Down syndrome include upward-slanting eyes; small, malformed ears; large, protruding tongue; broad hands and feet; and some degree of mental disability.
- Ethnic background. Several genetic disorders occur with higher frequency in certain groups. Anyone can be a carrier of Tay-Sachs disease, but the disease is most common among the Ashkenazi Jewish population. The incidence of Tay-Sachs disease in this population is 1 in 3600 people. The carrier frequency for the general population for Tay-Sachs disease is 1 in 250 (National Tay-Sachs & Allied Diseases Association, 2023). Tay-Sachs is a genetic disorder caused by the absence of beta-hexosaminidase. This missing enzyme causes cells to be damaged, resulting in progressive neurologic disorders. Abnormal deposits of lipids (fats) in the cells of the cerebral cortex, spleen, liver, and lymph nodes are characteristic of Tay-Sachs disease. Rapid and progressive deterioration of the brain and nervous system ensues, with death typically occurring by age 6 years. An autosomal recessive gene transmits the disease. Blacks have a much greater chance of carrying the sickle cell trait than does the general population. **Sickle cell anemia** is an autosomal recessive condition that occurs in 1 in 500 African Americans and 1 in 1200 Hispanic Americans and causes severe hemolytic anemia crises. Sickle cell anemia affects millions worldwide. Approximately 100,000 Americans have sickle cell disease, which is a lifelong illness. One in 13 Black Americans carries the sickle cell trait (National Institutes of Health [NIH], 2020a).
- Family history. Certain diseases, such as Huntington chorea, hemophilia, and some forms of intellectual disability, are hereditary. Huntington chorea (an autosomal dominant disease involving the brain) is characterized by deterioration of intellectual functions and involuntary movements of the limbs, face, and trunk. Once symptoms have manifested themselves, a steady deterioration leads to death in approximately 20 years. Hemophilia is a sex-linked recessive coagulation disorder caused by a functional deficiency of a clotting factor; it leads to prolonged bleeding. There are several types, but hemophilia generally passes from an unaffected carrier to their male offspring. It affects 1 in 5000 male births. Approximately 400 babies are born with hemophilia each year in the United States, with approximately 20,000 people with it in the United States presently (CDC, 2023a).
- Reproductive history. Spontaneous abortions, stillbirths, and previous live-born children with birth defects or slow development may indicate an increased risk.
- Maternal disease. Several maternal disorders are associated with a higher frequency of birth defects, including diabetes mellitus, seizure disorder, mental disability, and phenylketonuria. Prenatal diagnosis offers the couple the option of aborting a fetus that has certain genetic disorders. For many people, however, this option is unacceptable. Chapter 16 discusses the various tests used for prenatal diagnosis.

The nurse's role throughout the genetic counseling process is to provide the vital link between the counseling team and the high-risk couple. Nurses need to understand not only the foundations of genetics and genomics but also the implications of these sciences for those for whom they provide care. The nurse is involved in case finding, referral, and family education. As a result of the new and expanding technology devoted to genetic and genomic research, a growing number of genetic tests are available for the screening, diagnosis, and treatment of rare and common diseases. All nurses will need to become knowledgeable about the basics of genetics and genomics and their applications to clinical care so that they can provide quality health care that is appropriate to their setting, population, geographical location, access, and coverage. During the genetic assessment process, nurses can help clients understand test results, provide support, explore implications for the family, and encourage compliance with screening and treatment recommendations. This knowledge will allow nurses to provide appropriate and accurate information to care recipients regarding genetic tests that are part of their own health care (International Society of Nurses in Genetics [ISONG], n.d.).

GORDON'S FUNCTIONAL HEALTH PATTERNS

Health Perception–Health Management Pattern

Health promotion is aimed at assisting the infant and the infant's family to change behavior to produce better physical and emotional health in adulthood. The old saying "an ounce of prevention is worth a pound of cure" has great merit, and if considered and acted on, this can be very effective in promoting an individual's health. To reach this goal, the nurse encourages childrearing practices that promote normal growth and development, fosters attitudes and values compatible with health, and teaches appropriate use of health services. Parents must be advised to factor health implications into all their decisions to prevent their infants from becoming ill and to protect them from injuries. Health-promotion measures by nurses aim to prevent and minimize ill health of all individuals and their families. Nurses provide a pathway to access health care, engaging people to stay healthy, share in decision-making concerning their own health, and to help families that need to negotiate the health care system (Phillips, 2019). The nurse promotes the infant's health through the parents, who determine the care practices for the dependent infant.

Health is largely a subjective judgment. Each person's perception of health is related to physical and mental capabilities, self-concept, relationships with others and the environment, and personal goals and values. Living a healthy lifestyle relates to making lifestyle choices that support an individual's physical, mental, spiritual, and emotional well-being (WHO, 2023b). With this understanding, the nurse uses every opportunity to convey confidence in the parents' health perception–health management pattern and to improve their ability to implement behaviors that promote the infant's health. When parents learn and adopt behaviors that improve their own health, they are more likely to ensure that the health needs of their infant are met. Parental modeling increases the chances that good health practices will be retained throughout the child's life.

The goals of nursing practice with infants and their families are to promote individual motivation for health, to assist the family in identifying health needs, and to develop problem-solving skills within the family unit using the family's own resources. To meet these goals, the nurse identifies the family's perception of good or bad health practices, which greatly influences participation in health-promoting activities. Age, sex, educational level, cultural orientation, financial status, and occupation combine to influence health perception. When parents believe that the infant is more susceptible to a health problem if promotional behavior is not enacted, they become more motivated to adopt the behavior.

The nurse's task helps the parents recognize their infant's susceptibility and the potential consequences when healthy practices are not instituted. The nurse works within the family's health perception framework to become acquainted with the characteristics that influence the infant's health. Unless caregivers meet their own personal needs, they will be unable to meet their infant's developmental needs. The empowerment and growth of parents is a key element in facilitating the successful development of their infants. Parents with higher levels of education have healthier children. Supportive households and communities are vital to ensuring that parents and their infants have full access to the opportunities they need to realize their full potential (US Agency for International Development [USAID], 2023). The nurse supports the parents, strengthening their parental confidence and self-esteem, providing information on meeting their infant's needs, and reinforcing their health perception–health management pattern.

Nutritional-Metabolic Pattern

One of the most important aspects of health promotion in the infant is nutritional status. Many opinions have been expressed about the infant's nutritional needs. As research in this area continues, recommendations and opinions will change; however, some basic facts about nutrition remain consistent. Breast/chest milk or formula will provide practically every nutrient the infant needs for the first year of life. Infant nutritional requirements are based on what is considered necessary to support life, provide for growth, and maintain health.

Essential Nutrients

During infancy, a period of rapid growth, nutrient requirements per pound of body weight are proportionally higher than at any other time in the life cycle. Water, proteins, fats, carbohydrates, vitamins, and minerals are the essential nutrients in any diet. Each infant is unique. Infants differ in the amount of nutrients ingested and stored, their body composition, growth rates, and physical activity levels. Because the first year of life is a period of rapid growth, nutritional needs during this period are especially important and always changing. Water is vital to survival. A person can live for several weeks without food but can survive only a few days without water. Because the infant's body weight is approximately 75% water, the baby must consume large amounts of fluid to maintain water balance. Under normal circumstances, the water requirements of healthy infants who are fed adequate amounts of breast/chest milk or properly reconstituted infant formula are met by the breast/chest milk or infant formula alone. Supplemental water is not necessary, even in hot, dry climates (US Department of Agriculture [USDA], 2019). The sources of water are fluids (primarily milk) and food; most strained foods are 75% to 85% water. Most infant diets, without supplementation, meet the basic water requirement.

The infant must also consume sufficient high-quality protein to facilitate growth and development. The recommended daily protein requirements are 9.1 g during the first 6 months and 11 g during the second 6 months. No more than 20% of an infant's daily energy requirement should come from protein because infants are not able to process and excrete the excess nitrogen from higher-protein diets (USDA, 2019).

Carbohydrates should supply 30% to 60% of the energy intake during infancy. Approximately 37% of the calories in human milk and 40% to 50% of the calories in commercial formulas are derived from lactose or other carbohydrates (USDA, 2019).

For infants, 31 g of fats per day for the first 6 months of life and 30 g of fats per day during the second 6 months of life (40% to 50% of the calories) are recommended. These quantities are present in human milk and in all formulas prepared for infants. Breast/chest milk and formulas provide approximately 50% of their calories as fat. Significantly lower intakes, such as in skim milk feedings, can result in an inadequate nutritional intake (USDA, 2019).

Vitamins are essential nutrients in the infant's diet that regulate metabolism and allow more efficient use of carbohydrates, fats, and proteins within the body. Although most infants receive adequate vitamin intake through iron-fortified formula, breast/chest milk, and food, recent research has raised a concern about a vitamin D deficiency in infants who receive only breast/chest milk. Vitamin D deficiency is quite common among US infants. Because human milk does not contain enough vitamin D, all breast/chest fed infants should receive a minimum intake of 400 international units (IU) of vitamin D per day starting soon after birth. The formula-fed infant does not need additional supplementation (USDA, 2019). Minerals are found in relatively small amounts in the infant's body but are vital elements in body structure and control of certain body functions. Mineral intake for infants appears to be adequate, except for iron and fluoride.

The full-term infant is born with stores of iron adequate to meet the needs for hemoglobin production for approximately 4 to 6 months. After this time, body stores may need to be replenished. Although iron in human milk is bioavailable, both breast/chestfed and formula-fed infants should receive an additional source of iron by 6 months of age. Iron-fortified formula and cereals are the most commonly used food sources. It is important to note that vitamin C helps a food's natural iron remain absorption friendly and helps enhance the iron's uptake by the body cells.

Fluoride, concentrated in the bones and teeth, helps reduce dental caries. Although fluoride is important for strong tooth development, it is not recommended during the first 6 months of life. Supplementation is necessary only when the diet contains insufficient fluoridated water.

A review of these requirements shows that milk (breast/chest or formula) meets most of the infant's nutritional needs when consumed in adequate amounts, plus vitamin D supplementation for the high-risk infants. The AAP recommends starting solid food at 6 months old and states that solids should not begin before 4 months old (AAP, 2023b)

If the parents choose to formula-feed versus breast/chestfeed their infant, the nurse should educate the parents about safe preparation of infant formula as follows:

- Check the expiration date and condition of each container of formula.
- Wash the top of the container with soap and water before opening it.
- Wash hands thoroughly before preparing infant formula.
- Prepare the bottle by washing it with soap and water or in the dishwasher.
- Follow the manufacturer's instructions for how much water to use.
- Use prepared formula within 2 hours of preparation and within 1 hour from when feeding begins.
- Throw out any infant formula that is left in the bottle after a feeding. The combination of formula and the infant's saliva can foster bacterial growth.
- Warm the formula by placing it in warm water, never in a microwave oven.
- Shake the bottle well and feed the formula to the infant.

Formula Shortage. In February 2022, the United States' largest formula supplier, Abbott Nutrition, shut down their Michigan plant and voluntarily recalled their formula products due to contamination with *Cronobacter sakazakii* or *Salmonella*. This shutdown and recall lead to a formula shortage that continued for over a year and a half. The average out-of-stock rate for formula reached a nationwide high of 70% in May of 2022, and some states, such as California, saw an out-of-stock rate up to 80%. The formula shortage created immense stress and uncertainty for families whose infants relied on formula for nutrition. Most concerning, the shortage disproportionately affected families of low income as Abbott Nutrition supplies formula for the governmental program Women, Infants, and Children (WIC; Jung et al., 2022). In response to this unprecedented event, it is important to consider what planning and recommendations should be in place should something like this occur in the future. The current recommendations focus on consumer awareness of potential shortages, prevention of contamination events, and support for breast/chestfeeding families (Abrams & Duggan, 2022). Even with these recommendations, consideration must be given to those who cannot or choose not to breast/chestfeed, particularly those of low socioeconomic status.

Food Additives

In addition to their questionable nutritional value, additives in commercial baby food can negatively influence an infant's health status. The purposes of food additives differ, including adding nutritional value; preserving or extending shelf life; facilitating preparation; improving flavor, color, and texture; and keeping flavors and textures consistent (WHO, 2023a).

Commercially prepared baby foods are generally safe, nutritious, and high quality. In response to consumer demand, baby food manufacturers have removed much of the added salt and sugar that their products once contained and have eliminated most food additives.

Nutrition problems include undernutrition, in which infants do not receive an adequate supply of an essential nutrient, and overnutrition, in which they receive more of a certain nutrient than is needed for healthy growth and development. Rapid weight gain in infancy over and above the average weight gain by WHO growth charts has consistently been associated with increased subsequent obesity risk in later years by several studies (Koletzko, Godfrey, & Poston et al., 2019). For infants in the United States, both problems are present. A parent who wants the infant to have family foods rather than commercial baby food can provide a small portion of table food at each meal. This choice necessitates cooking without salt or sugar, which is the practice of baby food manufacturers. Making baby food is easy and economical. Written resources are available for parents who are interested in more details about home food preparation for infants.

Parents should be encouraged to read baby food labels carefully. Nurses can obtain lists of baby foods and their ingredients from the manufacturers. The best overall recommendation that nurses make to parents is to provide their infants with a well-balanced diet and avoid excesses.

Breast/chestfeeding

The AAP recommends breast/chestfeeding for the first 6 months of life. Breast/chestfeeding should be continued for at least the first year of life and beyond for as long as mutually desired by the parent and child (AAP, 2019a). Both the American Dietetic Association and the AAP have released position statements in support of breast/chestfeeding. This has influenced several health-promotion strategies in the United States. The Healthy People 2030 objectives do address breast/chestfeeding (US Department of Health and Human Services [USDHHS], 2023; Box 17.2: Evidence-Based Practice). Efforts to promote breast/chestfeeding must be strengthened in hospitals, health maintenance organizations, private health care offices, and public health clinics. The federal law, Providing Urgent Maternal Protections (PUMP) for Nursing Mothers Act, requires all employers to provide a private place and breaktime for breast/chestfeeding employees (US Department of Labor, 2024).

While breast/chestfeeding is recommended as the optimal source of nutrition for an infant, it is important to note that parents may choose not to breast/chestfeed for a multitude

BOX 17.2 EVIDENCE-BASED PRACTICE

Skin Care Interventions in Infants for Preventing Eczema and Food Allergy (Kelleher et al., 2022)

Skin care lotions to protect and moisturize have been sold for over 100 years. Today, there are numerous products that claim to be for sensitive skin, have protective barriers, relieve eczema, and contain a wide array of products. Some products such as oils may be used in infant bath water.

Eczema and food allergies are common health conditions that typically start in early childhood and often occur in the same individual. An allergy is an overreaction of the body's immune system to a specific substance, such as skin products or food. The results can be mild or serious. Eczema is a topical skin allergy that causes dry, itchy, cracked skin on various parts of the body. The objective of this study was to evaluate the effects of skin care interventions, such as emollients, to prevent eczema and food allergies in infants. Several studies searched databases to identify randomized controlled trials on this topic, in addition to contacting field experts to find unpublished or incomplete trials. Many smaller studies tested the use of moisturizers and others used bathing and cleaning products on the infant's skin. In the first study, 33 studies involving 25,827 infants were found to meet the criteria, and 17 were used in the analysis (Kelleher et al., 2022). Skin care was compared against no skin care or standard care as usual. Most of the study data came from children's hospitals. The effects of interventions were not influenced by infant age, duration of intervention, or hereditary risk of developing eczema. The second study was an update of the first.

Skin care interventions, such as the application of emollients, bathing, or cleaning agents, did not demonstrate eczema prevention in healthy infants during their first year of life and may have contributed to an increased risk of skin infections. The study findings were inconclusive about how skin care interventions affected the development of food allergies.

Based on the findings of this study, nurses can discourage the use of skin emollients on infants for the purpose of eczema or food allergy prevention. It is even possible that the risk of skin infections might be increased with daily use of these agents. In addition, an allergic reaction to lotion moisturizers that have many ingredients may develop. As infants must be held, using moisturizers may also contribute to the increased risk of infant slippage. The authors concluded that more evidence to define the risks might become available in future research studies.

of reasons. In these cases, these parents should be supported in their informed decision-making process. The decision to breast/chestfeed is complex and depends on multiple factors—demographic, biologic, psychological, social, and educational.

"Chestfeeding" is a term that is used by some individuals who identify as transgender or nonbinary to describe how they feed their baby. The use of the word "chestfeeding" to describe how an individual feeds their baby does not indicate whether that individual has had breast/chest tissue removal surgery. Transgender individuals may need support in inducing lactation if they choose to breast/chestfeed or in suppressing their milk supply if they have chosen not to breast/chestfeed (La Leche League International, 2024). An individual does not need to have physically given birth to choose to breast/chestfeed their infant. Lactation can be induced for a multitude of reasons including in the cases of adoption and surrogacy.

WHO, the United Nations Children's Fund (UNICEF), and Healthy People 2030 have adopted the Baby-Friendly Hospital Initiative to establish a global effort to increase breast/chestfeeding (Baby-Friendly USA, 2023a). To become a baby-friendly health care facility, the 10 steps to successful breast/chestfeeding must be implemented, as shown in Box 17.3.

BOX 17.3 Baby-Friendly Hospital Initiative Breast/Chestfeeding Guidelines

- Have a written breast/chestfeeding policy that is communicated routinely to all health care staff.
- Train all health care staff in the skills necessary to implement this policy.
- Inform all pregnant people about the benefits and management of breast/chestfeeding.
- Help initiate breast/chestfeeding within 30 minutes after birth.
- Show birthing parents how to breast/chestfeed and how to maintain lactation even when they are separated from their infants.
- Give newborn infants no food or drink other than breast/chest milk unless medically indicated.
- Practice rooming-in; allow parents and infants to remain together 24 hours a day.
- Encourage breast/chestfeeding on demand.
- Do not give pacifiers to breast/chestfeeding infants.
- Foster the establishment of breast/chestfeeding support groups and refer to these groups upon discharge from the hospital or clinic.

Baby-Friendly USA (2023b)

A birthing parent's decisions on whether to breast/chestfeed can be influenced by information they receive from their health care providers (March of Dimes, 2020b). Guidance given to parents on breast/chestfeeding in the postpartum period increases their knowledge of the subject and, consequently, the prevalence of this practice for a longer period. Nurses need to provide parents with guidance and congruent, sensitive, effective, and beneficial support for them to be successful with the breast/chestfeeding experience (Brown & Jones, 2020). Low levels of actual or perceived professional support and lack of knowledge, support, and measures needed to cope with breast/chestfeeding difficulties are found to be associated with lower breast/chestfeeding rates. In one study done in Sweden, mothers often perceived a lack of support from pediatric nurses, while nurses felt that adequate support had been given. Mothers who perceived low support felt that the efforts were superficial and often contradictory (Ranch et al., 2019). Because of the important role of the parent's choice of infant feeding, nurses can be instrumental in working toward the national goal to increase breast/chestfeeding by supporting and educating all parents about the advantages of the practice (Box 17.4). Community nurses who are caring for breast/chestfeeding parents stress the following tips to increase the duration of this activity:

- Drink 1 quart of fluids daily to produce a sufficient quantity of breast/chest milk.
- Watch the infant, not the clock. Look for early signs of wanting-to-feed behaviors.
- Sunlight is the principle source of vitamin D, so a supplement might be needed.
- Try to rest when the infant sleeps, so you do not become overtired.
- Consume 300 to 400 kcal/day above the prepregnancy energy intake to avoid excessive weight loss.

BOX 17.4 Advantages of Breast/Chestfeeding

Human Milk

- Has the correct balance of all essential nutrients for infants
- Is full of immunologic agents to protect against disease
- Has a composition that changes to meet the growing infant's needs
- Is easier to digest than is formula
- Contains antiinflammatory properties
- Promotes growth of *Lactobacillus bifidus*
- Reduces risk of childhood obesity, ear infections, and diabetes
- Reduces risk of asthma and respiratory viruses

Breast/chestfeeding

- Assists in the process of uterine involution
- Decreases postpartum vaginal bleeding
- Reduces childhood obesity
- Strengthens the immune system of infants
- Reduces incidence of pneumonia, colds, and viruses
- Releases oxytocin, which promotes better healing in the postpartum period
- Protects infants against developing allergies
- Decreases costs for public health programs (e.g., WIC)
- Decreases SIDS rate, overweight, and obesity in adulthood
- Decreases environmental burden for disposal of formula cans and bottles

SIDS, Sudden Infant Death Syndrome; *WIC,* Women, Infants, and Children.
Brown & Jones (2020); March of Dimes (2020b)

- Learn the appropriate interventions for engorged breasts, sore nipples, plugged ducts, infection, and leaking nipples.
- Expose nipples to air after each feeding and allow some breast/chest milk to dry on nipples for its lubricating and antiinfective properties.
- Learn about the use of breast/chest pumps and milk storage.
- Join breast/chestfeeding support groups for continued help within the community.
- Learn about the effects of drugs, environmental pollutants, alcohol, and nicotine on breast/chest milk (Brown & Jones, 2020).

Introduction of Solid Foods

The timing of the first introduction of solid food during infancy may have potential effects on lifelong health. No scientific evidence is available on the best time to introduce solid foods during infancy. At approximately 4 to 6 months of age, the infant is usually physiologically and developmentally ready to have solid foods, either commercial or home prepared. The infant should be able to do the following developmental tasks before solid foods are introduced: sit with little or no support, have good head and neck control, push up with straight elbows from a lying face-down position, lean forward and open mouth when interested in food, and turn away when not hungry. The AAP and WHO recommend that waiting until the child is 6 months old to introduce solid food decreases the tendency for the child to develop food allergies and reduces the risk of childhood obesity. The introduction of various foods is recommended to supply a more appealing, diversified diet for the infant; supply energy, iron, and vitamins; and provide needed trace elements (CDC, 2023b). The decision to start solid foods earlier than 6 months of age is based more on neuromuscular and developmental readiness of the infant than on any hard scientific data, but research does validate the lowered risk of developing food allergies if solid foods are not introduced until 6 months of age. It is now thought that early introduction of highly allergenic foods, such as eggs, peanuts, tree nuts, and fish, can actually decrease the risk of allergy. Peanut allergy is a growing public health problem and the leading cause of death related to food-induced anaphylaxis in the United States. Infants with severe eczema, egg allergy, or both are at high risk for the development of peanut allergy. Early introduction of peanut-containing foods will result in the prevention of peanut allergy in many infants (National Institute of Allergy and Infectious Diseases [NIAID], 2018).

TABLE 17.4 First Food Options for the Infant

Age (Months)	Addition
4–6	Iron-fortified cereal, followed by other cereals
5–7	Strained vegetables and fruits and their juices
6–8	Protein foods (cheese, meat, fish, chicken, and yogurt)
9	Finely chopped meat, toast, teething crackers
10–12	Whole egg, whole milk (allergies less likely now)

US Department of Agriculture (n.d.); Brown (2019)

All infants develop according to their own schedules, and some are ready to start eating solid foods earlier than other infants. The addition of foods should be governed by an infant's nutritional needs and readiness to handle different forms of foods (Kliegman et al., 2020). The order of food introduction and the specific amounts to be given are based on tradition rather than on scientific fact. Few scientific studies have been performed to determine whether a specific order of infant food introduction is necessary or the amounts needed for optimal development. The sequence of solids typically recommended by the AAP is cereal (oatmeal, barley, grain), fruits, vegetables, and meats (Table 17.4). Certain foods to avoid for any infant younger than 12 months include whole cow's milk; foods that could cause choking—nuts, grapes, raw carrots, or candy; and honey. Cow's milk is not recommended because it does not contain adequate iron; honey is not recommended because of the potential risk of exposure to a harmful bacteria toxin—botulism poisoning. Honey can contain botulism spores; these spores release a toxin that can poison an infant. The typical sequence in which foods are introduced is shown in Box 17.5. A few tips to assist parents in making the introduction of solid foods a smooth transition are listed in Box 17.6.

Weaning

Weaning is a gradual, caring process that introduces the infant to a cup, which replaces the bottle or breast/chest. The biologic norm and desired method for weaning is to allow the infant to self-wean. Weaning should be started when the infant is ready. Developmentally, the infant can usually learn to use a cup by age 5 to 6 months; however, many children continue to nurse after they start using a cup. The infantile extrusion reflex needs to be absent. This reflex is present in very young infants and involves the tongue pushing out any material in the mouth

BOX 17.5 Solid Food Introduction Sequence

- Cereals (avoid large amounts of rice cereal due to high levels of arsenic); consider oat, barley, and multigrain
- Fruits such as peaches, pears, and applesauce
- Vegetables, with yellow vegetables (squash and carrots) given before green vegetables (peas or beans)
- Strained meats, such as nonallergenic lamb or veal

CDC (2022a)

BOX 17.6 Tips for Introducing Solid Foods

Assess the Infant's Readiness to Consume Solid Foods First

- The infant can sit up (with support) and can hold her/his head and neck up well.
- The infant is interested in what you are eating and may even try to grab food from your plate.
- The infant can keep food in her/his mouth rather than letting it dribble out.
- The infant shows signs of being hungry by wanting to nurse more often.
- If readiness is validated, then begin with the following:
  - Introduce only one new food at a time and in small amounts for 3–5 days. When the new food is not tolerated or the infant is allergic to it, the new food can be identified quickly and discontinued.
  - Initially, foods that are mashed, pureed, or strained and very smooth in texture should be provided as it can take time for infants to become used to new textures.
  - Introduce potentially allergenic foods when other foods are introduced including: cow's milk products, eggs, fish, shellfish, tree nuts, peanuts, wheat, soy, and sesame. Drinking cow's milk or fortified soy beverages is not recommended until your child is older than 12 months.
  - The infant must learn how to handle solid foods. Because infants use sucking movements, part of the food is ejected from the mouth. With time and practice, the infant learns how to take solid food from a spoon.
  - Always feed the infant with the infant in an upright position; do not feed the infant solids from the bottle.
  - Until the infant is 1 year old, feed the infant milk before solid foods.
  - Look at, smile at, and talk to the infant during feeding.
  - Do not give honey to infants younger than 12 months because of the risk of infant botulism.
  - Respect the infant's likes and dislikes; rejected foods may be reintroduced later.
  - Introduce peanut-containing foods early to avoid allergies later in life.

US Department of Agriculture (2023); CDC (2023b)

not associated with sucking. The safety advantages of this are obvious, but weaning cannot be commenced until the infant has matured sufficiently for the reflex to be absent. In addition, weaning should not be started until the infant can sit only slightly supported and turn away his/her head to indicate food refusal. The AAP recommends breast/chestfeeding for at least the first year of life. WHO and UNICEF suggest that the health benefits of breast/chest milk are important throughout the second and third years of life and that breast/chestfeeding should be continued. However, because breast/chest milk is very low in iron content, there has been concern about the possible effect of this advice on the development of anemia, a condition that if left untreated could cause irreversible developmental delays. The iron in human milk is absorbed more efficiently (60%) than the iron in cow's milk (4%), partly because of the high amount of vitamin C in human milk (Brown, 2019; Box 17.7: Quality and Safety Scenario)

Some infants accept the cup readily; other infants are extremely reluctant to give up the bottle, especially the bedtime bottle. Allowing infants to sleep with propped bottles can lead to aspiration if the milk flows too rapidly or the infant becomes too sleepy to coordinate sucking and swallowing. Another potential problem is baby-bottle tooth decay, of all upper teeth and some of the lower posterior teeth, from direct contact with sugar, syrup, honey-sweetened water, or fruit juice. When the infant falls asleep and stops sucking on the bottle, the sugary solution pools around the infant's teeth and remains there for long periods. The carbohydrate in the solution is fermented into organic acids that demineralize the teeth until they decay. By not using the bottle as a pacifier, parents can prevent this condition.

Some additional tips for counseling parents are as follows:

- Keep a calm, relaxed attitude throughout the weaning process.
- Let the child lead the way; it could take days, weeks, or months.
- Anticipate the previous feeding times and offer a cup or snack instead.
- Do not force an infant to use a cup; it is more detrimental to wean an infant sooner than later.
- Introduce the cup for one feeding per day and progress.
- Introduce one new food at a time.
- Start iron-containing foods (meat, iron-supplemented cereals).
- Continue breast/chest milk to 12 months of age, then cow's milk can be substituted.
- Give no more than 24 oz/day of cow's milk when substituted.
- Avoid fluids other than breast/chest milk, formula, and water.
- Avoid sugar-sweetened beverages; discourage fruit juices.
- Drop a feeding out every few days until the evening feeding is the last one left.
- Be sure the infant is getting enough nutrition from other sources.
- Put only purified tap water into the bottle and give the infant juice and milk from a cup.
- Remember that infants enjoy the accomplishment of using a cup; it is one of their first steps toward independence.
- Make sure to make up the bonding time with your infant by holding and cuddling the infant throughout the day (Duryea & Fleischer, 2023; Kliegman et al., 2020).

Anticipatory Guidance

The infant progresses from a diet of breast/chest milk or formula alone to a diet of milk and solid foods within a short period. Understanding the infant's nutritional needs and developmental capabilities, the nurse can guide the parents in meeting them and in the process, foster healthy family-infant relationships. Recent positive changes and advice for parents include increased duration of breast/chest feeding to 12 months, delayed introduction of complementary foods, and avoidance of juice consumption.

BOX 17.7 QUALITY AND SAFETY SCENARIO

How to Hold Your Infant for Feedings

- Sit or lie down comfortably with your back supported.
- Make sure the infant has one arm on either side of the breast/chest.
- Use firm pillows or folded blankets under the infant as a means of support during the feeding. As the infant gets older, the extra support will likely be unnecessary.
- Support the infant's back and shoulders firmly.
- Do not push on the back of the infant's head.
- Ensure correct positioning to enable good attachment.
- Ensure the infant is at a 90-degree angle, with his/her nose meeting the nipple.
- Pull the infant quickly to the breast/chest after the infant's mouth is open wide.

Three Common Breast/Chestfeeding Positions

Football

- Hold the infant's back and shoulders in the palm of your hand.
- Tuck the infant up under your arm, keeping the infant's ear, shoulder, and hip in a straight line.
- Support the breast/chest. After the infant's mouth is open wide, pull him/her quickly to you.
- Continue to hold your breast/chest until the baby feeds easily.

Lying Down

- Lie on your side with a pillow at your back and lay the infant such that you are facing each other.
- To begin, prop yourself up on your elbow and support your breast/chest with that hand.
- Pull the infant close to you, lining up his/her mouth with your nipple.
- After the infant is feeding well, lie back down. Hold your breast/chest with the opposite hand.
- Cradle the infant in the arm closest to the breast/chest with his/her head in the crook of your arm.
- Have the infant's body facing you, tummy to tummy.
- Use your opposite hand to support the breast/chest.

Across the Lap

- Lay your infant on firm pillows across your lap.
- Turn the infant, facing you.
- Reach across your lap to support the infant's back and shoulders with the palm of your hand.
- Support the breast/chest from underneath to guide it into his/her mouth.

Signs Breast/Chestfeeding Is Successful:

- Your infant is feeding approximately eight times in 24 hours for 30–40 minutes at each feeding. Some infants need to eat more frequently until they learn to breast/chestfeed efficiently. Other infants gain weight although they feed less often.
- At least one side of the breast/chest softens well at each feeding.
- You feel a tug, but not pain, when they suck.
- The infant's arms and shoulders are relaxed during the feeding.
- The infant has bursts of 10 or more sucks and swallows at the beginning of each feeding.
- As your breast/chest softens, the infant slows down to two to three sucks and swallows at a time.
- Your infant is content when you finish breast/chestfeeding.
- By the time the infant is 4 days old, you should see at least six wet diapers and two bowel movements every 24 hours.
- Signs that a good latch has been made are:
  - The infant's nose is free from the breast.
  - The infant's chin is firmly pressed against the breast/chest.
  - The infant has round cheeks.
- If any areola is visible, it should be more above the top lip versus the bottom lip.

Lauwers & Swisher (2016)

Overconsumption of complementary foods can lead to excessive weight gain in infancy, leading to an increased risk of obesity in child and adulthood. The health-promotion activity used in meeting proper infant nutrition focuses on parent education and positive reinforcement of parenting abilities.

Elimination Pattern

The infant develops an elimination pattern by the second week of life, usually associated with the frequency and amount consumed at feedings. Both breast/chestfed and bottle-fed infants progress to a pattern of fewer stools per day after the first few months of life.

A breast/chestfed infant's stools have a mushy golden-yellow color and a seedy, even consistency, with a slightly sour but clean smell, dissimilar to stools passed later in life. A bottle-fed infant's stools are firm, pasty, and smellier and resemble those of an infant eating solid food. The breast/chestfed infant has many daily stools during the first and second months of life, progressing to one stool per day or even one stool every 4 to 5 days in the later months before solid foods are introduced. The bottle-fed infant has two to four stools per day during the first month, tapering to one a day or even fewer at the end of infancy (Brown, 2019).

For the first year of life, an infant cannot control the bowels. Bowel evacuation remains under involuntary, reflexive control until myelination of the spinal cord is complete, usually by 14 to 18 months of age (Kliegman et al., 2020). Experts advise the delay of toilet training until the infant is developmentally ready. The stress in American culture on daily bowel movements makes many parents concerned about their infant's elimination patterns. The breast/chestfed infant may go for several days without having a bowel movement, which is usually not a problem. When the infant's behavior and feeding and sleeping patterns are normal, no elimination problem exists. A breast/chestfed infant rarely becomes constipated when consuming adequate amounts of breast/chest milk. Usually, the nurse only has to reassure the parents and discuss normal elimination patterns. Urination increases as fluid intake increases. An infant who voids 6 to 12 times a day during the first few months of life is usually healthy and well-hydrated. The color of urine should be light to dark yellow. Voiding is involuntary until sometime during the second year of life, when bladder sensation develops. Irregular patterns of voiding characterize the remaining period of infancy.

Anticipatory Guidance

Anticipatory guidance and health promotion concerning elimination patterns of the infant consist of parental teaching and reassurance, with special emphasis on good hygienic practices.

Reassuring the parents about the infant's inability to control elimination is important so that their expectations are realistic.

Activity-Exercise Pattern

Physical activity and exercise contribute to development and coordination throughout the life span; infants receive their exercise through play. Initially, infants engage in play with themselves with their hands or feet, by responding to various sounds, and by rolling and getting into various positions. By manipulating objects and achieving pleasurable sensations, infants learn about themselves and the objects in the environment.

Activity Through Play

Play is the chief way that infants learn how to move, communicate, socialize, and understand their surroundings. Play is crucial for an infant's social, emotional, physical, and cognitive growth. Exploration is the heart of play, as it is how infants learn about their body and the world around them. Although the word *play* suggests physical activity, the infant's first play is actually an exercise of the senses. The infant's first toys are visual. Through play, infants learn to hone their senses, to exercise their physical abilities, and to relate to other people. Most of the infant's play is solitary and repetitious. As each discovery is made, self-confidence and pride in the achievement are reinforced (as is the skill) through repetition.

As the infant enters the second half of the first year and becomes mobile, the family should provide the infant with increasing opportunities for spontaneous play and exploration. A planned play period in a safe environment should be established. The infant should have unrestrictive clothing so that movement can be free and unhampered. The caregiver should not interfere directly with the play but should be attentive to the infant's needs.

An important nursing role is assisting parents to promote play, stressing the importance of providing opportunities that are appropriate for the infant's age. Buying expensive toys is unnecessary; common household items, such as pots, pans, lids, and spoons, provide excellent objects for play purposes. Parents should be instructed to talk and read to their infants. Infants learn by interacting with their caretaker.

Activity Through Stimulation

Parental stimulation of the infant is an important developmental technique; the infant needs stimulation to learn about the world. This activity does not require expensive objects, but rather involves experiences of sight, sound, and touch that are free and can be provided by any parent (Fig. 17.1). Examples of stimulating experiences for infants include the following:

- Having lullabies sung to them
- Listening to tape recordings of a heartbeat
- Seeing colorful mobiles in the crib
- Being rocked in a rocking chair
- Having a familiar face smiling close by
- Receiving a soothing massage, which can reduce infant's stress and improve their self-regulation ability
- Having space to wander when developmentally ready
- Looking at themselves in mirrors
- Listening to music

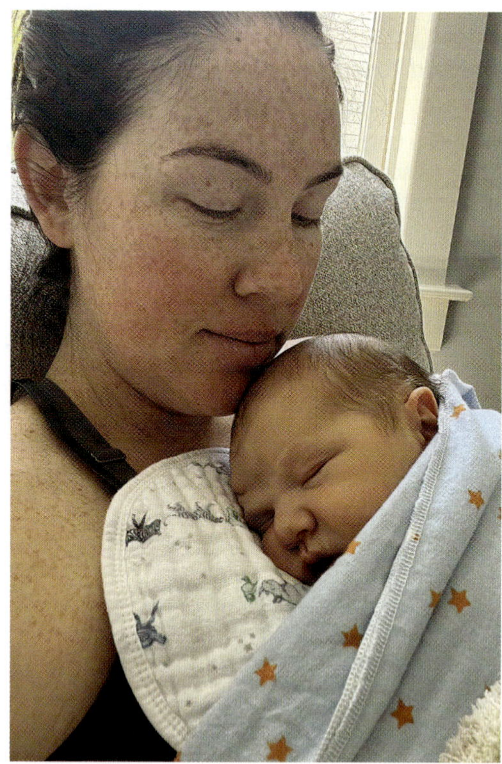

FIG. 17.1 The mother provides an infant with comfort by her closeness.

Anticipatory Guidance

Knowledge of developmental landmarks allows the nurse to guide parents in proper play and stimulation for infants. Handing a 15-month-old child a ball and placing the child in a fenced-in backyard to play is not enough. These activities must provide interpersonal contact, activity, and exercise. Activity and exercise through stimulation and play are extremely important for adequate and healthy development (Berk, 2019).

Sleep-Rest Pattern

Sleep is a developmental process and infant's sleep patterns are individualized. The amount of sleep that infants need is closely related to their rate of growth. Initially, infants sleep approximately 80% of the time, as demanded by their rapid growth. As growth begins to slow toward the middle of the first year of life, less sleep is needed. The 12-month-old infant sleeps for only 12 of 24 hours, a pattern that remains essentially unchanged through the second year. Many new parents think that there is a link between the amount of food fed to their infant and sleep duration. Recent studies indicate that infants who received more milk or solid feedings during the day were less likely to feed at night but not less likely to wake (Olsen, Ammitzboll, Olsen, & Skovgaard, 2019). The findings have important implications for nurses who support new parents with infant sleep and diet in the first year. Increasing infant calories during the day may reduce the likelihood of night feeding but will not reduce the need for parents to attend to the infant in the night. To assist parents in understanding normal sleep and rest patterns, the nurse stresses that no set schedule exists (Table 17.5).

TABLE 17.5 **GROWTH AND DEVELOPMENT**

Normal Sleep Patterns for Infants

Age (Months)	Hours in 24-hour Period
2–3	Low: 10 Average: 16.5 High: 23
3–4	Low: 8–10 nightly High: 11–12 nightly (two or three naps daily)
6–12	11–12 nightly (two or three naps daily)
12–18	8–12 nightly (one or two naps daily)

Kliegman et al. (2020); Arora (2019)

Anticipatory Guidance

Infant sleep patterns are a common concern for new parents. Health-promotion activities can also help parents determine the individual needs of their infant. The nurse stresses that longer sleep patterns are signs of maturation and that sleep and rest are recognized as having a significant influence on the infant's growth and development. Sleep problems are highly prevalent in early childhood. Frequently, parents seek professional help when they suspect their child has a sleep problem. The nurse may offer the parents helpful comments for promoting infant sleep patterns, such as the following:

- Provide a quiet room for the infant that is separate from the parents' room.
- Learn behavioral clues that signal that the infant is going to sleep and is not interacting socially.
- Have a set bedtime and bedtime routine for the infant.
- Make the hour before bedtime quiet time; avoid any screen time during this hour.
- Keep the infant's bedroom quiet and dark.
- Realize that periodic, brief arousals at night are normal for infants.
- Establish a bedtime routine and a consistent sleep schedule.
- Learn to become sensitive to sleep cycles and rest periods that the infant is establishing, and base care accordingly.
- Attempt to schedule feeding times during wakeful rather than drowsy periods.
- Learn that certain cycles are intrinsic to infants and that each infant is unique.
- Learn about normal development of infants' sleep and napping patterns.
- Review safe sleep practices (sleeping position, surface, environment).
- Perform rituals for the infant, such as rocking or reading a bedtime story, to provide comfort and security and to let the infant know the expected behavior (Kliegman et al., 2020).

If parents express a sleep concern, the nurse assesses their reactions, considers their definition of the concern, assesses the sleep environment, and observes the infant's own unique sleep patterns. Only then can the nurse's health-promotion approach be individualized to assist the family in caring for the infant.

Sudden Infant Death Syndrome

Sudden infant death syndrome (SIDS) is defined as the sudden death of an infant younger than 1 year old during sleep that is unexpected and unexplained after a thorough postmortem examination including autopsy, a thorough history, and scene evaluation. SIDS is the only cause of death derived by exclusion of other causes. The incidence of SIDS has decreased significantly in the past 20 years, largely because of the Safe to Sleep campaign. This campaign focuses on actions parents can take to promote sleep safety and reduce the risk of SIDS in their infants. One consequence of the Safe to Sleep campaign is a significant increase in occipital flattening. Infants who develop a flat spot should be placed with the head facing alternative directions each time they are put to bed. Supervised prone positioning when the infant is awake, avoiding excessive use of carriers, and upright positioning when the infant is awake are also recommended (NIH, 2024). Despite declines in prevalence during the past two decades, SIDS continues to be the third leading cause of infant death in the United States, accounting for approximately 7% of all infant deaths. Most SIDS deaths occur before the infant reaches 6 months of age (NIH, 2019). SIDS is a complex, multifactorial disorder, the cause of which is still not fully understood. Behavioral risk factors identified in epidemiologic studies include prone- and side-sleeping positions, preterm birth and/or infant low birth weight, smoke exposure, soft bedding, bed sharing, not breast/chestfeeding, and overheating. Risk-reducing measures include use of a firm, flat crib mattress covered by a fitted sheet, with no stuffed toys, crib bumpers, or blankets; placing infant on his/her back to sleep or nap; avoiding any smoking around the infant; breast/chestfeeding; keeping vaccinations up to date; avoidance of overheating due to over-bundling; avoidance of soft bedding and objects in the crib; encouragement of supervised "tummy time" when the infant is awake; and consideration of the use of a pacifier during sleep once breast/chestfeeding is established (NIH, 2019; Box 17.8). These factors may also be associated with sleep disorders in infants, principally with bedtime problems, abnormal night awakenings, and arrhythmic sleep. Although SIDS affects infants from all social strata, lower socioeconomic status, younger maternal age, inadequate prenatal care, and lower maternal education level are consistently associated with SIDS. The incidence of SIDS has varied over time and among nations. SIDS still accounts for 3600 cases of infant death in the United States annually and is the third leading cause of death among infants beyond 1 month of age (CDC, 2023c). By definition, the cause of SIDS is not known.

In a recent NIH study (2020b), it was found that infants born to parents who both smoked and drank beyond the first trimester of pregnancy had a 12-fold increased risk for SIDS compared with those unexposed or only exposed in the first trimester of pregnancy. Preconception counseling on the use of alcohol and tobacco is a preventative measure for SIDS.

Parents should be instructed to allow supervised tummy time when the infant is awake and should be cautioned about the amount of time their infant spends in a car seat. Delayed gross motor development can be prevented by reduction of the amount of time the infant spends in the supine position.

BOX 17.8 Safe to Sleep Public Education Campaign

The Safe to Sleep campaign aims to educate parents, caregivers, and health care providers about ways to reduce the risk of SIDS and other sleep-related causes of infant death.

Safe to Sleep is an expansion of the original Back to Sleep campaign, which started in 1994. Back to Sleep was named for its recommendation to place healthy babies on their backs to sleep, the most effective action that parents and caregivers can take to reduce the risk of SIDS. Since that campaign started, the percentage of infants placed on their backs to sleep has increased dramatically, and the overall SIDS rates have declined by more than 50%.

The expanded Safe to Sleep campaign builds on the success and reach of the Back to Sleep campaign. In addition to strategies for reducing the risk of SIDS, Safe to Sleep also describes actions that parents and caregivers can take to reduce the risk of other sleep-related causes of infant death, such as suffocation.

Safe to Sleep campaign collaborators include the Eunice Kennedy Shriver National Institute of Child Health and Human Development; the Maternal and Child Health Bureau of the Health Resources and Services Administration; the CDC, Division of Reproductive Health; the AAP; the American College of Obstetricians and Gynecologists; First Candle; and the Association of SIDS and Infant Mortality Programs.

The safe sleep strategies outlined in Safe to Sleep materials and publications are based on recommendations defined by the AAP Task Force on SIDS. More information about these recommendations is available at the Eunice Kennedy Shriver National Institute of Child Health and Human Development website.

Based on the AAP Task Force on SIDS recommendations, parents and caregivers can make changes to their babies' sleep environment to make it safer and to reduce the risk of SIDS and other sleep-related causes of infant death.

AAP, American Academy of Pediatrics; *CDC,* Centers for Disease Control; *SIDS,* sudden infant death syndrome.
Eunice Kennedy Shriver National Institute of Child Health and Human Development (n.d.)

Tummy time is the key intervention in preventing gross motor delays in infants. This prone position provides infants with increased physical challenges and gives them a chance to begin developing head control by strengthening neck muscles. Nurses should educate the parents to introduce prone positioning for short periods several times a day. As infants get stronger, they will use arm muscles to lift themselves and aid them to reach for toys or other objects. This strengthening is essential in assisting them in rolling over, crawling, pulling themselves up to stand, and developing fine motor development, including coordination and sensory processing.

When an infant dies suddenly, unexpectedly, and for no apparent reason, a family crisis occurs. The parents are devastated and completely unprepared for the shock, reacting with intense guilt, blaming themselves and each other, and agonizing over the part they may have played in the infant's death. Because many unanswered questions remain, these feelings are universal. Parents think there is something they could have done to prevent the tragedy. In most cases, nothing could have been done. Too frequently, the first sign that something was wrong is death. The nurse is in an excellent position to help the family through this crisis. Dealing with the family's grief is very difficult. Many families find strength in their faith to help them through this difficult time. Other family members and close friends can assist the family in their grieving process. Many receive solace and support from talking to other parents who have lost an infant to SIDS. Several parent groups are available from local chapters of the SIDS Foundation; the nurse can refer them to their local chapter.

The nurse's main supportive role for families coping with SIDS is listening and offering compassionate guidance through the weeks and months that follow. The nurse encourages parents to talk about their infant. Too soon, family and friends expect the surviving family to "get over it." A parent, however, is never able to "get over it"; it is only put in perspective and not so near the surface. Nurses need to actively participate in helping parents through their grieving process and remember that a standard time frame is not applicable (Newberry, 2019).

Nursing assessment of the infant at risk of SIDS includes observing the infant for apneic episodes. Usually, however, nursing assessment occurs after death and consists of support and providing appropriate resources for the family. Nurses must also consider a family's cultural background when educating and supporting them through this challenging time. Nursing diagnoses for sudden infant death might include the following:

- Spiritual distress related to coping with death
- Ineffective family coping related to the loss of an infant
- Dysfunctional grieving related to the parents' inability to cope

Nurses also discuss with the family feelings about caring for future children. Life can appear out of control, and parents may believe that they cannot care for another infant. These feelings must be resolved before another pregnancy is contemplated. When dealing with the families of SIDS infants, nurses can feel uncomfortable and helpless. As health professionals, they might speak in terms of easing the pain or alleviating the guilt of these families, but many times simple nonverbal human contact is sufficient to express concern and understanding.

Cognitive-Perceptual Pattern

Cognition is the process by which an individual recognizes, accumulates, and organizes the knowledge of the environment, beginning with the perception or recognition of an event within that environment. Cognitive development is concurrent with biologic, adaptive, and psychosocial achievement. The infant's biologic and cognitive developmental patterns (Piaget's Sensorimotor Period) were discussed earlier in this chapter. The focus of this section is on the infant's sensory and language development and the importance of stimulation of both developmental areas. From birth, infants possess sensory capabilities; all sensory organs are well-developed and functioning. As the infant is cared for and handled, the special senses become organized neurologically into a pattern of behavior that will greatly influence subsequent development.

Vision

Sight is the least developed sense at birth. The infant's initial visual impressions are unfocused, bizarre, unfamiliar, and meaningless. The visual system of the newborn infant takes

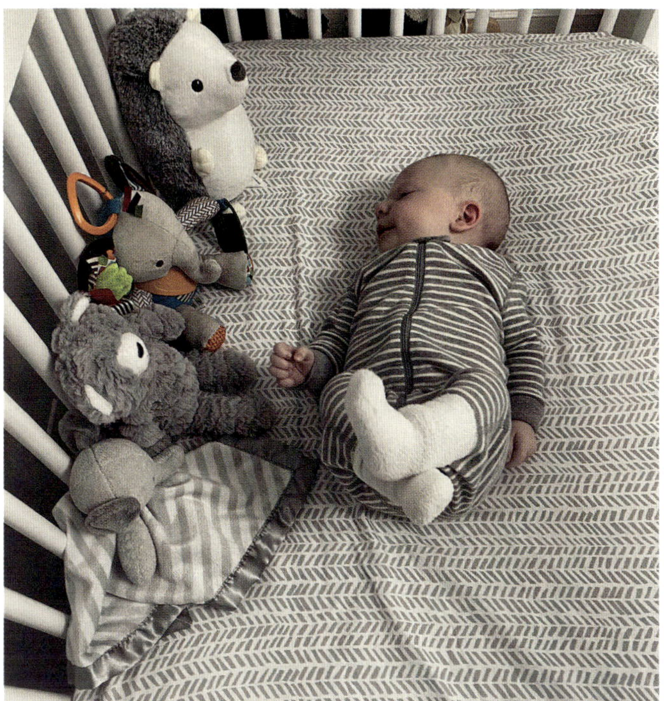

FIG. 17.2 An infant observes toys during supervised playtime.

TABLE 17.6 GROWTH AND DEVELOPMENT
Visual Development During Infancy

Age (Months)	Behavior That Indicates Vision
1–3	Fixes gaze on object 12–24 inches away Takes interest in bright colors and faces Follows objects in field of vision
3–6	Begins to show interest in hands Follows in range of 90 degrees Recognizes familiar objects Able to see full color by now
6–9	Visual scanning becomes more integrated Capable of organized depth perception Begins to perceive distances accurately Both eyes should focus equally now
9–12	Able to look for concealed items Converges on objects in close proximity Peripheral vision is well developed Judges distance well
12–18	Eye-hand coordination develops Depth perception more refined Ability to identify forms and shapes

American Optometric Association (2019); Ruffin (2019)

several months to develop. The infant's eyes are not very sensitive to light in the first month of life, so it is okay to leave a light on in the nursery—it will not affect the infant's ability to sleep. Because everything is new and only somewhat significant, visual stimuli must be moving, bright, or flashing to capture the infant's attention. To help stimulate the infant's vision, decorate their room with bright, cheerful colors and hang a brightly colored mobile above the crib that has a variety of shapes and colors (Fig. 17.2). Keep reach-and-touch toys within your infant's view of 8 to 12 inches, encourage them to crawl to objects just out of reach, and talk to the infant as you walk around the room so that they will follow the direction of the sound. The infant's eyes are well-developed at birth, but the muscles that attach the eyes to their sockets are weak. This weakness may be stressful to parents because the infant's eyes do not appear to function simultaneously. Parents can be assured that most infants coordinate their eye movements by the age of 3 months; by 6 months this function is mature. Table 17.6 summarizes visual developmental milestones.

Hearing

After the amniotic fluid has drained from the middle ear several days after birth, the infant's hearing becomes acute. Hearing is one of the better-developed senses in the infant; the fetus can even hear in utero and responds to loud sounds. The newborn can distinguish sound frequencies and turns toward a voice or another sound. The infant may be familiar with their parent's voice early in life. Sounds gradually gain significance and meaning when they are associated with caregivers, food, and pleasure.

The ability to listen and discriminate among sounds is an important task during infancy. Caretakers should talk to their infants, sing nursery songs, and make faces so the infants develop language and social skills. The use of baby rattles and musical mobiles is also a good way to stimulate the infant's hearing. The closer the infant is to the sound, the more easily the sound can be discriminated. The groundwork for verbal ability begins to develop long before words appear, and many believe that infants whose parents talk to them tend to speak earlier than infants who are not exposed to these sounds (March of Dimes, 2020a). Table 17. 7 summarizes the infant's auditory development.

Smell

The ability to smell is fully developed at birth. The senses of smell and taste are very closely connected. The infant has many receptors in the nose, but it lacks the cilia that line the inside of the adult's nose. As a result, the infant has a keen sense of smell because odors reach the receptor cells easily. Within 2 weeks after birth, an infant can differentiate the odor of the parent's milk from other sources of milk, an ability developed when the infant is held closely (Berk, 2019). At this time, the infant begins associating the parents with their body odors, a perception that is important for infant-parent bonding.

Taste

Taste buds in newborns can be found on the tonsils and the back of the throat, as well as on the tongue. Infants use their sense of smell from the start and can localize odors by turning their heads in the direction of the odor. The sense of taste begins to develop around 7 to 8 weeks of gestation. The sense of taste is present at birth, and salivation begins at approximately 3 months of age. The four primary sensations are sour, salty, sweet, and bitter. The taste buds for sweet tastes are more

TABLE 17.7 GROWTH AND DEVELOPMENT
Normal Development of Hearing

Age (Months)	Behavior That Indicates Hearing
1–3	Is startled by loud noises Stops activity when spoken to Turns head toward sound and knows caretaker's voice
3–6	Turns eyes and head toward sound Responds to mother's voice Imitates own noises: "ooh" and "ba-ba"
6–9	Responds to own name, telephone ringing Looks toward sounds Knows words for common things and makes babbling sounds Recognizes familiar sounds
9–12	Points to familiar objects or people Imitates simple words and sounds Locates a sound in any direction
12–18	Follows simple spoken directions Distinguishes between sounds Spoken words are well on their way Knows 10–20 words

National Institute on Deafness and Other Communication Disorders (2017); Kliegman et al., (2020)

abundant during early life than they are in later life, which may account for the preference for sweets that is characteristic of infants and children. An infant's reaction to salty foods does not come until approximately 4 to 5 months of age.

Touch and Motion

Touch is by far the most developed of all the infant's senses, as it is the main way in which infants learn about their environment and bond with other people. The skin is the sensory organ for touch. Tactile sensation is well-developed at birth, particularly on the lips and tongue. Perceptions of motion and touch are perhaps the most important of all senses. Rocking and other motions are sensations of equilibrium picked up by the middle ear. Skin-to-skin touching should be performed regularly; evidence shows that touch helps relieve the unspent tensions that infants develop and accelerates neuromuscular development (CDC, 2023d). Infants respond with pleasure to rocking and other motions and to tactile sensations of warmth, closeness, and cuddling.

Language Development

Language development, an important aspect of the infant's cognitive and perceptual pattern, is affected by development of the intellect, maturation of the central nervous system, development of the organs of speech, and exposure to human verbalization.

As in other areas of development, language acquisition follows a definite sequence. During the first 2 months, most of the infant's sounds are vowels and are made primarily in the front part of the mouth (CDC, 2023d). Crying is the major means of communication during this period. Cooing sounds are heard at approximately 2 to 3 months, usually in response to an adult's voice. By 6 months, babbling sounds are heard, and by 9 to 10 months, the infant forms two-syllable sounds. By 12 months, words such as "ma-ma," "bye-bye," and "da-da" are emerging. From 15 to 18 months, expressive jargon with rhythmical intonations develops, but words are recognized only rarely. The infant uses jargon along with pointing to express wishes.

Anticipatory Guidance

The nurse's knowledge and understanding of an infant's cognitive and perceptual behavior facilitates interaction with infants and serves as a guide in parental counseling. The main focus centers on stimulation, because each of the infant's senses is receptive to environmental stimulation. This activity helps the infant learn from the environment. When an infant is exposed to appropriate sensory stimulation, greater curiosity, improved mental capabilities, accelerated neuromuscular growth, enhanced gastrointestinal functioning, quicker weight gain, more rapid language development, and pleasing parent-infant interactions are likely to occur (Phillips, 2019).

Parents are the primary providers of pleasurable and stimulating experiences for the infant. The nurse assists them by offering suggestions about suitable stimuli for each sensory modality.

Self-Perception–Self-Concept Pattern

Self-perception has a pervasive influence on all aspects of life. Self-concept consists of a set of attitudes regarding what each person thinks, believes, and feels about the self. These attitudes form a personal self-belief that is an abstraction referred to as "me." Many researchers believe that the infant determines self-existence by first noting that actions such as crying or smiling have an effect on others, which depends on receiving feedback (Malik & Marwaha, 2022). Studies confirm that infants can identify themselves and therefore form a self-concept. Infants at 4 months of age were found to be particularly fascinated with their images in mirrors and smiled more at themselves than they did at pictures of other infants. Self-awareness is the realization that the infant is separate from others. Once this has been achieved, the infant can move toward understanding social emotions such as guilt, shame, and embarrassment, as well as sympathy or empathy (Children's Bureau, 2019).

As the infant continues to grow and mature, many circumstances combine to influence self-concept. How others relate to the infant's body and the messages that the infant receives from the body lead to knowledge of a physical self. The ability to use the body to influence others can lead the psychological self to conclude that someone cares about the infant (Ruffin, 2019).

The infant's development of body image is gradual. At birth, the infant has diffuse feelings of hunger, pain, anger, and comfort, but no body image. Initially, the infant knows only the self and regards the external world as an extension of the self. Only when infants begin to experience the environment through sensory modalities are they able to distinguish their bodies from animate and inanimate objects.

Nursing Suggestions

The nurse plays a vital role in assisting parents to foster the development of a positive self-concept and a good body image in their infant. Socialization is unique and begins in infancy. Parenting skills and style have a strong influence on outcomes of integrated socialization as infants develop. The nurse first identifies personal self-concept and how it influences individuals (CDC, 2023d). The nurse stresses that the way in which parents treat the infant influences the infant's self-concept. Basically, infants and young children incorporate their parents' interactions with them (good or bad) into their own view of self. What the infant knows and later believes about the self will affect all interactions with others, and by influencing what the infant will later attempt, the self-concept may have broad effects on the development of new skills. The mental state or the idea of "me" is that part of the self that makes reference to itself. This mental state develops over the first 2 years of life and is a function of both brain maturation processes and socialization (Levine & Munsch, 2020).

Roles–Relationships Pattern

What happens during the first few months of an infant's life matters a great deal because this period of life provides a blueprint for adult well-being and sets the foundation for what follows. Researchers have explored extensively the effect of early bonding between parents and their infants, emphasizing that this initial attraction sets the stage for the later development of love and affiliation. The bonding experience that occurs between a parent and their infant has been shown to have a positive effect on neurobehavioral responses. The bonding process has many other implications for the infant's future development as well (Hill & Flanagan, 2019).

Attachment and Bonding

The attachment relationship is a vital bond between the infant and the caregiver that, when secure, facilitates physical and psychological well-being.

Various theories have attempted to explain the basis for attachment behavior. Freudian psychoanalytic theory emphasizes that the bond between the child and the birthing parent develops as a result of the parent's fulfillment of the infant's innate desire to socialize and the physical requirements for survival. Social learning theory contributes the principles of reinforcement to the attachment process; as the parent meets the infant's needs, discomfort is reduced or removed. The infant associates the pleasurable feeling of being satisfied with the parent, who becomes a significant other in the infant's life. The bonding process is the basis for the parent-infant relationship, which, in turn, forms the basis for the interdependence that is necessary for the infant's psychological and physical development. All infants are born with the building blocks that develop into attachment behaviors, and thus all infants have the ability to form an attachment relationship with their primary caregiver (Oliveira & Fearon, 2019).

Just as the infant's behavior influences attachment, it also continues to influence the evolving parental-infant relationship as the infant develops. Studies have shown that if the process of attachment is encumbered, later problems are more likely to occur, such as child abuse, **poor growth** (formally termed *failure to thrive syndrome*), and behavior problems. Poor growth is a physical sign that an infant is receiving inadequate nutrition for optimal growth and development. Poor growth generally describes an infant whose current weight, or rate of weight gain, is significantly below that expected of similar infants of the same age and sex (Kliegman et al., 2020).

Many factors are present when a relationship is being established and maintained. Because the parents' self-esteem is associated closely with their infant's interactions and accomplishments, when parents' self-esteem is low, disappointment, anger, and a disturbance in the relationship with their infant can occur. In some instances, this disturbed parent-infant relationship is short-lived and nothing harmful develops. When a disturbed parent-infant relationship continues, however, the infant is at risk of abuse and behavior problems (Box 17.9: Best Practice).

The prevalence of **infant/child abuse** is difficult to estimate, partly because, like an iceberg, it is mostly hidden. Infant/child abuse is an important cause of pediatric morbidity and death and is associated with major physical and mental health problems that can extend into adulthood. Infant and child abuse, as defined by the WHO, constitutes all forms of physical and/or emotional ill-treatment, sexual abuse, neglect or negligent treatment, or commercial or other exploitation resulting in actual or potential harm to the infant/child's health, survival, development, or dignity (WHO, 2023c). The family traditionally has been considered a safe place for its members, but many infants are at risk of maltreatment. Infant and child abuse has always been a part of human history. Acceptable behavior toward

BOX 17.9 BEST PRACTICE

The Touchpoints Model

The birth of a baby is a life-changing event for a couple and family. Although most infants develop through predictable yet individual patterns of development, parents, especially first-time parents, are usually unaware of these patterns or have difficulty assessing their infant's progress and problems. All of these processes can be stressful for the parents, the entire family, and the infant.

The Touchpoints Model Program at Children's Hospital in Boston, Massachusetts, delivers a training model for practitioners, emphasizing the building of supportive alliances between parents and professionals around key points in the development of young children. The model is an outgrowth of Brazelton's classic book *Touchpoints* and research at Boston Children's Hospital. The Touchpoints model provides a form of outreach through which multidisciplinary practitioners can engage parents around important, predictable phases of their baby's development. The Touchpoints model stresses preventive health through development of relationships between parents and providers; acknowledges that developing and maintaining relationships is critical to appreciating cultural, religious, and societal family dynamics; and encourages the practitioner to focus on strengths in individuals and families. Touchpoints is not a stand-alone model; it is intended to be integrated into ongoing pediatric, early childhood, and family intervention programs.

Contact Information

Brazelton Touchpoints Center
Child Development Unit
Boston Children's Hospital
1295 Boylston Street
Boston, MA 02215

Brazelton (2023)

infants is largely a learned phenomenon; the art of parenting is not instinctively acquired, as many people believe. Abusing parents are seldom "monsters"; they are merely individuals ineffectively coping with the demands of parenthood, for which there is little or no preparation, as well as other life stressors.

The scope of child abuse is extensive: estimates indicate that one in seven infants and children in the United States are victims of abuse annually, and more than 1700 children die of abuse or neglect. Infants from birth to 2 years of age are the most vulnerable to abuse and neglect (CDC, 2022b). Brain and head injuries are the most common cause of traumatic death in children less than 2 years old. Abusive head trauma carries with it the highest mortality rate (Joyce & Huecker, 2023). Children younger than 2 years of age are the most frequent victims. Females are more frequent abusers than are males because they are often the primary caregivers. Males abuse more severely and commit sexual abuse more frequently. Child abuse does not discriminate among children; it occurs in families of every race, creed, and socioeconomic class.

Child-abuse syndrome is a clinical condition in infants who have suffered serious active or passive abuse at the hands of their parents or other caregivers. Physical trauma is not the only facet, but it is the most overt indicator of a dysfunctional family unit and a disturbed parent-infant relationship. Bruising is the most common sign of physical abuse but is missed as a sentinel injury in most. Infants tend to have increased morbidity and mortality with physical abuse (Gonzalez & McCall, 2024).

Active manifestations of abuse include the following:

- Brain injuries, subdural hematomas, and skull fractures
- Soft-tissue injuries, such as bruises, lacerations, or burns
- Fractures of the long bones and ribs; multiple fractures in various stages of healing
- Sexual abuse manifested by genital tissue injury, sexually transmitted infections
- Bullying manifested by intentional, aggressive behaviors toward others

Passive manifestations of abuse include the following:

- Poor nutrition, failure to thrive, and severe malnutrition
- Poor physical condition: neglected safeguards against disease, poor skin condition, and lack of medical attention
- Emotional neglect: rejection, indifference, and deprivation of love
- Moral neglect: allowing the infant or child to remain in an immoral atmosphere
- Spiritual abuse: incorporating religion into abuse of a child (Boy Scouts of America, 2018)

Abusing parents often have common patterns of behavior. As children, their own parents may have abused them. In this way, child abuse is cycled from generation to generation. The development of the maternal role on which the infant depends for health, progress, and survival begins during the parent's early childhood. Unless they receive love and proper nurturing, they will have difficulty with a relationship that entails the complete dependency of another person. She may find the relationship with her own infant to be unrewarding, threatening, and frustrating. Feelings of inadequacy and guilt in the parental roles compound the problems.

Abusing parents are often socially isolated and have few people to whom they can turn during times of crisis; they also cannot support one another emotionally. If parents grew up with harsh methods of discipline, they may be prone to violence with their own children. These parents may view the infant as the person who can provide the love, support, and nurturing that is lacking in their own lives. When the infant does not fulfill their expectations, the risk of abuse increases (AAP, 2022b).

The abused infant or child is frequently singled out as someone who is different. This infant may be chronically ill, may have been born prematurely, may be hyperactive, may have been the product of a difficult and complicated pregnancy, or may have an obvious anomaly. Early bonding disturbances (inadequacies in feeding, holding, and caring for the infant) are characteristic signals.

The long-term effects of child abuse are profound. They can result in detrimental societal effects, including high costs for health services and increased involvement in the juvenile and criminal justice systems. The victims lack basic trust (a major task of infancy) and confidence and self-worth. These deficits follow the victims into adulthood and parenthood, and the vicious cycle continues. One of the discouraging findings is that infants and children who were abused frequently grow up to be abusing parents (Child Welfare, 2019).

There is great interest in identifying parents during prenatal and perinatal periods who have significant potential for child abuse. Nurses play a critical role in recognizing infants who have been intentionally harmed, because they are often the first to begin taking a history of the infant. The role of the nurse may include identifying abused infants with suspicious injuries who present for care, reporting suspected abuse to the child protection agency for investigation, supporting families who are affected by infant abuse, coordinating with community agencies to provide immediate and long-term care to the victimized infant, providing court testimony when necessary, providing preventive care and anticipatory guidance in the health care setting, and advocating policies that support and protect vulnerable infants (Gosselin, 2019). Nurses work collaboratively with community agencies to provide follow-up care for the infant in danger of continued abuse. Nurses take appropriate action if they suspect an infant is at risk. Some of the biggest challenges of child protection come from our own internal reluctance to act, but doing nothing is not an option. The following measures have been undertaken to help prevent child abuse:

- Predictive questionnaires to be given to parents on postpartum units
- Recognition of parents who have difficulty relating to their infants through body language clues or verbalizations
- Closer follow-up during the postpartum period by the public health nurse
- Crisis hotlines made available to parents in distress

Nurses can encourage parental-infant bonding from birth and can offer rooming-in, which could increase breast/chest-feeding significantly and decrease the incidence of failure to thrive, abuse, neglect, and abandonment of infants. Most communities are seeking ways in which child abuse can be prevented through educational efforts, improved agency coordination, and development of new collaborative efforts and services for parents and infants. Laws for reporting abuse have been enacted in every state. Reporting all cases of suspected abuse and neglect is mandatory. Everyone must assist in this endeavor to prevent continued abuse. It takes a community effort to address the problem.

Sexuality–Reproductive Pattern

An infant's identity begins at birth, when the gendered child is identified, and caretakers behave a certain way toward the infant because of its sex. The infant's sexuality gives direction to its physical, emotional, social, and intellectual responses throughout life. Infants have a great oral sensitivity, enjoy skin-to-skin contact, and explore their own bodies for pleasure during the first year of life. A healthy, accepting attitude by caretakers is important in an infant's evolving sexual development.

Coping–Stress Tolerance Pattern

The term "*stress*" implies intense reaction to an experience and changes in usual behavior. Stress is a normal phenomenon that occurs throughout the life span, as, for example, when an individual experiences a developmental or situational crisis.

Developmental Crisis

Developmental crises are turning points or periods of great change. Most stressors that an infant experiences are a necessary part of growth and development. For example, learning new skills creates stress. The infant who is unable to move forward while learning to crawl experiences stress. The infant expresses this stress by crying for help. Other stressors are more psychosocial in nature, such as being left with a babysitter or in an unfamiliar place.

Situational Crisis

Situational crises are not anticipated easily and do not occur necessarily as part of the normal growth and development process. One major situational crisis during infancy is separation from the significant other. Separation anxiety is a normal stage in an infant's development from about 8 months, as they begin to understand that a parent can be out of sight right now but will return later. The following three distinct phases are evident in the reaction to separation (Conci, 2019):

- Protest. Infant cries loudly, screams for the parent, and refuses attention of the substitute caregiver.
- Despair. Infant stops crying and becomes less active, withdraws, and becomes apathetic.
- Withdrawal. Infant takes an interest in the surroundings but tends to ignore or reject the parent when they return, because they failed to meet the infant's needs.

Initially, with no time framework and no understanding of waiting, the infant has little ability to cope with stress. As maturity and a sense of security provided by the caregiver increase, the infant begins to wait a short time to have its needs met without protest. An infant who experiences stress reacts by crying, the main tool of communication. The infant gradually learns to tolerate greater stress with time.

Nursing Interventions

Every family needs good information, concrete resources, and consistent support to thrive. By allaying anxiety in the infant's caregiver, the nurse facilitates coping behaviors in the infant. The stressful situation and problem-solving activities can be turned into growth-producing experiences for the family, with coping capacities strengthened for the future.

Values–Beliefs Pattern

Values are goals and beliefs that establish a behavior and provide a basis for decision-making. A value is a standard or principle that reflects a person's judgment on what is important in life. When people communicate, they send both the content message of the spoken words and the unspoken message of who they are and what they believe. Values are pervasive and important and give a focus to both individuals and groups within a particular culture. Because values are attitudes learned especially from significant others within the environment, the parents' values–beliefs pattern greatly influences the care and development of the infant.

Nursing Activities

By understanding and respecting the parents' value system, the nurse works within their framework of values in the counseling situation. The nurse communicates personal values to the family. To work successfully within a different value system, the nurse incorporates the following attitudes concerning the values–beliefs pattern into the nursing process (Stanhope & Lancaster, 2020):

- Believe in the ultimate worth of the infant and the family, regardless of their behavior or situation.
- Use the family's value system as a core guide to all nurse's actions.
- Grant families the freedom to make their own informed choices and to experience the responsibilities and consequences of their decisions.
- Recognize and acknowledge the beliefs, values, and culture that influence the family.
- Use knowledge of the family's value system in specific ways to reward and reinforce positive health practices.
- Value the growth potential inherent in developmental and situational crisis situations.
- Recognize your own value system and its influence on your behavior.
- Work with families without applying your personal value system in judging their behavior.
- Broaden your value system by accepting lifestyles different from your own.

The nurse influences the behavior of the parents, who have the greatest influence on their infant's values–beliefs pattern. The nurse accomplishes this task by modeling (living congruently with professed values), acting as a consultant by sharing pertinent information with parents, and modifying their own values. Nurses can anticipate a family crisis of values and can help to promote positive coping and effective use of social supports (Sue et al., 2019).

Modeling can be a potent influence on another individual's behavior. In the counseling situation, the family looks to the nurse for guidance and assistance in promoting healthy childrearing practices. The methods by which the nurse interacts with the infant, listens to the parents' concerns, and demonstrates respect for the family unit are influencing factors in changing behavior.

Second, the nurse acts as a consultant to influence values. Advice on childrearing practices is overwhelming to parents; everyone has opinions. The nurse listens before giving advice to determine whether parents will accept the advice and to allow parents to decide whether the advice can be useful. Repeated attempts to convert parents to the nurse's value system can make them defensive and resistant to the advice.

Third, by expressing values and attitudes but remaining open to other approaches, the nurse influences the values–beliefs pattern. Parents can realize that they are free to change and are not bound to values that others outside their value system express. Nurses need to listen to, understand, and respect client values, opinions, needs, and ethnocultural beliefs. By integrating these elements into the plan of care, nurses are supporting their clients to meet their specific health care goals (Brooks, Manias, & Bloomer, 2019). Communication skills can more effectively promote the health of the infant and the family.

ENVIRONMENTAL PROCESSES

Physical Agents

This section discusses various factors within the environment that can affect the infant's health status. The entire realm of accident prevention and safety promotion is applicable here.

According to the CDC (2023e), unintentional injuries, including motor vehicle traffic crashes, falls, poisonings, suffocations, drownings, and fires/burns, are the leading cause of death for people aged 1 to 44 years and the third leading cause of death for people of all ages. Beyond the emotional damage that accompanies such tragedies, the CDC (2023f) reports that unintentional injuries cost the United States more than $700 billion per year.

One of the overall goals for the Quality and Safety Education for Nurses (QSEN) project is to meet the challenge of preparing future nurses who will have the knowledge, skills, and attitudes necessary to continuously improve the quality and safety of the health care systems within which they work. One of their competencies promotes safety within the environment.

Some areas applicable to this competency of safety for infants would be the use of flame-retardant sleepwear, car seats, and crib mattresses, and knowledge of measures to promote crib safety and toy safety.

Sleepwear made for infants aged 9 months or younger can be flame resistant or non–flame resistant. Flame-resistant clothing is usually labeled as such and is either a synthetic fiber or treated cotton. Parents should not select flame-resistant sleepwear for their infant; if they use it, they should follow the laundry instructions. Snug-fitting clothing that conforms to the body has less opportunity to ignite when exposed to a flame than loose-fitting clothing. Smaller sizes are not required to be snug fitting, because a smaller infant is less likely to be mobile enough to expose himself/herself to a fire hazard.

All new cribs are required to meet strict safety standards; however, if parents accept a secondhand crib, they need to be advised to check the following:

- The slats should be no farther than 2.375 inches apart. Slats with wider gaps could allow an infant's head to become trapped between them.
- There should be no decorations or projections that could snag an infant's clothes. Avoid cribs with decorative cutouts in the headboard or footboard.
- Some older cribs were painted with lead-based paint, which could poison an infant who mouths or chews the wood. If unsure, strip the old paint and repaint it with new lead-free enamel.
- No screws and bolts that hold the crib together should be missing, and all should be tight. Avoid cribs with drop side rails. If a drop side rail detaches or becomes loose, an infant may become trapped between the mattress and the railing.
- The crib mattress should be firm and should fit very snugly, with no room for the baby to become trapped between the mattress and the crib. Do not cover the mattress with plastic or a quilt, which can suffocate a baby.

Never put an infant to sleep on a waterbed, pillow, quilt, beanbag chair, or sofa. All these surfaces increase the chance that a baby could suffocate or get his/her head or another part of his/her body trapped in the furniture. Car seats are an unsafe place for infants to sleep for long periods of time because their heads can fall forward, restricting their airways and causing them to stop breathing. Limit the time that the infant is strapped into the car seat and remove them when the destination is reached.

Do not put pillows or stuffed animals in an infant's crib, because they can cause suffocation. Crib quilt bumpers also pose a risk for suffocation and should not be used. When your infant learns to sit, lower the mattress so they cannot fall out of the crib. Remove mobiles, and make sure draperies and window blind cords are well out of his/her reach.

Anticipatory guidance to promote infant toy safety would include instructions for parents purchasing new toys to follow the age guidelines on the packaging. Infant toys should have no tiny parts that pose choking hazards, and nothing on the toy should be sharp or detachable. Infants explore objects with their mouths, so anything they pick up should be too big to swallow. The more chewable and unbreakable a toy is, the safer it will be.

Accidents are always unexpected and, in retrospect, could usually have been prevented. Unintentional injuries are the leading cause of death for children in the United States and globally. The leading cause of injury death for children less than 1 year old is suffocation. For children less than 1 year of age, falls account for over 50% of nonfatal injuries (CDC, 2022d). Adults are living in a world designed by adults for adults, and they take that world's safety for granted. They must remind themselves constantly that infants also live in this complex world and that they learn at a remarkable rate, primarily by exploring and playing in the environment. These experiences render them extremely vulnerable to accidents; this is a major problem and presents a challenging field for preventive measures.

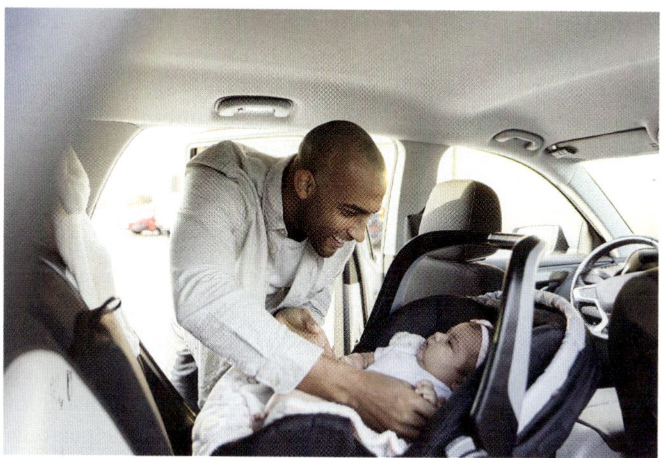

FIG. 17.3 Injury prevention for infants in their car seats includes the use of safety belts. (From iStock.com/SDI Productions)

Accidents occur in many situations: in the home, outside, on the playground, and in automobiles. The use of safety belts prevents infant injury (Fig. 17.3). Most accidents, however, occur in the home. Their number and seriousness are closely linked to the infant's developmental stage. Accidents tend to increase with the mobility of the infant, but even a 2-month-old infant can wiggle or fall from a high place. Keeping the environment free from hazards and ensuring caregiver supervision are crucial for this age group.

Nurses have the opportunity to help parents and caregivers anticipate and understand the common hazards of early life and provide specific guidance for accident prevention.

Unintentional Injuries

Falls. Falls are most common after 4 months of age, when the infant has learned to roll over, but they can occur at any age. Falls involving infants happen more often in the home environment, on stairs, from furniture, and out of windows. The best advice is never to place an infant unattended on a raised surface that has no type of guardrail. When in doubt, the safest place is the floor. Parental supervision is the key prevention strategy to prevent falls (CDC, 2020). Safety tips to assist parents in preventing falls are listed in Box 17.10.

Burns. In the United States, burns are the third leading cause of unintentional injury or death in children aged 1 to 14 years, accounting for more than 600 deaths per year in children from birth to 19 years of age. Every day, more than 300 children aged 0 to 19 years are treated in emergency departments for burn-related injuries and two children die because of being burned (CDC, 2021b).

Burns are the most frequent and frightening of all accidents during infancy. Most fire deaths occur in the home, and most victims die because of smoke or toxic gases and not because of the burns (CDC, 2021b). Because nearly all burns are preventable, the attendant caregiver can experience severe guilt.

Fire from matches or other sources, hot liquids, ultraviolet light from the sun, electricity or electrical outlets, and heating elements such as radiators, registers, and floor heaters can all cause burns. Do not leave the child unattended in the tub, even for a moment. Place the child at the end of the tub away from the faucet. Use safety outlet covers throughout the home (AAP, 2023c).

Foreign Objects. Choking occurs when a foreign object becomes lodged in the throat, blocking air flow (National Safety Council, 2023). Choking is the fourth leading cause of unintentional death in infants. At least one child is killed by choking on food every week in the United States (AAP, 2019b). Any small object that an infant puts in the mouth has the potential to be swallowed and choked on. More than 65% of deaths from foreign-body aspiration occur in infants. Liquids are the most common cause of choking in infants, whereas balloons, small objects, and foods are the most common causes of foreign-body airway obstruction in children (Duckett & Roten, 2022). Parents should be advised that objects such as safety pins, nuts, beads, coins, hot dogs, paper clips, corn, buttons, popcorn, chips, apple with peel, and parts of broken toys are frequently swallowed. Many objects can fit into this category and into the infant's mouth. The carelessness of a caregiver, relative, friend, or babysitter in leaving small objects available and within reach, or giving toys unsuited to the infant's stage of development, frequently causes these accidents.

When choking occurs, the adult should place the infant across the adult's knees and deliver five back blows (slaps) followed by five chest thrusts repeatedly until the object is expelled or the infant becomes unresponsive. Abdominal thrusts are not recommended for infants because thrusts in the abdominal area could potentially damage the relatively large and unprotected liver. Cardiopulmonary resuscitation should be performed if the infant becomes unresponsive (American Heart Association, 2021).

The entire balance of safety for infants depends on allowing them plenty of opportunity to explore and play within the environment while protecting them from harmful agents.

BOX 17.10 Safety Tips to Prevent Falls

- Keep sides of the crib up and firmly secured when the infant is in the crib.
- Place the infant seat on a stable surface, preferably the floor. The infant should be strapped in securely.
- Check highchairs, strollers, and carriages for safety, and restrain the infant who is active.
- All windows above the first floor should be locked and have operable window guards.
- Clean up food or liquid spills immediately from the floor.
- Remember that polished floors are hazardous, especially when throw rugs are present.
- Close off stairways with doors or properly installed gates, at the top and bottom.
- To prevent falls, set the crib mattress at the lowest adjustment level after the infant can pull himself/herself up and stand.
- Place furniture away from windows and anchor pieces to the wall.
- Avoid the use of baby walkers.
- Secure TVs, bookcases and furniture to the wall using mounts, brackets, braces, anchors, and wall straps to prevent tip-overs.
- Never leave an infant alone on a bed, changing table, shopping cart, or piece of furniture.
- Avoid bringing strollers onto escalators.
- Best fall prevention is to watch, listen, and always stay near the infant.

Data from Safe Kids Worldwide (2023a)

BOX 17.11 Home Childproofing Tips

- Remove any heavy, sharp, or breakable objects from tables and low shelves.
- Bolt bookcases to the wall and remove heavy books to prevent falls.
- Test floor and table lamps to make sure they cannot be pulled over.
- Avoid placing toys, blankets, pillows, or bumper pads in the crib.
- Disconnect unused appliances and wrap up cords.
- Secure all other cords to prevent appliances from being pulled down.
- Safely discard unused and unneeded medicines.
- Avoid referring to medicines as candy.
- Post the National Capital Poison Center telephone number (1-800-222-1222) nearby.
- Store potentially toxic substances out of sight and reach.
- Close reachable outlets with safety covers.
- Avoid leaving an infant unattended in the bathtub, even for a moment.
- Avoid using tablecloths that can be pulled down by a crawling infant.
- Tie drapery and blind cords out of the infant's reach.
- Choose stair gates with openings too small for an infant's head and child-resistant fasteners such as pressure bars.
- Avoid accordion or expandable gates with openings that can trap an infant's head.
- Install smoke detectors and check the batteries at least once a month.
- Use sturdy screens in front of fireplaces.
- Place crib, playpen, and highchair well away from heaters, fans, and electrical outlets.
- Install childproof latches on drawers and cupboards. Store all cleaning compounds and detergents in a high, locked cupboard.
- Keep plants out of an infant's reach, as some are poisonous.
- Buy all medicines in bottles with childproof lids and keep them in their original labeled containers for identification in case of accidental ingestion.
- Install lids on garbage pails and never leave any harmful materials in them, such as sharp can lids or spoiled food.
- Place furniture away from windows and anchor pieces to the wall, such as TVs.
- Check the floor regularly for objects small enough to be swallowed.
- Cut blind cords into two pieces.

CDC (2023g)

According to the AAP, the greatest threat to the health of infants is not illness but injuries, many of which can be prevented. The nurse informs the infant's parents, babysitters, family friends, and day care workers about the need to childproof their environments when an infant is present. The nurse can explain ways to promote the safety of these varied environments (Box 17.11).

Biologic Agents

The fetus is partially protected from some biologic agents in the environment by the placental barrier and the birthing parent's defense system. After birth, however, the infant is thrust into an environment that is filled with infectious, disease-causing agents. These bacterial or viral organisms can be found in food, cribs, the air, pets, parents, and siblings—literally everywhere. Common sources of indoor air pollution include combustion sources such as oil, gas, kerosene, coal, wood, and tobacco products, wet or damp carpet, household cleaners, central air, and humidification devices. Infants are more susceptible to the effects of contaminated air because they breathe in more oxygen relative to their body weight than adults (Environmental Protection Agency [EPA], 2023). Even the healthiest environment harbors disease-causing agents. Although the infant cannot escape exposure to these pathogens without being completely isolated, immunizations are given to assist the infant's defense against some communicable diseases.

Acquired Immunodeficiency Syndrome

Human immunodeficiency virus (HIV) is a retrovirus and can be transmitted vertically, sexually, or via contaminated blood products or intravenous drug abuse. Acquired immunodeficiency syndrome (AIDS) is spread by contact with HIV through blood and body secretions. HIV becomes established in cells of the host's immune system, called "*T cells*." The T-helper cells are sometimes referred to as "*CD4+*" cells because they have a glycoprotein on their surfaces. CD4+ T-helper cells recognize HIV, but if the CD4+ T-helper cells are low as with infection with HIV, they cannot coordinate an immune response to the HIV virus. The infant with HIV infection is unable to resist normal infections. Transmission of HIV from birthing parent to infant is the most likely cause of childhood HIV infection. Transmission can occur during pregnancy, at childbirth, or during breast/chestfeeding. HIV can definitively be diagnosed through the use of virology assays with perinatal exposure by age 2 months and in virtually all infants with HIV infection by age 4 to 6 months. For 4 weeks after birth, infants born to HIV-positive individuals receive antiretroviral medications to protect them from infection with any HIV that may have been passed during the birthing process. In addition, because HIV can be spread in breast/chest milk, individuals with HIV who live in the United States are encouraged not to breast/chestfeed (Vijayan et al., 2021; see Chapter 16). There is no immunization against HIV infections currently, but frequently preventive options are offered, and babies are usually delivered by cesarean delivery. Antiretroviral drugs reduce viral replication and can decrease birthing–parent-to-child transmission of HIV, either by lowering plasma viral load in pregnant individuals or by providing postexposure prophylaxis in their newborns. In developed countries, antiretroviral therapy (ARV), which usually comprises three drugs from at least two classes, has reduced the transmission rates to approximately 1% to 2%, but ARV medications are not always available in developing countries (Vijayan et al., 2021).

Although signs and symptoms of illness can occur at any time, they usually begin during the first year of life. In infants, the symptoms of the disease include growth failure, oral candidiasis, recurrent bacterial infections, pneumonia, recurrent fungal infections, chronic diarrhea, and delays in reaching important milestones in motor skills and mental development such as crawling, walking, and speaking. Early recognition and triaging of infants suspected of having HIV infection provide an opportunity for early diagnosis and treatment, which could prevent the adverse effect of rapidly progressive HIV disease (CDC, 2023h).

HIV continues to be a major global public health issue, having claimed more than 32 million lives thus far. WHO recommends preexposure (PrEP) prophylaxis as a preventive measure for high-risk HIV-negative people. Postexposure prophylaxis (PEP) is another ARV drug used within 72 hours of HIV exposure to prevent infection. In response to the urgent need to reduce the number of new HIV infections globally, the WHO and the Joint United Nations Program on HIV/AIDS (UNAIDS) funded research to determine whether male circumcision should be recommended for the prevention of HIV infection (WHO, 2023d). Based on the research findings presented, experts recommended that use of condoms and voluntary medical male circumcision be recognized as important interventions to reduce the risk of heterosexually acquired HIV infection in males. There is strong evidence that medical male circumcision reduces the acquisition of HIV in heterosexual males by approximately 60%. The incidence of adverse events is very low, indicating that male circumcision, when conducted under these conditions, is a safe procedure. Inclusion of male circumcision into current HIV prevention measure guidelines is warranted, with further research required to assess the feasibility, desirability, and cost-effectiveness of implementing the procedure globally. Currently, voluntary medical male circumcisions are being implemented in several sub-Saharan African countries to prevent HIV spread (WHO, 2023d). Parents must weigh their decision to circumcise their male infant based on their own values, religious backgrounds, and culture in light of this new information.

Nursing assessment focuses on a careful and complete history of the infant and parents, signs and symptoms of the disease, growth and development history, and psychosocial concerns. Parents are assessed carefully to determine their level of anxiety; knowledge of the disease process, including prognosis, treatment, and transmission; and awareness of resources, support systems, coping strategies, and the infant's needs.

No other disease causes as much public awareness and panic as does AIDS. Part of this behavior is ignorance. Nurses play a major role in educating the public about the disease process, its mode of transmission, and most of all, preventive measures. Preventive education should begin with young children. Most school health programs include information on HIV/AIDS. School nurses can contribute to the success of these programs, as can nurses working in prenatal clinics, to spread information on the importance of prevention. Nurses in all settings can engage in research related to HIV/AIDS to gather further clarification of this fatal disease.

Although the infant is not an active participant in the spread of HIV, parents should understand how the virus is transmitted and not allow their infant to become a passive participant because of their own high-risk behaviors.

Immunization

Disease prevention by immunization is a public health priority in Healthy People 2030 and society as a whole. Progress continues toward the goal of protecting children from serious disease through immunizations. The most recent schedule recommends the rotavirus vaccine in a three-dose schedule at ages 2, 4, and 6 months. The influenza vaccine is now recommended as an annual vaccine for all children aged 6 to 59 months, as well as for pregnant individuals. In addition, varicella vaccines should be administered at age 12 to 15 months, and a newly recommended second dose should be administered at age 4 to 6 years (CDC, 2023i). For current-year immunizations, see https://www.cdc.gov/vaccines/imz-schedules/index.html.

The two types of immunization are active and passive immunization. In **active immunization**, the individual is exposed to a disease organism that triggers the immune system to produce antibodies against that disease. Exposure can occur through having the actual disease or the introduction of a killed or weakened form of the disease through a vaccination (vaccine-induced immunity) (AAP, n.d.). Examples of active immunization include diphtheria, tetanus, and acellular pertussis vaccine; inactivated polio vaccine; and measles, mumps, and rubella vaccines. Active immunity is relatively long-lasting, waning over several years if at all.

Passive immunization is accomplished by injection of blood from an actively immunized person or animal rather than through the patient's own immune system After an individual has been exposed to a disease, a passive immunization is given to prevent the disease from developing. Passive immunizations provide a short immunity, usually a few weeks or months, which will protect the person until the danger of contracting the disease has passed. Passive immunization also helps reduce the severity of the disease when it is contracted. Because of the short duration, active immunization is still needed for a person to remain permanently immune. Passive immunity occurs naturally in newborns when maternal antibodies are passed through the placenta or in breast/chest milk.

Immunization provides one of the most cost-effective means of preventing infection in infants. Immunizations not only help protect those receiving the vaccinations from developing potentially serious diseases but also help protect entire communities by preventing and reducing the spread of infectious agents. Immunization is additionally important because antibiotics cannot destroy viruses; therefore, immunization offers the only means of control of viral illnesses. Nurses have a special responsibility to keep informed of the recommendations and document all vaccinations given. Emphasis must be placed on educating parents about the importance of immunization. Children need a series of vaccinations, starting at birth, to be fully protected against potentially serious diseases. To motivate parents to have their infants immunized, the nurse can work toward increasing health education to achieve greater health maintenance knowledge; send reminders for upcoming visits and needed immunizations; vigorously advocate that all infants should receive comprehensive health care, including immunizations; provide health services that make immunizations feasible and available; develop a close relationship with the family; and continue surveillance of the immunization status of every infant in the health care system.

Chemical Agents

Drugs

Despite advances such as childproof caps on medications, childproof packaging, increased educational efforts, and increased awareness of commonly ingested substances, deaths attributable to unintentional poisonings still occur. Medicines are the leading cause of child poisoning (Safe Kids Worldwide, 2023b). Unintentional poisonings are an unfortunate and usually preventable cause of death and disability in infants and children. The very nature of a young child predisposes the child to explore the surrounding environment. As children grow and learn to become independent, they are compelled to investigate new and interesting items, places, and objects, such as medications. Based on calls to the US poison control centers, each year more than 1 million children younger than 5 years, or one child every 10 minutes, ingests toxic substances. Eighty-four percent of those children were under the age of 3. More than 90% of poisoning exposures occur in homes (Kelly, 2023).

Recent changes in packaging and limits on the number of tablets contained in each bottle have reduced deaths resulting from overdose. Drug manufacturers are using childproof caps increasingly as a safety measure. Despite a concerted effort by manufacturers, childproof bottle caps differ in effectiveness (Kliegman et al., 2020). Frequently, the safety caps are adult-proof, although children can readily open bottles that have them.

This accessibility points to the dangers of medications, regardless of the bottle. All medications must still be secured in a safe place when infants are in the home or visiting other homes. Some additional guidelines to help prevent accidents involving drugs include the following:

- Use a prescription drug only for the purpose and the person for whom it is intended. Do not use medication prescribed for someone else for a similar condition in the infant.
- Discard unused drugs by taking them to dump into trash on toxic dump days; many infants have been poisoned by eating tablets found in the trash at home.
- Request safety caps on all prescription drugs.
- Keep all medicines under lock and key.
- Educate grandparents and visitors about being mindful with their medicines and pillboxes.
- Use the dosing device that comes with the medicine.
- Consider products not thought about as medicine—diaper rash remedies, eye drops.
- Have the telephone number of the nearest poison control center readily available.

The main points to be emphasized in giving parents guidance in accident prevention are to eliminate access to specific environmental hazards, such as drugs, for exploring infants and to supervise infants while they play, gradually replacing supervision with safety training (Safe Kids Worldwide, 2023b).

Plants

Colorful, interesting-looking houseplants add beauty to our homes, but they are often an irresistible attraction to a young infant or child. Infants and small children have a curious nature and cannot keep their hands out of dirt-filled plant pots or resist the temptation to eat leaves from the plant. Houseplants are a source of poison if ingested or can cause rashes if they come in contact with a child's skin. Most people fail to think of houseplants as potentially poisonous because people do not consider eating them. However, infants test almost everything by putting things in their mouths, and a number of plants can be deadly when eaten. As a result, plants are one of the leading sources of poisoning of infants, and amateur foragers frequently learn the hard way that not everything that looks good can be eaten. Most plants, however, have an unpleasant taste, and therefore are consumed only in small amounts. The effects of unintentional poisonings are typically dose-dependent; therefore, as children age and their sense of taste becomes more defined, the risk of large-dose unintentional poisonings decreases because children are better able to discriminate the unpleasant taste. Household plants are frequently placed on the floor, where the leaves or flowers are easy to pull off and taste. The best intervention for plant poisoning is prevention, which, in this case, means previous knowledge.

The most prominent groups of plants involved in exposures are those containing oxalates, and the most common symptom is gastroenteritis. The top 13 identified plants (in descending order) nationally are *Spathiphyllum* species (peace lily), *Philodendron* species (philodendron), *Euphorbia pulcherrima* (poinsettia), *Ilex* species (holly), *Phytolacca americana* (pokeweed), *Toxicodendron radicans* (poison ivy), capsicum (pepper), ficus (rubber tree, weeping fig), *Crassula argentea* (jade plant), *Dieffenbachia* (dumb cane), *Epipremnum aureum* (pothos), *Aconitum napellus* (monkshood), and *Schlumbergera bridgesii* (Christmas cactus; National Capital Poison Control Center, 2024a).

The American Association of Poison Control Centers (AAPCC) (n.d.) lists plants as the third most commonly ingested poison, after aspirin and household cleaning agents. Safety education is stressed at all well-baby visits beginning in the first 6 months of life. Prevention of plant poisoning and other accidents depends on a reciprocal relationship between protection and education that must be related to age. Keep all poisonous substances, medicines, cleaning agents, health and beauty aids, paints, and plants locked in a safe place out of an infant's sight and reach. Find out the names of all the plants in and around the house because if someone ingests one of them, the poison control center will need to know what it is when it is called. Never store poisonous substances in containers other than original ones (e.g., empty jars or soda bottles). Safe behavior is a learned behavior, gradually acquired in a progressive process with increasing age.

When parents are being taught, anticipatory guidance should include ways to prevent ingestions, the phone number for the National Capital Poison Center (800-222-1222), early recognition of common signs and symptoms of poisoning, and the importance of never giving remedies before the poison control center has been contacted. It is also important to discuss with parents and caregivers the importance of storing these medications out of the reach of infants and children, using safety locks on cabinets, and keeping purses (or any other places of storage of these medications) out of the reach of infants and children who are at risk of unintentional poisoning. When parents are provided with anticipatory guidance, particular emphasis must be placed on the prevention of unintentional poisonings (National Capital Poison Control Center, 2024b).

Education is part of the nursing role. Talking with parents outside the health care arena is a great place to start. Girl Scout meetings, meetings of parent-teacher associations, church

BOX 17.12 Nursing Interventions to Prevent Plant Poisoning in Infants

- Keep plants out of reach of infants and young children.
- Never eat any part of a plant except the parts that are grown or sold as food.
- Keep jewelry made from unknown seeds or beans away from exploring infants.
- Learn to identify poisonous plants around your house and garden.
- Do not use unknown plants as medicines or teas.
- Pay close attention to infants at play inside and outside.
- Seek help whenever anyone chews or swallows a poisonous plant.
- Be aware that infants are more susceptible than are adults to the effects of poisonous plants.
- Keep the National Capital Poison Center telephone number handy (1-800-222-1222).

National Capital Poison Control Center (2024b); Association of Poison Control Centers (n.d.)

gatherings, day care centers, and other community-based activities can provide a forum for teaching and learning, and such training sessions could also provide an opportunity for questions to be answered.

Box 17.12 lists specific safety measures for parents to prevent plant poisoning of infants (AAPCC, n.d.; National Capital Poison Control Center, 2024b).

Toxins

Susceptibility to environmental toxicants depends on the child's developmental stage and interactions within the physical, biologic, and social environment. Infants are at particular risk of exposure to toxic factors in the environment; as dependent, developing organisms, they are inherently vulnerable. Generally, the exposure of infants to potential toxins is quite different from that of adults because of differences in physical environment, activities, and diet. Daily activities of infants, such as proximity to the floor or carpet inside the home and the lawn or soil outside, hand-to-mouth behaviors, and smaller body size and composition, place them at great risk of exposure to environmental toxins. The floor inside the home is an important microenvironment for infants because their breathing zones are low, and many chemicals are concentrated near the floor. Ingestion, inhalation, and dermal exposure can occur. Infants are exposed to a host of environmental pollutants on a regular basis. These exposures occur through all possible environmental media: air, water, soil, and food. Infants have a unique exposure pattern and unique vulnerabilities. For example, some studies identify that the infant's oral habits and unique diet (ingesting more fruits, vegetables, and water than do adults) magnify their exposure to certain agents. Finally, because infants have a longer life span, toxins that have a long latency or cumulative toxicity (such as certain carcinogens) pose a greater risk to them than to adults (Kliegman et al., 2020).

Pesticides are internationally used harmful chemicals that are used to control pest attacks on crops. Commonly, pesticides are used to kill insects (insecticides), weeds (herbicides), fungi (fungicides), and rodents (rodenticides). Some pesticides that are used to control insects that feed on cereal grains, fruits, and vegetables are notorious for their slow accumulation in human tissue. Produce washes are available now to rid vegetables and fruits of these potential toxins. Over sufficient time, exposure to relatively small amounts of pesticides can result in the buildup of toxic quantities and lead to chronic disease in humans. Pesticides pollute water sources and agricultural products, and consumption of their residues by drinking water or the eating of foods may lead to serious health risks (National Pesticide Information Center [NPIC], 2023). All pesticides have the ability to harm infants if they are exposed to them. The essence to decreasing the health hazards of pesticides is to limit exposure by use of precautionary measures and to have knowledge of their chemistry to decrease their hazards. The following are pesticide safety tips: read the label and follow directions when using; store pesticides in their original containers, out of sight of children; and when adding water to dilute pesticides, never use spoons or cups that are used for food (NPIC, 2023).

Lead is another environmental toxin that has no known physiologic role in the human body. Lead exposure can cause serious damage to infants' developing brains. Lead exposure is a public health concern, especially in early childhood, because young children are more prone to practice hand-to-mouth activity and absorb lead. Lead exposure can slow mental development and cause lower intelligence later in childhood. The effects of lead are more toxic on developing nervous systems of infants and young children than on a mature brain (AAP, 2021b). Although lead is essentially a contaminant, most people absorb a certain amount through exposure to lead-based paint in older homes, contaminated soil, household dust, drinking water, lead crystal, and lead-glazed pottery. Before 1950, lead-based paint was used on the inside and outside of most homes. It was used to make several colors, including white, and was known to dry to a hard, durable surface. In 1977, federal regulations banned lead from paint for general use. However, homes built before 1977 are likely to contain lead-based paint. Studies have revealed a high lead content in drinking water, dirt, old toys, imported toys, lead-glazed pottery, household dust, and soil. Lead in the air comes primarily from automobile emissions (National Institute of Environmental Health Sciences [NIEHS], 2019a). Absorption of lead is closely related to particle size. Airborne lead of small particle size is readily absorbed through the lungs, whereas larger particles fall to the ground. Lead affects practically all systems within the body. At high levels, lead can cause convulsions, coma, and even death. Lower levels of lead can adversely affect the brain, central nervous system, blood cells, and kidneys.

Infants are vulnerable to lead exposure for several reasons. In proportion to their weight, infants inhale more air and more lead than adults (EPA, 2018). Additionally, infants breathe closer to the ground, where a higher concentration of lead is located. Their dust-raising play and habit of putting their hands in their mouths add to their lead consumption; they also have a greater rate of gastrointestinal absorption of lead and other chemicals than do adults. Both exercise and blockage of the nasal passages increase mouth breathing, and the mouth is a far less capable filter than the nose. Mouth breathing, coupled with infants' greater frequency of respiratory tract infections, exposes them to a greater amount of environmental toxins. The growing prevalence of asthma is also evidence of environmental exposure to lead and other pollutants.

Asthma is an inflammatory disease of the lung. Approximately 1 in 12 children have asthma; it is the leading chronic disease in children (Asthma and Allergy Foundation of America [AAFA], 2023). Asthma rates have doubled in the last decade, and death rates from asthma have increased in recent years. The reality is that we do not know why asthma is becoming more prevalent, but air pollution is a contributing factor. A few select steps to decrease indoor allergens to prevent asthmatic attacks include vacuuming carpets and upholstered furniture weekly; washing sheets, blankets, and towels in hot water weekly; avoiding second-hand smoke; pet dander, mold, cockroach elimination; and placing allergen-impermeable covers on pillows, box springs, and mattresses (NIEHS, 2019b).

Human potential and development are clearly important natural resources, and a growing body of evidence now links increased lead exposure to impaired intellectual performance and potential. Clinical lead poisoning affects many children, but it is preventable; excess lead in the infant's environment is made by, and should be eliminated by, human beings. Childhood lead exposure has been linked to numerous health problems, including learning disorders, attention deficit disorder, and hearing loss. Researchers suspect that there is no threshold of exposure to lead for many of these adverse outcomes, especially as a neurotoxicant (NIEHS, 2019a). Progress has been made in reducing blood lead levels in infants and young children. But still today, more than 300,000 American children remain at risk of lead exposure. Many infants and young children live in poverty and inhabit old, rented dwellings, which can lead to or exacerbate the effects of lead exposure.

Parents need education regarding measures that can reduce their infant's exposure to lead:

- Keep areas in which the infant plays as dust-free and clean as possible.
- Do not remove lead paint yourself.
- Wash hands and toys often with soap and water.
- Use contact paper or duct tape to cover chipping or peeling paint.
- Wash the child's hands and face before meals.
- Regularly wet-mop floors and wet-mop window components.
- Remove shoes upon entering the house to prevent tracking in lead-contaminated soil.
- Prevent children from playing in bare soil outside.
- Change clothes and bathe before entering the environment of infants (e.g., day care centers) if work or a hobby involves lead.
- Do not burn painted wood in a fireplace.
- Eat a balanced diet rich in calcium, iron, and vitamin C.

Infants do not necessarily escape noxious chemicals when they are indoors. The levels of contaminants that cause air pollution are approximately the same indoors as they are outdoors, with perhaps higher indoor concentrations of carbon monoxide, nitrogen dioxide, and various hydrocarbons from tobacco smoke; poorly ventilated heating and cooking equipment; and aerosol sprays. There are radon checks and carbon dioxide detectors that can be used to assess the presence of these contaminants. Many consequences of exposure to air pollution may not be observed during infancy but can surface as problems that affect both physical and mental well-being over a lifetime.

Among the acute illnesses of infancy, respiratory disease is ranked first, representing between 50% and 75% of all childhood diseases (NIEHS, 2019c). In addition to the inconvenience and incapacity induced by respiratory diseases, medical costs are high. Dirty air aggravates and, in some cases, causes nearly all respiratory problems. Infants with chronic respiratory disease can become adults with respiratory problems.

Water pollution can cause gastrointestinal disturbances in the infant. Parents and health care providers are quick to blame food, teething, or a virus for simple diarrhea, when the underlying cause may come from the kitchen tap. Numerous strong chemicals are used today to purify drinking water. These chemicals can irritate the delicate lining of the gastrointestinal tract and cause disturbances. Nurses encourage parents to boil all water for 20 minutes before they give it to their infant to help eliminate any potential problems.

Toxicants are widely dispersed throughout the environment of infants. It is essential for nurses to understand the potential routes of exposure, toxic effects, and strategies for prevention of exposure to provide anticipatory guidance to parents and family members.

Motor Vehicles

This section considers the effects of motion or action of forces on the infant; the focus here is on motor vehicle accidents.

Automobiles present a danger to people of all ages, but especially to infants. Motor vehicle injuries are the leading cause of death among children ages 1 to 13 in the United States, but most of them can be prevented (CDC, 2023j). Usually, an infant is injured because of improper restraint inside the automobile. Many parents have been misled by thinking that it is better to be thrown clear of an accident than it is to be restrained. Many also think that it is safer to hold an infant on the lap in the front seat rather than to have the infant restrained in the back seat. On the contrary, these practices increase the probability of a fatality. A free-moving child not only distracts the driver but also means the child is in a more vulnerable position for being thrown.

Adult seat belts are unsuitable for infants or children younger than 4 years because their pelvic structure is small; the AAP (2022a, 2023d) recommends that safety car seats for infants be used. The AAP and the National Highway Traffic Safety Administration (NHTSA) recommend four evidence-based sequential steps to properly protect infants and children in passenger vehicles for children from birth through adolescence: rear-facing car safety seats with harnesses for most infants as long as possible, until they reach the highest weight or height allowed by the seat manufacturer; forward-facing car safety seats with harnesses for most children for as long as possible, until they reach the height and weight limits for their seats; belt-positioning booster seats used with a three-point belt restraint for most children through 8 to 12 years of age; and lap-and-shoulder seat belts for all who have outgrown booster seats. In addition, a fifth evidence-based recommendation is for all children younger than 13 years to ride in the rear seats of vehicles (NHTSA, n.d.-a). All children should be in the back seat because of the potential danger posed by air bags. Infant safety in motor vehicles depends entirely on the responsible adults.

Each year some infants die of heat stroke after being left unattended in motor vehicles or getting into unlocked vehicles. More than half these deaths are of children younger than 2 years. On days when ambient temperatures exceed 86°F, the internal temperature of a vehicle quickly reaches 120°F to 140°F (NHTSA, n.d.-b). At those temperatures, children are at great risk: such temperatures can lead to fever, dehydration, seizures, stroke, and death.

Even at relatively cool ambient temperatures, the temperature can rise inside the vehicle to more than 100°F, which places the infant at risk of hyperthermia. Vehicles heat up rapidly, with most of the temperature rise occurring within the first 15 to 30 minutes. A child's body overheats three to five times faster than an adult body. Leaving the windows opened slightly does not significantly slow the heating process or decrease the maximal temperature attained (Kids & Cars, n.d.).

Nurses can take the lead in increasing public awareness and improving parental education regarding heat rise in motor vehicles. The take-home message here is never to leave an infant alone in a motor vehicle. Make "look before you leave" a routine whenever you get out of the car. The nurse can also suggest the automobile safety precautions listed in Box 17.13. Much of automobile safety is common sense, but the nurse must cover all areas in anticipatory preventive teaching. Children have died in hot cars on days when the outside temperature was in the 50s—it doesn't have to be hot outside for this to happen. The importance of automobile safety cannot be overemphasized.

BOX 17.13 Automobile Safety Precautions

- Be a good role model. Make sure you always wear your seat belt.
- Never leave a child unattended in a parked car or around cars.
- Never hold a child in the lap in the front seat.
- Look before you lock the car to make sure no child is left behind.
- Always use an infant car seat that is properly installed by following the manufacturer's instructions.
- Keep car doors and windows locked, even in driveways or garages.
- Use safety restraints for passengers and the driver.
- Do not be distracted by an infant while driving.
- Continue to use car seats as directed by the manufacturer; then use seat belts.
- Never place an infant in a rear-facing car safety seat in the front seat of a vehicle that has a passenger air bag.
- Make sure the seat belt is routed through the correct belt path for adult seat belts.
- Always lock your car and secure the keys so that children cannot access keys.
- Install a trunk release mechanism so that children will not be trapped in the trunk.
- Take the child out of the car seat first, and then worry about getting other items (e.g., groceries) out of the car.
- If you see a child alone in a car, get involved. Call 911 immediately and get the child out of car immediately. It may save the child's life.

National Highway Traffic Safety Administration (2019); CDC (2023j)

Radiation

Radiation exists all around us. People are exposed to varying amounts of radiation from outer space, rocks and soil, food, water, air, airline travel, medical procedures, fallout from past nuclear weapons testing, and radiation emergencies. In its broadest sense, radiation means the transfer of electromagnetic waves or energy through space (CDC, 2022c). Radiation of all types presents a potential hazard in the infant's environment. The risk level depends on the amount of radiation and the length of exposure and on the particular tissues involved. The infant's rapidly growing and immature cells are especially vulnerable.

The infant is exposed to two basic categories of radiation: natural background radiation, which comes from cosmic rays and radioactive material existing naturally in the soil, water, and air, and human-made radiation, which includes x-rays and radiation from nuclear power plants, microwave ovens, and other electronic devices found in the home (CDC, 2022c). Infants have a developing immune response. As their immune system develops, immunity occurs in response to external factors such as the environment. Their exposure to ultraviolet radiation alters the development of the immune system, leading to long-term implications for suppression of immunity in adulthood (Kliegman et al., 2020).

DETERMINANTS OF HEALTH

Social Factors and Environment

Community and Work

As infants grow and develop, their boundaries extend beyond the home environment. Many parents of infants return to the workforce, placing the infants in community day care centers.

Today, few young families can escape financial burdens. With more than half of all American parents working outside the home, the need for childcare service is growing. Childcare quality is of great concern to parents, yet the quality of childcare varies widely, and the current supply is inadequate to meet the needs. This situation is usually an emotional issue for families; the separation process can be traumatic for both the infant and the parent.

Findings from social science research regarding the effects of day care on an infant's development and health can be summarized as follows: little evidence suggests that day care permanently enhances or slows intellectual development; day care can be used, even from earliest infancy, without damaging the parent-infant relationship; and day care can lead to a slight increase in minor illnesses, but excluding ill infants from the center is not an effective means of reducing the spread of illness. The day care environment must promote and positively support the infant's development and the infant's interaction with space, materials, and people (Office of Child Care, 2023).

The question of how old an infant should be before being placed in day care is frequently asked of health professionals. Many experts believe that the parents and infant should have

4 to 6 months together before the parent returns to work. Brazelton and Sparrow (2015) outline the case for parent/infant transitioning through four stages of attachment together before the parent returns to work:

- In the first stage, which takes 10 to 14 days, the infant learns to be attentive to the parent, and the parent learns cues from the infant about being both ready for and tired of attentiveness.
- The second stage, which lasts 8 weeks, is a stage of playful interaction, when the parent learns how to recognize the infant's nonverbal cues and helps the infant maintain the alert state.
- The third stage, from the 10th week to the fourth month, is when the parent and infant learn to play games together.
- During the fourth stage, which occurs in the fourth month, infants rapidly learn about themselves and their world. A parent, when possible, should spend the first 4 months with their new infant (Brazelton & Sparrow, 2015).

The nurse has a vital role in assisting families with infants who need day care. Many factors are reviewed when a family is looking for an appropriate day care program; the nurse can counsel and guide the family in its search. The means by which the nurse counsels and guides the family in selecting a day care center are as follows:

- Promote awareness of the three types of day care available in their local communities.
- Counsel parents on questions to ask employees of a prospective day care facility (Building Blocks, 2023; Box 17.14).

BOX 17.14 Prospective Day Care Facility Questions

- Is the center currently licensed by the state?
- Is the day care facility open all year?
- Ask for recommendations from other parents.
- Are all children required to have immunizations before they begin?
- What are the qualifications and credentials of the staff here?
- What hours is it open?
- Do extensive research on the potential childcare facility.
- How long has the center been in business?
- What is the center's licensed capacity?
- How flexible are you with pickup and drop-off times?
- How many children are present at the center?
- What is the age range of children at the center?
- What is the teacher-to-child ratio? (For infants, 1:3 is recommended.)
- Describe the day care program.
- What meals are served?
- What is the cost?
- Are there openings?
- Do you have webcam capability so I can view my infant during the day?
- What are the qualifications of the caregivers?
- Are the caregivers happy and interacting with the infant?
- Are infants content?
- What supplies would I need to bring for my infant?
- Are parents welcome to drop in?

Office of Child Care (2023)

- Help parents learn ways to cope with the separation behaviors manifested by their infant:
  - Remain calm in the situation.
  - Attempt to reduce the number of adults who interact with the infant and always introduce them.
- Instruct parents to ask the question: Where do the infants sleep and are they separate from older children? Exposure to older children increases the risk of infection.
- Encourage the parents to bring an infant's special cuddly toy from home to the day care facility to promote security.
- Listen to the parent's understanding of the separation and expected behaviors.
- Reassure parents that it takes time for the infant to make the transition from the parent to another caregiver and vice versa.
- Emphasize that at certain developmental levels stranger anxiety may be heightened (8 months), and separation behaviors of crying and clinging may be repeated.
- Work toward promoting a good relationship among parents, the infant, and the caregiver by providing opportunities for open discussions of concerns.

Culture and Ethnicity

Culture is defined as a set of learned values, beliefs, attitudes, and practices that are passed from generation to generation (Purnell & Fenkl, 2019). Culture plays an important role in influencing an infant's development, and what is considered "normal" development differs greatly from one culture to the next. Child development is a dynamic, interactive process. Parents worldwide have universal feelings of love, hope, and care for their infants. Culture can influence parenting styles, which can vary significantly and affect children's development. Culture defines how health care information is received, how rights and protections are exercised, what is considered to be a health problem, how symptoms and concerns about the problem are expressed, who should provide treatment for the problem, and what type of treatment should be given. In short, culture is the lens through which one views the world, affecting everything that an individual and that individual's family perceive and do.

The developing infant is subject to the influences of culture from the moment of conception. Partly because of the long dependency period, the family environment is the setting within which the infant experiences overall cultural attitudes. The lives of infants tend to be more under the direct control of parents or other caregivers than the lives of older children, who are often actively involved in selecting their own environments through contacts with peers, teachers, and other adults. The special demands of infancy require extensive and specific caregiving routines across cultures. Effective parenting styles also vary as a function of culture. The parents' perceptions of illness, wellness, roles, childrearing practices, religious values, language, and health practices are all modeled for the infant. To summarize, culture helps form the infant's view of the world. While children are unique and develop at their own pace, the cultural influence on their development is considerable (Huang, 2019).

BOX 17.15 Factors That Facilitate Multicultural Health Care by Nurses

- Self-exploration of values and beliefs concerning other cultures and their beliefs
- Knowledge of the historical experience, recent and long term, of ethnic groups that live in the community
- Demographic data that include family size, socioeconomic status, and future expectations that are characteristic of diverse ethnic groups
- Understanding and sensitivity to cultural health care practices different from their own
- Recognition of folk beliefs and cultural attitudes toward health and illness
- Awareness of the nature of problems encountered by ethnic group members when they enter the health care system, including fear and distrust of health care professionals, language barriers, and discrimination by caregivers

The family's ethnicity includes ideas about health, illness, food preferences, moral codes, and family life that persist across generations and survive even the upheaval of coming to a new country. All cultural groups confront repeated challenges as they transfer their families from familiar to unfamiliar surroundings. Infants are exposed to an appropriate mode of behavior that is in accordance with their family's cultural standards. By observing and imitating family members, infants take cues for behavior. These perceptions are then incorporated into their own self-concepts (Kersey-Matusiak, 2019).

To assess and plan appropriate interventions for different ethnic groups, nurses must be aware of their own cultural values and beliefs. An important consideration is to examine all customs and values in relative terms, seeing none as either good or bad (Box 17.15). Change is inevitable in family life, whether it is resisted or welcomed. An important function of the nurse is to help families monitor the rate of change that is acceptable to various members and reach a consensus.

The need for culturally appropriate nursing care was identified as a key area of intervention by WHO (2023e). Research has identified several strategies that nurses can use that improve communication and reduce stress for culturally diverse populations: answering questions carefully, teaching by demonstration, and taking time to explain in plain language. In addition, if individuals felt that the staff truly cared for their infant, this facilitated communication across multiple barriers because they "felt safe to ask questions" or express needs (Kersey-Matusiak, 2019). Thus nurses who are mindful of the specific views of a culture respect the boundaries of the particular cultural perceptions, beliefs, and practices. Culturally competent nurses have achieved efficacy in communication skills and incorporate health care practices and beliefs of a particular culture in health care plans. Furthermore, respect for the individual's cultural values is viewed as essential if the nurse is to successfully help the family achieve a state of health and wellness. The nurse assesses the cultural groups' practices and beliefs before planning interventions. Improving the quality and safety of nursing care for culturally diverse individuals globally should be the primary goal of all perinatal nurses. Approaches to infant care

BOX 17.16 HEALTH AND SOCIAL DETERMINANTS/HEALTH EQUITY

Quick Guide for Cross-Cultural Nursing Care

The dominant American attitudes about infants and approaches to infant care have undergone many changes in the past several years. Cultural beliefs and practices are continually evolving and changing. Nurses acknowledge and explore their meanings with all the families they meet. All behavior must be evaluated from within the context of the family and the family's cultural background and experience.

Nurses must facilitate health-promoting attitudes and practices and show empathic concern and respect for individuals of all cultural backgrounds. By incorporating the assessment of cultural beliefs and practices into the individual's plan of care, nurses can demonstrate respect and take a step forward in developing culturally appropriate patterns of caring.

The family is the primary health care provider for the infant. The family determines health promotion for the family, including when an infant is ill. Nurses are cautious in imposing their own values, beliefs, and attitudes on others. Rather than judging people, the nurse ascertains how each family's values and beliefs influence health outcomes.

The nurse remembers that all behaviors must be evaluated from within the context of the family's cultural background and experiences. Nurses who strive to foster health-promoting attitudes and behaviors begin at the most basic level: empathic concern and respect for the individual. By incorporating the assessment of cultural beliefs and practices into the infant's plan of care, nurses demonstrate respect, reduce alienation, and take a step toward developing culturally appropriate patterns of health promotion.

practices differ among cultural groups (Box 17.16: Health and Social Determinants/Health Equity).

Levels of Policy Making and Health

Legislation

Enormous strides have been made in infant health in the past decade: many common, lethal infections have been eradicated (smallpox), and infant mortality rates continue to decline.

One of the concerns of federal legislation is infant health. The goal, as described by the USDHHS (2023), is to "improve the health and well-being of women, infants, children and families."

The infant mortality rate has been on a steady decline since the turn of the century, a result of better infant nutrition, improved technology, improved housing, and improved prenatal, obstetrical, and pediatric care (USDHHS, 2023). To meet the goal of improving infant health, major health problems in this age group must be reduced. A major hazard for infants is low birth weight. To address this problem, factors that increase the risk of low birth weight in infants must be identified (Kliegman et al., 2020).

Many of these factors can be prevented, or risks can be identified early and managed to prevent low birth weight in infants. The major focus for prevention is prenatal care for all individuals.

Another major threat to infant survival is congenital disorders, such as malformations of the brain and spine (e.g., microcephaly and myelomeningocele), congenital heart defects (e.g., ventricular septal defects), and combinations of genetic anomalies, such as Down syndrome or Tay-Sachs disease. Although some congenital abnormalities cannot be prevented, others can be detected by performing prenatal screening and promoting research to determine their cause.

Other factors identified by the USDHHS (2023) and Healthy People 2030 that contribute to the high infant mortality rate are injuries at birth, SIDS, accidents, respiratory distress syndrome, and inadequate parenting.

The federal government's plans to attain the goal of healthy infants are as follows:

- Promote family planning services such that all pregnancies are planned, and all infants are wanted.
- Provide pregnancy and infant care services to high-risk populations through Maternity and Infant Care (MIC) projects. The Special Supplemental Nutrition Program, WIC, improves the nutritional status of both the birthing parent and the infant.
- Encourage educational efforts by schools, health providers, and the media to promote prenatal care.
- Promote massive immunization efforts such that each infant is protected from communicable disease.

Nursing's Role. Nurses have important roles in promoting change in response to a continually expanding knowledge base, consumer health care needs, and governmental legislation. By actively participating in groups involved with health planning, the nurse helps make governmental policy more responsive to infants' health care needs. Health promotion essentially relates to collective or population well-being, which is wholly compatible with all nurses' roles. Nurses need to work together with other professionals, agencies, and local people to improve the health and well-being of infants. Informed and focused nurses work together to shape health care policies that positively affect clients and their families. A coordinated effort is needed to be most effective in advancing major health policy issues (American Association of Critical-Care Nurses [AACN], 2019).

Economics

Many health problems are found more frequently in segments of the population with low incomes than in high-income groups. The infant mortality rates in low-income families remain significantly higher than those in high-income families, despite an overall decrease in the infant mortality rate nationally (CDC, 2022d; USDHHS, 2023).

In the United States, roughly 45% of children are born into poor or low-income families, and their health suffers when basic needs such as food, housing, health screening, and vaccinations are not met. Developing effective behavioral interventions requires better understanding of parent characteristics and needs (AAP, 2019c). Parents with low incomes might be unaware of their infant's developmental needs; they are frequently faced with many environmental and social stresses that demand their time, energy, and other resources (AAP, 2019c). Many parents have so many unfulfilled needs of their own that they cannot meet their infants' needs. In many cases, infants from families in poverty have delayed language development. With limited educational and life experiences, their parents are often unable to be ideal models for language development. Infants learn early language sounds from their parents, but their attempts at language must be reinforced.

Armed with the knowledge of how economics can affect the infant's growth, development, and health status, the nurse, before deciding on interventions, assesses the family situation by performing the following tasks:

- Establish a relationship with the family to obtain pertinent information.
- Evaluate the home environment in which the infant interacts.
- Elicit the parents' health perceptions about their own health and that of the infant.
- Offer assistance for the family to navigate the health care system for their infant
- Complete a thorough physical examination of the infant to identify any problem areas.
- Identify community resources that are available to the low-income family.

Through assessment of need and the identification and implementation of available resources, nurses can be a driving factor in limiting the exposure to poverty and its health consequences.

Health Services/Delivery System

The US health care delivery system is diverse and large; many different sectors merge to provide infant care. Within this enormous, multidisciplinary system, the nurse is an advocate who facilitates the family's passage through the many facets of care.

The value of health promotion and preventive health care has been validated; it is cost-effective and is here to stay. As nurses' roles continue to expand within the various parts of the health care system, their duty is to keep pace with the needs, concerns, and available strategies (Stanhope & Lancaster, 2020). Because many conditions that cause morbidity or death in infants are preventable when health-promotion practices are used, nurses have the mission of working within the health care system to promote infant health (USDHHS, 2023).

NURSING APPLICATION

Nurses can promote health to all their clients by improving public knowledge about health and empowering people to make positive choices for themselves and their families so that communities can be transformed. Nurses can do more to ensure the health of our youngest and most vulnerable population. It is the responsibility of all nurses to make health-education and health-promotion activities an integral part of their professional role. The primary role of the nurse in promoting the health of an infant is to provide the family with education during the most critical developmental period. Initial health-promotion efforts should focus on the nutritional needs of the infant during the first 18 months of life. Basic principles of biologic growth and development set the stage for appropriate developmental tasks and psychological growth in the coming months. Nurses can make a difference in the lives of infants and their families by encouraging early and adequate prenatal care for the birthing parent, supporting the transition from the hospital to the home, providing increased access to infant care services, and supporting childhood health surveillance.

The nurse promotes the health of the infant through their interactions with the parents, as the infant is dependent on them for care. The nurse is in a position to encourage practices in the home that create the optimal conditions for normal growth and development. An important starting point for the nurse is to teach new parents about the nutritional value of breast/chestfeeding and to encourage those efforts. Professional support and education play a vital role in increasing the rates of breast/chestfeeding individuals.

Following a routine immunization and well-child health visit schedule is another aspect of health promotion for the infant. Nurses play a role in this task by educating parents about the importance of immunization. In addition, nurses should remain informed about the immunization recommendations and assist the family in maintaining documentation of vaccines administered. If cost or access to care is a factor, families can be referred to free or low-cost vaccination clinics.

Essentially, health promotion should be viewed as an umbrella concept, encompassing all health-related activities that contribute to the formation of a state of health in that individual or community. It should include education, disease-prevention, and environmental-health promotion measures. The health-promotion goals of the nurse working with infants are met through the family. The nurse must ascertain the health perceptions and motivation of the family, including the use of good or bad health practices. The family must be motivated to provide good health practices for the infant. As the nurse plans health-promotion activities for families of infants, it is imperative that factors influencing health perception are identified. The ability of the nurse to provide a supportive relationship with the parents is a key element in facilitating successful infant development. The nurse working with this population has a unique opportunity to influence the health status of both the infant and the family for years to come.

The leadership of nurses in collaboration with other health care professionals will be key to improving the health of future generations. Whereas there is still room for improvement in the United States, many of the existing pediatric programs of care offer solutions that improve infants' health. It is essential that nurses continue to support these evidence-based models of care.

CASE STUDY

Homelessness: Homeless Minority Infants

As a community health nurse in an inner-city health center, you are increasingly aware that the homeless population in your city appears to be the forgotten aggregate. Your community health center provides primary care to a culturally diverse and indigent population. As a nurse, you believe that the homeless population within your city has numerous health needs. Beyond the basic requirements, many homeless people have mental health conditions and substance abuse disorders, a deficiency in life skills, and poor family support, and most of all lack access to child health services.

Although there are several glaring concerns, you plan to focus your attention on securing immunizations for the homeless infants and obtaining formula for them.

Reflective Questions

- What barriers to accessing health care for minority infants confront the homeless family?
- How can you overcome some of the barriers in developing your plan for health care?

Recognizing and Analyzing Cues

In planning health services for this special population, what facts do you need to know? The following are some of the first questions that might be asked:

- How many homeless minority infants are in this aggregate?
- Where are they?
- How can they access health care in the city?

To answer these questions, it might be prudent to collaborate and partner with other health and social service agencies, local hospitals, and the state health and human services agency. Collaboration and partnering can bring in additional resources and reduce duplication and gaps in services.

What barriers to accessing health care for infants confront the homeless family?

- Lack of transportation
- Lack of trust in the medical establishment
- Judgmental care on the part of health care providers and nurses
- No health insurance to cover medical visits
- Preventive care, such as immunizations, not a priority when you are hungry
- No money to get prescriptions filled or transportation to get to pharmacies
- Waiting until the condition is serious before seeking treatment

How can you overcome some of the barriers in developing your plan for health care?

- Provide health care in the city shelters for use by homeless minority families.
- Set up a mobile health care team and visit the shelters to provide care.
- Offer free immunizations for all family members.
- Establish educational sessions within the shelters to provide information.
- Stress the importance of preventive measures to reduce illness in infants.
- Obtain free formula from companies or hospitals to give to homeless infants.
- Work closely with other health care interests within the community.

SUMMARY

- Health promotion has long been a central part of nursing practice, but at this juncture it is increasingly vital for all nurses to play an active role in promoting the health of individuals, families, communities, and nations.
- Nurses must have evidence-based understanding of the significant effect that can be made through health-promotion interventions and communicate this understanding to families they care for.
- Families today want more information and knowledge, and they demand that health care professionals be more responsive to their needs. Their demand has been a catalyst for the nurse's expanded health care role and responsibility for health promotion.
- Health promotion by nurses is associated with common universal principles of health education.
- Nurses should be able to plan, implement, and evaluate health-promotion interventions for infants and their families to improve their health outcomes.

EVOLVE CHAPTER FEATURES

http://evolve.elsevier.com/Edelman/

- Study Questions

REFERENCES

Abrams, S. A., & Duggan, C. P. (2022). Infant and child formula shortages: Now is the time to prevent recurrences. *The American Journal of Clinical Nutrition, 116*(2), 289–292. https://doi.org/10.1093/ajcn/nqac149

American Academy of Pediatrics [AAP]. (2019a). *Breastfeeding success: helping families get the support they need.* https://www.aap.org/en/news-room/aap-voices/breastfeeding-success/

American Academy of Pediatrics [AAP]. (2019b). *Choking prevention.* https://www.healthychildren.org/English/health-issues/injuries-emergencies/Pages/Choking-Prevention.aspx

American Academy of Pediatrics [AAP]. (2019c). *Early cognitive and language development: what low-income parents of newborns know and do.* https://pediatrics.aappublications.org/content/144/2_MeetingAbstract/53

American Academy of Pediatrics [AAP]. (2021a). *Toy buying tips for babies and young children.* https://www.healthychildren.org/English/ages-stages/baby/Pages/What-to-Look-for-in-a-Toy.aspx

American Academy of Pediatrics [AAP]. (2021b). *Lead exposure in children.* https://www.aap.org/en/patient-care/lead-exposure/

American Academy of Pediatrics [AAP]. (2022a). *Child passenger safety.* https://publications.aap.org/pediatrics/article/142/5/e20182460/38530/Child-Passenger-Safety?autologincheck=redirected

American Academy of Pediatrics [AAP]. (2022b). *Healthy children: child abuse and neglect.* https://www.healthychildren.org

American Academy of Pediatrics [AAP]. (2023a). *2023 recommendations for preventive pediatric health care.* https://publications.aap.org/pediatrics/article/151/4/e2023061451/190849/2023-Recommendations-for-Preventive-Pediatric

American Academy of Pediatrics [AAP]. (2023b). *Infant food and feeding.* https://www.aap.org/en/patient-care/healthy-active-living-for-families/infant-food-and-feeding/

American Academy of Pediatrics [AAP]. (2023c). *Burn treatment and prevention tips for families.* https://www.healthychildren.org/English/health-issues/injuries-emergencies/Pages/Treating-and-Preventing-Burns.aspx

American Academy of Pediatrics [AAP]. (2023d). *Car seats: information for families.* https://www.healthychildren.org/English/safety-prevention/on-the-go/Pages/Car-Safety-Seats-Information-for-Families.aspx

American Academy of Pediatrics [AAP]. (n.d.). *Red Book Online: immunization schedules for 2024.* https://redbook.solutions.aap.org/SS/Immunization_Schedules.aspx

American Association of Critical-Care Nurses [AACN]. (2019). *Policy & advocacy.* https://www.aacn.org/policy-and-advocacy

American Association of Poison Control Centers [AAPCC]. (n.d.). *Prevention & education: in the home.* https://www.aapcc.org/prevention/home

American Heart Association. (2021). *2017 infant CPR and choking fact sheet.* https://cpr.heart.org/-/media/cpr-files/courses-and-kits/resources-for-infant-cpr-anytime-kits/2017-infant-cpr-and-choking-fact-sheet-ucm_495372.pdf?la=en&hash=EA373CE77F94FA8D8F9AC20B126061F035957B80

American Optometric Association. (2019). *Ways to help infant vision develop.* https://www.aoa.org/patients-and-public/good-vision-throughout-life/childrens-vision/infant-vision-birth-to-24-months-of-age/ways-to-help-infant-vision-development

Arora, T. (2019). Sleep routines in children. *Journal of Clinical Sleep Medicine, 15*(6), 821–822.

Asthma and Allergy Foundation of America [AAFA]. (2023). *Asthma facts and figures.* https://www.aafa.org/asthma-facts/

Babakr, Z., Mohamedamin, P., & Kakamad, K. (2019). Piaget's cognitive developmental theory: Critical review. *Education Quarterly Reviews, 2*(3), 517–524.

Baby-Friendly USA. (2023a). *The Baby-Friendly Hospital Initiative.* https://www.babyfriendlyusa.org/about/

Baby-Friendly USA. (2023b). *The guidelines & evaluation criteria.* https://www.babyfriendlyusa.org/for-facilities https://doi.org/10.31014/aior.1993.02.03.84/practice-guidelines/

Berk, L. E. (2019). *Exploring child development.* New York, NY: Pearson.

Boy Scouts of America. (2018). *How to protect your children from child abuse: a parent's guide.* https://filestore.scouting.org/filestore/pdf/100-014_WEB.pdf

Brazelton, T. B. (2023). *Brazelton Touchpoints Center.* https://www.brazeltontouchpoints.org/

Brazelton, T. B., & Sparrow, J. A. (2015). *Discipline: The Brazelton way* (2nd ed.). Old Saybrook, CT: Tantor Media.

Brooks, L. A., Manias, E., & Bloomer, M. J. (2019). Culturally sensitivity communication in health care: A concept analysis. *Collegian, 26*(3), 383–391.

Brown, A., & Jones, W. (2020). *A guide to supporting breastfeeding for the medical profession.* Boca Raton, FL: Taylor & Francis.

Brown, J. (2019). *Nutrition through the life cycle* (7th ed.). Boston, MA: Cengage Learning.

Building Blocks. (2023). *Choosing a quality child care provider.* https://penfieldbuildingblocks.org/early-education/choosing-quality-child-care-provider/

Center for Parenting Education. (2023). *The tasks of infants through 18 months old.* https://centerforparentingeducation.org/library-of-articles/child-development/developmental-tasks/#infants

Centers for Disease Control and Prevention [CDC]. (2019). *Use and interpretation of the WHO and CDC growth charts for children from birth to 20 years in the United States.* https://www.cdc.gov

Centers for Disease Control and Prevention [CDC]. (2020). *Fall prevention.* https://www.cdc.gov/vitalsigns/childinjury/index.html

Centers for Disease Control and Prevention [CDC]. (2021a). *Infants: positive parenting tips.* https://www.cdc.gov

Centers for Disease Control and Prevention [CDC]. (2021b). *Burn Institute Teaches Kids Burn Prevention, Fire Safety.* https://blogs.cdc.gov

Centers for Disease Control and Prevention [CDC]. (2022a). *Infant and toddler nutrition.* https://www.cdc.gov/nutrition/InfantandToddlerNutrition/index.html

Centers for Disease Control and Prevention [CDC]. (2022b). *Preventing child abuse and neglect.* https://www.cdc.gov

Centers for Disease Control and Prevention [CDC]. (2022c). *Radiation.* https://www.cdc.gov/nceh/radiation/default.htm

Centers for Disease Control and Prevention [CDC]. (2022d). *Promoting health for infants.* https://www.cdc.gov

Centers for Disease Control and Prevention [CDC]. (2023a). *Data and statistics on hemophilia.* https://www.cdc.gov/ncbddd/hemophilia/data.html

Centers for Disease Control and Prevention [CDC]. (2023b). *When, what, and how to introduce solid foods.* https://www.cdc.gov/nutrition/infantandtoddlernutrition/foods-and-drinks/when-to-introduce-solid-foods.html

Centers for Disease Control and Prevention [CDC]. (2023c). *Sudden unexpected infant deaths: data and statistics.* https://www.cdc.gov/sids/data.htm

Centers for Disease Control and Prevention [CDC]. (2023d). *CDC's developmental milestones.* https://www.cdc.gov/ncbddd/actearly/milestones/index.html

Centers for Disease Control and Prevention [CDC]. (2023e). *Accidents or unintentional injuries.* https://www.cdc.gov/nchs/fastats/accidental-injury.htm

Centers for Disease Control and Prevention [CDC]. (2023f). *Cost of injury data*. https://www.cdc.gov/injury/wisqars/cost/index.html

Centers for Disease Control and Prevention [CDC]. (2023g). *Information on safety in the home and community for parents with infants and toddlers (ages 0-3)*. https://www.cdc.gov/parents/infants/safety.html

Centers for Disease Control and Prevention [CDC]. (2023h). *HIV and pregnant women, infants, and children*. https://www.cdc.gov

Centers for Disease Control and Prevention [CDC]. (2023i). *Child and adolescent immunization schedule by age - recommendations for ages 18 years or younger, United States, 2024*. https://www.cdc.gov

Centers for Disease Control and Prevention [CDC]. (2023j). *Child passenger safety: get the facts*. https://www.cdc.gov/transportationsafety/child_passenger_safety/index.html

Child Welfare. (2019). *Long-term consequences of child abuse and neglect*. https://www.childwelfare.gov/pubPDFs/long_term_consequences.pdf

Children's Bureau. (2019). *Social connection on child development*. https://www.all4kids.org/social-connection-on-child-development/

Clarke, A. (2020). *Harper's practical genetic counseling* (8th ed.). Boca Raton, FL: CRC Press.

Conci, M. (2019). Childhood, attachment, separation, and trauma. *International Forum of Psychoanalysis*, *28*(3), 125–126.

Duckett, S. A., & Roten, R. A. (2022). *Choking*. StatPearls. https://www.ncbi.nlm.nih.gov/books/NBK499941/

Duryea, T. K., & Fleischer, D. M. (2023). *Patient education: starting solid food during infancy*. UpToDate. https://www.uptodate.com/contents/starting-solid-foods-during-infancy-beyond-the-basics

Environmental Protection Agency [EPA]. (2018). *Protecting children from lead exposures*. https://www.epa.gov/sites/production/files/2018-10/documents/leadpreventionbooklet2018-v11_web.pdf

Environmental Protection Agency [EPA]. (2023). *Resources about indoor air quality for parents*. https://www.epa.gov/indoor-air-quality-iaq

Eunice Kennedy Shriver National Institute of Child Health and Human Development. (n.d.). *About SIDS and safe infant sleep*. https://safetosleep.nichd.nih.gov/safesleepbasics/about

Gonzalez, D., & McCall, J. D. (2024). *Child abuse and neglect*. StatPearls. https://www.ncbi.nlm.nih.gov/books/NBK459146/

Gosselin, D. K. (2019). *Family & intimate partner violence: Heavy hands* (6th ed.). New York, NY: Pearson

Hill, R., & Flanagan, J. (2019). The maternal-infant bond: Clarifying the concept. *International Journal of Nursing Knowledge*, *31*(1), 14–18.

Huang, C. Y. (2019). *How culture influences children's development*. https://thesector.com.au/2019/06/07/how-culture-influences-childrens-development/

International Society of Nurses in Genetics [ISONG]. (n.d.). *What is a genetics nurse?* https://www.isong.org/page-1325051

Joyce, T., & Huecker, M. R. (2023). *Pediatric abusive head trauma (shaken baby syndrome)*. StatPearls. https://www.ncbi.nlm.nih.gov/books/NBK499836/

Jung, J., Widmar, N. O., & Ellison, B. (2022). The curious case of baby formula in the United States in 2022: Cries for urgent action months after silence in the midst of alarm bells. *Food Ethics*, *8*(1), 4. https://doi.org/10.1007/s41055-022-00115-1

Kelleher, M., Phillips, R., Brown, S. J., Cro, S., Cornelius, V., Carlsen, K., et al. (2022). Skin care interventions in infants for preventing eczema and food allergy. *Cochrane Database Systematic Reviews*, *11*(11):CD013534. doi:10.1002/14651858.CD013534.pub3

Kelly, N. R. (2023). *Prevention of poisoning in children*. UpToDate. https://www.uptodate.com/contents/prevention-of-poisoning-in-children?search=prevention%20of%20poisoning%20&source=search_result&selectedTitle=1~47&usage_type=default&display_rank=1

Kersey-Matusiak, G. (2019). *Delivering culturally competent nursing care: Working with diverse and vulnerable populations* (2nd ed.). New York, NY: Springer Publisher Company.

Kids & Cars. (n.d.). *Hot cars resources*. https://www.kidsandcars.org/hot-cars/media-resources

Kliegman, R. M., St. Geme, J. W., Blum, N. J., Shah, S. S., Tasker, R. C., & Wilson, K. M. (2020). *Nelson textbook of pediatrics* (21st ed.). Philadelphia, PA: Elsevier.

Koletzko, B., Godfrey, K. M., Poston, L., & Zalewski, B. M. (2019). Nutrition during pregnancy, lactation, and early childhood and its implications for maternal and long-term child health: Early nutrition project recommendations. *Annals of Nutrition & Metabolism*, *74*, 93–106

La Leche League International. (2024). *Support for transgender & non-binary parents*. https://llli.org/breastfeeding-info/transgender-non-binary-parents/

Lauwers, J., & Swisher, A. (2016). *Counseling the nursing mother: A lactation consultant's guide*. (6th ed.). Burlington, MA: Jones & Bartlett Learning.

Levine, L. E., & Munsch, J. (2020). *Child development: From infancy to adolescence* (2nd ed.). Thousand Oaks, CA: SAGE Publications.

Malik, F., & Marwaha, R. (2022). *Developmental stages of social emotional development in children*. StatPearls. https://www.ncbi.nlm.nih.gov/books/NBK534819/

Malik, F., & Marwaha, R. (2023). *Cognitive development*. StatPearls. https://www.ncbi.nlm.nih.gov/books/NBK537095/

March of Dimes. (2020a). *Hearing loss and your baby*. https://www.marchofdimes.org/complications/hearing-loss-and-your-baby.aspx

March of Dimes. (2020b). *Breastfeeding is best*. https://www.marchofdimes.org/baby/breastfeeding-is-best.aspx

National Academies of Sciences, Engineering, and Medicine. (2019). *Fostering health mental, emotional, and behavioral development in children and youth: A national agenda*. Washington, DC: The National Academies Press.

National Capital Poison Control Center. (2024a). *Poisonous plants*. https://www.poison.org/articles/plant#poisonousplants

National Capital Poison Control Center. (2024b). *Poison & prevention information: infants*. https://www.poison.org/poison-prevention-tips-by-age/infants

National Highway Traffic Safety Administration [NHTSA]. (n.d.-a). *Car seats and booster seats*. https://www.nhtsa.gov/equipment/car-seats-and-booster-seats#age-size-rec

National Highway Traffic Safety Administration [NHTSA]. (n.d.-b). *Too many children dying in hot cars*. https://www.nhtsa.gov/child-safety/help-too-many-children-are-dying-hot-cars

National Institute of Allergy and Infectious Diseases [NIAID]. (2018). *Guidelines for the prevention of peanut allergy in the United States: Report of the NIAID-sponsored expert panel*. https://www.niaid.nih.gov/sites/default/files/addendum-peanut-allergy-prevention-guidelines.pdf

National Institute of Environmental Health Sciences. (2019a). *Lead poisoning*. https://kids.niehs.nih.gov/topics/pollution/lead/index.htm

National Institute of Environmental Health Sciences. (2019b). *Asthma and allergies and their environmental triggers*. https://kids.niehs.nih.gov/topics/pollution/asthma-and-allergies/index.htm

National Institute of Environmental Health Sciences. (2019c). *Environmental pollution health problems*. https://kids.niehs.nih.gov/activities/stories/mama-didnt-know/environmental-health-problems/index.htm

National Institute on Deafness and other Communication Disorders [NIDCD]. (2017). *Your baby's hearing and communicative development*. https://www.nidcd.nih.gov/health/your-babys-hearing-and-communicative-development-checklist

National Institutes of Health [NIH]. (2019). *Fast facts about SIDS*. https://safetosleep.nichd.nih.gov/safesleepbasics/SIDS/fastfacts

National Institutes of Health [NIH]. (2020a). *Sickle cell disease*. https://ghr.nlm.nih.gov/condition/sickle-cell-disease

National Institutes of Health [NIH]. (2020b). *Combined prenatal smoking and drinking greatly increases SIDS risk*. https://www.nih.gov/news-events/news-releases/combined-prenatal-smoking-drinking-greatly-increases-sids-risk

National Institutes of Health [NIH]. (2024). *Ways to reduce the risk of SIDS and other sleep-related causes of infant death*. https://safetosleep.nichd.nih.gov/reduce-risk/reduce

National Pesticide Information Center [NPIC]. (2023). *Pesticides and children*. http://npic.orst.edu/health/child.html

National Safety Council. (2023). *Choking prevention and rescue tips*. https://www.nsc.org/home-safety/safety-topics/choking-suffocation

National Tay-Sachs & Allied Disease Association. (2023). *Tay-Sachs disease*. https://www.ntsad.org/index.php/tay-sachs

Newberry, J. A. (2019). Creating a safe sleep environment for the infant: What the pediatric nurse needs to know. *Journal of Pediatric Nursing*, *44*, 119–122.

Office of Child Care. (2023). *Ensuring safe and healthy childcare*. https://www.childcare.gov/consumer-education/ensuring-safe-and-healthy-childcare

Oliveira, P., & Fearon, P. (2019). The biological basis of attachment. *Adoption & Fostering*, *43*(3), 274–293.

Olsen, A. L., Ammitzboll, J., Olsen, E. M., & Skovgaard, A. M. (2019). Problems of feeding, sleeping and excessive crying in infancy: a general population study. *Archives of Disease in Childhood*, *104*(11), 1034–1041.

Phillips, A. (2019). Effective approaches to health promotion in nursing practice. *Nursing Standard*, *34*(4), 43–50.

Purnell, L.D., & Fenkl, F. A. (2019). *Handbook for culturally competent care*. Cham, Switzerland: Springer Publishers.

Ranch, M. M., Jamten, S., Thorstensson, S., & Ekstrom-Bergstrom, A. C. (2019). First-time mothers have a desire to be offered professional breastfeeding support by pediatric nurses: An evaluation of the mother-perceived-professional support scale. *Nursing Research and Practice*, *2019*, 8731705.

Ruffin, N. (2019). *Understanding growth and development patterns of infants*. https://www.pubs.ext.vt.edu/350/350-055/350-055.html

Safe Kids Worldwide. (2023a). *Fall prevention for little kids*. https://www.safekids.org/safetytips/field_age/little-kids-1–4-years/field_risks/falls

Safe Kids Worldwide. (2023b). *Medication safety*. https://www.safekids.org/medicinesafety

Stanhope, M., & Lancaster, J. (2020). *Public health nursing: population-centered health care in the community* (10th ed.). St. Louis, MO: Mosby Elsevier.

Sue, D. W., Sue, D., Neville, H. A., & Smith, L. (2019). *Counseling the culturally diverse: Theory and Practice* (8th ed.). Hoboken, NJ: John Wilen & Sons.

University of Vermont Health Network. (2022). *Air travel with children: how to use car seats on airplanes*. https://www.uvmhealth.org/healthsource/air-travel-children-how-use-car-seats-airplanes#:~:text=The%20Federal%20Aviation%20Administration%20(FAA,from%20being%20injured%2C%20or%20worse

US Agency for International Development [USAID]. (2023). *Promoting gender equality and women's empowerment*. https://www.un.org/sustainabledevelopment/gender-equality/

US Department of Agriculture [USDA]. (n.d.). *USDA MyPlate: Infants*. https://www.myplate.gov/life-stages/infants

US Department of Agriculture [USDA]. (2019). *Infant nutrition and feeding*. https://wicworks.fns.usda.gov/sites/default/files/media/document/infant-feeding-guide.pdf

US Department of Health and Human Services [USDHHS]. (2023). *Healthy People 2030 objectives*. https://health.gov/healthypeople

US Department of Labor. (2024). *FLSA protections to pump at work*. https://www.dol.gov/agencies/whd/pump-at-work

Vijayan, V., Naeem, F., & Veesenmeyer, A. F. (2021). Management of infants born to mothers with HIV infection. *American Family Physician*, *104*(1), 58–62. https://www.aafp.org/pubs/afp/issues/2021/0700/p58.html

Webster, S., Morris, G., & Kevelighan, E. (2018). *Essential human development*. Hoboken, NJ: John Wiley & Sons.

World Health Organization [WHO]. (2023a). *Food additives*. https://www.who.int/en/news-room/fact-sheets/detail/food-additives

World Health Organization [WHO]. (2023b). *What is the WHO definition of health?* https://www.who.int/about/frequently-asked-questions

World Health Organization [WHO]. (2023c). *Child maltreatment (child abuse)*. https://www.who.int/violence_injury_prevention/violence/child/en/

World Health Organization [WHO]. (2023d). *HIV/AIDS*. https://www.who.int/news-room/fact-sheets/detail/hiv-aids

World Health Organization [WHO]. (2023e). *The global strategic directions for strengthening nursing and midwifery*. https://www.who.int

18

Toddler

Diane Marie Welsh and Carol Anne Martin

http://evolve.elsevier.com/Edelman/

OBJECTIVES

After completing this chapter, the reader will be able to:

- Identify key physical growth and developmental and maturational changes that occur during the toddler period.
- Examine the recommended health-promotion and disease-prevention visits for the toddler with the appropriate topics for anticipatory guidance for the parents.
- Compare and contrast developmentally appropriate approaches to toddlers at different ages.
- Analyze the factors that contribute to the heightened vulnerability of toddlers to injury and abuse.
- Develop a plan to reach the Healthy People 2030 target objectives specific to toddlers.

KEY TERMS

Adverse childhood experiences
Amblyopia
Autism spectrum disorders
Autonomy
CDC growth charts
Child abuse
Conditioned-play audiometry
COVID-19
Doubt
Egocentrism
Masturbation
Night terrors
Object permanence
Otitis media
Parallel play
Poisoning
Preoperational stage
Rituals
Sensorimotor stage
Shame
Strabismus
Styes
Temperament
Toilet training
Visual-reinforcement audiometry
World Health Organization growth charts

THINK ABOUT IT

Reframing the Terrible Twos

A young mother tells the nurse that she is convinced her 22-month-old child, who used to have the sweetest disposition, has entered what must be the terrible twos. She reports that her child's favorite words include "mine" and "no," with "no" responses to every request the mother makes. In addition, the child is becoming increasingly stubborn and just threw her first public temper tantrum. The mother says that she is tired of saying and hearing "no" and turns to the nurse for help.

- How does the nurse explain the relationship between the child's stage of psychosocial development and the meaning behind the child's behaviors?
- What suggestions can the nurse provide the mother to help her respond sensitively to her child's evolving need for independence while balancing her own need to provide for and protect her child?

Having spent their first year of life getting to know and trust their parents and other childcare providers and their immediate environment, toddlers' increasing mobility now allows them to begin to expand their worlds, bringing excitement and challenges to themselves and their parents. Toddlers are ready to develop a sense of self and separate from their parents, and understanding and respecting this evolving independence is a common parental challenge. Extensive research conducted by Phillippe Rochat (2021) identified and established a theory surrounding the five stages of self-awareness (Rochat, 2015; Table 18.1). In this theory, Rochat outlined how children learn to identify themselves and the caregivers in their lives as separate, distinct entities. Instilling children's independence from an early age is one of the main keys to success that is useful for children's lives in the future. One way to promote independence is to give children choices. Children who have an independent attitude will find it easier to deal with diversity and social dynamics (Chasani & Izzaty, 2019). Toddlers gain their independence by feeding themselves and playing independently with their toys (Meylia et al., 2020).

Nurses explain to parents and other primary care providers the many physical and developmental changes that occur in toddlers and describe how these changes contribute to children's vulnerability to injury and overall health, as well as to the health and vulnerability of the family unit (Centers for Disease Control [CDC], 2019a).

Unfortunately, the recommended schedule for health-promotion and disease-prevention visits for this age group advocates fewer contacts than during infancy. Parents may begin to fall into a pattern of illness care, missing the continued opportunity to receive anticipatory guidance and health-promotion

TABLE 18.1 Rochat's Layer Theory of Self	
Birth+	Starting state: Differentiating the self from the world via rooting
2 m/0+	Capable of mapping own body space
3 years+	Birth of "Me" extending over time; recognizing self as extending over time rather than a third party
6 years+	Meta-cognitive knowledge: hold multiple representations and perspectives on objects and people

Adapted from Rochat (2021)

information until they are required by preschool or school prerequisites. Health professionals are well positioned to counsel parents to support children's development, identify developmental concerns, identify family and social assets and risks that often affect development, and link families to early intervention and other community resources (Inkelas & Oberjklaid, 2018). The nurse plays an integral role in encouraging health-promotion efforts and behavior (Hockenberry et al., 2024).

BIOLOGY AND GENETICS

Growth Patterns

The toddler period begins at 12 months and extends to 36 months (Hockenberry et al., 2024). According to Chiocca (2019), the assessment of a child's growth and development helps evaluate the child's physical growth and progress toward maturity, provides clues to health conditions that impede physical growth, shows cognitive delays, and may point out abuse or neglect. The overall growth rate slows significantly, and the increasingly active toddler begins the process of shedding baby fat and straightening their posture. Toddlers have a protuberant abdomen and a characteristic gait, in which their feet are planted wide apart and appear flat because of an extra fat pad in the instep for stability.

A slow, steady growth in height of 2 to 4 inches per year and in weight of 4 to 6 pounds per year occurs during toddlerhood, and growth remains steady until puberty. Birth weight usually quadruples by 2.5 years of age, and the toddler's height at age 2 years is approximately 50% of the final adult height (Hockenberry et al., 2024). Growth charts are used to determine the parameters within which an individual toddler's growth lies for head circumference, height, and weight. The CDC recommends that health care providers use the 2022 World Health Organization (WHO) growth charts to monitor growth for infants and children up to 2 years of age in the United States, and then use the 2000 revised CDC growth charts for US children aged 2 to 20 years (CDC, 2022a; American Academy of Pediatrics [AAP] & Healthy Children, 2020). The toddler's height may be measured with the toddler in a recumbent position for length, as in infancy, or in a standing position for stature. When the CDC growth charts for toddlers aged 2 years or older are being used, measure the height with the toddler in a standing position to obtain the toddler's stature, and then use the appropriate chart based on stature.

The nurse continues to measure head circumference throughout the toddler period. The anterior fontanel usually closes by 18 months, the skull begins to thicken, and by 24 months, it is 80% of its adult size (Hockenberry et al., 2024).

Body Systems

The kidneys are well differentiated by the toddler years, and specific gravity and other urine findings are similar to those of adults. The daily excretion of urine for the 2-year-old child is 500 to 600 mL, increasing to 750 mL for the 3-year-old child. Toddlers empty their bladders less frequently than infants and begin to develop voluntary control of urination. However, full bladder control comes later and begins after 18 to 24 months, when the toddler first becomes physiologically able to control the bladder.

The toddler's gastrointestinal tract also reaches functional maturity, although it continues to grow into adulthood. Toddlers tend to need meals and snacks more frequently than an older child or adult. Most toddlers develop sufficient voluntary control of internal and external anal sphincters to accomplish successful bowel training. Bowel control usually occurs before urinary control.

Lung capacity continues to increase as the toddler grows, and the respiratory rate decreases from a mean of 30 breaths per minute at 1 year of age to 25 breaths per minute at 3 years. The diameter of the toddler's upper respiratory tract is small compared with that of an older child or adult, and this may lead to mouth breathing when the nose is obstructed with mucus (Fig. 18.1). This small diameter, coupled with the toddler's exploratory nature and lack of judgment in deciding what to

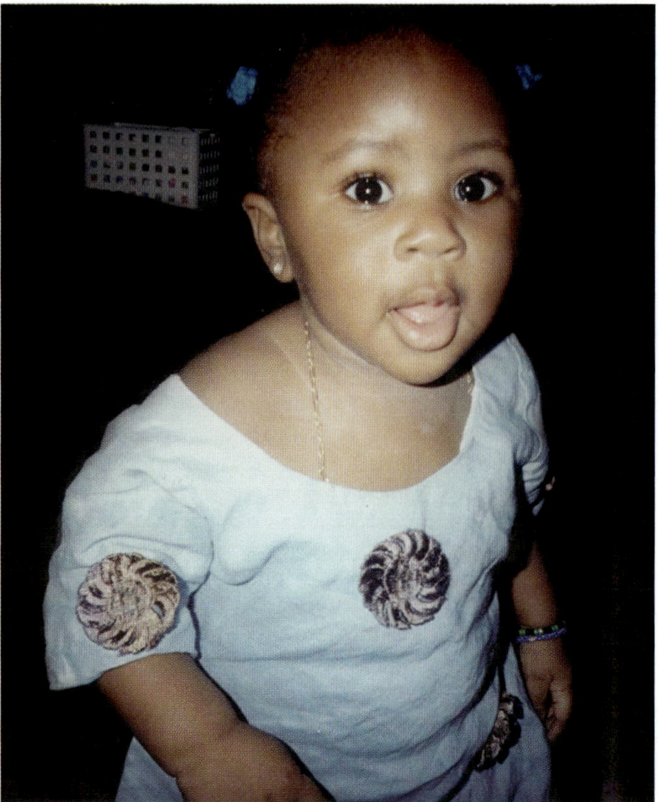

FIG. 18.1 Toddler demonstrates mouth breathing.

place in the mouth, can result in accidental airway obstruction, which demands emergency action. The eustachian tube connects the middle ear with the nasal passages and helps balance air pressure in the middle ear with that in the environment. In older children and adults, the tube is relatively vertical, wide, and rigid, and secretions that pass into it from the nasal passages drain easily (Shah, 2022). The proximal anatomy of the ear, eustachian tube, and nasal pharynx continue to resemble those of the infant more closely than those of the adult, continuing the risk of otitis media. Enlarged tonsils and adenoids in children may result from infections but may be normal. Enlargement usually causes no symptoms but can occasionally cause difficulty breathing or swallowing and sometimes recurring ear or sinus infections or obstructive sleep apnea (Shah, 2022).

With the exception of reproductive functions, most endocrine organs become functionally mature during the toddler and preschool years, although function continues at a minimum. The production of glucagon and insulin can be limited or labile, producing variations in blood glucose levels throughout early childhood. The production of cortisol, aldosterone, and deoxycorticosterone by the adrenal cortex remains somewhat limited, but they appear to function effectively in protecting the young child from the hazards of fluid and electrolyte imbalance well-known in infancy. Secretion of epinephrine and norepinephrine from the adrenal medulla increases sufficiently to perform homeostatic functions of the autonomic nervous system and to mediate certain aspects of increased emotional components of behavior. Regulation of growth during early childhood remains one of the most important functions of the endocrine system.

Changes in the circulatory system include a decrease in heart rate, an increase in blood pressure, and a change in vascular resistance in response to growth in the size of various blood vessel lumens. The toddler's heart rate ranges from 80 to 120 beats per minute, and the mean blood pressure is 90/56 mm Hg. Getting the toddler to sit still for blood pressure reading can be difficult, but it is worth the effort to obtain several baseline readings for future reference.

The capillary beds gradually increase their capacity to respond to heat and cold in the environment, providing the toddler with more effective thermoregulation. Toddlers can also begin to take voluntary measures to relieve the discomfort of heat or cold. For example, the older toddler can put on clothing or move to warmer or cooler areas, assisting physiologic efforts to maintain a constant internal thermal environment.

The immune response continues to mature (Pai et al., 2018). As toddlers expand their worlds through play groups and day care centers, exposure to new and different organisms is greatly increased. They may experience a period during which they appear to succumb to many minor respiratory tract and gastrointestinal tract infections. As immunity begins to develop against the organisms in their new environments, their resistance similarly increases.

Passive immunity to communicable disease acquired through transfer of maternal antibodies during fetal life has disappeared, and active immunity through the initial immunization series is usually completed by the age of 18 months. The next scheduled immunizations do not occur until age 4 to 6 years, before the toddler enters kindergarten. If a toddler is behind in the initial immunization series, a separate schedule is available that provides a catch-up schedule and minimal intervals between doses (CDC, 2019b, 2023a). For updated CDC immunization schedules and the latest guidance, refer to the CDC website at http://www.cdc.gov/vaccines/schedules/.

All 20 primary or deciduous teeth (Fig. 18.2) erupt by the end of toddlerhood (US Preventive Services Task Force [USPSTF], 2021). The timing of these eruptions can differ widely,

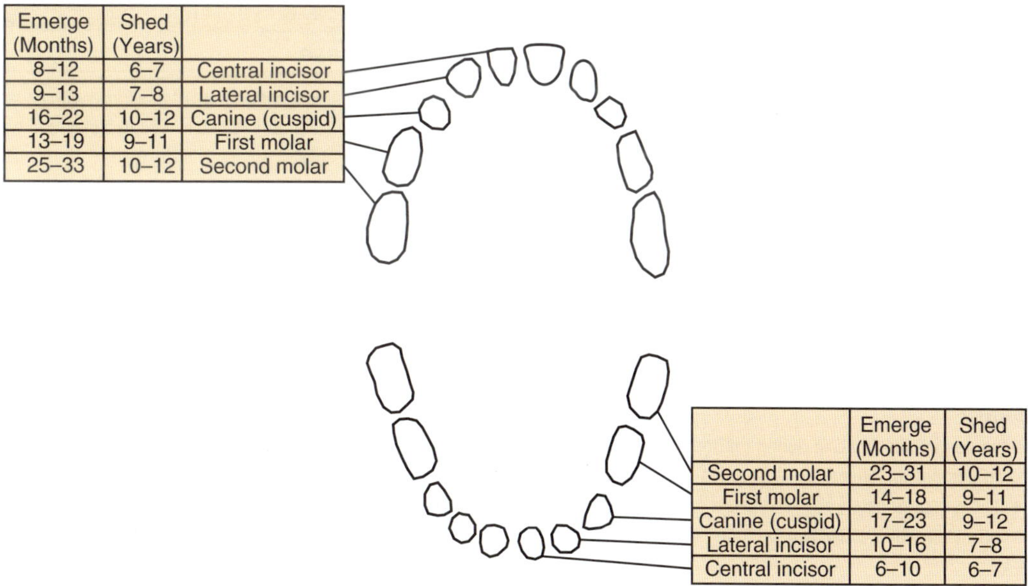

FIG. 18.2 Eruption (and shedding) of primary teeth.

but a variation in the sequence alerts the nurse to inquire about early trauma to the mouth or familial traits for nonsequential tooth eruption. Application of fluoride varnish to primary teeth is recommended shortly after the teeth erupt through the gum. The important aspects of dental care at this age are included in health teaching and are listed in Box 18.1: Nursing Interventions to Promote Dental Health Care for Toddlers (USPSTF, 2021).

A mature swallowing pattern using the tongue rather than the cheeks has not yet developed, and toddlers continue to be at risk of choking. Toddlers who are mouth breathers rather than nose breathers because of ongoing respiratory illness or allergies may have an underdeveloped palatal arch. With normal breathing, the tongue rests on and naturally widens the palate; however, when the child is forced to breathe through the mouth, the tongue rests in the lower jaw, not on the palate. This resultant narrowing of the palatal arch predisposes these toddlers to dental crowding when the permanent teeth erupt (Guilleminault et al., 2019). During sleep, a child should be able to manipulate their tongue by the age of 3 to decrease their chances of sleep apnea later in life. Children should be able to perform requested tongue maneuvers and have oral form recognition (Guilleminault et al., 2019).

An increase in the size and strength of muscle fibers continues. During toddlerhood, as in infancy, the use of muscle tissues is the primary stimulus for increased size and strength necessary for gross and later fine motor movement. Myelination of the corticospinal tract is functionally sufficient to support most movement, but achievement of full control does not occur until much later in life. Throughout early childhood, voluntary motor movement is often accompanied by involuntary movements on the opposite side of the body. This mirroring of action is more pronounced in children who have some damage to the central nervous system, but the mechanisms by which this occurs are unknown. Usually, the toddler does not show complete dominance of one side of the body and may still switch hands when eating, throwing a ball, or engaging in other-handed activities.

Genes are passed from each parent to the child, and great similarities may show between the generations. Most genetic syndromes and disease entities are diagnosed either during the prenatal period or during infancy. However, some genetic syndromes and diseases are not detected until the toddler years or even later. The most common initial sign is either a change in growth pattern or developmental delays. As an example, celiac disease may develop any time after wheat or other gluten-containing foods are introduced into the diet, typically after 6 to 9 months of age (Box 18.2: Genomics; Celiac Disease Foundation [CDF], 2018).

Developmental delays are often not diagnosed during infancy because subtle language, motor, or cognitive deficiencies do not interfere with the expected performance and behavior of the infant as they do with those of the more actively developing toddler.

BOX 18.1 Nursing Interventions to Promote Dental Health Care for Toddlers

Brushing

- When teeth are present, begin to use a soft-bristled brush. The finger-wrapped gauze method used during infancy is no longer adequate because the teeth are too close together to reach all tooth surfaces.
- Introduce only a moist toothbrush at first. After the toddler has accepted the toothbrush, begin using toothpaste. A pea-sized amount is adequate. If the child does not like the taste of the toothpaste, use plain water.
- Toothpaste should contain supplemental fluoride if not in water supply. The US Preventive Services Task Force (2021) recommends that primary care clinicians prescribe oral fluoride supplementation starting at age 6 months if the water supply is not fluoridated.
- Toddlers do not have the motor coordination to brush their own teeth. They may enjoy imitating parents and putting the toothbrush in their mouths, but an adult should be responsible for the actual brushing.
- Brush daily; for many toddlers, this practice becomes part of the bedtime routine. If the child appears too tired to cooperate in the evening, the parent should choose some other time of day when this important task will not be so difficult.

Foods

- Limit intake of foods high in sugar because they contribute to dental caries.
- When the young toddler still drinks from a bottle, only plain water should be given. Milk and juices should be offered by cup. If milk or juice is given in a bottle, this should never be done at naptime or bedtime.

Visits to the Dentist

- The first visit to the dentist should occur during the toddler years. Many dentists suggest an introduction-orientation, inspection-consultation type of visit when the child is approximately 18 to 24 months of age. This type of visit provides an early, enjoyable introduction to professional dental health promotion and care.
- Once the primary teeth of infants and children have erupted, the US Preventive Services Task Force (2021) recommends the application of fluoride varnish to the primary teeth.

BOX 18.2 GENOMICS

Celiac Disease

- Immune-mediated disorder that affects those with genetic susceptibility to it. When gluten (a protein found in wheat, barley, and rye) is consumed, the individual gets sick.
- Infants and toddlers tend to have more obvious symptoms, which usually manifest in the gastrointestinal tract. Symptoms include, but are not limited to vomiting, bloating, irritability, poor growth, abdominal distention, diarrhea with very foul stools, and malnutrition.
- Affects 0.6% to 1.0% of the population worldwide, with prevalence differing regionally for unknown reasons.
- Certain genes are seen in individuals with celiac disease. Although not causal, it appears that *HLA-DQ2* and *HLA-DQ8* haplotypes are largely expressed in individuals with celiac disease.
- For disease diagnosis, serologic testing of antibodies IgA and IgE is performed. Further testing involves biopsies of the intestines, which measures expression of haplotypes *HLA-DQ2* and *HLA-DQ3*.
- Treatment for children with celiac disease is a completely gluten-free diet. As a result of the recent increased awareness around gluten allergies, there are more gluten-free food choices available at the grocery store.

Ig, Immunoglobulin.
For more information on celiac disease, visit http://www.celiac.org.

GORDON'S FUNCTIONAL HEALTH PATTERNS

Health Perception–Health Management Pattern

Toddlers may eventually learn that being sick means feeling bad or having to stay in bed, but they have little, if any, understanding of the meaning of health. They may perform requested health-promotion activities, such as brushing teeth, but they may simply brush their teeth as part of their bedtime ritual and not because they know this activity will prevent dental caries. Toddlers depend on their parents for health management, and their overall health will be greatly influenced by their parents' health perceptions and health-management priorities (Box 18.3: Healthy People 2030).

Toddlers identify with parents, caregivers, and other important role models, internalizing a wide range of lifestyle attributes. Parents' and caregivers' health perceptions and health behaviors should model the perceptions and behaviors desired for health promotion. Toddlers whose parents eat a variety of foods are more likely to try new foods. Such modeling increases the likelihood that good practices will be retained throughout the toddler's life. The nurse's task is to help parents strengthen their confidence and self-esteem as parents and provide them with the information needed to anticipate and meet the developmental needs of their toddler as they develop as a family.

 BOX 18.3 ***HEALTHY PEOPLE 2030***

Selected Health-Promotion and Disease-Prevention Objectives for Toddlers

Symbol	*Healthy People 2030* Objectives
EH-04	Reduce blood lead levels in children aged 1–5 years
EH-09	Reduce exposure to mercury among children 1–5 years, as measured by blood or urine concentrations of the substance or its metabolites
IID-06	Increase the vaccination coverage level of four doses of the DTaP vaccine among children by age 2 years
IID-03	Maintain an effective vaccination coverage level of one dose of MMR vaccine among children by age 2 years
IID-02	Reduce the percentage of children in the United States who receive 0 doses of recommended vaccines by age 2 years
IID-09	Increase the percentage of noninstitutionalized persons aged 6 months and older who are vaccinated annually against seasonal influenza
MICH-18	Increase the proportion of children with ASD enrolled in special services by 48 months of age
MPS-01	Reduce emergency department visits for medication overdoses among children <5 years of age
NWS-16	Reduce iron deficiency among young children aged 1–2 years
RD-02	Reduce emergency department visits for children with asthma under 5 years

ASD, Autism spectrum disorder; *DTaP,* diphtheria-tetanus-acellular pertussis; *MMR,* measles-mumps-rubella

From Healthy People 2030 (http://www.healthypeople.gov); US Department of Health and Human Services, Office of Disease Prevention and Health Promotion (https://health.gov/healthypeople/objectives-and-data/browse-objectives)

Nutritional-Metabolic Pattern

For the best health outcomes, the AAP (2022a) recommends exclusive breastfeeding for approximately 6 months followed by continued breastfeeding with complementary foods for at least 2 years and beyond as mutually desired. Adequate iron intake must be ensured as the toddler changes from breast milk or iron-fortified formula and cereal to whole cow's milk, which is low in iron. Whole cow's milk also interferes with the absorption of iron from other food sources. A toddler who continues to ingest whole milk from a bottle tends to drink up to 32 ounces per day. This practice blunts the child's appetite at mealtimes and can lead to an exclusion of foods that contain iron in the diet, particularly during the first 12 months of life (AAP, 2019), requiring iron from fortified foods or supplements. Cow's milk is a key component of a child's diet. Although the consumption of even trace amounts of cow's milk can result in allergy to its proteins and/or hypolactasia, excessive cow's milk consumption can result in numerous health complications, including iron deficiency, due to the diet being improperly balanced (Graczykowska et al., 2021). The AAP recommends that children stay on whole milk until they are 2 years of age, unless there is a reason to switch to low-fat milk sooner (AAP, 2022b).

Fruit juice and other drinks are often overconsumed because they taste good, are conveniently packaged, are easily carried around by the toddler, and most are viewed as nutritious. Most toddlers consume a sweet snack, a sugar-sweetened beverage or dessert daily, and one-third consume salty snacks. However, the AAP (2019) cautions parents to limit all juice consumption and that children aged 1 to 3 years should have a maximum of 4 ounces daily. It further states excessive consumption of juices may be associated with malnutrition, diarrhea, and tooth decay. Fruit juice has no nutritional advantage as compared with fruit and lacks the fiber contained in whole fruit (CDC, 2023b; AAP, 2019).

A decrease in the growth rate during toddlerhood results in a decrease in appetite. Parents need to be reminded of this if they begin to worry about their toddler's nutritional intake (AAP, 2022b; Healthy Children, 2022). A daily record kept over a 3- to 5-day period presents a better picture of a child's intake and is a useful teaching tool for this age group. The combination of diet, exercise, and physiologic and psychological factors are important factors in the control and prevention of childhood obesity. Primary prevention methods should be aimed at educating the child and family about appropriate diet and exercise from a young age through adulthood while secondary prevention should be targeted at lessening the effect of childhood obesity by preventing the child from continuing unhealthy habits and obesity into adulthood (Sanyaolu et al., 2019). In addition to main meals, snacks provide important nutrients for toddlers and a further opportunity to develop preferences for nutritious foods. As a result, experts recommend serving fruits or vegetables at most snacking occasions while avoiding highly processed foods, including salty snacks and snacks with added sugar (Harris et al., 2023).

Toddlers use mealtimes as an occasion to assert individuality and control as well as exploration. Families will differ in their expectations of eating behavior and mealtime routines. The nurse's

BOX 18.4 Nursing Actions to Promote Healthy Eating in Toddlers

- Recognize that routines are important to toddlers. Serve scheduled meals and snacks. Parents are responsible for what, when, and where the toddler eats. The toddler decides whether to eat and how much.
- Schedule meals and sleep periods such that the child is awake and alert during mealtime.
- Turn off the television. Mealtimes should be a relaxed and pleasant time, free of distractions.
- Serve small portions and let your toddler ask for more.
- Offer simple, single foods because mixtures of foods are often rejected.
- Serve your toddler's favorite foods along with new ones. Several introductions may be necessary before the toddler accepts a new food. Make sure you eat it too.
- Encourage the use of utensils but accept that toddlers still often need to use their fingers.
- Do not use food to bribe, reward, or punish your toddler.
- Avoid foods that may cause choking, such as hard candy, mini marshmallows, popcorn, pretzels, chips, spoonfuls of peanut butter, nuts, seeds, large chunks of meat, hot dogs, raw carrots, dried fruits, and whole grapes.
- Recognize that drinking more than 24 ounces of milk per day can reduce your child's appetite for other healthy foods. For those younger than 2 years, do not use reduced-fat, low-fat, or fat-free (skim) milk because children younger than 2 years need the extra fat for their developing nervous systems.

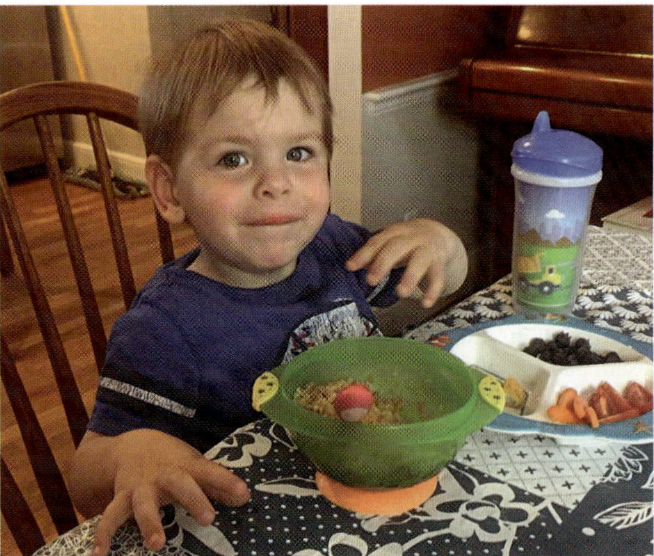

FIG. 18.3 Toddlers need healthy, age-appropriate food choices.

best guide for parents of toddlers is to remind them that parents are in charge of what food is offered, when it is offered, and where it is offered (Nuzzi et al., 2022; Shuya et al., 2022). According to various sources (CDC, 2023b; Hodder et al., 2019; Verhage et al., 2018), early childhood represents a critical period for the establishment of dietary habits that track into adulthood (Box 18.4: Promoting Healthy Eating). Interventions to increase consumption of fruit and vegetables in early childhood may therefore be an effective strategy to reduce future disease burden. However, it is up to the toddler to decide the amount to eat. Periodically, a toddler may even refuse a meal altogether. Parents need to be encouraged to offer healthy, age-appropriate food choices (Fig. 18.3). Toddlers will eat them, if they do not fill up on empty calories from juice and high-carbohydrate snacks that are often given to children "so they eat something." Furthermore, parents should not focus too much attention on food intake or punish children for refusing food. Toddlers may learn how easily parents can be controlled by their behavior around food intake and may then continue the behavior for the attention alone.

Maintaining a record of food intake over time, the nurse can demonstrate the adequacy of the nutrients that the toddler is already receiving during mealtimes. Nurses can help parents develop a plan to offer more of the essential foods during meals, which can play a role in reducing childhood obesity (Verhage et al., 2018). Children with inadequate nutrition are predisposed to impaired immune systems, leading to infections and delayed healing and recovery. They are also predisposed to depletion of muscle mass, leading to diminished functional capacity (Box 18.5). According to Cohen et al. (2021), nutrition is critical in supporting healthy brain development early in life, with long-lasting and often irreversible effects on an individual's cognitive development and life-long mental health. Cohen et al. (2021) reviewed recent human and preclinical evidence on the role of nutrition, with particular focus on newly discovered nutrients, in neurocognitive development in healthy infants and children aged 0 to 59 months. In addition, although this is inadequately understood, nutrients and neurotropic factors interact with one another for brain and behavioral development (Cohen et al., 2021).

BOX 18.5 EVIDENCE-BASED PRACTICE

Asthma, Diet, and Toddlers—A Cure?

There is observational evidence that Mediterranean diet exposure, assessed through the Mediterranean diet index, is associated with a lower prevalence of asthma in children. One possible explanation for the observed beneficial effects is that the Mediterranean diet is characterized by low consumption of red meat and saturated fat and a high intake of fruits, vegetables, whole grains, legumes, fish, and olive oil, which are rich in antioxidants, micronutrients, and vitamin D. These compounds limit the inflammatory response in the airways, thereby possibly reducing the risk of asthma (Nuzzi et al., 2022). Conversely, the Western dietary pattern, characterized by increased consumption of foods rich in AGEs, that is, meats and saturated fats, may promote activation of the toll-like receptor pathway and NF-κB inflammatory cascade, thereby contributing to airway inflammation and asthma pathogenesis. Indeed, higher meat consumption and increased AGE intake are associated with childhood wheezing. A recent cohort study demonstrated that a proinflammatory diet is associated with increased wheezing in atopic children. These findings support the epidemiological association between fast food consumption and the increasing prevalence of asthma but are in contrast with the results of the Dutch research study, where an association between a healthy dietary pattern in early life and a lower risk of childhood asthma was not found (Nuzzi, et al, 2022).

AGE, Advanced glycation end product; *NF-κB*, nuclear factor kappa-light-chain-enhancer of activated B cells

The family who has a vegetarian or vegan diet may need some assistance from the nurse or a dietitian to assess a child's intake of vitamins and other nutrients (Nuzzi et al., 2022).

Food Allergies

Approximately 5% of children under the age of 5 years have food allergies. From 1997 to 2007, the prevalence of reported food allergies increased 18% among children under the age of 18 years. Although most children "outgrow" their allergies, allergy to peanuts, tree nuts, fish, and shellfish may be lifelong (John Hopkins Medicine, n.d.). The exact reason for this phenomenon is unclear (Mathias et al., 2019). Despite lack of clear evidence for why allergies are developing in infants, there are some allergies that are common enough that health care providers should be aware of them, including peanut and other tree nut allergies, gluten, eggs, milk, fish, and soy (Renz et al., 2018; Samady et al., 2020). Food allergies present differently in each person; thus, it is important to ensure that parents know frequent allergy symptoms to monitor in their child. Food allergy symptoms can include gastrointestinal distress like vomiting or diarrhea, hives, itching, swelling, tightness of the throat, and wheezing (Stanford Medicine, Childrens Health, n.d.). Although early recognition of signs and symptoms by parents is important, being able to act quickly and administer epinephrine within the first few minutes of a reaction is more lifesaving. Upon diagnosis of anaphylaxis, physicians often prescribe epinephrine injection (Rahman et al., 2022). The pediatric EpiPen dose is fixed and depends on the weight of the child, which makes it easier to use: EpiPen Junior Auto-Injector 0.15 mg is for children 15 to 30 kg and the EpiPen Regular Auto-Injector 0.3 mg is for children 30 kg or more. According to DiGrazia & Anstrom (2023), parents should be advised to seek emergency services immediately should symptoms develop after their infant or toddler tries new food.

Elimination Pattern

Toilet training is often a major parental concern during toddlerhood. The nurse anticipates this developmental stressor and initiates discussion with the parents to determine their understanding of the child's signs of developmental readiness and their attitude and commitment to establishing a toileting pattern for their toddler. Emotional and physiologic readiness for toilet training rarely develops before 18 months of age. Parents who begin before their child is ready usually experience frustration. Most healthy children are ready to begin toilet training between 18 to 24 months due to the ability to gain physical control of the bladder and bowel sphincters. Healthy children acquire toilet training without the need for medical intervention. During frequent health visits in the first year of life, the pediatric nurse can assess the child's temperament, the family's coping ability, and the child-rearing technique, so they can give individual guidance about toilet training techniques for each child and family (Boyraz et al., 2018).

Nursing Interventions for Elimination Pattern

By suggesting the sequence in Box 18.6: Initiating a Toileting Program, the nurse assists parents with toilet training. The parent who can approach toilet training with a relaxed attitude, accepting some delays and frustrations, will have a better chance of success and a more positive outcome for the toddler.

BOX 18.6 Initiating a Toileting Program for Toddlers

Interest in and awareness of bowel and urinary elimination usually begin by 18 months of age.

- Before beginning toilet training, parents should check their toddlers for the prerequisite skills, which include being able to walk well, stoop and recover, stay dry for at least 2 hours during the day, and communicate sensation before elimination, as well as the discomfort of wet or messy pants and the need for assistance.
- When these prerequisites are present, introduce the child to a potty seat or chair. The potty chair should provide secure seating with the child's feet touching the floor. The potty seat should be used with a small step stool to create the same effect.
- Because of the gastrocolic reflex, bowel elimination is more likely after a meal, so this is a good time to place the toddler on the potty. When a pattern of bowel or urinary elimination is noticed, use this pattern as a guide for placing the child on the potty.
- The toddler should be encouraged to stay on the chair for 2 to 3 minutes and always explain what to do ("Go potty") rather than what not to do ("Don't wet your pants"). Do not refer to elimination as dirty or yucky. Remember this is your child's first creation.
- The child should be praised for desired behavior. Introduce underwear as a badge of success. Ignore undesired behavior and never punish the child by scolding the child, spanking the child, or other punitive measures.

Remember that daytime dryness is usually achieved by 3 years of age and ahead of nighttime dryness, where the need to wear a diaper remains.

Activity-Exercise Pattern

Toddlers are always busy—emptying wastebaskets and drawers; building and destroying towers; throwing, kicking, and chasing after balls; or dressing and undressing. Many of their activities are repeated over and over, providing practice opportunities for their newly realized skills. The various toys designed for toddlers capitalize on this ability to explore and imagine with laptop trainers, electronic coloring tablets, musical instruments, and books with accompanying audiovisual disks.

During the toddler period, children will advance from taking their first step to running, climbing stairs, and even pedaling a tricycle. They enjoy pushing and pulling, whether it is an unsuspecting laundry basket or a push-pull toy made for the job. They scribble spontaneously, usually with vigor, and will emerge from toddlerhood capable of copying a circle and creating tadpolelike figures. They learn to use a spoon and a fork with fairly good success and to wash their hands. They also advance from being dressed by others to dressing themselves with assistance, although at times they resist it.

Toddlers spend most of their waking hours at play—exploring their expanding environment, imitating others' actions, and creating a safety net of **rituals** around the routines of eating, sleeping, and everything in between. In their enthusiasm to try many activities, toddlers invariably take on tasks that are beyond their abilities, which can result in frustration and an occasional well-known temper tantrum. Their exploratory nature and limited but advancing skills also make them vulnerable to injury.

Most toddlers are interested in playing around other children. However, this interest is limited because toddlers, although ready to be with other children, are not ready to share. Successful social encounters with toddlers are best described as "parallel play," where children play side by side, doing similar things with similar toys, but each working independently (Scott & Cogburn, 2023). This playtime with other children helps toddlers develop social skills. Playing has a very important role in children's lives. It contributes to the development of cognitive, motor, and psychosocial, emotional, and linguistic skills. It also has a key role in raising self-confident, creative, and happy children. The profession of the child is the game he plays. Similar to adults' need for their coworkers, children feel a need for their playmates. The skills learned while playing will have an important function for that child throughout life. While playing games, they learn to deal with difficulties, mutual respect, and sharing (Dag et al., 2021).

Nursing Interventions for Activity-Exercise Pattern

When parents inquire about what toys and activities to provide for their toddler, the following are suggested:

- Provide toys that challenge the child to develop new skills: toys that require skills slightly above the child's present level but not so advanced that the child cannot achieve some success.
- Provide opportunities for new learning. This may be as basic as a book with pictures of new animals or a walk through the produce section of the grocery store to point out fruits and vegetables.
- Provide opportunities for social encounters with other children, but do not force playing together. Creating separate yet parallel space, with the use of small mats or hula-hoops as boundaries, is recommended.
- Follow the child's lead. Let the toddler choose and explore new toys or objects, within safe limits.
- Make sure the toy is safe for the toddler and does not have any parts that can be removed and swallowed, does not have lead paint, and cannot cause harm to the curious toddler.

The desire of some parents to raise the smartest, most coordinated, or most musically talented children often begins during the toddler period. It is interaction with parents and others in their environment that provides the advantage in cognitive development. AAP calls for no screen time at all for children until 18 to 24 months, except for video chatting, and states children aged 2 to 5 should get no more than an hour of screen time per day (McHarg et al., 2020). For interactive computer games that may include touch screens (on smartphones and tablets), the parent needs to be there with the toddler so that two-way conversation occurs. Ideally, children should be allowed to explore their interests, with parents responding to their cues. Past research associated television watching by toddlers with interference at a critical time when language development occurs and suggested that this can cause a delay in that process. According to Karani et al. (2022), the influence of screen time is multifactorial and includes both positive and negative influences on children's language development. A majority of the studies analyzed indicate that an increase in the amount of screen time and an early age of onset of viewing have negative effects on language development, especially for children under the age of 2, with older age of onset of viewing showing some benefits. Research indicates that audible television is loud enough to decrease the child's exposure to discernible adult speech, and decreased child vocalizations lead to delayed speech development. Kirkorian et al. (2019) published findings that revealed an indirect negative effect of background television volume (BTV) on the proportion of time that 12- and 24-month-old children played with toys, which was completely mediated by parents' active engagement in their child's play. According to Salunkhe et al. (2021), the prolonged duration of electronic media for more than 3 hours is associated with speech and language delay in children. Mobile media provides more interaction than passive television viewing, and the risk of speech delay is greater in prolonged television viewing. Hyperactivity (attention-deficit hyperactivity disorder [ADHD]) is seen more in children using electronic media (Salunkhe et al., 2021). Increased screen time at age 1 was associated with developmental delays in communication and problem-solving at ages 2 and 4 years, according to study findings reported in *JAMA Pediatrics* (Takahashi et al., 2023). For more information on helping parents support their toddler's activity, use of technology, and exploration in a safe and educational way, visit the Zero to Three website at http://www.zerotothree.org. Television viewing and computer use are modifiable, highly prevalent, and related to increased body fat because they are often sedentary, making these behaviors a promising intervention target (Zink et al., 2023). By 2030, an estimated 39% of children and 46% of adolescents will be overweight or obese. Other markers of adiposity, such as percent body fat and fat mass index (FMI; defined as fat mass divided by height-squared), are also on the rise (Zink et al., 2023).

Sleep-Rest Pattern

The National Sleep Foundation (NSF) recommends toddlers 1 to 2 years old sleep 11 to 14 hours per 24-hour day. The NSF recommendations do not provide any additional detail on the proportion of sleep that should come from daytime naps compared with nighttime sleep, although most children under 2 years of age partake in daytime naps in addition to sleeping at night (Bucko et al., 2023). One of the naps is usually replaced by quiet time, a brief period to unwind from a busy or noisy activity. Occasionally, the parents or caregivers need these rest breaks as much or more than the toddler. Sitting together in a rocking chair for a soothing song or quiet music or reading side by side or together can be suggested by the nurse.

The toddler may be involved in an activity and not be aware of fatigue, especially when visitors are in the home or some interesting new toys have been discovered. All parents are familiar with the child who is overtired but unable to relax enough to sleep. Parents can potentially avoid this dilemma by scheduling naps and quiet time even when there are houseguests or holidays that preempt the toddler's routine.

Rituals are characteristic of this age, and most toddlers have a nap and bedtime ritual. The following might be a typical pattern: eating a nutritious snack, followed by bathing, brushing teeth, listening to a story, getting a kiss, and having overhead lights turned off and the night light turned on. Following this ritual is important because the toddler gets a sense of security when ending the day. Changing this ritual can be upsetting. The nurse encourages parents to establish and follow the bedtime ritual as closely as possible, even when visitors, family illness, or travel makes the routine more difficult. In addition, incorporate rituals as much as possible when the toddler stays outside the home; for instance, staying overnight at their grandparent's house or during a hospitalization.

Usually, toddlers will try to delay sleep by calling for water, another story, or another kiss, or by making other requests. Parents should be certain that the toddler has ample opportunity for interaction with them during the day, follow the usual bedtime ritual, and be firm and consistent in resisting any requests for attention after the final good nights have been said. Encouraging toddlers to use transition or security objects, such as stuffed animals or blankets, helps them to self-quiet and console themselves both at bedtime and in new situations (Fig. 18.4).

Night terrors may begin in toddlerhood (Boyden et al., 2018). Night terrors are different from nightmares, which usually begin at a later age and result in the child awakening and being able to recall the frightening dream. The child who experiences night terrors does not awaken completely but cries out, looks terrified, and cannot be aroused for several minutes. Eventually, usually after 5 to 10 minutes, the child falls back into a quiet sleep. Parents need to be reassured that these episodes will become less frequent as the child develops. The parents should talk in a soothing voice but should not try to awaken the child. If the child does awaken, the parents should then provide comfort and tuck the child back into bed.

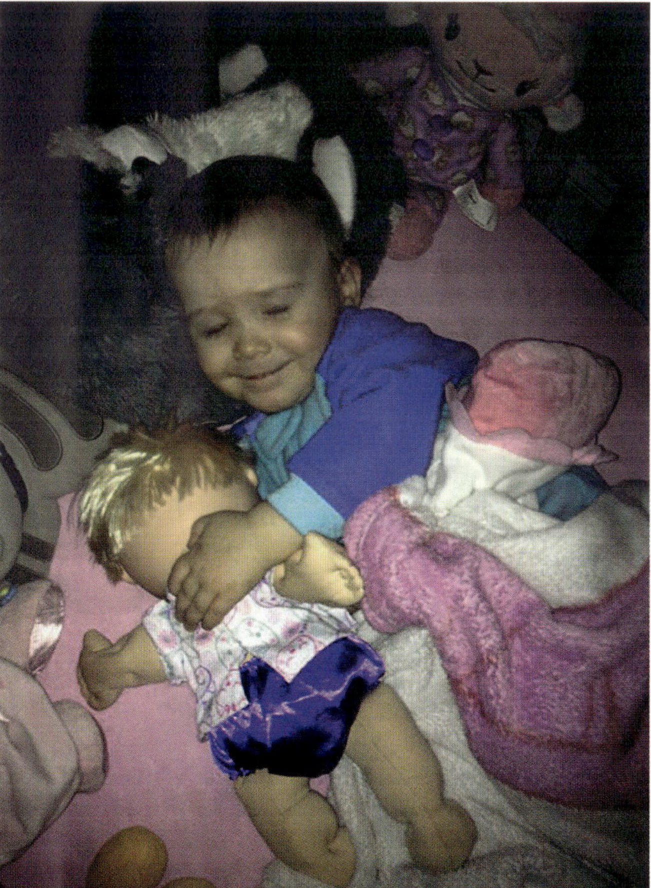

FIG. 18.4 Toddlers need adequate sleep for healthy growth, and their stuffed toys can help them feel more secure.

Cognitive-Perceptual Pattern

Toddlers who experienced the security of a nurturing and reliable source of protection and attachment during infancy have a strong base from which to begin to explore and learn about their expanding world. They begin toddlerhood in Piaget's **sensorimotor stage** of cognitive development and start moving to the **preoperational stage**. Their advancing thought-processing skills and abilities to use the language are heralded by the development of **egocentrism**, an inability to put oneself in another's shoes. Toddlers who come running into a room asking their parents "Where is it?" are confused when parents respond, "Where is what?" They assume their parents and all others share the same thoughts and cannot understand why they do not.

Toddlers interpret and learn about objects and events, not in terms of general properties but in terms of their relationship with them or their use of them. Their thoughts are dominated by what they see, hear, or otherwise experience, and they want to experience everything. Their two- to three-word phrases are most often related to present events, describing an action, a desire, or a possession (e.g., "Mommy, me up!").

Both receptive and expressive language skills are developing rapidly in toddlers; however, their receptive language skills far outweigh their expressive language ability, and toddlers often use gestures until words are found to represent the meanings already acquired. Toddlers also learn the use of inflection. "Mommy" may mean "Pick me up" on one occasion and "I'm scared" or "Where are you?" on another. Often frustrated by their limited repertoire of expressive language, which usually includes approximately 400 words, young toddlers default to using "no" as a method of gaining control over a situation or expressing themselves (see the Think About It box at the beginning of this chapter).

By age 3 years, children have mastered the basics of language function, form, and content, and these fundamentals will continue to be refined throughout childhood and adolescence (Hockenberry et al., 2024; Rochat, 2021). Table 18.1 outlines the landmarks of speech, language, and hearing ability for this age group. There is extensive research on bilingual home environments. According to Grosjean (2021), half of the world's population uses two or more languages. In the United States, more than 67 million people speak a language other than English at home according to the 2018 American Community Survey (ACS) from the Census Bureau. English-Spanish bilinguals represent 61% of all bilinguals in the United States, making Spanish the second-most frequently spoken language in the country (Grosjean, 2021). Research findings by Gámez et al. (2023) suggest that children's dual language development may depend on their exposure to a diverse set of words, not only the amount of language exposure, as well as warm interactions with caregivers.

Attention span increases in the toddler phase. The capacity to keep out-of-sight objects in mind, the gradual appreciation of **object permanence**, is a key achievement of the sensorimotor stage (DeWolfe, 2023). Many toddlers will sit patiently in front of the washing machine while a favorite blanket is laundered or stare out of a front window awaiting a parent's return. They can inadvertently put themselves in harm's way as they pursue an object or person.

The toddler period is dominated by play, often referred to as "child's work," which is repetitive and ritualistic. When toddlers bounce a ball repeatedly they are not trying to drive their parents crazy. They are trying to learn about balls, and repetition is the best teacher. Toddlers' ritualistic behaviors help them master skills and decrease anxiety, and the addition of a seemingly endless string of questions to these behaviors can test the limits of the most patient parents. These queries, however, must be acknowledged and answered in a manner that not only provides solutions but also validates and reinforces the toddler's burgeoning curiosity. The nurse explains the "terrible twos" by teaching parents and caregivers that toddlers might better be viewed as "young scientists" in need of a safe "laboratory" in which to conduct their trial-and-error research. This period of exploration mirrors the development period of adolescence; however, it is different in that toddlers can be closely monitored compared with adolescents who are often outside of the home and out of proximity to their parents.

Autism spectrum disorder (ASD) is usually diagnosed between the ages of 18 and 24 months, and over the years there has been an increase in its prevalence. The global number of old and new cases of ASD has increased from 0.62% in 2012 to 1.0% in 2021 (Okoye et al., 2023). ASDs are defined as pervasive developmental disorders with onset in infancy or childhood and characterized by impaired social interactions, impaired communications, significantly restricted activities and interests, and difficulties with sleep behaviors (Healthy Children, 2023; Reynolds et al., 2019). There is no known cause. The current prevalence is 1 in every 59 American children (CDC, 2018). There is not a single treatment that works for all children with autism; however, there are many options available, including applied behavior analysis. This involves the principle that positive reinforcement increases the frequency of the desired behavior. It is best to implement treatment early in the child's development. See http://www.autismsociety.org and http://www.myautism.org for more information.

Hearing

The ability to hear and listen to others is critical for speech and language development. Listening includes attending to what is heard, discriminating among the various qualities of sound, cognitively associating what is heard with previously learned experiences, and remembering what is heard. During the first 3 years of life, as the brain undergoes dramatic growth, children begin to develop speech and language. Hallmarks of this progression are seen when children reach developmental milestones, forming the foundation of language (Del Tufo et al., 2019). Expressive language milestones, such as the production of a child's first word, are delayed in 5% to 8% of children. Although delays in reaching these milestones are harbingers of developmental disorders for some children, for others expressive language delays appear to be resolved. Toddlers often seek repetition of auditory input, as observed in their seemingly endless repetition of sounds, words, and combinations of words. Young children are likely to have evolving abilities to exploit word repetition and continuity of reference as they learn new information from the environment, and individual differences in this evolution are likely to depend on the specifics of caregivers' naturalistic use of discourse cues in the home. This repetition is their way of practicing and organizing new language (Schwab & Lew-Williams, 2020; Slomian et al., 2019; Table 18.2).

Approximately 1.3 million American children under the age of 3 have hearing loss. Even temporary or treatable forms of hearing loss, such as fluid in the ears, can cause speech delays if they are experienced by a child who is learning to understand language and to speak. Impaired social skills may also occur in children with hearing loss. Additionally, many children with hearing loss experience difficulty in areas of academic achievement (Hayes & Carew, 2019). Health care providers need to continue to monitor, screen, and refer children for formal audiologic evaluation if they develop signs of identified risk factors for hearing loss. The timing and number of hearing reevaluations for children with risk factors should be individualized. Infants who pass the neonatal screening but have a risk factor should have at least one diagnostic audiology assessment by 24 to 30 months of age (AAP, 2018a). Early and more frequent assessment may be indicated for children with cytomegalovirus infection, syndromes associated with progressive hearing loss, neurodegenerative disorders, head trauma, or culture-positive postnatal infections associated with sensorineural hearing loss (e.g., herpes viruses); for toddlers who spent more than 5 days in a neonatal intensive care unit at birth or who received extracorporeal membrane oxygenation, exchange transfusions, or chemotherapy; and for toddlers where there is a family history of hearing loss (Subbiah et al., 2018).

Younger toddlers are screened with the use of **visual-reinforcement audiometry**, in which stimulus tones and visually animated reinforcers (e.g., a lighted toy) are paired and presented together. After the toddler has been conditioned to expect this relationship, the visual reinforcer is withheld, and the sound is presented alone. The toddler looks for the visual reinforcer in response to the sound, and the visual reinforcer is then presented as a reward. **Conditioned-play audiometry** is used for older toddlers and preschool children. The child is first taught to play listening games, using blocks or rings. The child learns to wait and listen for a sound and then performs a motor task (e.g., places a block, a bucket, or a ring on a stacking stick) in response. The motor task is followed by social reinforcement. Noncalibrated toys or noisemakers and signals that lack frequency specificity are inappropriate screening methods and should be used only as gross indicators for monitoring.

Otitis media, or middle ear infection, is one of the leading causes of visits to health care providers during the toddler years and the primary reason for which antibiotics are prescribed for these children. Discussing the current literature and evidence-based reports and recommendations often helps parents understand the proper use of antibiotics, which is also imperative in preventing antibiotic resistance. When it is deemed necessary to use an antibiotic, nurses teach how to administer the medication safely and stress the importance of taking the medication at the prescribed time and for the full duration of the course,

TABLE 18.2 Growth and Development Landmarks of Speech, Language, and Hearing Ability During the Toddler Period

Age (Months)	Receptive Language	Expressive Language	Related Hearing Ability
18	Up to 50 words; recognizes between 6 and 12 objects by name, such as "dog," "cat," "bottle," "ball"; identifies three body parts, such as eyes, nose, mouth; understands simple, one-step commands such as "give me the doll," "open your mouth," "stick out your tongue"	Up to 20 words; jargon and echolalia are present; uses names of familiar objects and one-word sentences, such as "go" or "eat"; uses gestures; uses words such as "no," "mine," "eat," "good," "bad," "hot," "cold" and expressions such as "oh-oh," "what's that," "all gone"; use of words can be quite inconsistent; 25% of speech intelligible	Has begun to develop gross discrimination by learning to distinguish between highly dissimilar noises, such as doorbell and train, barking dog and automobile horn, and mother's and father's voices
24	Up to 1200 words; knows "in," "on," "under"; identifies dog, ball, engine, bed, doll, scissors, hair, mouth, feet, nose, cup, spoon, car, key; distinguishes between one and many and formulates a negative judgment (a knife is not a fork); understands simple stories; follows simple, two-step directions; is beginning to make distinctions between you and me	Up to 270 words; jargon and echolalia almost gone; average 75 words per hour during free play; talks in words, phrases, and two- to three-word sentences; averages two words per response; first pronouns appear, such as "I," "me," "mine," "it," "who," "that"; adjectives and adverbs are only beginning to appear; names objects and common pictures; refers to self by name, such as "Katrina go bye-bye"; uses phrases such as "I want," "go bye-bye," "want cookie," "ball all gone"; 60% of speech intelligible	Refinement of gross discriminative skills
30	Up to 2400 words; identifies action in pictures and objects by use; carries out one- and two-part commands, such as "pick up your shoe and give it to mommy"; knows what is used to drink liquids, what goes on the feet, what is used to buy candy; understands plurals, questions, difference between young male and young female; the concepts one, up, down, run, walk, throw, fast, more, my	Uses up to 425 words; jargon and echolalia no longer exist; averages 140 words per hour; knows words such as "chair," "can," "box," "key," "door"; repeats two digits from memory; average sentence length is approximately 2.5 words; uses more adjectives and adverbs; demands repetition from others, such as "do it again"; nearly always announces intentions before actions; begins to ask questions of adults; 75% of speech intelligible	—
36	Up to 3600 words; understands "both," "two," "not today;" what to do when thirsty (hungry, sleepy); why people have stoves; understands "wait," "later," "big," "new," "different," "strong," "today," "another," and taking turns at play; carries out two-item and some three-item commands, such as "give me the ball," "pick up the doll," and "sit down"; identifies several colors; is aware of past and future	Up to 900 words in simple sentences, averaging three to four words per sentence; averages 170 words per hour; uses words such as "when," "time," "today," "not today," "new," "different," "big," "strong," "surprise," "secret"; can repeat three digits, name one color, say name, give simple account of experiences, and tell stories that can be understood; begins to use more pronouns, adjectives, and adverbs; describes at least one element of a picture; is aware of past and future; uses commands such as "you make it" and expressions such as "I can't," "I don't want to"; verbalizes toilet needs; expresses desire to take turns; communication includes criticisms, commands, requests, threats, questions, answers; 85% of speech intelligible	Starts to distinguish dissimilar speech sounds, such as the difference between "ee" and "er," although there may be some difficulty with the concepts of same and different

Adapted from Hockenberry et al. (2024)

which is indicated by an empty container of medication and not by the absence of initial symptoms.

Vision

Toddlers' visual acuity is usually approximately 20/40, although gaining their cooperation for screening is often difficult and not recommended unless parents, caregivers, or health care providers identify a concern. Depth perception is still immature, although more developed than in infancy.

Amblyopia is one of the major health care concerns for this age group and occurs in 2 to 3 of every 100 children (National Eye Institute, 2019). It is defined as diminished, or loss of, vision in an eye that has not received adequate use. The eye looks normal, but it is not being used normally. Because the brain favors the other eye, the term "lazy eye" is often used. The most common cause of amblyopia is strabismus, but it may also occur when one eye is more nearsighted, farsighted, or astigmatic than the other. Occasionally, amblyopia is caused by other eye conditions such as cataract.

Amblyopia is preventable and treatable, especially if detected early. The earlier detection of amblyopia will contribute to the greater chance for a complete recovery. The AAP and the American Academy of Ophthalmology strongly recommend that children have their eyes examined at the following times: newborn period, 6 months, 3 years, and before starting school (American Association for Pediatric Ophthalmology and Strabismus [AAPOS], 2022; National Center for Children's Vision and Eye Health at Prevent Blindness, 2020).The USPSTF 2017 guidelines recommend vision screening for children aged 3 to 5 years of age for the purpose of detecting amblyopia or risk factors for amblyopia. Management of amblyopia depends on the cause and may include surgery or paralytic, autonomic, and centrally acting pharmacologic agents. However, no matter what the cause, management will involve making the child use the lazy eye, the eye with reduced vision. There are two ways to accomplish this: use of atropine eye drops or patching the stronger eye (AAPOS, 2022). If glasses are worn with the patch, the nurse will help the parents secure them with the active toddler. Not all children benefit from eye drop treatment for amblyopia. When the stronger eye is nearsighted, the atropine eye drops may not be as effective (AAPOS, 2022; Box 18.7: Best Practice).

Strabismus is a deviation of the line of vision from the midline resulting from extraocular muscle weakness or imbalance and is commonly referred to as "crossed eye." One or both eyes may turn in, out, up, or down, and this can be constant or intermittent. Marked or continuous strabismus is usually noticed early by the parents and health care providers and is therefore treated early; the subtler deviations are often unnoticed until older toddlerhood or the preschool years. Every toddler should be screened for strabismus as part of the routine eye examination that is performed by the physician or nurse practitioner during well-child visits.

Other signs of vision problems that the nurse observes or parents report in their toddlers include the following red flags:

- Rubs eyes excessively
- Shuts or covers one eye, tilts head, or looks sideways to view an object
- Has difficulty or is irritable when doing close work
- Blinks, squints, or frowns when viewing objects
- Holds books close to eyes
- Has red, encrusted, or swollen eyelids
- Has red, inflamed, or watery eyes
- Develops recurring **styes** (swelling at the edge of the eyelid)

> **BOX 18.7 BEST PRACTICE**
>
> ***The Eye Patch Club***
>
> It is estimated that 2% to 5% of all children have amblyopia. Prevent Blindness America created a support group in 2012 called the Eye Patch Club for families coping with a child's amblyopia treatment. The Eye Patch Club News is a newsletter featuring tips and techniques for promoting adherence; stories from and about children whose eyes are patched; and professional advice from optometrists, ophthalmologists, and orthoptists. Each issue also includes a Kid's Page, and there is a classroom guide for teachers with explanations for the classroom, as well as activities for everyone to learn more about their eyes. An Eye Patch Club calendar and stickers that allow children to track their patch-wearing activity, a refrigerator magnet with helpful hints, and pen pal opportunities are also available. For more information on children's eye health and safety, local financial resources for eyecare, or to sign up for The Eye Patch Club, call Prevent Blindness Northern California at (415) 567-7500 or visit www.eyeinfo.org. To learn more about Prevent Blindness America and for resources for parents, visit the website at https://nationalcenter.preventblindness.org/small-steps-for-big-vision/.

Taste and Smell

Toddlers are beginning to take control of their world and have the capacity to taste and smell, new skills that are rapidly used. Toddlers often refuse to even taste something that looks or smells displeasing to them or to eat something that they recall as tasting terrible. They can react accurately to a sensation that a taste or smell arouses in them, and they begin to learn conditioned association between certain smells and culturally acceptable values. Foods and smells found in one family or culture become palatable and accepted, and those that are unacceptable become displeasing. Many of our adult eating habits, food likes and dislikes, and visceral responses to odors have their roots in this period.

Self-Perception–Self-Concept Pattern

According to Erikson (1995, 1998), the developmental task of toddlers is to acquire a sense of **autonomy** while overcoming a sense of **doubt** and **shame**. To exert autonomy, toddlers must relinquish the dependence on others that was enjoyed during infancy. Continued dependency has the potential to create a sense of doubt in toddlers about their ability to take control of, and take responsibility for, their own actions. Toddlers seem to thrive when parents can accommodate their increasing autonomy yet maintain a strong parenting presence that includes a full measure of patience, enough parental self-confidence to set appropriate limits, and the ability to realize that their toddler's negative behavior is not directed at them and their egocentrism is not a reflection on them.

The toddler must explore the world, not only the physical aspects but also the interpersonal aspects of relationships, to develop a true sense of autonomy. Exploring the physical world involves poking into, climbing onto, crawling under, tasting, smelling, and taking apart the objects encountered. The child explores relationships with others by searching for the limits of the child's power: If a "no" or a temper tantrum means control of another person's behavior, the child learns that one's own self is more powerful than the other person's self. The toddler continually practices separateness to develop a sense of autonomy.

This process can be frustrating and confusing for parents. The toddler may say a vehement "no" when offered a drink and then scream and cry when the drink is taken away; the parents may wonder whether the toddler wants the drink. Likely the answer is "yes," but the toddler may also need to express autonomy by refusing it. Occasionally, the same toddler who displays a strong need for autonomy spontaneously cuddles or even clings to a parent. These conflicting desires can be confusing to both the parent and the toddler. The toddler's need for more autonomy may conflict with parental expectations, safety limits, or the rights of other children or adults. Any of these conflicts result in feelings of frustration. A typical toddler response to frustration is the well-known temper tantrum.

Potential Nursing Actions for Self-Perception/Self-Concept Patterns

The nurse assesses the toddler-parent relationship to determine the following:

- How is the toddler expressing the need for autonomy?
- How do the parents perceive these actions?
- How does the toddler respond to frustration in exploring the environment or controlling personal and others' actions?
- How do the parents respond to the toddler's display of frustration?
- What provisions are the parents making to allow safe choices for the toddler?

The nurse's teaching focuses on the aspects that are troublesome for the toddler-parent relationship. The following examples are some general concepts to include:

- Match the environment to the child's needs and abilities. Childproof the home such that the child can explore safely. Provide toys that the child can master. Give opportunities to play with more challenging toys, but do not make these toys the rule.
- Give advance notice of a change in activity, such as lunch or nap time. Use transition rituals and objects.
- Do not offer a choice if there is not one. For example, rather than ask if the toddler wants to take a bath, say "It is time to take a bath, do you want to take it upstairs or downstairs" or "Do you want to start at the face and move down to the toes or start with the toes and wash the face last?" This allows the toddler to be in charge and the task of bathing to be achieved.
- Set and enforce consistent limits such that the toddler will come to develop control within these limits.
- Keep routines simple and consistent to prevent temper tantrums, set reasonable limits and give rationales, avoid "head-on clashes," and provide choices.
- Provide a safe environment for the toddler if temper tantrums occur. Identify the tantrum's cause, and help the toddler regain control. Do not reason, threaten, promise, hit, or concede. Respond consistently and follow through on discipline free of anger. Over-criticizing and restricting the toddler may dampen enthusiasm and increase feelings of shame and doubt.
- Praise the toddler's skills and abilities. Never miss an opportunity to catch your toddler being good. Be positive. Remember to say "yes" occasionally.

Roles-Relationship Pattern

According to Hay et al. (2018), toddler peer relationships are important for children's socialization and set the stage for later social, emotional, and cognitive development. Toddlers' capability for relationships is limited and usually reflects their egocentric approach. Parents and siblings' roles are understood in terms of how those roles relate to the toddler. One family member may be the fixer of toys or the comforter of bruises, another the troublemaker who takes away toys.

Toddlers are interested in everything, and their parents' and siblings' activities and possessions are often imitated and preferred. Frequently, the desire to be like or have something that belongs to a sibling creates sibling rivalry. This happens between toddlers and their older siblings but even more when a new, younger sibling is introduced (Fig. 18.5). A new baby who is

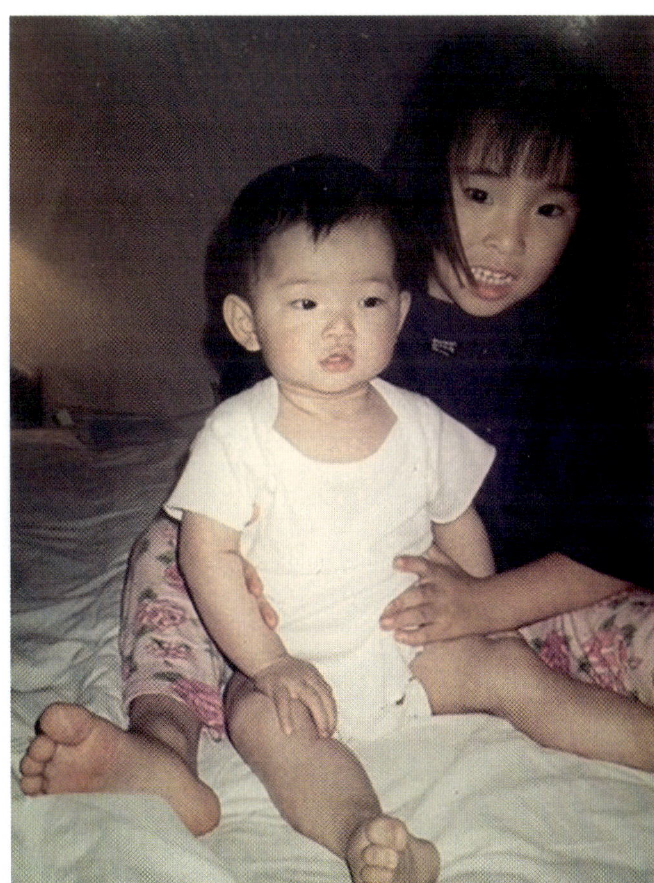

FIG. 18.5 It is a big change for a toddler when a new baby is introduced to the family.

often loud, unable to play, unable to be touched or explored too vigorously, and demands and gets too much parental attention quickly becomes a nuisance to toddlers, who have been known to inform their parents that they can "take the new baby back where it came from now." Realizing the new sibling is here to stay, toddlers often regress, reverting to earlier, previously abandoned infantile behavior such as losing toileting skills, wanting to be fed or dressed, or even communicating by "baby talk." They are usually trying to retain or regain a sense of mastery and, once reassured, will progress. This process is not the end of sibling rivalry but only the beginning of what will assume many forms and require ongoing negotiation from all family members. Parents cannot stop siblings' fighting by forbidding it, but reasonable limits can be established. One way to deescalate fighting is to remove the reward of the fight. The desired outcome in the toddler's mind is to see the self rewarded and the sibling punished. When parents do not reward the toddler or punish the sibling or when they do not take sides, the gain is missing and fighting becomes less satisfactory. This approach does not mean that all fighting will stop, but the child will look for other ways of getting approval.

Child-externalizing behavior problems often emerge during the toddler years and are associated with increased parenting stress. Family stress theory posits that resources (e.g., social support) may buffer the effects of stressors such as child behavior concerns (Schellinger et al., 2020). The quality of the early parent-child relational context has emerged as a particularly important moderator of those paths. Across several studies, broadly ranging measures, correlational and experimental designs, and child ages, the maladaptive sequelae of early child difficulty have been consistently shown to unfold in insecure or suboptimal relationships but not in those that were secure (Kochanska et al., 2019). Parents may also engage in other behaviors, which indirectly influence sibling relationship dynamics, including marital and broader home environment behaviors, which serve as a model for children for use in their own sibling engagement (Milevsky, 2018).

Sibling relationships and parent-child relationships can be difficult subjects for parents to discuss. It was found that the more authoritarian style of parenting that parents demonstrated with their children, the more harmonious sibling relationships were. In an indulgent parenting style, researchers discovered that the score of sibling conflicts was high (Liu & Rahman, 2022). The nurse includes normal family development and role relationships as part of the anticipatory guidance given during the toddler years. Toddlers really begin to show their different emotions at this age. Anger and frustration are two main emotions that toddlers tend to display pretty frequently. They also can be very possessive and become excited over certain objects or people. It is normal to experience temper tantrums at this age because of all these really big emotions that the child does not really know how to express properly yet (Healthy Children, 2022).

Early identification of potential risks to children's health and development is a critical component of an effective early childhood system of care that promotes health equity and mitigates the damaging and lasting effects of poverty, racism, and other stressors experienced during early childhood (Boone et al., 2021).

Adverse childhood experiences (ACEs) are defined as early exposure to maltreatment and household dysfunction. Researchers have demonstrated the link between ACEs and negative psychological, behavioral, interpersonal, and health outcomes (Rowell & Neal-Barnett, 2021). Children exposed to invalidating environments often develop a negative internal working model of their attachment figure that predicts their beliefs about the self and the world. If the internal working model is comprised of an abundance of poor parent-child interactions, the child is likely to have emotion regulation problems, view others as untrustworthy and unavailable, and consider themselves to be unworthy of love and acceptance (Cooke et al., 2019). When parental anger, depression, and parental conflict (Harold & Sellers, 2018) go unchecked, physical and emotional abuse can occur.

Child Abuse

Child physical abuse is an extensive public health problem because of its high prevalence and its associations with adverse health outcomes. There is a great amount of research showing that there are strong enduring effects of physical abuse and other adverse childhood experiences on mental and/or physical health in adulthood (Annerbäck et al., 2018). The effect of child abuse on health cannot be explained by a single cause because health depends on a complex web of different factors. However, these effects are more likely to occur with a major change or turmoil (CDC, 2022c) in the family and when parental role models were abusive. Over the long term, children who are abused or neglected are also at increased risk for experiencing future violence victimization and perpetration, substance abuse, sexually transmitted infections, delayed brain development, lower educational attainment, and limited employment opportunities (CDC, 2022b). The risk for child abuse and neglect perpetration and victimization is influenced by many individual, family, and environmental factors, which interact to increase or decrease risk over time and within specific contexts. According to data from the National Child Abuse and Neglect Data System (NCANDS), the federal database tracking involvement in state child welfare systems for allegations of child abuse or neglect, approximately 4.4 million referrals were screened-in for investigation in fiscal year (FY) 2019 (U.S. Department of Health and Human Services [USDHHS], 2021). Toddlerhood is a time that tries the patience of most parents, and nurses are alert to family changes and stresses as well as to warning signs of abuse (Box 18.8). Many injuries are difficult to differentiate from accidental injury and, at times, may even be confused with culturally appropriate healing practices (Box 18.9: Health and Social Determinants/Health Equity). However, the toddler years have the greatest incidence of child maltreatment, with 27% of nonfatal cases reported for children aged 3 years or younger and 70% of deaths from child maltreatment occurring in children younger than 3 years (CDC, 2019b, 2022b,c). Nonfatal cases appearing in emergency departments, pediatrician offices, and day care centers may be the only opportunity for health care providers to prevent later death from continued child maltreatment.

Typically, parental responses to childhood injuries include a spontaneous reporting of the details of the illness or injury accompanied by concern, questions about progress and

BOX 18.8 Warning Signs of Child Abuse

Any nurse that is working with children under the age of 18 is considered a mandated reporter. This means that it is the law to report possible child abuse or neglect to authorities. This can be done by referring to each state's child abuse department by going to the following website: https://www.childwelfare.gov/.

There are warning signs that can be identified by health care professionals that include the following:

- Parental delay in seeking medical help
- Inconsistencies in the history of how the injury occurred
- Injury inconsistent with the history or the child's developmental capability
- Old, unexplained fractures evident on radiographs
- Repeated dental fractures or head traumas
- Bruises confined to back surface of the body—neck to knees
- Bare spots and broken hair
- Pattern of injury or bruising descriptive of object used to inflict injury (belt or belt buckle, hand, cigarette, hot water)
- Burns with sharply demarcated edges or circumferential patterns
- Perineal injuries of any kind
- Poor hygiene

For more information about recognizing signs of child abuse, visit the Child Welfare Information Gateway at https://www.childwelfare.gov/pubs/usermanuals/childcare/.

BOX 18.9 SOCIAL DETERMINANTS/ HEALTH EQUITY

Evaluating a Child for Child Abuse With Cultural Sensitivity

Nurses are required by law to report cases of suspected child abuse to Child Protective Services. The nurse who takes a careful health history may discover that what might appear to be characteristic burns or bruises associated with child abuse may instead be the product of a traditional culturally appropriate healing practice. The following are two examples of healing practices found in the Pacific Islander and Asian populations that might create such confusion.

Coining (Cao Gio)

Coining is a common healing practice used among Pacific Island and Asian families within the United States. Traditionally, coining is used for conditions associated with "wind" illnesses, as well as a wide variety of febrile illnesses. The lesions seen from coining are produced by rubbing a warm oil or balm on the skin and firmly abrading the skin with a coin or special instrument. The practice produces linear petechiae and ecchymosis on the chest and back that often resemble strap or belt marks. The appearance of the deep red-purple skin color is confirmation that the person had bad wind in the body.

Cupping (Ventouse)

Cupping involves the creation of a vacuum inside a special cup or glass by burning the oxygen out of it and then promptly placing it on a person's skin surface. Cupping draws blood and lymph to the body surface that is under the cup or glass, increasing local circulation. The purpose for doing this is to remove cold and damp "evils" from the body or to assist blood circulation, or both. The procedure is frequently used to treat lung congestion. The resulting circular ecchymoses marks are approximately 2 inches in diameter and resemble nonaccidental trauma.

discharge, difficulty in leaving the child, and an attempt to identify with the child's feelings. These parents may also experience guilt for not protecting the child from the accident and may offer gifts to compensate for these feelings of guilt. In contrast, neglectful or abusive parents are often hesitant to provide information about illness or injury; they may be evasive or even contradict themselves, irritated by the inconvenience of being asked questions. Abusive parents may not exhibit guilt feelings and often contend that the toddler was solely responsible for the injury.

Although these signs of potential abuse are certainly not present in all abusive parents, their presence alerts the nurse to assess and observe further. The nurse also remembers that some of these signs may be found in nonabusive parents, and that the presence of these signs serves only as a cue for further assessment. All nurses are required by law to report all suspected child abuse to the local child protective services agency.

Childhood Trauma

Trauma experienced during toddlerhood can have long-term effects on childhood behavioral and academic outcomes in development (McKelvey et al., 2018). Examples of ACEs can include witnessing domestic violence, community violence, and overdose and/or suicide of a family member. A number of checklists and assessment tools for ACEs are available to nurses and should be used when working with young children and families so that treatment plans can be devised.

Sexuality-Reproductive Pattern

The toileting process, during which attention is focused on the genital area, may precipitate the toddler's curiosity about genital organs. The nurse includes this aspect when teaching about toilet training, giving parents time to consider their feelings and decide on their approach to genital exploratory behavior and **masturbation**. Some parents accept the child's curiosity, whereas others see this as an opportunity to introduce their own sexual values and taboos (Healthy Children, n.d.). Masturbation is an aspect of childhood sexuality that parents find hard to respond to comfortably and appropriately. Part of the difficulty may be the need to acknowledge that children are sexual beings. The misunderstandings and secrecy about masturbation add to parent and child discomfort (Healthy Children, n.d.).

The nurse encourages parents to approach this curiosity and exploration, as well as masturbation, as a normal developmental process. These behaviors provide toddlers with an opportunity to become better acquainted with their bodies. Many parents are uncertain about the vocabulary they should use and often create cute, unrelated words rather than provide the correct anatomical terms. The use of cute alternative words is often a reflection of parental discomfort or embarrassment. Using correct terms will help toddlers develop accurate knowledge about sexuality and communicate more effectively if inappropriate touching by others occurs. For example, initially day care providers ignored a young male because he said an older male ate his "pickle." After repeated episodes, the parents were contacted because the child seemed so upset (even though day care workers gave him a new pickle to eat). The parents shared that "pickle" was their name for penis.

Coping–Effective/Ineffective Stress Tolerance Pattern

Perceptions of events and reactions to them are filtered through children's developing cognitive, emotional, and social capacities. The relevance of life events and the child's vulnerability to their effect depend on the given developmental period (see the Case Study and care plan at the end of this chapter). A child's **temperament**, which is defined as an individual's style of emotional and behavioral response across situations, especially those involving change or stress, serves as a foundation for coping (Garzon et al., 2019). Thomas and Chess (1986) originally described three common temperament patterns that they believe are innate: the easy child, the difficult child, and the slow-to-warm-up child. The easy child is cuddly, affectionate, and easy to manage. Children with a difficult temperament, however, are less adaptable, are more intense and active, and have more negative moods. Although temperament is generally accepted as inborn, it is influenced by environmental characteristics and exerts an influence on psychosocial adjustment by way of its effect on parent-child interactions. Nurses assist parents in recognizing their toddler's innate behavioral qualities as expressions of temperament and in developing management strategies. According to Chess & Thomas (1991), using the goodness-of-fit interactive model of temperament, adults can accommodate their demands and expectations in ways that match the child's behaviors, including learning strategies to help toddlers adapt positively to social expectations.

Toddlers develop new ways to cope with the myriad of new stresses that come with being a toddler. Coping is egocentric and reflective of their need for autonomy. Typical stressors include new siblings, babysitters, day care, toilet training, parental limit setting, and an endless string of tasks involving skills they have yet to develop.

Toddlers often imitate their parents' behavior, which includes their methods of dealing with stress. When overwhelmed, they regress until they regain some sense of mastery. Parents can help to anticipate and prepare toddlers for stressful experiences before they happen. However, they need to remember that toddlers' sense of time and ability to recall are limited. Preparations should be honest, simple, and focused on what the toddler will experience. Enough time should be allowed for the toddler to rehearse the coping behavior with the parent, but not so early before the event that the toddler forgets.

For children deemed to be at high risk for toxic stress responses, potential barriers to relational health need to be identified and addressed through team-based care (Westphaln et al., 2022). These additional interventions are supplemental and do not replace universal primary preventions. The nurse helps the parents anticipate developmental stressors and suggests age- and temperament-appropriate coping behaviors for toddlers. Early efforts at dealing with stress are an essential step to more mature coping responses as the child grows (Garner & Yogman, 2021). Promoting emotional support for parents may bolster family resilience and help young children to flourish despite adversity (Westphlan et al., 2022).

Values-Beliefs Pattern

Healthy behaviors are expressions of positive values and beliefs. Values and beliefs are learned, and their recognition and acceptance are fundamental to the integrity of the child. According to Kohlberg (1981), toddlers believe rules are absolute and behave out of a fear of punishment. However, toddlers' environments should help them become aware of right and wrong and contribute to their sense of security, belonging, and autonomy. Development of moral integrity is enhanced if toddlers believe they are valued.

Most toddlers develop values and beliefs based on their interactions with their parents. Thus, the nurse's assessment questions are often directed to the parent or caregiver. Some questions include the following:

- What are the family's values and beliefs about right and wrong?
- How does the parental approach to limit setting reflect these values and beliefs?
- What religious, spiritual, or cultural traditions and activities does the family have?
- How is the toddler included in traditions and activities?

During toddlerhood, children are exposed to, participate in, and imitate their family's religious rituals and practices. They are taught prayers and religious songs that are tied to family beliefs of right and wrong. Toddlers may be able to learn the words to simple prayers and songs, but parents should be cautioned that knowing the words does not mean that toddlers understand the full meaning of what is said. This early introduction into the family's religious beliefs is important as a socialization factor but should not be assumed to produce a good child.

The development of values and beliefs in young children is related to their developmental stage and is reflected in their behaviors. An important aspect of teaching young children what is right and wrong involves stating what acceptable behavior is and then reinforcing the behavior when it occurs. Parents often address toddlers only when they are misbehaving. In this scenario, toddlers receive no attention for acceptable behavior but gain their parents' attention when they misbehave. The nurse can remind parents to pay equal attention when their child behaves well.

ENVIRONMENTAL PROCESSES

Physical Agents

Accidents

If a disease were killing our young children in the proportions that injuries are, people would be outraged and demand that this killer be stopped.

C. Everett Koop, MD, Former Surgeon General

Toddlers are at high risk of accidental injury because they lack judgment and experience and have only rudimentary problem-solving skills, limited physical coordination, and a heightened level of curiosity about their environment. Unintentional injuries are the leading cause of death in children aged 1 to 4 (Childstats.gov, 2023; CDC, 2022d). Injuries in children are preventable and there is a huge potential to save children's lives by concerted public health action (WHO, n.d.). Irdawati et al. (2023) identified that most parents think that it is natural for children to get hurt and that childhood injuries are just a part of growing up. However, most injuries are predictable and preventable and can cause disabilities requiring long-term care. In summary, home-based injuries cause more deaths than all childhood diseases combined.

According to the CDC (2021), between 2018 and 2019, child unintentional injury death rates were highest among male children, babies under 1 year old, and those children who identified as American Indian, Alaska Native, and Black children. Motor vehicle crashes caused more deaths than other causes of unintentional injury. Male toddlers tend to have more injuries than females, but the overall numbers of accidental injuries peak during toddlerhood for both. Major causes of accidental injury in toddlers involve structural hazards, drowning, burns, motor vehicles, and poisoning.

Although overall injury rates for young children have decreased in the past 20 years, injury mortality rates remain higher in Black American and American Indian/Alaskan Native children (Khan et al., 2018). These children are at higher risk for injury and death, suggesting that new approaches are needed to address such racial disparities.

Structural Hazards

Houses and other buildings can be hazardous for toddlers. Toddlers' desire for exploration lures them to dangerous areas. They will climb onto furniture or fixtures, out of windows, or into small spaces. Resulting injuries can range from minor scrapes and bruises to fatal head injuries. Ideally, homes are "baby-proofed" before the infant begins scooting and crawling and toddler-proofed before the toddler becomes increasingly mobile. Parents should reassess the safety of their home as their child acquires new skills. Injuries to toddlers occur most often when they fall from furniture, highchairs, changing tables, stairs, windows, and playground equipment. When the child or family visits the home of a friend or relative, it must be inspected for hazards, or the toddler must be confined to one safe room. Many injuries occur in unfamiliar environments.

Preventive measures for structural hazards include the following:

- Do not leave a toddler unattended.
- Use gates at the top and bottom of stairways and at doors.
- Keep chairs away from countertops and tables to prevent toddlers from climbing.
- Securely anchor large television screens and other electronic equipment that can fall onto toddlers.
- Lock doors to dangerous areas and use gates and window guards.
- Store guns in a locked, safe area out of reach.

Toys

Toys commonly found in homes are another source of injury. Parents should inspect not only the toys that are in their own homes but also those outside the home that are given to the toddler by relatives, friends, babysitters, or day care personnel (see the Case Study and care plan at the end of this chapter). Many toys that are likely to be safe for older children are extremely hazardous for toddlers, such as those with small, removable parts, magnets and batteries, toxic paint or stuffing, sharp edges, and flammable material.

Sports Equipment

Although sporting and recreational equipment is recognized as a major source of accidents in older children and adolescents, parents and health care personnel occasionally forget that this equipment can be dangerous to toddlers. Improper storage of this equipment is a primary danger. Firearms that are left loaded and unlocked are deadly hazards, and bodybuilding weights and other heavy equipment can easily overwhelm toddlers, who may pull these objects down on themselves. Toddlers should always be supervised closely, especially in new environments or on playground equipment.

As toddlers become more mobile, they are introduced to riding toys, scooters, tricycles, and bicycles. Nurses remind parents about the need for, and in most states the requirement for, bicycle helmets that are fitted properly and worn every time the toddler rides or is a passenger on a bicycle.

Drowning

Children between the ages of 1 and 3 years are at the highest risk of drowning because most do not know how to swim and do not have the skills to keep their heads above water or to get out of the water. Toddlers can drown in water just deep enough to cover their noses and mouths. Although swimming pools and other natural bodies of water are a big part of the problem, even pails of water, toilets, bathtubs, and wading pools are dangerous. When toddlers fall into a pail of water or a toilet, it is hard for them to straighten up because all their weight is forward. Toddlers should never be left unattended—even for a few seconds—near a bathtub, hot tub, wading or swimming pool, toilet, pail of water, or small creek. All swimming pools should be fenced and have self-closing gates and latches. Toddlers must be supervised constantly and competently whenever they are near any body of water, regardless of its size, and should be fitted properly with personal flotation devices whenever they are on a boat.

Burns

There has been an increase in emergency room visits related to burns in pediatric patients over the past few years (Lee & Monuteaux, 2019; National Center for Health Statistics, 2021). Hot tap water, boiling water, coffee, tea, and food are the most common sources of scalds. These very painful and often debilitating injuries often occur as toddlers begin to gain mobility and explore their environments, inadvertently touching hot surfaces or spilling hot liquids on themselves. They may also put their mouths on live electrical cords or their fingers into electrical sockets and become seriously burned. Toddlers may fall into or against fireplaces or woodstoves.

The nurse's role is to educate parents regarding the following:

- Never eat, drink, or carry anything hot while holding a child.
- Lower the water heater temperature to between 120°F and 125°F.
- Never leave hot beverages or foods within a child's reach.
- Put children in a playpen while cooking.
- Never leave a toddler unattended in the bathtub. It takes only a moment to turn on the hot water.
- Put screens around fireplaces or woodstoves.
- Do not let children touch food taken directly from the microwave oven.
- Use burners at the back of the stove and turn pot handles in toward the stove.
- Install and maintain smoke detectors and replace batteries annually.

Motor Vehicles

Motor vehicle–related injuries include both passenger and pedestrian injuries. Primary forms of injury in children from 1 to 4 years of age often involve the lack of use or misuse of child safety seats. When child safety seats are properly installed and used, there is a reduced risk of death and serious injury to children. Improper installation and use of child safety seats, including both rear-facing and forward-facing seats, are widespread problems, with some experts reporting that more than 46% of them are misused in some way (CDC, 2023c). Certified child passenger safety technicians are trained in installing car safety seats properly and can help parents make sure their children are as safe as possible in the car. To find the closest inspection station, the nurse can visit or direct parents to visit https://www.nhtsa.gov/equipment/car-seats-and-booster-seats.

The rear-facing child safety seat supports a young child's head, neck, and spine, reducing stress to the neck and spinal cord in a crash. When children reach 2 years of age and are at the upper weight and height of the child safety seat, the nurse confirms with the parents that they can switch to forward-facing child safety seats. All children 12 years of age and younger should be seated in the rear seat of the vehicle because it is safer than the front seat (AAP, 2018b). Both rear-facing and forward-facing child seats should always be placed in the rear seat of the car (see https://exchange.aaa.com/safety/child-passenger-safety/car-seat-safety/).

During the toddlerhood years, it is safest to keep the child in a forward-facing rear seat with a harness until they reach the seat's maximum height of 4 feet 9 inches. Children can use a booster seat when they have outgrown the height limit of their forward-facing harnesses. At this stage, children are not yet ready for adult safety belts and should use belt-positioning booster seats until they are at least the required height and between 8 and 12 years old (AAP, 2018b). Safety belts are designed for 165-pound male adults; thus, it is no wonder that research shows that poorly fitting adult belts can injure children. According to the AAP (2018b), when a child can sit with his or her back straight against the vehicle seat back cushion and with knees bent over the seat edge without slouching, and they are 13 years old, it is time to switch to an adult safety belt (see https://www.aap.org/en/patient-care/early-childhood/early-childhood-health-and-development/safe-environments/child-passenger-safety/; http://exchange.aaa.com/safety/child-passenger-safety/). The nurse can provide a list of approved car seats and local retail outlets or agencies that sell, lend, or rent car seats.

Parents should be warned that toddlers may be injured or killed when they are hit by drivers backing up in their own driveways and often by members of their family or nearby neighbors. They are too small to be seen by a driver backing up and are quick to run after a departing parent or relative who thinks they are still safely inside.

Biologic Agents

Children are especially at risk of these bacterial hazards because of their physiology. Compared with adults, they have a faster respiratory rate, increased skin permeability, higher skin-to-body mass ratio, and less body fluids (AAP, 2023). Nurses provide information that can assist parents in dealing with their toddlers' and their own fears.

Nurses encourage parents to:

- Talk about their fears and worries.
- Stick to family diet routines that help toddlers maintain a varied and nutritious diet.
- Educate themselves, the best protection against unnecessary fear. Toddlers will be less fearful if they see that their parents are not afraid.

Many parents feel that toddlers, because of their immature immune systems and varied diet, are especially vulnerable to certain agents such as *Escherichia coli*. Parents might request antibiotics when they hear of an *E. coli* outbreak, just to be certain their child does not get sick, despite confirmation the child was never exposed to contaminated food. The nurse should reassure parents and explain that giving children antibiotics when they are not needed can do more harm than good. Many antibiotics, especially those identified for *E. coli* management, have serious side effects, and use of them when they are not needed can lead to the development of drug-resistant forms of bacteria.

COVID-19

In 2019, the CDC recommended that adults and children aged 2 and older wear a mask (Fig. 18.6) for protection against the COVID-19 virus (Høeg et al., 2023). During the pandemic, Mulkey et al. (2023) identified how the COVID-19 pandemic had significant indirect effects on multiple areas of child development, school readiness, educational attainment, socialization skills, and mental health, in addition to risks based on social determinants of health. The childhood experience of the COVID-19 pandemic relates to the child's age at the time of this experience, their family support structure, overall health, opportunities for e-learning and learning at home, and their community environment. Pediatricians and primary care physicians, teachers, and other health care professionals need to consider the child's "COVID-19 pandemic experience" as one of the important factors that can affect their neurodevelopment,

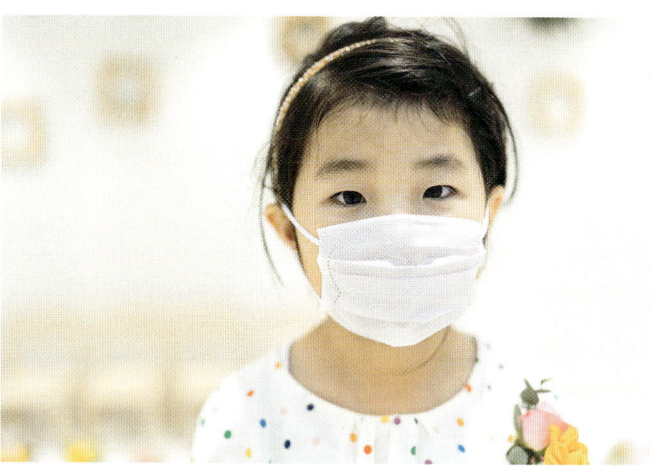

FIG. 18.6 Toddler wearing facemask during COVID-19. (From iStock.com/recep-bg)

academic performance, and physical and mental health. With the pandemic experience in mind, we must support children's development, as their needs may be different than those of prior generations (Mulkey et al., 2023).

To date, there is a lack of studies showing the effect of long-term masking of children. Previously, no society had engaged in such an experiment. Høeg et al. (2023) documented negative effects of mask wearing on children such as shortness of breath, impaired recognition of emotions and facial expressions (most pronounced in 3–5 year olds), reported negative effects on learning ability, increased anxiety, and decreased word identification, which will likely disproportionately affect children with decreased hearing and nonnative speakers.

Chemical Agents

Poisoning

Poisoning happens 10 times more often among young children aged 1 to 4 years than in their older counterparts. Toddlers aged 1 to 2 years are at the greatest risk. They are becoming more mobile, enabling them to explore and discover poisonous substances in the home. These include prescription and over-the-counter medications, alcohol, household products, plants, cosmetics, lead-based paint, and cigarettes (Box 18.10: Quality and Safety Scenario). They are also at risk because they still use their mouths as a way of exploring. Although many parents take precautions against poisoning in their own homes, some forget that toddlers can be poisoned away from the home, while visiting grandparents or other relatives (see the Case Study at the end of this chapter).

Due to the toddlers' limited experiences and functioning cognitive level, they are unaware that these items are harmful. Many emergency department calls and visits are precipitated by a toddler's ingestion of a potentially harmful substance. These incidents are likely to occur in the kitchen, bathroom, bedroom, or work area, and are usually discovered by a parent or caretaker who finds an open or empty container or a half-eaten leaf or other substance. Recent concerns with toddler poisoning relate to accidental access to vaping liquids that older siblings and parents might leave out; children are reported to have died from liquid nicotine poisoning (Healthy Children, 2019).

When parents or caregivers suspect that a toddler has ingested a poisonous substance, they should call the poison control center at 1-800-222-1222 or refer to the website (https://www.poison.org/), even if the child appears perfectly healthy. Each center is part of a nationwide effort to provide immediate information about poisonings. Parents should not attempt to induce vomiting without specific instructions from the center. Vomiting can cause further harm if the child is drowsy, unconscious, or convulsing, or if the substance ingested is corrosive, such as lye or a strong acid. When vomiting is recommended by the poison control center, instructions are often given to use ipecac syrup to stimulate the vomiting rapidly. This medication should be stored as carefully as any other medication or hazardous household product and replaced often because of its short shelf life.

Chronic poisonings, such as lead poisoning, are often undetected until irreversible damage has occurred (Mayans, 2019). Primary prevention involves teaching parents about risk factors and dangers of lead poisoning and the importance of a diet that encourages decreasing fat intake, because lead is retained in fat. Vitamin C, calcium, and iron intake reduce lead levels in the body. Secondary prevention involves performing periodic screening of blood lead levels in all young children identified as at risk. Consumer protection laws in the United States require that all toys and furniture manufactured for small children be free of lead-based paint products. However, imported toys and older family furniture or older houses may have been painted with a lead-based product.

BOX 18.10 QUALITY AND SAFETY SCENARIO

Preventing Accidental Poisonings in the Home

- Keep all household, garden, and car products out of reach.
- Keep medications and all household cleaning products out of reach in locked cabinets.
- Use childproof caps on medication.
- Keep all products and medication in their original containers for easy identification.
- Do not keep poisonous plants in the house. A list, which includes poinsettia, amaryllis, aloe vera, English ivy, mistletoe, chrysanthemums, and spider plants, is available from local poison control centers.
- Avoid outdoor plants and shrubs that are poisonous, including azaleas and chrysanthemums.
- Supervise the toddler's activity at all times.
- Post the National Capital Poison Center telephone number (1-800-222-1222) next to every telephone, and program it into each family member's cell phone. The National Capital Poison Center offers assistance 24 hours daily, 7 days each week. Their website is located at https://www.poison.org/about-poison-control.

Day Care

During the toddler years, many parents return to work or decide that an experience in a group setting would be beneficial for their child. The nurse can provide counseling about the decision to place a child in day care and the resulting emotions, as well as guidelines for selecting a safe childcare or day care provider (Goodhue et al., 2019).

The USDHHS Administration for Children and Families recommends a four-step approach as a guideline for selecting a childcare provider or day care center (see https://www.childcareaware.org/starting-child-care-search/). The parents should do the following to find the best facility for their toddler:

- Interview potential childcare providers and observe the program or setting.
- Ask about cost, enrollment, ages served, daily activities, accreditation and licensing regulations, caretaker credentials and experience, and policies about visiting, illness, and nutrition.
- Observe provider-child interactions, safety, and the quality of the learning material and toys.
- Check references.
- Talk to parents with children in the center or parents with children being cared for by the provider about discipline and responsiveness to parents, and talk to local childcare resources, referral agencies, and licensing offices.
- Think about safety, values, overall comfort level for you and your toddler, and affordability.
- Talk to the provider regularly about how your child is doing, to your child about what the children are doing each day, and to other parents.
- Visit often, announced and unannounced and at various times of the day.

Many organizations have developed guidelines and checklists on choosing childcare. Child Care Aware (https://www.childcareaware.org/) is a national initiative designed to improve the quality of care and increase the availability of high-quality childcare in local communities. Services include helping to find childcare and connecting parents with local childcare resources and referral agencies. Their brochure, Give Your Child Something That Will Last a Lifetime—Quality Child Care, outlines the steps to finding childcare and includes an observation checklist.

Regardless of the reasons for the parents wanting or needing day care for their child, the traditional expectation of caring for the young child at home continues to influence the parents' concept of what they should do for their child.

Culture and Ethnicity

Culture influences everything we do, know, and believe. Each culture possesses its own values, attitudes, and practices regarding family and childrearing. Toddlers continue to be shaped by the cultural values and beliefs of their parents and families, these being the first of many socializing forces they will encounter. As the toddlers' world expands, they will encounter many other forces, including peers, media, and schools.

Unlike older children, toddlers do not question the cultural practices of the family. The toddler who refuses to do certain expected things usually does so out of a need for autonomy and control rather than a questioning of beliefs. However, nurses remind parents of this because parents may be feeling the pressure of cultural norms and expectations. This is especially true for families who have recently emigrated.

Nurses must be prepared to provide culturally sensitive and competent care. Knowledge of and respect for various cultural world views, customs, values, and traditions are needed to negotiate different approaches in developing a health-promotion plan with families. Health care practices are culturally influenced. For example, if a culture views immunizations as dangerous or unnecessary, the toddler may be unprotected from certain communicable diseases. Incorporation of knowledge, respect, and negotiation facilitates the development of a therapeutic relationship.

Levels of Policy Making and Health

A lack of economic resources can affect the toddler's health and well-being. According to the Children's Defense Fund (2023), about one in seven children—nearly 10.5 million—were poor in 2019. Almost half of these children lived in extreme poverty at less than half the poverty level. Seventy-one percent of poor children were children of color. More than one in four Black and one in five Hispanic and Indigenous children were poor compared with 1 in 12 White children. Across all racial and ethnic groups, the youngest children were the poorest. Nearly one in six children under 6 lived in poverty during their years of greatest brain development.

Toddlers who live in poverty have higher mortality rates, poorer health, poorer growth, and more physical morbidity from diet tract infections, gastrointestinal tract infections, anemia, asthma, dental caries, otitis media, and visual loss, as well as higher rates of accidental injury and psychological and developmental disorders (Garzon et al., 2019; Box 18.4: Asthma, Diet, and Toddlers—A Cure?).

Legislation

Local and state legislation pertaining to toddlers is directed primarily toward safety and injury prevention. Many states have passed laws requiring the use of child safety seats, bicycle helmets, and temperature limits for household hot water heaters.

Each state has passed laws that provide protection for children that define abuse and neglect requiring a report to a designated agency. If there is an actual or suspected case of abuse or neglect, there are defining responsibilities to be performed by the protecting agency. These laws also provide for a central registry of reported cases of abuse. Nurses are required by law to report suspected child abuse and should familiarize themselves with the child abuse and neglect laws in their states.

The nation's 1600 Head Start and Early Head Start (collectively, "Head Start") programs serve as a ready-built solution in all 50 states and territories to support at-risk young children aged birth to 5 years through comprehensive health, education, and family support. National Head Start's 2020 issue described 12 state policies—six that promote Head Start access and six that promote Head Start quality—with broad support, identification, and treatment for infants and toddlers at risk for poor development. This also includes building a state-wide policy framework in every state, an infant and early childhood mental health infrastructure to become a comprehensive system of care, which will finally be adequate to meet the needs of children, adolescents, and their families (National Head Start Association, 2020).

Another legislative issue affecting toddlers is the Education of the Handicapped Act amendment of 1986 (Public Law 99-457). This law created programs that assist states in planning, developing, and implementing systems within states for handicapped children from birth to 3 years of age. Nurses who work with young children with disabilities should investigate and familiarize themselves with the programs in their states.

Health Services/Delivery System

The health of toddlers is significantly affected by the health care delivery system in the place where they live (Garzon et al., 2019). Private physicians, nurse practitioners, and public well-child clinics are the most frequently used resources for ongoing health maintenance or illness care for toddlers. Health professionals specializing in pediatrics coordinate their efforts to provide optimal health care for young children. For young children who do not receive routine health care, some public clinics sponsor special immunization days. Retired health care professionals may donate their time at free dental clinics for children.

Each health care visit includes an interval history, assessment of growth and development, physical assessment, discussion of age-appropriate developmental concerns, and anticipatory guidance. Immunizations are given according to the current CDC (2023) Recommended Immunizations for Children From Birth Through 6 Years Old. Provider and parent schedules are easily found on the CDC website (http://www.cdc.gov/vaccines/schedules). The nurse informs parents that they can anticipate and keep track of their toddler's immunizations with the CDC Childhood Immunization Schedule. Recently, there has been controversy about the relationship between childhood immunizations and ASD. Some parents are choosing not to vaccinate their children as recommended by the CDC, which has resulted in multiple measles outbreaks in regions of the United States (Hester et al., 2019). Despite what beliefs are held by certain groups of people, there is no research indicating that vaccinations contribute to development of autism (Mayo Clinic, n.d.; Destefano & Shimabukuro, 2019).

Toddlers need to explore their environment to master it, and this includes their encounters with health care. As their parents interact with health care providers, they may need to listen, observe, be introduced to and allowed to manipulate examination equipment. Nurses should provide them with simple explanations and choices so they can maintain a sense of control. Taking the time to enlist the cooperation of a toddler can make the health care visit more productive and conducive to information exchange and health care teaching.

NURSING APPLICATION AND ACTIONS

In addition to educating the parents, the nurse can begin to teach some health-promotion activities to the toddler. Examples of this type of toddler education are nutrition and oral hygiene. At this stage of development, it is crucial that caregivers model healthy behaviors and eating patterns. Parents may need education from the nurse about providing age-appropriate food choices while discouraging the intake of empty calories.

The nurse and the family can engage in screening activities. Assessments can be performed to evaluate the toddler for hearing loss and vision disturbances. Some vision and hearing conditions can be treated if detected early.

As toddlers begin to explore their autonomy, they become at risk for accidental injury. Parents should be educated about objects on which the child may climb, possibly leading to a crush or entrapment injury. They should be aware of hazardous toys, sports equipment, drowning, burns, poisoning, and motor vehicle safety. The nurse must remain alert to the potential for child abuse and report any suspicious injuries.

Another essential component of health promotion with the toddler age group is educating parents about routine health examinations and the childhood immunization schedule. Nurses must be informed about changes in immunization recommendations and educate families as these changes occur. They also should remain knowledgeable about the resources available in the community that may provide free or low-cost injections.

CASE STUDY

Grandparents Provide Care: Dante

Maria and José are the parents of 18-month-old Dante. Maria is 25 and will be starting her new job as a preschool teacher in 2 weeks. José is 26 and works in construction. As they both will be working full-time, they wanted to take time away for a week-long vacation before Maria starts her new job. They plan to leave Dante with José's parents, who are in their 70s and live in a second-floor condominium. The grandparents have two small dogs in their home. Because Dante is the first grandchild, the older couple is eager to spend time with him, but they have expressed concern about caring for a toddler.

Reflective Questions

- What do the parents need to discuss with the grandparents concerning safety issues in the home?
- What psychosocial issues of a toddler are important for both the parents and the grandparents to consider?
- What resources are available for grandparents?

SUMMARY

- Toddlerhood development can be an exciting and challenging time for toddlers and their parents.
- Parents who have encouraged their toddler's desire to explore can now delight in their developing sense of adventure as they enter their preschool years.
- The world is a wonderful place for the toddler who has known and experienced support, affection, and protection.

EVOLVE CHAPTER FEATURES

http://evolve.elsevier.com/Edelman/

- Study Questions

REFERENCES

American Academy of Pediatrics (AAP). (2018a). *Ages & stages: listen up about why newborn hearing screening is important*. https://www.healthychildren.org/

American Academy of Pediatrics (AAP). (2018b). Policy statement—child passenger safety. *Pediatrics, 127*(4), 788–793.

American Academy of Pediatrics (AAP). (2019). Fruit juice in infants, children, and adolescents: current recommendations. *Pediatrics, 139*(6), e20170967.

American Academy of Pediatrics (AAP). (2022a). *American Academy of Pediatrics calls for more support for breastfeeding mothers within updated policy recommendations*. https://www.aap.org/

American Academy of Pediatrics (AAP) & Healthy Children. (2022b). *Feeding and nutrition: your two-year-old*. https://www.healthychildren.org/English/ages-stages/toddler/nutrition/Pages/Feeding-and-Nutrition-Your-Two-Year-Old.aspx

American Academy of Pediatrics (AAP). (2023). *Children's environmental health: the biological remembrance of things past to inform the future*. https://publications.aap.org/pediatrics/resources/26225/Children-s-Environmental-Health-The-Biologic

American Academy of Pediatrics, Healthy Children (AAP). (2020). *How to read a growth chart: percentiles explained*. https://www.aap.org/en/search/?context=Healthy%20Children&source=Healthychildren.org&lang=English&k=growth%20charts&s=

American Association for Pediatric Ophthalmology and Strabismus. (2022). *Vision screening for infants and children*. https://www.aao.org/education/clinical-statement/vision-screening-infants-children-2022#Approvedby

Annerbäck, E. M., Svedin, C. G., & Dahlström, Ö. (2018). Child physical abuse: Factors influencing the associations between self-reported exposure and self-reported health problems: A cross-sectional study. *Child and Adolescent Psychiatry and Mental Health, 12*, 38. https://doi.org/10.1186/s13034-018-0244-1

Boone Blanchard, S., Ryan Newton, J., Didericksen, K. W., Daniels, M., & Glosson, K. (2021). Confronting racism and bias within early intervention: the responsibility of systems and individuals to influence change and advance equity. *Topics in Early Childhood Special Education, 41*(1), 6–17. https://doi.org/10.1177/0271121421992470

Boyden, S. D., Pott, M., & Starks, P. T. (2018). An evolutionary perspective on night terrors. *Evolution, Medicine, and Public Health, 2018*(1), 100–105. https://doi.org/10.1093/emph/eoy010

Boyraz, G., Yıldız, D. B., & Fidancı, B. E. (2018). Current approaches and nursing practice related to toilet training. *Guncel Pediatri Dergisi, 16*, 247–260.

Bucko, A. G., Armstrong, B., McIver, K. L., McLain, A. C., & Pate, R. R. (2023). Longitudinal associations between sleep and weight status in infants and toddlers. *Pediatric Obesity, 18*(8), e13056. https://doi.org/10.1111/ijpo.13056

Celiac Disease Foundation (CDF). (2018). *Celiac disease in children*. https://celiac.org/about-celiac-disease/celiac-disease-in-children/

Centers for Disease Control and Prevention. (2018). *Data & statistics on autism spectrum disorder*. https://www.cdc.gov/ncbddd/autism/data.html

Centers for Disease Control and Prevention. (2019a). *Learning the signs, act early: developmental milestones*. http://www.cdc.gov/ncbddd/actearly/milestones/index.html

Centers for Disease Control and Prevention. (2019b). *Immunization schedules*. https://www.cdc.gov/vaccines/schedules/index.html

Centers for Disease Control and Prevention. (2021). Q & A with author: rural-urban differences in unintentional injury death rates among children aged 0–17: United States, 2018–2019. https://blogs.cdc.gov/nchs/2021/10/27/6157/.

Centers for Disease Control and Prevention. (2022a). *National Center for Health Statistics*. https://www.cdc.gov/growthcharts/

Centers for Disease Control and Prevention. (2022b). *Child maltreatment: risk and protective factors*. https://www.cdc.gov/violenceprevention/childabuseandneglect/riskprotectivefactors.html.

Centers for Disease Control and Prevention. (2022c). *Fast facts: preventing child abuse & neglect*. https://www.cdc.gov/

Centers for Disease Control and Prevention. (2022d). *National Center for Health Statistics: child health*. https://www.cdc.gov/nchs/fastats/child-health.htm

Centers for Disease Control and Prevention. (2023a). *Vaccines for your children. Vaccines at 12 -24 month*. https://www.cdc.gov/vaccines/by-age

Centers for Disease Control and Prevention. (2023b). *Food and drinks to avoid or limit*. https://www.cdc.gov/nutrition/InfantandToddlerNutrition/foods-and-drinks/foods-and-drinks-to-limit.html

Centers for Disease Control and Prevention. (2023c). *Child passenger safety: get the facts*. https://www.cdc.gov/transportationsafety/child_passenger_safety/cps-factsheet.html

Chasani, M. F., & Izzaty, R. E. (2019). Model team teaching dalam meningkatkan keterampilan sosial anak melalui pemanfaatan lingkungan alam. *JPPM (Jurnal Pendidikan Dan Pemberdayaan Masyarakat), 6*(1), 76–87. https://doi.org/10.21831/jppm.v6i1.21871

Chess, S., & Thomas, A. (1991). Temperament and the concept of goodness of fit. In J. Strelau & A. Angleitner (Eds.), *Perspectives on individual differences. Explorations in temperament: international perspectives on theory and measurement* (pp.15–28). Plenum Press. https://doi.org/10.1007/978-1-4899-0643-4_2

Children's Defense Fund. (2023). *Children's health coverage in the United States*. https://www.childrensdefense.org/

Childstats.gov. (2023). *America's children: key national indicators of well-being, 2023-physical environment and safety child injury and mortality*. https://www.childstats.gov/

Chiocca, E. M. (2019). *Advanced pediatric health assessment* (3rd ed.). New York: Springer.

Cohen Kadosh, K., Muhardi, L., Parikh, P., Basso, M., Jan Mohamed, H. J., Prawitasari, T., et al. (2021). Nutritional support of neurodevelopment and cognitive function in infants and young children—an update and novel insights. *Nutrients, 13*(1), 199. http://dx.doi.org/10.3390/nu13010199

Cooke, J. E., Racine, N., Plamondon, A., Tough, S., & Madigan, S. (2019). Maternal adverse childhood experiences, attachment style, and mental health: Pathways of transmission to child behavior problems. *Child Abuse & Neglect, 93*, 27–37. https://doi.org/10.1016/j.chiabu.2019.04.011

Dag, N. C., Turkkan, E., Kacar, A., & Dag, H. (2021). Children's only profession: Playing with toys. *Northern Clinics of Istanbul, 8*(4), 414–420.

Del Tufo, S. N., Earle, F. S., & Cutting, L. E. (2019). The impact of expressive language development and the left inferior longitudinal fasciculus on listening and reading comprehension. *Journal of Neurodevelopmental Disorders, 11*, 37. https://doi.org/10.1186/s11689-019-9296-7

DeStefano, F., & Shimabukuro, T. T. (2019). The MMR vaccine and autism. *Annual Review of Virology, 6*(1), 585–600. https://doi.org/10.1146/annurev-virology-092818-015515

DeWolfe, T. E. (2023). *Developmental stages*. Salem Press Encyclopedia of Science.

DiGrazia, S., & Anstrom, C. (2023). Introducing various foods during infancy and the development of food allergies during toddler/preschooler years...Academy of Nutrition and Dietetics, Food & Nutrition Conference & Expo, October 7-10, 2023, Denver, Colorado. *Journal of the Academy of Nutrition & Dietetics*, *123*(9), A68. https://doi.org/10.1016/j.jand.2023.06.234

Erikson, E. H. (1995). *Childhood & society* (35th anniversary ed.). New York, NY: Norton.

Erikson, E. H. (1998). *The life cycle is completed*. New York, NY: Norton.

Gámez, P. B., Palermo, F., Perry, J. S., & Galindo, M. (2023). Spanish-English bilingual toddlers' vocabulary skills: The role of caregiver language input and warmth. *Developmental Science*, *26*(2), e13308. https://doi.org/10.1111/desc.13308

Garner, A., & Yogman, M. (2021). Committee on Psychosocial Aspects of Child and Family Health, section on developmental and behavioral pediatrics, Council on Early Childhood. Preventing childhood toxic stress: Partnering with families and communities to promote relational health. *Pediatrics*, *148*(2), e2021052582. https://doi.org/10.1542/peds.2021-052582

Garzon, D. L., Starr, N. B., Brady, M. A., Gaylord, N. M., Driessnack, M., & Duderstadt, K. G. (2019). *Pediatric primary care* (7th ed.). Philadelphia: Saunders.

Goodhue, C. J., Rickenback, T., Hays, S., & Donohoe, M. (2019). NAPNAP position statement on pediatric-focused advanced practice registered nurses' role in disasters involving children. *Journal of Pediatric Health Care*, *33*(1), A16A18. https://doi.org/10.1016/j.pedhc.2018.09.004

Graczykowska, K., Kaczmarek, J., Wilczyńska, D., Łoś-Rycharska, E., & Krogulska, A. (2021). The consequence of excessive consumption of cow's milk: Protein-losing enteropathy with anasarca in the course of iron deficiency anemia-case reports and a literature review. *Nutrients*, *13*(3), 828. https://doi.org/10.3390/nu13030828

Grosjean, F. (2021). *Life as a bilingual: knowing and using two or more languages* (pp. 27–39). Cambridge University Press. https://doi.org/10.1017/9781108975490.003

Guilleminault, C., Huang, Y. S., & Quo, S. (2019). Apraxia in children and adults with obstructive sleep apnea syndrome. *Sleep*, *42*(12), zsz168. https://doi.org/10.1093/sleep/zsz168

Harold, G. T., & Sellers, R. (2018). Annual research review: Interparental conflict and your psychopathology: An evidence review and practice focused update. *The Journal of Child Psychology and Psychiatry*, *59*(4), 372–402. https://doi.org/10.1111/jcpp.12893

Harris, J. L., Romo-Palafox, M. J., Gershman, H., Kagan, I., & Duffy, V. (2023). Healthy snacks and drinks for toddlers: A qualitative study of caregivers' understanding of expert recommendations and perceived barriers to adherence. *Nutrients*, *15*(4), 1006. https://doi.org/10.3390/nu15041006

Hay, D. F., Caplan, M., & Nash, A. (2018). The beginnings of peer relations. In W. M. Bukowski, B. Laursen, & K. H. Rubin (Eds.), *Handbook of peer interactions, relationships, and groups* (2nd ed.; pp. 200–221). Guilford.

Hayes, K., & Carew, J. (2023). *Hearing loss and developmental delay in children*. https://www.verywellhealth.com/hearing-loss-and-developmental-delay-4125686

Healthy Children. (n.d.). *Ages & stages: Masturbation*. https://www.healthychildren.org/ Accessed September 10, 2023.

Healthy Children. (2019). *Liquid nicotine used in e-cigarettes can kill children*. https://www.healthychildren.org/English/safety-prevention/at-home/Pages/Liquid-Nicotine-Used-in-E-Cigarettes-Can-Kill-Children.aspx

Healthy Children. (2022). *Emotional development: 2-year olds*. https://www.healthychildren.org/English/ages-stages/toddler/Pages/emotional-development-2-year-olds.aspx

Healthy Children. (2023). *Early signs of autism*. https://www.healthychildren.org/English/health-issues/conditions/Autism/Pages/Early-Signs-of-Autism-Spectrum-Disorders.aspx

Healthy People 2030. (2023). https://health.gov/healthypeople/search?query=children

Hester, G., Nickel, A., LeBlanc, J., Carlson, R., Spaulding, A. B., Kalaskar, A., et al. (2019). Measles hospitalizations at a United States Children's Hospital 2011-2017. *The Pediatric Infectious Disease Journal*, *38*(6), 547–552. https://doi.org/10.1097/INF.0000000000002221

Hockenberry, M. J., Duffy, E. A., & Gibbs, K. (2024). *Wong's nursing care of infants and children* (12th ed.). Elsevier Health Sciences.

Hodder, R. K., O'Brien, K. M., Stacey, F. G., Tzelepis, F., Wyse, R. J., Bartlem, K. M., et al. (2019). Interventions for increasing fruit and vegetable consumption in children aged five years and under. *The Cochrane Database of Systematic Reviews*, *2019*(11), CD008552. https://doi.org/10.1002/14651858.CD008552.pub6

Høeg, T. B., González-Dambrauskas, S., Prasad, V. (2023). The United States' decision to mask children as young as two for COVID-19 has been extended into 2023 and beyond: The implications of this policy. *Paediatric Respiratory Reviews*, *47*, 30–32. https://doi.org/10.1016/j.prrv.2023.04.004

Inkelas, M., & Oberklaid, F. (2018). Improving preventive and health promotion care for children. *Israel Journal of Health Policy Research*, *7*(1), 62. https://doi.org/10.1186/s13584-018-0259-3

Irdawati, I., Ramadhanni, J., & Syaiful, A. R. (2023). An overview of parents' knowledge about accident prevention in toddler. *Jurnal Berita Ilmu Keperawatan*, *16*(1), 47–52. https://doi.org/10.23917/bik.v16i1.1014

Johns Hopkins Medicine. (n.d.). *Food allergies in children*. https://www.hopkinsmedicine.org/health/conditions-and-diseases/food-allergies-in-children. Accessed October 20, 2023.

Karani, N. F., Sher, J., & Mophosho, M. (2022). The influence of screen time on children's language development:A scoping review. *The South African Journal of Communication Disorders* = Die Suid-Afrikaanse tydskrif vir Kommunikasieafwykings, *69*(1), e1–e7. https://doi.org/10.4102/sajcd.v69i1.825

Khan, S. Q., Berrington de Gonzalez, A., Best, A. F., Chen, Y., Haozous, E. A., Rodriquez, E. J., et al. (2018). Infant and youth mortality trends by race/ethnicity and cause of death in the United States. *The Journal of the American Medical Association Pediatrics*, *172*(12), e183317. https://doi.org/10.1001/jamapediatrics.2018.3317

Kirkorian, H., Choi, K., & Anderson, D. R. (2019). American parents' active engagement mediates the impact of background television on toddlers' play. *Journal of Children and Media*, *13*(4), 377–394. https://doi.org/10.1080/17482798.2019.1635033

Kochanska, G., Boldt, L. J., & Goffin, K. C. (2019). Early relational experience: A foundation for the unfolding dynamics of parent-child socialization. *Child Development Perspectives*, *13*(1), 41–47. https://doi.org/10.1111/cdep.12308

Kohlberg, L. (1981). *The philosophy of moral development* (*Vol. 1*). San Francisco: Harper & Row.

Lee, M., & Monuteaux, M. C. (2019). Trends in pediatric emergency department use after the Affordable Care Act. *Pediatrics*, *143*(6), e20183542.

Liu, C., & Rahman, M. N. A. (2022). Relationships between parenting style and sibling conflicts: A meta-analysis. *Frontiers in Psychology*, *13*, 936253. https://doi.org/10.3389/fpsyg.2022.936253

Mathias, J. G., Zhang, H., Soto-Ramirez, N., & Karmaus, W. (2019). The association of infant feeding patterns with food allergy symptoms and food allergy in early childhood. *International Breastfeeding Journal, 14*, 143. https://doi.org/10.1186/s13006-019-0241-x

Mayans, L. (2019). Lead poisoning in children. *American Family Physician, 100*(1), 24–30.

Mayo Clinic. (n.d.). *Link between autism and vaccination debunked.* https://www.mayoclinichealthsystem.org/hometown-health/speaking-of-health/autism-vaccine-link-debunked. Accessed October 19, 2023.

McHarg, G., Ribner, A. D., Devine, R. T., & Hughes, C. (2020). Infant screen exposure links to toddlers' inhibition, but not other EF constructs: A propensity score study. *Infancy, 25*(2), 205–222. https://doi.org/10.1111/infa.12325

McKelvey, L. M., Edge, N. C., Mesman, G. R., Whiteside-Mansell, L., & Bradley, R. H. (2018). Adverse experiences in infancy and toddlerhood: Relations to adaptive behavior and academic status in middle childhood. *Child Abuse & Neglect, 82*, 168–177. https://doi.org/10.1016/j.chiabu.2018.05.026

Meylia, K. N., Siswati, T., Paramashanti, B. A., & Hati, F. S. (2020). Fine motor, gross motor, and social independence skills among stunted and non-stunted children. *Early Child Development and Care, 192*, 95–102. https://doi.org/10.1080/03004430.2020.1739028

Milevsky, A. (2018). Theoretical and clinical foundations of siblings in therapy: Use of parental context in adult sibling discord. *The American Journal of Family Therapy, 46*, 1–17. https://doi.org/10.1080/01926187.2018.1558423

Mulkey, S. B., Bearer, C. F., & Molloy, E. J. (2023). Indirect effects of the COVID-19 pandemic on children relate to the child's age and experience. *Pediatric Research, 94*(5), 1586–1587. https://doi.org/10.1038/s41390-023-02681-4

National Center for Children's Vision and Eye Health at Prevent Blindness. (2020). *Small steps for big vision: an eye health information tool kit for parents and caregivers.* https://nationalcenter.preventblindness.org/small-steps-for-big-vision/

National Center for Health Statistics. (2021). *Emergency department visits within the past 12 months among adults aged 18 and over, by selected characteristics: United States, selected years 1997–2019.* https://www.cdc.gov/nchs/data/hus/2020-2021/EdAd.pdf

National Eye Institute. (2019). *Results—amblyopia treatment study (ATS I), background.* https://www.nei.nih.gov/research/clinical-trials/results-amblyopia-treatment-study-ats-i-background

National Head Start Association. (2020). 12 No-Cost or Low-Cost State Policies to Support Head Start Access and Quality. https://nhsa.org/wp-content/uploads/2022/03/2020-12-State-Policies.pdf

Nuzzi, G., Di Cicco, M., Trambusti, I., Agosti, M., Peroni, D. G., & Comberiati, P. (2022). Primary prevention of pediatric asthma through nutritional interventions. *Nutrients, 14*(4), 754. https://doi.org/10.3390/nu14040754

Okoye, C., Obialo-Ibeawuchi, C. M., Obajeun, O. A., Sarwar, S., Tawfik, C., Waleed, M. S., et al. (2023). Early diagnosis of autism spectrum disorder: A review and analysis of the risks and benefits. *Cureus, 15*(8), e43226. https://doi.org/10.7759/cureus.43226

Pai, U. A., Chandrasekhar, P., Carvalho, R. S., & Kumar, S. (2018). The role of nutrition in immunity in infants and toddlers: An expert panel opinion. *Clinical Epidemiology and Global Health, 6*(4), 155–159. https://doi.org/10.1016/j.cegh.2017.11.004

Rahman, S., Elliott, S. A., Scott, S. D., & Hartling, L. (2022). Children at risk of anaphylaxis: A mixed-studies systematic review of parents' experiences and information needs. *PEC Innovation, 1*, 100018. https://doi.org/10.1016/j.pecinn.2022.100018

Renz, H., Allen, K. J., Sicherer, S. H., Sampson, H. A., Lack, G., Beyer, K., et al. (2018). Food allergy. *Nature Reviews. Disease Primers*, 4, 17098. https://doi.org/10.1038/nrdp.2017.98

Reynolds, A. M., Soke, G. N., Sabourin, K. R., Hepburn, S., Katz, T., Wiggins, L. D., et al. (2019). Sleep problems in 2- to 5-year-olds with autism spectrum disorder and other developmental delays. *Pediatrics, 143*(3), e20180492. https://doi.org/10.1542/peds.2018-0492

Rochat, P. (2015). Layers of awareness in development. *Developmental Review, 38*, 122–145. http://doi.org/http://dx.doi.org/10.1016/j.dr.2015.07.009

Rochat, P. (2021). Clinical pointers from developing self-awareness. *Developmental Medicine and Child Neurology, 63*, 382–386. https://doi.org/10.1111/dmcn.14767

Rowell, T., & Neal-Barnett, A. A. (2021). Systematic review of the effect of parental adverse childhood experiences on parenting and child psychopathology. *Journal of Child and Adolescent Trauma, 15*, 167–180. https://doi.org/10.1007/s40653-021-00400-x

Salunkhe, S., Bharaswadkar, R., Patil, M., Agarkhedkar, S., Pande, V., & Mane, S. (2021). Influence of electronic media on speech and language delay in children. *Medical Journal of Dr. D.Y. Patil Vidyapeeth, 14*(6), 656–661. https://doi:10.4103/mjdrdypu.mjdrdypu_636_20

Samady, W., Warren, C., Wang, J., Das, R., & Gupta, R. S. (2020). Egg allergy in US children. *The Journal of Allergy and Clinical Immunology Practice, 8*(9), 3066–3073.e6. https://doi.org/10.1016/j.jaip.2020.04.058

Sanyaolu, A., Okorie, C., Qi, X., Locke, J., & Rehman, S. (2019). Childhood and adolescent obesity in the United States: a public health concern. *Global Pediatric Health, 6*, 2333794X19891305. https://doi.org/10.1177/2333794X19891305

Schellinger, K., Murphy, L., Rajagopalan, S., Jones, T., Hudock, R., Graff, C., et al. (2020). Toddler externalizing behavior, social support, and parenting stress: examining a moderator model. *Family Relations, 69*(4), 714–726. https://doi.org/10.1111/fare.12478

Schwab, J. F., & Lew-Williams, C. (2020). Discontinuity of reference hinders children's learning of new words. *Child Development, 91*, e29–e41. https://doi.org/10.1111/cdev.13189

Scott, H. K., & Cogburn, M. (2023). Peer play. In: *StatPearls*. Treasure Island (FL): StatPearls Publishing. https://www.ncbi.nlm.nih.gov/books/NBK513223/

Shah, U. K. (2022). *Communication disorders in children.* https://www.merckmanuals.com/professional/pediatrics/endocrine-disorders-in-children/hyperthyroidism-in-infants-and-children

Shuya, S., Guizhen, C., & Litao, Z. (2022). The prevention effect of probiotics against eczema in children: an update systematic review and meta-analysis. *Journal of Dermatological Treatment, 33*(4), 1844–1854.https://doi.org/10.1080/09546634.2021.1925077

Slomian, J., Honvo, G., Emonts, P., Reginster, J. Y., & Bruyère, O. (2019). Consequences of maternal postpartum depression: A systematic review of maternal and infant outcomes. *Women's Health (London, England), 15*, 1745506519844044. https://doi.org/10.1177/1745506519844044

Stanford Medicine, Childrens Health. (n.d.). *Food allergies in children.* https://www.stanfordchildrens.org/en/topic/default?id=food-allergies-in-children-90-P01993. Accessed October 23, 2023.

Subbiah, K., Mason, C. A., Gaffney, M., & Grosse, S. D. (2018). Progress in documented early identification and intervention for deaf and hard of hearing infants: CDC's hearing screening and follow-up survey, United States, 2006-2016. *Journal of Early Hearing Detection and Intervention, 3*(2), 1–7. https://doi.org/10.26077/6sj1-mw42

Takahashi, I., Obara, T., Ishikuro, M., Murakami, K., Ueno, F., Noda, A., et al. (2023). Screen time at age 1 year and communication and problem-solving developmental delay at 2 and 4 years. *The Journal of the American Medical Association Pediatrics, 177*(10),1039–1046.

Thomas, A., & Chess, S. (1986). The New York longitudinal study: From infancy to early adult life. In R. Plomin & J. Dunn (Eds.), *The study of temperament. Changes, continuities, and challenges* (pp. 39–52). Hillsdale, NJ: Erlbaum.

U.S. Department of Health and Human Services. (2021). *Child maltreatment 2019*. https://www.acf.hhs.gov/sites/default/files/documents/cb/cm2019.pdf

U.S. Preventive Services Task Force. (2017). *Final recommendation statement: vision in children ages 6 months to 5 years: screening*. https://www.uspreventiveservicestaskforce.org/uspstf/recommendation/vision-in-children-ages-6-months-to-5-years-screening

U.S. Preventive Services Task Force. (2021). *Final update summary: dental caries in children from birth through age 5 years: screening*. https://www.uspreventiveservicestaskforce.org/uspstf/recommendation/prevention-of-dental-caries-in-children-younger-than-age-5-years-screening-and-interventions1

Verhage, C. L., Gillebaart, M., van der Veek, S. M. C., & Vereijken, C. M. J. L. (2018). The relation between family meals and health of infants and toddlers: A review. *Appetite, 127*, 97–109. https://doi.org/10.1016/j.appet.2018.04.010

Westphaln, K. K., Lee, E., Fry-Bowers, E. K., Kleinman, L. C., & Ronis, S. D. (2022). Examining child flourishing, family resilience, and adversity in the 2016 National Survey of Children's Health. *Journal of Pediatric Nursing, 66*, 57–63. https://doi.org/10.1016/j.pedn.2022.05.014

World Health Organization (WHO). (n.d.). *Preventing child injuries*. https://www.who.int/

Zink, J., Liu, B., Yang, C. H., Herrick, K. A., & Berrigan, D. (2023). Differential associations between television viewing, computer use, and adiposity by age, gender, and race/ethnicity in United States youth: A cross-sectional NHANES analysis. *Pediatric Obesity, 18*(10), e13070. https://doi.org/10.1111/ijpo.13070

19

Preschool Child

Kevin K. Chui, Sheng-Che Yen and Daniele Piscitelli

http://evolve.elsevier.com/Edelman/

OBJECTIVES

After completing this chapter, the reader will be able to:

- Explain the physical and psychosocial changes occurring during the preschool years that influence child and family health needs.
- Discuss the concepts of cognitive development of preschoolers using Piaget's theory.
- Review the *Healthy People 2030* concepts that pertain to preschool children and their families.
- Describe family teaching and nursing support for the typical sleep disturbances of the preschool years.
- Describe current recommendations for developmental screening and surveillance for health care professionals.
- Outline the primary prevention immunization requirements for preschoolers.
- Identify the major causes of injuries during the preschool years.

KEY TERMS

Acute lymphocytic leukemia
Amblyopia
Asthma
Centering
Deduction
Developmental screening
Developmental surveillance
Doll or puppet play
Early and periodic screening, Diagnosis, and Treatment
Eccrine sweat gland function
Egocentrism
Expressive language
Heterophoria
Heterotropia
Homeostasis
Induction
Induction explanation
Initiatives
Irreversibility
Ishihara test
Lactose intolerance
Mnemonic techniques
Mutual storytelling
Myopic vision
Neuroblastoma
Nightmares
Night terrors
Otitis media
Parental divorce
Preoperational stage
Quiet
Receptive language
Refractive errors
Retinoblastoma
Snellen Screening Test
Strabismus
Transductive reasoning
Wilms tumor

THINK ABOUT IT

Aggressive Behavior

Phillip, aged 4 years, started preschool 2 weeks ago after spending his early years at home with his mother and his 18-month-old sister. His mother intended for Phillip to start preschool earlier; preschool classes were canceled due to the COVID-19 pandemic. His mother also recently returned to her office job as an accountant, works 9 hours a day, and is fatigued when she picks up Phillip at 5:00 p.m. Phillip's father travels for his job but is home on weekends to spend time with his family. Although Phillip's mother always believed that Phillip was shy because he was **quiet**, during the last week he started hitting his peers and becoming loudly vocal at story time. His mother, believing that Phillip's behavior is related to her return to office work, feels embarrassed and frustrated by his behavior, especially because she enjoys returning to office work and the extra income.

- What factors might be contributing to Phillip's changed behavior?
- How might you define Phillip's temperament? Why?
- What discussions might you have with Phillip's parents to help them understand, respond to, and change their son's behavior for the better?
- How did the COVID-19 pandemic affect child development, such as learning and socialization?

The preschool child (aged 3–6 years) has a more developed body structure, an ability to control and use the body, and a facility with language that more closely resembles that of the adult than that of the toddler. The major psychological thrust of this period of development is mastery of self as an independent human being, with a willingness to extend experiences beyond those of the family. Although historically the end of early childhood in the Western world was marked by entrance into the formalized educational system, increasing numbers of children in the United States begin formalized schooling during their preschool years. Box 19.1: *Healthy People 2030* presents the objectives related to this developmental stage (https://health.gov/healthypeople).

BOX 19.1 *HEALTHY PEOPLE 2030*

Select National Health-Promotion and Disease-Prevention Objectives for Preschool Children

- PA-09 Increase the proportion of children who do enough aerobic physical activity
- PA-13 Increase the proportion of children aged 2 to 5 years who get no more than 1 hour of screen time a day
- EMC-03 Increase the proportion of children who get sufficient sleep
- NWS-01 Reduce household food insecurity and hunger
- NWS-04 Reduce the proportion of children and adolescents with obesity
- MICH-03 Reduce the rate of deaths in children and adolescents aged 1 to 19 years
- MICH-17 Increase the proportion of children who receive a developmental screening
- MICH-18 Increase the proportion of children with autism spectrum disorder who receive special services by age 4 years
- EH-04 Reduce blood lead levels in children aged 1 to 5 years
- OH-02 Reduce the proportion of children and adolescents with active and untreated tooth decay
- V-01 Increase the proportion of children aged 3 to 5 years who get vision screening

US Department of Health and Human Services. (2024). *Healthy People 2030*. Office of Disease Prevention and Health Promotion. https://www.health.gov/healthypeople/objectives-and-data/browse-objectives.

BIOLOGY AND GENETICS

The protuberant abdomen of the toddler disappears during the preschool years as the pelvis begins to straighten and the abdominal muscles develop. The hips gradually rotate inward, replacing out-toeing with straight or slight in-toeing. Mild in-toeing may remain during the preschool years, but anything beyond a mild level should be investigated and treated. At around 4 to 5 years of age, children may demonstrate knock knees and flat feet; however, this typically resolves by 6 years of age.

Growth rates remain steady from age 3 to 6 years. Average preschoolers gain approximately 2 kg (4.4 lb) of body weight and 7 cm (2 in) of height each year, whereas head circumference increases by less than 2 cm during the entire preschool period. During early childhood, skin matures in its ability to protect the child from outer invasion and loss of fluids. The skin's capacity to localize infection increases but remains less than that of a mature person. Negligible secretion of sebum makes the skin fairly dry. **Eccrine sweat gland function**, part of the body's heat-regulation mechanism, gradually matures, but the quantity of eccrine sweat produced in response to heat or emotion remains minimal. Apocrine sweat glands, located primarily in the axillae, areolas of the breast, and the anal area, remain nonsecretory during this period.

The kidneys reach full functional maturity by the end of infancy and early toddlerhood, with only their size changing during the preschool years. By the end of the preschool years, urine excretion ranges from 650 to 1000 mL (22 to 34 ounces). Under normal homeostatic conditions, the preschooler's renal system conserves water and concentrates urine on a level that approximates adult abilities. Under conditions of stress, however, the kidneys lack the ability to respond fully and to maintain **homeostasis** when compared with the more rapid response of the adult renal system.

Growth of gastrointestinal organs continues through the preschool years without functional changes. Children achieve full voluntary control of elimination. **Lactose intolerance**, intolerance to milk products manifested by diarrhea, often appears during the preschool years. This condition, more common in Black, Asian American, and Native American children, can be managed successfully by elimination of lactose from the diet.

Lung capacity continues to increase, with a gradual decrease in respiratory rate. Respiratory rate for preschoolers ranges from 20 to 25 breaths/min (Cleveland Clinic, 2022). Preschoolers make better decisions than toddlers about objects they place in their mouths, resulting in fewer instances of choking and obstruction. A gradual increase in the size and shape of the ears coincides with decreases in the incidence of **otitis media** (middle ear infection). Tonsils and adenoids are large compared with the throat, which may contribute to noisy breathing and upper respiratory tract infection in preschoolers.

The cardiovascular system enlarges in proportion to general body growth. Heart rate for preschoolers ranges from 70 to 115 beats/min, with blood pressure ranging from 95 to 110/60 to 75 mm Hg (Cleveland Clinic, 2022). Early hypertension develops in some children during the preschool years; therefore, routine measurement of blood pressure is indicated, particularly in children with a strong family history of hypertension (see Chapter 20). Preschool children maintain adequate hemoglobin levels when dietary intake is sufficient. Bone marrow of the ribs, the sternum, and the vertebrae become fully established as primary sites for red blood cell formation. The liver and spleen continue to form erythrocytes and granulocytes.

The immune system continues to develop. Preschoolers boost their immune response to common pathogens as exposure occurs. Group activities, such as joining preschool or play groups, increase exposure and subsequently escalate the incidence of common contagious illnesses regardless of the child's age. Initial encounters with such group activities usually result in increases in illness. Later these children may be less prone to common contagious diseases because of their early exposure to infectious illnesses and their consequent immunity.

Musculoskeletal and neurological development reaches a level that allows seemingly effortless walking, running, and climbing. Older preschoolers' ability to copy figures and draw recognizable pictures indicates their advancing fine motor abilities, and they are eager to demonstrate these skills to others. Advances in fine motor, gross motor, cognitive, communicative, and social-emotional skills are outlined in Table 19.1.

TABLE 19.1 GROWTH AND DEVELOPMENT

Developmental and Behavioral Milestones for Preschool Children

Age (yr)	Expectations
3	At this age, the typical child: • Builds a tower of six to eight cubes • Throws ball overhand, rides tricycle, walks up stairs alternating feet • Has self-care skills (self-feeding, self-dressing) • Knows own name, age, and sex • May comprehend cold, tired, hungry; may understand the prepositions *over* and *under*, differentiates bigger and smaller; can convey the use of scissors, key, and pencil • Copies a circle; draws a person with two body parts (head and one other part) • Engages in imaginative play that becomes more elaborate with specific themes or story lines demonstrated; enjoys interactive play • Speech is understandable 75% of the time; names a friend; carries a conversation with two or three sentences spoken together • Is toilet trained during the daytime for both bowel and bladder
4	At this age, the typical child: • Alternates feet when descending stairs; jumps forward; hops on one foot and can stand on 1 foot for up to 5 sec • Using overhand toss can hit target from 5 feet • Builds a tower of eight blocks • Copies a cross • Holds and uses a pencil with good control • Cuts paper into two pieces • Pours, cuts, and mashes own food • Brushes own teeth • Dresses self, including buttons • Gives first and last name • Engages in conversational give-and-take • Knows what to do if cold, tired, or hungry • Sings a song or says a poem from memory • Talks about daily experiences and things that are used at home (food, appliances) • Can name three or four primary colors • Is aware of sex (of self and others) • Plays board/card games • Draws a person with three parts • Tells you what he/she thinks is going to happen next in a book • Describes features of themselves, including sex, age, interests, and strengths • Engages in fantasy play
5	At this age, the typical child: • May be able to skip; can walk on tiptoes; makes broad jumps • Folds paper parallel; colors between vertical lines • Ties a knot, has mature pencil grasp • Names four or five colors and can identify coins • Tells a simple story and knows several nursery rhymes • Dresses and undresses without supervision • Prints some letters and numbers; is able to copy a square and triangle from an illustration • Draws a person with at least six body parts • Begins to understand right and wrong, fair and unfair • Engages in dramatic make-believe and dress-up play during which the child assumes a specific role; engages in domestic role-playing and dressing up • Enjoys the companionship of other children; plays cooperatively • Has good articulation; uses appropriate tenses and pronouns • Can count to 10
6	At this age, the typical child: • Bounces a ball four to six times; throws and catches • Skates • Rides a bicycle • Ties shoelaces • Counts up to 10; prints own first name; prints numbers up to 10 • Understands right from left • Draws a person with six body parts, with the figure depicted wearing clothing

Modified from American Academy of Pediatrics. (n.d.). *Bright futures*. https://www.aap.org/en/practice-management/bright-futures

Primary teeth finish erupting by late toddler or early preschool years. Initial permanent teeth generally erupt toward the end of the preschool period. Permanent teeth tend to erupt approximately 6 months earlier in females than in males. Older preschoolers usually take responsibility for dental hygiene, although all children need gentle guidance about proper brushing and appropriate nutritional intake for healthy teeth. Parents should continue to assist with brushing and supervise flossing and fluoride intake. Use of fluoride toothpaste is effective in caries prevention (Jullien, 2021; Walsh et al., 2019), however, risk of fluorosis exists in children younger than 6 years and is influenced by both the dose and the frequency of exposure to fluoride during tooth development. Considerations in balancing the risk of too much fluoride to prevent caries depends on a child's probability of caries development and assessment of the amounts of fluoride the child receives from other sources. Fluoride sources include public water supply in some regions, foods, drinks, combustion of coal, fluoride supplements, and occasionally accidentally swallowed toothpaste (American Dental Association, 2023; Zhang et al., 2023). Because the preschool period is an age of caries formation, regular dental checkups are essential. The American Dental Association Council on Scientific Affairs (2014) recommends fluoride toothpaste for young children to prevent caries: a smear (the size of a grain of rice) of toothpaste for children up to age 3 years and a pea-sized amount for children 3 to 6 years. Fluoride varnish is recommended in the primary care setting every 3 to 6 months starting at tooth emergence. Over-the-counter fluoride rinse is not recommended for children younger than 6 years because of the risk of their swallowing higher-than-recommended levels of fluoride. Nurses assess whether the child is receiving preventive dental care, and parents should be encouraged to begin or maintain this care. Suggestions for promoting good oral hygiene as part of general health-promotion teaching can be found in Chapter 20.

Gender

Males tend to experience more childhood illnesses than do females from 3 to 6 years of age. Preschoolers are more aware of their gender identity than are toddlers and may imitate societal stereotypes more closely. Traditionally males have been encouraged to take more risks, and they have more accidents than do preschool females, who may have been encouraged to choose more sedentary activities. In today's society, males and females have more opportunities to choose the same activities, but preschool activities can also be geared to be gender neutral to encourage more female participation. Gender-neutral activities such as tag; hide and seek; kick ball; duck, duck, goose; Red Rover; and obstacle courses may encourage physical activity for both males and females. Two separate studies completed by Nilsen et al. (2019) investigated sex differences and environmental factors that may affect physical activity levels in Norwegian preschoolers. One study found that males were consistently more active than females and that physical activity increased with age (Nilsen et al., 2019). The second study's findings were consistent with the prior studies but also found that the preschool environment was beneficial for males to increase their level of moderate to vigorous physical activity (Nilsen et al., 2019).

A study in China examined preschool children aged 3 to 6 years and compared sedentary time and physical activity levels between sexes of the same age (Ma & Luo, 2023). Six-year-old males had significantly less sedentary activity and more physical activity at all intensity levels compared with females. Five-year-old males had significantly less sedentary activity and more low-intensity physical activity compared with females. Three- and 4-year-old males had significantly more moderate to vigorous and vigorous physical activities compared with females. A study in the southwestern region of the United States objectively examined the physical activity of preschool children using an accelerometer and found several demographic differences (Lee et al., 2022). Females, Hispanic/Latinx preschool children (see later section on race), and those with an at-risk weight level and/or below-average motor development engaged in less physical activity and more sedentary behavior while in a Head Start program.

Race

As is the case at all ages, the social construct of race, with related economic and cultural issues, may influence health care practices of preschool children. In a systematic review of outdoor play and time among children aged 3 to 12 years across 29 countries, common correlates included sex and race/ethnicity (Lee et al., 2021). This study used a socioecological modeling framework and found that female sex (see previous section on gender) was negatively correlated with outdoor play/time. However, membership in the dominant race/ethnic group was positively correlated with outdoor play/time (Lee et al., 2021).

Genetics

The signs and symptoms of most genetic problems appear during infancy or the toddler years, whereas other genetic problems will be noted during adolescence. Those most likely to appear during the preschool years are cystic fibrosis, Duchenne muscular dystrophy, fragile X syndrome, Williams syndrome, and autism, which is generally considered a genetic disorder with a high degree of heritability. In a recent summary of meta-analyses and systematic reviews, results consistently found that another genetic variant (MTHFR C667T) was a risk factor for autism spectrum disorder (Wei et al., 2021).

However, current research has only identified some genetic conditions that present with diagnosable early symptoms. Genetic conditions (Box 19.2: Genomics), if diagnosed early in life, can affect the child's health and well-being. Nursing strategies focus on continuing parent education, assessing the child's development, and providing interventions to support family coping.

BOX 19.2 GENOMICS

The field of cystic fibrosis (CF) has benefited from developments and advancements in genomics in terms of detection, understanding, and monitoring of the disease state. Infants with CF are structurally normal at birth; however, they have an inability to control bacterial infection, which plays a key role in early CF lung disease pathogenesis. Research and application of novel molecular techniques to explore the human microbiome has helped develop an understanding of CF airway microbiology and how it differs from those airways without the disease. The drug Ivacaftor was approved by the Food and Drug Administration (FDA) in 2012 for the treatment of patients with CF carrying at least one copy of the G551D mutation in the CF transmembrane conductance regulator gene (CFTR) (Silva, 2019). CF is caused by one of several defects in the CF transmembrane conductance regulator gene, which regulates fluid flow within cells and affects the components of sweat, digestive fluids, and mucus. The G551D mutation, in particular, is characterized by a dysfunctional CF transmembrane conductance regulator that cannot transport chloride through the ion channel. Ivacaftor increases the transport of chloride through the ion channel by binding and thus for the first time is able to treat the underlying cause of CF instead of its symptoms.

Since its initial approval by the FDA, Ivacaftor has been approved for use in patients 6 months and older for 9 specific genetic mutations and patients 18 years and older for 38 mutations as of May 2019. A recent meta-analysis of 57 studies from multiple countries on the effectiveness of Ivacaftor treatment in people with CF reported significant improvements in lung function, nutrition, and quality of life (Duckers et al., 2021). Additional positive findings include decreases in hospitalization, decreases in infection, reduced mortality, and reduced organ transplantation. The authors concluded that Ivacaftor treatment results in highly consistent and sustained benefits in people with CF across pulmonary and nonpulmonary outcomes.

GORDON'S FUNCTIONAL HEALTH PATTERNS

Health Perception–Health Management Pattern

Preschoolers have a fairly accurate perception of the external parts of their own bodies based on what they can see and do; they may be extremely curious about the body of a member of the opposite sex. Their concepts of what is inside the body and how its internal functions operate are vague and inaccurate. Most preschoolers can name one or two items inside the body (blood, bones). Many of their questions involve body functions. Anxiety surrounding the body and fear of mutilation and death pervade the children's concerns. Preschooler body size as compared with that of adults produces a sense of vulnerability and fear of loss of control.

By age 4 or 5 years, children have amassed their beliefs about health from the family. They begin to understand that they play a role in their own health. The preschooler often becomes upset over minor injuries. Pain or illness may be viewed as a punishment. The preschooler's declaration "If you don't put your seat belt on you will get in an accident" is a statement that reflects the idea of expected immediate and absolute cause and effect. The preschooler may not understand that the purpose of the seat belt is to prevent injury in the event of an accident, not prevention of the accident itself.

Although preschoolers are not completely responsible for their own health management, they positively contribute by brushing their teeth, taking medication, wearing appropriate clothing for inclement weather, and performing other actions. Childhood is an important time to learn healthy habits to establish a strong foundation for lifelong health and well-being (US Department of Health and Human Services [USDHHS], 2018).

Reinforcement of health-promotion activities, which occurs in the home and childcare environments, helps instill behaviors that affect self-esteem, safety, and an individual's overall balance with life. Adults play an important role in laying the foundation for lifelong, health-promoting physical activity by providing age-appropriate opportunities for physical activity (USDHHS, 2018). The National Association of Pediatric Nurse Associates and Practitioners (NAPNAP, 2006) published the Healthy Eating and Activity Together Clinical Practice Guideline (CPG), which provides family-centered recommendations to promote healthy weight in children and continues to be consistent with newer CPG recommendations focused on reducing childhood overweight and obesity (Davis et al., 2021; Gooey et al., 2022; Polfuss et al., 2020). NAPNAP further developed training resources to implement the CPG into practice for clinicians to engage families in health-promoting behaviors.

Policies and characteristics of the preschool environment, in addition to the type of physical activity encouraged, influences health-promotion activities for many children in this age group. Children who attend preschools with larger playgrounds with less fixed playground equipment and more portable playground equipment tend to use less electronic media and are more likely to be involved in moderate and vigorous activities. Frank et al. (2018) compared physical activity during free play and structured play recess periods and found that both conditions equally promoted increased levels of physical activity in preschoolers overall. However, they found that structured play may have limited the amount of physical activity for children who were highly active during free play but had a positive effect on children who were less active during free play. There is a need for health-promotion advocacy and policy development focused on the preschool playground environment. Many community bookstores carry health-promotion–focused books appropriate to the preschool population; these references provide information for discussion among parents, caregivers, and children on the importance of healthy behaviors for success in life.

Nutritional-Metabolic Pattern

Establishing healthful nutritional and physical activity behaviors begins during childhood. The 2015–2020 Dietary Guidelines for Americans released by the USDHHS outlines five guidelines and provides key recommendations for Americans of all ages to promote a healthy eating pattern (see Chapter 11). The following key recommendations should also be applied in conjunction with the *Physical Activity Guidelines for Americans, 2nd edition* (USDHHS, 2018) to help promote overall health. Children should consume a healthy eating pattern that accounts for all foods and beverages within an appropriate calorie level. Children aged 3 to 5 years old should receive 1000 to 1600 calories/day depending on their activity level and sex (US Department of Agriculture & USDHHS, 2015). According to the key recommendations, a healthy eating pattern includes a variety of vegetables from all of the subgroups—dark green, red and orange, legumes, starchy, and other; fruits, especially whole fruits; grains, at least half of which are whole grains; fat-free or low-fat dairy, including milk, yogurt, cheese, and/or fortified soy beverages; a variety of protein, including seafood, lean meats and poultry, eggs, legumes, nuts, seeds, and soy products; oils; and limited saturated fats and trans fats, added sugars, and sodium. Guidance for these recommendations along with the types and amounts of foods based on age, sex, and activity level is depicted in the system called *MyPlate* (US Department of Agriculture, n.d.) (https://www.myplate.gov). Healthy meal and snack ideas, tips for picky eaters, physical activity recommendations, and food safety tips can also be found on the MyPlate website to assist families in promoting healthy eating and activity habits. Information on healthy eating is also available for each age group on the Life Stages tab, from infants to older adults, as well as for pregnancy and for families.

Specific issues that affect the preschool age include bone growth, iron-deficiency anemia, milk intake, salt intake, sugar intake, and dentition. For bone growth, children aged 1 to 8 years require a calcium intake of approximately 700 to 1000 mg. Although the frequency of iron-deficiency anemia is decreasing generally, it is more prevalent in vulnerable populations. Iron deficiency is associated with behavioral and cognitive deficits, and iron supplementation may improve cognitive development in children aged 2 to 5 years old. Salt and sugar intake should be moderated to be consistent with the well-established association of sugar intake to dental caries. Two recent meta-analyses found that children with caries had significantly greater odds of iron-deficiency anemia (Easwaran et al., 2022; Ji et al., 2021).

Nutrition and dentition affect health at all ages. Pain from dental caries, infection, and poorly maintained teeth affects appetite and chewing ability, with a subsequent effect on future nutritional status. The frequency of dental caries in children has declined dramatically in recent years because of preventive measures, such as use of fluoride toothpaste, fluoridation of community water supplies, implementation of sound dietary practices, and use of dental sealants. Many studies have shown the strong relationship between low socioeconomic status and prevalence of dental caries in children. In addition, food insecurity is associated with dental caries in children, further supporting the effect of nutrition on oral health. Therefore public health **initiatives** should include nutrition-focused social and behavioral interventions as well as reinforcement of preventive oral health behaviors for vulnerable populations. A recent study by Sanjeevi et al. (2023) found that the Special Supplemental Nutrition Program for Women, Infants, and Children (WIC) mitigated the negative effects of food insecurity on oral health in preschool-aged children. Children in homes with food insecurities that were eligible for, but did not participate in, WIC had significantly higher odds of dental caries. In contrast, this relationship was not observed in children who participated in WIC, which suggests that supplemental nutrition programs can improve the oral health of children with food insecurities. Two recent meta-analyses also reported higher odds of dental caries in children with food insecurities (Bahanan et al., 2021; Sabbagh et al., 2023). The American Dental Association (2023) provides community resources (www.mouthhealthy.org) to educate families on proper nutrition to promote oral health and recommendations for home and professional dental care. Nurses interface with families in a variety of settings and are therefore in an ideal position to affect dental health promotion.

As early childhood progresses, intense food preferences can emerge. This behavior is a natural outgrowth of the increased physical capacity to react to the taste and textures of foods and the realization that expressing an opinion about food is a way to control the environment. Older preschoolers frequently refuse to try new foods. Favorite foods for this age are meat, cereal grains, baked products, fruits, and sweets. Parents should provide nutritious foods, avoiding salty and sweet foods. Examples of appropriate nutritional foods include cheese, crackers, small pieces of meat, and celery stuffed with cheese or peanut butter. Selecting finger foods that facilitate independence helps the preschooler learn to eat without assistance. Parents should encourage good nutritional habits to help establish healthy eating behaviors. Increased consumption of fats and processed foods along with diminished physical activity has contributed to a significant increase in the frequency of obesity and type 2 diabetes in children and adolescents. Family tolerance for individual food preferences differs, and children differ in their tendency to develop strong likes and dislikes. When families have extreme differences over food preferences, major conflicts may arise, requiring insightful counseling to achieve a mutually satisfying solution. For example, some families may institute a "take a little taste before you refuse" standard for foods at the preschool age. Nurses collaborate with families to discover comfortable approaches to maintaining nutritional adequacy of foods that children prefer. Community nurses use a variety of approaches and recognize the wide range of possibilities that exist for families of differing cultures.

Preschoolers begin to eat meals away from home more often than toddlers. Minimal standards require licensed childcare centers and preschools to serve foods using recommended dietary allowances of basic nutrients. Parents should communicate regularly with agency personnel about foods eaten at home and away from home to provide healthy food variety. Communication about nutritional intake habits reinforces positive behaviors and discourages negative habits at home. Preschoolers in group settings learn both positive and negative eating habits and food preferences from care providers and other children. School settings are ideal for community health nurses to affect the nutritional patterns of the preschool child.

Preschoolers struggle with the intricacies of using utensils. In the later years of the preschool period, children attain skill with spoons, demonstrate fair proficiency with forks, and manage knives for spreading soft foods on bread or crackers. Most preschool children, however, need help cutting meat and pouring liquids from large, heavy containers. Preschoolers enjoy helping prepare family meals and may be capable of simple tasks, such as washing fruits and vegetables. Involving young children in meal preparation teaches them about healthy nutrition and how to serve safe food (US Department of Agriculture, n.d.). Sharing important family functions nurtures self-esteem and a sense of value.

In a study of parent-reported childhood food allergies, the prevalence of food allergy in children in the United States was estimated at 7.6%, with 11.4% of parents believing that their child has a food allergy (Gupta, et al., 2018). Furthermore, approximately 42.3% of food-allergic children reported a severe reaction. Peanut, milk, egg, and tree nut allergies were the most prevalent allergies. There was also a difference reported between race and/or ethnicity, with African American children having significantly higher odds of confirmed food allergies compared with non-Hispanic White children (Gupta et al., 2018). A recent review on food allergies across the globe found that the incidence/prevalence is increasing in select regions of the world (Sampath et al., 2021).

A study by Du Toit et al. (2015) found that introduction of peanut-containing foods between 4 and 11 months of age in high-risk infants actually reduced the prevalence of peanut allergy at 5 years of age to a greater extent than avoidance of the allergen. Previous recommendations to avoid allergenic foods were withdrawn in 2008 (Du Toit et al., 2015). Caretaker and teacher education should include emphasizing symptoms that warrant treatment with epinephrine—for example, using EpiPen autoinjectors. Clear food labeling and education are essential for allergic reaction prevention. Many preschools have banned foods such as peanut products as a precautionary measure. Parents may need help identifying potential hazardous situations and communicating their child's needs to agency personnel. A food allergy action plan that includes a written emergency plan should be developed for parents to use to facilitate communication regarding their child's allergies.

Elimination Pattern

Toilet training is an important milestone in child development, as it is often the first opportunity for a child to independently manage an activity of daily living (American Academy of Pediatrics, 2018b). Children need to be developmentally ready for toilet training, both physically and emotionally, with multiple studies in the literature describing readiness signs, though there is no consensus on which signs to use. The American Academy of Pediatrics has developed an educational resource to assist families with toilet training, which includes articles such as "Toilet Training: 12 Tips to Keep the Process Positive" and "Create a Potty Training Plan for Your Child" among others on the subject matter (https://healthychildren.org/English/ages-stages/toddler/toilet-training/Pages/default.aspx).

Older preschool children are capable of and responsible for independent toileting. As their verbal skills have developed to better communicate their needs, they begin to insist on performing this skill independently, and they are proud of their accomplishments. They may forget to flush the toilet or wash their hands when they are rushed, but they have the physical ability to perform the skills. Preschoolers should not be teased or punished when they are unable to perform toileting independently. If their clothing becomes soiled, they should be responsible for changing their clothes and reminded gently and encouragingly of ways to avoid problems in the future. (Enuresis and encopresis are discussed in Chapter 20.)

Activity-Exercise Pattern

Play continues to be the primary activity for preschoolers as well as for toddlers; however, preschoolers explore intently and demonstrate increased coordination and confidence in motor activities. Preschoolers enjoy using language skills to tell stories and ask questions. Their physical capabilities include balancing on one foot, jumping, and running. In general, most 4-year-old children separate easily from their parents, play simple interactive games, dress themselves, copy a number of basic geometrical figures well, and draw recognizable people. At this age many activities involve other children (Fig. 19.1) and involve modeling behavior. Particularly in group care settings, children should be monitored for safe activities that enhance gross and fine motor skills while promoting engagement and movement. Generally, preschoolers appreciate an audience, enjoy practicing new skills, and demonstrate mastered skills to others.

Play is essential for development by promoting social-emotional, cognitive, language, and self-regulation skills that are important to build executive functioning skills. Play also promotes problem-solving, collaboration, and creativity. It provides children with the opportunity to have fun while taking risks, experimenting, and testing boundaries, allowing them to actively engage in meaningful discovery (Yogman et al., 2018). For preschoolers, play constitutes an important part of their cognitive, social, physical, and psychological development. Play offers a vehicle that allows them to explore while experimenting with who they are, who they might become, and how they relate to others socially. The drama of play allows preschoolers to view themselves from another perspective. Play often reveals the child's reality and complex perception of the world.

Children mimic the behavior of people familiar to them, expanding their representation beyond self and rehearsing what has been demonstrated to them as appropriate behavior. Young children seldom assume the role of a younger child or infant while playing. They usually assume adult roles and use a doll for the younger child. Through play preschoolers learn to exert control over their own behavior. Assuming an adult role in play allows children to consciously adopt more mature behaviors.

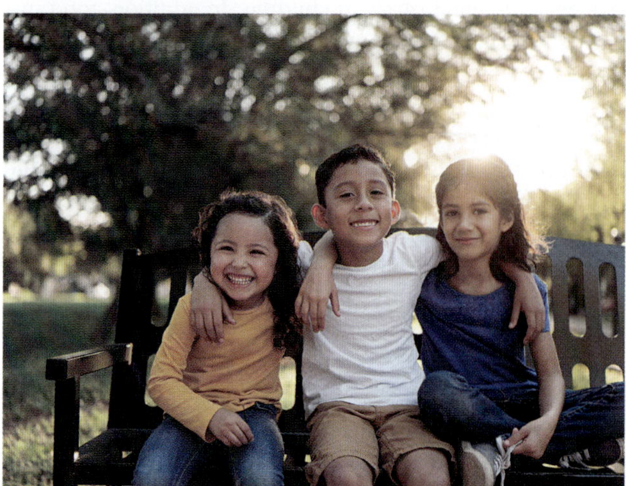

FIG. 19.1 Preschool children can enjoy activities with other children. (From iStock.com/aldomurillo)

Patterns of behavior used in play can be transferred to actual situations. For example, children who express their anger in a play situation aggressively by vocalizing their distress, scolding the offending party, or using withdrawal of attention are likely to respond with aggression or tantrum behavior when facing frustration or anger in real-life situations.

Preschool children engage in more interactive play, particularly dramatic play, than at any other age. Two or more children may become involved in an imaginary plot, especially when toys and equipment support a particular scenario, such as toy kitchen equipment. Patterns emerge in the interactive processes of play: initiating, deciding with whom to play, play themes/roles/rules, and finally enactment or collaborative pretending. This pretend play encourages self-regulation because through this process children must collaborate on the imaginary environment and agree about pretending and conforming to roles (Yogman et al., 2018).

Observing children at play reveals natural physical capacities of children better than observation in an examination or testing environment and provides further evidence of the child's social and inner development. Observing symbolic play and pretend play in peer groups helps nurses assess social competency as the children's perceptions unfold. In addition, much of the preschooler's play involves fantasy and imaginative play. The young child frequently invents an imaginary companion who plays, eats, and sleeps with the child. The Cognitive-Perceptual Pattern section addresses more fully the aspects of fantasy during the preschool stage; however, the goal of symbolic or pretend play is to derive meaning from the play experience using the knowledge and skills acquired. The play is a way to integrate previously learned ideas and skills.

Most preschoolers spend some time in a group setting each week. Ground rules at these facilities govern sharing, quiet times, and group activities. Although time orientation remains incompletely developed in preschoolers, they have some concept of past and future. They enjoy planning activities with their parents for the future. Visiting the library to review books about wild animals, packing lunches, and choosing what clothes to wear may preface a trip to the zoo.

The preschooler regulates body activities with more purpose and copes with limit setting better than the toddler but has much energy and requires outlets for this energy throughout the day. The young child requires physical activity for energy expenditure. Physical activity in the preschool child is not typically structured exercises. Children do not usually need formal muscle-strengthening programs, such as lifting weights. Younger children usually strengthen their muscles through play activities, such as climbing on a jungle gym or trees; riding a balance bike, bicycle, or tricycle; playing ball; and running/jumping with parents and peers. Becker and colleagues (2014) investigated whether active play during recess was associated with self-regulation and academic achievement in prekindergarten children. The results revealed that higher active play was associated with better self-regulation and higher scores on early reading and math assessments. Nurses should encourage parents to engage the preschool child in active, locomotor, and rough-and-tumble play. Parents and childcare directors/school administrators should also encourage physical activity and work together to overcome perceived barriers that might limit the young child's ability to access physical activity.

In 2018 the USDHHS released the *Physical Activity Guidelines for Americans, 2nd edition*, which was revised to include physical activity recommendations for the preschool child. Box 19.3: Best Practice outlines these recommendations and provides play activity ideas to promote muscle strengthening and bone strengthening, as well as examples of moderate- and vigorous-intensity aerobic activity.

Despite the recommendations and reported benefits of physical activity, many preschoolers spend long periods each day in front of a screen while immersed in electronic media (watching television, watching videos, playing electronic games, and using smartphone/tablet applications). Although there are some excellent television, video, and electronic game programs and applications available for preschoolers, use of these forms of media often encourages passivity rather than active learning and socially interactive play. Young childcare specialists tend to agree that social media, electronic games, television, videos and other types of digital entertainment disengage the child's mind and contribute to less learning (see Chapter 20).

BOX 19.3 BEST PRACTICE

Physical Activity Guidelines for Americans, 2nd Edition: Recommendations for the Preschool-Aged Child

Key Guidelines for Preschool-Aged Children

- Preschool-aged children (ages 3 through 5 years) should be physically active through the day to enhance growth and development.
- Adult caregivers of preschool-aged children should encourage active play that includes a variety of activity types.

Preschool-aged children should be encouraged to move and engage in active play as well as structured activities. It is recommended that preschoolers engage in about 3 hours of activity per day, to include light, moderate, and vigorous intensity, in an effort to improve bone health and avoid excess fat. Activities should be age appropriate, with examples in the following list:

Moderate- and vigorous-intensity aerobic activity:

- Games such as tag or follow the leader
- Playing on the playground
- Tricycle or bicycle riding
- Walking, running, skipping, jumping, dancing
- Swimming
- Playing games that require catching, throwing, and kicking
- Gymnastics or tumbling

Muscle-strengthening activity:

- Games such as tug of war
- Climbing on playground equipment
- Gymnastics

Bone strengthening activity:

- Hopping, skipping, jumping
- Jumping rope
- Running
- Gymnastics

Modified from US Department of Health and Human Services (USDHHS). (2018). *Physical activity guidelines for Americans, 2nd edition.* https://www.health.gov/our-work/physical-activity/current-guidelines

Yogman et al. (2018) described research comparing the skills of preschoolers who played with blocks independently with preschoolers watching Baby Einstein tapes. They found that those children actively engaged in play developed better language and cognitive skills. In addition, many electronic entertainment options focus on adult themes and violence. Parents should remember that preschoolers who rely on television, videos, and electronic games for entertainment do not have enough life experiences to interpret many of the issues presented in adult shows (violence, interpersonal relationships, moral decisions) and cannot judge which shows are appropriate for them. Parents should choose which electronic devices and activities are appropriate for their child, limiting time and promoting physical activity in lieu of screen time and sedentary play. A recent meta-analysis found that higher levels of screen time in the evening was associated with shorter sleep duration, later bedtime, and lower quality of sleep in preschool children (Janssen et al., 2020). Furthermore, taking time to share activities provides the child with an opportunity for discussion and for the child to ask questions. Nurses should explain to parents and preschoolers the relationship between watching television/screen time and lack of physical activity that leads to health problems such as obesity. Family support for engaging in physical activity has been shown to affect children's health-promoting behaviors. In a longitudinal childhood obesity prevention study of children aged 2 to 5 years, researchers examined the effects of screen time parenting practices on the weight status of their children (Neshteruk et al., 2021). There was an association between parents who limited/monitored screen time and weekly viewing time (decreased) and body weight (i.e., decreased BMI and smaller waist circumference). These findings suggest that screen time parenting practices can reduce screen time and promote healthy weight in children.

Sleep-Rest Pattern

The National Sleep Foundation (2023) and American Academy of Sleep Medicine (Paruthi et al., 2016; Ramar et al., 2021) recommend that preschoolers sleep 10 to 13 hours per 24-hour period (including naps) on a regular basis to promote optimal health. Electronic device use can have a negative effect on children's sleep, with those children who spend a lot of time in front of a screen tending to go to bed later, take longer to fall asleep, and sleep fewer hours. On average children lose about 26.4 minutes of sleep per hour of tablet device use (National Sleep Foundation, 2023). Regularly sleeping less than the recommended duration is associated with attention, behavior, and learning difficulties, while regularly sleeping the recommended duration is associated with better health outcomes. These outcomes include improved attention, behavior, learning, memory, emotional regulation, quality of life, and mental and physical health.

A nap may not be necessary for many older preschoolers, as 50% of children stop napping by age 4 and 70% by age 5 (National Sleep Foundation, 2023). Instead of napping, the National Sleep Foundation encourages quiet time, which can provide a welcome respite for the parent and a chance for the active preschooler to relax before afternoon activities. Many childcare/preschool environments routinely provide quiet time, enhancing rest and relaxation with soft music and a story. An afternoon rest also gives the young child energy for the evening routine, when family members have other duties beyond work and school.

Sleep time habits, falling asleep, and waking up during the night present challenges for families with preschool children (National Sleep Foundation, 2023). The preschooler's expanded imaginative play and increased physical activity during the day may provoke nighttime fears, **nightmares**, sleepwalking, and sleep terrors, which are at a peak during this stage of development (National Sleep Foundation, 2023).

Bedtime Ritual

Preschoolers usually require a routine at bedtime to move from playing and being with others to being alone and falling asleep. Bedtime routines provide a sense of predictability that helps with these transitions and moderates impulsivity and self-regulation. Bedtime routines should not last longer than 30 to 45 minutes; however, preschool-age children prolong bedtime routines more often than toddlers. They insist on sleeping with the light on or taking a treasured object to bed, request parental attention after being told good night, and experience delays falling asleep. Bedtime routines typically involve the same few relaxing activities with parents honoring reasonable rituals, but repeated requests for attention afterward are handled firmly and consistently. Consistent sleep hygiene, which includes bedtime routine, is associated with less resistance at bedtime and may reduce resistance in children with difficult temperaments. Vigorous resistance to bedtime challenges parents more during the preschool period than at any other developmental stage. Behavioral insomnia in children occurs when this resistance is associated with a negative association with sleep (Owens et al., 2017). Preschoolers learn to use the behaviors that meet their needs and control the family regardless of the disruption created.

Nursing Interventions

When a demanding bedtime behavior extends beyond 1 year or an episode persists longer than 1 hour, the nurse explores the family situation. A comprehensive assessment in this case includes the following elements:

- Description of early episodes
- The manner in which these early episodes were managed and the progression of events since then
- Current bedtime behaviors of the child and siblings
- Identification of parental temperament and the resulting responses of the parents and family members
- Feelings of the parents and child about each other and about the bedtime situation
- Stressful events and changes that have occurred in the past several years
- Behavior of the child at other times of the day
- Parents' thoughts about the reasons why these episodes continue
- Parents' ideas about strategies to use now

The nurse observes interactions within the family. A home visit at mealtime provides an excellent method to observe active interaction. In the office or clinic setting, the nurse can ask a parent to teach the child a task or give directions. The nurse remains as unobtrusive as possible while observing the interaction. The first-hand observation of parent-child interaction, along with the detailed history, usually provides the nurse with adequate baseline information to decide whether to manage the situation in the primary care setting or to refer the family to a child behavior specialist. Laukkanen et al. (2014) examined the association between children's temperament and mothers' parenting styles and found that difficult temperaments affected maternal well-being, which subsequently affected the mothers' parenting styles. This potential effect is important to note when observing interactions within the family. Parents may benefit from education on their child's temperament characteristics and strategies to handle their behaviors in adaptive ways (Laukkanen et al., 2014). Parents' psychological well-being is also important in preventing dysfunctional parent-child interactions. The findings from a study of more than 1500 children by Prior et al. (2011) support that temperament in children may be somewhat modifiable and that parents may consider strategies to influence their preschooler's behavior that focus on their temperament. Sharing recent literature about management techniques for children with differing temperaments helps families understand more about the behaviors. Research-based strategies should be used to help parents reach their goals related to managing bedtime concerns.

Sleep Disturbances

Night terrors (or sleep terrors) and nightmares characterize the nighttime wakening problems that generally occur during the preschool years. Night terrors are most common in children aged 4 to 12 years old and manifest themselves as frightening dreams that cause fear, agitation, and confusion, with children misperceiving and unresponsive to their environment. The child may sit up in bed, scream, stare at an imaginary object, breathe heavily, perspire, and appear in obvious distress (see Chapter 18). The child, not fully awake, may be inconsolable for 10 minutes or more before relaxing and returning to a deep sleep. In most cases the child does not recall the dream and in the morning does not remember the incident. A review by Leung et al. (2020) summarizes the recent evidence on the clinical manifestations, diagnosis, and management of night terrors. **Nightmares** (anxiety dreams) are a more common cause of night wakening. Although infants and toddlers likely have nightmares, their limited verbal skills hinder their relating of details of the incidents. After age 3 years, nightmares occur more frequently, occurring in 1.9% to 3.9% of preschool-age children (Bathory & Tomopoulos, 2017). Dreams frighten preschoolers as they connect to the larger world with their active imaginations and fantastic ideas. These children can waken fully and feel fearful and helpless. Usually they provide vivid descriptions at the time, and they frequently remember the event the following morning. Consolation can be given by a parent who sits with the child, listens to descriptions and fears about the dream, and reminds the child that dreaming is natural and sleep will soon return. Management may include avoidance of frightening television shows, games, books, or movies, as well as maintaining good sleep hygiene with regular routines and adequate sleep.

Helping children appreciate the meaning of the words *pretend* and *real* facilitates growth during this phase of childhood. When the parent reads a story to the child or the child tells a make-believe tale, the parents can specify that these are "pretend" and did not really happen. The parent relating a true event can say, "This is real." Children differentiate between the two concepts as they develop cognitively. This differentiation may help parents console a child following a nightmare.

Recommendations

Parents of a preschooler can benefit from knowing the following:

- Bedtime routines of 30 to 45 minutes are common for preschoolers. These routines, because of their importance to children, should be respected within reasonable limits. Maintaining a regular, consistent, and relaxing routine facilitates sleep and encourages good sleep hygiene (National Sleep Foundation, 2023).
- Limit overall daily screen time, and power off electronic devices at least an hour before bedtime (National Sleep Foundation, 2023).
- Night-wakening events are common during the preschool years. A consistent sleep environment with the same bed in a room that is cool, quiet, and dark without a television promotes sleep (National Sleep Foundation, 2023). Children who waken at night are reassured and encouraged to return to sleep.
- Parents have clear rules about children sleeping with them if the children will not stay in their own beds.
- Restricting the watching of frightening television shows and the reading of frightening stories and discussing "real" versus "pretend" ideas and stories can help lessen the incidence of nightmares.

Cognitive-Perceptual Pattern

During the preschool years, children cultivate their conceptual and cognitive capacities. The quality of the child's care environment enhances these gains. Family and cultural values influence preschoolers' perceptions of and reactions to events. Internalization of family rules has been associated with social competency in this age group. Preschoolers gradually differentiate today from yesterday and define tomorrow and the future more clearly as concepts of time emerge. The child becomes more oriented in space and develops an awareness of the location of the home within the neighborhood. The child also begins to structure daily activities and to value certain activities, objects, and people above others.

Piaget's Theory

The older toddler enters the first substage of the **preoperational stage** described by Jean Piaget (1950, 1959). The hallmark of this preconceptual substage includes the ability to function symbolically using language. The preschool child demonstrates increased symbolic functioning during the intuitive substage, from 4 to 7 years of age. The predominant feature of this and the following period is the concrete thought process, as compared with adult abstract thinking. As they experience symbolic mental representations, preschoolers process mental symbols as though they were actually participating in the event. Adults analyze and synthesize symbolic information without concrete connections between the mental process and the actual event. At this stage, mental abstraction, such as skipping from one part of an operation to another, reversing the operation mentally, or thinking of the whole in relation to the parts, is not feasible.

The **egocentrism** that is characteristic of the preschool years exemplifies this concept of concrete thinking. At this stage, children concentrate solely on their own perspective. They consider only their own personal meanings for symbols. The preschooler wonders why another person fails to follow these idiosyncratic communications.

Furthermore, attention focuses solely on one part of an object without shifting. This behavior, termed **centering** by Piaget, illustrates the child's inability to consider more than one factor at a time when solving simple problems. For example, a child can be given two identical cups containing equal amounts of water and asked which cup contains the greater amount of water. During the preoperational stage, the child responds that they contain the same amount of water. The child is then asked to pour the water from each cup into two different containers (one flat and wide, the other tall and narrow). When asked which container has more water, the child always identifies one. The child usually selects the taller, narrower container with water at the higher height. When the water is again transferred to the identical cups and the experiment is repeated, the child returns to the original conclusion that the amounts are equal.

This experiment also illustrates the trait of **irreversibility**. The child is unable to connect the reversible operation, the transfer of the water back into the original cup, to reach the logical conclusion that the differently shaped containers may hold the same amount of water. The child cannot mentally associate that the transformation from one state to another relates to the shape of the container, not the amount of the water.

Finally, Piaget (1959) describes the preoperative stage of thinking as **transductive reasoning**. The child cannot proceed from general to particular (**deduction**) or from particular to general (**induction**); rather, the child moves only from particular to particular in making associations and solving problems. For example, Piaget relates an association made by one of his children between being hunchbacked and being ill. When a hunchbacked neighbor was unable to visit one day because he had a communicable illness, the child understood that the neighbor was ill. However, when the child was told later that the neighbor was better and that she could go see him, her conclusion was that now his hunched back was straight and well. She thought in terms of the male being well or ill, but she placed the male in one or the other category and assumed that he possessed all the attributes and meanings that she linked symbolically with either trait.

The cognitive development of preschoolers is reflected in their symbolic games, which become significantly more orderly and representative of reality (Box 19.4). They begin to incorporate the reality of the world as it exists outside the self. They increasingly seek play objects that represent models of authentic objects in their environment. Preschoolers increasingly imitate social rules in their play. Social interactive play predominates as the young child develops a more secure sense of self.

BOX 19.4 Play as a Method of Learning: Preschool Child

Throughout life, play develops cognitive, affective, and psychomotor skills that are important for the effective performance of life skills. For the preschool child, the following play activities provide the foundation for later competency and socialization-skill refinement:

- Arts and crafts (jewelry making, painting, drawing, ceramics, printmaking)
- Group sports (softball, volleyball, soccer, swimming)
- Skating, skateboarding
- Bicycling
- Puzzles
- Gymnastics
- Games (board, card, knock-knock jokes, computer)
- Secret clubs
- Imaginary play (being in playhouse productions)
- Horseback riding

Preschoolers may have one or more imaginary companions (or friends) who exist for differing periods. These fantasy companions assume the form of another child, an animal, or some other friendly or fearsome creature. Preschoolers may save special chairs, insist that an extra place be set at the table, and talk at length to this companion. Imaginary companions serve an important function; they are controlled totally by the child and are not a threat. In this way the preschooler practices social interactions, controls a fearsome beast, or blames someone for naughty behavior without fear of being scolded, shamed, or attacked. Imaginary companions do and say only what the child wills.

Vision

Vision capabilities, which are well developed by 2 years of age, continue to undergo refinement during the early childhood period. By approximately age 6 years, the child should approach a 20/20 visual acuity level. The possibility of developing **amblyopia** (or "lazy eye" when vision in one or both eyes does not develop properly during childhood) decreases; it appears most frequently during infancy through approximately the fourth year. Depth perception and color vision become fully established, and the child recognizes subtle differences in color shading by the sixth year. Maximal visual capability is usually achieved by the end of the preschool years.

Visual capacity throughout the rest of life deteriorates rather than improves. This phenomenon relates partly to changes in the refractive power of the lens and developmental changes that occur in the shape of the eyeball. In the normal sequence of growth, the eyeball becomes increasingly spherical, losing the short shape typical of infancy and progressing to the point at which light converges accurately on the surface of the retina. This change occurs at approximately 6 years of age. When this change occurs before the sixth year, growth continues past the point of ideal light conversion, the eyeball lengthens, and the child may develop early **myopic vision**, which will progress with age. Glasses are always indicated for the child who develops myopia before approximately age 8 years.

Early detection requires regular screening with standardized tests such as the Denver Eye Screening Test or the **Snellen Screening Test**. The Snellen Screening Test, when administered under standardized procedures, has the advantage of rendering a reliable estimate of actual visual acuity (Hockenberry et al., 2024). The child must be able to understand the test requirements of either pointing in the direction of the *E* or naming the letters. The Denver Eye Screening Test was designed for preschool children and includes detection of commonly occurring visual problems, such as **refractive errors**, **strabismus** (crossing of the eyes), and amblyopia.

The Prevent Blindness organization recommends regular vision screening of children by health care providers, educators, or public health programs (Prevent Blindness, n.d.). It is not recommended that parents take on the role of vision screener. Children who do not pass a vision screen should be taken to an optometrist or ophthalmologist for examination. The pupillary light reflex provides a screening approach for **heterotropia**, a condition in which the child's eyes do not focus together to transmit effective, coordinated binocular vision. When the child has heterotropia, the light from a penlight held approximately 20 inches from the eyes reflects off the pupil slightly off center. Consistent and observable strabismus may be noted. The cover test provides further evidence of a tendency for the child's eyes to cross, known as **heterophoria**. The child focuses on a spot 14 inches away, then 20 feet away. As the child gazes at the designated spot, one eye is covered completely for several seconds (the eye and eyelashes must not be touched), and then the cover is removed abruptly. If the covered eye moves from the line of vision of the uncovered eye, that eye has a tendency toward muscle imbalance and must be evaluated further.

Color blindness presents a particular problem for younger children because many cues encountered at school depend on the child's ability to distinguish colors. With early detection the child is able to receive assistance to interpret visual cues, thus minimizing the disadvantage of being color blind. The nurse screens the child for certain types of color discrimination difficulties by asking the child to respond to various colors in the environment; however, accurate testing for all types of color blindness requires a specialized tool, such as the **Ishihara test**, which uses a series of cards with color-tinted letters and figures.

Preschoolers may be aware of some discomfort or limitations with vision. The nurse gathers the history from the parents, including the questions listed in the Vision section in Chapter 18, about signs of eye problems.

The preschooler is asked questions to elicit information about the following symptoms:

- Itching, burning, or "scratchy" eyes
- Poor vision
- Dizziness, headaches, or nausea after close eye work
- Blurred or double vision

Refractive error can be significant in the preschool child. The prevalence of refractive errors (5%–7%) and amblyopia (2%–4%) in preschool children places vision loss as an important public health concern. Screening tests, while important, are not able to diagnose a vision disorder or create a treatment plan (Prevent Blindness, n.d.). Children younger than 7 years with amblyopia demonstrate significant improvement in vision when treated, providing a rationale for early screening and recognition programs. The American Academy of Pediatrics (AAP) online resources supply information for nurses and families and can be accessed at http://www.healthychildren.org.

Sensory Perception

Sensory abilities contribute to preschoolers' skills of perceiving and interacting with the world. Both sensory acuity and sensory perceptual abilities mature during the preschool years. The nature of the visual stimulus determines the response. Preschoolers respond powerfully to visual illusions and have difficulty discriminating between right and left mirror images. Confusion commonly occurs with the letters *b*, *d*, *p*, and *q*.

Hearing

Hearing sounds and words has profound implications for children's development. During the preschool years, hearing develops to the level of an adult, when the ability to attend to and interpret what is heard becomes more refined. Preschoolers with normal hearing will respond when a parent or caregiver calls from another room and to environmental sounds (e.g., phone notifications, water turning on, birds chirping). Hearing loss can lead to speech and language delays, academic problems, and difficulty making friendships (Findlen et al., 2019). It is generally accepted that the hearing ability of preschoolers can be hindered by repeated middle ear infections (otitis media). Otitis media with effusion can occasionally result in temporary hearing loss. Parents who notice language delays because of ear infections should be referred to their health care provider for appropriate follow-up care for their children (Hockenberry et al., 2024). Parental reports of difficulty should be taken seriously. If families express concerns about their child's hearing, they should be referred for a hearing test (Findlen et al., 2019). Hearing screenings may be available through local early intervention programs or health departments (American Speech-Language-Hearing Association, 2024).

Audiometric methods most accurately measure the child's ability to hear. Preschool children possess the developmental capability to perform the standard audiometric test (e.g., pure tone test). The child can follow directions by this age, and most preschoolers enjoy demonstrating their abilities and cooperate easily during vision and hearing screening examinations (Hockenberry et al., 2024).

To ensure success, the nurse encourages a positive experience by adhering to the following points:

- Use equipment skillfully.
- Use age-appropriate language.
- Avoid the word test to limit anxiety or fear of failure.
- Encourage the child to ask questions and scrutinize the equipment.
- Perform screening before other intrusive or painful procedures.

- Perform screening in a quiet, private area without distractions.
- Praise the child for cooperating.
- Allow rest periods when the child becomes distracted or tired.
- Discuss results with the child in age-appropriate language.

Language

Speech Sound Development. During the preschool period, there is a wide range in children's ability to articulate different speech sounds. Families may express concern regarding their children's ability to articulate or pronounce certain words, but some articulation errors are developmental and can resolve without intervention. By age 3, 90% of children use the following sounds correctly: "m," "h," "w," "p," and "b." By age 4, 90% of children use the following sounds correctly: "n," "t," "d," "k," "g," and "f." By age 6, 90% of children use the following sounds correctly: "v," "th," and "l." Other single sounds and sound blends continue to develop during preschool ages and early school age. Speech sound disorders are developmental disorders consisting of articulation or phonologic impairment that impedes a child's ability to be understood by adults and is not due to cognitive, sensory, physical, or motor impairments. Nearly 1 in 12 (7.7%) US children aged 3 to 17 years has had a disorder related to voice, speech, language, or swallowing in the past 12 months (NIDCD, 2024). If a child's articulation errors persist beyond the developmental norms listed previously or affect their ability to be understood, refer the child for a speech-language evaluation.

Receptive and Expressive Language. Children continue to develop their **receptive language** skills, or their ability to understand and comprehend spoken language, during the preschool period. Receptive language skills are important to the development of the preschool child's social, academic, and literacy skills. Their receptive vocabulary is larger than their expressive vocabulary, or the words they use when communicating with others. Preschoolers can also follow instructions with two or three steps ("Go get your pajamas and put them in the hamper"). By age 5 they will be able to understand most of what they hear at home and at school (ASHA, 2020). As children's vocabularies and receptive language skills develop, they can attend to longer stories and conversations with adults. Table 19.2 outlines the receptive and **expressive language** skills of preschoolers. Preschool-aged children begin to express themselves with longer and more grammatically complex sentences. They will use pronouns (*I*, *you*, *me*, *we*) and plural words. They can tell short stories and have conversations with other children and adults.

Many children who exhibit early delays during toddlerhood may catch up with their peers during the preschool period. Although children's language skills have wide variability during the preschool years, it is critical for nurses to continue to monitor developmental delays such as difficulty understanding simple instructions or identifying common objects and actions in pictures. As nurses help parents provide anticipatory guidance for language development, they should maintain vigilance to identify those children who are not outgrowing their language difficulties. These children encounter lifelong obstacles with learning and socialization. Suggestions for nurses to assist parents and to facilitate preschoolers' language development are listed in Box 19.5.

Memory

Memory plays an important role in language development and learning in general. At the preschool level, children label pictures, group objects, and mimic others as ways to aid memory, performing these tasks with less precision than the older child. Younger children benefit from suggestions about how to group items using characteristics to remember. Preschoolers remember pictures better by saying the names of pictures rather than by simply hearing the name of a picture when it is first shown. Preschoolers do not spontaneously use rehearsal or other **mnemonic techniques** for remembering, but they do use and benefit from rehearsal when it is suggested. The nurse tests memory by asking the child to repeat an arbitrary sequence of numbers. By approximately age 5 years, children are able to repeat four consecutively named numbers easily.

Developmental Surveillance and Screening. Early identification of developmental and emotional disorders is critical to the well-being of children and is an integral function and appropriate responsibility of all pediatric health care professionals. Approximately 10% to 20% of children aged 3 to 17 in the United States have one or more developmental or behavioral disabilities (Ogundele, 2018). Although there has been significant progress in the early identification and treatment of children with developmental and behavioral disorders in the past decade, many children with developmental disabilities are still not identified until they are in school and therefore miss the opportunity for early intervention. High-quality early intervention for children with developmental delay or who are at risk for delay can reduce the incidence of future problems with a child's learning, behavior, and health. It is recommended that children who may need services be identified as early as possible to provide intervention when the brain is developing and most capable of change. This has the potential to positively influence the child's developmental trajectory and improve outcomes for families, children, and communities (CDC, 2020a; Center on the Developing Child at Harvard University, 2010).

The AAP recommends a system of regular **developmental surveillance** and periodic **developmental screening** of all children to identify neurodevelopmental and behavioral conditions that may affect a child's early and long-term development. *Developmental surveillance* is defined as "the process of recognizing who may be at risk for developmental delays" and is recommended as part of every well-child visit. Surveillance is a collaborative process that should involve communication with early childhood professionals. Developmental screening is a more formal process that is defined as "the use of standardized tools to identify and refine that recognized risk." It is recommended that screening take place as part of the 9-, 18-, and 30-month well-child visits. In addition, specific screening for autism spectrum disorder (ASD) should be performed at the 18- and 24-month visits. Surveillance should continue through childhood, and it is recommended that surveillance occur at the 4- and 5-year well-child visit, as it may be particularly important before entry into elementary education.

TABLE 19.2 **Landmarks of Speech, Language, and Hearing Ability During the Preschool Period**

Age (Months)	Receptive Language	Expressive Language	Related Hearing Ability
42	Up to 4200 words; knows words such as *what, where, how, funny, we, surprise, secret;* knows number concepts to two; knows how to answer some questions accurately, such as: Do you have a dog? Which is the girl? What toys do you have?	Up to 1200 words in mostly complete sentences averaging four to five words per sentence; uses all 50 phonemes; 7% of sentences are compound or complex; averages 203 words per hour; rate of speech is accelerating; relates experiences and tells about activities in sequential order; uses words such as *what, where, how, see, little, funny, they, we, he, she, several;* can recite a nursery rhyme; asks permission; 95% of speech is intelligible	
48	Up to 5600 words; carries out three-item commands consistently; knows why people have houses, books, umbrellas, keys; knows nearly all colors; knows words such as *somebody, anybody, even, almost, now, something, like, bigger, too,* full name, one or two songs, number concepts to four; understands most preschool stories; can complete opposite analogies such as brother is a boy, sister is a girl and in daytime it is light and at night it is dark	Up to 1500 words in sentences averaging five to six words per sentence; averages 400 words per hour; counts up to three, repeats four digits, names three objects, repeats nine-word sentences from memory; names the primary colors, some coins; relates fanciful tales; enjoys rhyming nonsense words and using exaggerations; demands reasons why and how; questioning is at a peak, up to 500 questions a day; passes judgment on own activity; can recite a poem from memory or sing a song; uses words such as *even, almost, something, like, but;* typical expressions might include "I'm so tired," "You almost hit me," "Now I'll make something else"	Begins to make fine discriminations among similar speech sounds, such as the difference between "f" and "th" or "f" and "s"; has matured enough to be tested with an audiometer; formal hearing testing can usually be done; not only has hearing developed to its optimal level, but listening has also become considerably refined
54	Up to 6500 words; knows what materials a house, window, chair, and dress are made of and what people do with eyes and ears; understands differences in texture and composition, such as hard, soft, rough, smooth; begins to name or point to penny, nickel, dime; understands *if, because, why, when*	Up to 1800 words in sentences averaging five to six words; now averages only 230 words per hour—is satisfied with less verbalization; does little commanding or demanding; likes surprises; approximately 1 in 10 sentences are compound or complex, and only 8% of sentences are incomplete; can define 10 common words and count up to 20; common expressions are "I don't know," "I said," "tiny," "funny," "because"; asks questions for information and learns to manipulate and control people and situations with language	
60	Up to 9600 words; knows number concepts to five; knows and names colors; defines words in terms of use, such as a *bike* is to *ride*; defines *wind, ball, hat, stove*; understands qualifiers such as *if, because, when;* knows purpose of horse, fork, and legs; begins to understand *left* and *right*	Up to 2200 words in sentences averaging six words; can define *ball, hat, stove, policeman, wind, horse, fork*; can count five objects and repeat four or five digits; definitions are in terms of use; can single out a word and ask its meaning; makes serious inquiries—"What is this for?" "How does this work?" "Who made those?" "What does it mean?"; language is now essentially complete in structure and form; uses all types of sentences, clauses, and parts of speech; reads by way of pictures, and prints simple words	

Modified from Hockenberry, M. J., Duffy, E., & Gibbs, K. (2024). *Wong's nursing care of infants and children* (12th ed.). Elsevier.

BOX 19.5 Nursing Suggestions to Encourage Language Development in Preschoolers

- Read to the child. Encourage the child to be an active listener. Pause during the story to ask questions, such as "What do you think will happen next?" "Why do you think the boy said that?" and "What would you do now?" Praise the child's storytelling and creativity with stories.
- Always respond to the child's questions. Occasionally a response must be delayed; for example, when the parent is driving in heavy traffic and the child asks a question that requires a complex answer, the parent might say, "That's a very good question; let's talk about that as soon as we get home." The parent should remind the child of the question later and respond if the child still expresses interest.
- Never tease or criticize a child about speaking style. If the child speaks so fast as to be fumbling over words, then the parent might say, "I can't listen that fast. Slow down a little for me." This is much more encouraging than is the statement "You talk too fast. No one can understand you."
- Play language-focused games, such as naming the colors of houses or kinds of flowers as parent and child walk to the store.
- Look at pictures from magazines, books, or personal photos and encourage your child to make up a story.

If any developmental concerns emerge with surveillance at any point, screening should be performed with a standardized tool, or the child should be referred to developmental and/or medical specialists for further evaluation. Early developmental intervention/early childhood services should also be initiated if necessary. Formal evaluation by developmental and/or medical specialists are needed to identify and diagnose specific developmental conditions (Lipkin & Macias, 2020; CDC, 2020b; CDC, 2020c). The AAP's *Bright Futures, Fourth Edition* outlines how to provide surveillance and screening throughout the first 5 years of life (Hagan, et al., 2017). The AAP's Screening Technical Assistance Resource Center (STAR) (AAP: STAR Center, 2024) has more information about how health care professionals can use evidence-based screening tools to review the child's development in a more systematic way (https://www.aap.org/en/patient-care/screening-technical-assistance-and-resource-center). Additionally, the CDC's "Learn the Signs. Act Early" campaign provides additional tools for parents and professionals to track healthy child development (CDC, 2020g) (https://www.cdc.gov/ncbddd/actearly/index.html).

Autism Spectrum Disorders. ASD describes a group of conditions that are characterized by challenges with social interaction and communication, restricted interests, and repetitive behaviors. In 2013, the *Diagnostic and Statistical Manual of Mental Disorders (DSM-5)* merged four distinct diagnoses under the umbrella diagnosis for all subtypes: autistic disorder, childhood disintegrative disorder, pervasive developmental disorder (not otherwise specified), and Aspergers syndrome (Academic Pediatric Association [APA], 2013). The DSM-5 describes the criteria for ASD and core symptoms which are divided into two domains (social communication and social interaction; restrictive, repetitive patterns of behavior). To receive a diagnosis of ASD, a child must display all three symptoms of social affective difference in addition to at least two of the four symptoms related to restrictive and repetitive behaviors. Children should be monitored for red flags or early symptoms that could indicate a child is at risk for ASD (CDC, 2022b). Box 19.6 lists some of the possible early symptoms.

The reported prevalence of ASD has increased from 6.7 per 1000 in 2000 to 14.7 per 1000 in 2010 and to 27.6 per 1000 in 2020; ASD currently affects more than five million Americans (CDC, 2023). ASD occurs in all racial, ethnic, and socioeconomic groups (Baio et al., 2018). In 2020, the male (prevalence of 43.0 per 1000)-to-female (11.4 per 1000) ratio for ASD was 3.8 among children aged 8 years in the United States (Maenner et al., 2023). In addition, there were differences in the prevalence of ASD between different races and ethnicities of 8-year-old children: Asian or Pacific Islander (prevalence of 33.4 per 1000), Black (29.3 per 1000), and Hispanic (31.6 per 1000) had higher rates than White (24.3 per 1000) and two or more races (22.9 per 1000). Children with ASD may also have cooccurring developmental conditions, a psychiatric diagnosis, or a neurologic diagnosis. Among 8-year-old children, there were differences in the prevalence of intellectual disability (proportion of the sample

BOX 19.6 Autism Spectrum Disorders: Possible Early Symptoms

Developmental surveillance and screening for autism spectrum disorders (ASDs) can help identify children who are at risk for ASDs. It is important to note that some individuals *without* ASDs might have some of these symptoms. For children with ASDs, their symptoms interfere with their function. To receive a diagnosis of ASDs, children must have a formal evaluation by qualified professionals to determine if they meet the criteria described in the DSM-5.

Possible "Red Flags" in the Preschool Child

Social Skills

- Not responding to their name
- Avoiding eye contact and wanting to play alone
- Having flat or inappropriate facial expressions
- Not understanding personal space boundaries
- Avoiding physical contact
- Having difficulty understanding other people's feelings or talking about their own feelings

Communication

- Delayed speech and language skills
- Repeating words or phrases over and over (echolalia)
- Responding to questions with unrelated answers
- Not pointing at objects or not looking at objects when another person points at them
- Using few or no gestures (e.g., does not wave goodbye)
- Talking in flat, robot-like, or sing-song voice
- Not pretending in play
- Not understanding jokes, sarcasm, or teasing

Unusual Interests and Behaviors

- Lining up toys or other objects
- Playing with toys the same way every time
- Having obsessive interests
- Needing to follow routines and getting upset by minor changes
- Flapping their hands, rocking their body, or spinning in circles
- Having unusual reactions to the way things sound, smell, taste, look, or feel

Modified from Centers for Disease Control and Prevention (CDC). (2022b). *Signs and symptoms of autism spectrum disorders.* https://www.cdc.gov/ncbddd/autism/signs.html

with an IQ ≤70) by race and ethnicity: Asian or Pacific Islander (41.5%), Black (50.8%), Hispanic (34.9%), White (31.8%) and two or more races (37.8%) (Maenner at al., 2023). Furthermore, there were significant differences in the proportion of intellectual disabilities between the following races and ethnicities: Black and White, Black and Hispanic, White and Asian or Pacific Islander, and Black and Asian or Pacific Islander. It is recommended that health care professionals screen for possible cooccurring conditions when evaluating children with ASD (Hyman et al., 2020). Although the exact causes of ASD remain unknown, it appears to be a result of both genetic and environmental factors. Although the genetic foundation is highly variable, ASD is associated with both inheritable and de novo mutation genes (Ghafouri-Fard et al., 2023). Additional potential risk factors associated with ASD are increased parental age, prematurity, maternal infection during pregnancy, and prenatal exposure to thalidomide and valproic acid (Hodges et al., 2020). Children conceived using assisted reproductive technology are two times more likely to be diagnosed with ASD; however, this appears to be largely due to higher rate of adverse prenatal and perinatal outcomes and multiple births (Fountain et al., 2015; Kissin et al., 2015). There is no evidence that ASD is associated with childhood vaccinations (Hviid et al., 2019). Advances in technology and biologic research have helped to identify some of the genetic markers associated with ASD. Chromosome microarray analysis is a promising technology that has helped to identify several sites that are associated with increased risk of ASD (Hodges et al., 2020). Although genetic tests may help explain the cause of a child's ASD, they are not diagnostic. A recent review by Yoon et al. (2020) summarizes the environmental, genetic, and epigenetic risk factors associated with the different phenotypes of ASD.

A reliable diagnosis of ASD can be made as early as 2 years of age, although it may be detected at 18 months or younger. The AAP recommends starting to screen for ASD at the 18- and 24-month well-child visits. The Modified Checklist for Autism in Toddlers, Revised with Follow-Up (M-CHAT-R/F) is the most studied screening tool for ASD in preschoolers and is validated for children aged 16 to 30 months (Robins et al., 2014). A recent analysis by Wieckowski et al. (2023) found the M-CHAT-R/F to be a sensitive and specific instrument. An electronic web-based version of the M-CHAT-R/F has also been validated for ASD screening (Attar et al., 2023).

For children older than 30 months, there are currently no recommended validated screening tools and therefore no current recommendations for screening for ASD in this age group from the AAP. Children who are found to be at risk for ASD by surveillance or screening should be referred for further diagnostic evaluation and early intervention or school-based services, depending upon the age of the child. A diagnosis is made by assessing clinical symptoms and using the DSM-5 criteria and is typically assessed by a specialist such as a developmental pediatrician, psychologist, or neurologist (Hyman et al., 2020). Interestingly, a sensorimotor component of postural control may be impaired in children with ASD (Perin et al., 2020). More information on screening and diagnosis can be found on the CDC (2020f) website at https://www.cdc.gov/autism/screening.html#ref.

In 2016, a population-based ASD surveillance study was published that looked at the characteristics and prevalence of ASD in 4-year-old children (Christensen et al., 2016). The study authors concluded that when compared with diagnosis in 8-year-old children, ASDs were diagnosed in 4-year-olds approximately 5 months earlier (27 months compared with 32 months, respectively), demonstrating improved methods of early identification. They also found that 4-year-old children with ASD were more likely to have intellectual disability than 8-year-old children in the same communities. Lastly, they concluded that among 4-year-old children, females and White children were more likely to receive their first comprehensive developmental evaluation by age 3 years compared with males and Black children, demonstrating that although there have been improvements in early diagnosis, at-risk populations still exist for later diagnosis/identification. It is critical that ASD and developmental delay be detected early to minimize delay, improve outcomes for children, and reduce educational costs.

School Readiness. School readiness includes readiness in the child, the school's readiness for children, and the ability of the family and community to support the child's early development (Williams & Lerner, 2019). The US Department of Education outlines five Essential Domains of School Readiness: 1) language and literacy development, 2) cognition and general knowledge (including early mathematics and early scientific development), 3) approaches toward learning, 4) physical well-being and motor development, and 5) social and emotional development (2011). School readiness is greatly influenced by a child's environment during early childhood and the health and well-being of the families in the child's community. Many children within the United States enter school with limitations in their social-emotional, cognitive, or motor development that could have potentially been reduced with early identification and support services. When used appropriately, school readiness testing can help provide information about how well communities and states are meeting the needs of young children. Although there have been some national initiatives for standardization, testing approaches for school readiness and how the testing results are utilized varies greatly within and among states (Williams & Lerner, 2019). One program, Race to the Top-Early Learning Challenge (RTT-ELC) (Office of Early Childhood Development, 2019), is a state-level grant competition focused on building and enhancing early learning and development systems for children from birth through age 5 (to date, 20 states have received this grant across three phases). RTT-ELC focuses on reforming the five following areas: 1) establishing successful school systems, 2) defining high-quality and accountable programs, 3) promoting early learning and development outcomes for children, 4) supporting a great early childhood education workforce, and 5) measuring outcomes and progress (e.g., using the Kindergarten Entry Assessment). Since the start of the program, and in the states that have received the grant, there have been enrollment increases in the number of children with high needs in high-quality preschool programs (263%), high-quality childcare programs (86%), and Early Head Start or Head Start programs (189%).

The Early Childhood Education State Collaborative on Assessment and Student Standards recommends that assessments of school readiness take place over time, using a variety of tools if there are multiple purposes, and that information should be collected from multiple sources. Assessments should address multiple developmental domains and diverse cultural contexts and should align with early learning guidelines and common core standards. Additionally, the data collected should not be used inappropriately, such as to label a child or limit entry into kindergarten. Health care professionals can support school readiness by monitoring the health and well-being of the child and family, identifying and addressing risk factors, and connecting families to community services when warranted.

Self-Perception–Self-Concept Pattern

During the preschool years, basic self-concept emerges from the child's personal struggle for autonomy. As children develop beyond the toddler years, they refine their sense of self through both task-oriented and socially oriented experiences. By reinforcing skills and successfully accomplishing tasks, preschoolers build self-esteem, enhancing overall health. Social acceptance helps children feel successful in their role as a child, sibling, and friend. Preschoolers investigate roles through rich imagination. Pretending to be the parent or baby allows preschoolers to imagine the experiences and feelings of others (i.e., empathy) and to safely experiment with new ideas.

Preschool children learn about their roles in their childcare environments and learn that being dependable within their world is important. When children perceive their value in improving the world in which they live, they experience good feelings about themselves and, ultimately, demonstrate improved mental and physical health. Many simple ways of improving the environment are available, and when children learn ways to contribute to environmental health, they often reinforce these behaviors in their parents (Box 19.7: Quality and Safety Scenario).

Erikson's Theory

Preschoolers develop a sense of initiative through their vigorous motor activity and active imagination (Fig. 19.2). Erikson (1995, 1998) views this growth as the most central developmental task in the emerging self-concept of the preschool years. By praising preschoolers' efforts and providing opportunities for new experiences, parents promote the development of initiative. More current research suggests that learning can be enhanced, and independent exploration encouraged, when adults successfully scaffold skills without being intrusive. Rather than requiring a particular behavior, caregivers should provide avenues for experimentation while scaffolding foundational skills to help children develop decision-making and problem-solving skills (Yogman et al., 2018).

Roles-Relationships Pattern

Family members continue to play a vital role in the preschooler's life, but peers become increasingly significant as development progresses. Research shows that play affects the developing brain structure and function both directly and indirectly.

 BOX 19.7 **QUALITY AND SAFETY SCENARIO**

Health Promotion With Preschoolers: Environmental Accountability

Rationale for Teaching Preschoolers About Environmental Protection

- Environmental education at an early age will produce environmental practitioners of the future.
- Preschoolers can learn basic concepts of environmental accountability and gain a sense of empowerment when they perceive that they make a difference to the future world.
- Health care providers, in consultation with childcare providers, can promote environmental education that is based on their knowledge of child growth and development and concerns about overall health.

Basic Ways for Preschoolers to Help the Environment and Promote Overall Societal Health

- Use water wisely.
- Use electricity only when necessary.
- Recycle.
- Avoid using balloons.
- Plant trees, protect plants, and grow a garden.
- Create a compost pile.
- Care for birds.
- Clean up the neighborhood.
- Decrease the amount of trash; say "no" to Styrofoam and plastic garbage bags, and use paper cups and reusable cloth bags for groceries.
- Recycle old toys by giving them to others.
- Buy and use only Earth-friendly school supplies.
- Walk rather than ride in the car.
- Use live Christmas trees and replant them.

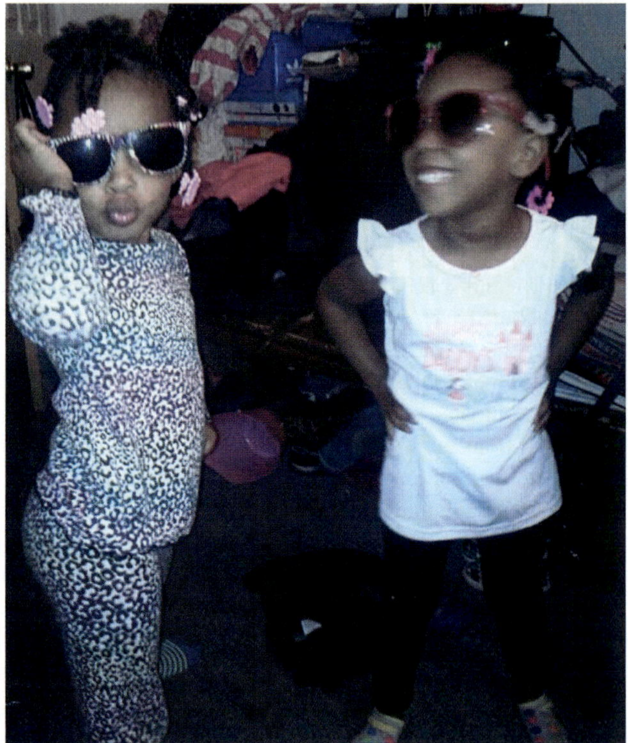

FIG. 19.2 Two preschoolers using their imagination in being movie stars.

Developmentally appropriate play with parents and peers helps build executive functioning across three dimensions: cognitive flexibility, inhibitory control, and working memory. As a result, play can help children develop essential adaptive behaviors, such as sustained attention, the ability to filter through distracting information, improved self-regulation and self-control, improved cognitive and language skills, and mental flexibility. These skills are essential for school readiness for adult success (Yogman et al., 2018) and support maturing relationships. The Center on the Developing Child at Harvard University's resource on play and executive functioning (Bowne, 2015) provides ideas for specific activities to promote executive functioning skills in children (https://harvardcenter.wpenginepowered.com/wp-content/uploads/2015/05/Enhancing-and-Practicing-Executive-Function-Skills-with-Children-from-Infancy-to-Adolescence-1.pdf).

Preschoolers receive ideas and information from peers. They may subsequently question rules or expectations at home, comparing them with their friends' situations. Parents and caregivers should be aware of the powerful influence that the environment has on role perceptions (Brown et al., 2009). Preschoolers experiment through play, including by adopting family roles. These roles differ depending on the family structure and function. Discussion about family values and behaviors that are acceptable in one place but not another helps them understand differences. Furthermore, play represents an important strategy for preschoolers to use for stress reduction and experimentation with new roles. By playing different roles, children safely experience the effects of their behavior and understand others' roles more clearly. Parents also better understand the effects of their own actions when they observe the behaviors of their child.

Social interaction during the preschool period allows children to experiment with different social roles. As children play with their peers, they learn to negotiate "the rules" and thus learn how to negotiate and cooperate. Through experience within the family, with peers, and with other adults, the child acquires readiness to interact in group situations, follow directions, take turns, recognize others' rights, channel energy toward an assigned activity, and demonstrate increasing independence (Yogman et al., 2018). Health care professionals who see the child repeatedly in an office, clinic, or group care or preschool setting should help monitor a child's social-emotional development as part of performing developmental surveillance and screening, as was described earlier in this chapter.

Parental divorce commonly creates disruption in family relationships. Children's responses to changes in family circumstances depend on their developmental stages and their relationships before the change. Divorce represents a final decision, usually culminating from a period of conflict, stress, and changing relationships. Preschool-aged children often cannot comprehend the performance of divorce. They may exhibit behavioral challenges, sleeping and eating problems, or regression in developmental skills. They commonly start to test boundaries with each parent and question differences in limit setting (Cohen, 2016). Although preschoolers can sense stress in the home, they often cannot articulate their feelings or determine their origin. Children react to changes in various ways, including regression, confusion, or irritability. Asking the same questions repeatedly—such as "Is Daddy coming home for supper tonight?" or "Why doesn't Daddy stay here anymore?"—can be a child's way of expressing difficulty in coping with or comprehending the situation.

Parents in the midst of marital problems or divorce frequently lack the psychological energy or patience to deal with questions and altered behavior. Nonetheless, their children need closeness, patience, and consistent responses from their parents. As parents develop skills to explain situations, they may realize that children are deeply affected during times of family disruption, regardless of their behavior. Parents need to connect emotionally with their children to demonstrate that love will continue for the child despite dissolution of the marriage. The AAP (2020) provides information on how health care professionals can help support children and families during divorce and during stressful events.(https://www.healthychildren.org/English/healthy-living/emotional-wellness/Building-Resilience/Pages/When-Things-Arent-Perfect-Caring-for-Yourself-Your-Children.aspx)

Child Abuse and Neglect

A child's early childhood experiences can have a significant effect on their well-being throughout their life. Early negative events, known as adverse childhood experiences (ACEs), are defined as potentially traumatic events that occur in childhood and can be found in adults regardless of race and ethnicity, socioeconomic status, or education (Hustedde, 2021). These events include experiencing violence, abuse, or neglect or growing up in an environment with mental health or substance use problems. Approximately one in six adults report four or more types of ACEs. ACEs are linked to changes in brain development, may affect how the body is able to respond to stress, and have significant long-term effects on health throughout the life span. Children who experience ACEs are at greater risk for childhood obesity (Schroeder et al., 2021) and are more likely to experience chronic health problems, chronic pain and pain-related disability, mental illness, and substance misuse as adults (Bhutta et al., 2023; Bussières et al., 2023; Jones et al., 2020). There are four types of abuse and neglect: physical abuse, sexual abuse, emotional abuse, and neglect. During the federal fiscal year of 2021, the National Child Abuse and Neglect Data System (USDHHS, 2023) reported the following data: a) 40.7 children per 1000 received an investigation report or alternative response, b) 8.1 children per 1000 were victims of child abuse and neglect, and c) 2.46 children per 100,000 were victims who died from abuse and neglect. Victims experienced neglect (76.0%), physical abuse (16.0%), sexual abuse (10.1%), and sex trafficking (0.2%). From 2017 to 2021, the national rate of children who received an investigation or alternative response decreased from 47.1 to 40.7 per 1000 children, and the rate of child victimization decreased from 9.1 to 8.1 per 1000. Unfortunately, the national fatality rate increased in 2017 from 2.28 children per 100,000 to 2.46 children per 100,000 in 2021. By sex, the rate of victimization is higher for females than males (8.7 vs. 7.5 per 1000). By age, the rate of child victimization is highest for those less than 1 year old at 25.3 per 1000, and in general this rate decreases with age. The rate of victimization for-,

4-, and 5-year-old children is 9.1, 8.6, and 8.5 per 1000, respectively. American Indian or Alaska Native (15.2 per 1000), African American (13.1 per 1000), and multiracial individuals (10.3 per 1000) had the highest rates of victimization, followed by Native Hawaiian or Pacific Islander (8.5 per 1000), Hispanic (7.7 per 1000), White (7.1 per 1000), and Asian (1.4 per 1000) (USDHHS, 2023).

Children living in poverty are five times more likely to experience abuse and neglect (CDC, 2020d). Although it is important for families to begin teaching children about how to respond to strangers, child abuse in general—and sexual abuse in particular—occurs more often within a family than with a stranger as the perpetrator. Most children are abused by someone who is familiar to them. In 2021, 90.6% of child victims had a parental relationship with their perpetrator (USDHHS, 2023). The two most common caregiver risk factors for child abuse are drug abuse (26.1%) and domestic violence (28.2%) (USDHHS, 2023). The social processes within families and communities that create child abuse are multifaceted and complex. Research focuses on the complexity of the abuse cycle and the challenges involved in resolution. Prevention of ACEs and child neglect and abuse is the focus of many health-promotion programs. Effective primary and secondary prevention interventions involve promoting awareness of violence as a social problem, promoting social norms that protect against violence, strengthening economic support to families, ensuring a strong start for children, teaching children skills, connecting children to caring adults and activities, and intervening to reduce immediate and long-term harm (CDC, 2020d). Health care professionals can help recognize signs of child abuse and neglect and are mandated to report suspected abuse or neglect (Tufford & Lee, 2018). Most reports (67%) of alleged child abuse or neglect are submitted by professionals, with the next-highest percentages coming from legal and law enforcement personnel (21.8%), education personnel (15.4%), and health care professionals (12.2%) (USDHHS, 2023). In addition, health care professionals can help prevent abuse and neglect. The AAP (2021) has helpful information for health care professionals on how to help recognize and prevent child abuse and neglect (https://www.aap.org/en/patient-care/child-abuse-and-neglect/).

The American Psychological Association (2009) also provides helpful information about abuse for families at https://www.apa.org/pi/families/resources/understanding-child-abuse.

Sexuality-Reproductive Pattern

At birth, gender, or sex, is assigned as male or female based on physical characteristics. Gender identity is defined as "a person's internal sense of being female, male, a combination of both, somewhere in between, or neither, resulting from a multifaceted interaction of biologic traits, environmental factors, self-understanding and cultural expectations" (Rafferty, 2018, p. 2). Gender identity develops over time and in stages. By 2 years of age, children are often aware of the physical differences between sexes. By 3 years of age, most children label themselves as either a boy or a girl. Most children have a more stable sense of their gender identity by age 4 years (AAP, 2018a). Through play, children explore gender roles and learn gender role behavior during the preschool years. Appropriate and positive representations of both sexes on television and in role models, such as working mothers, allow preschoolers to interpret gender roles broadly and define their own roles more realistically (Hockenberry et al., 2024). Body image, a part of gender identity, also includes perception of sex organs. Preschoolers develop curiosity at this age, including inquisitiveness about bodies and sexual functions of others. Questions should be answered simply and factually. Teasing preschoolers about this interest or implying that sexual information is unacceptable or naughty promotes negativity. Positive feelings about all aspects of the self (including gender role) create positive self-esteem. Many children's books address self-esteem in young children and provide interesting and informative approaches to nurturing overall health promotion in this age group.

Coping–Stress Tolerance Pattern

Play Approaches

Assessing self-concept in preschool children who struggle to articulate their feelings presents a challenge for the health professional. Play can elicit behaviors that indicate a sense of self and self-esteem, future success or failure, a sense of acceptance, and competence. **Doll or puppet play** provides valuable insight into a child's sense of self. Dolls or puppets, including those representing a young child of the same sex, race, and cultural background as the preschooler, should be available (Hockenberry et al., 2024). If the child spontaneously begins to engage the dolls or puppets in imaginary activity, no further guidance may be needed. With a reluctant child, an adult can help model how to pretend, using examples for the child, such as going to the store, moving the dolls through the related activities, and then involving the child. Frequently preschoolers continue the scenario to tell their personal stories.

A related technique is **mutual storytelling**. The nurse begins a story for the child to finish. The nurse might begin with a standard line, such as "Once upon a time there lived a (girl, boy, cow, monkey, etc.) who…." The nurse then pauses for the child to continue. If the child hesitates, the nurse resumes the story for another sentence or two and asks what the figure in the story is doing. As the child supplies details, the nurse offers encouragement to continue, asking questions such as "And then what happened?" or "How did the child feel?"

The child's inner nature can be explored along several dimensions. The emotional theme of the story is noted and should be congruent with the child's tone and expression. For example, a child who centers on a theme of aggression and destruction but describes the character's anger in a monotone is demonstrating incongruence between content and expression. The child's emotionless response suggests difficulty with expressing feelings. At the conclusion of the story, possible meanings can be revealed by the nurse asking whether the child feels similar to any of the characters or would like to be any of the characters.

Although these dimensions may be explored for meaning, interpretation of a child's behavior in these play situations remains highly speculative. Determining possible themes or estimating the child's self-esteem requires several encounters. Additionally, the nurse's personality and approach influence the child's spontaneity and ability to tell a story. Observed behavior and responses without associated interpretation should be recorded for future reference. Interpretations are avoided until validated by a specialist.

Coping Mechanisms

Preschoolers use coping mechanisms similar to those of the toddler (separation anxiety, regression, denial, repression, and projection). Protest behavior in the form of temper tantrums normally disappears as a stress response in the older preschooler. Temper tantrums that persist through the fifth year indicate a lack of mature coping responses. The child uses tantrums and continues to gain the desired result.

Preschoolers lack cognitive awareness, social abilities, and motives for communication like those of adults and older children. Through positive interactions with parents and caregivers, preschoolers frequently learn how to organize their bodies, abilities, and environment to move successfully to the next stage of development. A positive relationship between the child's temperament and the demands of the environment (also known as goodness of fit) can be attained by social interaction, which in turn prevents the development of problem behaviors later (Box 19.8: The Challenge of Temperament and Preschoolers).

Preschoolers possess a considerable range of experiences and memories; therefore, they respond more maturely to stress than do toddlers. Positive coping resources are determined by some of the following variables:

- Availability of emotional comfort and the child's inner resilience
- Ability to work on task
- Availability of play materials and toys
- Opportunity to engage in activities

Preschoolers use many of the coping mechanisms developed during their toddler years, but they generally show greater ability to verbalize frustration, have fewer temper tantrums, and display more patience in experimentation to resolve difficulty than the typical toddler. Preschoolers refine their problem-solving skills. Through fantasy play, they investigate solutions or responses to stressful events and find inner control for challenging situations.

Occasionally projection and fantasy lead parents to consider their child dishonest. When faced with the question "Did you break this dish?" the preschooler might respond, "No, Teddy did it." The child might even relate a detailed story of the toy bear mishap. Preschoolers tend to project blame. Active fantasies help tell the story. Parents should not accuse the preschooler of lying, but rather the adult should help the child decide whether the story is pretend or real. The concepts of pretend and real help encourage children to discuss nightmares, television shows, stories, and their own active imaginations.

Compared with toddlers, preschoolers better perceive their ability to control and manage situations. Strict adherence to rituals or game rules controls situations. As discussed, preschoolers have longer and more rigid bedtime rituals than those of toddlers. Preschoolers also dislike losing games and may structure the rules to ensure they win. Older children and adults may be able to accept these structures, but these controlling behaviors frustrate other preschoolers because they also need to win. Gentle, consistent direction by parents and caregivers about how to play games fairly and how to move toward positive group outcomes helps preschoolers develop a sense of morality, which is important for later life success and happiness. See the case study and care plan at the end of this chapter for an example of ineffective coping in a preschool child.

> **BOX 19.8 The Challenge of Temperament and Preschoolers**
>
> Temperament describes the way in which an individual behaves or responds to new situations and to life occurrences and has consistently been associated with psychopathology and family function since the early work of pediatrician Terry Brazelton on maternal attachment in 1978 (Brazelton Touch Points Center, 2024). Most children can be defined as *easy, difficult,* or *hard to warm up to* on the basis of how they react to their surroundings and to people. Temperament and parental stress are linked; however, many other factors influence interactions between the parent and the child, including the child's own temperament. The challenge in parenting is to learn how to work with a child's temperament, which can differ from the parents' or other children's temperaments, in efforts to achieve family happiness. Education on their child's temperament characteristics and adaptive strategies to handle their behaviors may be beneficial for parents. Education in coping skills and stress management for families, particularly those with children defined as difficult, may improve overall family function. Parents' psychological well-being is important in managing and preventing dysfunctional parent-child interactions (Brazelton Touch Points Center, 2024).

Values-Beliefs Pattern

Preschoolers, like toddlers, lack fully developed consciences; however, at age 4 to 5 years, these children do demonstrate some internal controls on their actions. Immaturity limits the consistency and effectiveness of these internal controls. With the child's concrete perspective, the internal controls may be rigid; therefore, a preschooler may feel overwhelming guilt when behavior and internal controls conflict. Cognitive developmental level determines, for the most part, preschoolers' maturity and their feelings about their behavioral fluctuations. Cognitive development continues with dramatic transformation during these years, explaining the differences not only among children but also for different times in the same child. Modeling and **induction explanation**, moving from specific to general, influence moral behaviors appreciably. Modeling stems from many sources, not all of which leave positive impressions. Parents affect the availability of models by screening television shows, carefully selecting childcare situations, and monitoring play sessions. Responsible parents verify the suitability of the models. More detailed inductive explanations, based on the child's cognitive level, are generally comprehended by the preschool population.

Preschoolers control their behavior to retain parental love and approval. From their perspective, parental disapproval represents a decrease in the child's importance from the parent's viewpoint. The child therefore suffers a decline in self-esteem, which motivates a change in behavior. Guilt results from perceived reduction of self-esteem, a critical step in the development of conscience.

Moral actions are demonstrated in simple activities, such as taking turns and sharing. These actions stem from the assumption that other people have rights and desires that are as important as the rights and desires of preschoolers.

Preschoolers frequently express their values by stating who or what they like or what they want to be when they become adults. These values change frequently, even within a few minutes. Preschoolers occasionally use statements of value as punishment for playmates or family members and display insensitivity to the effect of their remarks on others. Preschoolers ask endless questions. When they ask these questions about moral actions or feelings, they may simply be asking "How does this work?" and not questioning the underlying parental value. The same intent exists when the child asks about the spiritual values that the parent may be teaching. Parents may enroll their child in faith-oriented classes or activities. The preschool child generally enjoys the social aspects of these activities and receives some important modeling of values from the involved adults and from working with peers as they struggle to develop morality.

Life beginnings and death concepts fascinate preschoolers. Because of their limited emotional experiences with death, some ask about dead insects and the process of death with great interest, occasionally with insensitivity. Others become upset with the idea of dying, assuming that when someone becomes angry and wishes them dead, they will cease to exist. Many children worry about who will care for them if their caregivers die, whether pain comes with death, what causes death, and what happens after someone dies. Children who actually lose a loved one to death can experience sleep disturbances and other behavioral changes as part of the grieving process. Parents, on the basis of their own religious and cultural values, should respond to children in a supportive and open manner to provide an accurate interpretation of death. In some cases, counseling may be needed if the parents are unable to cope with their duties or if the child has significant behavioral problems as a result of the family disruption. Assessment using the preschooler's drawings in such situations provides an accepted method of exploring their perceptions about family relationships, death, and the afterlife.

ENVIRONMENTAL PROCESSES

Physical Agents

For many children, physiologic, psychosocial, and environmental factors create health problems that interfere with the physical, social, and educational activities of normal development (Hockenberry et al., 2024). Major disruptions limit fulfillment of the child's potential in adulthood. The environmental processes that affect toddlers also affect preschoolers. Occurrence rates and outcomes of health problems differ in this age group, likely because of developmental differences. Preschoolers have more refined problem-solving skills, are more coordinated, and have more experience with a variety of situations than do toddlers. Although preschoolers recognize and avoid some environmental hazards, they remain impulsive and immature. Population-based programs ensure that screening occurs at the most developmentally appropriate time (Box 19.9: Evidence-Based Practice).

BOX 19.9 EVIDENCE-BASED PRACTICE

Association of Parent Training With Child Language Development: A Systematic Review and Meta-analysis

Roberts and colleagues (2019) conducted a systematic meta-analysis of 76 studies with 5848 participants aged 0.2 to 5.0 years (mean 3.53 years) of which 64% were male. Studies examined participants with autism spectrum disorder (n=27), developmental language disorder (n=10), and those at risk (n=34). The majority of the studies were conducted in the United States or Canada (57%). Parent training consisted of responsive and naturalistic strategies in 63 studies or a dialogic reading approach in 16 studies. Results from the meta-analysis show a large association between parent training and their use of language support strategies. Results also show moderate associations between parent training and outcomes including child communication, engagement, and language. These findings demonstrate the association between training parents and 1) increased parent use of language and communication strategies and 2) improved child outcomes for communication, engagement, and language (Roberts et al., 2019).

Because many preschoolers attend childcare programs, many have been trained to use 911 and can access help in emergencies when a phone exists. At this age a child needs to know their name, address, and how to say "no" to strangers.

Injuries

Although death among children and adolescents is relatively rare, accidents and injuries are often predictable and preventable (Cunningham et al., 2018). As preschoolers become more independent, causes of injury change; they may chase a ball into a busy street or suffer from sports-related injuries. Preschoolers continue to need supervision to prevent injury related to their developmental age. Nurses guide families to provide a safe environment for preschoolers with opportunities to explore without negative consequences (Box 19.10).

Of all injuries, two-thirds occur in children and adolescents. According to the Web-based Injury Statistics Query and Reporting System (WISQARS, 2023), the rate of death from all intents injuries is increasing in the United States for children aged 3 to 6 years (in 2011 the crude rate was 6.64 per 100,000, and in 2021 the crude rate had increased to 7.48). The death rate for males is consistently higher than for females (in 2021 the crude rate was 9.14 per 100,000 for males and 5.75 per 100,000 for females). For both sexes, the crude rate consistently decreases each year between the ages of 3 and 6 years old (WISQARS, 2023).

Death rates due to motor vehicle crashes and firearms continue to be higher than in other high-income countries (Cunningham et al., 2018). Although preschoolers have fewer accidents than toddlers, accidental (unintentional) injury continues to be a predominant cause of morbidity in this age group. WISQARS (2023) indicates the leading causes of death in preschool children in 2021 were due to unintentional injury by motor vehicle traffic, drowning, fire/burns, firearms, suffocation, and pedestrians. Preschoolers are most likely to sustain nonfatal unintentional injuries from falls, "struck by/against," "foreign body," "cut/pierce," "other bite/sting," and "dog bite" more than any other accidental causes; however, as the child's

BOX 19.10 Injury Prevention for Preschoolers

A safe and developmentally stimulating environment allows children of all ages to explore without negative consequences. When teaching parents how to modify their homes for preschoolers, the nurse should consider the following requirements for child safety.

Safe Sleep Environment

Provide beds with guardrails (as needed), soft corners, and appropriate bedding to prevent suffocation.

Well-Ventilated but Optimal-Temperature Environment for Play

Provide safe play areas by using electrical outlet covers, handrails in stairwells, nonslip floor materials, well-anchored furniture, and appropriate soft ground coverings and padding for outdoor play equipment.

Burn Prevention

Use only a cool mist humidifier for management of upper respiratory tract infections; dress child only in flame-retardant clothing, particularly at bedtime.

Appropriate Installation and Use of Emergency Home Equipment

Discuss the importance of properly operating smoke detectors and fire extinguishers and practicing a plan for escape from the home in case of emergency.

Connection to Emergency Services

Post 911 on all phones; teach the child how to use 911 and how to report the child's name and address over the phone; parents should be trained in cardiopulmonary resuscitation and the use of abdominal thrusts.

Prevention of Aspiration

Monitor use of balloons and eating habits of preschoolers.

Safe Daily Home Environment

Close doors of the dishwasher, oven, washer, and dryer; mark all glass doors with decals to delineate doors; use gates at the top and bottom of stairs for the younger child; set water heater temperature at a maximum of 120°F to avoid burns; store all poisonous substances out of the reach of children; discourage running in the house; avoid using throw rugs on bare floors.

Prevention, Recognition, and Management of Poison Ingestion or Exposure

Know how to use syrup of ipecac and have the nearest poison control center phone number within easy access; learn how to evaluate burns or blisters around the mouth, odor of poisons, empty containers around the child, stomach distress, or changes in normal activity level that might indicate poison ingestion.

Water Safety

Monitor bathtub and pool activity; teach preschooler swimming skills (usually by age 4 years); ensure that all pools are fenced.

Bicycle Safety

Ensure that the child is riding a developmentally appropriate bicycle with a federally approved safety helmet and is schooled in the rules of riding in the street and interacting with strangers.

Lead Concerns

Avoid exposure to items with a high lead content in the home (paint, wrapping paper, earthenware, colored newspaper); ensure that children are monitored when lead exposure is a concern.

Environmental Contaminants Hazardous to the Child's Health

Avoid exposure to tobacco smoke, nitrous oxide from wood-burning stoves, asbestos, pesticides, radiation, and factory-produced irritants.

Hockenberry, M. J., Duffy, E., & Gibbs, K. (2024). *Wong's nursing care of infants and children* (12th ed.). Elsevier.

age increases toward school age, these injuries begin to decline in number.

Motor vehicle accidents consistently remain the top-ranked reason for death attributable to injury in the preschool age group (WISQARS, 2023). Consequently, the *Healthy People* initiative has an objective of reducing motor vehicle crash-related deaths and reducing the proportion of passenger vehicle occupant deaths that were known unrestrained (*Healthy People 2030:* Objectives 5 and 6, respectively). Being an occupant in a motor vehicle was also the eighth most common cause of nonfatal injuries in children 3 to 6 years old (WISQARS, 2023). An analysis of 2021 data from the National Survey of the Use of Booster Seats revealed that unfortunately 13.2% of children 1 to 3 years old were not being properly restrained (a decrease from 16.3% in 2019) and 26.7% of children 4 to 7 years old were not being properly restrained (a decrease from 30.4% in 2019). In fact, in 2021, 6.3% of children 1 to 3 years old and 10.6% of children 4 to 7 years old were unrestrained (WISQARS, 2023).

According to the Fatality Analysis Reporting System (a database maintained by the National Highway Transportation Safety Administration [NHTSA], 2023), in 2011 there were 358 fatalities of children aged less than 5 years and 344 fatalities of children aged 5 to 9 years. These numbers changed to 355 fatalities of children aged less than 5 years and 366 fatalities of children aged 5 to 9 years in 2021. The NHTSA provides Car Seat Recommendations for Children, which describes proper usage of a rear-facing car seat, forward-facing car seat, booster seat, and seat belt. According to the NHTSA, children from birth to 3 years should remain in a rear-facing car seat with a harness for as long as possible, up to the highest weight and height allowed by the car seat manufacturer. Children should then transition to a forward-facing car seat with a harness and tether up to the highest weight and height allowed by the car seat manufacturer. Next the child can transition to a booster seat, still in the back seat, until they are big enough to properly fit a seat belt. A seat belt fits properly when the lap belt lies across the upper thighs and the shoulder belt lies across the shoulder and chest. When the lap belt lies across the stomach or the shoulder belt lies across the neck or face, the belt does not fit properly. The NHTSA website has a tool that recommends which type of car seat to use based on the child's age, height, and weight.

Children may transition out of a belt-positioning booster seat typically when they have reached 4 feet 9 inches in height and are between 8 and 12 years of age. Federal investigations concluded that children younger than 13 years should ride in the back seat of a motor vehicle, particularly because of potential injury or death from a passenger seat airbag that could inflate in a severe car accident. In 2013, changes were made by car manufacturers regarding the use of LATCH (Lower Anchors and Tethers for Children) for older children using child restraints. This is important in the preschooler because per the new guidelines, in general, if the combined weight of the car seat and child is more than 65 pounds, LATCH should not be used. Instead of LATCH, the seat belt should be used. Each car seat and car manufacturer has slightly differing regulations, so parents are encouraged to have a certified car seat technician install their child's seat to ensure proper and safe installation. It is important to note that each state has differing laws regarding child safety restraints. However, these laws are often minimum requirements, not updated often, and not always reflective of best practice.

Nurses actively participate in health-promotion programs in communities and emergency departments that help families use car restraints correctly. In a recent randomized controlled trial on the effects of car seat education, video-based social learning was compared with didactic teaching, and both methods significantly improved proficiency in child passenger restraint (Kuroiwa et al., 2018). When families must consider financial constraints to comply with the requirements to restrain their children, nurses are often the first line of information. Nurses provide information about resources available locally through agencies such as hospitals, physicians' offices, insurance companies, United Way, Safe Kids Worldwide (2024), the fire department, and other community organizations.

Household furniture and fixtures also remain a hazard for preschoolers, as do structural features such as stairs and windows. A meta-analysis found that home safety interventions were effective in significantly increasing the proportion of families with fitted stair gates (Kendrick et al., 2013). A more recent study found reduced stair fall injury risk in children with the use of stair gates, keeping stair gates closed, and having carpet on stairs (Kendrick et al., 2016). Nursery and toy injuries decrease during the preschool years. Sports and recreational injuries increase markedly. This elevated incidence likely reflects a change in many preschoolers being involved in group sports, riding bicycles, and using playground equipment (WISQUARS, 2023). Preschoolers need a broad range of play areas and experiences. Conscientious parents supply age-appropriate limits and supervision. Preschoolers lack the skill or judgment to ride bicycles in the street. They need instruction about safe use of playground equipment. Adult supervision of most preschooler activities—group sports in particular—is required to prevent injury.

Preschoolers begin to safely handle basic tools, kitchen equipment, and cleaning supplies. Children at this age take pride in participating in household projects with a supervising parent. They spend much of their time in the home and in the preschool or childcare center. These facilities pose the same potentially harmful environmental conditions as the home, as well as some additional threats to safety (WISQUARS, 2023).

In response to concern about firearm safety in homes with small children, most states have passed child access protection (CAP) legislation to encourage safe storage of firearms. For young children, CAP results in a decline in the rate of deaths attributable to firearms. The risk of death increases in the mere presence of the firearm. Preschool children are physically capable of pulling a trigger before they are able to cognitively depict the cause and effect of their actions. Even if there is gun safety training, most curious children will handle firearms given the opportunity, which may give families a false sense of security (Children's Defense Fund, 2020).

To appreciate the magnitude of the problem, in 2017 the number of children under 5 years of age killed by firearms (93) was more than twice the number of law enforcement officers killed by firearms (42) (Children's Defense Fund, 2020). More recent data from WISQARS (2023) reports 289 unintentional firearm deaths, which represents 3.13% of all unintentional deaths of children aged 3 to 6 years in the United States from 2011 to 2021 (range 38 to 87 deaths per year). Most deaths from firearms are preventable when adults take responsibility for storing and minimizing access to firearms. A recent review of the effectiveness of interventions to promote safe firearm storage found that safe storage device provision, with or without counseling, significantly improved firearm storage practices (Rowhani-Rahbar et al., 2016).

Burns

Scalds and direct flame burns are major hazards for preschoolers. With 96 deaths in 2021, thermal injury (unintentional fire/burn) ranks as the third-highest cause of death from injuries in US children from 3 to 6 years of age (WISQARS, 2023). Thermal injury also ranks as the 12th highest cause of nonfatal injury in US children from 3 to 6 years, with 14,315 cases in 2021. The number of deaths of preschool children in house fires is nearly double that of children of other ages. Children of this age experiment with matches and fire, and they may be unable to escape from a fire once it starts. The measures discussed in Chapter 18 to reduce scald burns in the home apply to this age group as well. Preschoolers should be taught about the dangers of matches, open flames, and hot objects. Parents and caregivers should model appropriate use of active and potentially dangerous burning devices. In a study of five emergency departments, the majority (58%) of thermal injuries were scalds from beverages (49.6%), domestic water (37.6%), and food (12.7%) most frequently caused by pull-down (48%) and spill (32%) mechanisms (Kemp et al., 2014). A meta-analysis found that home safety interventions were effective in significantly increasing the proportion of families with safe hot tap water temperatures, functional smoke alarms, and a fire escape plan (Kendrick et al., 2013).

Drowning

Children older than 3 years are at lower risk of drowning in the bathtub but at greater risk of drowning in a swimming pool than toddlers. With 276 deaths in 2021, drowning was the second highest cause of death from injuries in US children 3 to 6 years of age (WISQARS, 2023). Drowning also ranks as the 17th highest cause of nonfatal injury in US children from 3 to 6 years. Preschool children aged 1 to 4 years are at highest risk of drowning, with two near-drowning episodes for every fatality. Most children are close to safety when drowning occurs. With this in mind, it is important to supervise young children when they are near a body of water, to install fencing to isolate a residential pool from the house, to have young children use personal flotation devices (PFDs) while playing near a natural body of water, and to teach children how to swim and that swimming alone is unsafe. Preschoolers should receive instruction in water safety and swimming and should always be supervised by a trained adult or older person. Following less educational outreach during the pandemic, the AAP suggests that all children aged 4 years or older should receive swimming lessons (AAP, 2022). It is reasonable to encourage parents and pool owners to learn poolside cardiopulmonary resuscitation and lifesaving strategies.

Preschoolers have the cognitive ability to learn water survival. They should always wear a PFD (i.e., life jacket) when they are on boats, even when they know how to swim, and they must be supervised when near water, even shallow water. The AAP recommends the following strategies to prevent drownings: adult supervisors, pool fencing, pool alarms, lifeguards, cardiopulmonary resuscitation training, swimming instructions and water-survival training, and PFDs (Denny et al., 2021). Safety campaigns provide one effective measure for preventing unnecessary injury and death (Children's Defense Fund, 2019; USDHHS, 2024). To summarize the importance of safety water education, each year, over 4000 unintentional drowning deaths occur in the United States, and more children aged 1 to 4 die from unintentional drowning than from any other cause except birth defects. Drowning is the second-leading cause of unintentional injury-related death among children aged 5 to 14 (WISQARS, 2023).

Mechanical Forces

Bicycle accidents become a greater source of injury during the preschool years. Many bicycle accidents involve automobiles, and most of these accidents result from the child's errors. Parents should set reasonable and age-appropriate limits on bicycle use. In 2021, the crude rate of nonfatal emergency department visits due to bicycle use was 65.88 per 100,000 for 3-year-olds, almost doubling to approximately the same rates for 4- (113.41), 5- (114.34), and 6-year-olds (112.24) (WISQARS, 2023). In 2021, bicycle use was the 10th most common cause of a nonfatal emergency department visit for children 3 to 6 years. From 2009 to 2018, the crude rate for bicycle-related traumatic brain injuries was 15.3 per 100,000 for children less than 4 years old and 35.2 per 100,000 for children 5 to 9 years old (Sarmiento et al., 2021). During this same period, the rate of bicycle-related traumatic brain injuries decreased by almost half for children ≤17 years.

A study by McAdams et al. (2018) examined bicycle-related injuries in the emergency department among children aged 5 to 17 years, and the most common injuries included contusion and abrasion (29.1%), laceration (23.4%), fracture (21.7%), strain and sprain (11.5%), and traumatic brain injury (10.7%). The most common body regions injured included the upper extremity (36.2%), lower extremity (24.9%), face (15.4%), head and neck (14.9%), and trunk (8.4%). The majority of injuries occurred on the street (47.9%) or at home (36.6%), did not involve a motor vehicle (92.5%), were sustained by males (71.6%), and happened while the child was not wearing a helmet (72.8%). For children 5 to 9 years, there was a ratio of no helmet use to helmet use slightly greater than 2:1. After adjusting for age and sex, helmet use resulted in lower odds of sustaining head and neck injuries, sustaining a traumatic brain injury, or requiring hospitalization.

Federally approved bicycle helmets are effective in reducing head trauma, a major cause of death among young children. Preschoolers, as passengers or pedestrians, are at great risk of an automobile-related accident. At this age, pedestrian injury is more likely to occur than is passenger injury. Preschoolers should be taught proper street-crossing techniques and, generally, should be supervised when crossing streets. Schwebel et al. (2012) discuss risk factors for child pedestrian injuries, which include developmental factors (cognitive and perceptual), distraction, temperament and personality, social influences (parents and peers), environmental risks, attention-deficient/hyperactivity disorder, and sleep and fatigue. The prevention strategies reviewed include parental instruction, school-based instruction (including crossing guards), street-side training, technology-based training, and community-based training.

Biologic Agents

Preschoolers seem healthier than toddlers, with fewer illnesses of the respiratory and gastrointestinal tracts. They have developed antibodies to many common organisms through exposure. Children usually become ill more often when they enter their first group situation, where they may be exposed to new organisms. This concerns parents and should be discussed by the nurse before the child begins attending a group setting. Childcare settings provide instruction to children about appropriate handwashing techniques to decrease disease transmission and provide relevant health-promotion teaching.

Immunization recommendations are reviewed annually and updated with professional educational tools and parent-friendly resources. These resources for professionals and families can be found in a variety of formats, in both Spanish and English, at https://www.cdc.gov/vaccines/index.html. The CDC's updated vaccine recommendations in 2023 and information for children 18 years and younger can be found at https://www.cdc.gov/vaccines/hcp/imz-schedules/child-adolescent-age.html.

The AAP also publishes the most current recommendations annually, with a particular focus on the immunization needs of children. The 2023 recommendations can be found at https://www.healthychildren.org/English/safety-prevention/immunizations/Pages/Recommended-Immunization-Schedules.aspx with a downloadable table covering birth to 6 years (https://downloads.aap.org/HC/EN/childvaccineschedule.pdf).

The child with a full course of immunizations as an infant receives repeated doses of diphtheria, tetanus, and acellular pertussis; measles, mumps, and rubella; and varicella vaccines between the fourth year and the sixth year (CDC, 2020f). Many states require that all children in a school setting be fully immunized. Parents who choose not to immunize their children usually make this choice for religious reasons, but some parents worry about the risk of the immunization itself. Although vaccines provide an extremely safe way to combat communicable disease, issues about safety do arise. Individual health providers should develop strategies to impart evidence-based information and participate in professional and public educational campaigns to disseminate the information widely. Because autism is often diagnosed around the same time a child is vaccinated, some parents have connected the onset of their child's autism with the vaccine. The CDC (2021) emphasizes the safety and importance of vaccines (https://www.cdc.gov/vaccines/hcp/conversations/provider-resources-safetysheets.html) and clearly states that vaccines and vaccine ingredients do not cause autism (https://www.cdc.gov/vaccinesafety/concerns/autism.html).

The risk of the consequences of the disease itself far outweighs any vaccine risk, but without first-hand experience with vaccine-preventable diseases such as measles, *Haemophilus influenzae* type b, or polio, families today may minimize their severity. Nurses must remain informed about recommended vaccines, their schedule, and their risks and benefits to provide accurate, evidence-based information to families.

Nurses who remain informed about the reasons for avoidance of immunization will be better able to increase parents' understanding of the possible consequences of omitting doses or not following vaccination schedules. Incomplete immunization may also occur as a result of parental forgetfulness or procrastination. Mandatory immunization for school entry provides an effective incentive for these parents. Although immunization rates are increasing, disparities exist in certain regions of the United States and are associated with race, poverty, and insurance coverage (Hill et al., 2016). Advances on the horizon include more combination vaccines to decrease the cost of administration. Noninjectable vaccines that could be inhaled or eaten would greatly enhance pediatric immunization programs with ease of administration and simplified storage.

Continued efforts to vaccinate all children are needed, especially children living in poverty, particularly in large cities, where they are traditionally undervaccinated. Nurses use immunization registry programs to consolidate records, to remind parents, to evaluate the person's scheduled program, and to investigate particular population problems. Registry programs avoid duplication and are valuable for the preschool age group that may not be involved in day care or preschool with mandated immunizations. The CDC publishes recommendations for individuals who have omitted doses. These alternative schedules are updated regularly along with the routine schedules and are available at the CDC website (https://www.cdc.gov/vaccines/schedules/hcp/imz/child-adolescent.html). When immunizations have been omitted or delayed, the immunization schedule continues from the last vaccine dose. Parents should be fully informed about the potential side effects of immunizations. In most office and clinic settings, parents sign state-developed informed consent documents that describe potential side effects. The CDC also provides resources for Caring for Children in a Disaster, Specific Threats, Biological Threats (https://www.cdc.gov/childrenindisasters/biological-threats.html).

Chemical Agents

Preschoolers face exposure to environmental pollutants, especially those that live below the federal poverty level and in homes built before 1978. A young child's skin area relative to body mass is twice that of an adult's; this increases the risk of toxicity. Young children also tend to put their hands or other objects into their mouths. Due to the unique vulnerability of a child's brain to chemicals, environmental exposure has been implicated in the increased prevalence of learning disabilities. Other reported health effects include lower intelligence quotient (IQ) scores, attention-related health problems, antisocial behavior, delayed puberty, reduced postnatal growth, and hearing loss.

Disparities exist among populations with regard to their risk. Ethnicity, socioeconomic status, and geographical location all have an effect on the risk of exposure. In particular, lead poisoning and elevated blood lead levels are an ongoing concern in children younger than 5 years. Health care professionals should perform targeted screening for lead poisoning in children who are Medicaid enrolled or Medicaid eligible, foreign born, or identified as high risk by the CDC location-specific recommendations or by a personal risk questionnaire. A carefully collected finger-stick sample is an acceptable method for measuring blood lead levels. In 2021 the CDC lowered the blood lead reference value from 5.0 to 3.5 micrograms per deciliter (μg/dL) based on NHANES data to identify children who have been exposed to lead and require intervention. In fact, according to the Childhood Blood Lead Surveillance System, of the children less than 72 months of age tested in 2018, 2.6% were confirmed with blood lead levels greater than 5 μg/dL (down from 5.2% in 2012), and 0.41% were confirmed with blood lead levels greater than 10 μg/dL (down from 0.58% in 2012) (CDC, 2022a).

Lead is found in old paint and its dust, toys, jewelry, and imported candles, among other sources. Lead is also found in products used in folk remedies. In the preschool group, lead may be found in products used to treat upset stomach *(empacho)*, constipation, diarrhea, and vomiting. In Hispanic traditional medicine, these products, known as *greta*, *azarcon*, *alarcón*, *coral*, *luiga*, *maría luisa*, or *rueda*, may contain extremely high lead contents. Lead has also been found in traditional remedies from cultures other than the Hispanic group. For example, *ghasard*, an Indian traditional tonic, and *ba-baw-san*, a Chinese herbal remedy for colic, has also been found to contain lead. Sources of lead other than those found in traditional medicine include pottery, cosmetics, and food additives. The CDC has a Childhood Lead Poisoning Prevention website that provides information on sources of lead, at-risk populations, blood lead levels in children, health effects, and lead FAQs (https://www.cdc.gov/nceh/lead/prevention/default.htm). The CDC stresses that "lead poisoning is 100% preventable."

Most poisonings in the US occur in the home. In 2021, unintentional poisoning was the 14th leading cause of nonfatal emergency department visits for children aged 3 to 6 years, with a total of 8983 cases and a crude rate of 56.46 per 100,000 (WISQARS, 2023). In 2021, there were also 15 deaths of children aged 3 to 6 due to poisoning. Parents should teach children about the four forms of poison, which are solids (air fresheners, pills, vitamins, aspirin, lipstick), liquids (cleaning products, fuel, alcohol), sprays (furniture polish, oven cleaner, room deodorizer), and invisibles (carbon monoxide, space heater fumes). Communication with parents about environmental dangers remains a major role of the childcare provider. Even though manufacturers enclose many children's medications in childproof packaging, the product may be administered incorrectly by the caregiver, or the child may experiment with another family member's colorful pills.

Many household products, drugs, carbon monoxide, pesticides, lead, mercury, polychlorinated biphenyls, ethers, and poisonous plants pose hazards to preschoolers. Secondary smoke and lead exposure also represent negative chemical influences on the growing child.

Preschoolers should receive verbal explanations about poisonous or dangerous substances, but parents cannot rely on preschoolers to remember instructions. A poison control program from the University of Pittsburgh introduced a character called *Mr. Yuk* in 1971, and this symbol has continued to be used to increase awareness and access to poison control centers (https://www.chp.edu/injury-prevention/teachers-and-parents/poison-center/mr-yuk). The ability to identify warning symbols such as Mr. Yuk helps preschoolers remain safe. Preschools and childcare facilities often incorporate topics about environmental pollutants and dangerous substances into their curricula to promote the health of preschoolers. Information about poison control is widely available online (https://www.aapcc.org/). The CDC provides resources for poisoning prevention (https://www.cdc.gov, search for child poisoning. The Children's Safety Network also provides resources on poison prevention (https://www.childrenssafetynetwork.org/child-safety-topics-terms/poison-prevention). The CDC also provides resources for parents by age groups (ages 0–3 and 4–11) on Safety in the Home & Community, including topics on different types of poisoning including carbon monoxide, environmental contamination, lead, and medicine (https://www.cdc.gov/parents/index.html).

Cancer

Overall cancer mortality in children aged 0 to 14 years from every major racial and ethnic group continued to decrease in the US from 2015 to 2019, while the overall incidence remained stable (Cronin et al., 2022). In 2001, 2011, and 2021, the cancer death rates for children aged 0 to 4 years were 2.52, 2.10, and 1.77 per 100,000, respectively (Curtin et al., 2023). In 2001, 2011, and 2021, the cancer death rates for children aged 5 to 9 years were 2.44, 2.17, and 1.71 per 100,000, respectively. According to WISQARS (2023), in 2021, malignant and benign neoplasms were the 2nd and 10th most common causes of death in children aged 3 to 6 years old, respectively. Unfortunately, disparities in survival attributed to race, ethnicity, poverty, and lack of health insurance exist (Delavar et al., 2020; Penumarthy et al., 2020).

From 2014 to 2018, the overall incidence of all sites of cancer was 17.8 per 100,000 in children ages 0 to 14 years. The three most common types of cancers in children are leukemia (5.3 per 100,000), brain and other nervous system (3.8 per 100,000), and lymphoma (1.7 per 100,000); unfortunately, there was a significant increasing trend in the occurrence of these three cancers from 0.7% to 0.9% per year, on average, from 2001 to 2018. For all types (sites) of cancer, the death rate from 2015 to 2019 was 2.0 per 100,000, and during this time frame there was a significant average annual percent change of -1.5% (National Cancer Institute, 2023). More specifically, the death rate due to brain and other nervous system cancers was 0.7 per 100,000 and due to leukemia was 0.5 per 100,000; fortunately, there was a significant decline in the occurrence of these two cancers of 0.4% for brain and other nervous system cancers and 2.9% for leukemia, per year, on average, from 2001 to 2019 (National Cancer Institute, 2023).

Remarkable advances in long-term survival of children with cancer have occurred. For example, the 5-year relative survival for all types of cancer increased from 58.0% in 1975 to 1977 to 83.1% % from 2000 to 2019 for children aged less than 15 years (National Cancer Institute, 2023). Early detection remains key to successful treatment; therefore, aggressive efforts have been invested in detection programs. Some of the increases in the rates of diagnosis may be attributed to improved imaging techniques and early detection.

Leukemia

According to the National Cancer Institute (2023), the 2016 to 2020 age-adjusted incidence rate for leukemia for both sexes aged 1 to 4 years and 5 to 9 years was 9.4 per 100,000 and 4.6 per 100,000, respectively. The rate for males aged 1 to 4 years (10.1 per 100,000) was higher than for females (8.6 per 100,000). Similarly, the rate for males aged 5 to 9 years (5.0 per 100,000) was higher than for females (4.1 per 100,000). Acute lymphocytic leukemia (ALL) is the most common, with an incidence rate of 7.8 per 100,000 for children aged 1 to 4 years and 3.8 per 100,000 for children aged 5 to 9 years. The dominant signs and symptoms of ALL appear suddenly, but often the child demonstrates a prodromal period of weakness, malaise, anorexia, fever, and tachycardia. Bone pain, petechiae, and hemorrhages after minor procedures such as dental extractions are frequently encountered. When an unexplained infection does not respond to management, suspicion should arise. Early detection and treatment of ALL has resulted in a marked increase in 5-year survival rates. Survival depends on the age at diagnosis, with the best survival rates occurring when diagnosis occurs during the preschool years (Hockenberry et al., 2024).

With suspected leukemia, the nurse institutes secondary prevention strategies with an assessment that includes the following parameters:

- Examination of the cervical and peripheral lymph nodes
- Palpation and percussion of the liver and spleen
- Inspection of the skin for systemic signs of leukemia, such as pallor, purpura, petechiae, and chloroma, which is a localized tumor mass that has a greenish appearance and may be found in the skin, orbits, or other tissues in granulocytic forms of leukemia
- Inspection of the mouth for enlarged tonsils; hyperplasia of the gums; and red, friable gingivae
- Palpation of the sternum, bones, and joints for tenderness and pain

The rate of leukemia is higher in children with Down syndrome; therefore, school nurses and public health nurses should monitor these children for early signs of the disease.

Wilms Tumor

Incidence rates from 2016 to 2020 for renal tumors range from 2.0 per 100,000 for children aged 1 to 4 years to 0.7 per 100,000 for those aged 5 to 9 years (National Cancer Institute, 2023). Furthermore, from 2013 to 2019, the 5-year relative survival for children aged <15 years was 92.0%. Most cases of Wilms tumor, the most common childhood malignant renal tumor, occur before 5 years of age. A strong correlation exists between Wilms tumor and several congenital malformations. Genetic links may contribute to its occurrence in children with bilateral tumors and those who have family members with the disorder. When Wilms tumor, aniridia (a congenital malformation of the iris of the eye), genitourinary malformations, and intellectual disability occur together, the genetic association strengthens. However, survivors of Wilms tumor that is unilateral at diagnosis possess a low risk of producing a child who will develop the disease. Information about the risk factors for Wilms tumor is not definitive. The 5-year survival rates for children with this disease are excellent (Hockenberry et al., 2024).

Retinoblastoma

Incidence rates from 2016 to 2020 for eye and orbit tumors range from 0.9 per 100,000 for children aged 1 to 4 years to 0.1 per 100,000 for those aged 5 to 9 years (National Cancer Institute, 2023). Furthermore, from 2013 to 2019, the 5-year relative survival for children aged <15 years was 96.0%. Genetic mutations contribute to the incidence of retinoblastoma, usually causing the bilateral form of the disease. Even though the tumor is uncommon, the scientific work surrounding its diagnosis and management has resulted in many of the methods used for treatment of other cancers. Survival rates are excellent (Hockenberry et al., 2024). The child's history usually reveals a slow symptom progression. To determine risk factors, the following questions should be asked:

- Do tumors of the eye run in your family?
- If tumors of the eye run in your family, which relatives were affected, and how were they treated?
- Have you noticed that your child has eye problems (crossed or lazy eyes or difficulty seeing)?
- Have you noticed any changes in your child's eyes?
- Screening eye examinations for high-risk children include the following:
  - Visual acuity
  - Red reflex, which appears whitish with retinoblastoma (cat's eye reflex)
  - Ophthalmoscopic findings
  - Lid lag, which is found with exophthalmos
  - Strabismus, by doing the cover-uncover test

The cat's eye reflex and strabismus are the most common signs of retinoblastoma. Any suspicious findings indicate referral for further evaluation.

Neuroblastoma

Neuroblastoma, a cancer of the sympathetic nervous system, begins in the abdomen, primarily in the adrenal gland, approximately 70% of the time. The remaining 30% of cases originate in cervical, thoracic, or pelvic areas. Maternal characteristics and perinatal factors have been reported with this type of cancer. The incidence rates from 2016 to 2020 for brain and other nervous system range from 4.1 per 100,000 for children aged 1 to 4 years to 3.3 per 100,000 for those aged 5 to 9 years (National Cancer Institute, 2023). Furthermore, from 2016 to 2020, the 5-year relative survival for children aged less than 15 years was 74.9%. Unfortunately, many of the children have metastases when the cancer is identified. Frequently, symptoms of secondary distribution bring the child to the health professional. The survival rate for children in whom neuroblastoma is diagnosed during the preschool years is increasing, but in other age groups it has remained static. There is little convincing evidence of specific risk factors. Cancer in a child can be frightening to parents, particularly if there is a strong family history of cancers of any kind. Early detection continues to be associated with increased survival rates. Secondary prevention programs should include the warning signs of cancer in children.

Asthma

Based on 2022 data from the National Center for Health Statistics (CDC, 2020e), about 9.9% of children less than 18 years have asthma, with the prevalence varying by age group (0–4 years = 3.2%, 5–11 years = 10.6%, 12–17 years = 13.9%). It is more common in males (11.4%) than females (8.2%) less than 18 years, and the prevalence increases as the poverty level increases. For example, children less than 18 years old with family incomes below 100% (10.5%) and below 200% (11.1%) of the federal poverty level have higher rates of asthma than children with family incomes above 200% (9.2%) of the federal poverty level. Similar differences are seen with other socioeconomic variables, such as parental employment, parental education, and health insurance coverage. There are also prevalence differences by race and ethnicity: Black = 15.9%, Hispanic or Latino = 9.8%, White = 8.9%, and Asian = 6.0% (data were unreliable for American Indian or Alaska Native and Native Hawaiian or Pacific Islander). The death rate in 2021 for children less than 18 years varied by age group (0–4 years = 1.4 per million; 5–11 years = 2.4 per million; 12–17 = 2.0 per million), was higher in males than females (2.4 vs. 1.6 per million), and varied by race and ethnicity (Black = 7.7, Hispanic = 1.4, White = 1.0 per million) (CDC, 2023).

Inflammation in this disorder contributes to a hyperresponsive airway, limited airflow, and respiratory symptoms including breathlessness, wheezing, cough, and chest tightness. The causes include genetic predisposition, allergens such as animal dander or dust mites, and nonspecific precipitants such as infections, exercise, weather, or stress. Poverty and social determinants of health contribute significantly to asthmatic illness, disability, and death (Federico et al., 2020; Stern, Pier, & Litonjua, 2020).

Multiple factors contribute to exacerbation of asthma symptoms. High levels of exposure to tobacco smoke, pollutants, and allergens contribute. In addition to the generally known allergens of house mite dust and pet and rodent dander, cockroach particles have been implicated. Access to quality medical care, financial resources, and social support to manage the disease on a long-term basis exist in significantly different proportions from one population to another in the United States.

DETERMINANTS OF HEALTH

Social Factors and Environment

Some preschoolers by the age of 3 years become involved with groups outside their families in childcare settings, faith-based

BOX 19.11 Evaluating a Childcare Setting

Childcare that meets the needs and expectations of parents will most likely ensure a happy preschooler as well. The questions that parents should consider in evaluating and choosing a childcare setting include the following:

- Will my needs and those of my child be best met with a caregiver in a family home, commercial center, or preschool, or by having a person come to my home to care for my child?
- What kinds of backup plans will I need or will be available if the provider becomes ill?
- What are my standards for nutrition, safety, sanitation, and health, and can these standards be met at the chosen childcare facility?
- How important is it to my child to be with other children? How many children would be ideal for my child's socialization needs?
- What personality attributes and educational preparation do I desire in my child's caregivers? What attributes do I dislike, and how will I deal with these attributes to maximize the care given to my child? How important is caregiver stability to me? Can I comfortably communicate with the staff to collaborate with my child's learning?
- What educational philosophy do I want in the setting? What involvement do I wish to have in the educational mission of the facility?
- Do the hours of the facility meet my personal and professional needs? Is close access to my job or home important to me?
- How are the children grouped, and what is the caregiver-to-child ratio?
- Does the cost of the service meet my financial needs? Can I pay part-time fees during vacation or when my child is ill for a lengthy period?
- Is accreditation of the facility mandatory for me to use it?
- What is my internal response or my general feelings about the setting when I visit it before my child's enrollment? Are the caregivers interacting with and responsive to the children? Are the children happy and interactive? Are the children's individual needs addressed appropriately? Is the environment supportive of my child's care? Is discipline appropriate?

groups, or family involvement in other activities. Other children of the same age experience little outside contact. A preschool setting introduces the child to a wider social arena. Parents learn to release their child to encourage independent activity in a safe, supervised setting. Preschoolers test their independence, interactive skills, and self-discipline as they learn to function in a group. Preschool provides a transition to kindergarten and first grade, where group interaction skills are expected. Parents often select a preschool based on geographical closeness to their home or a friend's recommendation, using the most practical approach (Box 19.11). With many childcare facilities and options now available, parents may visit and evaluate several settings to determine the one most appropriate for their needs.

Culture and Ethnicity

Family cultural heritage continues to shape preschoolers and influences their overall health. Nutrition and activity patterns are not only determined by the child but influenced by the family and community in which they live. Health-promotion assessment and intervention should adapt to cultural differences to promote a positive effect and understand the differences in disease prevalence among different groups. For example, children of African American and Hispanic cultures are at an increased risk for being overweight or obese, and the prevalence of type 2 diabetes in children is consistently higher in Native American, Hispanic, African American, and Southern Asian ethnic groups. Barkin et al. (2012) found that implementation of a culturally tailored, family-centered behavioral obesity intervention was effective in promoting short-term improvements in reducing the overall BMI in Latino-American preschool children. Their approach supports other studies that demonstrate the importance of including parent-child dyads for effectiveness of intervention in early childhood and also explores the effects of social networks in disseminating health behaviors and health outcomes within communities.

Culture and family traditions influence the child's understanding of community and society. Unlike toddlers, preschoolers frequently ask why the family follows certain practices. These young children notice differences from one family to another. Their playmates may celebrate different holidays or practice family rituals that are different from their own. As preschoolers experience more activities outside their home, differences become more apparent. Preschoolers also notice ethnic differences in appearance and pronounce skin colors, eyes, and hairstyles as "pretty" or "ugly." Mass media influences on physical attractiveness also contribute and become more significant to the adolescent. The socialization process forms presumptions similar to those of their family or playmates. Parents and caregivers who teach and role model positive behaviors allow children to see differences in others as being positive rather than negative. Discussion about the strength of cultural differences provides an excellent learning opportunity for the preschool child and family (Boyle et al., 2024).

Certain cultures have higher demands for children to assume responsibility for younger siblings or household tasks. Confusion develops in preschoolers when the family's culture differs from that of most playmates. Disciplinary approaches differ from culture to culture. Uncertainty also results when parents integrate their cultural background into the community standards, but the grandparents may adhere to traditional cultural practices, rituals, and childrearing preconceptions.

Levels of Policymaking and Health

Many safety-focused legislative bills have affected preschoolers (see Chapter 18). School issues, as discussed in Chapter 20, also affect this age group. With current concerns about health care costs, financial programs that focus on children may lose when competing with the whole of health care. If overall funding for vulnerable populations such as the homeless and the poor decreases, child health care in general in the United States suffers. Historical poverty data from the US Census Bureau (2023) shows that poverty has declined from 2012 to 2022, that racial and ethnic differences persist, and that there are geographic differences.

In 2022, 10.8 million people in the United States under 18 years old were in poverty, representing 28.4% of the population in poverty. These numbers were down from 2012 when there were 16.1 million people under 18 in poverty, representing 34.6% of the population in poverty. In 2022, there were also differences in the percentage of those under 18 years old in poverty by race and ethnicity: White alone = 13.5%, Black alone = 22.3%, Asian alone = 8.8%, American Indian or Alaska Native alone = 37.1%, and Hispanic (any race) = 21.7%. In fact, the percentage of those under 18 in poverty for all races fell from

2012 (White alone = 18.5%, Black alone = 37.9%, Asian alone = 13.8%, American Indian or Alaska Native alone = 45.1%, and Hispanic [any race] = 33.8%). In 2022, 15.0% of males and 14.9% of females under 18 years old were in poverty, an improvement from 2012, when 21.3% of males and 22.3% of females were in poverty. The percentage of related children under 6 years old in poverty was 15.9% in 2022, an improvement from 24.4% in 2012. By region and in 2022, the South had the highest percentage of people below poverty at 13.2%, followed by the Northeast (10.8%), West (10.7%), and Midwest (9.8%). Compared with 2012, the poverty level in all regions went down, and there was a change in the order (South = 16.5%, West = 15.1%, Northeast = 13.6%, and Midwest = 13.3%) (US Census Bureau, 2023).

The social circumstances in which people live and work significantly influence their health and development, especially for children growing up in poverty. Child health clinicians are in a position to provide surveillance and screening to address these social determinants of health to help prevent their affect on the child, however, clinicians often lack the training, tools, and resources to address these issues (Chung et al., 2016). The APA and AAP authorized task forces to address childhood poverty, with the work group of the APA Childhood Poverty Task Force Health Care Delivery Committee publishing guidelines that provide an evidence-based, practical approach to the aspects of surveillance and screening that apply to children and families living in poverty (Chung et al., 2016). These social determinants of health are outlined in Box 19.12: Health and Social Determinants/Health Equity, with the published guide for clinicians assisting in their ability to work one-on-one with families to address the issues that may be affecting overall health and well-being. Clinicians should work in collaboration with other health care providers and community resources while building on identified family strengths and assets. By working one-on-one with families in surveillance, screening, and referral to resources, health care clinicians can affect the effects of childhood poverty and maximize child health and well-being (Chung et al., 2016).

Economics

Poverty influences preschoolers as it does any child. Unlike toddlers, preschoolers become more aware of family economic status. A preschooler may know that the family lacks money for toys but recognizes less the limits to resources that influence the family lifestyle. In some cases, the family's financial history prevents attendance at preschool or influences exposure to expanded learning activities. Preschoolers realize money acquires food, toys, and clothes, but they do not yet have a concept of economic values. The child might trade an expensive item for a trinket that looks more interesting. A child who uses the earnings to buy something realizes that more must be earned to buy more things. The child thus begins to learn the concepts of earning and spending.

Health Services/Delivery System

Access to health care resources for preschoolers is the same as that for toddlers. When preschoolers enter a school setting, admission may require that a health care worker screen them physically and developmentally. For indigent children, **Early and Periodic Screening, Diagnosis, and Treatment** (EPSDT), a Medicaid program, may fund the visit. Screening for individuals younger than 21 years who meet the economic criteria for Medicaid occurs in private offices, local health departments, and community clinics. Medicaid provides one screening examination per year, which includes the following elements:

- Medical history
- Assessment of physical growth, nutritional status, and mental development
- Inspection of ears, eyes, nose, mouth, teeth, and throat
- Vision screening
- Auditory screening
- Screening for cardiac abnormalities
- Screening for anemia
- Screening for the sickle cell trait
- Urine sampling
- Blood pressure reading
- Assessment and updating of immunizations
- Tuberculosis screening, when indicated
- Referral to a dentist for diagnosis and treatment for children aged 3 years or older

Referral for a complete physical examination addresses any health or developmental concerns identified during this

BOX 19.12 HEALTH AND SOCIAL DETERMINANTS/HEALTH EQUITY

Social Determinants of Health Among Children and Families Living in Poverty

A workgroup of the Academic Pediatric Association Childhood Poverty Task Force Health Care Delivery Committee (Chung et al., 2016) identified and published the following social determinants of health that affect children and families living in poverty. The published guidelines provide an overview of these social determinants of health and provide health care clinicians with practical screening tools and resources.

- Child Maltreatment
- Childcare and Education
- Family Financial Support
- Physical Environment
- Family Social Support
- Intimate Partner Violence
- Maternal Depression and Family Mental Illness
- Household Substance Abuse
- Firearm Exposure
- Parental Health Literacy

The guide outlines the following core components for surveillance and screening:

1. Eliciting and attending to parents' concerns by asking general questions at routine visits.
2. Identifying the presence of risk factors and protective factors.
3. Screening for specific social issues at periodic visits.
4. Referring patients and families with identified needs to professionals in the appropriate disciplines and community agencies that provide direct assistance and resources.

The guide also outlines specific principles that inform screening:

1. Screening should be tailored to address the most commonly identified issues in the community served.
2. Screening should be appropriate for the child's developmental stage.
3. Screening for specific issues should ideally be implemented after available resources to address the issues are identified.

BOX 19.13 Health-Promotion Screening for Preschool Children

Annually
- Health history
- Height and weight
- Blood pressure
- Vision screening (age 3–4 years)
- Developmental and behavioral assessment
- Physical examination

Periodically
- Immunizations based on recommended schedule
- Ensure currency
- Diphtheria, tetanus, acellular pertussis
- Oral poliovirus
- Pneumococcal
- Measles, mumps, rubella
- *Haemophilus influenzae* type b
- Hepatitis B
- Varicella
- Hematocrit or hemoglobin level at least once after age 9 months
- Urinalysis at 5 years old

Screenings for High-Risk Children
- Lead
- Tuberculosis
- Cholesterol

Anticipatory Guidance
- Injury prevention
- Child safety car seat (through at least 4 years)
- Belt-positioning booster seat with lap and shoulder belt (through at least 8 years)
- Use helmet and avoid traffic when bicycling
- Smoke detectors, flame-retardant sleepwear
- Hot water temperature less than 120°F
- Window and stair guards, pool fence
- Safe storage of drugs, toxic substances, firearms, matches
- Close availability of syrup of ipecac, poison control phone number
- Parents and caretakers trained in cardiopulmonary resuscitation
- Violence prevention
- Nutrition and exercise
- Limit saturated fats; maintain caloric balance; and emphasize grain, fruit, vegetable intake
- Regular fun physical activity
- Tobacco
- Effects of passive smoking
- Antitobacco messages
- Dental health
- Floss, brush with fluoridated toothpaste at least daily
- Regular visits to dentist

screening. Eligible children receive EPSDT as a comprehensive service administered by Medicaid (https://www.medicaid.gov/medicaid/benefits/early-and-periodic-screening-diagnostic-and-treatment/index.html). Enactment of the Affordable Care Act in 2010 ensured health coverage for all children and free immunizations, affecting preschool children's health and health promotion (https://www.healthcare.gov/health-care-law-protections).

NURSING ACTIONS AND APPLICATION

Preschoolers show much interest in the tools and procedures of a health screening examination (Box 19.13). Preschoolers may observe and play with the stethoscope, otoscope, and other diagnostic instruments. The nurse explains the tests in age-appropriate terminology and expects the child to cooperate for most of the visit. Preschoolers may show self-control during injections but definitely need a parent close by to offer support and encouragement. The nurse includes the preschooler in the history inventory by directing questions about dietary intake and health practices, such as tooth brushing, favorite activities, and friends. At this age, children begin taking some interest in health, developing cognitive maturity to learn many health-promotion skills that they will use for the rest of their lives.

CASE STUDY

Preschool Child: Ricky

Ricky, aged 4 years, arrives at the clinic with his mother. Ricky lives with his mother and father, who both work full-time, and his infant sister. Their extended family lives in a different state more than 100 miles away. Ricky has just started preschool for part of the week, as preschool classes were canceled during the COVID epidemic. Ricky's mother mentions that Ricky often expresses frustration, particularly in regard to food. Conflict over food occurs every day. Mealtime is a battle to get him to eat unless his mother feeds him. Ricky's baby sister seems to tolerate all baby foods but requires her mother to spoon-feed. Ricky's mother is quite frustrated and concerned that he will become malnourished.

Analyzing Cues and Reflective Questions
- What additional assessment information would you collect?
- What questions would you ask and how would you further explore this issue with the mother?
- In what ways does the distance of the extended family influence this family's approach to health promotion?
- What factors would you consider to determine whether malnourishment is a factor in this family?

SUMMARY

- Schedules for preventive health care during the preschool years include visits at 4 and 5 years of age.
- Each visit includes an ongoing history; growth, physical, and developmental assessment; and discussion of age-appropriate developmental concerns.
- Early exposure to and reinforcement of health care information as part of preschool education lays a foundation for later healthy lifestyle habits, which influence overall societal health.
- Health as a curricular subject during the school-age years continues this focus. The school nurse's role in health promotion and prevention of illness is discussed in Chapter 20.

EVOLVE CHAPTER FEATURES

http://evolve.elsevier.com/Edelman/
- Study Questions

REFERENCES

American Academy of Pediatrics (AAP). (2018a). *Gender identity development in children.* https://www.healthychildren.org/English/ages-stages/gradeschool/Pages/Gender-Identity-and-Gender-Confusion-In-Children.aspx

American Academy of Pediatrics (AAP). (2018b). *Toilet training.* https://publications.aap.org/patiented/article-abstract/doi/10.1542/peo_document105/80105/Toilet-Training?redirectedFrom=fulltext

American Academy of Pediatrics (AAP). (2020). *How to support children after their parents separate or divorce.* https://www.healthychildren.org/English/healthy-living/emotional-wellness/Building-Resilience/Pages/How-to-Support-Children-after-Parents-Separate-or-Divorce.aspx

American Academy of Pediatrics (AAP). STAR Center. Developmental Surveillance and Screening Resources for Pediatricians. (2024). *Screening tools.* https://www.aap.org/en/patient-care/developmental-surveillance-and-screening-patient-care/developmental-surveillance-resources-for-pediatricians/?srsltid=AfmBOooynRr1KkBeQyotJlvZ9UEO7HRrk21F9YUXGPEIlUljCeqv995J

American Academy of Pediatrics (AAP). (2021). *Child abuse and neglect.* https://www.aap.org/en/patient-care/child-abuse-and-neglect/

American Dental Association. (2023). *Mouth healthy.* www.mouthhealthy.org

American Dental Association Council on Scientific Affairs. (2014). Fluoride toothpaste use for young children. *The Journal of the American Dental Association, 145*(2), 190–191.

American Psychiatric Association. (2013). *Diagnostic and statistical manual of mental disorders. 5th Edition: DSM-5.* American Psychiatric Publishing.

American Psychological Association. (2009). *Understanding and preventing child abuse and neglect.* https://www.apa.org/pi/families/resources/understanding-child-abuse

American Speech-Language-Hearing Association. (2024). *How does your child hear and talk?* https://www.asha.org/public/speech/development/chart.htm

Attar, S. M., Bradstreet, L. E., Ramsey, R. K., Kelly, K., & Robins, D. L. (2023). Validation of the electronic modified checklist for autism in toddlers, revised with follow-up: A nonrandomized controlled trial. *The Journal of Pediatrics, 262,* 113343. https://doi.org/10.1016/j.jpeds.2022.11.044

Bahanan, L., Singhal, A., Zhao, Y., Scott, T., & Kaye, E. (2021). The association between food insecurity, diet quality, and untreated caries among US children. *Journal of the American Dental Association, 152*(8), 613–621. https://doi.org/10.1016/j.adaj.2021.03.024

Barkin, S. L., Gesell, S. B., Po'e, E. K., Escarfuller, J., & Tempesti, T. (2012). Culturally tailored, family-centered, behavioral obesity intervention for Latino-American preschool-aged children. *Pediatrics, 130*(3), 445–456.

Bathory, E., & Tomopoulos, S. (2017). Sleep regulation, physiology and development, sleep duration and patterns, and sleep hygiene in infants, toddlers, and preschool-age children. *Current Problems in Pediatric and Adolescent Health Care, 47*(2), 29–42.

Becker, D. R., McClelland, M. M., Loprinzi, P., & Trost, S. G. (2014). Physical activity, self-regulation, and early academic achievement in preschool children. *Early Education and Development, 25*(1), 56–70.

Bhutta, Z. A., Bhavnani, S., Betancourt, T. S., Tomlinson, M., & Patel, V. (2023). Adverse childhood experiences and lifelong health. *Nature Medicine, 29*(7), 1639–1648. https://doi.org/10.1038/s41591-023-02426-0

Boyle, J. S., Collins, J. W., Andrews, M.M., & Ludwig-Beymer, P. (2024). *Transcultural concepts in nursing care* (9th ed.). Philadelphia, PA: Wolters Kluwer.

Brown, W. H., Pfeiffer, K. A., McIver, K. L., Dowda, M., Addy, C. L., & Pate, R. R. (2009). Social and environmental factors associated with preschoolers' non-sedentary physical activity. *Child Development, 80*(1), 45–58.

Bowne, J. (2015). *Enhancing and practicing executive function skills with children from infancy to adolescence.* Center on the Developing Child, Harvard University. https://harvardcenter.wpenginepowered.com/wp-content/uploads/2015/05/Enhancing-and-Practicing-Executive-Function-Skills-with-Children-from-Infancy-to-Adolescence-1.pdf

Brazelton Touch Points Center. (2024). https://www.brazeltontouchpoints.org/newborn-behaviors/

Bussières, A., Hancock, M. J., Elklit, A., Ferreira, M. L., Ferreira, P. H., Stone, L. S., Wideman, T. H., Boruff, J. T., Al Zoubi, F., Chaudhry, F., Tolentino, R., & Hartvigsen, J. (2023). Adverse childhood experience is associated with an increased risk of reporting chronic pain in adulthood: a systematic review and meta-analysis. *European Journal of Psychotraumatology, 14*(2), 2284025. https://doi.org/10.1080/20008066.2023.2284025

Centers for Disease Control and Prevention (CDC). (2020a). *Creating positive childhood experiences.* https://www.cdc.gov/

Centers for Disease Control and Prevention (CDC). (2020b). *Data and statistics on autism spectrum disorder.* https://www.cdc.gov/ncbddd/autism/data.html

Centers for Disease Control and Prevention (CDC). (2020c). *Developmental monitoring and screening for health professionals.* https://www.cdc.gov/

Centers for Disease Control and Prevention (CDC). (2020d). *Preventing adverse childhood experiences.* https://www.cdc.gov/violenceprevention/childabuseandneglect/aces/fastfact.html

Centers for Disease Control and Prevention (CDC). (2020e). *National Center for Health Statistics. Percentage of ever having asthma for children under age 18 years, United States, 2019–2022.* National Health Interview Survey. https://wwwn.cdc.gov/NHISDataQueryTool/SHS_child/index.html

Centers for Disease Control and Prevention (CDC). (2020f). *Screening and diagnosis of Autism spectrum disorder.* https://www.cdc.gov/autism/diagnosis/index.html

Centers for Disease Control and Prevention (CDC). (2020g). *Why act early if you're concerned about development?* https://www.cdc.gov/ncbddd/actearly/whyActEarly.html

Centers for Disease Control and Prevention (CDC). (2021). *Autism and vaccines.* https://www.cdc.gov/vaccinesafety/concerns/autism.html

Centers for Disease Control and Prevention (CDC). (2022a). *National childhood blood lead surveillance data.* https://www.cdc.gov/nceh/lead/data/national.htm

Centers for Disease Control and Prevention (CDC). (2022b). *Signs and symptoms of autism spectrum disorders.* https://www.cdc.gov/ncbddd/autism/signs.html

Centers for Disease Control and Prevention (CDC). (2023). *Most recent national asthma data.* https://www.cdc.gov/asthma/most_recent_national_asthma_data.htm

Center on the Developing Child. (2010). *The foundations of lifelong health are built in early childhood.* https://developingchild.harvard.edu/

Children's Defense Fund. (2019). *Protect children not guns 2019.* Washington, DC: Children's Defense Fund.

Children's Defense Fund. (2020). *Gun violence protection.* Washington, DC: Children's Defense Fund.

Christensen, D. L., Bilder, D. A., Zahorodny, W., Pettygrove, S., Durkin, M. S., Fitzgerald, R. T., Rice, C., Kurzius-Spencer, M., Baio, J., & Yeargin-Allsopp, M. (2016). Prevalence and characteristics of autism spectrum disorder among 4-year-old children in the Autism and Developmental Disabilities Monitoring Network. *Journal of Developmental and Behavioral Pediatrics, 37*(1), 1–8.

Chung, E. K., Siegel, B. S., Garg, A., Conroy, K., Gross, R. S., Long, D. A., Lewis, G., Osman, C. J., Messito, M., Wade, R., Yin, H. S., Cox, J., & Fierman, A. H. (2016). Screening for social determinants of health among children and families living in poverty: A guide for clinicians. *Current Problems in Pediatric and Adolescent Health Care, 46*(5), 135–153.

Cleveland Clinic. (2022). *What you need to know about infant and children's vital signs.* https://health.clevelandclinic.org/pediatric-vital-signs

Cronin, K. A., Scott, S., Firth, A. U., Sung, H., Henley, S. J., Sherman, R. L., Siegel, R. L., Anderson, R. N., Kohler, B. A., Benard, V. B., Negoita, S., Wiggins, C., Cance, W. G., & Jemal, A. (2022). Annual report to the nation on the status of cancer, part 1: National cancer statistics. *Cancer, 128*(24), 4251–4284. https://doi.org/10.1002/cncr.34479

Cunningham, R. M., Walton, M. A., Carter, P. M. (2018). The major causes of death in children and adolescents in the United States. *N Engl J Med, 379*(25), 2468–2475. doi:10.1056/NEJMsr1804754

Curtin, S. C., Anderson, R. N. (2023). *Declines in cancer death rates among youth: United States, 2001–2021.* NCHS Data Brief, no 484. Hyattsville, MD: National Center for Health Statistics. https://dx.doi.org/10.15620/cdc:134499

Davis, R. L., Quinn, M., Thompson, M. E., Kilanowski, J. F., Polfuss, M. L., & Duderstadt, K. G. (2021). Childhood obesity: Evidence-based guidelines for clinical practice-part two. *Journal of Pediatric Health Care: Official Publication of National Association of Pediatric Nurse Associates & Practitioners, 35*(1), 120–131. https://doi.org/10.1016/j.pedhc.2020.07.011

Delavar, A., Barnes, J. M, Wang, X., & Johnson, K. J. (2020). Associations between race/ethnicity and US childhood and adolescent cancer survival by treatment amenability. *JAMA Pediatrics, 174*(5), 1–9.

Denny, S.A., Quan, L., Gilchrist, J., McCallin, T., Shenoi, R., Yusaf, S., Weiss, J., & Hoffman, B., & COUNCIL ON INJURY, VIOLENCE, AND POISON PREVENTION. (2021). Prevention of drowning. *Pediatrics, 148*(2), e2021052227. https://doi.org/10.1542/peds.2021-052227

Du Toit, G., Roberts, G., Sayre, P. H., Bahnson, H. T., Radulovic, S., Santos, A. F., Brough, H. A., Phippard, D., Basting, M., Feeney, M., Turcanu, V., Sever, M. L., Gomez Lorenzo, M., Plaut, M., & Lack, G. (2015). Randomized trial of peanut consumption in infants at risk for peanut allergy. *The New England Journal of Medicine, 372*(9), 803–813.

Duckers, J., Lesher, B., Thorat, T., Lucas, E., McGarry, L. J., Chandarana, K., & De Iorio, F. (2021). Real-world outcomes of ivacaftor treatment in people with cystic fibrosis: A systematic review. *Journal of Clinical Medicine, 10*(7), 1527. https://doi.org/10.3390/jcm10071527

Easwaran, H. N., Annadurai, A., Muthu, M. S., Sharma, A., Patil, S. S., Jayakumar, P., Jagadeesan, A., Nagarajan, U., Pasupathy, U., & Wadgave, U. (2022). Early childhood caries and iron deficiency anaemia: A systematic review and meta-analysis. *Caries Research, 56*(1), 36–46. https://doi.org/10.1159/000520442

Erikson, E. H. (1995). *Childhood and society* (35th anniversary ed.). New York: Norton.

Erikson, E. H., & Erikson, J. M. (1998). *The life cycle completed.* New York: Norton.

Federico, M. J., McFarlane, A. E., Szefler, S. J., & Abrams, EM. (2020). The impact of social determinants of health on children with asthma. *Journal of Allergy and Clinical Immunology: In Practice, 8*, 1080–1814.

Findlen, U. M., Hounam, G. M., Alexy, E., & Adunka, O. F. (2019). Early Hearing Detection and Intervention. *Ear and Hearing, 40*(3), 651–658.

Fountain, C., Zhang, Y., Kissin, D. M., Schieve, L. A., Jamieson, D. J., Rice, C., & Bearman, P. (2015). Association between assisted reproductive technology conception and autism in California, 1997–2007. *American Journal of Public Health, 105*(5), 963–971.

Ghafouri-Fard, S., Pourtavakoli, A., Hussen, B.M., Taheri, M., Ayatollahi, S.A. (2023). A review on the role of genetic mutations in the autism spectrum disorder. *Mol Neurobiol, 60*(9), 5256–5272. https://doi.org/10.1007/s12035-023-03405-9

Gooey, M., Skouteris, H., Betts, J., Hatzikiriakidis, K., Sturgiss, E., Bergmeier, H., & Bragge, P. (2022). Clinical practice guidelines for the prevention of childhood obesity: A systematic review of quality and content. *Obesity Reviews: An Official Journal of the International Association for the Study of Obesity, 23*(10), e13492. https://doi.org/10.1111/obr.13492

Gupta, R. S., Warren, C. M., Smith, B. M., Blumenstock, J. A., Jiang, J., Davis, M. M., & Nadeau, K. C. (2018). The public health impact of parent-reported childhood food allergies in the United States. *Pediatrics, 142*(6), e20181235.

Hagan, J. F., Shaw, J. S., & Duncan, P. M. (2017). *Bright futures: Guidelines for health supervision of infants, children, and adolescents.* Elk Grove Village, IL: Bright Futures/American Academy of Pediatrics.

Hill, H. A., Elam-Evans, L. D., Yankey, D., Singleton, J. A., & Kang, Y. (2016). Vaccination coverage among children aged 19–35 months — United States. *MMWR. Morbidity and mortality weekly report, 66*, 1171–1177.

Hockenberry, M. J., Duffy, E., & Gibbs, K. (2024). *Wong's nursing care of infants and children* (12th ed.). Elsevier.

Hodges, H., Fealko, C., & Soares, N. (2020). Autism spectrum disorder: Definition, epidemiology, causes, and clinical evaluation. *Translational Pediatrics, 9*(S1), S55–S65.

Hustedde, C. (2021). Adverse childhood experiences. *Primary Care, 48*(3), 493–504. https://doi.org/10.1016/j.pop.2021.05.005

Hviid, A., Hansen, J. V., Frisch, M., & Melbye, M. (2019). Measles, mumps, rubella vaccination and autism. *Annals of Internal Medicine, 170*(8), 513.

Hyman, S. L., Levy, S. E., & Myers, S. M. (2020). Identification, evaluation, and management of children with autism spectrum disorder. *Pediatrics, 145*(1), e20193447.

Janssen, X., Martin, A., Hughes, A. R., Hill, C. M., Kotronoulas, G., & Hesketh, K. R. (2020). Associations of screen time, sedentary time and physical activity with sleep in under 5s: A systematic review and meta-analysis. *Sleep Medicine Reviews, 49*, 101226. https://doi.org/10.1016/j.smrv.2019.101226

Ji, S. Q., Han, R., Huang, P. P., Wang, S. Y., Lin, H., & Ma, L. (2021). Iron deficiency and early childhood caries: A systematic review and meta-analysis. *Chinese Medical Journal, 134*(23), 2832–2837. https://doi.org/10.1097/CM9.0000000000001729

Jones, C. M., Merrick, M. T., & Houry, D. E. (2020). Identifying and preventing adverse childhood experiences: Implications for clinical practice. *JAMA, 323*(1), 25–26.

Jullien, S. (2021). Prophylaxis of caries with fluoride for children under five years. *BMC Pediatrics, 21*(Suppl 1), 351. https://doi.org/10.1186/s12887-021-02702-3

Kemp, M. A., Lawson, Z., & Macguire, A. S. (2014). Patterns of burns and scalds in children. *Archives of Disease in Children, 99*(4), 316–321.

Kendrick, D., Young, B., Mason-Jones, A. J., Ilyas, N., Achana, F. A., Cooper, N. J., Hubbard, S. J., Sutton, A. J., Smith, S., Wynn, P., Mulvaney, C., Watson, M. C., & Coupland, C. (2013). Home safety education and provision of safety equipment for injury prevention (review). *Evidence-Based Child Health: A Cochrane Review Journal, 8*(3), 761–939.

Kendrick, D., Zou, K., Ablewhite, J., Watson, M., Coupland, C., Kay, B., Hawkins, A., & Reading, R. (2016). Risk and protective factors for falls on stairs in young children: Multicentre case–control study. *Arch Dis Child, 101*, 909–916.

Kuroiwa, E., Ragar, R. L., Langlais, C. S., Baker, A., Linnaus, M. E., & Notrica, D. M. (2018). Car seat education: A randomized controlled trial of teaching methods. *Injury, 49*(7), 1272–1277.

Laukkanen, J., Ojansuu, U., Tolvanen, A., Alatupa, S., & Aunola, K. (2014). Child's difficult temperament and mothers' parenting styles. *Journal of Child and Family Studies, 23*, 312–323.

Lee, E. Y., Bains, A., Hunter, S., Ament, A., Brazo-Sayavera, J., Carson, V., Hakimi, S., Huang, W. Y., Janssen, I., Lee, M., Lim, H., Silva, D. A. S., & Tremblay, M. S. (2021). Systematic review of the correlates of outdoor play and time among children aged 3-12 years. *The International Journal of Behavioral Nutrition and Physical Activity, 18*(1), 41. https://doi.org/10.1186/s12966-021-01097-9

Lee, J., Keller, J., & Zhang, T. (2022). Relation between demographics and physical activity among preschoolers attending Head Start. *Journal of Child and Family Studies*, 1–11. Advance online publication. https://doi.org/10.1007/s10826-022-02468-x

Leung, A. K. C., Leung, A. A. M., Wong, A. H. C., & Hon, K. L. (2020). Sleep terrors: An updated review. *Current Pediatric Reviews, 16*(3), 176–182. https://doi.org/10.2174/1573396315666191014152136

Lipkin, P. H., & Macias, M. M. (2020). Promoting optimal development: Identifying infants and young children with developmental disorders through developmental surveillance and screening. *Pediatrics, 145*(1), e20193449.

Ma, F. F., & Luo, D. M. (2023). Relationships between physical activity, fundamental motor skills, and body mass index in preschool children. *Frontiers in Public Health, 11*, 1094168. https://doi.org/10.3389/fpubh.2023.1094168

Maenner, M. J., Warren, Z., Williams, A. R., et al. (2023). Prevalence and characteristics of autism spectrum disorder among children aged 8 years — Autism and Developmental Disabilities Monitoring Network, 11 sites, United States, 2020. *Morbidity and Mortality Weekly Report. Surveillance Summaries (Washington, D.C.: 2002), 72*(No. SS-2):1–14. https://dx.doi.org/10.15585/mmwr.ss7202a1

McAdams, R. J., Swidarski, K., Clark, R. M., Roberts, K. J., Yang, J., & Mckenzie, L. B. (2018). Bicycle-related injuries among children treated in US emergency departments, 2006-2015. *Accident Analysis and Prevention, 118*, 11–17.

National Association of Pediatric Nurse Practitioners (NAPNAP). (2006). Healthy eating and activity together clinical practice guidelines: Identifying and preventing overweight in childhood. *Journal of Pediatric Health Care, 20*, s1–s63.

National Cancer Institute. (2023). https://www.cancer.gov/

National Highway Transportation Safety Administration. (NHTSA). (2023). *FARS data table, people, all victims.* https://www-fars.nhtsa.dot.gov/People/PeopleAllVictims.aspx

National Institute on Deafness and Other Communication Disorders (NIDCD). (2024). *Quick statistics about voice, speech, language.* https://www.nidcd.nih.gov/health/statistics/quick-statistics-voice-speech-language#:~:text=5%25%20of%20U.S.%20children%20ages,during%20the%20past%2012%20months.&text=The%20prevalence%20of%20speech%20sound,children%20is%208%20to%209%25

National Sleep Foundation. (2023). https://www.sleepfoundation.org

Neshteruk, C. D., Tripicchio, G. L., Lobaugh, S., Vaughn, A. E., Luecking, C. T., Mazzucca, S., & Ward, D. S. (2021). Screen time parenting practices and associations with preschool children's tv viewing and weight-related outcomes. *International Journal of Environmental Research and Public Health, 18*(14), 7359. https://doi.org/10.3390/ijerph18147359

Nilsen, A., Anderssen, S. A., Resaland, G. K., Johannessen, K., Ylvisaaker, E., & Aadland, E. (2019). Boys, older children, and highly active children benefit most from the preschool arena regarding moderate-to-vigorous physical activity: A cross-sectional study of Norwegian preschoolers. *Preventive Medicine Reports, 14*, 100837.

Nilsen, A., Anderssen, S. A., Ylvisaaker, E., Johannessen, K., & Aadland, E. (2019). Physical activity among Norwegian preschoolers varies by sex, age, and season. *Scandinavian Journal of Medicine & Science in Sports, 29*(6), 862–873.

Owens, J. A., & Moore, M. (2017). Insomnia in infants and young children. *Pediatric Annals, 46*(9), e321–e326. https://doi.org/10.3928/19382359-20170816-02

Ogundele, M. O. (2018). Behavioural and emotional disorders in childhood: A brief overview for paediatricians. *World Journal of Clinical Pediatrics, 7*(1), 9–26. https://doi.org/10.5409/wjcp.v7.i1.9

Piaget, J. (1950). *The psychology of intelligence*. London: Routledge and Kegan Paul.
Piaget, J. (1959). *Language and thought of the child*. New York: Routledge.
Paruthi, S., Brooks, L. J., D'Ambrosio, C., Hall, W. A., Kotagal, S., Lloyd, R. M., Malow, B. A., Maski, K., Nichols, C., Quan, S. F., Rosen, C. L., Troester, M. M., & Wise, M. S. (2016). Recommended amount of sleep for pediatric populations: a consensus statement of the American Academy of Sleep Medicine. *Journal of clinical sleep medicine: JCSM: Official Publication of the American Academy of Sleep Medicine*, *12*(6), 785–786.
Penumarthy, N. L., Goldsby, R. E., Shiboski, S. C., Wustrack, R., Murphy, P., & Winestone, L. E. (2020). Insurance impacts survival for children, adolescents, and young adults with bone and soft tissue sarcomas. *Cancer in Medicine*, *9*(3), 951–958.
Perin, C., Valagussa, G., Mazzucchelli, M., Gariboldi, V., Cerri, C. G., Meroni, R., Grossi, E., Cornaggia, C. M., Menant, J., Piscitelli, D. (2020). Physiological profile assessment of posture in children and adolescents with autism spectrum disorder and typically developing peers. *Brain Science*, *10*(10), 681. https://doi.org/10.3390/brainsci10100681
Polfuss, M. L., Duderstadt, K. G., Kilanowski, J. F., Thompson, M. E., Davis, R. L., & Quinn, M. (2020). Childhood obesity: Evidence-based guidelines for clinical practice-part one. *Journal of Pediatric Health Care*, *34*(3), 283–290.
Prevent Blindness. (n.d.). *Vision screenings and eye exams*. https://preventblindness.org/vision-screenings-and-eye-exams/
Prior, M., Bavin, E., Cini, E., Eadie, P., & Reilly, S. (2011). Relationships between language impairment, temperament, behavioural adjustment and maternal factors in a community sample of preschool children. *International Journal of Language & Communication Disorders*, *46*(4), 489–494.
Rafferty, J. (2018). Ensuring comprehensive care and support for transgender and gender-diverse children and adolescents. *Pediatrics*, *142*(4), e20182162.
Ramar, K., Malhotra, R. K., Carden, K. A., Martin, J. L., Abbasi-Feinberg, F., Aurora, R. N., Kapur, V. K., Olson, E. J., Rosen, C. L., Rowley, J. A., Shelgikar, A. V., & Trotti, L. M. (2021). Sleep is essential to health: An American Academy of Sleep Medicine position statement. *J Clin Sleep Med*, *17*(10), 2115–2119.
Roberts, M. Y., Curtis, P. R., Sone, B. J., & Hampton, L. H. (2019). Association of parent training with child language development: A systematic review and meta-analysis. *JAMA Pediatrics*, *173*(7), 671–680. https://doi.org/10.1001/jamapediatrics.2019.1197
Robins, D. L., Casagrande, K., Barton, M., Chen, C. A., Dumont-Mathieu, T., & Fein, D. (2014). Validation of the modified checklist for autism in toddlers, revised with follow-up (M-CHAT-R/F). *Pediatrics*, *133*(1), 37–45.
Rowhani-Rahbar, A., Simonetti, J. A., & Rivara, F. P. (2016). Effectiveness of interventions to promote safe firearm storage. *Epidemiologic Reviews*, *38*(1), 111–124.
Sabbagh, S., Mohammadi-Nasrabadi, F., Ravaghi, V., Azadi Mood, K., Sarraf Shirazi, A., Abedi, A. S., & Noorollahian, H. (2023). Food insecurity and dental caries prevalence in children and adolescents: A systematic review and meta-analysis. *International Journal of Paediatric Dentistry*, *33*(4), 346–363. https://doi.org/10.1111/ipd.13041
Safe Kids Worldwide. (2024). *Car seat safety tips*. https://www.safekids.org/car-seat
Sampath, V., Abrams, E. M., Adlou, B., Akdis, C., Akdis, M., Brough, H. A., Chan, S., Chatchatee, P., Chinthrajah, R. S., Cocco, R. R., Deschildre, A., Eigenmann, P., Galvan, C., Gupta, R., Hossny, E., Koplin, J. J., Lack, G., Levin, M., Shek, L. P., Makela, M., Renz, H. (2021). Food allergy across the globe. *The Journal of Allergy and Clinical Immunology*, *148*(6), 1347–1364. https://doi.org/10.1016/j.jaci.2021.10.018
Sanjeevi, N., Freeland-Graves, J. H., & Wright, G. J. (2023). Food security status, WIC participation, and early childhood caries in a nationally representative sample of children. *Journal of the Academy of Nutrition and Dietetics*, *123*(2), 276–283. https://doi.org/10.1016/j.jand.2022.06.223
Sarmiento, K., Haileyesus, T., Waltzman, D., & Daugherty, J. (2021). Emergency department visits for bicycle-related traumatic brain injuries among children and adults - United States, 2009-2018. *Morbidity and Mortality Weekly Report*, *70*(19), 693–697. https://doi.org/10.15585/mmwr.mm7019a1
Schroeder, K., Schuler, B. R., Kobulsky, J. M., & Sarwer, D. B. (2021). The association between adverse childhood experiences and childhood obesity: A systematic review. *Obesity Reviews: an Official Journal of the International Association for the Study of Obesity*, *22*(7), e13204. https://doi.org/10.1111/obr.13204
Schwebel, D. C., Davis, A. L., & O'Neal, E. E. (2012). Child pedestrian injury: a review of behavioral risks and preventative strategies. *American Journal of Lifestyle Medicine*, *6*(4), 292–302.
Silva, P. (2019). *Kalydeco (ivacaftor) for cystic fibrosis*. Cystic Fibrosis News Today. https://www.cysticfibrosisnewstoday.com/kalydeco-ivacaftor/
Stern, J., Pier, J., & Litonjua, A. A. (2020). Asthma epidemiology and risk factors. *Seminars in Immunopathology*, *42*, 5–15.
Tufford, L., & Lee, B. (2018). Decision-making factors in the mandatory reporting of child maltreatment. *Journal of Child & Adolescent Trauma*, *12*(2), 233–244. https://doi.org/10.1007/s40653-018-0211-2
US Census Bureau. (2023). *Historical poverty tables: People and families - 1959 to 2022*. https://www.census.gov/data/tables/time-series/demo/income-poverty/historical-poverty-people.html
US Department of Agriculture, & US Department of Health and Human Services (USDHHS). (2015). *2015–2020 dietary guidelines for Americans* (8th ed.). Washington, DC: US Government Printing Office. https://health.gov/sites/default/files/2019-09/2015-2020_Dietary_Guidelines.pdf
US Department of Agriculture. (n.d.). *Choose my plate*. https://www.myplate.gov
US Department of Education. (2011). *Race to the top - early learning challenge*. https://www.ed.gov/
US Department of Health and Human Services (USDHHS). (2018). *Physical activity guidelines for Americans, 2nd edition*. https://www.health.gov/our-work/physical-activity/current-guidelines
US Department of Health and Human Services (USDHHS). (2024). *Healthy People 2030. Office of Disease Prevention and Health Promotion*. https://www.health.gov/healthypeople/objectives-and-data/browse-objectives
US Department of Health & Human Services (USDHHS), Administration for Children and Families, Administration on Children, Youth and Families, Children's Bureau (USDHHS). (2023). *Child maltreatment*. https://www.acf.hhs.gov/cb/data-research/child-maltreatment
Walsh, T., Worthington, H. V., Glenny, A. M., Marinho, V. C., & Jeroncic, A. (2019). Fluoride toothpastes of different concentrations for preventing dental caries. *The Cochrane Database of Systematic Reviews*, *3*(3), CD007868. https://doi.org/10.1002/14651858.CD007868.pub3

Wei, H., Zhu, Y., Wang, T., Zhang, X., Zhang, K., & Zhang, Z. (2021). Genetic risk factors for autism-spectrum disorders: a systematic review based on systematic reviews and meta-analysis. *Journal of Neural Transmission (Vienna, Austria: 1996)*, *128*(6), 717–734. https://doi.org/10.1007/s00702-021-02360-w

Wieckowski, A. T., Williams, L. N., Rando, J., Lyall, K., & Robins, D. L. (2023). Sensitivity and specificity of the modified checklist for autism in toddlers (original and revised): A systematic review and meta-analysis. *JAMA Pediatrics*, *177*(4), 373–383. https://doi.org/10.1001/jamapediatrics.2022.5975

Williams, P. G., & Lerner, M. A. (2019). School Readiness. *Pediatrics*, *144*(2), e20191766.

WISQARS™ (Web-based Injury Statistics Query and Reporting System: Data and Statistics- WISQARS). (2023). *Centers for Disease Control and Prevention (CDC)*. https://www.cdc.gov/injury/wisqars/index.html

Yogman, M., Garner, A., Hutchinson, J., Hirsh-Pasek, K., & Golinkoff, R. M. (2018). The power of play: A pediatric role in enhancing development in young children. *Pediatrics*, *142*(3), e20182058.

Yoon, S. H., Choi, J., Lee, W. J., & Do, J. T. (2020). Genetic and Epigenetic Etiology Underlying Autism Spectrum Disorder. *Journal of Clinical Medicine*, *9*(4), 966. https://doi.org/10.3390/jcm9040966

Zhang, K., Lu, Z., & Guo, X. (2023). Advances in epidemiological status and pathogenesis of dental fluorosis. *Frontiers in Cell and Developmental Biology*, *11*, 1168215. https://doi.org/10.3389/fcell.2023.1168215

20

School-Age Child

Maureen McDonald and Helen Bellenoit

http://evolve.elsevier.com/Edelman/

OBJECTIVES

After completing this chapter, the reader will be able to:

- Identify expected physical and developmental changes occurring in the school-age child.
- Explore stages of cognitive development of the school-age child, particularly their relation to academic skills and performance.
- Appraise relevant health-promotion needs and common health risk factors found in the school-age child.
- Analyze the influence of culture, society, peers, and stress on development in the school-age child.
- Describe common developmental problems that occur in the school-age child including ways to assist parents in the management of these common problems.
- Select strategies for family (parents) to improve child's **self-concept**, **socialization** abilities, and stress reduction in the school-age child.

KEY TERMS

Anxiety
Asthma
Astigmatism
Attention-deficit/hyperactivity disorder (ADHD)
Auditory acuity
Auditory learners
Bullying
Child abuse
Chronic serous otitis media
Classifying and ordering
Concrete operation
Conservation
Coping strategies
Dental caries
Depression
Discipline
Disorders of arousal
Dyslexia; Encopresis
Enuresis
Gastroenteritis
Genomics
Healthy People 2030 initiatives
Human papillomavirus
Hyperopic (farsighted)
Hypertension
Individualized educational plan
Individuals with Disabilities Education Act (IDEA)
Industry versus inferiority
Intelligence
Intelligence quotient (IQ)
Kinesthetic learners
Latchkey children
Learning disability
Lice
Limit setting
Malocclusion
Menarche
Meningococcal vaccination
Moral development
Myopia (nearsightedness)
No Child Left Behind Act of 2001
Obesity
Orthodontic care
Ossification
Overweight
Pediculosis
Peer groups
Phonics
Preconventional level
Puberty
Public Law 94-142 (Education for All Handicapped Children Act)
Scabies; Section 504 of the Rehabilitation Act of 1973, Amendment Act of 2008
Self-concept
Self-discovery
Self-esteem
Sexual abuse
Sleep apnea
Sleep talking
Sleepwalking
Socialization
Somatization
Standardized growth charts
State Children's Health Insurance Program (SCHIP)
Talismans
Tooth eruption
Tympanograms
Vision screening programs
Visual learners

THINK ABOUT IT

School-Age Bullying

Raja is 9 years old and has recently started demonstrating withdrawn behavior. His mother reports "he used to enjoy school." Recently, he has mentioned wanting to stay home from school and has become apathetic regarding participating in school-related activities. Two weeks ago, his mother reports she began driving him to school. "He hasn't wanted to walk to school with his friends lately. I don't understand what is going on; he tells me 'It's nothing.'" He was performing well in school until this most recent grading period. As a result of COVID closing down his school classes for over a year, the classmates are fully online and sharing details about each other's situations. Since he returned to school, there have been drills about school shootings and protection of the classroom environment. He may be behind in math and reading. His teacher has voiced concern that Raja seems "distracted" and doesn't want to participate in group work conducted in class. Raja's father has voiced frustration that he seems to be "losing" things too. "Earlier this week he lost his backpack. Last week it was a jacket."

- Is Raja's behavior typical for a 9-year-old male child?
- How might a 9-year-old female child's behavior differ from Raja's in this situation?
- As a health care professional, how might you guide this family in finding ways to address Raja's behavior and possibilities of online **bullying**?
- How might you assist/counsel Raja on developing skills associated with resilience?
- Are there any further underlying issues that may be contributing to Raja's behavior?

TABLE 20.1 Growth and Development: Motor Development of the School-Age Child

Age (yr)	Gross Motor	Fine Motor
5	Dresses independently Runs well and jumps	Prints letters Ties shoes, buttons Draws triangle, square
6–8	Balances on one foot for 10 seconds Can perform tandem gait Pedals a bicycle Is skilled in physical activities, running, skipping	Spreads with knife Holds pencil with fingertip Draws a person with three to six parts Cuts and pastes Aligns letters horizontally Knows right from left
8–10	Has good body balance Enjoys vigorous activities Has increased coordination	Spaces words and letters with writing Draws a diamond Has better eye-hand coordination Bathes self Sews and builds models
10–12	Balances on one foot for 15 steps Catches a fly ball May experience clumsiness from prepubertal growth spurt Possesses all basic motor skills similar to adult	Writes well Has skills similar to those of an adult

The school-age years is a span of time between a child's entrance to kindergarten and the beginning of adolescence, a range from 6 to 10 years of age. During this period, observable differences in growth, development, and cognitive ability are prominent. Consider how different the child entering kindergarten is from the preadolescent, particularly the differences in size as well as mental ability. Children grow (physically) much more slowly during this period as compared with growth during infancy and adolescence. Fine and gross motor skills are being perfected, and mental abilities grow tremendously as the child learns to read, write, and compute mathematics, in addition to other topics of interest (Table 20.1). Relationships outside the family, including **peer groups**, are also developing during this phase of growth and development.

Most children are relatively healthy during this period. Health-promotion and health-maintenance strategies are important. During this period of development, children learn to accept personal responsibility and participate in the management of self-care tasks in the areas of personal hygiene, nutrition, physical activity, sleep, and safety. Nurses fill a significant role in the facilitation of parental roles and child roles in meeting growth, developmental, and self-care aspects of the school-age child (Centers for Disease Control and Prevention [CDC], n.d.-a,-o,-p; Luster, 2018).

BIOLOGY AND GENETICS

A child's growth and development are influenced by genetic inheritance, nutrition, and the physical-sociocultural environments in which the child lives. The school-age child has an overall slimmer appearance as compared with the preschool child. Their legs are longer as compared with the rest of the body, allowing greater strength, balance, coordination, and fluidity of motion in running, jumping, climbing, throwing, and riding a bicycle (Graber, 2023).

Most body systems reach adult level of function during the school-age years. Before 6 years of age, children use the diaphragm as the primary breathing muscle. After 6 years of age, thoracic muscles develop, and the respiratory rate slows to 14 to 22 breaths/min (Mersch, n.d.). The school-age child's head circumference continues to grow. However, after age 5 years, head growth slows until **puberty**. Head circumference and the brain are most of the adult size by age 7 years (Graber, 2023). The heart slowly grows in size, and the heart rate slows to an average rate of 60 to 95 beats/min, approaching that of an adult. Mean blood pressure is lower in this age group than in adults and ranges from 95 to 119 mm Hg systolic and from 60 to 76 mm Hg diastolic (Mersch, n.d.). The gastrointestinal system is maturing with increased stomach capacity, resulting in less need for snacks and decreased calorie needs as compared with the preschooler. Bladder capacity increases. The immune system is better able to produce an antibody-antigen response (Savoy, 2023). By puberty, the endocrine system (with the exception of reproductive function) approaches adult capacity and function.

Elevated Blood Pressure

The long-term effects of elevated blood pressure, **hypertension**, in adults are well known and documented. The realization that adult hypertension often begins in childhood has encouraged efforts to screen young children for elevated blood pressure. The American Academy of Pediatrics (AAP) and the National Heart, Lung, and Blood Institute recommend that children have their blood pressure measured annually, beginning at 3 years of age (CDC, n.d.-l; Flynn et al., 2017. This recommendation emerged from concerns of higher blood pressures in children over the past several decades, demonstrating risk of cardiovascular disease. Approximately one in every seven children aged 12 to 19 years has high blood pressure (CDC, n.d.-l). Blood pressure measures among school-age children may differ greatly depending on the height and weight of the child. A family history of hypertension or identification of an elevated blood pressure in a child mandates close monitoring and assessment of cardiovascular risk factors at well-child checkups during the school-age years (Flynn et al., 2017; American Heart Association [AHA], 2023). Differentiation between primary and secondary hypertension should be determined in any school-age child with elevated blood pressure (AHA, 2023). Risk factors for childhood hypertension include obesity, high sodium intake, and increased calories. Low birthweight, food insecurity, and higher BMI can lead to higher blood pressure in children. Childhood perception of threats to safety or security of the child's bodily integrity and family and social structures may influence hypertension (Falkner et al., 2023).

Physical Growth

Although many children have "spurts" of growth alternating with periods of minimal growth, height and weight growth velocities assume a slower and steadier pace as compared with earlier years of growth. The school-age child gains approximately 7.6 cm (<3 in) in height per year and 2 to 3 kg (4.4 to 6.6 lb) in weight per year until puberty, at which time growth rates increase (Graber, 2023). Black American children tend to be slightly larger and Asian American children tend to be somewhat smaller than their Caucasian counterparts, as plotted on growth charts that are believed to be standardized for various ethnic groups (Williams, 2016). Before the onset of puberty there is little difference in size between young males and females. However, toward the latter part of this developmental stage, females tend to grow more rapidly in height and weight (Graber, 2023). A preadolescent increase in height and weight tends to occur at approximately 10 years of age in females and 12 years of age in males. However, maturation rates differ, resulting in a wide range of sizes in both males and females, particularly among those aged 10 to 12 years (Perng et al., 2019; Isong et al., 2018).

Black American and Mexican American children mature earlier than Caucasian children (Perng et al., 2019). Black American children are often taller and heavier than their Caucasian counterparts. They also tend to have longer and denser bones, slimmer hips, more muscle, and less fat on their limbs than on their central body as compared with Caucasian children. Females tend to mature, enter puberty, and stop growing earlier than males. From birth, females tend to have more fat than males, and after puberty females have a greater percentage of body weight derived from fat. Adiposity has a direct correlation to puberty onset in females yet conversely relates to a delayed pubertal onset in males (Perng et al., 2019).

School-age children tend to be concerned about their rate of growth, weight, time of **menarche**, and final height. These children need to understand that the timing and extent of their physical changes usually reflect their genetic inheritance. When one is assessing a child's height and weight, and before referring to **standardized growth charts**, the height of the child's family must be taken into consideration (CDC, n.d.-g). More recently, the growth charts have also been adjusted to reflect higher BMI and weight (for more information, see https://www.cdc.gov/growthcharts/clinical_charts.htm). For example, the child whose height is in the third percentile may have parents who are shorter than average. Shorter height can be expected because of the family's genetic composition. Earlier menarche is frequently associated with a redistribution of body fat and increase in weight. Although the average age of menarche is approximately 12.5 years in Caucasian females and 12.0 years in Black American females, many females experience their menarche at approximately the same age their mothers reached menarche (American College of Obstetrics & Gynecology [ACOG], 2019; Perng et al., 2019). A higher gain in BMI during childhood is related to an earlier onset of puberty, and females can have their first menstrual period as early as 11 years of age and still be considered normal. Due to better nutrition and differences in lifestyle, females appear to experience menarche earlier than did females of 30 years ago (ACOG, 2019). During the COVID epidemic more young females experienced earlier puberty (Fava et al., 2023). Although the school-age child experiences numerous physical changes before adolescence, changes in three physical areas are of particular interest: oral development, lymphoid tissue, and motor skills development.

Oral Development

Teeth enable a person to speak, chew, and smile. They also help give the face shape and form. The school-age child appears to be constantly losing or gaining a tooth. Deciduous, or baby, teeth are usually lost in the same order in which they initially erupted. School-age children begin shedding their first teeth when they are approximately 6 to 7 years of age, and the process is complete with the loss of the second molars at 11 to 13 years of age. The first permanent teeth, the 6-year molars, erupt at 6 to 7 years of age and continue to erupt until the third molars (wisdom teeth) appear at approximately 17 to 22 years of age. The child aged between 6 and 13 years loses and gains approximately four teeth per year. A 13-year-old child should have 28 teeth, having lost 20 deciduous teeth (Freidman, 2019). When deciduous teeth erupt, only the crown is lost; the root is reabsorbed by the developing permanent tooth. As the child's mouth is filled with the larger, permanent teeth, the shape of the jaw and the facial appearance normally change. Females tend to experience permanent tooth eruption earlier than do males (Freidman, 2019).

Dental problems, primarily **dental caries** (cavities), periodontal disease, and **malocclusion**, are among the most common health problems in school-age children today. It remains the most common chronic disease of children 5 to 17 years of age, four times more prevalent than asthma (CDC, n.d.-f). Half of children aged 6 to 11 and more than half of children aged 12 to 19 are affected by tooth decay (American Academy of Pediatric Dentistry [AAPD], n.d.). School dental programs are necessary to educate school-age children on proper care and maintenance of their teeth. School-based oral health education programs and sealant programs are in line with the **Healthy People 2030 Initiatives** and interventions for reducing dental caries among children (Office of Disease Prevention and Health Promotion, 2020c). In the past decade of Healthy People initiatives, it has been determined that community-based and school-based sealant programs can reduce new cases of tooth decay in 2- to 5-year-old high-risk children by up to 60% after a single application (AAPD, n.d.). According to the midway report, a reduction in the proportion of children (6–9 years) experiencing dental caries has been demonstrated (Office of Disease Prevention and Health Promotion, 2020b). These programs demonstrate an area in which child oral health affects the overall health of children in the United States.

The rapid change in the number and type of teeth and the uneven growth in the child's jaw may cause malocclusion, an unacceptable relationship of the teeth in one jaw to those in the other (Friedman, 2019). Dentists evaluate children with overbites, gaps between teeth, and other alignment problems that may influence speech and eating (AAPD, n.d.). Some children will grow out of these problems, but others may need **orthodontic care** and appliances (braces) to correct problems or improve their appearance. Peer reaction to braces is addressed as part of the teaching about body changes; this teaching may decrease problems with the child's self-concept or body image because of looking different. School dental programs include education about conscientious tooth care for the child who wears braces, because these frequently make brushing and flossing more difficult, especially for the school-age child who lacks manual dexterity.

Lymph Tissue

Lymph tissue grows rapidly throughout childhood, reaching maximal size before puberty, after which it begins to decrease in size, most likely due to changes in the concentrations of sex hormones. The amount of lymphoid tissue of a child up to 10 years of age often exceeds that of an adult (Weinstock et al., 2018). This is often reflected in the size of the child's tonsils. Tonsils that appear pathologically enlarged to a parent can be normal for the child's age. Additional lymphoid tissue during the school-age period generally helps this group to have a stronger immune response than do younger and older children. This is a result of the immune system being activated by environmental antigens and exposure to common organisms (Weinstock et al., 2018).

Motor Skills Development

Neurologic, skeletal, and muscular changes combine to increase the child's overall motor abilities. With maturation of the nervous system by age 7 or 8 years, the brain's two hemispheres articulate to allow the child more control over and coordination with motor tasks.

The child grows taller because of lengthening of the long bones that continues into adolescence. **Ossification**, replacement of cartilage with bone, occurs throughout childhood but is not complete until adulthood (National Institute of Arthritis and Musculoskeletal and Skin Diseases, 2023). Special attention must be paid to well-fitting shoes, appropriately sized chairs and desks, and backpack loads to avoid strain on an developing musculoskeletal system . Children at this age also need protective sports equipment and conditioning exercises before sports to prevent sports fractures (National Institute of Arthritis and Musculoskeletal and Skin Diseases, 2023). However, the child builds new bony tissue during the entire period of childhood, which generally allows rapid healing of fractures. **Overweight** children typically have greater bone density as compared with their normal-weight peers. Although they have greater bone density, this does not translate into reduced risk of fractures and joint pain. Overweight children are more likely to experience bone fractures and more joint and muscle pain than their normal-weight counterparts (Dimitri, 2019). The reason for this finding is not clearly understood at this time.

Muscle mass also increases with muscle strength. During the school-age years, physically active males are slightly stronger than females, but this difference is not significant until adolescence. With these changes the child has the potential to perform more complex fine motor and gross motor functions but must practice to perfect these skills. Children willingly exercise their newfound skills and feel pride when others see their improved skill level when bike riding, tying shoes, and engaging in team sports, for example.

GORDON'S FUNCTIONAL HEALTH PATTERNS

The school nurse can be an integral and influential person for the school-age child. The school nurse provides the infrastructure for the health of the student. Gordan's Functional Health Patterns can be used to comprehensively assess the school-age child.

Health Perception–Health Management Pattern

The school-age child understands an abstract definition of health and sometimes the factors causing illness, but this understanding differs from that of an adult. Most school-age children perceive symptoms and show an ability to participate in health-promoting behaviors. Health-promoting behaviors taught at school and home must meet the school-age child's cognitive level (**concrete operation**) and moral level (external rules and forces) to be effective. Teaching strategies using cognitive, psychomotor, and affective senses can help children learn responsibility for their own health (Chatterjee, n.d.). This knowledge provides an excellent foundation for health-promotion behaviors during the school years.

School-age children's understanding of illness is directly correlated with their cognitive development and follows a direct sequence of developmental stages. It is important for nurses to integrate the child's developmental views on illness because this has direct implications for plans related to health education. When specifically asked about their ideas on causes of illness, school-age children usually state the germ theory, the punishment theory, or the external forces theory. Although many younger school-age children know that germs play a role in illness, they have limited understanding of how germs work (Nemours TeensHealth & Durani, 2024b). They may believe that a misdeed or misbehavior caused their illnesses.

Various cultural influences may also contribute to a child's understanding of illness. Hinduism ascribes to the theory of karma (law of cause and effect). People create their own destiny by thoughts, words, or deeds (White et al., 2017). Illness, accident, or injury results from the karma one creates and is often seen as a means of purification. Belief in the "evil eye," another cultural influence, occurs in many cultures and manifests itself in slightly different ways depending on where it arises. Most cultures believe that the victims are primarily babies or young children because they are so often praised and commented on by strangers. The evil eye is thought to be based on jealousy and can have significant implications for the health of the victim (White et al., 2017). This belief is strongest in Middle Eastern countries, Asia, Latin America, and Europe. Attempts to ward off the curse have led to the use of a number of **talismans** within the various cultures. It is important to be aware of such cultural and developmental beliefs of the school-age child when one is defining strategies for teaching health promotion.

School-age children face challenges in meeting health-promotion goals as defined by Healthy People 2030 (US Department of Health and Human Services, 2024). The Healthy People 2030 initiative presents selected objectives related to this age group (Box 20.1: Healthy People 2030). However, people in the school-age child's life can facilitate attainment of these goals. Parents, caregivers, school nurses, and teachers teach health-promotion concepts, and they spend time monitoring and reinforcing preventive health practices, such as personal hygiene, dental care, and good nutrition. Role-playing, reading age-appropriate books, and modeling of health-promotion behaviors (e.g., washing hands) may also help children make the link between behavior and improved health. Unfortunately, by imitating some caregivers, children can become passive health care consumers, asking few questions, doing as told, and perpetuating poor choices. These responses may be due to children's developmental and cultural obligation to obey authority figures. Parents, caregivers, school nurses, and teachers need to make commitments to demonstrate and teach healthy behaviors at home and in school; this helps children develop health values as part of their educational process toward reaching a healthy adulthood.

Counseling the child and the child's family on a broad definition of health, one that includes personal and environmental health and safety, requires an awareness of the school-age child's normal perceptions of health (National Association of School Nurses [NASN], 2024). The school nurse, in consultation with teachers, is in a prime position to use such information to present content in a manner beneficial to the school-age child's level of understanding. Topics may include some of the following content areas: cultural difference of causes and management of illnesses, causes of personal and environmental health problems, and critical issues affecting the school-age child's general health (NASN, 2024). All these issues can be integrated into general academic studies to establish a foundation for teaching prevention as well as to help the school-age child develop advocacy skills to become an assertive health care consumer.

Nutritional-Metabolic Pattern

School-age children, like all people, need a well-balanced diet. An average of 1200 to 1600 calories per day is recommended to meet growth requirements (based on sedentary behavior; AHA, n.d.). Usually these calories are consumed in three daily meals and one or two snacks. School-age children often eat foods low in iron, calcium, and vitamin C and foods that have a higher fat and sodium content than foods their parents ate when they were this age. There is a disjuncture between current dietary practices and recommended dietary intake of children. These behaviors place children at risk of poor nutritional habits, **obesity**, iron-deficiency anemia, and chronic illnesses such as diabetes and hypertension (AHA, n.d.; CDC, n.d.-d; Just, 2019). The school nurse can be an integral component and assume a leadership role in the education of school-age children on the health and cognitive benefits of consuming nutritional, sound foods (NASN, 2024).

Factors Influencing Food Intake

Access to food, the influence of mass media, and contemporary busy lifestyles play a role in poor food choices. Although food insecurity rates have continued to fall since 2011, 35% of low-income (>185% below federal poverty level homes with children were food insecure in 2017 (Thomas et al., 2019). Federal food assistance programs are in existence to assist in the continued improvement of these initiative targets.

A multitude of television and billboard messages pressure children to eat certain foods, many of which contain large

BOX 20.1 *HEALTHY PEOPLE* 2030 OBJECTIVES

EMC-01	Increase the proportion of children and adolescents who communicate positively with their parents
EMC-03	Increase the proportion of children who get sufficient sleep
EMC-04	Increase the proportion of children and adolescents with ADHD who get appropriate treatment
EMC-DO1	Increase the proportion of children who are developmentally ready for school
HOSCD-04	Reduce frequent ear infections in children
MHMD-D01	Increase the number of children and adolescents with serious emotional disturbances who get treatment
NWS-03	Reduce the proportion of children and adolescents with obesity
OH-10	Increase the proportion of children and adolescents who have received dental sealants on one or more permanent molar tooth
PA-02	Increase the proportion of parents who follow recommendations on limiting screen time

ADHD, Attention-deficit/hyperactivity disorder.
US Department of Health and Human Services (2024)

amounts of salt, sugar, and calories. These messages constitute the bulk of food commercials seen by children. Unfortunately, children are now being exposed to food and beverage marketing through social media at alarming rates (Kent et al., 2019). The majority of nonprogram content time is devoted to food-related advertisements. Frequent and lengthy watching of television and exposure to food-related advertisements are linked to childhood obesity (Shakir et al., 2018). In 2015, American children (eight to 12 years) watched an average of 4 hours, 36 minutes of television daily (Common Sense Media, 2020). This increase in media exposure worsens children's exposure to unhealthy food and beverage options. On a typical day, 33% of children consume food from a fast-food restaurant (Ali, 2022). In 2016, 91% of parents reported purchasing a meal for their child from one of the top four fast food restaurants (McDonalds, Burger King, Wendy's, or Subway) within the previous week (Harris et al., 2018). These behaviors contribute to childhood obesity and more consumption of food with poor nutritional quality. These behaviors are in direct disagreement with the Healthy People 2030 objectives of Nutrition and Weight, which call for a reduction in added sugar, saturated fats, and dietary sodium consumption by children in the United States (see Box 20.1). Healthy food often costs more and may be less accessible than unhealthy food (Robinson & Segal, 2024).

Cultural factors, as well as food access, influence poor nutrition among the homeless and children in childcare centers and may contribute to the high level of obesity, especially among Hispanic, Black American, and Native American children (Ricketts, 2018). These groups often lack access to safe and nutritious food. Thus, successful interventions for school-age overweight and nutrition must focus on economic, social, and cultural factors that influence access to and use of food (Méndez et al., 2019). School nurses are in a position to affect intervention strategies because of their familiarity with community needs, local cultural norms, and available resources (CDC, n.d.-k).

Although some school-age children willingly try new foods, many continue to dislike vegetables, fruits, casseroles, spicy foods, and iron-rich foods and prefer a small range of foods. Some children may eat only raw vegetables and fruits and go through a phase of eating only one food at lunch, such as a peanut butter sandwich. These practices seldom hurt the child nutritionally.

Children frequently make their own after-school snacks and need supervision regarding the content. Daily consumption of foods high in vitamins A and C, fruits, and vegetables should be encouraged. With parental, caregiver, or teacher help and positive reinforcement, school-age children can learn to calculate nutrition needs, plan family meals, and eat better for their overall health. These activities also assist school-age children in developing wise decision-making practices, feelings of empowerment about health, and healthy food habits for the rest of their lives.

American families have such busy lives that they eat few meals together. A positive environment for nutrition and socialization during a shared mealtime is important. Parents encourage positive food habits for each family member, and pressure to eat certain foods is avoided to prevent power struggles between the parent or caregiver and the child. A child's nutritional pattern usually reflects family patterns (Robinson & Segal, 2024). For example, parents who skip breakfast tend to have trouble convincing their children to eat breakfast. Educating children as a group to eat healthy foods can be successful because of the powerful influence of a peer group (people of the same age, experience, and usually sex). The child whose friend is eating a candy bar usually prefers the same rather than an apple for a snack.

Nutrition Education

Nutrition education incorporated into the general curriculum of school-age children throughout their educational experience is important. Despite evidence that the school can serve as an environment for nutritional health-promotion education, not all schools require nutrition education from kindergarten through 12th grade (NASN, 2024). School nurses and teachers, as part of core concepts usually taught in school, teach students about choices related to weight control and health and help them understand the role of the media and culture in nutritional choices (Hewett, 2019; NASN, 2024). Teachers and school personnel also serve as role models for optimal eating and exercise habits for children in their charge. Lunch and breakfast programs exist in most schools and meet guidelines established by the US Department of Agriculture (USDA) (2023). Many of these programs continue in after-school programs and during the summer when school is out of session to support needs for quality food intake in 31 million US children (NASN, 2024; USDA, 2023).

The AAP and the AHA have established dietary guidelines for children and adolescents. Current guidelines align with Healthy People 2030 objectives Nutrition and Weight Status. Current objectives include increased consumption of fruits, increased total vegetable consumption (including dark green, red, and orange vegetables), and increased consumption of whole grain foods (see Box 20.1). The daily nutritional needs of a child who is 9 to 14 years old include the following (AHA, n.d.; Fig. 20.1):

- Milk group: 3 cups (24 oz total) of fat-free milk
- Meat group: 5 oz of lean meat, beans, or equivalent combinations of these foods
- Vegetable group: 2 to 2.5 cups of vegetables daily

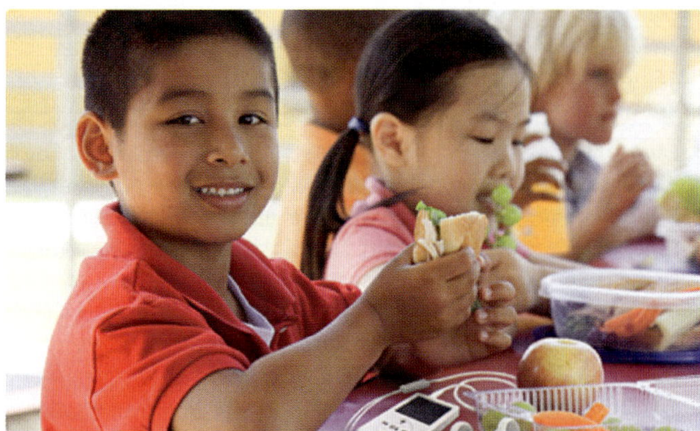

FIG. 20.1 Children 9 to 13 years old should eat two or more portions of vegetables and fruit totaling three to four cups daily.

- Fruit group: 1.5 cups of fruit
- Grains group: 4 to 6 oz daily, of which half should be whole-grain items (AHA, n.d.)

Overweight and Obesity

Overweight and obesity are major nutritional problems that have reached alarming proportions among adults and children in the United States. The Expert Committee on the Assessment, Prevention, and Treatment of Child & Adolescent Overweight and Obesity lists the following definitions for use in children and adolescents (CDC, n.d.-h):

- Individuals 2 to 18 years of age with a BMI greater than the 95th percentile for age and sex or a BMI exceeding 30 kg/m^2 (whichever is smaller) should be considered obese.
- Individuals with a BMI greater than the 85th percentile, but less than the 95th percentile, should be considered overweight.

The problem of overweight and obesity in children and adolescents has increased significantly in the last 50 years (APA, 2021c; Hewitt, 2019). Childhood obesity is now the number one concern for parents, surpassing drug abuse and smoking. In the United States, 20.7% of children 6 to 11 years of age are obese (CDC, n.d.-b). Unfortunately, this demonstrates movement away from the Healthy People 2020 initiative target of 14.5% (Office of Disease Prevention and Health Promotion, 2020a). Evidence suggests that adult obesity begins in infancy or childhood and results from both genetic and environmental factors. For example, a child whose overweight parents constantly use food as a reward faces a greater risk of obesity than does a child of thin parents who do not reward the child with food. Excessive food intake and lack of physical activity also lead to obesity, and once overweight these children tend to exercise even less. Obesity occurs more in Hispanic and Black American children than in Caucasian children (26.2%, 24.8%, and 16.6%, respectively; CDC, n.d.-b).

Overweight and obesity increases the risk of hypertension, diabetes, **sleep apnea**, orthopedic problems, and heart disease. Experts believe that overweight and sedentary behaviors are the primary risk factors for the development of insulin resistance, hyperlipidemia, hypertension, type 2 diabetes, and heart disease (American College of Cardiology, 2018). There is also evidence that postprandial hyperinsulinemia may result in excessive weight gain. In addition, hormones released during the pubertal years make the situation worse in that these hormones cause the body to use insulin less effectively, leading to insulin resistance and thus increasing the risk of development of type 2 diabetes (Cardenas-Vargas et al., 2018).

Current evidence suggests that overweight is associated with obstructive sleep apnea (Hanlon et al., 2019). Whether each disease state increases the expression of the other is unclear (ACC, 2018; CDC, n.d.-e). The potential association between short sleep duration and childhood overweight is described in the literature (Venkatapoorna et al., 2020). Longer sleep durations are associated with higher degrees of activity, which may assist with weight loss. Recent findings support the proactive approach of ensuring adequate sleep in the prevention of overweight in children.

BOX 20.2 Nursing Interventions to Prevent Overweight/Obesity During the School-Age Years

- Incorporate discussion of healthy food intake and daily activity into daily school life.
- Encourage parents to be a role model for their child—be active; plan physically active family outings.
- Make activity fun!
- Limit the amount of time spent watching television, playing video games, and using the computer/internet.
- Discourage eating while watching television or using tech devices.
- Encourage parent(s) to consider cultural influences on dietary intake. Evaluate snacking habits and food choices. Balance healthy foods with ethnic food choices.
- Encourage the family to assess "fast food" consumption and explore/develop eating habits that support a healthier diet as defined by the food-guide pyramid.
- Encourage child to participate in food/meal selection and preparation.
- Support lunch choices that meet overall healthy nutrition intake.

The overweight and obese child faces ridicule by peers and discrimination later in life. These responses reinforce an already low **self-esteem** and poor body image and cause a cycle of personal isolation that influences a child's success, current and future (AAP, 2021c;). Helping the overweight and obese child change lifestyle patterns requires intensive intervention, including the support of parents. Even with these interventions, few overweight children achieve or maintain significant weight loss because of the complexity of factors (environmental, cultural, economic, and psychological) involved. Some success has been achieved by programs that include implementation of reasonable caloric restriction; eating a variety of low-fat and low-cholesterol foods; and use of diet support groups, physical exercise, peer counseling groups, and habit changes (AHA, n.d.; NASN, 2024). However, intervention sometimes fails because some school-age children do not show concern about being overweight. Nursing suggestions for parents who are interested in preventing obesity in their school-age children are given in Box 20.2.

Elimination Pattern

Most children have full bowel and bladder control by 5 years of age. Control involves the ability to undress and dress, to wipe and flush, and to clean hands. The child's elimination patterns are similar to the adult's, with urination occurring six to eight times a day and bowel movements averaging one or two times a day. For some school-age children, however, elimination continues to be a problem.

Enuresis

Involuntary urination at an age when control should be present is called **enuresis** (AAP, 2019; Tu et al., 2022). Children with primary enuresis have never achieved bladder control, and those with secondary enuresis have periods of dryness and recurrent enuresis. Involuntary nocturnal urination (bedwetting) that occurs at least once a month is nocturnal enuresis, and wetting during the day has been termed *diurnal enuresis*. Enuresis should be considered a variation of normal development.

Enuresis affects 16% of children at 5 years of age and 5% of children at 10 years of age (Tu et al., 2022).

Nocturnal enuresis causes disruption for both the child and the family. The child may frequently experience teasing from classmates and siblings. It can have profound effects on life socially, emotionally, and behaviorally. A night away from home might appear impossible because of fear of wetting. Parents may be angry about the frequent bed changes and laundering and may try punishments, thinking that the child should be able to control the problem. Parental stress places additional pressure on the child, who may already have low self-esteem and lack self-confidence as a result of a perceived inability to control the problem (Tu et al., 2022).

Often because they lack information, frustrated families seek help. Many therapies exist yet require a high degree of motivation from the child and parents. Their views must be taken into consideration when one is considering various treatment options. In addition to providing information, the nurse provides active support to facilitate coping. If a child does not have a urinary tract infection, various forms of management may be considered. These include wet alarm systems, bladder training and retention control, waking schedules, drug therapy, and hormone therapy. Each method has advantages, disadvantages, and cost considerations, but all require consistency and time from the child and parents, as well as positive reinforcement by the parents, to reach a successful outcome (Tu et al., 2022).

Diurnal enuresis is often called "daytime dribbling." This term describes a urinary pattern most often seen in school-age females. These children demonstrate "holding on" behaviors, including not voiding first thing in the morning, voiding minimal times a day, or voiding exceptionally quickly (Urology Care Foundation, n.d.). It is not clear why children delay urination or empty their bladders only partially, thus promoting overflow incontinence. Evaluation of these children begins with a urine culture to rule out urinary tract infection. If no infection exists or symptoms persist after treatment, then the intervention is focused on increasing fluid intake to prevent "holding" and establishing a voiding routine of every 2 hours, with a conscious effort to empty the bladder completely. The nurse can be instrumental in helping the child and parents understand the problem and its management.

Encopresis

Another elimination problem that may occur in children is **encopresis**, defined as the persistent voluntary or involuntary passing of stool into the child's underpants after age 4 years (Fife & Hawkins, 2019). In most cases the problem has no discernible physiologic cause and is not related to laxative use. There may be a history of inconsistent toilet training or early life stress in affected children. Encopresis is a common complication of chronic constipation. More than 90% of children with encopresis have a history of recent constipation and/or painful bowel movements (Stein et al., 2017). Once children become constipated or have hard and painful stools, they begin to hold their bowel movements to prevent further pain, which may lead to fecal impaction and rectal distention. Stool then begins to leak around the impaction and leaks through the child's rectum, often without the child's knowledge. In most cases, soiling occurs during the day when the child is awake and active. Soiling at night is uncommon.

Encopresis is often associated with recurrent abdominal pain and, for many, enuresis as well. Often these children have emotional difficulties that began before or resulted from encopresis (Inannelli, 2023; Stein et al., 2017). They experience poor peer relationships and self-esteem, perhaps attributable to their offensive odor. Awareness of this childhood problem is necessary to appropriately identify the affected child, refer the child for treatment, and support the child and the family during a bowel management program and counseling.

Activity-Exercise Pattern

Physical activity in children is an important aspect of health and an integral component of health promotion. Childhood is considered to be a critical time in which regular physical activity behaviors are acquired and fostered (Fig. 20.2). Generally, the school-age child is naturally active, although many do not meet current activity recommendations (CDC, n.d.-r). Young males are typically more active than young females (Fig. 20.3).

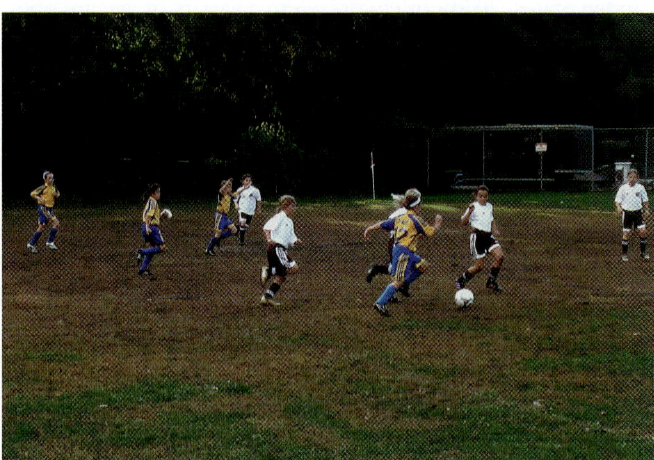

FIG. 20.2 Peer play is important during the school-age years.

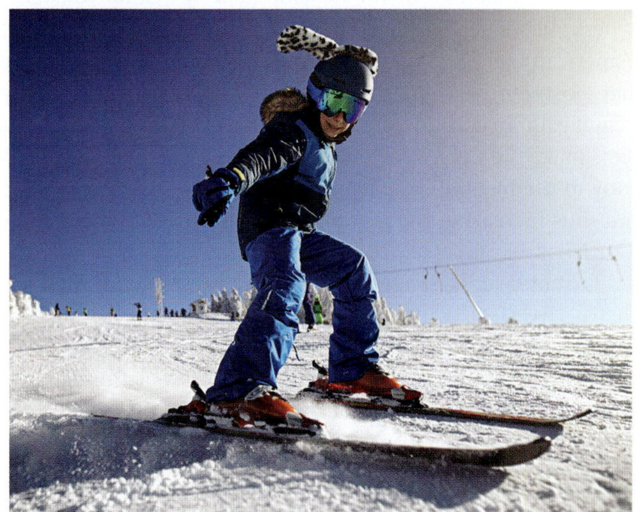

FIG. 20.3 Males are typically more active than females. (From iStock.com/Imgorthand)

In addition, those who perceive their neighborhood as unsafe or do not have at least one parent who exercises are less likely to exercise themselves. Physical activity and participation in sport activities tends to decrease with age, particularly among females.

As previously discussed, impressive changes in motor skills occur between the ages of 6 and 12 years, allowing the child to engage in many activities that develop strength, balance, and coordination (see Table 20.1). Exercise typically occurs through group activities and organized sports such as Little League baseball and soccer; through individual activities such as gymnastics and ballet; and through unorganized play such as bike riding, sledding, rollerblading, and imaginary play. Play provides important learning and health promotion skills and should be encouraged consistently during the school-age years. For many children, involvement in physical activities is fun and connects them to their peers, family members, and other important people in their lives. Play is such an integral part of child development, Healthy People 2030 objectives on physical activity propose an increase in proportion of children 6 to 17 years who participate on a sport team or take sport lessons after school or on the weekend (see Box 20.1).

Play activities promote social, personal, and cognitive development. School-age children frequently prefer interacting with peers rather than with the family. This desire for peer interaction, usually with one of the same sex, extends beyond school and carries over to play and outside activities. A child's skill in motor tasks wins the respect of other children and provides a feeling of self-accomplishment (CDC, n.d.-o). Organized sports such as baseball teach team cooperation, competition, and other social skills. Concerns exist that young children have experienced too much physical and psychological pressure to perform in sports. This has generated a renewed commitment by many parents to focus more on the fun of sports than on the winning of games (Nemours TeensHealth & Schilling, n.d.). Organized activities such as Scouts and 4-H clubs teach children about group functioning, processes involved in performing a task, and the power of social relationships to create change. These lessons can prepare them for the **discipline** needed for a job later in life. Overall, children who perform well in these activities feel good about themselves and their competency and have an enhanced sense of industry. Parents and teachers who compliment children when they perform well enhance self-esteem.

As part of play, school-age children incorporate new cognitive skills, including the ability to count and sort objects. Children of this age express pleasure in their collections of stamps, rocks, or other objects. Understanding the concepts of fair and consistent rules found in games requires cognitive skills of memory, logical reasoning, and the desire to work with others. Many children like to read, which provides ideas about life and cultures that differ from their own, thereby enhancing their acceptance of human diversity. The nurse helps parents promote healthy play activities for children by doing the following (CDC, n.d.-n):

- Encouraging family activities that focus on physical activity and togetherness between parents or caregivers and children
- Encouraging use of a library card to encourage reading on a variety of topics and to teach responsibilities involved with borrowing
- Encouraging the monitoring of daily television and computer use that detracts from physical activity and more active mental activities
- Encouraging both group and solitary activities to support the child's overall development

Sleep-Rest Pattern

Sleep Patterns

Most school-age children have no difficulties with sleep. Generally, their sleep requirements and patterns are more similar to those of an adult than those of a younger child. Individual needs vary based on activity, age, and state of health, but most school-age children sleep between 10 and 12 hours a night without naps during the day (CDC, n.d.-u). Unlike younger children, school-age children experience less difficulties with going to bed. Most children and parents can agree on a bedtime with some flexibility on nonschool nights and adhere to that agreement. When problems arise regarding bedtime, children may be testing parents who have not been clear and firm about their expectations for their children going to bed or have not been willing to discuss the arrangement with their children (National Sleep Foundation, 2023). Although most Americans accept the idea that school-age children should sleep in their own beds, some Black American, Hispanic, Chinese, and Japanese families may encourage the family or siblings to sleep together (National Sleep Foundation, 2023). In the younger child, bedsharing may result in shorter overnight sleep and shorter sleep periods in general (Mason et al., 2021) However, in the school-age child, bed-sharing may not have any effect on sleep patterns or show long-term effects on health, positive or negative.

Sleep Disturbances

The most common sleep problems (Anwar et al., 2018) that occur during the preschool and early school-age years are night terrors (see Chapter 19), **sleepwalking**, **sleep talking**, and enuresis. As a group, these disturbances have been called **disorders of arousal** (National Sleep Foundation, 2023) and share the following characteristics:

- They occur immediately before a rapid eye movement state of sleep.
- Most occur 1 to 2 hours after going to sleep.
- There is a family history of sleep problems; males experience more sleep problems than females.
- Problems reflect normal central nervous system immaturity of the child.
- Problems may be influenced by fatigue and stress within the child.
- Problems do not involve the respiratory system.

Approximately one in six children (15%) aged between 5 and 12 years has sleepwalked at least once, but far fewer children walk in their sleep persistently. Sleepwalking is most likely due to the brain's inability to regulate sleep-wake cycles because of immaturity of the central nervous system. It occurs more often in males and often occurs with enuresis (Nemours TeensHealth & Durani, 2024a). Shortly after going to sleep, the child may suddenly sit up in bed, make repetitive finger and hand movements, or walk, usually for a short time. In most cases, however, the child stays in bed. The child may mumble when talking to a parent or other person (sleep talking). The words tend to be simple but unclear to the listener. Often the child falls back to sleep quickly after talking or walking (Nemours TeensHealth & Durani, 2024a).

Parents who are concerned about sleepwalking or sleep talking need to know that most children outgrow these episodes with central nervous system maturation. However, parents should protect their child from injury by placing gates at the top of stairs and removing sharp objects from the child's path. Most parents find that the easiest solution is to direct the sleepwalker back to bed, where the child returns to a normal sleep. Occasionally, parents can intervene effectively by implementing relaxation techniques for their child before bedtime, avoiding stressful and fatiguing situations, and providing consistency with sleep preparation patterns (Nemours TeensHealth & Durani, 2024a). If a child has many episodes of sleepwalking or sleep talking, or if parents express particular concern, he or she may need further evaluation and treatment by health care professionals.

Cognitive-Perceptual Pattern

The school-age child spends extensive time in settings that require mastery of new ideas and concepts. The child's basic **intelligence**, heredity, and environment encourage or discourage learning. Mastery of ideas and learning requires intact senses, such as vision, hearing, language, and memory capabilities that allow cognitive development and acquisition of skills needed for later life success (Kaneshiro, 2022). Unfortunately, many children in society lack these capabilities and will have learning problems if issues are not identified early through parental awareness, school observations, or routine health care assessments.

Piaget's Theory

Piaget's theory of cognitive development refers to the age span of 7 to 11 years as the period of concrete operation, a stage when children learn by manipulating concrete objects and lack the ability to perform thinking operations that require abstraction. During this period the child moves from egocentric interactions to more cooperative interactions and increased understanding of many concepts gained through environmental connections (McLeod, 2023b). Children increasingly change their reasoning from intuitive to logical or rational operations (rule-governed actions) and engage in serial ordering, addition, subtraction, and other basic mathematical skills. The operations of this period are termed *concrete* because the child's mental operations or actions still depend on the ability to perceive specific examples of what has happened. Older school-age children use both concrete and recently acquired abstract operations, which add flexibility and control to their thinking and meet developmental needs of adolescence. Unlike the egocentric preschooler, a school-age child begins to consider another's point of view. This trait does not emerge suddenly. The new skill appears occasionally and then more frequently as the child's mental capacity and experience grow.

During the school-age period, the child understands a number of expanding concepts regarding objects, including the concept of **conservation** of substance (McLeod, 2023a). When asked if a difference exists for liquid poured into two glasses of different shapes, the preschool, preoperational child focuses on the different shapes and says "yes." The concrete operational school-age child realizes that no change has occurred for liquid despite the change in shape. Conservation of numbers, weight, volume, and quantity, required to understand basic mathematics, sequentially develops as the school-age child gains chronologic age and experience.

The concept of time also develops during this period. Children begin to learn to tell time and understand the passage of time. By age 8 years, most children understand the difference between past and present, and history becomes meaningful. The concept of human aging becomes increasingly understandable, and the child can comprehend the difference between an 18-year-old person and an 80-year-old person.

Two major operations of the school-age period are **classifying and ordering**. The child classifies or groups objects by their common elements and understands the relationship between groups or classes. For example, when given 12 wooden beads, some brown and some white, the child understands that the beads can be grouped by their color and by their material. Conversely, the preschool child focuses only on one property of the beads, such as color. The newfound ability to classify objects shows in the school-age child's interest in collections, such as stamps or coins (McLeod, 2023a). Children in school frequently "order" their world; they line up in school according to height, they repeat numbers and letters in their classic order, and they receive numbers in school to reflect an alphabetized surname. These two operations (classifying and ordering) must exist to learn to read, understand the concepts of numbers, and learn subjects based on relations, such as history (the relation of events in time) and geography (the relation of places in space).

Vision

The child's sensory abilities continue to develop during the school-age years. Visual capacity should reach optimal function by the sixth or seventh year (American Optometric Association, 2020). Peripheral vision and the ability to discriminate fine color distinctions are fully developed. Although many 4-year-olds have 20/20 vision, a school-age child should have a visual acuity of at least 20/30 in each eye, as measured by the Snellen chart, an assessment tool for children who can read some letters (American Optometric Association, 2020).

Physiologic changes occur in the eye during the school-age years. Eyes in the preschool years are normally **hyperopic (farsighted)**, a condition in which the visual image of an object falls behind the retina. However, unlike older individuals, preschool children do not need glasses because their eyes normally accommodate by adjusting their lenses. For most children, vision becomes normal as the shape of the eye changes and lengthens with maturation. However, many school-age children need visual correction to prevent academic difficulties, headaches, and dizziness when reading or doing close work. The peak incidence of hyperopia diagnosis in school-age children is at approximately 6 years of age (American Optometric Association, 2020).

Twenty-five percent of school-age children have visual problems. Unfortunately, nearly one in five children 6 to 11 years of age did not receive their annual checkup in the previous year. This is a missed opportunity for an eye exam or visual screening (Gracy et al., 2018; American Optometric Association, 2020). **Vision screening programs** for schoolchildren help identify those children who have or may potentially have a vision problem that may affect physiologic or perceptual processes of vision or interfere with school performance. Vision screenings are not diagnostic, nor do they determine treatment, but rather indicate a potential need for further evaluation. The school nurse is in an optimal position to ensure eye screenings, and the nurse encourages parents of children with deficits to seek further optometric care. Correcting visual defects can help children learn more effectively.

Two visual problems are common in the age group of the school-age child. Many school-age children inherit **myopia (nearsightedness)**, a condition in which the visual image of an object falls in front of the retina, causing the child to have difficulty seeing distant objects. The other condition, **astigmatism**, causes blurred vision because the image is focused poorly on the retina because of changes in the surface of the cornea or lens (Debrowski, 2019). Eyeglasses correct the defects, but the problem must be identified before it can be solved. For example, a child with myopia may not realize that his visual images are impaired. Children with corrective lenses often express delight and surprise when they first see the fully focused, rich detail of the world after experiencing less refined visual acuity for some time.

Hearing

The child's hearing ability (**auditory acuity**) is nearly complete by 7 years of age, although some maturation continues into adolescence. Hearing deficits occur less frequently than visual deficits, but hearing loss affects 5 out of every 1000 children aged 3 to 17 years in the United States (Victory, 2022a). Having a deficit in hearing compromises learning in school and important socialization with peers. **Chronic serous otitis media**, or long-term fluid in the middle ear, remains a common cause of hearing deficit in both the preschool years and the early school-age years (CDC, n.d.-t). Several environmental factors place a child at risk for hearing loss. There is growing concern about the potential for long-term hearing loss due to ear bud use, loud music, or exposure to other loud environmental noises (Victory, 2022a,b).

All school-age children, especially those with a history of environmental noise exposure, recurrent ear infections, or fluid behind the eardrum, should have periodic hearing evaluations (CDC, n.d.-t). Hearing screenings are part of a health-promotion program in most schools and are required by many states. Work continues on a vaccination for prevention of otitis media infections. Recent reports have found the administration of the influenza vaccine may help to reduce ear infection rates and antibiotic use in children (Norhayati et al., 2017). **Tympanograms**, used to measure the sensitivity of the tympanic membrane to vibrations induced by pressure and sound waves, help detect and monitor hearing problems as part of well-child and ill-child care (Victory, 2023). By providing education on hearing protection for school-age children, the school nurse plays an important role in the maintenance of this important sense for the future.

Sensory Perception

Children learn simultaneously through many senses, and most teaching approaches incorporate this concept (Only About Children, 2024). For example, young school-age children see a letter, hear its sound, and feel its shape. With this approach, children learn a number of ways to interpret an event. For example, some children learn best by listening (**auditory learners**), others by doing (**kinesthetic learners**), and others by engaging all sensory modalities (auditory, kinesthetic, and **visual learners**). Because no two children have exactly the same sensory acuity, sensitivity, or discrimination, all children build slightly different perceptions and conceptions of the world around them and do not follow the same timetable to grasp concepts (Joseph, 2019). Therefore, teaching approaches must be individualized to meet the learning needs of most children.

Of all the senses, visual perception has been studied the most, primarily because of its role in helping children learn to read. Studies have examined children's abilities to discriminate parts of a picture (to see a figure within a picture). Children usually progress from the preschool stage, during which they perceive visual stimuli more as a whole, to the school-age stage, during which they perceive more details, and finally to the point at which they perceive and integrate both. This process helps children recognize letters, the first step needed for reading. Children may first be able to differentiate between obviously different letters, such as "h" and "o," but may have difficulty with letters similar in appearance, such as "b" and "d," until they can distinguish details more effectively.

Language develops rapidly during the school years. Most school-age children enter this period with an ability to understand and speak a language, but with only a basic knowledge of reading and writing. By the end of the school-age period, most children have acquired at least a functional ability in both areas. Language development mandates that a child have visual perception for reading, auditory acuity, perception for understanding spoken language, and fine motor skills for both articulation and handwriting.

The full capacity to imitate sounds develops during the childhood years. Between 6 and 7 years of age, the child shows the ability to produce proper articulation for most vowel and consonant sounds (US Department of Health and Human Services [USDHHS], 2022). However, some have difficulty expressing sounds for "s," "l," "z," "sh," "ch," and "r." By 7 years of age, the child should be able to articulate all sounds for speaking and by age 12 years has a vocabulary of approximately 4000 words. Understanding of the syntax (grammar) and semantics (meaning) of language continues to develop. The child uses more complex sentences and understands multiple meanings for the same word and metaphors. The child should be able to recognize and correct spelling and grammatical errors by 8 or 9 years of age. The capacity to learn foreign languages is at an optimal level at this stage and provides the rationale for foreign language instruction during the school-age years. Foreign language instruction also provides children with information about other cultures and an opportunity to understand people who are different from themselves.

Much of the child's time in school focuses on learning to read and write. Learning to read is a complex process, beginning with letter and sound recognition (Reade & Sayko, 2017). Letters combine to form words that the child must learn to decode. Words combine to form sentences, and so on. Most children need help from teachers, peers, parents, or older children to learn to read effectively. Some researchers believe that children learn best by sounding out the individual letters of a word (**phonics**), whereas others think that learning the word as a whole unit is better. Both processes have value, and likely a combination of both is most effective (Reade & Sayko, 2017). Considering the wide range of processes that support development of reading skills (conceptual, perceptual, verbal, and motor), it is not surprising that most children experience some difficulty in learning to read (Hamilton, 2023).

Handwriting requires eye-hand coordination, motor control, and perceptual abilities (National Handwriting Association, 2024; Understood, n.d.). Primarily a motor skill, handwriting does not reflect mental capacity. Many bright children and adults have poor handwriting and vice versa. Males tend to have more problems with legible handwriting than do females. Writing style does not approach adult-level maturity until the end of late childhood, but the handwriting should reflect the child's handedness. No reversal of letter outlines should occur by age 7 or 8 years, and the relative size of letters should be uniform. By age 8 or 9 years, letter strokes should be firm, even, and flow with ease (Bonneton-Botté et al., 2023; James, 2017). The individual who has difficulty with handwriting may use a typewriter, computer, or graphics to produce a satisfactory written product. Tutoring by a handwriting specialist can help children with **dyslexia,** a term defining the tendency to reverse the normal appearance of letters and numbers in writing.

Memory

Memory abilities, both short-term and long-term, improve for school-age children. Strategies such as organizing, classifying, and labeling information help them retain information. Rehearsal, repeating an item to be learned, is also a helpful memorization strategy. At age 5 years, children use rehearsal when someone suggests or models it; at age 10 years, they rehearse spontaneously. Memory abilities improve with practice and through various strategies, such as placing the words that need to be remembered in a song or by rhyming words (Wang & Gülgöz, 2019).

Intelligence

Intelligence tests assess a person's mental abilities and compare them with the abilities of other people using numerical scores. Although the term *intelligence* is used as if there is agreement on what it means, in reality there is much debate as to how this term should be and has been defined. For example, debate has surrounded whether intelligence should be considered an inherent cognitive capacity, an achieved level of performance, or a qualitative construct that cannot be measured. Psychologists have debated whether intelligence is learned or inherited, culturally specific or universal, or one or several abilities (Cherry, 2022b). Although these debates are ongoing, evidence is increasing that traditional intelligence tests measure specific forms of cognitive ability that are predictive of school functioning but do not measure the many forms of intelligence that are beyond these more specific skills, such as music, art, and interpersonal and intrapersonal abilities.

The concept of intelligence usually conveys an ability to think and process information learned earlier in life. Scores on an intelligence test should measure the child's basic abilities as compared with those of others of the same age and experience level and, ideally, should predict performance in school or society. However, this is not always the case. Intelligence test scores tend to differ because each test, or each form of the same test, measures slightly different samples of abilities and reflects the test author's philosophy on intelligence. It is important to note that some intelligence tests may be culturally insensitive (Martschenko, 2018). For example, the protectionism of the Asian culture may cause lower test scores on self-help skills and socialization among Asian children, who demonstrate in other ways that they are good students. Furthermore, words on the test may not be part of an ethnic group's usual vocabulary, causing children to miss these items on an intelligence test.

Children also take achievement tests that measure the amount of information learned in a specific area and offer insight into a child's overall intelligence. Although intelligence and achievement tests should measure different issues (basic ability versus learned achievement), their results correlate well. Some researchers believe this correlation exists because both tests actually measure the same thing (achievement, notability).

Reports from intelligence and achievement testing differ. Intelligence tests usually provide a number that represents **intelligence quotient (IQ)**. An IQ of 90 to 110 is considered average (Kerry, 2024). Achievement tests compare the child's performance with that of other children and report scores as percentiles. For example, a score in the 20th percentile of a test means the child scored better than only 20% of other children of the same age in that skill. Current beliefs accept that people inherit some of their intelligence but that environmental factors also influence opportunities for learning and overall intelligence. Most likely the greatest environmental influence is socioeconomic, reflected in the correlation in scores: children from low-income families tend to score lower on intelligence tests than do children from middle-income or high-income families. The reason for this probably relates to many sub-factors, such as nutrition, language, parental reinforcement and encouragement, and sociocultural environmental stimuli. Social programs such as the federal Special Supplemental Nutrition Program for Women, Infants, and Children and preschool stimulation programs such as Head Start have attempted to address these sub-factors to improve the potential of young children from diverse populations. Many people have suggested less focus on IQ tests, primarily because they label children early in life and influence, often negatively, their self-perception and their performance.

Learning Disabilities

Educators estimate that 15% of children 6 to 17 years of age have a **learning disability** (National Center for Education Statistics, 2023). Many terms and definitions describe the impairments of children who have normal or above-normal intelligence and usually do not have visual, hearing, or motor handicaps or emotional problems yet have difficulties in school learning (CDC, n.d.-n). Some children have minor, almost unnoticeable difficulties, whereas other children are so impaired that they appear to be significantly disabled until their impairment has been diagnosed and treated. An individual child may have more than one developmental disorder. Some children will develop behavior and self-esteem problems as a response to their inability to function satisfactorily (Silver, 2020).

One well-known condition that causes difficulty in the child's adjustment to the school setting is **attention-deficit/hyperactivity disorder** (ADHD), a disorder that reflects developmentally inappropriate degrees of inattention, impulsiveness, and hyperactivity (CDC, n.d.-n; Farrone & Larsson, 2019). ADHD is the most common neurobehavioral disorder of childhood and among the most prevalent chronic health conditions affecting school-age children. Frequently, these children have high energy, intuitiveness, and creativity, personal characteristics that help them succeed in some facets of their lives. The problem has been difficult to assess, primarily because the child manifests symptoms in varying degrees in different settings and with different people (Box 20.3: Diagnostic Criteria for Attention-Deficit/Hyperactivity Disorder). Because ADHD often affects a child's learning (Healthy People 2030 Objective EMC-04), early middle childhood is a period to increase the proportion of children aged 4 to 17 years with ADHD who receive an age-specific recommended treatment, including medication and/or behavioral therapy (Box 20.1: Healthy People 2030). There have been possible links to chromosomal patterns (16 chromosome) in individuals with ADHD, and some associated symptoms are linked to changes to the *DRD4* gene (Faraone & Larsson, 2019). Treatment of ADHD in children includes behavior management, family counseling, classroom management, nutrition therapy, and medication. However, with the use of **genomics**, new treatments and therapies may better match the individual needs of the child with ADHD (Box 20.4: Genomics).

BOX 20.3 Diagnostic Criteria for Attention-Deficit/Hyperactivity Disorder

Consider a criterion met only if the behavior occurs more frequently than noted in most people of the same mental age as the child.

- A disturbance of at least 6 months exists during which at least six of the criteria for either inattentive behavior or hyperactivity-impulsivity behavior are met.
- Some inattentive or hyperactive-impulsive symptoms that cause impairment existed before age 7 years.
- Some impairment for the symptoms exists in two or more settings (at school or at home).
- Clear evidence of clinically significant impairment exists in social or academic functioning.
- The symptoms do not occur only with a pervasive developmental disorder, schizophrenia, or other psychotic disorder and do not support another mental disorder (mood disorder, anxiety disorder, dissociative disorder, or personality disorder).

BOX 20.4 GENOMICS

Medicine in Children

Clinical genome and exome (coding portion) sequencing technologies are promising tools for determining genetic causes of childhood diseases, including sickle cell anemia, cystic fibrosis, asthma, autism spectrum disorders, and childhood cancers. The use of genomic tests aids in discovery of genetic mutations that drive various diseases; the objective is to yield new targets for the development of novel therapies (Kent, 2018; de Wert et al., 2021). The next generation of medical treatments and therapies is being designed to better improve outcomes for many childhood conditions. There is controversy about who should be tested and whether the genomic analysis should be restricted to only the presenting problem or whether testing should also take a wider view to secondary or opportunistic findings (de Wert et al., 2021). Nurses are well positioned to incorporate genetic and genomic information across all aspects of health care. This translation of science, clinical, and medical research technologies into practice is not without challenges. Nurses have an opportunity to close the gap between research and therapeutic developments.

There are two laws protecting children with disabilities, including those with ADHD: the **Individuals with Disabilities Education Act** (IDEA) of 1997 and **Section 504 of the Rehabilitation Act of 1973**, **Amendment Act of 2008** (Wrightslaw, 2018). The IDEA is a special education law, whereas Section 504 is a civil rights statute. Both guarantee qualified students a free and appropriate public education and instruction in the least restrictive environment. This means that students are to be instructed among those who are not disabled and to the maximal extent appropriate for the student's needs.

The nurse plays a vital role in promoting the school-age child's overall cognitive and perceptual health, helping to prevent problems in these areas. The nurse must talk to parents and school administration personnel about any child who has language articulation problems beyond 6 or 7 years, because further evaluation is necessary. The nurse helps parents understand their child's level of cognitive and sensory abilities so that learning expectations are realistic. Through educational materials and counseling provided during school meetings, the nurse may address the socialization needs and development of school-age children with learning disabilities (National Center for Learning Disabilities, 2024). The nurse may also advocate for the school-age child believed to have a learning disability, ensuring underlying health problems, general immaturity, or an environmental deficit (poverty or divorce) is not the result of the perceived learning deficiencies.

Self-Perception–Self-Concept Pattern

Through each of the developmental processes of physiologic growth, cognitive development, and social development, children progressively engage in an important process of **self-discovery**. Through these processes, children actively build and create their own personalities, develop relationships with others, and expose themselves to a wide range of experiences that influence their behavior, attitudes, and values.

Erikson's Theory

The stage of personality development described by Erikson for the school-age child is **industry versus inferiority**. The major task to be accomplished is full mastery of whatever the child is doing (sense of industry). The child focuses on success in personal and social tasks and avoidance of a sense of inferiority. Inferiority occurs with repeated failures at attempted tasks and with little encouragement or trust from people important to the child. With mastery of the tools of the culture in relation to those of the peer group, a sense of worth and understanding of the self develops (Erikson, 1995: Erikson & Erikson, 1998)

Self-Concept

Self-concept develops over time and through a variety of experiences and relationships. For example, by being responsible for a pet's care and by showing love to this animal, the older school-age child nurtures a positive self-concept. The way in which others, especially peers, view the child influences the sense of self. Increasing cognitive abilities facilitate better understanding of the identifying factors of others (race, ethnicity, disability, or gender) and how those others compare with the child. Self-concept includes self-esteem, sense of control, and body concept (Kaneshiro, 2022).

Self-Esteem. Self-esteem has been defined as the extent to which an individual believes oneself to be capable, significant, successful, and worthy (McLeod, 2023a). The younger school-age child has a limited self-concept, but one that develops with successful completion of the tasks of this period (Erikson's Sense of Industry). Although engaged in more activities outside the home, the child still depends on the family, as defined by one's culture, to develop high self-esteem. In school, teachers or group leaders frequently reward those who have succeeded in a task with badges, stars, or privileges (tangible objects that validate success).

The peer group's influence on the school-age child's self-esteem is unquestionable. Acceptance by a peer group contributes to feelings of self-worth and a sense of belonging to a desired group. Competition or collaboration with peers in school, clubs, and activities also influences feelings of adequacy and feelings of success (Nemours KidsHealth, n.d.-b). Parents must be encouraged to expose their school-age children to interesting activities of their choice, involving peers, to nurture their self-esteem and sense of uniqueness.

Gender differences and self-esteem in early childhood may exist (Nemours KidsHealth, n.d.-b). There is evidence of other variables that may play a larger role in self-esteem (Magee & Upenieks, 2019). Studies that are more recent show a positive correlation between child self-esteem and academic achievement. This relationship between positive self-esteem and higher academic achievement is regardless of gender. Children tend to have positive self-esteem if they perceive parental warmth and involvement that supports a perception of balance within themselves and promotes their emotional health (Leung Ling et al., 2020).

In encouraging development of self-esteem in all school-age children, the nurse remembers that a child needs to experience success with tasks; completely structured activities may not provide this opportunity for some children. A child who succeeds in some things and receives acceptance by peers gains a sense of competence and worth, is self-confident, and has high self-esteem, which are important qualities for life survival.

Sense of Control. As the school-age child matures and makes choices, a sense of control develops about the self and the environment. Self-control allows children to manage their thoughts, emotions, and behavior, demonstrating a degree of executive functioning (Griffin, 2024.). Older children and females tend to have a more internalized locus of control than do younger children and males. Children with an internal locus of control believe they are responsible for their behavior and accomplishments and tend to have higher levels of achievement than do children who believe in an external locus of control. The latter think that fewer reasons exist for them to try hard at a task, because others or fate determines life results. Cultural contexts may play a role in a child's development of self-control. Hispanic and Black American cultures may more often support an external locus of control based on a strong belief that God determines one's outcome. Socioeconomic status may also play a role. Those with lower socioeconomic status may perceive they lack the ability to control their life in the presence of negative environmental influences (CogniFit, 2019).

Body Concept. The school-age child's concept of the body and its functioning also changes from the preschool period and adds to overall self-concept. By age 8 to 11 years, children know that parts of the body constitute a related whole. The 11-year-old child can name twice the number and functions of internal body structures that a 6-year-old child can and frequently understands the functions of the cardiovascular, musculoskeletal, and nervous systems. For example, the 7-year-old child knows that the heart is important and that it beats, whereas the 13-year-old child knows that the heart pumps blood. Changes or differences in the body may frighten the school-age child until the child understands normal developmental processes, such as losing deciduous teeth. Physical differences, such as freckles, can provoke ridicule and isolation. Children in this age group frequently feel threatened by others with deformities. Children with chronic illness worry that their peer relationships will be negatively influenced if others know about their illness. Children who learn about body differences, by meeting people with chronic health problems as well as by reading and discussion of **anxiety** about differences, increase their knowledge of the body and ways to maintain health. They also gain an understanding of the value of each person, despite their differences.

Roles-Relationships Pattern

The family environment provides a sense of security that allows the school-age child to cope with uncertainties in the external environment (Fig. 20.4). Although many live in single, divorced, mixed-race, or same-sex parenting households, the family structure generally encourages a child's cognitive growth through exposure to a variety of experiences that bolster the desire to achieve and develop positive self-esteem.

Parents, caregivers, and children interact in a variety of ways to show love and companionship for each other. Caregivers, such as grandparents or extended family members, protect the dependent child and teach the learning child. The caregiver-child relationship is not equal, primarily because caregivers and parents serve as authority figures that establish the rules needed for the functioning of the family and safe growth of the child.

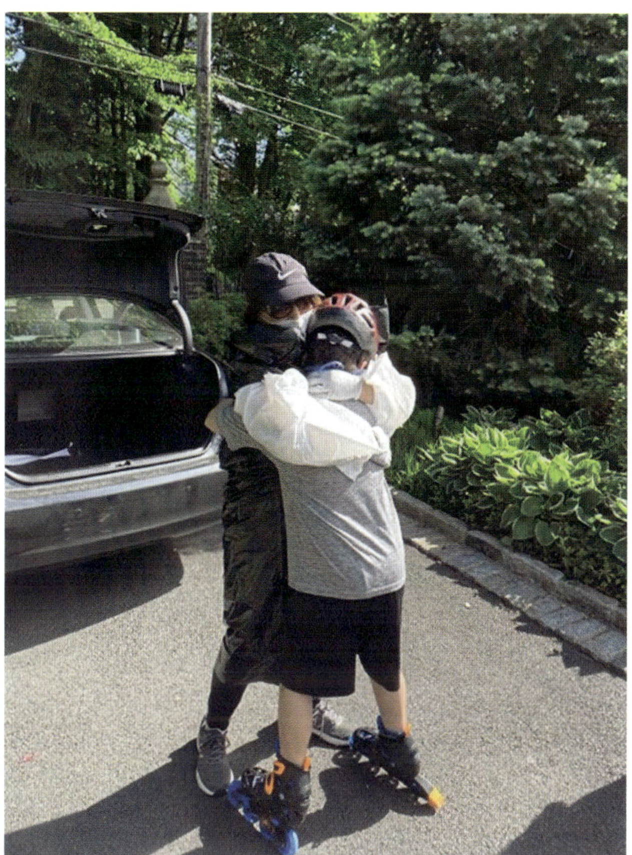

FIG. 20.4 Grandmother and grandchild hugging with protective gear during COVID-19 pandemic.

During the school-age years, the child's increasing maturity, independence, and responsibility begin to reduce the amount of parental authority and structure needed. With increasing independence, the child prioritizes school and peer group relationships to develop socialization skills and understand group social mores. These connections will help prepare the child for future relationships.

School-age children also begin to broaden their interests outside the home, often encouraged by parents. The child's changing world frequently alters family schedules and patterns, supporting studies that have found that parents express the least amount of parental satisfaction when their oldest child is between 6 and 13 years of age. The relationships between siblings differ, depending on birth order, culture, sex, age differences, and perceived power of siblings. Siblings interact with one another in a number of roles, such as playmates, teacher-learner, protector-dependent, and adversaries, based on feelings of jealousy and rivalry that often occur in families. School-age children cope with these feelings better than do preschool children because they have outlets outside the family, including school and friends. Parents can minimize conflicts by recognizing each child's needs and level of maturity and by providing guidance and support.

As children mature, they assume more responsibilities within the family and the community. School-age children learn responsibility for allowance, household chores, self-care, and pets and acquire a sense of empowerment as an integral part of the family. School-age children learn valuable life lessons by earning and spending their allowances.

Children learn socially accepted behaviors when their parents engage in **limit setting** (defining expected behavior and consequences when limits are not honored). Violent behavior must be discouraged, and nonviolent methods to reach resolutions for personal problems should be encouraged (Box 20.5). Parents who express their feelings, explain why things happen, and listen to their children while setting limits encourage the development of self-control and positive self-esteem. Some families with school-age children find it helpful to have periodic family meetings during which everyone discusses family issues, rules, and responsibilities. Behavior contracts between the parent and the child provide direction and may also encourage improved behavior by delineating favorable consequences when the terms of the contract are followed.

Child Abuse

Child abuse (physical, sexual, or emotional exploitation of children) and neglect (lack of adequate food, shelter, or emotional support) continue to be significant societal problems (Administration for Children and Families, 2025). More than 4.1 million cases of abuse or neglect in children are reported annually in the United States. Abused children have an increased likelihood of becoming violent adults and of abusing their own children. The factors that increase the risk of abuse include family poverty, culture, limited maternal education, needy child syndrome, presence of a stepfather, single-parent status,

BOX 20.5 The School-Age Child: Points for Effective Discipline

Effective discipline is essential to family harmony and individual child growth and reflects cultural beliefs. The goal of discipline is to encourage and reinforce positive child behaviors, eliminate inappropriate child behaviors, improve parent-child communication, and meet parental needs (Sege & Siegel, 2018). Effective discipline requires the essential components of a positive, supportive, loving relationship between the parent and the child. Positive reinforcement strategies are used to increase desired behavior and reduce/eliminate undesired behaviors.

Specifics of discipline strategies may include the following:

- Ignoring the misbehavior and acknowledging the appropriate behavior
- Using distraction or substitution to avoid a problem situation
- Offering choices to prevent inappropriate behavior such as whining or emotional outbursts
- Using humor to decrease the intensity of a situation
- Modeling the appropriate behavior
- Setting age-relevant limits
- Giving specific and clear commands for behavior appropriate to the child's age
- Talking calmly, being a good listener, and encouraging negotiation, perhaps in a family meeting, to promote problem resolution
- Limiting a child's environment (distractions such as music and television)
- Setting clear and consistent consequences for misbehavior (withholding privileges, using contracts)
- Providing one-to-one time, focusing on positive attention
- Finding time for oneself to replenish one's energies as a parent and as an individual

parental drug addiction, and teenage parenthood (Sege et al., 2017, 2018). However, child abuse also occurs in families that do not have these risk factors. Cultural factors must be considered in detecting abuse. For example, coin rubbing of the chest (used in the Asian ethnic group for treatment of respiratory tract infections) leaves abrasions that may be perceived as abuse by a nurse assessing an ill child. National governmental agencies and professional organizations require that health care providers report suspected abuse and participate in preventing, assessing, and treating victims. State nurse practice acts require nurses to report suspected cases of abuse. Ultimately, nurses help interrupt the vicious cycle of abuse by becoming involved in community coalitions and innovative evidence-based programs that prevent and intervene in child and family abuse.

Unfortunately, relationships between children and adults are not always positive. **Sexual abuse**, use of a child for sexual exploitative purposes, has become a more common but often hidden problem for a variety of reasons (AAP, 2021b). The child may be too frightened to talk about the situation, families and society do not want to admit its existence, internet traffic supports pornography and pedophilia, and fewer agencies exist to respond to these cases. Many victims know their abusers (many are parents), and people in positions of authority (e.g., teachers, coaches, or clergy members) may be abusers. The child may comply for a variety of reasons, such as a need to be good or a need to keep the family together. Emotions are complex and change as the child grows, but they often lead to adult anxiety, **depression**, and physical symptoms and illnesses. Males less often report sexual abuse but are more likely than females to suffer negative emotional effects from incest, a form of sexual abuse.

As in any type of suspected abuse, nurses assist these children by recognizing those at risk and those experiencing abuse and referring them to relevant resources. All people who work with young children must acknowledge the warning signs of abuse (Box 20.6). When sexual abuse is suspected, a specially trained, multidisciplinary team that is sensitive to the needs of the child and can validate the abuse must conduct an in-depth interview and examination. Most authorities believe that children who describe sexual abuse are telling the truth because the details are usually specific and trauma is evident. Therefore, a child's story should be believed unless it is disproved.

BOX 20.6 Selected Warning Signs of Child Abuse

- Physical evidence of abuse or neglect, including previous injuries
- Conflicting stories about the "accident" or injury from the parents or others
- Injury or complaint inconsistent with the child's history or developmental level (e.g., the child received a concussion and broken arm from falling off a bed)
- Signs and symptoms consistent with signs of abuse and inconsistent with history, vague recall of event (e.g., chief complaint is a cold when there is evidence of first-degree and second-degree burns)
- Inappropriate response of caregiver, such as an exaggerated or absent emotional response, refusal to give consent for additional tests or agree to necessary treatment, excessive delay in seeking treatment, or absence of the parents
- Inappropriate response of child, such as little or no response to pain, fear of being touched, excessive or lack of separation anxiety, or indiscriminate friendliness to strangers
- Child's report of physical or sexual abuse
- Previous reports of abuse in the family
- Repeated visits to emergency facilities with injuries

Administration for Children and Families (2025); Smith et al. (2024)

Sexuality-Reproductive Pattern

The preschool child learns about sex differences and begins to model the general societal behaviors expected of a female or male child. The child enters the school-age years with a strong identification with the parent of the same sex. The child continues to learn the concepts and behavior of the gender role and incorporate these into the self-concept. This challenge is significant for all children (Rafferty, 2022a). Societal stereotypes related to gender roles continue to influence the school-age child's ideas of male and female roles. Some children have a gender identity different from their gender assigned at birth. Many children have interests or hobbies that may align more with the other gender. Fortunately, most children receive early teaching about gender roles that emphasizes that sex does not determine one's choices, personality, or behavior. Because of this teaching, children increasingly choose activities based on their skills and interests, rather than on what appears appropriate because of their sex (Rafferty, 2022b).

The school-age child's increasing awareness of the body, its functioning, and a need for sexual identity combine to foster a desire for knowledge about the biologic aspects of sexual function. Late in the school-age period, when the physical changes of puberty have begun, concern and curiosity about sexual issues frequently develop. A child may become extremely attached to another of the same sex, and they may explore one another's sexual organs. This is common exploratory behavior and does not reflect true homosexuality, even though parents and children may express concerns about it. With the advent of physical changes of puberty, the school-age child desires more privacy in a bedroom shared with no one. As noted earlier, the physical changes of puberty appear gradually over several years (Rafferty, 2022b).

Children frequently share questions about sexual matters with their peer group. Parents are often uncomfortable or unsure of what sexual information to give to their children and when to give it. Many health care agencies sponsor short programs to educate parents and older school-age children, in a supportive environment, about body and mental changes during preadolescence and puberty. An increasing number of age-appropriate books that focus on emotional and body changes can be used at home and in school to increase children's understanding. Particularly because menstrual cycles start earlier now than they did 50 years ago, education about body changes and puberty appears appropriate as part of later school-age education.

The nurse plays an important role in sex education in health care and education settings. This professional should be receptive to answering questions in this area and at each health care visit. The nurse employed in the school is in an ideal position to teach group sex education programs using literature and games. Children at this age appear to respond most favorably with sex-segregated classes because of their general discomfort with sexual topics and unique needs and questions. Some schools appropriately incorporate these classes into school curricula as part of a health-promotion curriculum. Other schools have special programs focused only on sex education based on parental desires or school board policies. Most school-age children have the cognitive skills to respond to programs on responsible sexuality, including discussions on abstinence and condom use, pregnancy, sexually transmitted diseases, and the human immunodeficiency virus (NASN, 2024). The nurse also wants to include program content specific to disabled children, who face unique body changes and concerns and need to understand ways others can express affection to them without causing accusations of abuse.

Coping–Stress Tolerance Pattern

The school-age child must learn to cope with stress as part of the developmental process. Through a health-promotion program, children can learn to identify symptoms of stress (pounding heart, stomach "butterflies," and sweaty hands) and ways to cope with these perceived stresses (e.g., deep breathing and walking) before they cause illness. The child actually faces many stressful experiences in life, including competition, homework deadlines, failure at home or school, and decisions whether to cheat, steal, or even join an unpopular peer group. The young school-age child may never have shared his or her life with other children the same age, and cultural values learned earlier in life may not be reflected in school or in peer relationships. Threats to the child's security (e.g., bullying) cause feelings of helplessness and anxiety that may affect the ability to function successfully (Nemours KidsHealth, n.d.-a). Grief over the death of a loved one, parental divorce, loss of a favorite activity because of misbehavior, or expulsion from a favorite peer group may cause negative behavior. Parents need to provide appropriate discipline in responding to this behavior but should also listen and analyze factors related to the problem to increase the child's feelings of control and decrease stress for the family.

Children use a variety of **coping strategies**, healthy behaviors intended to buffer perceived stressful events. However, in a very stressful situation or many stressful situations, a child may be unable to move beyond the coping behaviors. In conversations with teachers and parents, the nurse may offer a variety of strategies for coping with a school-age child's problems, enabling the child to cope and learn from others (Table 20.2). These strategies may involve role-playing or referral to literature on the problem topic to interrupt the child's negative behavior cycle and improve family health (Table 20.2). The nurse may also refer a child to relevant religious and spiritual leaders, based on school-age children's belief that prayer will help them cope with an otherwise uncontrollable situation.

Parental Divorce

More than half of all marriages end in divorce, leaving many school-age children to face stress related to their parents' separation. Often children experience a feeling of loss, although they may hope that their parents will reunite at some point. Box 20.7 discusses the effects of divorce on a school-age child. Children's responses vary with their level of development (American Association for Marriage and Family Therapy, n.d.). Factors such as economic security; availability of both of their parents, other family, church, and school supports; and quality of interactions with their parents can influence the child's ability to cope with divorce. Unfortunately, many parents become so immersed in their own feelings that they fail to support their children. Conflicts over custody, child support, and visitation rights add to the child's difficulty in coping. In some cases, the school system becomes the child's advocate to encourage the parents to

TABLE 20.2 The School-Age Child's Coping Strategies and Nursing Interventions to Promote Coping

Strategies	Nursing Interventions
Use of defense mechanisms (regression, denial, repression, projection, displacement, sublimation)	Accept child's use of defense mechanisms as temporary, healthy coping responses; provide child with options for moving to more age-appropriate ways of responding to stressors
Cognitive mastery (problem-solving, communication)	Ask children what they know of the situation and how they might handle it; encourage questions; use diagrams and models to help explain; encourage child to verbalize feelings and use past successful strategies that might help deal with present stressors; try personalized approaches, such as books, puppets, and manipulation of equipment, to increase feelings of control when faced with a stressful situation; encourage praying and other communications to a chosen deity as appropriate
Controlling, holding behaviors	Encourage child to participate and to make decisions; accept child's need to direct as appropriate; set consistent age-appropriate limits; respond to signals for help; let child be responsible for self-care
Use of repetition	Use books, games, and other communication media to work through feelings; emphasize "ok" for child to continue to ask questions and to receive answers that assist in coping
Use of humor	Be a good listener and participate in riddles and jokes used by child; be a good sport with school-age children's desire to play jokes on each other; share stories and cartoons with child
Motor activity, aggression, protest behavior	Encourage physical activity to deal with stress; accept appropriate behavior; establish limits on behavior for group safety
Withdrawal (resurgence of separation anxiety)	When child is separated from the family, child may have separation anxiety; encourage close emotional contacts between child and significant others (friends, family, church members); allow favorite objects from home to be brought to the hospital or a new environment for child

BOX 20.7 Selected Strategies for Managing the Effects of Divorce on the School-Age Child

School-age children tend to view life in black and white and are likely to blame one parent for a marriage breakup. Males, especially, mourn the loss of their fathers and frequently express anger at their mothers. Both males and females have great difficulty accepting their parents' new dates. Crying, daydreaming, and problems with friends and school are common divorce-related behaviors in children of this age (Kemp et al., 2023).

Some suggestions that might help the school-age child cope with divorce of parents are the following:

- Discourage reconciliation fantasies.
- Have parents avoid dinners, outings, or holiday celebrations with the ex-spouse. This only fuels the child's fantasies. Instead, emphasize the finality of divorce.
- Make sure the child has the phone number of the absent parent.
- Encourage both parents to allow the child easy access and frequent conversations with the noncustodial parent.
- Do not allow the child to manipulate the parents into buying more possessions.
- Realize that school-age children are likely to feel deprived. Although they may intensify requests for playthings or other possessions, do not try to retain child's affection through material objects. Even children of divorce need to be told "No!"
- Talk to the child's teachers or school counselors about the divorce.
- Realize that school personnel may better understand possible learning or behavioral problems and will likely offer extra support.

provide a supportive environment during divorce proceedings. Despite this intervention, some children do not cope well with divorce and have emotional consequences that result in juvenile behavior problems or require long-term counseling (see the Case Study and care plan at the end of this chapter).

Somatization and Depression

Children, like adults, use defense mechanisms to cope, with various degrees of success. Two strategies used by the school-age child to respond to uncontrollable situations are **somatization** and depression.

Some children respond to a stressful situation by transferring their feelings to a physical problem (somatization). In this phenomenon, school-age children, unable to discuss their concerns, complain of stomach aches or headaches, symptoms reflective of functional or psychogenic pain. These children may also develop discrete, repetitive movement habits called *tics*. In many cases the child with these problems must be evaluated to determine whether an underlying physiologic cause exists. The child and the family will then need assistance in understanding the child's concerns to define successful ways to cope with the behavior.

Depression occurs in up to 2% to 3% of school-age children (Anxiety and Depression Association of America, 2021) and more often in males than in females during the school-age period. Depression reflects a disturbance of mood, when a child displays sadness, guilt, or worthlessness and other unusual behaviors that disengage the child from peers and the family. In defining depression in children, most authors emphasize that they are referring to a more long-term syndrome in which the child's normal development and functioning become impaired, not a periodic sadness that all children occasionally experience. The factors that place a child at risk of depression include homelessness, death of a parent or significant other, divorce, long-term hospitalization, chronic illness, learning problems, and emotional turmoil at home. Parents and teachers look for symptoms of depression, including anorexia, sleeplessness, lethargy, changed affect, aggressive behavior, frequent crying, and withdrawal from previously enjoyed activities.

Although it has been concluded that there is insufficient evidence to routinely screen all school-age children for depression, the nurse can serve an important role in identifying any child who appears to be depressed and in notifying parents about the need for further assessment. Depending on the child and the situation, differing amounts of counseling and individual child guidance may be required. Nurses in schools and outpatient settings are often the ideal helpers because they have the skills and time needed to help a child cope with a helpless feeling and its cause.

Values-Beliefs Pattern

Children make decisions related to moral and ethical issues every day. Should they tell the teacher which classmate broke the rule? Should they share their candy with a younger sibling? For these situations, the child makes a decision based on the level of **moral development**. Moral development involves choosing the most appropriate behavior based on one's values and feelings related to the situation. Environmental factors and culture strongly influence a child's moral development, as do the type of family discipline, role models, people with whom the child identifies, and the child's rehearsal and practice of moral behavior.

Kohlberg's Theory

Most researchers agree that the younger school-age child is at the **preconventional level**, a level of moral development characterized by self-interest only. The child continues to do many things simply to avoid getting in trouble and does not understand the reason for rules but also performs actions that will benefit the self (Cherry, 2022a). During later childhood (10 to 13 years) most children progress to the conventional level, a stage of moral development defined by concern about group interests and values. The conventional level of moral judgment involves the child looking to others for approval and to societal authority for a definition of rules. Children aged 10 to 12 years judge behavior in terms of the intention of the offender, understand the "golden rule" concept, and engage in behavior that maintains a valued relationship. The conventional level coincides with Piaget's Cognitive Level of Concrete Operations, when the child has increased social involvement with people outside the home (Cherry, 2022b).

Moral Behavior Problems

Some moral behavior problems, such as lying, stealing, or cheating, are common during the school-age years. Cultural, religious, and parental values influence a child's moral development, concept of right and wrong, and consequences of not demonstrating moral behavior. Preschool and younger school-age children frequently lie because of fantasy, exaggerations, or inaccurate understanding. As children mature, they may use the defense mechanism of denial to block upsetting situations and maintain self-esteem. The lie then becomes an unconscious act. Older children often lie because they fear punishment or ridicule. Children may cheat because of a desire to win, do well in competitive society, or "look good" for their peers. Children usually steal when they think they will not be caught, and they think that there is no other way to get what they want (Powel, 2019). Although these actions can be quite upsetting for parents, they are common developmental behaviors. Parents frequently need reassurance that their child is normal and will probably outgrow the behavior with parental assistance. They may need help in developing fair rules for behavior and communicating their expectations for a child's behavior to meet parental and cultural values. Therefore, the nurse encourages the parents to warn the child clearly not to steal, lie, or cheat; offer other, more socially acceptable ways to cope with the stressor causing the behavior; and then apply appropriate punishment congruent with an understanding of the event.

ENVIRONMENTAL PROCESSES

Physical Agents

School-age children, similarly to those of all other age groups, face daily exposure to environmental agents and factors that may cause injury, illness, or death. Many of these agents and factors are harmless if appropriately used or if there is minimal exposure. Examples include physical agents such as fires; mechanical agents such as bicycles, skateboards, and cars; biologic agents such as bacteria; chemical agents such as asbestos; and radiologic agents such as x-rays. Death rates from these agents differ among ethnic groups because of access to health care and environmental issues (Kids Count Data Center, n.d.).

Accidents

Accidents are the leading cause of death in children older than 1 year in the United States (CDC, n.d.-c,-q). Most accidents do not result in death, but many serious ones cause significant morbidity and disability. Because of this effect, the nurse has a significant role in educating parents and school personnel on ways to prevent dangers to school-age children and to become involved in public initiatives to create a safer society for them (Impact NW, 2024).

The agent, host, and environment must be considered when one is developing solutions to decrease the number of accidents. The type of agent varies with the child's age. Most fatal accidents during the school-age period occur from motor vehicle accidents when the child (host) is a passenger or pedestrian (walking or riding a bike). Other fatal accidents occur from fires and burns, riding bicycles, drowning, and use of firearms. Most common nonfatal accidents tend to be caused by simple agents that produce simple injuries. Despite helmet laws in several states, many school-age children continue to experience head injuries related to recreational equipment, such as bicycles, swings, skateboards, and trampolines (Brooks, 2024). Slightly older children have an increased number of accidents from contact sports, cuts, falls, burns, and injuries from firearms.

Specific accident factors relate to the host—the school-age child (Box 20.8: Quality and Safety Scenario). Children in this age group tend to become hurt because of their carefree attitude, curiosity, love of mimicking older people, and intense oral tendencies. Typically, school-age males have more accidents than school-age females, perhaps attributable to differences in personalities, societal expectations, childrearing practices, and increased propensity for risk-taking behaviors. The mechanism differs with the sex of the host. For school-age males, drowning is the most common fatal accident; for females, automobile accidents are the most common (CDC, n.d.-r,-v).

The physical environment of the child dictates the type or frequency of accidents that occur in the home, neighborhood, and school. Most accidents happen outdoors, which means that school-age children face greater risk of automobile or bicycle accidents than of poisoning or falls, indoor accidents that occur predominantly in younger children. More accidents (drowning and pedestrian-vehicle accidents) occur in the summer than in the winter because of children's outside play. Socioeconomic level affects children's physical environments and access to dangers. For example, space heaters place children of low-income families at risk of burns, whereas skiing places wealthier children at risk of injury.

The social environment, which includes the family, school, and playmates, also plays a role in accidents (AAP, 2022). Although little research has focused on the physical trauma caused by heavy backpacks that many school-age children use, these bags exert significant pressure against functionally immature muscles of the back and torso. Daily carrying of bulging backpacks causes muscle strain, headaches, improper posture, shoulder slouch, and other physical problems. Additionally, teachers' expectations that all textbooks be available both in the classroom and at home must be considered. At least one study has shown that children will change their backpack-carrying behaviors if they are involved in a school-based program focused on this topic (National Safety Council, n.d.).

As part of the social environment, the family may influence the rate of accidents in the school-age child (Kyu et al., 2018). Chronic familial stress (parental unemployment) or sudden acute stress (parental illness) may contribute to homicide as the fourth leading cause of death among children aged 5 to 14 years (CDC, n.d.-u). Homicide is a more common cause of death among Black American and Hispanic children than among White children. Children also face increased risk of accidents when parental supervision is limited, such as during holidays or a move to a new home.

Drowning

Fewer school-age children than infants and adolescents die of drowning. More Black American children of this age drown than do White American children (CDC, n.d.-i). Water safety measures can help reduce drowning, along with the many other injuries that occur around water, such as falls in slippery areas. Environment and safety teaching can influence the number of school-age children dying of drowning (CDC, n.d.-i).

Burns

Each year, many children become victims of house fires, many of which occur during the winter months from Christmas

BOX 20.8 QUALITY AND SAFETY SCENARIO

Safety Concerns Specific to School-Age Children

Because of increased independence, school-age children face significant exposure to situations threatening their health. Consequently, the parents of these children must be involved in community and legislative activities that provide safe school and play environments. Additionally, at appropriate health visits, health care workers should provide anticipatory guidance to parents in the following areas:

Bicycle Safety

Each child should have a well-maintained bicycle, ride only in safe areas approved by the parents, observe rules for vehicle traffic, ride on the side of the road with traffic, "bike defensively," and use a federally approved riding helmet.

Street Safety

Children should look right, left, then right again to check the safety of crossing a street; children should cross only at safe and well-monitored intersections, preferably with an adult present; ensure parental supervision when children play close to streets and heavy traffic areas.

Motor Vehicle Safety

Children should wear a seat belt or be in an age-appropriate booster seat as needed; older children should ride with a restraint system and in the back seat until age 12 years.

Pool Safety

All children should have swimming lessons and swim with a buddy or adult who swims well; all pools should have drain covers; children should avoid swimming after a heavy meal and avoid "roughhousing" behavior around the pool; children should be monitored by the parents during swimming.

Firearm Safety

Adults need to lock away guns and ensure gun safety locks are intact; parents need to educate children never to touch guns.

School and Playground Safety

Schools should follow state and federal recommendations for protection of students from outsiders who may want to injure them inside the school or in school areas. School shooting and lock-down education should occur regularly and be taken seriously. All playground equipment should meet federally approved standards; children should be trained on how to use equipment safely; equipment should be evaluated for safety and repaired before children use it.

Fire Safety

Working smoke detectors should be in place in the home and school; the family needs to have a fire evacuation plan and practice it; children need to wear fire-retardant clothing at night; children should not play with matches, open fires, fireworks, or open wires that can cause injury and fire.

Toxin Safety

Children should avoid insecticides, radiation sources, inappropriate use of medications, and pollution sources; parents need to store all known toxins, chemicals, and household cleaning agents in an adequately ventilated location that is inaccessible to children.

Stranger Safety

Children should play with friends, have a plan for returning home, know their home phone number and address, play in a safe and known area, and report any suspicious activity threatening their safety to an appropriate adult; children should know how to say "no" and how to locate assistance when in an unsafe situation.

Sports Safety

Children need to engage in age-appropriate activities and wear protective equipment relevant to the sport; parents need to ensure safety and maintenance of all sports equipment; parents need to caution children against hazardous sports, such as tramlining.

Animal Safety

Parents should teach children to avoid strange animals, especially sick or injured ones, and ensure that personal pets receive vaccinations; parents need to teach children not to mistreat pets and not to place their faces close to any animal.

Although nurses offer suggestions to parents to improve their children's play safety, studies have shown that few parents follow these suggestions. The reasons for this behavior include parental difficulty in assessing the safety of and age-appropriateness of play equipment, the amount of effort involved, and a lack of money to create a safe play area. The nurse helps parents respond to these perceived barriers. With more children using skateboards and rollerblades, the nurse also encourages the use of child safety helmets and knee, elbow, and wrist guards to prevent muscle sprains and bone fractures. The school offers an on-site opportunity for teaching children, teachers, and parents about accident prevention. In addition to providing this guidance, nurses can participate in legislative and educational actions to increase community consciousness about child safety.

trees, space heaters, and fireplace malfunctions. Many homes lack working smoke detectors because of incorrect installation or inadequate testing. If a fire occurs in a home with a smoke detector, the risk of death decreases by 40% to 50% (Ahrens, 2021). Most burned children survive, frequently with various degrees of physical and psychological scars. Children need to learn about fire safety, including the importance of avoiding situations involving fire and practicing fire drills routinely at school and at home. The nurse encourages parents to understand other practices to prevent fire-related problems, including parental purchase of flame-retardant sleepwear for children.

Firearms

People in the United States who use firearms frequently cause fatal injury through homicide, suicide, or accidents. Nearly 1300 children die and 5790 are treated for gunshot wounds each year in the United States (Fowler et al., 2017). A Healthy People 2030 Objective and injury, violence prevention goal is to reduce the number of firearm-related deaths and nonfatal firearm injuries (Box 20.1). With many US homes containing a handgun and because of recent shootings by adolescents, concern about children's safety remains well founded. Possibly, the best means of preventing accidents with firearms is to ban them from private ownership, as seen in England. However, because handgun ownership is an important individual right in the United States, several states have passed legislation that allows handguns for individual protection. Families with firearms in the home should store them in a locked area apart from ammunition and consider using nonlethal (wax) bullets. All family members should be knowledgeable about gun safety.

Much debate has been raised recently regarding the use of toy guns by children. Unlike video game use, the use of toy guns during childhood does not increase the likelihood of violent or aggressive behavior later in life. Unfortunately, there have been a number of deaths associated with police mistaking a toy gun used by school-age children for a firearm. These deaths have occurred in spite of mandatory markings on toy handguns.

Sports and Recreation

Accidents from sports and other recreational activities increase during the school-age years and include lacerations, contusions, hematomas, concussions, sprains, and fractures. Some evidence exists that adolescents now have more musculoskeletal injuries because of involvement in repetitive team sports earlier in their lives. This suggests that society needs to examine the current emphasis on initiating young children with musculoskeletal immaturity into team sports such as football, hockey, soccer, and basketball. Intense social pressure for children to participate in these sports means that parents and school systems must ensure that each child has protective body devices to prevent injuries, as well as psychological support to allow a child to benefit from the team sport. There is a further need to increase safety by ensuring that each child fits the sport, has adequate hydration during the game, and engages in conditioning exercises before and after the game for prevention of injuries. There is a societal need to focus more on the collaborative skills children learn by being part of a team rather than the intense focus-on-winning philosophy found in many school-age team sports.

Recreation area injuries may be prevented by several measures. The US Consumer Product Safety Commission released guidelines for playground safety in 1981 for home playground equipment, regulating objects such as sharp edges, moving parts, and equipment design. Nurses help prevent accidents by participating in decisions about school playground equipment and counseling families on a variety of issues.

Mechanical Forces

Motor vehicles and bicycles are the two most common mechanical agents that cause injury to school-age children.

Motor Vehicles. The leading cause of death in the United States in all individuals from ages 1 to 34 years is motor vehicle accidents (CDC, n.d.-c). Children die as passengers in cars, as pedestrians, and as bicycle riders. In the United States, more children die from pedestrian-related accidents than from passenger-related accidents (CDC, n.d.-q). Each year children are killed and injured because of bicycle-related accidents, head injuries accounting for a large part of the fatalities (Bicycle Helmet Safety Institute, 2023). Helmet use in children can reduce the risk of head injury by 45%. Although not all accidents result in death, children may also sustain injury that causes permanent disability because of motor vehicle accidents.

Automobile passenger injuries can be prevented, or the severity reduced, by alteration of some aspects of the child's environment. Lower speed limits, stricter enforcement of alcohol-related laws, better automobile and highway designs, improved door lock mechanisms, and more effective restraint system requirements in all states have reduced the severity and number of accidents and injuries. School-bus transportation is a risk for injury in the school-age child (US Department of Transportation, n.d.). The National Highway Traffic Safety Administration (NHTSA) reports children are safer on a school bus than traditional vehicle transportation to school. Debate exists related to the use of seat belts on school buses. The NHTSA reports school buses are the most highly regulated form of transportation and designed to be safer in preventing crashes and injuries (US Department of Transportation, n.d.). In response to community concerns and some school districts and states requiring safety restraint use in buses used to transport students, the NHTSA developed a comprehensive guide addressing school bus transportation (NHTSA, 2015).

Proper and consistent use of federally approved belt-positioned booster seats for children aged 4 to 7 years decreases the likelihood of child death and serious injury significantly (CDC, n.d.-m). However, one study showed that in 2017, of the children 12 years old and younger who died in a car crash (in which restraint use was known), 35% were not buckled up. Less than 10% of children needing the protection of a booster seat ride in one. Booster seat use can reduce risk for serious injury by 45% when compared with seat belt use alone (CDC, n.d.-c). Booster seat use is recommended for all children whose height or weight exceeds the forward-facing limits for their car safety seat. Use should continue until children are about 4 feet 9 inches in height and are 8 to 12 years of age (AAP, 2021a). The reasons given by parents and children for their not using seat belts or booster seats include forgetting to use the device, having difficulty reaching and fastening belts, feeling discomfort from wearing the belt or using the seat, and receiving misinformation about the need for the belt or seat for short trips. Clearly, consistent use of booster seats by young children and seat belts by older children and adults, who model seat belt behavior to their children, will occur only when legal enforcement occurs. Federal government and national professional groups recommend that all children younger than 13 years ride in the automobile's back seat in an appropriate restraint because of the potential for death from an air bag activated in a motor vehicle accident (AAP, 2021b). Many families have difficulty meeting this recommendation because of long-term acceptance of older children riding in the front seat after they have outgrown booster seats.

Urban children younger than 15 years old experience more than half of all pedestrian-automobile accidents. These occur when they are using rollerblades, skateboards, and skate scooters and tend to be more severe (head injuries) than passenger injuries. Many factors cause pedestrian accidents: children often have difficulty interpreting traffic signs and judging the speed of cars, and they forget to look carefully before crossing the street. Although overcrowding, poverty, high volume of traffic, stress, and unsafe play areas influence children's street safety, various principles can direct interventions to decrease the number of street dangers.

Bicycles and Motorized Vehicles. Many accidents occur each year with young children on bicycles, motorized skateboards, and all-terrain vehicles (ATVs). Most of these are not serious, but deaths occur among young children who have suffered head trauma or significant body injury from inappropriate use of this equipment. Jennissen (2022) recommends that only

BOX 20.9 Selected Nursing Actions to Prevent Accidents During the School-Age Period

Strategies for Counseling, Action, and Intervention

- Teach accident prevention at prime times, such as in the classroom or during pediatric or prenatal visits.
- Focus on the main concerns at the development level of the child as opposed to discussing many topics. For the school-age child, these topics usually include stranger, motor vehicle, water, fire, and bicycle safety (Box 20.8). School-age children are most at risk for extremity fractures around 8 to 12 years of age (Voth et al., 2022)
- Reinforce and repeat information at appropriate intervals.

Community Actions (Rushton et al., 2019)

- Use supplemental materials, such as pamphlets, pictures, and videos to reinforce verbal information.
- Support local or national legislation that sets standards for potentially harmful agents. Mandating standards is a successful accident preventive strategy, as seen with the Poison Prevention Packaging Act and the Flammable Fabrics Act.
- Encourage children to wear a helmet and other protective gear. Many nurses have been active in lobbying for state bicycle helmet requirements.
- Consult with manufacturers on safe designs of bicycles, scooters, ski equipment, rollerblades, and other exercise equipment used by children.
- Report objects that are potentially hazardous or broken.
- Participate in community events and activities that stress accident prevention.
- Educate groups such as schoolchildren and parent organizations.

people at least 16 years old ride ATVs and then only in rural areas with adult supervision. Bicycle accidents occur most frequently near the child's home and during the day and commonly involve injuries from the spokes when children ride behind the bike seat. More males than females experience these injuries from bicycles, motorized skateboards, and ATVs, perhaps because of their greater risk-taking behavior (Jennissen, 2022).

In response to children's developmental behavior related to bicycles, motorized skateboards, and ATVs, the nurse addresses safety issues (Jennissen, 2022). Additionally, nurses encourage parents to teach and reinforce safe bicycling habits to their children and should sponsor helmet and bike programs within the school (Box 20.9).

Biologic Agents

School-age children face constant exposure to bacterial, viral, and other biologic agents that pose threats to or improve their overall health (e.g., immunizations). Compared with the preschool child, the school-age child has fewer illnesses. The most frequent illness continues to be upper respiratory tract infections (URIs), illnesses shared among schoolchildren who fail to practice good handwashing techniques and avoidance of ill peers. These illnesses cause children to lose school days and learning opportunities. Most URIs result from viruses, but bacteria can play either a primary or a secondary role. Two problems associated with URIs are streptococcal infection ("strep throat") and otitis media.

Strep throat occurs frequently among school-age children. A child with an infection from group A *Streptococcus* may have a severe sore throat, fever, and malaise, or may have only a minor sore throat. A throat culture confirms the diagnosis, and antibiotic treatment typically cures the infection. Children are noninfectious after 24 hours of treatment and may return to school (CDC, n.d.-j). If not treated, the affected child may develop rheumatic fever or acute glomerulonephritis as a secondary infection following the sore throat. Greater transmission of streptococcal infection occurs in areas where there is close personal contact during colder weather. The school nurse's preventive efforts focus on teaching the children good handwashing techniques and identifying children who complain of sore throats. Children with throat infections caused by other strains of *Streptococcus*, such as group B, do not usually require treatment, because these infections generally do not cause the same serious complications.

Otitis media rates have subsided with the integration of the pneumococcal and influenza vaccines into the immunization schedule. Acute otitis media is often self-limiting and can often be regarded as a complication of a preceding or concomitant URI. Most cases of otitis media will resolve spontaneously. Without specific treatment, symptoms frequently abate within 24 hours and settle within 3 days (Donaldson, 2024). The nurse is in an integral position to help support the family and educate the family on risk factors associated with otitis media and nonpharmacologic therapies that may alleviate symptoms and discomfort during the course of illness.

The school-age child may experience other illnesses. The frequency of gastrointestinal tract infection (**gastroenteritis**) decreases during the school-age years but is still the second most common acute condition of childhood. Usually caused by a virus, gastrointestinal tract infections cause vomiting and diarrhea. Older and larger school-age children have little chance of rapid dehydration; they basically react to the illness the same as do adults and need to be treated similarly. Gastroenteritis is contagious, and therefore the nurse should monitor schoolchildren for symptoms of illness and encourage proper handwashing to prevent transmission of the virus from one child to another.

Scabies and **pediculosis** are common skin disorders among school-age children, involving extreme itchiness of either the body (scabies) or the head (pediculosis), and are easily spread to other children (Nemours Children's Health, n.d.). The nurse educates parents to visualize the mites and **lice** or use a lice comb to check their children for mites and lice when they complain of itchiness or seem to be constantly scratching their heads. Previously, children with lice could not come to school until they were lice-free, which isolated students from their peers and influenced state school funding based on student attendance. Nolt (2024) recommends that once children are undergoing treatment for the problem, they should be allowed in school.

Most states require that the child's immunizations be current before the child enters kindergarten or the first grade and that additional tetanus immunization be given every 10 years or when an unclean wound is acquired. Influenza vaccine is recommended annually beginning in October. Other immunizations recommended by the AAP include a **meningococcal vaccination** at age 11 or 12 years and the series of three injections for hepatitis B and **human papillomavirus** during the late school-age and early adolescent years (CDC, n.d.-s). If the child has no history of chickenpox, a varicella immunization is also recommended. In many states the school nurse has a responsibility to ensure that all students' immunizations are current, and if they are not current, the nurse informs the parents that the children may not attend school until their immunizations are up to date. Any child lacking age-appropriate immunizations can "catch up" according to a schedule developed by the AAP. Although most American children receive immunizations by school entrance time, increasing numbers of immigrants and transient workers have deepened concern about exposure of Americans to previously conquered diseases (e.g., tuberculosis). Strides toward meeting the Healthy People initiative targets related to immunizations continue to be made according to the 2030 objectives (USDHHS, 2024).

Chemical Agents

A number of potentially toxic chemical agents exist in the environment, and the child is exposed to these through inhalation, ingestion, or direct contact. Children are particularly susceptible to chemical hazards. Food and drugs are two sources of chemicals ingested by children on a regular basis, and some older school-age children ingest tobacco because of cigarette smoking. Although normally safe, some foods and drugs can be harmful when used inappropriately. Other environmental hazards include pollution, heavy metals (lead and mercury), and pesticides.

The nutritional needs of the school-age child were discussed earlier in this chapter. As stated, children frequently eat foods with large quantities of sugar, salt, and fat and with chemical additives. The effects of some of these additives have been questioned, and concern has been expressed about the effect of biochemically altered food on children and future generations. On a short-term basis, some foods may cause allergic reactions; on a long-term basis, some may contribute to the development of coronary disease, hypertension, and cancer. Nurses are aware that the child's diet may contribute to future health problems, and therefore assess intake and counsel the child and parents accordingly about ways to improve it (CDC, n.d.-d,-k).

The incidence of poisoning decreases during the school-age years as children become more aware of the appropriate uses of drugs and other agents. Childproof containers have decreased exposure of children to dangerous poisons and chemicals in the home. However, children continue to face exposure to drugs (alcohol and glue inhalants) because of less monitoring by working parents, and older school-age children face exposure to recreational drugs, primarily through their peers and older children. In the school environment, the nurse and school personnel need to encourage students to engage in wise decision-making about recreational drug use that will affect their future and overall health.

With pressure on older school-age children to smoke cigarettes, attention must be paid to effective strategies to prevent this behavior. Every day, more than 1600 school students try their first cigarette (CDC, n.d.-w). Most middle school students who smoke initiate their habit at approximately 11 years of age. White American students start smoking at a younger age than Black American students do. Males tend to begin smoking earlier than females; however, females catch up in smoking rates during the middle school years (National Institute on Drug Abuse, 2022). Children in growing numbers annually use e-cigarettes and vaping products (Nemours TeensHealth & Ben-Joseph, 2019). The Federal Tobacco Settlement Project provides funds to address the public health problem posed by tobacco smoke in the United States. Although funding for tobacco prevention and cessation programs has reached its highest level in 6 years, many states continue to fall short of the minimal recommendations (American Lung Association, 2023a). Attention to smoking as part of a health-promotion program seems merited because so many children begin smoking at a young age; in addition, because nicotine is highly addictive, many believe that this habit leads people to experiment with riskier drugs (cocaine and methamphetamines).

School policies have been instrumental in supporting a tobacco-free environment (American Lung Association, 2023b). To further assist in health-promotion efforts, many institutions require staff development and education programs related to the effects of tobacco use on health. There have been various governmental efforts to reduce exposure to environmental tobacco. For example, 40 states and numerous cities nationwide have enacted smoke-free laws (Campaign for TOBACCO-FREE Kids, 2024).

Pollution has become a fact of life for many Americans, particularly for the 25% of urban-dwelling children who must breathe air that exceeds federal government acceptable levels for ozone (American Lung Association, 2023a). Air pollution irritates the eyes and the respiratory tract, causing URIs, ear infections, and allergies. More children now experience asthma, and many inner-city children face higher rates of this disease because of poor air quality, including secondary and tertiary smoke. Knowing the negative effects of air pollution and smoking on their health, many school-age children participate in school projects to improve their environmental health.

Children also face exposure to various toxic materials in their environment. Progress has been made in the past decades to reduce children's exposure to chemical hazards. Lead, for example, has been removed from gasoline and paint. This in turn has resulted in significant reductions in children's blood lead levels. Lead exposure continues to exist. Children are exposed to lead through parents' clothes, shoes contacting lead-infused soil, lead in older residential water pipes, traditional medications in some cultures, and in school building structures. Children living in poverty receive high exposure from lead-based paint used on older and less expensive homes. The long-term effects of lead on children remain unclear, but some evidence indicates children suffer neurotoxic effects from this type of exposure. High lead levels in children contribute to dental caries and hearing loss.

Routine use of chemicals to control insects and undesirable weeds in landscaping has led to increasing concerns about children's exposure to these agents. With increased interest in more natural substances to control insects and gardening problems, perhaps less reliance will be placed on chemicals for these problems in the future. Knowing the primary source of exposure to the most hazardous materials and avoiding these materials are often sufficient to accomplish real risk reduction and offer substantial protection within the child's environment. Various behaviors can be implemented to create a safe environment and minimize health risks associated with hazardous chemical exposure. Nurses are instrumental in the assistance and support of parents, schools, and community agencies in the implementation of these behaviors, such as the use of nonhazardous cleaners and pesticide-free foods and further monitoring of the environment for hazardous materials.

X-ray Exposure

The child receives exposure from both naturally occurring radiation and human-made ionizing radiation. Exposure occurs in various degrees: radiographic examinations of teeth and bone, nuclear power plants and explosions, and in the management of many childhood cancers. Children exposed to high levels of radiation risk developing breast or thyroid cancer or leukemia and compromised growth. With little advocacy in this area, nurses and other professionals improve children's health by becoming active in initiatives that focus on prevention of chemical and radiation hazards.

Cancer

Leukemia is the most common form of childhood cancer. Of those younger than 5 years affected, 90% will be cured with current medical treatment. Among the 12 major types of childhood cancers, leukemia and cancers of the brain and central nervous system (second most common forms of childhood cancers) account for more than 50% of all new cases (CureSearch for Childhood Cancer, 2024). Lymphomas (Hodgkin disease and non-Hodgkin lymphoma) also affect school-age children and adolescents as the third most common group of malignancies. Non-Hodgkin lymphoma is more common during the school-age years, and males experience this malignancy three times more often than do females. A common presenting symptom is abdominal pain caused by intestinal obstruction or organ compression. With effective treatment regimens, children with limited disease may be cured but may experience side effects of treatment later in life (e.g., development of cataracts, dental problems, learning difficulties). Advances are being made with the use of genomic sequencing and the use of genomic medicine to explore novel treatments with the goal of improving childhood cancer outcomes (National Cancer Institute, 2024). Children with cancer present a challenge to the nurse because they are in various stages of recovery, may be developmentally delayed as a result of prolonged periods of absence from peer groups during therapy, and may fear a recurrence of their disease. The nurse provides psychological and emotional support to affected children and their families to help children develop peer relationships and meet developmental goals important to them during the school-age years.

DETERMINANTS OF HEALTH

The school-age child interacts daily with other children and adults to become more independent by age 12 years. Mutual problem-solving by the child and the parents or friends frequently occurs at this age related to a higher level of maturity in social relationships and concerns. Exposure to a variety of social roles and expectations of others strengthens the process of socialization so that the child develops social competence—the ability and skills to participate effectively in the social interactions of society. Social competence includes both the obvious social behaviors and an inner understanding of the appropriateness of behaviors.

Several elements play a role in the development of the child's social competence. The child's desire for a sense of industry encourages interactions, positive relationships, and accomplishments within society. Cognitive development supports understanding of relationships and effective problem-solving (Cherry, 2022a). Moral judgment helps the child understand consequences and fairness in relationships. Understanding and obeying authority help to maintain order in society. Social sensitivity is a result of social interactions and requires the child's ability to perceive the social cues of others, understand the roles of others, and communicate verbally with them. Social behaviors are also a part of social competence; these are learned most frequently through imitation, role-modeling, and reinforcement of others' behaviors. The interaction of all these elements produces a level of social competence and simultaneously plays a role in the child's self-perception. Individuals frequently see themselves as others see them.

Social Factors and Environment

Peers

The strongest relationships that school-age children develop outside their families are with their peers (other children encountered in the neighborhood and school). The peer group acts as a new social system, becoming increasingly influential in the child's life. All children continue to be influenced significantly by the family, the culture of the family, and many other environmental factors, but the peer group begins to influence lifestyle, habits, and speech patterns and formulate standards of behavior and performance. The standards of the peer group become vitally important, and children attempt to conform to its rules. Being accepted by the peer group becomes more important than being accepted by anyone else. Conforming to the pressures of peers becomes an issue, especially when it interferes with the parents' expectations. When children realize that their own goals, desires, and aspirations might be quite different from those held by the peer group or the school, they must find ways to cope and perform according to the new standards if they are to succeed. The degree to which children fit in socially, learn to cope, and receive satisfaction from the group is a powerful determinant of healthy socialization. Online chat rooms and social media may provide avenues for group classwork and outside socialization (AAP, 2021b) but can also provide opportunities for negative and bullying behaviors. A child may have one best friend or several important friends and a mutual understanding and willingness to help each other. Friendship groups that form during this age may change and become goal directed, such as groups composing a sports team. These groups frequently have set rules or rituals that connect the members. During the middle school years, friendships often revolve around same-sex relationships, videos, songs, books, and social media shared by the group. Later in the school-age years, the development of sexual relationships with the members of the opposite sex occurs during dating and mixed parties.

School-age children also become increasingly involved with adults outside the family, including teachers, coaches, and others who become role models, all of whom influence the child's view of the world and self. Although this influence may not be as significant as that of a child's peers, long-term ideas and beliefs frequently develop from these relationships. Children usually perceive some similarity between themselves and their models, those of the same sex with similar physical or behavior traits. During these years, children may not maintain a strong identification with the parent of the same sex, but they tend to adopt other adult models with whom they can identify.

Working Parents

Both dual-career couples and single-parent families influence their children's safety when no adult is present to monitor the environment after school. Many **latchkey children** who are left alone until their parents return from work follow directions given by their parents. These directions may include starting dinner in anticipation of their parents' return or completing homework while remaining inside the home with the doors locked.

Parents and school-age children often disagree about how old is "old enough" to be left at home alone or with an older sibling. Although the school-age child might consider being at home alone to be a real mark of maturity, children who look after themselves after school can become more isolated and miss peer relationships important to their development. Nurses give guidance to families who must cope with the issue of after-school care for school-age children to ensure that relevant and safe decisions are made.

Culture and Ethnicity

School-age children focus more on the influences of their culture on their lives than do younger children. Aspects of American culture that the child must confront include poverty and affluence, ethnic and racial differences, acceptance of these differences, and the power of media as a cultural phenomenon in American society.

Ethnic Groups

Preschool children may notice racial and ethnic differences, but school-age children increasingly show evidence of being aware of these differences. This is a time during which attitudes toward race develop on the basis of family and community attitudes. Although prejudice exists among some school-age children, they should be encouraged to view people from different cultures and ethnic backgrounds in a positive light. Many schools appropriately focus on the importance of other cultures by having multicultural awareness weeks. During these times, children dress, eat, and live as other cultures do, allowing them to recognize the uniqueness of individual cultural beliefs and values (Box 20.10: Health and Social Determinants/Health Equity).

BOX 20.10 HEALTH AND SOCIAL DETERMINANTS/HEALTH EQUITY

Promoting Educational Success: Social Emotional Learning

The school age years are an important time to acquire the ability to understand and manage emotions, set realistic and positive goals, demonstrate caring and concern to classmates, develop positive social relationships, and make sensible decisions. These skills are important for later success and are foundational to family life (Mahoney et al., 2021). Social emotional learning involves explaining behavioral management techniques such as breathing exercises to help relieve the stress associated with difficult or negative emotions; this allows a student to concentrate better on their studies. Children are taught to identify their emotions and approaches to calm themselves down. This is especially important when children bring different cultural values into the classroom. Consider some of the backgrounds of children in classes in the United States or globally. In the American Indian culture, the child is taught to respect elders, develop natural talents, and ask for assistance from family members not outsiders. The Mexican American child is taught to be obedient and respectful, and the next generation is expected to do better than the present. A Filipino child may be raised in a more protective environment where direct confrontation is avoided and education is valued for personal and financial gain. The Black American child has expectations to complete chores, focus on school, and project respectful behavior toward adults and elders. In the Chinese American family, the child is highly valued, especially if the child is male. The child is expected to honor elders and help with family needs, and attaining educational goals is seen as promoting family honor. These short examples over-simplify the differing values seen in the classroom environment.

With all of the nested values that the school-age child brings to the classroom, there is a need for education that helps children to promote positive relationships, manage emotions, regulate anger, solve conflicts, and look for areas of social agreement (Mahoney et al., 2021). Children need to learn to negotiate stressful experiences positively. In the instructional design of the classroom, there are many opportunities to apply social emotional learning techniques.

Television and Video and Computer Games

Television and video and computer games exert a major influence on ideas and behavior in American culture. Unfortunately, many television programs and video and computer games pose harm to children because of their messages and because such activities prevent children from engaging in physical activity. Advances in gaming offer an option for increased activity during gaming activities. Video games and gaming systems have been developed that encourage movement during gaming. Energy expenditure more than doubled when sedentary screen times were converted to active screen time.

Computers connected to the internet pose a danger unless locking devices have been installed to prevent school-age children from accessing inappropriate websites. Additional concerns have focused on the violent themes of programming, persuasive television commercials, unrealistic depictions of the world, unhealthy food intake, and the negative aspects of television viewing and video games (Children's Hospital Boston, 2022).

Television facilitates negative attitudes and values among children, increases their aggressive behavior, decreases their emotional sensitivity when aggressive acts occur, and leads them to accept aggressive acts. One positive note is that adults who discuss violence with children by pointing out that these acts are unacceptable and cause pain to others can help inhibit some childhood aggression. Discussion of recent acts of violence committed by young people in such a context also helps. Anger control programs, as part of school health-promotion programs, also help decrease societal violence and produce more collaborative workers needed for the future.

The average child views an overwhelming number of television commercials by age 18 years, and these commercials influence daily and future choices and behaviors. Many television commercials focus on sugary foods that cause damage to teeth, diminish overall healthy habits, and lead to increased rates of obesity. Young children cannot always separate the program from the commercials and believe that they must purchase products the television says to buy. Many childhood authorities question the ethics of exposing children to any type of advertising. Although concern about the effect of advertising has led to programming changes during children's watching time, more work is needed to send more socially responsible messages.

The world as presented on many television shows does not accurately reflect the real world. Despite an increasingly diverse and aging population, stereotypes of females and minority groups and a predominance of younger actors continue to make money for the media industry. Parents and health care providers should monitor television viewing to ensure the age appropriateness of the material, respond to television stations about inaccuracies in the content, and write letters to their newspaper or television networks to express concerns about the material presented. Parents may also participate with their children in responding to media presentations on learning and moral themes. Parents should follow recommendations from the AAP—limit television and media viewing to 2 hours per day, have media-free bedrooms, disallow television viewing while eating, and participate in national "Turn Off the Television Week" (AAP, 2021b).

Some positive aspects of television viewing exist. A number of children's programs, such as *Sesame Street, Wishbone,* and *Kratt's Creatures* for younger children and *Bill Nye, the Science Guy, Cyberchase,* and *Zoom* for older children, have been deemed developmentally appropriate for children (Public Broadcast Services, 2024). Likewise, there are excellent websites for school-age children that stimulate their learning and promote their health.

Increasingly, parents engage their school-age children in learning and playing on a home computer. Although this technology serves as a good resource for locating information, writing papers, and organizing information, parents must limit the time students spend on computers. Likewise, limitations must be put on use of computer games that detract from socialization with peers and the family and take time away from schoolwork.

Levels of Policy Making and Health

Throughout this chapter, laws that support the health and well-being of the school-age child have been discussed. These laws include guidelines for the safe use of products, use of flame-retardant clothes, mandates against tobacco advertisements, and nutritional guidelines for federally supported school lunch programs. Another important law is mandatory public education for disabled children. The Individuals with Disabilities Education Act, formally known as **Public Law 94-142 (Education for All Handicapped Children Act)**, established in 1977, states that any child with special needs (disabled) aged 5 to 21 years has the right to free appropriate public education in the least restrictive environment and evaluation by school or health professionals to identify learning needs. Disability includes having a limitation in one or more functional areas (Govtrack, 2019) and affects as many as 10% of children aged 5 to 17 years.

Many states begin educational services for affected children at 3 years of age based on an **individualized educational plan** (IEP) for that child and as mandated by law (Lee, n.d.). The school nurse is responsible for collaborating with other school personnel and parents in ensuring that the IEP, including the health care needs of the child and connection to resources addressing the unique learning needs, receives attention. However, some parents have expressed concern that their "normal" or "gifted" child receives less attention in school systems because of the cost and time expenditures associated with implementing IEPs for disabled children. To add further concern, with recent school budgetary shortfalls, people who have received less training than the school nurse often have responsibility for implementing IEPs. Despite these concerns, the value of Public Law 94-142 has been that disabled people have had their problems addressed in the educational arena.

To ensure access to educational opportunities for every individual, the US Department of Education was developed in 1980. Through the US Department of Education, President George W. Bush enacted the **No Child Left Behind Act of 2001**, aimed at improving the academic achievement of the disadvantaged (Chen, 2022). The No Child Left Behind Act of 2001 intended to help ensure that all children have the opportunity to obtain a high-quality education and reach proficiency on challenging state academic standards and assessments. As a result of the No Child Left Behind Act of 2001, more reading progress was made by 9-year-old children in 5 years than in the previous 28 years combined. Reading and math scores of 9-year-old children and fourth graders have reached all-time highs, and 46 states improved or held steady in all categories of students tested in reading and math (Chen, 2022).

Poverty, Environmental Conditions, and Safety

In the United States, 53% of ethnically and racially diverse students are taught in public elementary and secondary schools (Child Trends Databank, 2024). Among those diverse population groups, 50% of Black American, 30% of Hispanic, and an unknown percentage of migrant, indigenous, Native American children live in poor economic conditions that negatively influence their health. These conditions include unemployment, inadequate or crowded housing, poor sanitation, poor nutrition, low educational levels, and limited or sporadic access to health and social services perhaps attributable to lack of health insurance or contextual factors of these people's lives. The number of uninsured children continues to be high and limits the number of children and families receiving primary health care. The lack of primary care among Black American, Hispanic, and White American children in rural areas prevents needed asthma management, dictating an expanded role for health care providers to connect families to resources for more effective disease control.

Many homeless children face poor living conditions and high rates of depression related to few friends and poor health status. Migrant children face more diseases (e.g., tuberculosis, scabies, and ear infections), injuries, and dental caries, and pose treatment challenges because of their transient status. The effects of limited financial resources on children include higher mortality rates at all ages than in those who are not poor or migrant and more school days lost because of illnesses. Numerous problems exist for children in poverty, including greater developmental delay as a result of poor nutrition; increased peer rejection; poorer self-concept; increased risk of accidents, drug abuse, and abuse or neglect by parents; and greater overall poor coping abilities.

The nurse improves the overall health of poor children by encouraging relationships with appropriate role models and by reinforcing strong family relationships that help children develop resilient and positive self-images.

Family wealth may have a negative influence on the school-age child if there is frequent substitute caregiving of varying quality attributable to parental absence, extremely high or unreasonable parental expectations, availability of material possessions but little child awareness of relevant responsibilities, and easy access to drugs and alcohol and similar dangers. The nurse reinforces the need in wealthy families for consistent demonstration of parental love and support, firm limits on appropriate behavior, and the value of recognizing the child's unique abilities. The nurse also offers ideas that will help decrease risk-taking behavior (e.g., use of drugs) and increase parent-child connection until a parent is in the home.

When discussing children raised in poverty or affluence, the nurse remembers at least two points. First, many variables affect each child, often in different ways, to influence overall development. Second, although personality and support networks help a child in a socially poor environment to excel later in life, most authorities believe that problems of affluence are easier to overcome than are the all-pervasive problems of poverty.

Health Services/Delivery System

Well-Child Care

The AAP recommends that at least every 2 years children 6 years or older have a well-child examination by either a physician or a nurse practitioner. In the ideal situation, the child has a primary health care provider, one person or practice from which the child receives wellness and illness care coordinated by members of a health care team (AAP, 2023). Unfortunately, many American children still do not have this quality of care (see the earlier section on poverty). With increasing numbers living in poverty because of family violence, single parenthood, and divorce, many lack a primary care provider for their physical and emotional needs often because of a lack of health insurance. In this situation, they often receive emergency care only when they are very ill or injured.

The nurse encourages the school-age child and the parents to be active members of any health evaluation. Children may give some of their own history, answer questions, and discuss their health concerns. During the history taking, the child's privacy should be respected. Some children in this age group want a parent present during the examination; others do not. When possible, the nurse spends at least some time alone with the child to allow discussions that the child may not feel comfortable with when the parents are present. The examinations can also be a time for education on how the body works and ways to keep it healthy. Preventive information on diet and exercise can be offered relevant to prevention of obesity, cardiovascular disease, and diabetes. Information can also be obtained on school adjustment and performance, particularly because this is a major portion of the child's life. School performance can reflect the child's cognitive and general development. If there are any concerns, the nurse obtains more information through separate testing or discussion with school officials. Health education is directed to both the child and the parents for the best results. Activities that the child performs alone and with the family can give a picture of relationships and adjustments that relate to the child's health (see the Case Study at the end of this chapter).

A challenge for nurses who work with school-age children (NASN, 2024) is to maintain their normal healthy status and prevent illness. This task is accomplished through a variety of health-promotion mechanisms, such as examination, guidance, education, and legislation. Many professionals have noted that school-age children guided by the nurse generally seek health and use various resources to attain, maintain, or regain optimal health for their future productivity. Aspects of the nursing process are implemented when one is structuring a program to maintain the child's health (such as seen with an assessment of immunization status), promote health habits (seen with teaching bicycle safety), and prevent illness (seen by obtaining throat cultures to detect streptococcal infection).

Nurses have many opportunities and settings to help them implement their interventions as consultants, board members, and active providers of care. For example, nurses and school-age children interact during well-child evaluations and at school. Nurses in other roles, such as in public health positions and in hospitals, also play a role in health promotion, although these nurses must often focus more on helping the child and the family respond to an illness or a crisis. Local and national groups influence the health of children through their activities and regulations. These include organizations such as Boy Scouts and Girl Scouts, Big Brothers and Big Sisters, charities such as the Red Cross, and government agencies such as the Consumer Product Safety Commission.

As an integral part of the community, the school system has the responsibility to provide a healthy school environment and a comprehensive health-education program. In some areas, nurses, physicians, and other health care personnel work as a team in the school health program, which includes health care and maintenance and education. The nurse advocates and searches for resources so that each child has a source of health care, or the nurse is a nurse practitioner who delivers care. School health programs range from an occasional mention of body care and the changes of puberty to a full program that integrates physical and mental health principles into all aspects of the educational experience.

Comprehensive school health services require an interdisciplinary, coordinated effort between health care providers and educators. Recommendations state that each school should have an on-site nurse to conduct and mentor students and faculty in health-promotion areas (NASN, 2024). Nevertheless, many schools share nurses because of budgetary concerns. However, when available, nurses offer educational and interpersonal skills to initiate health-promotion teaching that improves the overall health of consumers (students, parents, teachers, community). Nurses have a wide scope of practice, including that of referring parents to relevant resources aimed toward activities that improve the school environment and its inhabitants.

The nurse's role in planning health maintenance for children of a school varies, depending on the type of health maintenance program. In one system, the school nurse may refer children to resources available to provide a source of health care, whereas in another system, the school nurse functions as a nurse practitioner. On the basis of the scope of practice and state legal requirements, the school nurse monitors and updates children's immunizations and identifies and intervenes with children who have acute or chronic health care problems, such as scoliosis, strep throat, common cold, or child abuse (NASN, 2024). Increasingly, school nurses provide sophisticated care according to evidence-based protocols for chronically ill school-age children who have been integrated into the regular academic environment. On the basis of state regulations, the nurse also engages in completing vision, hearing, and scoliosis screening at regular intervals. In most schools the nurse works with the school's physician, community physicians, and parents in meeting children's and community health needs.

For all school-age children, the school nurse plays a role in developing a healthy educational environment through promoting a comprehensive and age-appropriate health-education program focused on children becoming responsible for their own health. A program aimed at accident prevention in and around the school is part of the nurse's role. The program includes assessing the school for pedestrian and automobile traffic patterns, broken playground and classroom equipment, ice and snow dangers, poorly maintained toilet facilities, and inappropriately prepared food. Regular practice drills are held to acquaint teachers and students with emergency procedures (i.e., fire, bomb, or intruder threats. All people in the school are prepared to respond to chemical hazards. The nurse implements existing school-based programs on drug and alcohol abuse.

It is also important to consider the role of the nurse in fostering a healthy social environment in the school (NASN, 2024). The nurse examines the social interactions of the children and interacts with them to promote positive relationships. However, social problems continue to constitute a major concern for many children during this time. Children may experience difficulty in making the initial transition away from the family and gaining satisfaction from a group of peers. Children may make the initial adjustment but then have difficulties interacting with others (e.g., bullying). When problems such as these arise, the nurse, parents, and school system determine the reasons for this behavior and intervene appropriately.

NURSING APPLICATION

The nurse working with the school-age child has a unique and exciting opportunity to engage the child in health-promoting behaviors. Most school-age children are able to participate in the teaching strategies if the strategies are geared toward the child's appropriate cognitive ability. As the age range of the school-age child is from 5 to 12 years, the nurse must consider the mental ability and comprehension of each developmental stage. The COVID pandemic forced the closure of many schools and reduced on-site learning; it may be a long period before the full effects on children such as developmental and learning setbacks are fully understood (Busenbark, 2021).

Nurses can teach health-promotion behaviors directly to the child through spending time demonstrating, monitoring, and reinforcing preventive health practices such as handwashing, dental hygiene, nutrition, and physical activity. These activities can be taught through age-appropriate reading materials, modeling, and role-playing. Engaging the child in these practices may also help the child conceptualize the link between the behavior and disease prevention. The nurse must partner with parents to model healthy behaviors at home, at school, and in the community settings.

A variety of methods can be used to educate children on health and nutrition. Keeping culture, socioeconomics, and media influences in mind, the nurse should teach children concepts about food choices, exercise habits, and the ways overall health is affected by those choices. Nutrition education can be individualized to the age of the child through use of games, activities, colorful food guides, and simple cooking activities.

Physical activity in childhood is crucial in promoting healthy behaviors that continue into adulthood (USDHHS, 2019). Exercise for this age group is generally provided in group activities and sports. Physical activity provides the school-age child with peer interaction and social relationships. This aspect of health promotion should be encouraged by the nurse as well as the family.

As with younger age groups, health promotion of the school-age child focuses on education about routine health examination and the childhood immunization schedule. The nurse provides the families with immunization recommendations and must remain updated on current guidelines. The nurse also focuses on prevention of childhood injuries by educating them about seat belt and bicycle safety, as well as other things with a potential for causing injury.

Screening for health problems is another aspect of caring for the school-age child. Screenings are generally conducted for problems with vision, hearing, height, weight, and oral health. The nurse may be the first person to identify a potential issue with regard to an acute or chronic condition. At that time, he or she gathers assessment data to determine if the child needs immediate treatment or a referral to another provider. For the nurse working with school-age children and their families, the role is often one of providing education, case management, consulting, counseling, and community outreach (NASN, 2024).

CASE STUDY

Change in Usual Communication Pattern in School: Joey

Joey is an 8-year-old male in elementary school. His school lost almost 2 years of in-class attendance due to closures during COVID, so adapting to this year's classroom situation is new. His teacher has voiced a growing concern regarding his classroom behavior. In the past 2 months, Joey has become more withdrawn from his classmates and rarely participates in class discussion. This is a new behavior pattern. Two months before, he "used to talk all the time and raise his hand to answer questions in class." His teacher reports that they were discussing family and family roles in class this week. Joey became very aggressive and yelled, "My dad isn't at home anymore cause of my mom." He went on to say, "I really miss dad. My mom's new boyfriend isn't nice and won't buy me stuff, like my dad does." His teacher determines Joey's parents are separated. A parent-teacher conference has been scheduled to discuss Joey's behavior because it is now affecting his grades.

Analyzing Cues and Reflective Questions

- Is Joey's behavior appropriate for his age?
- Has the closure of schools during the COVID epidemic affected the behavior of school-age children?
- Joey's parents do not understand his change in behavior. His father yells, "If she would let me spend more time with my son, Joey wouldn't be having trouble with school. She doesn't care about my son now that she has her new boyfriend." How might the nurse respond to this situation?
- What interventions might be effective for Joey's parents and teacher in improving his classroom behavior and school performance?

SUMMARY

- Many changes occur in children during the exciting period of the school-age years.
- The child's development progresses from the immaturity of the preschooler to the beginning of adolescence and eventual adulthood.
- Cognitive abilities increase dramatically, adding to the desire to master tasks and the ability to develop moral judgment.
- The child's world expands beyond the family unit as school and peers begin to exert a major influence.
- Opportunities for nurses during this period occur primarily in ambulatory settings, with the school nurse frequently the most effective and influential health care provider for children of this age group and their families.

EVOLVE CHAPTER FEATURES

http://evolve.elsevier.com/Edelman/

- Study Questions

REFERENCES

Administration for Children and Families. (2025). *Child maltreatment.* https://acf.gov/cb/data-Hresearch/child-maltreatment

Ahrens, M. (2021). *Smoke alarms in US home fires.* https://www.nfpa.org/education-and-research/research/nfpa-research/fire-statistical-reports/smoke-alarms-in-us-home-fires?l=38

Ali, Y. (2022). *Fast food consumption by U.S. children.* https://www.verywellhealth.com/how-much-fast-food-do-us-children-eat-2509574. Accessed July 26, 2022.

American Academy of Pediatric Dentistry (AAPD). (n.d.). *State of little teeth two.* https://www.mychildrensteeth.org/state-of-little-teeth-two/

American Academy of Pediatrics (AAP). (2019). *Bedwetting in children & teens: nocturnal enuresis.* https://www.healthychildren.org/English/health-issues/conditions/genitourinary-tract/Pages/Nocturnal-Enuresis-in-Teens.aspx

American Academy of Pediatrics (AAP). (2021a). *Booster seats for school-aged children.* https://www.healthychildren.org/English/safety-prevention/on-the-go/Pages/Booster-Seats-for-School-Aged-Children.aspx

American Academy of Pediatrics (AAP). (2021b). *Media and children.* https://www.aap.org/en/patient-care/media-and-children/

American Academy of Pediatrics (AAP). (2021c). *The emotional toll of obesity.* https://www.healthychildren.org/English/health-issues/conditions/obesity/Pages/The-Emotional-Toll-of-Obesity.aspx

American Academy of Pediatrics (AAP). (2022). *School safety during an emergency or crisis: what parents need to know.* https://www.healthychildren.org/English/safety-prevention/all-around/Pages/Actions-Schools-Are-Taking-to-Make-Themselves-Safer.aspx

American Academy of Pediatrics (AAP). (2023). 2023 Recommendations for preventive pediatric health care [policy statement]. *Pediatrics, 151*(4), e2023061451. https://doi.org/10.1542/peds.2023-061451

American Association for Marriage and Family Therapy. (n.d.). *Children and divorce.* https://www.aamft.org/Consumer_Updates/Children_and_Divorce.aspx

American College of Cardiology. (2018). *Understanding the long-term effects of childhood obesity.* https://www.cardiosmart.org/News-and-Events/2018/05/Understanding-the-Long-Term-Effects-of-Childhood-Obesity

American College of Obstetrics & Gynecology (ACOG). (2019). *Menstruation in girls and adolescents: using the menstrual cycle as a vital sign [committee opinion].* https://www.acog.org/clinical/clinical-guidance/committee-opinion/articles/2015/12/menstruation-in-girls-and-adolescents-using-the-menstrual-cycle-as-a-vital-sign

American Heart Association (AHA). (n.d.). *Dietary recommendations for healthy children [position statement].* https://www.heart.org/en/healthy-living/healthy-eating/eat-smart/nutrition-basics/dietary-recommendations-for-healthy-children

American Heart Association (AHA). (2023). *High blood pressure in children.* https://www.heart.org/en/health-topics/high-blood-pressure/why-high-blood-pressure-is-a-silent-killer/high-blood-pressure-in-children

American Lung Association. (2023a). *Children and air pollution.* https://www.lung.org/clean-air/outdoors/who-is-at-risk/children-and-air-pollution

American Lung Association. (2023b). *Tips for talking to kids about smoking.* https://www.lung.org/quit-smoking/helping-teens-quit/tips-for-talking-to-kids

American Optometric Association. (2020). *School-age children: 6 to 18 years of age*. https://www.aoa.org/healthy-eyes/eye-health-for-life/school-aged-vision?sso=y

Anwar, A., Yingling, M. D., Zhang, A., Ramtekkar, U., & Nicol, G. E. (2018). Assessment and treatment of pediatric sleep problems: knowledge, skills, attitudes and practices in a group of community child psychiatrists. *Medical Sciences*, *6*(1), 18. https://doi.org/10.3390/medsci6010018

Anxiety and Depression Association of America. (2021). *Anxiety and depression in children*. https://adaa.org/living-with-anxiety/children/anxiety-and-depression

Bicycle Helmet Safety Institute. (2023). *Helmet statistics [summary: bicycle helmet and related statistics]*. https://helmets.org/stats.htm. Accessed October 2, 2023.

Bonneton-Botté, N., Miramand, L., Bailly, R., & Pons, C. (2023). Teaching and rehabilitation of handwriting for children in the digital age: issues and challenges. *Children*, *10*(7), 1096. https://doi.org/10.3390/children10071096

Brooks, A. (2024). *Tips to prevent sports injuries in children & teens*. https://www.healthychildren.org/English/health-issues/injuries-emergencies/sports-injuries/Pages/Sports-Injuries-Treatment.aspx? Accessed February 14, 2024.

Busenbark, M. M. (2021). *Seven effects of the COVID-19 pandemic on kids*. https://www.childrenshospitals.org/news/childrens-hospitals-today/2021/04/7-effects-of-the-covid19-pandemic-on-kids

Campaign for Tobacco-free Kids. (2024). *How schools can help students stay tobacco-free*. https://www.tobaccofreekids.org/assets/factsheets/0153.pdf. Accessed February 14, 2024.

Cardenas-Vargas, E., Nava, J. A., Garza-Veloz, I., Torres-Castañeda, M. C., Galván-Tejada, C. E., et al. (2018). The influence of obesity on puberty and insulin resistance in Mexican children. *International Journal of Endocrinology*, *2018*, 7067292. https://doi.org/10.1155/2018/7067292

Centers for Disease Control and Prevention (CDC). (n.d.-a). *Child health*. https://www.cdc.gov/nchs/fastats/child-health.htm

Centers for Disease Control and Prevention (CDC). (n.d.-b). *Child obesity facts*. https://www.cdc.gov/obesity/data/childhood.html

Centers for Disease Control and Prevention (CDC). (n.d.-c). *Child passenger safety: get the facts*. https://www.cdc.gov/transportationsafety/

Centers for Disease Control and Prevention (CDC). (n.d.-d). *Childhood nutrition facts*. https://www.cdc.gov/healthyschools/nutrition/facts.htm

Centers for Disease Control and Prevention (CDC). (n.d.-e). *Childhood obesity facts*. https://www.cdc.gov/obesity/data/childhood.html

Centers for Disease Control and Prevention (CDC). (n.d.-f). *Children's oral health*. https://www.cdc.gov/oralhealth/basics/childrens-oral-health/index.html

Centers for Disease Control and Prevention (CDC). (n.d.-g). *Clinical growth charts*. https://www.cdc.gov/growthcharts/clinical_charts.htm

Centers for Disease Control and Prevention (CDC). (n.d.-h). *Defining childhood BMI categories*. https://www.cdc.gov/obesity/

Centers for Disease Control and Prevention (CDC). (n.d.-i). *Drowning facts*. https://www.cdc.gov/drowning/

Centers for Disease Control and Prevention (CDC). (n.d.-j). *Group A streptococcal (GAS) disease*. https://www.cdc.gov/groupAstrep/index.html

Centers for Disease Control and Prevention (CDC). (n.d.-k). *Healthy eating learning opportunities and nutrition education*. https://www.cdc.gov/healthyschools/nutrition/school_nutrition_education.htm

Centers for Disease Control and Prevention (CDC). (n.d.-l). *High blood pressure in kids and teens*. https://www.cdc.gov/bloodpressure/

Centers for Disease Control and Prevention (CDC). (n.d.-m). *Keep child passengers safe on the road*. https://www.cdc.gov/injury/features/child-passenger-safety/index.html

Centers for Disease Control and Prevention (CDC). (n.d.-n). *Learning disorders in children*. https://www.cdc.gov/

Centers for Disease Control and Prevention (CDC). (n.d.-o). *Middle childhood (6-8 years of age)*. https://www.cdc.gov/

Centers for Disease Control and Prevention (CDC). (n.d.-p). *Middle childhood (9-11 years of age)*. https://www.cdc.gov/

Centers for Disease Control and Prevention (CDC). (n.d.-q). *Pedestrian safety*. https://www.cdc.gov/transportationsafety/pedestrian_safety/

Centers for Disease Control and Prevention (CDC). (n.d.-r). *Physical activity guidelines for school-aged children and adolescents*. https://www.cdc.gov/healthyschools/physicalactivity/guidelines.htm

Centers for Disease Control and Prevention (CDC). (n.d.-s). *Recommended vaccines by age*. https://www.cdc.gov/vaccines/vpd/vaccines-age.html

Centers for Disease Control and Prevention (CDC). (n.d.-t). *Screening and diagnosis of hearing loss*. https://www.cdc.gov/ncbddd/hearingloss/screening.html

Centers for Disease Control and Prevention (CDC). (n.d.-u). *Sleep and health*. https://www.cdc.gov/healthyschools/sleep.htm

Centers for Disease Control and Prevention (CDC). (n.d.-v). *Top 10 leading causes of death and injury*. https://www.cdc.gov/injury/wisqars/LeadingCauses.html

Centers for Disease Control and Prevention (CDC). (n.d.-w). *Youth and tobacco use*. https://www.cdc.gov/tobacco/data_statistics/fact_sheets/youth_data/tobacco_use/index.htm

Chatterjee, R. A. (n.d.). *Psychosocial development of middle childhood*. http://www.childhealth-explanation.com/psychosocial-development.html

Chen, G. (2022). *Understanding No Child Left Behind*. https://www.publicschoolreview.com/blog/understanding-no-child-left-behind

Cherry, K. (2024). *What is an IQ test?* https://www.verywellmind.com/how-are-scores-on-iq-tests-calculated-2795584

Cherry, K. (2022a). *Kohlberg's theory of moral development*. https://www.verywellmind.com/kohlbergs-theory-of-moral-development-2795071

Cherry, K. (2022b). *Theories of intelligence in psychology*. https://www.verywellmind.com/theories-of-intelligence-2795035

Child Trends Databank. (2024). https://www.childtrends.org. Accessed February 14, 2024.

Children's Hospital Boston, Digital Wellness Lab. (2022). *Family guide to video gaming*. https://digitalwellnesslab.org/family-guides/family-guide-to-video-gaming/

CogniFit. (2019). *Locus of control: internal or external?* https://blog.cognifit.com/locus-of-control/

Common Sense Media. (2020). *The common sense census: media use by kids zero to eight years, 2020*. https://www.commonsensemedia.org/research/the-common-sense-census-media-use-by-kids-age-zero-to-eight-2020

CureSearch for Childhood Cancer. (2024). Current childhood cancer statistics, statistics of number of diagnoses, cancer deaths per year, 5-year survival rate, average years of life lost to cancer, infographics. https://curesearch.org/Childhood-Cancer-Statistics. Accessed February 14, 2024.

Debrowski, A. (2019). *12 Hidden signs your child may need glasses*. https://www.allaboutvision.com/parents/schoolage.htm

de Wert, G., Dondorp, W., Clarke, A., Dequeker, E. M. C., Cordier, C., Deans, Z., et al. (2021). Opportunistic genomic screening.

Recommendations of the European Society of Human Genetics. *European Journal of Human Genetics, 29*, 365–377. https://doi.org/10.1038/s41431-020-00758-w

Dimitri, P. (2019). The impact of childhood obesity on skeletal health and development. *Journal of Obesity & Metabolic Syndrome, 28*(1), 4–17. https://doi.org/10.7570/jomes.2019.28.1.4

Donaldson, J. D. (2024). *Acute otitis media guidelines*. https://emedicine.medscape.com/article/859316-guidelines

Erikson, E. H. (1995). *Childhood and society* (35th anniversary ed.). New York: Norton.

Erikson, E. H., & Erikson, J. M. (1998). *The life cycle completed*. New York: Norton.

Falkner, B., Gidding, S. S., Baker-Smith, C. M., Brady, T. M., Flynn, J. T., Malle, L. M., et al. (2023). Pediatric primary hypertension: an underrecognized condition: a scientific statement from the American Heart Association. *Hypertension, 80*(6), e101–e111.

Faraone, S. V., & Larsson, H. (2019). Genetics of attention deficit hyperactivity disorder. *Molecular Psychiatry, 24*(4), 562–575. https://doi.org/10.1038/s41380-018-0070-0

Fava, D., Pepino, C., Tosto, V., Gastaldi, R., Pepe, A., Paoloni, D., et al. (2023). Precocious puberty diagnoses spike, COVID-19 pandemic, and body mass index: findings from a 4-year study. *Journal of the Endocrine Society, 7*(9), bvad094. https://doi.org/10.1210/jendso/bvad094

Fife, S. T., & Hawkins, L. G. (2019). Doctor, snitch, and weasel: narrative family therapy with a child suffering from encopresis and enuresis. *Clinical Case Studies, 18*(6), 452–467. https://doi.org/10.1177/1534650119866917

Flynn, J. T., Kaelber, D. C., Baker-Smith, C. M., Blowey, D., Carroll, A. E., Daniels S. R., et al. (2017). Clinical practice guideline for screening and management of high blood pressure in children and adolescents. *Pediatrics, 140*(3), e20171904. https://doi.org/10.1542/peds.2017-1904

Fowler, K. A., Dahlberg, L. L., Haileyesus, T., Gutierrez, C., & Bacon, S. (2017). Childhood firearm injuries in the United States. *Pediatrics, 140*(1), e20163486. https://doi.org/10.1542/peds.2016-3486

Friedman, M. (2019). *Dental health and your child's teeth*. https://www.webmd.com/oral-health/dental-health-your-childs-teeth

Govtrack. (2019). *S. 6 (94th): education for all handicapped children act*. https://www.govtrack.us/congress/bills/94/s6/summary

Graber, E. G. (2023). *Childhood development*. https://www.merckmanuals.com/professional/pediatrics/growth-and-development/childhood-development

Gracy, D., Fabian, A., Basch, C. H., Scigliano, M., MacLean, S. A., MacKenzie, R. K., et al. (2018). Missed opportunities: do states require screening of children for health conditions that interfere with learning? *PLoS One, 13*(1), e0190254. https://doi.org/10.1371/journal.pone.0190254

Griffin, M. J. (2024). *What is self-control?* https://www.understood.org/en/articles/self-control-what-it-means-for-kids. Accessed February 12, 2024.

Hamilton, S. S. (2023). *Reading difficulty in children: normal reading development and etiology of reading difficulty*. https://www.uptodate.com/contents/reading-difficulty-in-children-normal-reading-development-and-etiology-of-reading-difficulty. Retrieved November 28, 2023.

Hanlon, E. C., Dumin, M., & Pannain, S. (2019). Chapter 13 - Sleep and obesity in children and adolescents. *Global Perspectives on Childhood Obesity, 2019*, 147–178. https://doi.org/10.1016/B978-0-12-812840-4.00013-X

Harris, J. L., Hyary, M., Seymour, N., & Choi, Y. Y. (2018). *Parents' reports of fast-food purchases for their children: have they improved?* https://uconnruddcenter.org/wp-content/uploads/sites/2909/2020/09/272-10-Healthier-Kids-Meals-Parent-Survey-Report_Release_8_31_18.pdf

Hewitt, S. B. (2019). *School nursing interventions to prevent childhood obesity: integrative literature review*. https://via.library.depaul.edu/nursing-colloquium/2019/spring/8/

Impact NW. (2024). *Communities for safe kids*. https://impactnw.org/programs/youthfamily/communities-for-safe-kids/

Inannelli, V. (2023). *Diagnosis and treatment of encopresis in children*. https://www.verywellhealth.com/encopresis-and-children-diagnosis-and-treatment-2633457

Isong, I. A., Rao, S. R., Bind, M. A., Avendaño, M., Kawachi, I., & Richmond, T. K. (2018). Racial and ethnic disparities in early childhood obesity. *Pediatrics, 141*(1), e20170865. https://doi.org/10.1542/peds.2017-0865

James, K. H. (2017). The importance of handwriting experience on the development of the literate brain. *Current Directions in Psychological Science, 26*(6), 502–508. https://doi.org/10.1177/0963721417709821

Jennissen, C. (2022). *ATVs are not safe for children: AAP policy explained*. https://www.healthychildren.org/English/safety-prevention/at-play/Pages/ATV-Safety-Rules.aspx

Joseph, R. (2019). Learning styles of learners and its importance in instruction. *Journal of Applied Science and Research, 7*(1), 67–76. https://www.scientiaresearchlibrary.com/archive/JASR-2019-7-1-360-67-76.pdf

Just, D. (2019). *3 Ways nutrition influences student learning potential and school performance healthy food choices in school*. https://healthy-food-choices-in-schools.extension.org/3-ways-nutrition-influences-student-learning-potential-and-school-performance/

Kaneshiro, N. K. (2022). *School-age children development*. https://medlineplus.gov/ency/article/002017.htm

Kemp, G., Smith, M., & Siegel, J. (2023). *Helping a child through divorce*. https://www.helpguide.org/articles/parenting-family/children-and-divorce.htm

Kent, J. (2018). *Genomic medicine initiatives aid undiagnosed pediatric patients*. https://healthitanalytics.com/news/genomic-medicine-initiatives-aid-undiagnosed-pediatric-patients

Kent, M. P., Pauzé, E., Roy, E. A., deBilly, N., & Czoli, C. (2019). Children and adolescents' exposure to food and beverage marketing in social media apps. *Pediatric Obesity, 14*(6), e12508. https://doi.org/10.1111/ijpo.12508

Kids Count Data Center. (n.d.). *Child and teen death rate by race and ethnicity in United States (2018-2021)*. https://datacenter.aecf.org/data/tables/11053-child-and-teen-death-rate-by-race-and-ethnicity?loc=1&loct=2#detailed/2/2-52/false/2048,574,1729,37/10,11,9,12,1,13,185/21389,21390. Accessed November, 30, 2023.

Kyu, H. H., Stein, C. E., Pinto, C. B., Rakovac, I., Weber, M. W., Dannemann Purnat, T., et al. (2018). Causes of death among children aged 5–14 years in the WHO European Region: a systematic analysis for the Global Burden of Disease Study 2016. *The Lancet Child & Adolescent Health, 2*(5), 321–337. https://doi.org/10.1016/S2352-4642(18)30095-6

Lee, A. M. I. (n.d.). *Individuals with Disabilities Education Act (IDEA): what you need to know*. https://www.understood.org/en/articles/individuals-with-disabilities-education-act-idea-what-you-need-to-know

Leung Ling, M. T. W., Chen, H. F., & Chiu, K. C. N. (2020). Parental warmth and involvement and the self-esteem of young people in Hong Kong. *Child Indicators Research, 13*, 801–817. https://doi.org/10.1007/s12187-019-09645-3

Luster, S. (2018). *School nurses vital to student health, in and out of school*. https://www.nea.org/nea-today/all-news-articles/school-nurses-vital-student-health-and-out-school

Magee, W., & Upenieks, L. (2019). Gender differences in self-esteem, unvarnished self-evaluation, future orientation, self-enhancement and self-derogation in a US national sample. *Personality and Individual Differences*, *149*, 66–77. https://doi.org/10.1016/j.paid.2019.05.016

Mahoney, J. L., Weissberg, R. P., Greenberg, M. T., Dusenbury, L., Jagers, R. J., Niemi, K., et al. (2021). Systemic social and emotional learning: promoting educational success for all preschool to high school students. *American Psychologist*, *76*(7), 1128–1142. https://doi.org/10.1037/amp0000701

Martschenko, D. (2018). *The IQ test wars: why screening for intelligence is still so controversial*. https://theconversation.com/the-iq-test-wars-why-screening-for-intelligence-is-still-so-controversial-81428

Mason, G. M., Holmes, J. F., Andre, C., & Spencer, R. M. (2021). Bedsharing in early childhood: frequency, partner characteristics, and relations to sleep. *The Journal of Genetic Psychology*, *182*(4), 269–288. https://doi.org/10.1080/00221325.2021.1916732

McLeod, S. (2023a). *The concrete operational stage of cognitive development*. https://www.simplypsychology.org/concrete-operational.html

McLeod, S. (2023b). *Piaget's theory and stages of cognitive development*. https://www.simplypsychology.org/piaget.html

Méndez, R., Goto, K., Song, C., Giampaoli, J., Karnik, G., & Wylie, A. (2019). Cultural influence on mindful eating: traditions and values as experienced by Mexican-American and non-Hispanic white parents of elementary-school children. *Global Health Promotion*, *27*(4), 6–14. https://doi.org/10.1177/1757975919878654

Mersch, J. (n.d.). *Pediatric vital signs ranges and charts*. https://www.emedicinehealth.com/pediatric_vital_signs/article_em.htm

National Association of School Nurses (NASN). (2024). http://www.nasn.org. Accessed February 16, 2024.

National Cancer Institute. (2024). *Childhood cancer genomics (PDQ®)–Health professional version*. https://www.cancer.gov/types/childhood-cancers/pediatric-genomics-hp-pdq. Accessed February 16, 2024.

National Center for Education Statistics. (2023). *Students with disabilities*. https://nces.ed.gov/programs/coe/indicator/cgg/students-with-disabilities. Accessed November 30, 2023.

National Center for Learning Disabilities. (2024). *Social, emotional and behavioral challenges*. https://www.ncld.org

National Handwriting Association. (2024). *About handwriting*. https://nha-handwriting.org.uk/handwriting/

National Highway Traffic Safety Administration (NHTSA). (2015). *Child passenger safety restraint systems on school buses: national training*. https://www.nhtsa.gov/sites/nhtsa.dot.gov/files/documents/cps-restraint-school-buses-participant-manual-810906b.pdf

National Institute of Arthritis and Musculoskeletal and Skin Diseases. (2023). *Kids and their bones*. https://www.niams.nih.gov/health-topics/kids-and-their-bones

National Institute on Drug Abuse. (2022). *Tobacco, nicotine, and e-cigarettes research report: are there gender differences in tobacco smoking?* https://nida.nih.gov/publications/research-reports/tobacco-nicotine-e-cigarettes/are-there-gender-differences-in-tobacco-smoking

National Safety Council. (n.d.). *Backpack safety: it's time to lighten the load*. https://www.nsc.org/home-safety/safety-topics/child-safety/backpacks

National Sleep Foundation. (2023). www.thensf.org.

Nemours Children's Health. (n.d.). *Scabies*. https://kidshealth.org/en/parents/scabies.html

Nemours KidsHealth. (n.d.-a). *Anxiety disorders*. https://kidshealth.org/en/parents/anxiety-disorders.html. Accessed November 30, 2023.

Nemours KidsHealth. (n.d.-b). *Your child's self-esteem*. https://kidshealth.org/en/parents/self-esteem.html. Accessed November 30, 2023.

Nemours TeensHealth, & Ben-Joseph, E. P. (Reviewer). (2019). *What are the risks of smoking?* https://kidshealth.org/en/parents/smoking.html

Nemours TeensHealth, & Durani, Y. (Reviewer). (2024a). *Sleepwalking*. https://kidshealth.org/en/parents/sleepwalking.html

Nemours TeensHealth, & Durani, Y. (Reviewer). (2024b). *What are germs?* https://kidshealth.org/en/kids/germs.html

Nemours TeensHealth, & Schilling, E. M. (Reviewer). (n.d.). *Dealing with stress in sports*. https://kidshealth.org/en/teens/sports-pressure.html

Nolt, D. (2024). *Head lice: what parents need to know*. https://www.healthychildren.org/English/health-issues/conditions/from-insects-animals/Pages/Signs-of-Lice.aspx. Accessed February 16, 2024.

Norhayati, M. N., Ho, J. J., & Azman, M. Y. (2017). Influenza vaccines for preventing acute otitis media in infants and children. *Cochrane Database of Systematic Reviews*, (10), CD010089. https://doi.org/10.1002/14651858.CD010089.pub3

Office of Disease Prevention and Health Promotion. (2020a). *Child obesity*. https://www.healthypeople.gov/

Office of Disease Prevention and Health Promotion. (2020b). *Children with dental caries experience in their primary or permanent teeth (percent, 6–9 years)*. https://www.healthypeople.gov/

Office of Disease Prevention and Health Promotion. (2020c). *Early and middle childhood*. https://www.healthypeople.gov/

Only About Children. (2024). *Exploring the benefits of sensory play for children*. https://www.oac.edu.au/blog/sensory-play/. Accessed February 16, 2024.

Perng, W., Rifas-Shiman, S. L., Hivert, M. F., Chavarro, J. E., Sordillo, J., & Oken, E. (2019). Metabolic trajectories across early adolescence: differences by sex, weight, pubertal status and race/ethnicity. *Annals of Human Biology*, *46*(3), 205–214. https://doi.org/10.1080/03014460.2019.1638967

Powel, J. A. (2019). *Why children steal and what to do about it*. https://www.psychologytoday.com/us/blog/youve-had-baby-now-what/201905/why-children-steal-and-what-do-about-it

Public Broadcast Services. (2024). https://www.pbs.org. Accessed February 16, 2024.

Rafferty, J. (2022a). *Gender-diverse & transgender children*. https://www.healthychildren.org/English/ages-stages/gradeschool/Pages/Gender-Diverse-Transgender-Children.aspx

Rafferty, J. (2022b). *Gender identity development in children*. https://www.healthychildren.org/English/ages-stages/gradeschool/Pages/Gender-Identity-and-Gender-Confusion-In-Children.aspx

Reade, A., & Sayko, S. (2017). *Learning about your child's reading development*. https://improvingliteracy.org/. Accessed November 30, 2023.

Ricketts, D. (2018). *Influence of culture on nutrition with kids*. https://healthyeating.sfgate.com/influence-culture-nutrition-kids-9305.html

Robinson, L., & Segal, J. (2024). *Healthy eating*. https://www.helpguide.org/articles/healthy-eating/healthy-eating.htm. Accessed February 16, 2024.

Rushton, R., Bellis, M., & Haydock, D. (2019). *The role of the HV in accident prevention. Community Practitioner*, *91*(10), 45–47.

Savoy, M. L. (2023). *Passive immunization*. https://www.merckmanuals.com/professional/infectious-diseases/immunization/passive-immunization

Sege, R. D., Amaya-Jackson, L., American Academy of Pediatrics Committee on Child Abuse and Neglect, Council on Foster Care, Adoption, and Kinship Care, American Academy of Child And

Adolescent Psychiatry Committee on Child Maltreatment and Violence, & National Center for Child Traumatic Stress. (2017). Clinical considerations related to the behavioral manifestations of child maltreatment [clinical report]. *Pediatrics, 139*(4), e20170100. https://doi.org/10.1542/peds.2017-0100

Sege, R. D., & Siegel, B. S. (2018). Effective discipline to raise healthy children, council on child abuse and neglect. *Pediatrics, 142*(6), e20183112. https://doi.org/10.1542/peds.2018-3112

Sege, R. D., Siegel, B. S., Flaherty, E. G., Gavril, A. R., Idzerda, S. M., Laskey, A., et al. (2018). Committee on Psychosocial Aspects of Child and Family Health, & Council on Child Abuse and Neglect. Effective discipline to raise healthy children [policy statement]. *Pediatrics, 142*(6), e20183112. https://doi.org/10.1542/peds.2018-3112

Shakir, R. N., Coates, A. M., Olds, T., Rowlands, A., & Tsiros, M. D. (2018). Not all sedentary behaviour is equal: children's adiposity and sedentary behaviour volumes, patterns and types. *Obesity Research & Clinical Practice, 12*(6), 506–512. https://doi.org/10.1016/j.orcp.2018.09.001

Silver, L. (2020). *"I believe in you!" How to vanquish a child's low self-esteem*. https://www.additudemag.com/i-believe-in-you-how-to-vanquish-a-childs-low-self-esteem/

Smith, M., Robinson, L., & Siegel, J. (2024). *What is child abuse and neglect?* https://www.helpguide.org/articles/abuse/child-abuse-and-neglect.htm. Accessed February 13, 2024.

Stein, M., Benninga, M., Felt, B. (2017). An 8-year-old boy with treatment-resistant encopresis. *Journal of Developmental & Behavioral Pediatrics, 38*, S19–S22. doi:10.1097/DBP.0000000000000392

Thomas, M., Miller, D. P., & Morrissey, T. W. (2019). Food insecurity and child health. *Pediatrics, 144*(4), e20190397. https://doi.org/10.1542/peds.2019-0397

Tu, N. D., Baskin, L. S., & Arnhym, A. M. (2022). *Nocturnal enuresis in children: etiology and evaluation*. https://www.uptodate.com/contents/nocturnal-enuresis-in-children-etiology-and-evaluation?sectionName=EPIDEMIOLOGY%20AND%20NATURAL%20HISTORY&topicRef=2863&anchor=H2&source=see_link#. Accessed November 30, 2023.

Understood. (n.d.). *What is dysgraphia?* https://www.understood.org/en/articles/understanding-dysgraphia

Urology Care Foundation. (n.d.). *General pediatric incontinence*. https://www.urologyhealth.org/healthy-living/urologyhealth-extra/magazine-archives/summer-2019/general-pediatric-incontinence

US Department of Agriculture. (2023). *National school lunch program*. https://www.fns.usda.gov/nslp

US Department of Health and Human Services (USDHHS). (2019). *Children and activity & exercise, physical activity guidelines for Americans* (2nd ed.). https://health.gov/paguidelines/second-edition/pdf/Physical_Activity_Guidelines_2nd_edition.pdf

US Department of Health and Human Services (USDHHS). (2022). *Speech and language developmental milestones*. https://www.nidcd.nih.gov/health/speech-and-language

US Department of Health and Human Services (USDHHS). (2024). *Healthy People, 2030*. https://health.gov/healthypeople/objectives-and-data

US Department of Transportation. (n.d.). *School bus safety*. https://www.nhtsa.gov/road-safety/school-bus-safety

Venkatapoorna, C. M. K., Ayine, P., Selvaraju, V., Parra, E. P., Koenigs, T., Ramesh Babu, J., et al. (2020). The relationship between obesity and sleep timing behavior, television exposure, and dinnertime among elementary school-age children. *Journal of Clinical Sleep Medicine, 16*(1), 129–136. https://doi.org/10.5664/jcsm.8080

Victory, J. (2022a). *Hearing loss in children*. https://www.healthyhearing.com/help/hearing-loss/children

Victory, J. (2022b). *Middle ear infections*. https://www.healthyhearing.com/help/hearing-loss/middle-ear-infections

Victory, J. (2023). *What is tympanometry and how is it used?* https://www.healthyhearing.com/report/33583-What-is-tympanometry-and-how-is-it-used

Voth, M., Sommer, K., Schindler, C., Frank, J., & Marzi, I. (2022). Rise of extremity fractures and sport accidents in children at 8–12 years and increase of admittance via the resuscitation room over a decade. *European Journal of Trauma and Emergency Surgery, 48*, 3439–3448. https://doi.org/10.1007/s00068-021-01785-y

Wang, Q., & Gülgöz, S. (2019). New perspectives on childhood memory: introduction to the special issue. *Memory, 27*(1), 1–5. https://doi.org/10.1080/09658211.2018.1537119

Weinstock, M. S., Patel, N. A., & Smith, L. P. (2018). Pediatric cervical lymphadenopathy. *Pediatrics in Review, 39*(9), 433–443. https://doi.org/10.1542/pir.2017-0249

White, C., Baimel, A., & Norenzayan, A. (2017). What are the causes and consequences of belief in karma? *Religion, Brain & Behavior, 7*(4), 339–342. https://doi.org/10.1080/2153599X.2016.1249921

Williams, D. T. (2016). *Growth charts in an ethnically diverse refugee population*. https://med.virginia.edu/family-medicine/wp-content/uploads/sites/285/2017/02/Taylor-Williams-Refugee-Growth-Charts_Web.pdf

Wrightslaw. (2018). *IDEA 2004 statute and regulations*. https://www.wrightslaw.com/idea/law.htm

21

Adolescent

Susan Rowen James

http://evolve.elsevier.com/Edelman/

OBJECTIVES

After completing this chapter, the reader will be able to:

- Summarize the physical growth, developmental, and maturational changes that occur during adolescence.
- Discuss the recommended schedule of health-promotion and preventive health visits for adolescents and the appropriate topics for inclusion during each visit.
- Analyze factors that contribute to risk-taking behaviors and situations during adolescence.
- Develop a health teaching plan addressing some of the physical, emotional, social, and spiritual challenges facing adolescents.

KEY TERMS

Acne
Adolescence
Anorexia nervosa
Binge eating disorder
Body image
Bulimia nervosa
Depression
Egocentrism
Ejaculation
Emancipated minors
Formal operations
Genomics
Gynecomastia
Idealism
Identity
Introspection
Menarche
Menstruation
Nocturnal emissions
Obesity
Overweight
Peer group
Primary sexual characteristics
Puberty
Purge
Risk-taking behaviors
Role confusion
Scoliosis
Secondary sexual characteristics
Sexually transmitted infection (STI)
Tanner staging

THINK ABOUT IT

Risk Behaviors in Adolescents

The mortality rate for adolescents (aged 15–24 years) is more than six times higher than it is for school-age children (aged 5–14 years), representing a statistically significant increase (Xu et al., 2022). Unintentional injury, most specifically by falls and motor vehicles, is the leading cause of death in this age group (National Center for Health Statistics, 2023). Some factors contributing to this are the number of teens who drive at night, drive distracted, drive under the influence of alcohol, and do not use seat belts (Centers for Disease Control and Prevention [CDC] National Center for Injury Prevention and Control, 2023a). Homicide is the second leading cause of death in this age group followed by suicide (National Center for Health Statistics, 2023). The suicide rate among adolescents (aged 10–24) has increased 62% from 2007 to 2021, and the homicide rate has increased 60% between 2014 and 2021 (Curtin & Garnett, 2023). Nearly 21% of US adolescents report being currently sexually active, and of those who are sexually active, approximately 14% report not using any method of birth control (CDC, 2023f).

- What growth and developmental factors make adolescents susceptible to engaging in risky behaviors?
- What anticipatory guidance and strategies might be offered to adolescents and their families to prevent risky behavior?

The term **adolescence** refers to the psychosocial, emotional, cognitive, and moral transition from childhood to young adulthood. Many researchers and developmental specialists in the United States use the age span of 10 to 24 years as a working definition of adolescence. On the other hand, **puberty** refers to the development and maturation of the reproductive, endocrine, and structural processes that lead to fertility. The onset of puberty, which occurs at approximately age 11 to 13 years, signals the beginning of adolescence.

Rapid change in physical, psychosocial, spiritual, moral, and cognitive growth creates an extremely tenuous sense of balance. A pivotal developmental period, adolescence offers health care providers unique opportunities for providing health-promotion and preventive services to adolescents and their families. The CDC's Division of Adolescent and School Health (CDC, 2023) emphasizes that focusing on adolescent health promotion includes recognizing and enhancing protective factors against risk. These factors include positive parenting practices, such as monitoring and regular communication, parental engagement in the adolescent's education, and facilitating positive and mutual "connectedness" both at home and in the community.

BOX 21.1 *HEALTHY PEOPLE 2030*

Selected Health-Promotion and Disease-Prevention Objectives for Adolescents

AH-01	Increase the proportion of adolescents who had a preventive health care visit in the past year.
AH-02	Increase the proportion of adolescents who speak privately with a provider at a preventive medical visit.
AH-10	Reduce the rate of minors and young adults committing violent crimes.
EMC-DO4	Increase the proportion of children and adolescents who get appropriate treatment for anxiety or depression.
FP-04	Increase the proportion of adolescents who have never had sex.
LGBT-05	Reduce bullying of lesbian, gay, or bisexual high school students.
MICH-03	Reduce the rate of deaths in children and adolescents aged 1 to 19 years.
MHMD-02	Reduce suicide attempts by adolescents.
NWS-04	Reduce the proportion of children and adolescents with obesity.
PA-08	Increase the proportion of adolescents who do enough aerobic and muscle strengthening activity.
SU-05	Reduce the proportion of adolescents who have used drugs in the past month.

From US Department of Health and Human Services. (2023). *Healthy People 2030.* https://health.gov/healthypeople/objectives-and-data/browse-objectives

The US Department of Health and Human Services (USDHHS), Office of Disease Prevention and Health Promotion (2020), in its *Healthy People 2030* objectives for the United States, has many objectives specifically directed toward adolescent health (Box 21.1: *Healthy People 2030*). Progress on objectives is measured and compared with objectives from *Healthy People 2020;* there has been improvement in some areas, but worsening in others. These objectives can be used as references for nurses and health providers who are concerned about maintaining positive health and wellness for the adolescent population.

BIOLOGY AND GENETICS

Sex and Puberty

In contrast to the slow, steady growth of childhood, adolescents experience accelerated physical growth that dramatically alters their body size and proportions. Additionally, adolescents experience the onset of puberty. Changes associated with the onset of puberty occur in a predictable sequence, but the onset and duration of the sequence differ among individuals. Females usually begin puberty 1 to 2 years earlier than males and experience their growth spurt earlier. It is generally accepted that age of puberty onset is occurring at a younger age than in the past (10½ for girls, 11½ for boys). Contributing factors include both genetic and environmental influences, such as generally increased body weight, use of personal products containing substances that mimic estrogen, and increased stress (Harrington & Palmert, 2020). Demographic studies suggest that African American girls reach puberty earlier than White girls, which might be related to environmental or social factors (Osinubi, Lewis-de-los Angeles et al., 2022). Girls who have secondary sex characteristic development before age 8 years and boys before age 9 years should be referred to an endocrinologist for evaluation (Pediatric Endocrine Society, 2022). Although a delay in the onset of puberty is rare, adolescents who do not follow the normal sequence or who have not begun pubertal development by age 14 years for males and age 13 years for females should have an endocrine evaluation (Tang & Damian, 2019).

The physical changes experienced during adolescence are mediated primarily by the hormonal regulatory systems in the hypothalamus, pituitary gland, gonads, and adrenal glands (Fig. 21.1). The hypothalamus releases gonadotropin-releasing hormone (GnRH), which stimulates the anterior pituitary to release the gonadotropin hormones, luteinizing hormone (LH) and follicle-stimulating hormone (FSH) (Kahn, 2019; Van Every, 2019). In females, this stimulates development of the ovaries and estrogen production. Once sexual maturation is complete, the ongoing release of hormones controls menses, pregnancy, and lactation. In males, LH results in enlargement of the testes and the development of Leydig cells in the testes, which produce testosterone. FSH stimulates the development of the seminiferous tubules of the testes, leading to spermatogenesis and fertility.

During puberty, **primary sexual characteristics** begin to develop, and **secondary sexual characteristics** emerge. Primary sexual characteristics involve the organs necessary for reproduction, such as the penis and testes in boys and the vagina and uterus in girls. Secondary sexual characteristics are external features that are not essential for reproduction; however, because they are more obvious, they might signal the onset of puberty in the developing adolescent. Breast development, facial and pubic hair growth, and lowering of the voice are examples of

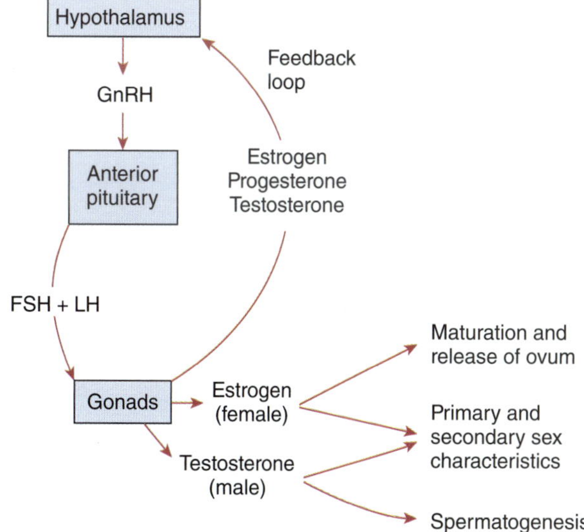

FIG. 21.1 Hormonal interaction among hypothalamus, pituitary, and gonads. FSH, Follicle-stimulating hormone; GnRH gonadotropin-releasing hormone; LH, luteinizing hormone. (From Hockenberry, M. J., Duffy, E., & Gibbs, K. (2024) *Wong's nursing care of infants and children* (12th ed.). St. Louis, MO: Elsevier.)

secondary sexual characteristics (Table 21.1). Estrogen produces all secondary sexual characteristics except axillary and pubic hair, which are controlled by adrenal androgens. Sexual maturity rating, also referred to as **Tanner staging**, is widely used to assess and monitor the degree of maturation of an adolescent's primary and secondary sexual characteristics. Each characteristic—breasts, pubic hair, and genitals—is staged separately (from 1–5) and compared with the expected sequencing (Fig. 21.2).

Breast development is usually confined to females; however, some degree of unilateral or bilateral breast enlargement, termed **gynecomastia**, may appear early in male puberty, just before the growth spurt. Gynecomastia is usually temporary and typically disappears. However, occasionally it persists and leads to body image problems, and it can be surgically reduced if psychological assessment warrants it. Gynecomastia is categorized as a benign breast condition in males (American Cancer Society, 2018b).

The first sign of puberty in males is a thinning of the scrotal sac and enlargement of the testicles. **Ejaculation** is considered a milestone of male puberty and precedes fertility by several months. **Nocturnal emissions**, or wet dreams, can concern adolescent males because they cannot control these events.

For females, the first sign of puberty is the appearance of breast buds, followed by the growth spurt. An area of possible concern for adolescent females is that during breast development, the breasts can be of different sizes; reassurance that this is not unusual can diminish anxiety. The onset of **menstruation**, or **menarche**, occurs approximately 2 years after the appearance of the breast buds and near the end of the growth spurt (Fig. 21.2).

Familiarity with the stages of development of sexual characteristics and their expected sequence helps the nurse monitor the adolescent's progression through puberty and detect any variations that might herald an alteration in normal growth and development.

Before the growth spurt, many adolescents experience a transient increase in the amount of body fat or adipose tissue. As puberty progresses the proportion of total body weight composed of fat usually declines, particularly in boys. Body fat begins to accumulate again in both sexes after their growth spurt, but at a slightly higher rate in females.

Other Physical Changes

The heart grows in size and strength. Blood volume and blood pressure increase, and the heart rate decreases to adult levels. These cardiovascular changes occur earlier in females, corresponding with puberty. Compared with adolescent males, adolescent females also generally have higher pulse rates and slightly lower systolic blood pressure. Normal blood pressure for an adolescent is considered to be a blood pressure of less than 120 mm Hg systolic over less than 80 mm Hg diastolic, or less than the 90th percentile (based on age, sex, height, and weight) (American Heart Association, 2023). Recent guidelines for the identification and management of hypertension in adolescents describe three stages of hypertension: elevated (systolic pressure of 120–129 mm Hg over <80 mm Hg diastolic), stage 1 (130–139 mm Hg systolic over 80–89 mm Hg diastolic), and stage 2 (>140 over 90 mm Hg) (American Heart Association, 2023). Because both children and adolescents can experience "white coat syndrome," or an artificially increased blood pressure due to anxiety from being in a medical facility, the American Heart Association recommends any adolescent that exceeds the 95th percentile should be evaluated using ambulatory blood pressure measurement, optimally over a 24-hour period (Flynn, 2022).

Respiratory rate decreases throughout childhood, reaching an average rate of 15 to 20 breaths per minute during adolescence. Respiratory volume and vital capacity increase, particularly in males. The larynx and vocal cords grow, producing the characteristic voice changes of puberty. Both male and female

TABLE 21.1 GROWTH AND DEVELOPMENT

Sexual Maturity Rating, Tanner Stages: Developmental Stages of Secondary Sexual Characteristics

Stage	Male Genital Development	Pubic Hair Development	Female Breast Development	Other Changes
1	Prepubertal	No distinction between hair over pubic area and hair over abdomen		
2	Initial enlargement of scrotum and testes; reddening and texture changes of scrotum	Sparse growth of long, straight, downy hair at base of penis or along labia	Enlargement of areolar diameter; small area of elevation around papillae (breast bud)	Usual time of peak height velocity for girls
3	Initial enlargement of penis, mainly in length; further growth of testes and scrotum	Hair becomes dark, coarse, and curly; spreads sparsely over entire pubic area	Further elevation and enlargement of breasts and areolas, with no separation of their contours	Usual time of menarche; facial hair begins to grow on upper lip and voice deepens in boys
4	Further enlargement of penile diameter, testes, scrotum, and glans	Further spread of hair distribution, not extending to thighs	Areolas and papillae project from breast to form secondary mound	Usual time of peak height velocity for boys; axillary hair begins to grow
5	Adult in size and contour	Adult in amount and type; spreads to inner surface of thighs	Adult, with projection of papillae only; recession of areolas into general breast contour	

Modified from Hockenberry, M. J., & Wilson, D. (2019). *Wong's nursing care of infants and children* (11th ed.). St. Louis, MO: Mosby.

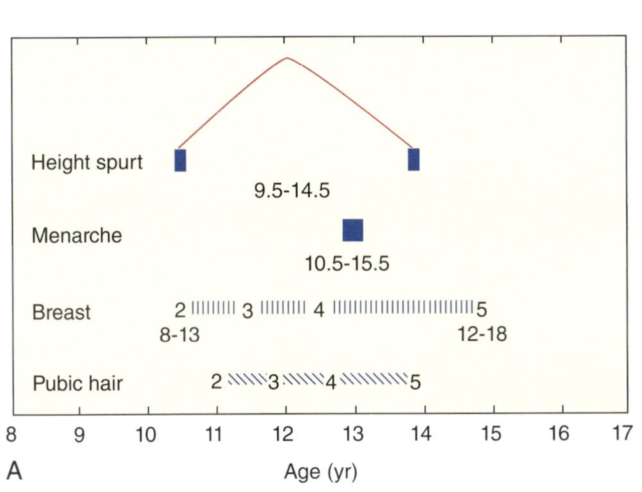

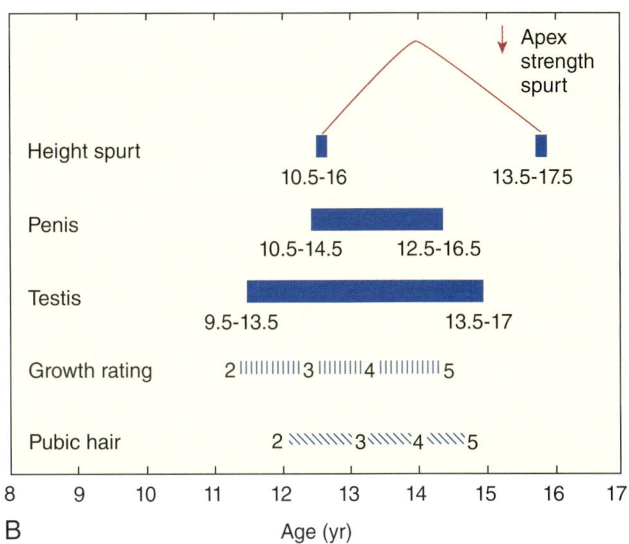

FIG. 21.2 Sequences of events at adolescence in girls (A) and boys (B). Single numbers (2, 3, 4, 5) indicate stages of development. The average is represented. A range of ages when each event may begin and end is indicated by inclusive numbers listed below each event. (Modified from Herman-Giddens, M., Slora, E. J., Wasserman, R. C., Bourdony, C. J., Bhapkar, M. V., Koch, G. G., Hassemeier, C. M. [1997]. Secondary sexual characteristics and menses in young girls seen in office practices: A study from the Pediatric Research in Office Settings Network. *Pediatrics, 99*[4], 505–512; Hockenberry, M. J., Duffy, E., & Gibbs, K. (2024). *Wong's nursing care of infants and children* (12th ed.). St. Louis, MO: Elsevier; Marshall, W., & Tanner, J. (1970) Variations in pattern of pubertal changes in boys. *Archives of Diseases in Childhood, 45*(239), 13–23.)

voices become deeper, and laryngeal cartilage enlarges, with both effects more pronounced in males.

Permanent teeth begin erupting at approximately 6 years of age, and all 32, except the third molars, or wisdom teeth, are in place by 13 to 14 years of age. Third molars are often pulled during adolescence to make space for the other permanent teeth. It is not uncommon for one or more of the third molars not to develop, and this lack of development (agenesis) is often familial.

The sweat and sebaceous glands both become more active during adolescence. The sweat glands are located primarily in the axillary, genital, and periumbilical areas and are the primary source of body odor. The sebaceous glands are located primarily on the face, neck, shoulders, upper back, chest, and genitals. They can become clogged and inflamed, leading to the common teenage condition called **acne**. It is estimated that in excess of 80% of all adolescents experience acne (Zimlich, 2022).

Scoliosis

During the growth spurt, adolescents may manifest signs of a common skeletal deformity called **scoliosis**, which is a lateral S-shaped curvature of the spine (Fig. 21.3). The curve is typically convex to the right. Classifications of scoliosis include secondary or functional; congenital, neuromuscular; constitutional; and idiopathic (no known cause), which has an infantile, juvenile, or adolescent onset. Most incidences of scoliosis in adolescence are idiopathic. Curves greater than 25 to 30 degrees are abnormal and can progress to significant curvature during the growth spurt (American Academy of Orthopedic Surgeons, 2022). Referral for orthopedic evaluation occurs when the curvature measures more than 7 degrees, measured

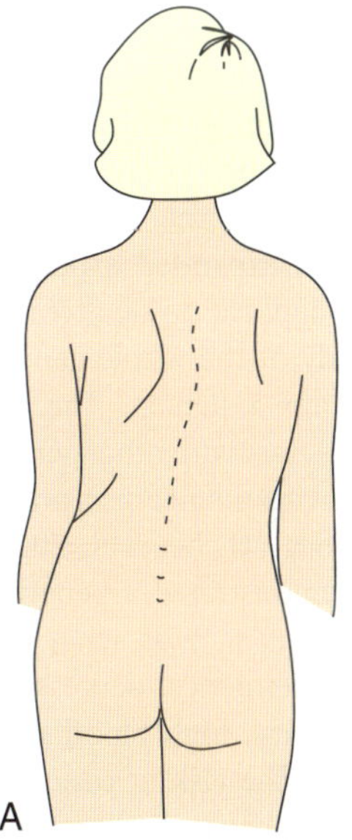

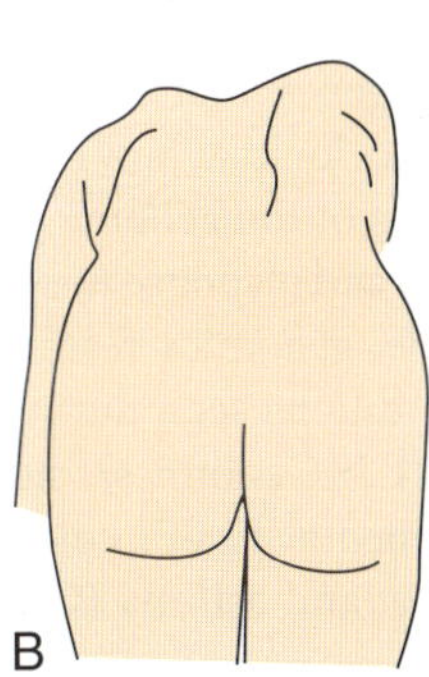

FIG. 21.3 Scoliosis screening. So that the entire back can be seen, the adolescent should remove all clothing from the upper body when being assessed for scoliosis. (A) While the adolescent stands up straight, check for any asymmetry; observe and palpate the body for differences in shoulder or scapular height, prominence of either scapula or hip, waist asymmetry, and misalignment of the spinous processes. Lateral curvature and thoracic convexity of the spine indicate scoliosis. (B) With feet together, legs straight, and arms hanging freely, the adolescent bends forward until the back is parallel with the floor. Check for prominence of the ribs, or rib hump, on one side only and hip and leg asymmetry. With scoliosis, the chest wall on the side of convexity is prominent, and the scapula on the side of convexity is elevated.

by a scoliometer when the adolescent is in the Adams position (Mistovich & Spiegel, 2020) (Fig. 21.3B).

Idiopathic scoliosis is significantly more prevalent in females. Early intervention is important because untreated scoliosis can result in disfigurement, impaired mobility, and cardiopulmonary complications. Evidence shows that early intervention in the form of scoliosis-specific physical therapy exercises or bracing can slow progression of curves and reduce the need for surgery, or, in children with mild scoliosis, reduce the need for bracing (DePaola & Cuddihy, 2020). A recent meta-analysis that looked at the effect of various forms of exercise (e.g., yoga, Pilates, scoliosis-specific exercise) on the angle of the curve demonstrated significant effects on the degree of curvature and possible reduction in the need for bracing (Chen et al., 2023).

Several years ago, the US Preventive Services Task Force (USPSTF) questioned routine scoliosis screening of older children and adolescents, which is done in either physicians' offices or through school-based preventive programs. On the basis of more recent information, however, the USPSTF is making no recommendation regarding screening, as there is not enough evidence to assess the balance of harm versus benefit (USPSTF, 2018).

Genetics

Most genetic problems are discovered during infancy and early childhood. Some syndromes, however, may not be diagnosed until adolescence. Turner syndrome in females and Klinefelter syndrome in males result from alterations in the X chromosome. These genetic disorders, which affect both physical and cognitive development, are frequently discovered during the assessment of an adolescent who has delayed or irregular pubertal development and require referral to an appropriate specialist.

Since the sequencing of the human genome, information on genetic predisposition to disease has expanded exponentially. Although genetics is the study and application of alterations in specific genes, **genomics** is the study of the whole genome, or all the genes that together make up a person. The field of **genomics** looks at how one's genes interact with other genes, relationships of the genome with the environment, susceptibility to disease, and response to pharmaceuticals (Lebet et al., 2019). For example, genomics research has demonstrated a genetic basis for conditions seen during adolescence, such as acne, scoliosis (Box 21.2: Genomics), substance dependence, depression and other mental health conditions, **obesity**, high blood pressure, diabetes, and asthma (CDC, 2023b). The risk of conditions of concern to adolescents, such as breast cancer, type 2 diabetes, and cardiovascular disease, can now be identified through genetic testing and early screening (CDC Public Health Genomics and Precision Health Knowledge Base, 2023). Routine genome screening is not yet recommended for adolescents; however, direct-to-consumer tests (e.g., Ancestry DNA, 23andMe) can provide analysis of genetic and genomic considerations. Furthermore, nontraditional health monitoring through devices that measure fitness status and other health issues are readily available to adolescents (Gangonil-Gagalang et al., 2023). Interpretation of these tests and devices can possibly be unreliable, so nurses need to be careful of discussing results with adolescents. There are also ethical considerations associated with genomic nursing, such as maintaining privacy, unauthorized release of information, and potential social, cultural, or religious discrimination (Laaksonen et al., 2023). Family history, however, can not only help physicians make a diagnosis if the adolescent shows signs of a disorder but also help reveal whether there is an increased risk of a disease for the adolescent (Box 21.3: Best Practice).

BOX 21.2 Scoliosis

For many years the cause of adolescent idiopathic scoliosis (AIS) has been elusive to determine. A body of research reveals that AIS is significantly more prevalent in girls than in boys, that AIS occurs in families, and that the condition is multifactorial (National Institutes of Health Genetic Home Reference, 2019; Menger & Sin, 2023). Multifactorial inheritance patterns suggest that a combination of genetics and environment affects the occurrence of a health condition. Genomic research findings suggest that there is no one cause of AIS. Instead, multiple genes influence its cause, severity, and progression. Genetic factors could include hormonal effects, defects in bone or muscle growth, or an altered neurologic system. Consistent with other genetic/genomic conditions, yet unidentified factors may contribute to its occurrence.

BOX 21.3 BEST PRACTICE

My Family Health Portrait

Interested teens can create a simple family pedigree with My Family Health Portrait (The Surgeon General, 2023) (https://cbiit.github.io/FHH/html/index.html). My Family Health Portrait is a downloadable, web-based tool for use on a personal computer. It helps individuals create their own family health history. Because it is web-based, teens may be the family member best prepared (or most technologically comfortable) to coordinate the input of data. With their family's help, teens gather their family health history and then, using any type of computer, build a drawing of their family tree and a chart of their family health history. Both the chart and the drawing can be printed and shared with other family members and health care providers. All information entered is kept private and confidential. It is suggested that families use holiday gatherings, when the family is present, to gather and record information for the family health history. The CDC has a website with various current genomic resources as well (https://www.cdc.gov/genomics/disease/genomic_diseases.htm).

GORDON'S FUNCTIONAL HEALTH PATTERNS

Health Perception–Health Management Pattern

Teens have fewer acute illnesses than younger children and fewer chronic illnesses than adults. They are seen in health care facilities less frequently than younger children and adults, and they are rarely hospitalized. Yet they need to be monitored, because adolescence is a pivotal developmental period with numerous physical, psychosocial, and spiritual changes. Box 21.4 lists interventions recommended for periodic health examinations for adolescents.

A crucial component for understanding adolescent health is an adolescent's own perceptions of health, illness, and health care services. Too often a sense of invincibility and "Peter Pan" ideology couples with typical adolescent experimentation and **risk-taking behaviors** to produce deleterious health care choices and outcomes. Caught somewhere between childhood and adulthood, teens may no longer feel as if they are being attended to by pediatricians, pediatric nurse practitioners, and pediatric

BOX 21.4 Interventions Recommended for the Periodic Health Examination

11 to 21 Years of Age

Screening—Physical[a]

- Height, weight, and body mass index
- Blood pressure
- Vision and hearing—screening or risk assessment
- Pubertal developmental status and other developmental surveillance
- Anemia screen or risk assessment
- Lipids
- Urinalysis
- Tuberculosis—if at risk
- STIs risk assessment
- Annual HIV risk assessment—screening once 15–21 years
- Hepatitis C screen—age 18 years
- Sudden cardiac risk assessment (see assessment questions)

Screening—Mental Health[a]

- Psychosocial and behavioral assessment/screening—individual and family (HEADSS questions)
- Substance use assessment
- Depression/anxiety/suicide risk screening

Prevention Guidance—Prevention of Injury

- Lap and shoulder belts in car
- No distracted driving or driving after using a substance
- Bicycle, motorcycle, all-terrain vehicle helmets
- Protective gear for sports, work, and other physical activities; know concussion protocol
- Learn first aid and cardiopulmonary resuscitation
- Skin cancer protection—avoid sun exposure (or exposure through tanning beds), use sunscreen with SPF 15 or higher
- Safe storage and use of firearms

Prevention Guidance—Substance Use

- Avoid tobacco, alcohol, and drug use
- Avoid alcohol or drug use while driving, swimming, boating, riding a bike or motorcycle, or operating farm equipment or other machinery
- Do not ride with a driver who has been using alcohol or other substancesNo vaping

Prevention Guidance—Sexual Behavior

- Abstinence, resisting sexual pressures, saying no, decreasing other risky behaviors
- STI prevention and protection
- Unintended pregnancy, contraception
- Avoiding and reporting date rape
- Assessment of sex trafficking victimization if appropriate

Prevention Guidance—Diet and Exercise

- Choose a variety of healthy foods
- Balance caloric intake and energy expenditure
- Limit fat and cholesterol; emphasize grains, fruits, and vegetables
- Consume adequate calcium, iron, and folic acid
- Recognize signs of disordered eating patterns
- Engage in moderate exercise 60 min. a day, muscle and bone strengthening three times a week

Dental Health

- Make regular (every 6 months) visits to dental care provider
- Brush teeth at least twice a day and floss daily
- Avoid tobacco products

Immunization[b]

- Tdap vaccine (tetanus, diphtheria, acellular pertussis) at age 11–12 years; Td vaccine (tetanus, diphtheria) every 10 years thereafter
- HPV vaccine; boys and girls at age 9–14 years old; two-dose series (initial, #2—6 to 12 months later); age 15–26; three-dose series (initial, #2—1 to 2 months later, #3—6 to 12 months after initial)
- Meningococcal vaccine; one dose at age 11–12 years, booster dose at age 16 years; influenza vaccine yearly
- Dengue at 9–16 years if previously infected and reside in endemic area
- Mpox at age 18 if at risk
- Catch-up vaccines (see recommended schedule)—hepatitis B (two or three doses depending on vaccine type); measles, mumps, rubella (two doses); varicella (two-dose schedule); hepatitis A (if indicated)

[a]Modified from American Academy of Pediatrics (AAP). (2023). *Bright Futures/AAP recommendations for preventive health care (periodicity schedule)*. www.aap.org; [b]Centers for Disease Control and Prevention (CDC), Advisory Committee on Immunization Practices (ACIP). (2023). *Recommended child and adolescent immunization schedule for ages 18 years or younger, United States, 2024.* http://www.cdc.gov

nurses—yet, at the same time, they are often misunderstood by adult health care providers. Health care services for adolescents that are available, visible, confidential, and flexible need to be developed. Unmet health care needs include lack of access to care that meets the adolescent's physical and emotional needs, poor coordination, and lack of attention to the adolescent's need for guidance and preventive counseling (Alderman et al., 2019). Unmet health care needs during adolescence can result in poor health outcomes during adulthood (Alderman et al., 2019). Contributing factors to unmet health care needs include lack of appropriate access, financial constraints, and adolescent attitudes that health is not important. Whereas adults search for health information using the Internet, adolescents are more likely to use social media (e.g., TikTok, Facebook, X, Instagram, Snapchat, online blogs) to obtain health information (Taba et al., 2022). Adolescents may make unintentional (e.g., clicking on links from friends) or intentional searches for information about particular health topics (Taba et al., 2022). Because these sites are not monitored for accuracy, nurses need to advise adolescents and their parents to verify information with their health providers. For information regarding health care services for adolescents, visit the National Adolescent and Young Adult Health Information Center (http://nahic.ucsf.edu).

Adolescents are in the process of developing healthy habits and patterns of problem-solving that are likely to last a lifetime. The cognitive and psychological changes they experience can affect their adherence to health-promotion and disease-prevention strategies. Teens do not always consider the health risks of their behavior and have an overall sense of invulnerability to illness or injury. Peer influence is primary, and parental input is often rejected. Parents need, however, to be vigilant to recognize when their adolescent needs assistance with avoiding situations that could lead to irreparable harm (CDC Adolescent and School Health, 2023). Parental monitoring, which involves knowing where the adolescent is, knowing with whom they are communicating, setting clear behavioral expectations, and being sensitive to behavioral changes, has been shown to be protective against adolescent risk behavior. Role modeling appropriate health behaviors is also a known protective factor against risk (CDC Adolescent and School Health, 2023). Parents, however, need to guard against overprotection, sometimes known as overparenting, because this behavior can lead to overdependence and a lack of confidence as the adolescent transitions to adulthood. Parents who are perceived by their children as being overly controlling (e.g., giving undue advice or assistance, being overly involved with the adolescent's activities, or failing to allow the adolescent to solve problems) can contribute to decreased self-confidence and self-esteem (Liu et al., 2019). Nurses can advise parents to strike a balance between desiring to overprotect their children and allowing their children increasing autonomy as they become increasingly capable of making independent decisions about their health behavior.

Parents, teachers, and health care providers will be more successful in assisting adolescents in managing their health needs wisely if they act as joint partners in planning the care for which the adolescents themselves will assume responsibility. Key components of successful health supervision include gradually facilitating adolescent independence and decision-making, involving parents and schools in a holistic approach to health promotion, and communicating effectively.

Nutritional-Metabolic Pattern

Although many adolescents gravitate to low-nutrient, processed foods, it is essential that they consume a well-rounded diet that provides a variety of high-nutrient, low-sugar, and low-fat foods and beverages (US Department of Agriculture [USDA] & USDHHS, 2020). Adolescents need to consume daily calorie amounts appropriate for their level of physical exercise (females—1800 to 2400 calories; males—2000 to 3200 calories) found primarily in vegetables, fruits, protein, whole grains, fish, and nuts. Nurses need to assist teens in following a healthy diet and educate them about the appropriate nutrients, such as protein (especially for vegetarians), calcium, and iron and folic acid (for females) (USDA & USDHHS, 2020). Recommending regular consumption of milk to prevent later osteoporosis is essential, especially for adolescent girls, as is avoidance of high-sugar and diet beverages. The nurse can encourage adolescents to eat breakfast every day to improve academic performance, or to carry protein snacks. Avoiding processed foods and reading food labels will assist with calorie planning. The risk of nutritional deficiencies during adolescence is high (USDA & USDHHS, 2020). An excellent resource for nurses and adolescents regarding dietary considerations is the MyPlate website (http://www.choosemyplate.gov/teens). There is also a nutrition calculator and individualized eating plan available through MyPlate.

Many teens have concerns about their body, proper nutrition, and exercise. The media not only portrays the ideal body as thin, lean, or muscular, but at the same time promotes access to unhealthy high-fat, high-sugar, processed foods. Asserting their newfound autonomy, teens may choose dietary intake as a mechanism to gain control over their changing bodies, exert independence, or experiment with a new **identity** or cause, such as becoming a vegetarian. All of this occurs as their body's nutrient and energy demands increase in preparation for and in response to the adolescent growth spurt. Teen activities, including sports and other vigorous extracurricular physical activities, can further increase these demands. Gymnasts, runners, bodybuilders, rowers, wrestlers, dancers, and swimmers are particularly vulnerable to eating disorders because their sports necessitate weight restriction. Complicating matters is teens' overwhelming desire to "fit in" with their peers, which often prevails and can lead to unhealthy dietary practices. The importance of healthy nutrition cannot be overemphasized. Recent research has demonstrated that healthy adolescent nutrition affects eventual height, adiposity, body composition, pubertal development, and risk for later health problems (Norris et al., 2022).

Eating Disorders

The occurrence of eating disorders results from a combination of genetic and environmental factors, mediated as well by internal and external factors prevalent during puberty (e.g., family, peer, and media influences) (Kreipe & Starr, 2020). In some cases, true eating disorders are preceded by what is called disordered eating, or eating patterns such as restricting food, using food to control one's emotions or environment, and irregular eating habits, among others. Recent research suggests that disordered eating relates to one's own perception of body size and weight (Lopez-Gil et al., 2023; Hahn et al., 2023). The current prevalence of disordered eating seen in adolescents in the United States is approximately 20%, with girls at a higher risk (National Association of Anorexia Nervosa and Associated Disorders [ANAD], 2023; Norris et al., 2022). The prevalence of adolescents with eating disorders is 2.2% in males and 4.9% in females (Chaves et al., 2023). Prevalence is also higher in the lesbian, gay, bisexual, transgender, queer, and questioning (LGBTQ+) populations as well as in adolescents of different races and ethnicities (ANAD, 2023). The incidence of various eating disorders increased during the COVID-19 pandemic (Radhakrishnan et al., 2022). Major eating disorders include **anorexia nervosa**, **bulimia nervosa**, and **binge eating disorder**. Many adolescents with eating disorders experience comorbid psychiatric conditions, such as anxiety, depression, or obsessive-compulsive disorder, and suicidal ideation is not uncommon (Kreipe & Starr, 2020). Adolescents who meet the criteria for eating disorders should be referred to an interdisciplinary team that is experienced and skilled in working with these disorders (Chew & Temples, 2022).

At one end of the eating disorder spectrum are anorexia nervosa and bulimia nervosa. At the other end is binge eating disorder. Adolescents with anorexia nervosa are typically female, perfectionists, and high achievers. Symptoms or warning signs include a relentless pursuit of thinness, self-starving with significant weight loss, lack of menstruation (in females) and decreased sexual interests (in males), compulsive physical activity, preoccupation with food, portioning food carefully, and eating small amounts of only certain foods.

The adolescent may also have brittle hair and nails; dry, yellowish skin; growth of fine hair over the body; constipation; mild anemia and muscle weakness; and often complaints of feeling cold. The severe restriction of food intake eventually contributes to dangerous malnourishment, and, in some cases, death. The onset of anorexia nervosa is typically in response to low self-esteem and real or imagined obesity.

Distorted **body image** is a hallmark of anorexia nervosa in both males and females. Body image specifically refers to the picture of and feelings about various characteristics of one's body. In females particularly, distorted body image may be related to self-objectification or to judging one's personality or character strictly by one's appearance, exclusive of other positive attributes. Adolescents who regularly access social media sites where photos of others are shared can begin to develop distorted ideas about their own body image (Hahn et al., 2023). Media images and positive or negative comments about appearance from others can contribute to self-objectification (Bell et al., 2018).

Bulimia nervosa has symptoms or warning signs that are different from those of anorexia nervosa. Teens with bulimia nervosa typically binge on huge quantities of high-calorie foods and then **purge** by self-induced vomiting and/or use of laxatives. Binge episodes may alternate with diets, resulting in dramatic weight fluctuations. These teens often try to hide the signs of vomiting by running water as a sound cover. Purging poses serious threats to the teen's health, including dehydration, sometimes fatal electrolyte imbalances, and erosion of tooth enamel.

Similar to the teen with bulimia nervosa, the teen with binge eating disorder frequently consumes large amounts of food while feeling a lack of control in overeating. However, this disorder is different from bulimia nervosa because these teens usually do not purge their bodies of the excess food they consume during their binge episodes. Adolescents who are binge eaters experience a lack of control in overeating, the inability to stop eating when full, social difficulties, altered mood, and decreased self-esteem (Marzilli et al., 2018).

Although technically not identified as an eating disorder, obesity is a concern for many adolescents and is viewed as a chronic illness (Hampi et al., 2023). The obese adolescent, whatever the underlying cause, consumes too many calories for the amount of energy expended. Obesity is more prevalent in adolescents who are Hispanic, Native American, and African American, partly related to their socioeconomic circumstances (CDC, 2022b; Hampi et al., 2023). Studies have shown a strong correlation between inactivity, such as viewing television, playing computer games, and Internet surfing, and the tendency to be **overweight**. Other research has identified depression as one of the strongest predictors of adolescent obesity. Obesity can be detrimental to the adolescent's self-esteem and social development because they often become trapped in a vicious cycle of social rejection, isolation, inactivity, and continued obesity. Adolescent obesity has a poor prognosis, with most obese adolescents becoming obese adults. In addition, obesity increases the risk and occurrence of type 2 diabetes mellitus along with the risk of later development of other diseases—most specifically, cardiovascular disorders.

School nurses may be the first to notice a possible eating disorder in students, often in conjunction with adolescents reporting instances of being bullied because of their weight (Hampi et al., 2023). The nurse can ask questions such as these: Do you have concerns about your weight or think you are fat? How often do you weigh yourself? How often do you exercise? Has your diet changed recently (become more picky with foods, not controlling eating, hiding food, counting calories excessively)? Are you still doing fun activities with friends?

Because of the multiple factors contributing to the occurrence of an eating disorder, there is no one method that can prevent its occurrence. However, when working with families of adolescents, nurses can recommend that the adolescent have access to nutritional foods and reduced access to sweets, that family members deemphasize the adolescent's body proportions or shape, model healthy eating, and encourage participation in regular exercise (Gahagan, 2020). Emphasizing the adolescent's positive and unique aspects can foster the adolescent's self-esteem.

Obesity, Type 2 Diabetes, and Teens

Soaring obesity rates are making type 2 diabetes, a disease that used to be seen mostly in adults older than 45 years, more common among teens and young people. Diabetes is a group of diseases marked by high levels of glucose in the blood, which, left unattended, lead to blindness, kidney failure, amputations, heart disease, and stroke. Type 2 diabetes, formerly called adult-onset diabetes, is the most common form. People can develop it at any age. However, being overweight and inactive increases one's risk. Teens can access information about weight control with the National Institute of Diabetes and Digestive and Kidney Diseases' *Take Charge of Your Health: A Guide for Teenagers* (http://www.win.niddk.nih.gov/publications/take_charge.htm). Furthermore, the National Diabetes Education Program (NDEP) has now developed a Tips for Teens series that includes a tip sheet on how to lower the risk of type 2 diabetes that is "teen friendly." Nurses can direct high-risk teens or teens with type 2 diabetes to visit the NDEP website at https://www.niddk.nih.gov.

More than anything, adolescents need reassurance about their bodies. Parents, teachers, and health care providers will be more successful in helping teens assume responsibility and manage their ongoing health needs if they approach and treat them as partners in planning their care. Assessment is of particular importance. Nurses working with adolescents need to be aware of the signs and symptoms that would suggest an eating disorder, such as preoccupation with food, dieting or skipping meals, heightened concern about weight or shape, inability to control eating, self-induced vomiting, and guilt associated with eating. Nurses can engage adolescents and help them create individualized wellness plans that address body image, diet, weight concerns, and physical activity.

Elimination Pattern

The renal and gastrointestinal systems are functionally mature by adolescence, and elimination patterns are consistent with those found in adults. Abnormal variation can occur in teens with eating disorders. It is important to remember that an adolescent's need for privacy or self-protection may inhibit normal elimination in public places, such as schools.

Activity-Exercise Pattern

During adolescence, alterations in body composition and growth of lean muscle mass allow the teen to experience increased physical strength and endurance. All adolescents should be taught that regular exercise can increase their endurance and improve their appearance and general state of health, and that these positive effects can extend into adulthood. Recommendations for exercise include 1 hour daily of moderate aerobic exercise, muscle strengthening three times a week, and three times a week of bone strengthening activities, which occur when participating in sports that involve running or jumping (CDC, 2022a; USDHHS, 2018).

Many teens participate in organized sports, and the preparticipation sports examination is one of the most common reasons adolescents seek primary care (Fig. 21.4). This examination offers an opportunity for nurses to identify adolescents at risk, evaluate their general state of health, and promote healthy lifestyle behaviors (Box 21.5).

Along with eating disorders related to maintaining or losing weight for sports participation, adolescent athletes are subject to a variety of injuries. Often these injuries are related to the specific sport in which the adolescent engages. The sports environment can contribute to or prevent overuse. Risk factors for sports injuries include lack of sleep, inappropriate use of correct athletic equipment, lack of pregame warm-up, and dehydration (American Academy of Orthopedic Surgeons, 2022). Overuse can occur if the adolescent plays the same sport throughout the year or has insufficient rest between sports. Nurses need to work closely with athletes and coaches to be sure the approach to sports participation is healthy and free of injury potential.

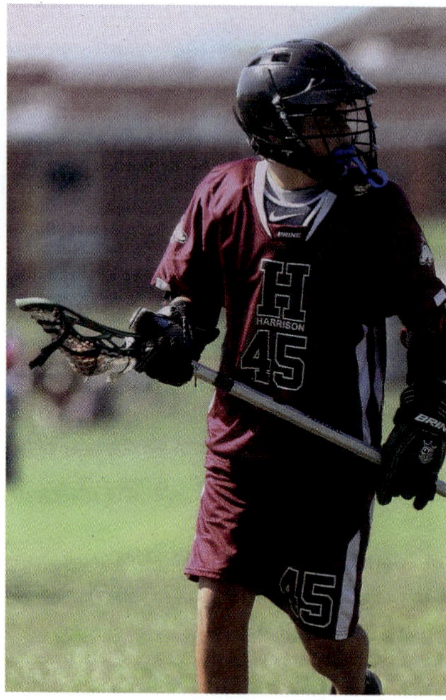

FIG. 21.4 Adolescents frequently participate in organized activities, especially sports.

BOX 21.5 Adolescent Preparticipation Sports Examination

Areas for Special Concern

- Previous trauma, including concussion
- Cardiovascular disease
- Hypertension
- Asthma
- Seizure disorder
- Splenomegaly, or enlarged spleen, often seen with infectious mononucleosis
- HIV infection
- Absence of paired organs: eye, kidney, testicle, or ovary

Sleep-Rest Pattern

During adolescence, the amount of time needed each night for sleep declines in comparison with earlier childhood needs. Although their sleep patterns differ greatly, adolescents need at least 8 to 10 hours of sleep per night (Juelich et al., 2023). Adolescents who are employed, those involved in extracurricular sports, and those who have "too much on their plate" are at increased risk of sleep deprivation. Research suggests that sleep quality and quantity have important effects on adolescent function. Positive sleep hygiene practices, such as maintaining a consistent routine, avoiding caffeine, and eliminating gaming before going to sleep, contribute to sleep quality (Juelich et al., 2023). Adolescents may stay up late and be forced to wake up before their sleep cycles have finished, given that the high school day has such an early start (Yip et al., 2022). Staying up late is also associated with increased snacking and food intake (Juelich et al., 2023). Adolescents without sufficient sleep can find it difficult to concentrate, learn, or even stay awake during classes (Cousins et al., 2019). Too little sleep can also contribute to mood swings and behavioral problems. Adolescents who drive when they are sleep deprived can cause accidents, which could lead to death. Nurses can suggest that adolescents keep their cell phones, computers, and other electronic devices out of their bedrooms at night. Nurses can also suggest strategies for daily living that help adolescents cope with the challenges of balancing their varied responsibilities while preventing exhaustion or burnout.

Cognitive-Perceptual Pattern

Piaget's Theory of Cognitive Development

Adolescence is characterized by a shift in cognitive abilities to Piaget's stage of **formal operations** (Piaget, 1969). Piaget's theory used the term *formal* to represent the emergence of ability to focus on the "form" of thoughts, objects, and experiences rather than on the exact content, which in turn lays the groundwork for abstract thinking. These new cognitive abilities are reflected in adolescent behaviors in several ways.

The first change is that, because of their new ability to "think about their thinking," adolescents become highly introspective. As introspection increases, they develop an internalized audience that provides them with a means to evaluate questions such as "Who am I?" "How do others see me?" and "Where am I going?" **Introspection** also combines with a reemergence of **egocentrism**, leading to their sense of being the primary focus—special, unique, and exceptional (Piaget, 1969). Adolescents think that nothing can happen to them, but only to others. This type of thought can contribute to the risk-taking behaviors for which adolescents are well known:

- I can get drunk on weekends and not develop a drinking problem.
- I won't get pregnant; I've had sex for 6 months and haven't gotten pregnant yet.
- I can take those turns at 60 miles per hour and not lose control.

Another behavioral manifestation of adolescents' formal operations is an intolerance of things as they are. They are able to conceptualize things as they might or could be, rather than how they are, and to think of elaborate means for achieving these changes immediately. With this newfound capability, they constantly challenge the ways things are and challenge themselves to consider the way things can or should be. Teens can be vehement in trying to convince others of their viewpoints and untiring in their support for causes that align with them. This **idealism** can lead to a rejection of family beliefs, religion, or social causes, which do not appear to the adolescent to be working quickly enough to solve the problems of society. Although this idealism appears to most adults to be a flight from reality, it is a necessary stage in formal thinking. Adolescents recognize reality, but only as a subset of many other possibilities that need to be aligned with their own thinking. Eventually, their thinking becomes less egocentric and omnipotent, giving way to an appreciation of differences in judgment between themselves and others (Piaget, 1969).

Erikson's Theory of Psychosocial Development

Erikson's theory of psychosocial development describes the central task of adolescence as being the establishment of identity, with the primary risk being **role confusion** (Erikson, 1968). Although it may appear that adolescents are involved in a final rather than a transient or initial stage of development, identity formation in adolescence provides a means of moving into and through what might be termed an identity crisis.

This crisis involves a restaging of each of the previous stages of psychosocial development (Erikson, 1968). Development of trust in self and others, as emphasized in infancy, is encountered again as the adolescent searches for people and ideologies in which to have faith. Toddlerhood, and its search for autonomy, is also revisited as adolescents search for independence from their primary family units. The preschooler's challenge, a sense of initiative rather than guilt, resurfaces as the adolescent searches for direction and purpose. The school-age child's developing sense of industry is carried into the adolescent period also, as teens make choices in social, recreational, volunteer, academic, familial, and occupational activities. Their confusion and hesitation in making these choices arise from fears of participating in activities that will not afford them the opportunity to excel or win the approval of their peers.

Erikson (1968) says that the extent to which these earlier tasks are accomplished successfully predicts the success of the current developmental stage, therefore influencing an adolescent's resourcefulness and success in experimenting with the new identity. When the threat of identity confusion is exceedingly great, delinquent behavior and alterations in mental health can occur. This threat is enhanced by conditions of poverty, racism, and other social inequities.

The pursuit of a meaningful ideology and an individual identity frequently creates a puzzling combination of shifting interests and sudden extremes in action. Erikson views this behavior as an attempt to try on various roles and to search for some stable principle that might last through the testing of extremes and be carried into adulthood. Reassuring parents that this behavior is normal during adolescence and encouraging them to maintain positive communication with their adolescents is an important nursing function.

Time Orientation

Adolescents look at time differently than they did as younger children. They realize that the response to a problem can, and sometimes should, be delayed in order to think through the possibilities for approaching the problem. Additionally, teens develop a future orientation and are able to delay immediate gratification to gain more satisfaction in the future.

Language

Advances in cognitive skills are reflected in an increased understanding of language. Formal operations and more abstract thought processes require expression in different words than did the more concrete thoughts of younger children. Adolescents give complex definitions, frequently including all possible meanings or uses. Interpretations of pictures or stories are intricate and abstract. Older teens are capable of using and understanding complex sentence structure, although they, like adults, may not use these complex sentences routinely in their speech.

Both receptive and expressive vocabularies increase during adolescence. As with all ages, receptive vocabulary far exceeds expressive vocabulary. The adolescent's vocabulary frequently includes slang. Slang may be centered on topics such as drug use, popular dress, music, and certain peer activities, or it may be more pervasive, in which case adults or "outsiders" may have difficulty following a conversation between two teens. The surge in cell phone use, instant and text messaging, and online social media has given rise to an entirely new set of communications to decipher (Table 21.2).

Self-Perception–Self-Concept Pattern

The term *self-perception*, which is often used interchangeably with the terms *self-concept* and *self-esteem*, refers to both the description of the self and to the evaluation of, or feelings about, that description. Tied together and brought to the forefront in adolescence, both self-perception and body image dominate,

TABLE 21.2 Deciphering and Conversing in the Latest Text Messaging Lingo

Message	Meaning
GR8	Great
LOL	Laughing out loud
BRB	Be right back
AFC/AFK	Away from computer/away from keyboard
POS/MOS/DOS	Parent over shoulder/Mom over shoulder/Dad over shoulder
9	Parent watching
99	Parent no longer watching
CD9	Code 9: parent watching or in room
RUOK	Are you ok?
XLNT	Excellent
F2F	Face to face
Zzz	Sleeping, bored, tired
Y	Why
B4N	Bye for now
YYSSW	Yeah yeah sure sure whatever
PCM	Please call me

influence, and are influenced by individual, peer, and societal norms and expectations.

Research suggests that having positive self-esteem during adolescence is related to positive physical and mental outcomes, goal achievement, and overall well-being (Arsandaux et al., 2021). Assessment, anticipatory guidance, education, and counseling are strategies the nurse can use to assist the adolescent in developing positive self-esteem. It is important for parents, teachers, and health care providers to remember to praise adolescents for who they are rather than for what they do, value each of them as unique, demonstrate belief in their abilities to grow and develop, and delight in their discoveries of themselves and their unique means of expressing this.

Acne

Teenage acne can influence self-perception, as it is a contributor to alterations in appearance. Most adolescents experience some degree of acne, especially during puberty, and they are typically concerned about their skin changes; in some cases, this can lead to mental health problems (Zimlich, 2022). The sebaceous glands increase production of sebum, a primary factor in the pathogenesis of acne. The sebaceous follicles become clogged with sebum and debris, forming open (blackheads) or closed (whiteheads) comedones. The incidence of acne within families suggests that hereditary factors are involved.

Taking a thorough history and performing an examination of the adolescent's skin might reveal contributing factors. Use of makeup and certain hair products can be problematic, as preparations, especially those with a fat base, when applied extensively over the face, prevent adequate exposure to light. Additionally, sports equipment, such as helmets, shoulder pads, and other types of padding, can contribute to acne because of rubbing and trapped moisture (American Academy of Dermatology [AAD], 2023c). A discussion of acne's affect on overall body image is necessary to determine appropriate management strategies. Intervention should include teaching the individual about the pathophysiologic nature of acne. Knowledge allows the adolescent to become instrumental in acne management and helps dispel common myths about acne and its care.

The approach to acne management is a stepwise approach according to severity; all recommended management strategies take between 6 and 8 weeks to be effective, followed by maintenance until clear (Kim, 2020). Gently washing the skin with mild soap and water two times a day is the best way to remove surface dirt and oil. Daily topical administration of a retinoid is recommended for all cases of acne. For mild acne, a combination of topical agents (retinoid, antibiotic) can be used. Should the condition worsen or be more severe than mild acne, management can include adding an oral antibiotic to the topical regimen (Thiboutot et al., 2020). For more severe acne, hormonal treatment along with topicals may be used. Systemic treatment with isotretinoin is used only for severe or moderate nonresponsive cases (Thiboutot et al., 2020). The adolescent should not attempt to remove the pustules and papules that form. Squeezing the lesion can result in further irritation of the gland and permanent injury to the tissue. Sunlight can have a beneficial effect on acne; however, prolonged exposure should be avoided. Stress can exacerbate acne in some adolescents. In these cases, stress-management techniques should be considered. The effect of diet on acne is a highly controversial issue. Evidence indicates that dietary restrictions specific to acne are unnecessary.

There are special considerations for adolescents of color (AAD, 2020). Because of deeper skin pigmentation, it might be more difficult to assess the extent and progress of acne lesions; this is especially important as scarring can be more prevalent. The adolescent of color needs to be gentle when washing the skin, be aware of how various skin and hair care products affect their skin, and avoid heavy makeup and use hair products that contain only water or glycerin (AAD, 2020). The adolescent of color needs to be particularly concerned with sun protection. Adolescents with acne need support and understanding. The nurse can help adolescents and their families understand that management does not result in immediate improvement. In fact, topical agents may make acne appear worse initially, with any improvement occurring slowly over several months.

Body Art and Piercing

Adolescence is a developmental period full of identity experimentation and risk-taking behavior. Body piercing and tattooing have become popular forms of expression of identity, particularly among adolescents, and are intimately related to self-perception. Each carries health risks and potentially fatal complications.

There are very few sites on adolescent bodies that have not been pierced. Ears, nipples, navels, noses, and eyebrows have all succumbed to metallic rings, rods, studs, and barbells. However, an adolescent who obtains a piercing is at risk for any number of associated complications. Most commonly these include localized infection, bleeding, dermatitis, and possible keloid formation. Intraoral soft tissue piercing of the lips, cheek, uvula, and tongue harbors additional and potentially fatal complications, including a constant risk of aspiration, hemorrhage, and swelling leading to airway compromise, nerve damage, keloid scar formation, abscess, and tetanus. There is also an increased risk of hepatitis and HIV infection, as well as tooth injury, gingival recession, and difficulty with speech, taste, and swallowing.

Tattooing carries similar risks of infection, with a heightened concern for the transmission of blood-borne diseases, including hepatitis and HIV infection, especially with colorful tattoos. The US Food and Drug Administration (FDA) has warned about possible contamination of colored ink leading to infection. Colored ink is expensive and is often reused to cut costs, increasing exposure risks. Other potential consequences from tattooing skin include allergic reaction and the masking of potentially cancerous skin lesions (Quinn, 2023). Tattoos are also permanent markings and may not age well. Despite the increase in the number of people who have tattoos, there may also be consequences for later employment. Nurses can explore with adolescents the reasons for acquiring body art and explain the potential short-term and long-term consequences to assist with their decision-making. To prevent infection from body piercing, the nurse needs to advise the adolescent to use meticulous handwashing when cleaning piercing sites. The sites should be cleaned with saline or antibacterial soap and protected from injury. Applying petroleum jelly (from a tube) around piercing sites keeps the skin intact for healing (AAD, 2023a). Adolescents with new tattoos need to avoid sun exposure and tanning beds as well as prolonged immersion in water, and they must apply water-based moisturizing cream to the site (AAD, 2023b). With both types of body art, adolescents should notify the provider of any signs of infection.

Roles-Relationships Pattern

Families

Until adolescence, the younger child is highly dependent on the parents and other adults. Striving for identity and increased independence, the adolescent begins to spend increased time away from the family. Parents sense a narrowing of their influence as their teen not only begins to prefer the company of peers and other adults but also begins to question familial beliefs and values. Parents may respond by setting unreasonably strict limits and asking intrusive questions about their teen's activities, friends, and ideas. With today's adolescents having access to smart phones that can track their whereabouts, parents are tempted to follow their child's every movement and action; this is referred to as overinvolvement or overparenting and can contribute to mental health issues such as anxiety and decreased coping skills for self-management (Jiao & Segrin, 2023). Another approach by a parent may be to decide to drop all rules and limits and assume that the adolescent can now manage alone. Neither of these approaches works well.

Whereas adolescents strive for a sense of identity and independence, their parents try to learn how to let go. Each is temporarily unsure of the relationship with the other, and the family unit may experience more stress than at any previous time. Furthermore, this period is often prolonged because more teens remain financially dependent on their families as they move into young adulthood.

Some families experience better outcomes than do other families. Families in which parents maintain a willingness to listen and demonstrate an ongoing affection for and acceptance of their adolescent, yet still maintain some consistent limits, experience more constructive, positive outcomes during this period. This situation does not mean that parents necessarily agree with their teen's ideas or actions, but rather that they are willing to hear what the adolescent has to say and to negotiate some limits. Parents may need assistance in determining negotiable versus nonnegotiable rules and in developing ways to voice their concerns in an honest, open way. Even when teens do not want to "discuss" a topic, they need to know why their parents are concerned.

Peers

Faced with the need to become autonomous, achieve identity, and become productive, the adolescent often turns from the family to the peer group to find a safe psychosocial shelter in which to develop. Belonging to an informally organized clique, crowd, gang, or group is the primary means with which to make the transition from the young child's allegiance to the family to a member of a group. Identification with a group is proclaimed through conformity to standards of clothing, behavior, language, and values. This feature of the adolescent subculture persists despite the strong inclination in society as a whole toward greater levels of individuality.

The **peer group** is a vehicle for disengaging from the family unit, and as such, it provides a means of achieving the goals of independence and individualization. Adolescents talk a great deal with their peers. Whether on the phone, online, or in person, adolescents can discuss situations for hours on end. This sharing of thoughts and impressions is important. The telephone or computer can provide a "safe" mechanism for the teen to interact with members of the opposite sex as they share intimate ideas and concerns and begin to experience the closeness and caring that develops into the capacity to form a future intimate relationship.

Adolescents in both urban and rural areas can have exposure to, and participate in, gangs. Gangs function as a peer group for adolescents who may feel they need protection from others, or, conversely, who may be perpetrators of violence and wish to identify with gang members (Vecchio & Carson, 2023). Major risk factors for gang engagement include living in disadvantaged neighborhoods that have increased incidence of crime, substance use, and exposure to violence. Having trouble in school, feeling isolated or bullied, and experiencing racial discrimination, hopelessness, and poor parental monitoring contribute to gang participation as well (Shelley & Petersen, 2019). Recent research findings suggest that early exposure to violence that results in posttraumatic stress disorder increases the risk for later gang membership (Mendez et al., 2023). Not all gangs exhibit delinquent behavior; however, there is a societal perception that violence is part of the gang culture. Nurses can alert parents to the signs that their adolescent may be associating with a gang; these include wearing symbolic clothing, new and extensive body art or specific hairdos, use of secret hand or verbal signals, withdrawal from family, secrecy about friends, worsening school performance, and possible substance use. Encouraging strong and positive relationships with friends during adolescence and increased vigilance by parents can be protective against gang membership (Seleckman et al., 2023).

Sexuality-Reproductive Pattern

Adolescent Sexual Issues

The emergence of secondary sexual characteristics increases adolescents' awareness of themselves as sexual human beings. They fantasize about relationships and sex and gradually experiment with dating and myriad coital and noncoital physical contacts. Adolescents become sexually active for a variety of reasons. They have sex for affection, because of peer pressure, as a symbol of maturity, as spontaneous experimentation, to feel close, or because it feels good or right. The overall prevalence of self-reported current adolescent sexual activity in the United States is 21%, a slight decrease over the last time data were collected. Only slightly more than half of those sexually active adolescents report using condoms; 13.7% use no method of pregnancy prevention (CDC, 2023a). At times, adolescents have intercourse without their consent. Approximately 8% of adolescents report forced intercourse, and approximately 11% report having been a victim of sexual violence (CDC, 2023f).

The technologic revolution has opened up a limitless world of unmediated information to adolescents and has led to increased issues of risky online behaviors. The use of online social networks such as Facebook, X, Instagram, Snapchat, and other messaging sites continues to expand rapidly among all age groups and segments of our society, presenting new opportunities for the exchange of sexual information as well as for potentially unsafe encounters between predators and the vulnerable or young. Additionally, adolescents who use the Internet to seek sexual information often receive conflicting messages and inaccurate facts. Sexting has been recognized as an increasing occurrence and is a global practice among teens and young adults. Sexting refers to sending a text message with sexually explicit content or a sexually explicit picture. This type of texting can cause emotional pain for the person in the picture, the sender, and the receiver. Nurses help adolescents understand that text messages should not contain pictures of naked people or of people kissing or touching each other, and that sending such a text message is considered a crime in some areas.

The importance of anticipatory guidance relative to sexual issues cannot be overemphasized. Adolescents ages 13 to 24 years account for 20% of HIV infections diagnosed in the United States and more than 50% of all sexually transmitted infections (STIs) (CDC, 2023f). Recent research demonstrates that discussions about sexual topics, other than pubertal changes, are not covered routinely in primary practice. Other important topics include sexual decision-making, gender identity, sexual orientation, and prevention of pregnancy and STIs (Sieving et al., 2021). Knowing adolescents are heavily invested in these and other sexual issues, nurses are capable of discussing and willing to discuss them with adolescents in a variety of settings, such as physicians' offices, clinics, and schools. Nurses need to be comfortable with their own sexuality; able to discuss the subject of sex and sexual orientation, contraception, and protection against STIs; and be aware of their own limitations, beliefs, and biases. Anticipatory guidance about the decision to become sexually active or not, to use contraception, and to obtain protection from STIs needs to be provided before adolescents encounter a situation in which they need this information (see Chapter 22). This is also a good time to introduce the adolescent to breast self-awareness and testicular self-examinations (Box 21.6: Quality and Safety Scenario).

School nurses are often leaders of, or participants in, school-based sex education programs. Depending on the philosophy of the educational district, sex education programs can be abstinence only or comprehensive, which combines abstinence with discussion of protective measures. Regardless of the focus of the school-based sex education program, it is only one factor that affects whether adolescents decide to become sexually active. Parental input is important as well. Nurses can work with parents, assisting them with techniques for addressing sexuality with their adolescents. Nurses also need to consider not only parental beliefs and values regarding the provision of

BOX 21.6 QUALITY AND SAFETY SCENARIO

Finding a change from "normal" is the first step toward an early detection of breast or testicular cancer, and early detection results in a more positive outcome. Patient-centered teaching can assist with identifying a problem early.

Breast Self-Awareness

Although breast cancer is rare in adolescents, adolescent females should develop an awareness of their breasts so that any changes can be recognized quickly. It is important for girls to become familiar with the size, shape, feel, and skin texture of their breasts, as these are features unique to each individual. Breast awareness will assist the adolescent in detecting any changes that might be indicative of a tumor or breast cancer. Changes to look for include feeling a lump in breasts, in armpits, or in the neck above the collar bone; unusual swelling; pain; and altered skin appearance of the nipple area (e.g., dimpling, unusual discharge). Any of these signs should be reported to the health provider right away.

Performing Testicular Self-Examination

Testicular self-examination (TSE) should be performed once a month so that teens become familiar with the usual appearance and feel of their testicles. This routine makes noticing any changes from one month to another easier. The best time for a TSE is during or immediately after a warm shower. The boy should:

- Hold the penis out of the way, and then cup or support the testicles with one hand and feel them with the other. Assess one testicle at a time.
- Gently roll each testicle between the thumb and fingers. There should not be any pain.
- Look at and feel each testicle for any firm lumps on the surface or changes in testicle size, feel or appearance. One may be slightly larger or lower than the other.
- Notice the tubelike structure, the epididymis, that is along the upper side of the testicle. Learn what it feels like.
- Contact a provider if any changes are noted.

American Cancer Society. (2022). *American Cancer Society recommendations for the early detection of breast cancer.* www.cancer.org. American Cancer Society. (2018a). *Can testicular cancer be found early?* www.cancer.org

sex education in schools but also regarding the optimal age for introducing information. In an attempt to increase adolescent confidence in resisting peer pressure and provide community support for the developing adolescent, some communities provide programs that emphasize community service along with a sex education curriculum (Breuner, 2020). Additional sources of sex information for adolescents are the Internet and social media sites; nurses can help adolescents discriminate between factual and exaggerated or inappropriate information, especially during a medical encounter or yearly physical. Special adaptations for adolescents with developmental disability are vitally important, as the risk for sexual abuse is high in this population (Murray, 2019). Finding creative ways to present information and using stories with which these adolescents can identify can increase their knowledge of positive, healthy, and safe relationships (Murray, 2019).

In the process of establishing a sexual sense of themselves, it is not uncommon for adolescents to question whether they are homosexual. Experimenting with same-sex physical intimacy does not necessarily predict future sexual orientation, but feelings associated with the possibility of homosexual identity can give rise to anxiety, mood disorders, feelings of isolation, and heightened risk of suicide in adolescents (Calvin et al., 2019; National Association of Pediatric Nurse Practitioners [NAPNAP] et al., 2019). The prevalence of adolescents in the United States who identify as gay or lesbian is 3%; 12% identify as bisexual, 5% are questioning, and 4% are not sure (Szucs et al., 2023). Approximately 22% of LGBTQ+ adolescents report being sexually active (CDC, 2023f). When developing *Healthy People 2030*, the USDHHS Office of Disease Prevention and Health Promotion (2020) proposed goals and objectives that include better identification of LGBTQ+ youth and addressing resulting issues such as bullying and increased risk for suicide in this population of adolescents. Associated with the purpose of these objectives is the recognition that many health providers, among others, may have a negative or biased attitude toward caring for individuals with gender differences (House et al., 2019). In addition to emotional issues associated with gender nonconformity, nurses need to educate themselves about health issues associated with adolescents in this population. As with adolescents who identify as heterosexual, there is a risk of acquiring a STI as well as a risk of pregnancy (NAPNAP et al., 2019). Dating violence is also heightened in this population, with nearly 23% of gay, lesbian, and bisexual adolescents reporting forced intercourse (CDC, 2023g).

LGBTQ+ adolescents make up a significant segment of the runaway and homeless teen population in the United States (Montano, 2019). Contributing factors to this include a lack of support or active hostility from family members, emotional difficulties such as mental illness and substance use, and stigmatization (Montano, 2019). In addition to the emotional and physical issues associated with gender nonconformity, unsafe conditions and instability associated with homelessness create additional risk.

When LGBTQ+ adolescents present for preventive or acute medical care, nurses and other health professionals need to be supportive and nonjudgmental. When taking a health history, for example, ask adolescents what name they would like to use for the visit (this might not be the name they were given by their families but a name they have chosen to match their gender identity). Using gender neutral and inclusive terms and pronouns, such as *they* rather than *he* or *she*, demonstrates unbiased support (Campanella Day, 2022). School nurses can encourage their school to establish a gay-straight alliance program and to set expectations of acceptance for both adults and students in the school environment (Calvin et al., 2019).

Transgender adolescents experience a persistent incongruence between their assigned birth sex and their gender identity (Rafferty, American Academy of Pediatrics [AAP] Committee on Psychosocial Aspects of Child and Family Health & Committee on Adolescence Section on Lesbian, Gay, Bisexual and Transgender Health and Wellness, 2023). Gender identity develops during childhood and can include actions that demonstrate different types of external mannerisms and appearances. It is estimated, however, that gender identity can be firmly established and recognized by the time children reach 8½ years old, even if they do not disclose this until years later (Rafferty et al., 2023). As with other LGBTQ+ groups, transgender adolescents are often subject to actions that adversely affect their mental health. These include altered relationships within the family; external violence, such as bullying; homelessness; and decreased access to medical and mental health care.

Care for transgender adolescents involves assessment at each well visit, using an accepting and nonjudgmental approach, using inclusive language, and facilitating access to medical, mental, and social support as well as other resources (Rafferty et al., 2023). It also addresses the supportive needs of parents and families. Although regret for transgender decision-making is rare, there are medical interventions that are reversible or partly reversible, including pubertal suppression and cross-sex hormonal therapy; surgical reconstruction is not reversible (Rafferty et al., 2023). Any of these interventions carries some risks. Several states in the United States have recently passed legislation that prohibits or restricts access to gender affirming care for minors, yet it is estimated that adolescents are capable of giving informed consent by the age of 16 years old (Roberts, 2022). This is an evolving issue as the incidence of individuals identifying as transgender is growing (Roberts, 2022). A complicating factor is that restricting puberty-suppressing medications can have adverse effects on children or adolescents who need them for other medical reasons.

Sex Trafficking. Sex trafficking can occur when the need for resources to survive pushes victims to exchange sex for money, food, or other essentials. Acquiring these basic necessities in this way increases vulnerability to exploitation by sex traffickers, whom victims may view as providing a measure of economic security and protection (Boswell et al., 2019). For adolescents, the risk is higher in the poor, homeless, or LGBTQ+ populations and often relates to forced isolation from usual supports as well as increased vulnerability to being manipulated psychologically and physically by others (Greenbaum et al., 2023). Sex trafficking can be domestic, occurring within the United States, or international, as might be seen in immigrant populations. Its prevalence affects millions of children and adolescents annually and is increasing (Greenbaum et al., 2023). Sex trafficking is illegal federally.

Identification and recognition of affected adolescents can occur in a multitude of health care, social service, and criminal justice settings, but indicators can be very subtle because of mistrust, reluctance to talk with a provider, concern about legal consequences, or fear of retaliation by the trafficker. The AAP recommends routine assessment for risks and signs of sex trafficking (Greenbaum et al., 2023). A variety of risks and symptoms might raise provider concerns. One of the most obvious is the presence of mental health problems, such as depression, anxiety, substance use, expressions of fear or shame, and demonstrated isolation from support systems (Gerassi et al., 2021). Physical indicators include signs of violence or trauma, diagnosis of STIs or pregnancy, and appearance of overall total neglect. Less-obvious signs are the presence of a controlling individual, indicators of possible gang involvement, history of contacts with the criminal justice system, and homelessness (Greenbaum et al., 2023; Gerassi et al., 2021).

The AAP recommends approaching these affected adolescents in a similar way as one would approach a victim of trauma. This would include building a trusting relationship, explaining all actions in a way the adolescent would understand, respecting privacy and confidentiality, and encouraging active participation in care and careful documentation, which could include taking photographs of areas of concern (Greenbaum et al., 2023). The provider needs to explain what information, if any, would need legal reporting, such as indicators of child abuse or violation of child labor laws. The approach to documentation is complicated and more sensitive if the victim is an immigrant or in the country illegally (Greenbaum et al., 2023). Making appropriate medical, psychological, and social referrals for follow-up care are essential. The National Human Trafficking Resource Center's phone number is 1-888-373-7888. The issue of human trafficking is complex, and the AAP has strongly recommended that all health professionals who work with children and adolescents acquire education that will enable them to identify the signs that an adolescent has become a victim of human trafficking and what resources to access to support them (Greenbaum et al., 2023).

Adolescent Pregnancy

For health care providers, adolescent pregnancy is viewed as a high-risk situation because of the serious health risks and potential complications for both the mother and the infant. For politicians and governmental agencies, it is a social problem that makes overwhelming demands on social and economic resources. For adolescents and their families, it may be seen as positive and normal or the worst disaster imaginable. No matter what the perspective, adolescent pregnancy represents myriad concerns with far-reaching social, educational, financial, and emotional effects.

Information from the National Center for Health Statistics (Ostermanet et al., 2023) reveals that births to girls aged 15 to 19 years in the United States number 146,973, or a birth rate of 13.9 per 1000. The overall teen birth rate has dropped dramatically for all racial and ethnic groups and is at its lowest level ever. Adolescent pregnancy has several possible negative outcomes for both the mother and the child. For the mother, these include a significant decline in future prospects, especially educationally and economically; single parenthood; reliance on government-sponsored assistance; and poverty (Schulkind & Sandler, 2019). Physical and emotional immaturity during adolescence increase the risk for pregnancy-related complications, and the incidence of low birth weight and neonatal death is higher for children born to adolescent mothers (Powers et al., 2021).

When pregnancy occurs, adolescents and their families deserve honest and sensitive counseling as well as access to the support systems available for them throughout the pregnancy, birth, and subsequent parenting. For the pregnant adolescent, early referral for prenatal care is essential, along with referral to supporting agencies for potential insurance, housing, nutrition and mental health needs (Powers et al., 2021). Nurses can provide support postnatally through referral for home visitation programs, assistance to mothers and fathers relative to parenting techniques, and monitoring infant development (Powers et al., 2021).

The American College of Obstetricians and Gynecologists (ACOG) has recommended that a girl's first gynecologic visit occur between the ages of 13 and 15 (ACOG, 2020). Although that may seem young, 3% of adolescent girls report having had sex before age 13 (CDC, 2023f). A visit dedicated to providing adolescent reproductive information can be used to emphasize positive and healthy sexual relationships (ACOG, 2020). One of the uncertain effects of the recent Supreme Court decision on *Dobbs v. Jackson Women's Health Organization* is access to reproductive care. For adolescents, fertility awareness and access to education about preconception information is essential for preventing unintended pregnancy. This has always been important but is now even more so given states' differences in access currently and potentially in the future (Wood & Stevenson, 2023). Nurses not only need to reinforce reproductive health-education efforts but also need to encourage adolescents to build on the strengths in their lives and opportunities available to them. (See Chapter 22 for additional information about pregnancy and contraception.)

Coping–Stress Tolerance Pattern

When all the changes that occur in adolescents align with their need to separate from their parents and gain a sense of their own independence, their ability to cope is put to the test over and over again. Common coping mechanisms, along with the strategies the nurse can use to encourage teens to use them in adaptive ways, are listed in Box 21.7.

However, too often adolescents are unable to balance stresses, lacking the appropriate skills and outlets, adequate support systems, or available mental health intervention. Depression, suicide, and substance abuse emerge as life becomes overwhelming and the future unimaginable.

Depression

As with many other diseases, the rate of **depression** increases with age, and the incidence continues to increase during adolescence. Approximately 20% of adolescents experience a major

BOX 21.7 Coping Mechanisms of Adolescents

Cognitive Mastery

The adolescent attempts to learn as much as possible about the situation or stressor. This strategy is common for the adolescent with a chronic illness. The nurse can assist by clarifying any misinformation, sharing research findings, and encouraging a discussion of feelings.

Conformity

The adolescent attempts to be a mirror image of peers, which includes dress, language, attitudes, and actions. The nurse must respect this need for sameness and can also encourage discussion of feelings about differences among teens.

Controlling Behavior

Adolescents must be in charge of some aspects of life and can no longer accept family and school rules without question as they did in the past. This need for control extends to health care. The nurse cannot simply give directions or instructions but rather should present the options and allow the adolescent to partner with the nurse to work out an acceptable plan.

Fantasy

The adolescent may use fantasy as a way to escape or experiment. The nurse can encourage the teen to use fantasy constructively to develop creative plans to deal with a stressful situation.

Motor Activity

Engaging in sports, dancing, running, or other physical activity can be an effective tension-releasing strategy and can also provide an instant peer group. The nurse can encourage physical activity and offer information about protective gear and injury prevention.

depressive disorder by age 18 years, with the prevalence in girls more than twice as high as in boys (Federal Interagency Forum on Child and Family Statistics, 2023). The prevalence of depression has increased over the past 10 years; every adolescent age group has been affected, although least so in the 12- to 13-year-old group. Approximately 40% of those affected, however, receive treatment (Federal Interagency Forum on Child and Family Statistics, 2023). The term *depression* includes both major depressive and persistent depressive disorders. Major depression is an alteration in mood that is disabling and interferes with normal activities for a minimum of 2 weeks, whereas persistent depression is a depressed or irritable mood that extends for more than 2 years but does not necessarily interfere with activities or performance (National Institute of Mental Health, 2023).

Depression is suspected when the adolescent uses words such as *down*, *sad*, *low*, *blue*, *hopeless*, *worried*, *bored*, or *discouraged* and exhibits several of the following symptoms:

- Change in weight or appetite
- Insomnia or hypersomnia
- Decreased energy or fatigue
- Loss of interest and pleasure in usual activities
- Out-of-proportion feelings of self-reproach or guilt
- Difficulty concentrating; declining school performance
- Preoccupation with death or suicidal ideation

The AAP has recommended routine screening for mental health disorders, particularly depression and suicide risk, in the primary care setting using a reliable and valid assessment instrument (AAP, 2022; Zucherbrot et al., 2018). The United States Preventive Services Task Force has recently supported this approach as providing reliable evidence that screening results in decrease in suicidal ideation and overall improvement in symptoms (Wenhua & Munoz-Laboy, 2023). The screening instrument most frequently used is the Patient Health Questionnaire-9, which is reliable and valid; it is a self-report of symptoms. Nurses need to lead the way in screening and assessing children and teens for depression and other mental health problems in a culturally sensitive way. Moreover, nurses may promote mental health in both children and teens by teaching them effective coping skills and stress-reduction techniques. One method recently proposed is developing an individualized adolescent depression plan. This is an approach that explains depression in terms the adolescent finds easily readable and that collaborates with the adolescent in achieving goals relative to eating, activity, and social relationships (Cucci et al., 2022). Because adolescents tend to discontinue treatment for depression, nurses can assist with ensuring that they are following their treatment plan appropriately (Cheung et al., 2018; Stafford et al., 2020).

Suicide

Adolescence is a period of considerable stress, and when coping mechanisms and social supports are inadequate, suicide may emerge as an outcome. Suicide has become the second leading cause of death among children and adolescents aged 10 to 14 and the third leading cause of death among adolescents aged 15 to 24 (CDC National Center for Injury Prevention and Control, 2023b). A national survey revealed that 22% of youths in grades 9 to 12 in the United States reported that they were seriously considering suicide and that 10.2% had attempted suicide during the previous year. Contemplation of suicide was twice as high in girls as in boys and approximately equal among Hispanic, Black, and White adolescents, while the reported incidence in Asian adolescents was lower. Adolescents who identified as gay, lesbian, or bisexual contemplated suicide at a percentage twice as high as their heterosexual counterparts (Gaylor et al., 2023). These figures may not even reflect the full scope of the problem because many suicides may be classified as accidental deaths. Along with well-known risk factors, such as depression, substance abuse, and adolescents identifying as LGBTQ+, the risk factors for suicide may be related to physical and cognitive developmental changes. Many researchers are convinced that suicide during adolescence is not an impulsive or spontaneous act; it is selected carefully only after other problem-solving methods have failed and suicide is viewed as the only option.

Adolescent suicide can be prevented. Distressed adolescents tend to give clues, both verbally and nonverbally. Any single clue may mean nothing, but when several clues are noted, they should be recognized as important warning signs. Box 21.8 outlines warning signs for parents, teachers, health care providers, and peers to watch for to prevent adolescent suicide. Any signs of suicide or threat to commit suicide should be taken seriously and require immediate intervention and referral. An adult should remain with the adolescent until medical assistance becomes available. Nurses can teach adolescents to be sensitive to signs that may indicate a friend is suicidal and to seek adult assistance immediately.

BOX 21.8 Warning Signs of Suicide Risk in Adolescents

Behavioral Changes

- Increased risk-taking
- Increased incidence of accidents
- Substance use and abuse
- Physical violence to self, others, or animals
- Decreased appetite
- Alienation from family or peer group
- Giving away personal items
- Writing letters or notes, essays, and poems with suicidal content

Cognitive and Mood Changes

- Expression of hopelessness
- Increasing rage or anger
- Dramatic swings in affect
- Sleep disorders
- Preoccupation with death
- Difficulty concentrating
- Hearing voices, seeing things or people
- Newfound interest in religion or cult

Another area of concern for adolescents is self-injury not associated with a suicide attempt (nonsuicidal self-injury [NSSI]). The National Center for Health Statistics (2023) reported 660,000 visits to emergency departments for treatment of self-injury during 2021, with prevalence higher in girls. Examples of NSSI include cutting, pinching, scarification, scratching, and burning, with cutting being the most frequently seen (Townsend et al., 2023). Several factors affect whether an adolescent will be a victim of NSSI: history of mental health issues (especially depression or anxiety), prior experiences of bullying or victimization, low perception of quality of life, family dysfunction, and isolation (Le et al., 2023; Townsend et al., 2023) Often adolescents try to hide what they are doing, and sometimes it is difficult for the nurse or other health provider to assess the behavior (Williams et al., 2018). Nurses can approach adolescents either with direct questions or indirectly, depending on the adolescent's age and the level of trust the adolescent has with the provider (Williams et al., 2018). Encouraging the adolescent to ask for help, assisting with developing a plan of action, and providing information about potential outcomes of behavior are all appropriate approaches. Should the situation become severe and out of the adolescent's control, referral to a mental health provider is necessary (Williams et al., 2018). Providing support to parents and family members is also essential, as research suggests that being positively connected with their child, including providing caring support, can mitigate the risk for NSSI as adolescents develop (Baher et al., 2023).

Values-Beliefs Pattern

Values and beliefs are learned phenomena that serve as guides for decision-making and actions. With the development of abstract thought, adolescents begin to expand their understanding of good and bad or right and wrong to include autonomous moral principles that have validity apart from the authority of a parent or society and instead are based on the individual's beliefs. Newly discovered maturity in moral reasoning is situational and relational and is often superseded by psychosocial developmental needs and influences. Adolescents may think or feel that something is wrong or bad yet may act contrary to that belief because of peer pressure or the need to declare their independence.

Adolescents often align their values and beliefs with a particular religion, philosophical school of thought, social movement or cause, or other formal system, using it to make decisions about what is right or wrong, best or worst, and important or trivial. During adolescence, these alignments can change drastically and often, causing strife and concern for parents yet providing the teen with different ranges of experience from which to base eventual and lasting choices.

Kohlberg's theory of moral development (Kohlberg, 1981) demonstrates that the adolescent begins to make the transition to the postconventional stage, equating what is right with the idea of justice and basing actions on the recognition of universal principles underlying laws and social agreements. Gilligan and colleagues (1990), who developed a parallel theory of moral development for females, propose that the female adolescent sees "good" as involving self-sacrifice and caring for the relationships in her life. They state that, as moral reasoning matures, the female adolescent learns to achieve a balance between what is good for her and what is good for others in her network of relationships (Gilligan et al., 1990).

As adolescents struggle with their journey to discover who they are, parents, teachers, and health care providers need to provide positive role modeling, reinforce positive behaviors, and remember the difficulty of their own journeys. It is often when we like them the least that they need us the most.

ENVIRONMENTAL PROCESSES

Because adolescents are in developmental transition, their lifestyle choices may have a significant effect on their current and future health. These choices are particularly sensitive to the immediate physical and social environments. These environmental influences include family members, friends, community, school, neighborhood, and work environments. Several critical types of adolescent health behaviors—including alcohol and drug use, injury and violence, tobacco use, nutrition, physical activity, and sexual behaviors—have been identified as contributing to the leading causes of death and disability among adults and youth.

Physical Agents

Unintentional Injury

Unintentional injury, along with suicide and homicide, remains the leading cause of death and injury during adolescence. Motor vehicle crashes are a major cause of unintentional deaths in adolescents of all ages (CDC National Center for Injury Prevention and Control, 2023a). Motor vehicle crashes are a significant cause of nonfatal injury as well. Whether drivers, passengers, pedestrians, or cyclists, few adolescents take measures to reduce their risk of injury, with nearly 40% of teens stating they do not always wear a seat belt when riding with others and 36% reporting that they have emailed or texted while driving a car (CDC, 2023f). Other contributing factors for motor vehicle injury include riding with someone who had been drinking alcohol (14%) and driving while drinking alcohol (4.6%) (CDC, 2023f).

Nurses talk to teens about the consequences of texting while driving and encourage teens to wear seat belts and to avoid driving or riding with someone who is under the influence of drugs or alcohol. The tendency to play loud music and change the song often, as well as the pressure to answer cell phones, can also be distracting, as can a car full of other teens. Recognizing this—and that teens have a much higher nighttime crash fatality rate—many states have enacted new driver restrictions and nighttime curfews.

Sports Injuries

Concussion. Organized sports in and out of school provide adolescents with experiences in competition, teamwork and effort, and conflict resolution. They also provide a valuable means for adolescents to develop self-esteem. However, adolescents are particularly vulnerable to sports injuries. Their coordination skills are developing, their judgment is often immature and inadequate, their epiphyses have not yet closed, and their extremities are poorly protected by stabilizing musculature. They can also become obsessed or driven to perform beyond their capabilities or to the exclusion of all other activities. The use of performance-enhancing substances, such as steroids, which has unfortunately been modeled by many professional athletes, can create another potential extreme scenario that places the adolescent at risk of injury.

Although mild traumatic brain injury (concussion) is caused by falls or other mechanical injuries, the most frequent contributing factor in children and adolescents is participation in sports (Halstead et al., 2018). Even a minor impact injury to the head or neck, with or without loss of consciousness, can result in long-term physical, emotional, and cognitive effects if it is not appropriately managed (Halstead et al., 2018; Hodges & Ameringer, 2019). The signs and symptoms of concussion in children include headache, deficits in cognition, altered neurological status, problems concentrating in school, emotional lability, and fatigue. Visual impairment is becoming a more frequently seen sign associated with concussion; nurses or providers need to assess visual acuity using an age-appropriate chart, as well as eye structures, visual tracking, and accommodation (Master et al., 2022). Evidence suggests that adolescents experience concussion symptoms and their affect on normal activities in different ways (Hodges & Ameringer, 2019). Traumatic brain injury should be managed by a provider who is experienced in recognizing the signs and symptoms and who is experienced in concussion management. Several reliable and valid assessment instruments are available to assist health care providers in diagnosis (Halstead et al., 2018). As a consequence of a body of evidence suggesting that traumatic brain injury effects can be more severe in children and adolescents, all states have enacted, to various extents, legislation related to concussion injuries in sports, which guides parents, coaches, and health providers in appropriate management. Related to sports participation for adolescents with a head or neck injury and signs of concussion, most applicable state laws provide for annual educational notice to parents of athletes, immediate removal from play, and return to play only with a signed medical release from a provider experienced with managing children with concussion (Halstead et al., 2018). Conservative management is essential and may involve restricting all or some physical activity and ensuring cognitive rest (no schoolwork; limitation of use of electronic devices, such as television, video games, computers, or phones) until the adolescent is no longer symptomatic (Halstead et al., 2018). Decisions regarding return to activity and school might be different for each affected adolescent, so individualized planning according to symptom experience is essential (Hodges & Ameringer, 2019).

Nurses work with adolescents and parents in carrying out the management plan. A successful plan would be one that facilitates adolescent autonomy, incorporates educating about the recovery course, and advises adolescents of strategies they can use, without focusing on what they should not be doing (Halstead et al., 2018; Hodges & Ameringer, 2019). The nurse advocates the proper use of protective gear during all activities and a thorough preparticipation sports examination, along with concussion training for coaches and parents. Strategies to prevent sports injury include using the right age-appropriate equipment, completing conditioning exercises, following all sports-related safety protocols, and maintaining hydration (Brooks, 2023). The nurse also monitors adolescents for overuse, overexertion, or overinvestment in a sport.

Sudden Cardiac Arrest (SCA). A rare but extremely serious condition in adolescent athletes is sudden cardiac arrest, which can be fatal. This can occur as a result of an underlying undiagnosed cardiac condition but has also occurred in individuals who have no underlying manifestations of disease. Cardiac risk factors include hypertrophic cardiomyopathy, ion channel defects, congenital heart disease, and abnormal electric pathways (Erickson et al., 2021). Sudden arrest during sports activities could result from what is called commotio cordis, which occurs after a small object, such as a baseball or hockey puck, causes a sudden hard impact to the chest, possibly triggering ventricular fibrillation (Erickson et al., 2021). This is a stunning event for all involved and requires an instantaneous response of cardiac resuscitation and defibrillation (Erickson et al., 2021; Fanous & Dorian, 2019). For prevention, the AAP currently recommends a routine cardiac assessment for all children and adolescents regardless of plans to participate in athletics. This could be done at the routine age-related check-up or during a preparticipation physical examination. Children and adolescents identified with underlying risk factors need to be referred to a pediatric cardiologist (Erickson et al., 2021). Screening questions can alert the nurse or provider to a possible underlying pathology; these are questions that assess for altered consciousness related to physical activity, exercise-induced pain or shortness of breath, and familial early cardiac death or identified electrocardiogram (ECG) abnormalities (Erickson et al., 2021; Fanous & Dorian, 2019).

Optimal management and prevention are the main approaches to managing or limiting SCA in athletes. Coaches, trainers, nurses, or spectators should intervene immediately with cardiac resuscitation and support, as these will make subsequent death less likely. For this to happen, there must be written action plans, increased training of personnel, and ready availability of automated external defibrillators (AEDs) at the scene (Erickson et al., 2021; Fanous & Dorian, 2019). There will be understandable and overwhelming anxiety and upset in parents, other team members, coaches, and spectators; support for them will be essential. Community participation in increasing the numbers of people knowledgeable about and capable of providing cardiopulmonary resuscitation (CPR) is the most important preventive measure.

Violence

Although the rate of adolescent victims of violence has decreased in the past 2 decades, adolescents still experience risk of injury and death from violence in their homes, schools, and communities. In the United States, the rate of adolescents aged 12 to 17 years who are victims of violent crime is four per 1000 adolescents (Federal Interagency Forum on Child and Family Statistics, 2023). Adolescents can be perpetrators of violence as well, and homicide is the third leading cause of death in adolescents older than 14 years (CDC National Center for Injury Prevention and Control, 2023). Fig. 21.5 outlines the interrelationships of internal and external precipitating factors that increase an adolescent's vulnerability to and for violent behaviors. Many teens report carrying weapons to protect themselves or intimidate others. Adolescents often report a fear of violence and try to avoid situations where they might be vulnerable to it, including at home or even in the bathroom at school. Victims of violent crime can experience both short-term and long-term physical and psychological health problems.

Becoming increasingly independent, adolescents test the limits of authority, experiment with a variety of roles, question adult values and authority, and look to peers for affirmation. They may feel pressure to join gangs or feel threatened by them. Many studies suggest that exposure to violence, whether in person or projected on television, in videos, or in movies, results in a higher incidence of aggressive or violent behaviors. Parental monitoring (e.g., knowing the adolescent's whereabouts and friends, gathering for family dinners) is protective against violent behaviors (Khurana et al., 2019).

Teenagers may be involved in physical or emotional bullying and/or electronic bullying via a variety of social media (cyberbullying). Bullying is the result of a purposeful intent to repeatedly harm or harass another who is perceived to be less powerful (Dow-Fleisner et al., 2023; Hornor, 2018). In a nationwide study, 17% of adolescents reported being bullied at school, and nearly 17% reported being cyberbullied, with the prevalence in girls twice as high as in boys and elevated in those who self-identify as being lesbian, gay, or bisexual (CDC, 2023g). In general, support and connectedness in the school setting can mitigate the extent of bullying. However, school nurses need to be aware that approaches to the problem must include interventions that will both increase school

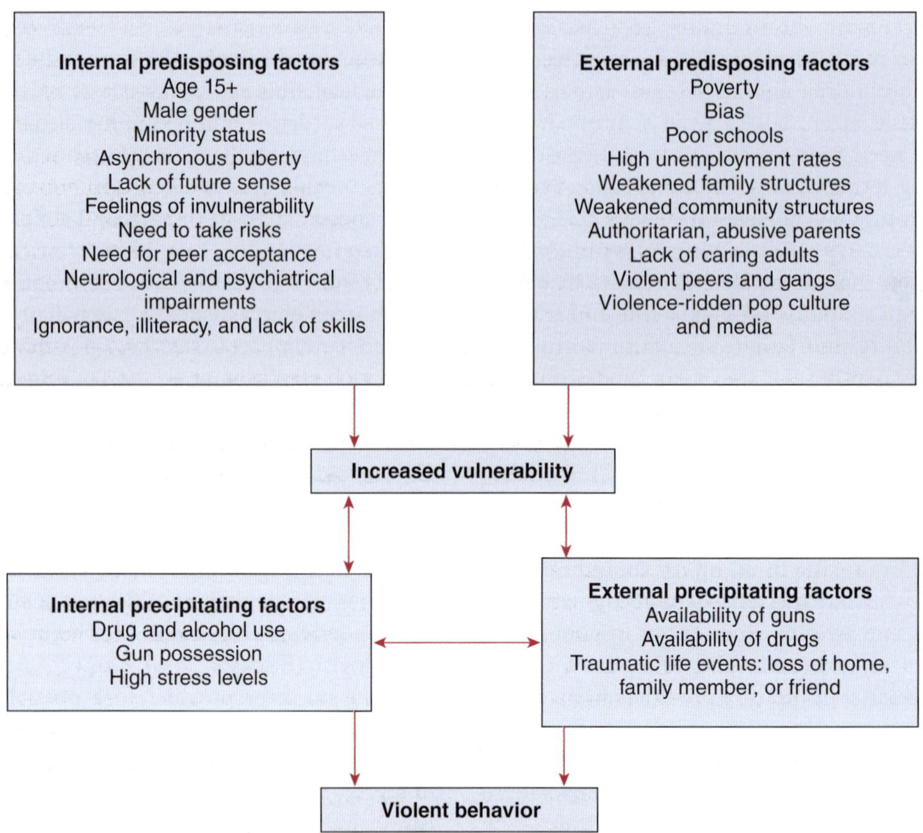

FIG. 21.5 Factors contributing to adolescent violence.

connectedness and support and decrease the level of bullying (Dow-Fleisner et al., 2023).

Electronic bullying can result in the development of mental health problems, which include self-injury and suicidal thoughts. The extent of bullying is positively related to the extent of health problems (Dow-Fleisner et al., 2023). As with any other form of bullying, receiving bullying text messages or being harassed on social media can make a teen feel insecure and may lead to school absences or serious emotional distress, including, in extreme cases, suicide.

Nurses engage adolescents, examining and realistically discussing the messages in videos, songs, movies, games, and television shows. Facilitating positive self-image and competency in peer relationships, along with helping adolescents access appropriate social supports, can be protective against adverse emotional experiences (Fredkove et al., 2019). Discussing their developing sense of self, their sense of belonging and where that sense is found, and their fears may help nurses to intercept adolescents who might otherwise turn to violence. Discussing frightening news events with adolescents in a realistic, contextual way might also help nurses mitigate fear and anxiety. Teens who are valued and nurtured by caring adults have the best chance of emerging from adolescence unscathed. Nurses may also discuss cyberbullying with adolescents, encourage them to talk to a trusted adult if they receive harassing text messages or to consider options such as rejecting texts from unknown numbers, and tell them that it is inappropriate to send harassing text messages to others. The warning signs of cyberbullying are similar to those that occur with any type of bullying and include changes in mood or behavior, decrease in school performance or reluctance to attend school, increased signs of stress, isolation from friends, unexplained injury, and altered sleep or eating patterns (CDC, 2023a).

Routine screening at well check-ups is essential to assess for bullying. Working with parents is important. Recent research suggests that parents are concerned about their child or adolescent using the Internet excessively (e.g., social media, streaming videos, gaming); they worry about social media misinformation, bullying, and Internet addiction. Conversely, some parents view access to the Internet as a positive influence on family relationships, connectedness and communication, and shared experiences (Kimball et al., 2023). Nurses can encourage parents to be vigilant regarding their adolescent's use of electronic media and work with them to set rules about use. These might include setting hourly limits; shutting off electronic media before bedtime; keeping devices out of the bedroom; encouraging other activities and hobbies; and arranging for regular device-free time together (AAP Center of Excellence on Social Media and Youth Mental Health, 2023; Astrop, 2020). If problems develop, parents might consider restricting access and using parental controls. Parents need to be aware of websites accessed by their adolescents, including YouTube sites, gaming sites, text messaging programs, and social media. Adolescents may be resistant to parental monitoring because of the perception that it invades their privacy; however, nurses can suggest that parents discuss these issues with teens before providing them with electronic access so that adolescents know from the outset that spot-checking will occur and there will be consequences for inappropriate use.

Biologic Agents

Infection

Infectious mononucleosis is a self-limiting viral infection transmitted by direct contact with body fluids, most frequently oropharyngeal secretions. It is prevalent among adolescents and is often referred to as the "kissing disease"; however, it can occur in younger children. It is caused by the Epstein-Barr virus. Typically, adolescents complain of a sore throat, lymph node enlargement, and lethargy. Both splenomegaly and hepatomegaly can occur, creating a risk of injury. The condition is self-limiting and resolves with symptomatic care and appropriate rest.

Meningococcal disease has declined considerably in the United States after the introduction of the preventive vaccine. The incidence remains highest in adolescents (age 16–23 years) compared with other age groups (CDC, 2023c). The CDC Advisory Committee on Immunization Practices (ACIP) (2023) recommends meningococcal vaccine administration to adolescents, with a first dose administered when the adolescent is 11 to 12 years old and a booster dose at 16 years old. Meningococcal B vaccine may be used for adolescents in certain high-risk groups (e.g., those with asplenia or sickle-cell disease).

Adolescents are at a stage of life with high sexual energy that may lead to high levels of risk-taking behaviors attributable to an increased sense of invulnerability. As adolescents experiment with and explore their sexual development and emerging independence, they engage in risky sexual behavior and expose themselves to increased risk of acquiring STIs. STIs most commonly include gonorrhea, syphilis, chlamydia, herpes simplex virus infection, human papilloma virus (HPV) infection, hepatitis B, and HIV infection. Approximately 50% of the newly diagnosed STI cases in the United States are among adolescents, and the incidence is higher in sexually active girls. Chlamydia, gonorrhea, and HPV are the infections most frequently seen (CDC, 2023e). The incidence of HPV infection has dramatically decreased since the introduction of HPV immunization for both females and males.

Many contributing factors have been identified and found to negatively effect this significant public and adolescent health problem. Nurses are aware of the cultural issues that may play a significant role in the prevention of STIs in adolescents. For example, there is a disparity in acquisition of STIs, with the incidence being higher in minority populations. This is not related to race but to adverse social environments that prevent access to education and treatment (CDC, 2023d). Factors such as inconsistent use of contraceptive and protective devices, increasingly earlier and more frequent sexual activity, lower self-esteem, depression, social and peer pressure, and an adolescent's sense of invincibility are related to higher risks of STIs. Lack of access to prevention measures or treatment in the adolescent population is also a major influence. Issues such as incongruence between the availability of medical professionals and adolescents' school or work, inability to pay for services, and concerns about confidentiality constitute barriers to access (CDC, 2021).

On the other hand, factors such as high self-efficacy, effective parent-child communications, parental monitoring, positive school relationships, and sexual knowledge could be significant protective factors to reduce the risk of STIs in adolescents (Hodder et al., 2018; Khurana et al., 2018). While nurses develop interventions for reducing STI-related sexual risk behaviors, they also take adolescents' cultural/ethnic backgrounds into consideration.

Several theories have been used to guide the practices of preventing sexual risk-taking behaviors in adolescents. The health-promotion model (Pender et al., 2010) has been used by nurses for the development of sexual risk-reduction interventions for adolescents, and these interventions were found to be effective. Most of the cognitive-behavioral interventions that stem from these theories report effectiveness in reducing the risk of HIV infection. Scientific studies show that well-designed and well-implemented HIV infection/STI prevention programs can decrease sexual risk behaviors among adolescents (Box 21.9: Evidence-Based Practice). Although adolescents can be evaluated and treated for STIs, the diseases must be reported, and the nurse needs to be aware of the government rules about reporting.

Cancer

Adolescents are affected by many of the same cancers as are younger children, such as leukemia, osteogenic sarcoma, lymphomas, and central nervous system tumors. Older adolescents are entering the period of their lives during which the risk for cancer of the reproductive and related organs is elevated. For females the focus is on cervical and breast cancer; for males, testicular cancer is of concern.

The peak incidence of breast and cervical cancer is during middle age, and breast and cervical cancers are actually rare in the teenage years. Risks for later development of these cancers can occur during adolescence, so prevention and surveillance are essential. Teaching females how to perform a regular breast self-examination is not currently recommended. Instead, recommendations emphasize focusing on breast self-awareness—knowing the normal size, shape, and feel of the breast to identify any observable abnormalities (American Cancer Society, 2022). Providers can encourage adolescent girls to become familiar with the normal appearance of their breasts and to report any changes of concern.

Cervical cancer is detected with a Papanicolaou (Pap) smear, obtained from the cervix during a pelvic examination; a test for HPV often is performed at the same time. Pelvic examinations are not performed on adolescents unless there is abnormal bleeding or vaginal discharge; however, all females should have a pelvic examination with a Pap smear beginning at age 21 years (ACOG, 2021, reaffirmed 2023). Factors that increase the risk of cervical cancer include early initiation of sexual intercourse (also applies to anal and oral sex), having multiple sexual partners or a sexual partner who has had many partners, any history of STIs in the adolescent or partner, smoking, and lack of condom use (American Cancer Society, 2020). Sexually active adolescents should be screened for STIs when taking a health history.

Administration of a vaccine to prevent cervical cancer and other diseases caused by certain types of genital HPV has been recommended by the ACIP (http://www.cdc.gov/hpv/). An HPV vaccination series is recommended for girls and boys at age 11 or 12 years (CDC ACIP, 2023). This is a two- to three-dose series, depending on age at first dose (younger or older than 15 years); recommendations are to begin the series with the first dose at 11 or 12 years (CDC ACIP, 2023). Ideally, females and males should get the vaccine before they are sexually active.

BOX 21.9 EVIDENCE-BASED PRACTICE

Adolescents' Sexual Health

Regardless of advances in prevention and treatment, sexual activity among adolescents increases risk for both unwanted pregnancy and acquisition of sexually transmitted infections (STIs). Finding ways of facilitating adolescents' commitment to avoid risk-taking sexual behaviors is considered a significant approach to encouraging sexual health in adolescents. One of the most effective approaches, aside from assisting parents with how to have sexual discussions with their teens, is including confidential and frank discussion with adolescents either at their regular well examination or through the school. Pertinent topics could include pubertal development, sexual orientation and identity, sexual activities, and healthy relationships.

Sieving and colleagues (2021) believed that these types of discussions occur rarely and wished to study the frequency of sexual health discussions between adolescents and providers. The goals of their research included identifying which topics are of most interest to both adolescents and their parents as well as assessing how often confidential discussions occur during health-promotion visits. Their probability sample consisted of 853 pairs of adolescents and matching parents identified through a confidential existing national survey; each pair accessed the research survey online. The survey asked about the importance of sexual topics that included puberty, safe dating, gender/sexual identity, STIs and HIV, birth control, sexual decision-making, and where to access appropriate services (Sieving et al., 2021). Questions also addressed whether these topics had been discussed or guidance provided at a previous health-promotion visit. The researchers restricted the sample to adolescents who had had a well visit during the previous 2 years to ensure adequate recollection.

Sieving and colleagues conducted multiple comparisons of the pairs in the sample: adolescent age (younger vs. older), sex, adolescents and parents, and perceived importance of topics versus actual experience of provider discussion (Sieving et al., 2021). Both parents and adolescents thought that the assessed topics are important to discuss at a well visit; the importance of topics differed somewhat depending on whether the adolescent was older or younger. Actual incidences of conversations reported to the researchers were exceptionally low. Much less than 50% of adolescents were asked about sexual activity or any of the other issues, except for puberty (Sieving et al., 2021).

Because adolescents are less likely to initiate conversations about these issues, Sieving and colleagues (2021) referred to their conclusions as a "missed opportunity" for providers to discuss important issues in a confidential setting. Nurses come in contact with adolescents in a variety of health care venues and have opportunities to begin these discussions confidentially. Offering support, clarifying misconceptions, and promoting preventive interventions will help adolescents navigate problems that could otherwise result in negative consequences.

Those who are sexually active may also benefit from the vaccine, but they may receive less benefit, because the vaccine will have no effect on HPV types they acquired before vaccine administration. The vaccine protects against HPV-related cancers in both boys and girls.

Testicular cancer is the number one cancer in adolescent and young adult males. Adolescent males should learn to perform a testicular self-examination and should continue this practice monthly (Box 21.6: Quality and Safety Scenario). Nurses introduce and teach methods of self-examination to adolescents, who naturally are interested in their developing bodies.

Chemical Agents

Substance Use and Abuse

Adolescents are influenced by a complicated interaction between biologic and psychosocial development, environmental messages, and societal attitudes regarding the use of substances such as alcohol, tobacco, or marijuana. Society as a whole is increasingly oriented toward using chemicals such as drugs, alcohol, and tobacco to feel better, look better, act more sociable, stay awake, sleep, be sexy or erect, or lose weight. Some of the most famous music, movie, and sports stars openly model substance use and abuse. It is no surprise that adolescents are making the choice to experiment with and use substances at younger and younger ages. Despite this, current use of substances (use within 30 days of assessment), especially alcohol and cigarettes, has significantly declined over the past 10 years (CDC, 2023f). Although 28% of adolescents report having tried marijuana, only 16% report current use (CDC, 2023f).

Alcohol is the substance used most frequently by adolescents who participated in the most recent Youth Risk Behavior Surveillance System survey (CDC, 2023f), with 23% reporting current use. Alcohol use is followed by marijuana use, misuse of prescription medications (12%), and use of inhalants (e.g., glue or other aerosols) (8%) (CDC, 2023f). Although overall heroin use has appeared to stabilize (1.3%), there are areas of the United States where heroin is readily available and current use would be higher. Heroin is particularly dangerous because it is purer than in the past and is also frequently laced with fentanyl, a potent painkiller.

The ready availability for sale and consumption of opioid prescription pain medications has led to a nationwide "opioid epidemic," which has affected people of all ages but particularly older adolescents and young adults. Opioid overdose, especially from synthetic opioids (e.g., fentanyl), is becoming a leading cause of death for people in these age groups. Poisoning from substance overdose is the second leading cause of death in the older adolescent population (CDC National Center for Injury Prevention and Control, 2023). Fentanyl overdoses represent 77% of total overdose deaths in adolescents (Hinckley, 2023). Illicitly manufactured fentanyl is readily available.

Evidence suggests that the misuse of prescription pain medications has caused many adolescents to become addicted through indiscriminate pain management of a musculoskeletal or other injury. This can occur in adolescents being seen in an emergency department, primarily for treatment of pain related to general surgical procedures, acute orthopedic injury, and dental pain (Hudgins et al., 2019). Contributing factors to this epidemic have included overprescribing, dispensing more doses than necessary, and lack of oversight (USDHHS, 2019).

Substance use is a precursor to substance abuse, which emphasizes the need for health care providers to be alert for and screen individuals for its presence. Identifying adolescent substance users or abusers requires a careful nursing assessment that is conducted in an accepting manner (Box 21.10) and referral for appropriate management. The AAP (2023) recommends that risk assessment for substance use be done at every well visit during adolescence. It is important to start prevention strategies early. Depending on the result of the screening, "brief interventions" such as health-promotion and substance-specific counseling are initiated to reduce risk; it is important to provide appropriate referral for those who have a significant problem (Camenga et al., 2022; Hinckley, 2023).

Substance use and abuse prevention and management require a community as well as an individual approach. For adolescent problem drinkers, Alcoholics Anonymous has pamphlets and other resources, including meetings, for young people who are

BOX 21.10 Major Signs of Substance Abuse

Nonspecific signs of substance abuse include the following:

- Disassociating from usual friends and peer groups; increased family problems
- Experiencing problems with grades and attendance in school
- Losing interest in formerly important recreational or other activities
- Lacking attention to activities of daily living and general appearance
- Getting in trouble with the law

Depending on the substance, the signs of abuse of the most commonly used substances can include the following:

- Agitation
- Altered sleep
- Appetite loss
- Blackouts
- Confusion
- Depression
- Diarrhea/nausea/vomiting
- Distorted perception
- Drowsiness/lethargy/slow reaction time
- Euphoria
- Hallucinations
- Itching
- Inability to concentrate or solve problems
- Memory loss
- Nausea or diarrhea
- Poor coordination
- Respiratory depression
- Unintentional injuries
- Weight loss

From National Institute on Drug Abuse. (2021). *What are the signs of having problems with drugs?* www.nida.nih.gov

ready to begin recovery. In response to the opioid epidemic, communities have supplied school, police, and emergency personnel with naloxone (Narcan) to be used for treatment of overdoses. Many states are approving legislation directed toward limiting the duration of individual pain medications, instituting prescription-monitoring programs, and facilitating the safe disposal of unused medications. Treatment equity is an important consideration, as a lack of or insufficient insurance coverage often prevents access to the necessary routine screening and counseling (Camenga et al., 2022). Some insurance companies are allowing patients to choose to receive fewer doses than prescribed and are increasing coverage for substance abuse treatment. Nurses need to be advocates for these and other approaches to this serious issue.

Tobacco Use

Although 6.3% of adolescents report beginning smoking at a young age, only 3.8% identify themselves as current frequent smokers. Smoking is more prevalent in White males and females than in Black or Hispanic populations (CDC, 2023f). Adolescents begin using tobacco for a variety of reasons, including wanting to appear older or wanting to imitate their friends, adult role models, or media images. Once they begin to smoke, many develop a nicotine addiction. Another less-used form of tobacco available is smokeless tobacco, such as chewing tobacco, snuff, or dip.

Over the past several years, adolescents have begun using electronic cigarettes (e-cigarettes, vaping devices) at an alarming rate, with 18% of adolescents reporting current use (CDC, 2023f). Vaping devices, some of which are as small as a computer thumb drive, are battery operated and vaporize flavored liquid for inhalation; there is no smoke involved. Originally designed to assist individuals with smoking cessation, vaping devices have become popular with adolescents, who, because of the device size, can conceal access during a school day. Not all adolescents who begin using a vaping device are cigarette smokers; however, because of the nicotine exposure, many can become smokers (Splete, 2019). This unique method of delivering nicotine has been used for other substances as well, most specifically the tetrahydrocannabinol (THC) component of marijuana. During 2019, users of vaping products began experiencing lung damage, leading to at least 68 confirmed deaths (CDC, 2020). Incidences occurred in nearly every state and have been linked to vaping THC. Research suggests that the lung injury is strongly correlated with vitamin E acetate used to assist with aerosolizing THC. As a result, the CDC recommends not using any vaping products containing THC, especially if purchased from individuals who cannot authenticate the safety of the product (CDC, 2020). Although many states forbid the sale of vaping products to adolescents and children younger than 18 years, 6.8% of adolescents in a nationwide survey reported having been sold products by a retailer (CDC, 2023f).

The nurse's primary prevention focus is on keeping nonsmokers from starting smoking and helping smokers to stop. Nurses can become actively involved in smoking-prevention programs through school districts or in the community. As with any other substance, health professionals can use the screening and brief intervention approach with adolescents.

DETERMINANTS OF HEALTH

Social Factors and Environment

School

Middle school, junior high, and high school bring new social experiences, introducing the adolescent to changing classes, multiple teachers and teaching styles, variable class schedules, homework load, and a variety of peer influences. School populations may be significantly larger than the child has experienced previously, and making and solidifying new friendships may be more difficult. Yet, despite these challenges, these school settings also provide meaningful in-school and after-school learning, peer contact, intellectual stimulation, and social or volunteer community service activities (Fig. 21.6).

Schools and peers, as opposed to home and parents, become the primary setting through which expectations are shared and standards communicated. During health-promotion visits, nurses ask adolescents about school and their friends and how they are doing with both. The nurse can also monitor adolescents as they prepare for and make the transition to their next social arena and role, whether it is college, vocational training, the military, or another career choice.

Culture and Ethnicity

Cultural and ethnic influences operate throughout childhood and continue into adolescence. The primary difference in adolescence is that teens might question, modify, or reject these influences, exchanging them for those of their peers or of the dominant cultural group. First-generation adolescents of immigrant parents have to negotiate two cultures, languages, and sets of expectations. These adolescents often live a double life that might result in increased stress. Adolescents from populations such as Black Americans, Hispanics, Asian Americans, Native Americans, Russian Americans, or Arab Americans

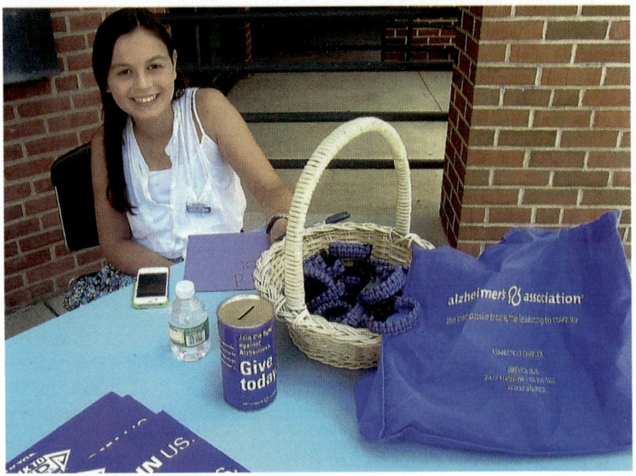

FIG. 21.6 Adolescents participate in school-sponsored community service.

might experience discrimination and rejection if they try to fit in to a middle class, White, Protestant culture. Advertising is directed to middle-class or affluent teens, not the economically depressed, and media images might not include attractive ethnic-looking models. Adolescents from different cultures might experience additional stress when their attempts to fit in to the dominant culture are contrary to the values and beliefs of their own culture.

The growing ethnic diversity in the adolescent population influences how adolescent health will be approached. The AAP has issued a policy guideline emphasizing the necessity for health professionals to become aware of and intervene in racial and cultural inequities from a health, education, and community perspective (Trent et al., 2019) (Box 21.11: Health and Social Determinants/Health Equity). With fast growth in the numbers of Hispanic and Asian American youth, cultural awareness of health care needs and increased attention to health disparities and academic outcomes are required, especially among adolescents from racial minorities and ethnic groups. It is essential for nurses to recognize their own biases to deliver culturally appropriate care. Nurses can become involved with community actions to provide safe spaces, education that helps adolescents achieve goals, access to nutritional food, and equality in housing (Trent et al., 2019). Nurses need to recognize the additional stresses experienced by adolescents and assess them for those stresses as they wrestle with not only their own identities but also their cultural identities.

BOX 21.11 HEALTH AND SOCIAL DETERMINANTS/HEALTH EQUITY

AAP Policy Statement on the Impact of Racism on Child and Adolescent Health

The American Academy of Pediatrics (AAP) (Trent et al., 2019) has identified racism as one of the most important predictors of a child or adolescent's overall physical, emotional, and social health. In general, when the social determinants of health (USDHHS, 2020) are considered, one thinks of such resource issues as accessing housing, education, nutritious foods, safe environment, employment, and health care, all of which affect quality of life and lifetime potential. It is not often that racism and freedom from bias, stereotyping, and discrimination are contemplated as social determinants of health. The AAP has issued an in-depth policy statement about racism's deleterious effects on children and adolescents and refers to racism as a "social disease." This phrase may be startling to some; however, in presenting the long history of the development of racism, the AAP describes scientific underpinnings that negate the biologic differences in humans based solely on superficial characteristics, most notably skin color. Instead, the AAP describes racism as the product of prolonged social, environmental, and educational marginalization based on overt and covert bias, combined with a cycle of diminished access to resources necessary for successful life outcomes. Not addressing racism for what it is will perpetuate disparities in health, educational attainment, employment potential, and economic stability (Trent et al., 2019).

As adolescents are developing a sense of identity, it is crucial for health care professionals to approach them in a culturally sensitive way. The AAP (Trent et al., 2019) states that providers of care need to set aside their own biases and stereotyping and assess adolescents for adverse effects of racism as an inclusive aspect of health assessment. These include such issues as victimization from bullying, increased stress, economic instability, and barriers to educational achievement (e.g., lack of diversity in educational systems, detention, suspension, missed school days, failure to graduate). Strong and positive identification with their specific culture and parental engagement are protective assets for adolescents to combat the effects of racism, as is diversity in social and educational settings. Other approaches include creating a climate of cultural acceptance in care, welcoming and providing high-quality care to everyone, and becoming community activists to reduce inequalities. Nurses can provide adolescents with strategies that assist them in recognizing racism, developing confidence to oppose it, accessing needed resources, and using positive actions to counter unfair treatment (Trent et al., 2019).

Levels of Policymaking and Health

Many laws and regulations are aimed at adolescents and deal with the minimum age at which they can assume adult responsibilities and decision-making. The rationale for these restrictions is that adolescents, although capable, lack the experience, perspective, and judgment to recognize and avoid choices that might be detrimental to them, so they require protection. A question raised frequently when minimum age is considered is whether strict age criteria are appropriate for any adolescent, particularly because development is variable, and experiences are diverse.

The restrictions that have recently been questioned most strongly deal with issues related to sexual activity. Variations that occur from state to state regarding access to and provision of contraceptive services and preconception education may become more of an issue as a result of the *Dobbs* decision. The nurse must be aware of legal age determinants as well as variations in definitions of **emancipated minors**.

The emancipated minor provision of certain laws recognizes that some adolescents become independent from their families at an early age and assume adult responsibilities. An emancipated minor is an adolescent who has not reached the standard legal age for certain activities, such as consenting to marriage or seeking certain kinds of health or illness care, but who is permitted to accept full responsibility for these decisions because the individual is economically and emotionally separate from the family.

Most often confidentiality is the more important issue for adolescents. The nurse can assure them that information shared will be kept confidential unless the teens pose a risk to themselves or others, or state or public health reporting mandates that the information be shared. For example, abuse must be reported, STIs need to be reported, and some states require adolescent sexual activity to be reported if an age difference of 3 years or more exists between the sexual partners. Nurses need to familiarize themselves with the legal rights of adolescents in their state and the resources available in their community.

Economics

Identification with peers, the essence of self-image during adolescence, includes dressing alike, having similar possessions, and doing similar activities, all of which require economic resources. This can cause a major conflict between parents and adolescents. Parents may think that they should have the power to decide how their adolescent spends money. Adolescents may believe, just as strongly, that they know the best ways to allocate resources and determine the amount of money they need.

Ideally, parents and adolescents should negotiate economic questions, with the parents becoming less controlling as the teen gains more experience and expertise in these matters. However, families with limited economic resources have fewer choices, and adolescents from these families may feel trapped by their circumstances. Poverty is particularly hard on children, and as they become adolescents, they often develop a fatalistic view of life.

Some adolescents seek employment to earn their own money and have control over it. Others work because their families need the income. It is important for the nurse to assess the economic resources of each adolescent's family and work within them when partnering with the adolescent in health care planning.

Health Services/Delivery System

Many health care resources are available to the adolescent. Teens can continue to see their child health care providers in a pediatric center as they did as younger children, but this setting is usually rejected because of the young-child atmosphere.

School-based clinics are frequently available in junior high and high school, and adolescent-focused clinics are available in many communities through both public and private agencies. Each of these clinics serves only adolescents, and the staff is oriented to the needs of this age group. Adolescents frequently have a stronger sense of comfort in these settings than in those in which young children or adults are also served.

Adolescents can also make use of services such as family planning clinics. These settings may designate certain days and hours for teens, whereas other facilities may integrate them into the adult-oriented protocols. Pregnant adolescents typically find prenatal care in an adult-focused setting, although more adolescent-specific programs are being developed. The physical needs of pregnant adolescents may be the same as those of pregnant adults, but the psychosocial needs are different and should be approached by a professional who has comprehensive knowledge of adolescent development and responses to stress.

The adolescent is a rapidly changing individual. The nurse who works in an adolescent-focused practice must be well prepared in adolescent health-promotion strategies. The nurse should have a thorough understanding of adolescent physical and psychosocial growth and development and should recognize each teen as a person.

Adolescents not only tend to be fearful of procedures or possible diagnoses but also have a desire to stay in control of situations. These conflicting feelings can be difficult to manage simultaneously. By establishing the adolescent as a partner with the health care providers in promoting good health and screening for health risks, the nurse facilitates the adolescent's sense of autonomy and control (Box 21.12).

BOX 21.12 HEEADSSS Assessment

The HEEADSSS assessment (Schmitt et al., 2021) provides a mnemonic that guides health care providers through an adolescent's psychosocial assessment. It is used both in community settings and in inpatient settings and is recommended for use by the AAP. Responses should be interpreted as those that are indicators of strengths or protection from risk and those that are indicators of risky behavior or situations.

Home
Education, employment, eating
Activities
Drugs
Sexuality
Suicide or depression
Safety

The adolescent's questions should be answered thoroughly and honestly. In many instances the adolescent is hesitant to voice concerns, so information is offered even when questions are not asked. An effective indirect approach to learning about adolescent concerns, especially about potentially embarrassing or stressful topics, is to say "Many teenagers ask me about [a topic]. Have you ever thought about this?" or "A lot of young people want to know about [a topic]."

Direct questions are also important, even about sensitive topics: "Have you ever thought about suicide?" "Are you depressed?" "Are you sexually active?" "If you are, do you use birth control and/or protection?" However, asking first about friends and the adolescent's feelings about them may be a good lead-in approach: "Are any of your friends doing drugs?" "How do you feel about it?" Vague or circuitous questions may be interpreted as a sign of discomfort or a lack of understanding and may cause the adolescent to be equally vague when responding.

Correct anatomical terms and descriptions of laboratory tests, disease processes, and possible outcomes are essential components in treating adolescents as individuals who are capable of being responsible for their own bodies.

NURSING APPLICATION

Adolescence is a period of rapid growth and development, with changes occurring physically and psychosocially. Nurses play a pivotal role in influencing adolescent health-promotion, preventive-screening, and disease-prevention activities. The primary responsibility for the nurse dealing with the important period known as the transition from childhood to adulthood is to provide education about some of its expected changes and how to deal with them.

Primary prevention methods are effective when the nurse is able to partner with adolescents in recognizing their specific health needs. Primary prevention is especially important for adolescents with special challenges and those with chronic illness (Alderman & Breuner, 2019). Treating teens in a respectful manner enables them to assume more responsibility. Nurses must remain sensitive to the changes the adolescent is encountering and understand the need for guided independence.

Teens are taught about the significance of their lifestyle choices with regard to future health. Poor nutrition, lack of exercise, drug and alcohol use, injury prevention, violence, infection risk, and tobacco use are all behaviors that are known to contribute to illness and death among teens. Nurses can use educational tools that appeal to the age group by conducting Internet searches for resources and recommending appropriate ones. Teens are able to relate to Internet resources, celebrities, and social media sites. Peers have the greatest influence on teenagers.

Nurses need to educate teens in partnership with their parents about the fact that unintentional injuries are the leading cause of death in the adolescent population. Nurses should reinforce research regarding seat belt use and the risks of distracted driving (e.g., texting or emailing while at the wheel, adjusting the radio, listening to loud music).

Adolescent girls are educated about breast self-awareness and the risks of engaging in sexual activity. Adolescent males are educated about testicular self-examination. Both sexes are encouraged to undergo physical examinations and follow the recommended vaccination schedule.

Various screenings are used by the nurse as a secondary prevention measure for the adolescent. Scoliosis screening is conducted in prepubertal and pubertal adolescents because early identification and treatment is important to prevent long-term disability or disfigurement. Nurses also screen adolescents for hypertension, eating disorders, type 2 diabetes, pregnancy, and STIs.

Adolescents respond better when they feel that they are regarded as young adults and partners in their health-promotion efforts. The nurse needs to become skilled at discussing difficult or embarrassing topics with teenagers. It is essential that adolescents feel they are treated with respect and regarded as individuals.

CASE STUDY

Drug-Facilitated Sexual Assault: Jessica

Jessica, a 16-year-old high school sophomore, arrives at the school nurse's office. She looks anxious and unsure of herself. She tells the nurse that she, along with several other girls her age, was invited to an overnight party at an older girl's house; they were driven there by a friend's parent. A group of high school boys were also at the party. The girl's parents were not at home, so there was alcohol available, and "everyone" was drinking. Jessica didn't like the way she felt but continued drinking to keep up with her friends. She wasn't due home until morning. Her concern in talking to the nurse is that she thinks someone might have had sex "without knowing it."

Knowing that sexual assault includes any type of sexual activity to which an individual does not agree, highlight any cues in Jessica's report that would be of concern to the nurse.

After analyzing the information Jessica has given, what action should the nurse take first?

What additional specific information will the nurse need to provide optimal care for Jessica?

SUMMARY

- Adolescence is a period of rapid change, when the integration of family, peer, educational, social, cultural, and community experiences begins to take form in the teen's sense of self.
- Many view adolescence as a construction site in its early stages. Onlookers assume that eventually a recognizable structure will emerge but have no idea what that structure will be.
- Although many parents, teachers, and health care providers may feel that hard hats and steel-reinforced shoes are needed, each is better equipped with an understanding of and respect for the adolescent's developmental struggles with physical and cognitive changes, autonomy, body image, peer relations, and identity.
- The goal is for the teen to emerge in young adulthood with a healthy body, mind, and spirit.

EVOLVE CHAPTER FEATURES

http://evolve.elsevier.com/Edelman/
- Study Questions

REFERENCES

Alderman, E., & Breuner, C., & AAP Committee on Adolescence. (2019). Unique needs of the adolescent. *Pediatrics, 144*(6), e20193150.

American Academy of Dermatology. (2020). *How to treat acne in skin of color*. www.aad.org

American Academy of Dermatology. (2023a). *Caring for new piercings*. www.aad.org

American Academy of Dermatology. (2023b). *Caring for tattooed skin*. www.aad.org

American Academy of Dermatology. (2023c). *Is sports equipment causing your acne?* www.aad.org/sports-equipment

American Academy of Orthopedic Surgeons. (2022). *A guide to safety for young athletes*. www.aaos.org

American Academy of Pediatrics (AAP). (2022). *Preventive care/periodicity schedule*. www.aap.org

American Academy of Pediatrics Center of Excellence on Social Media and Youth Mental Health. (2023). *How to build healthy digital habits: 5 tips for families*. www.healthychildren.org

American Cancer Society. (2018a). *Can testicular cancer by found early?* www.cancer.org

American Cancer Society. (2018b). *Risk factors for breast cancer in men*. https://www.cancer.org

American Cancer Society. (2020). *Risk factors for cervical cancer?* www.cancer.org

American Cancer Society. (2022). *American Cancer Society recommendations for the early detection of breast cancer*. www.cancer.org

American College of Obstetricians and Gynecologists (ACOG), Committee on Adolescent Health Care. (2020). *The initial reproductive health visit.* www.acog.org

American College of Obstetricians and Gynecologists (ACOG). (2021, reaffirmed 2023). *Updated cervical cancer screening guidelines.* www.acog.org

American Heart Association. (2023). *Understanding blood pressure readings.* www.heart.org

Arsandaux, J., Galéra, C., & Salamon, R. (2021). The association of self-esteem and psychosocial outcomes in young adults: a 10-year prospective study. *Child and Adolescent Mental Health, 26*(2), 106-113.

Astrop, J. (2020). Down with social media. *Community Practitioner,* 14–17.

Baher, A., Wallander, J., Elliott, M., & Schuster, M. (2023). Non-suicidal injury among adolescents: A structural model with socioecological connectedness, bullying, victimization, and depression. *Child Psychiatry and Human Development, 54,* 1190–1208.

Bell, B., Cassarly, J., & Dunbar, L. (2018). Selfie-objectification: Self-objectification and positive feedback ("Likes") are associated with frequency of posting sexually objectifying self-images on social media. *Body Image, 26,* 83–89.

Breuner, C. (2020). Adolescent pregnancy. In R. Kliegman, J. St. Geme, N. Blum, S. Shah, R. Tasker, K. Wilson, & R. Behrman (Eds.), *Nelson textbook of pediatrics* (21st ed., Chapter 144). St. Louis, MO: Elsevier.

Brooks, A. (2023). *Tips to prevent sports injuries in children and teens.* www.healthychildren.org

Boswell, K., Temples, H., & Wright, M. (2019). LGBT youth, sex trafficking and the nurse practitioner's role. *Journal of Pediatric Health Care, 33,* 555–560.

Calvin, S., Egan, J., & Coulter, R. (2019). School climate and sexual and gender minority adolescent mental health. *Youth and Adolescence, 48,* 1938–1951.

Camenga, D., Hammer, L., & AAP Committee on Substance Use and Prevention, Committee on Child Health Financing. (2022). Improving substance use prevention, assessment, and treatment financing to enhance equity and improve outcomes among children and adolescents. *Pediatrics, 150*(1), e2022057992.

Campanella Day, E. (2022). Communicating with LGBTQ adolescents: Preventing HIV and other STIs. *Pediatric Nursing, 48*(4), 163–166.

Centers for Disease Control and Prevention (CDC). (2020). *Outbreak of lung injury from use of e-cigarette use, or vaping.* www.cdc.gov

Centers for Disease Control and Prevention (CDC). (2021). *Sexually transmitted infections treatment guidelines, 2021.* www.cdc.gov

Centers for Disease Control and Prevention (CDC). (2022a). *Aerobic muscle-and bone-strengthening: What counts for school age children and adolescents.* www.cdc.gov

Centers for Disease Control and Prevention (CDC). (2022b). *Prevalence of childhood obesity in the United States.* www.cdc.gov

Centers for Disease Control and Prevention (CDC). (2023a). *Fast facts: Preventing bullying.* www.cdc.gov

Centers for Disease Control and Prevention (CDC). (2023b). *Genomics and health.* www.cdc.gov

Centers for Disease Control and Prevention (CDC). (2023c). *Meningococcal disease.* www.cdc.gov

Centers for Disease Control and Prevention (CDC). (2023d). *STD health equity.* www.cdc.gov

Centers for Disease Control and Prevention (CDC). (2023e). *STDs in adolescents and young adults.* www.cdc.gov

Centers for Disease Control and Prevention (CDC). (2023f). *Youth risk behavior surveillance – United States 2021 results: High school youth risk behavior survey.* nccd.cdc.gov/Youthonline

Centers for Disease Control and Prevention (CDC). (2023g). *Youth risk behavior survey data summary and trends report, 2011-2021.* www.cdc.gov

Centers for Disease Control and Prevention, Adolescent and School Health. (2023). *Parental monitoring.* www.cdc.gov

Centers for Disease Control and Prevention (CDC), Advisory Committee on Immunization Practices (ACIP). (2023). *Child and adolescent immunization schedule by age: 18 months to 18 years, 2024.* www.cdc.gov

Centers for Disease Control and Prevention (CDC), National Center for Injury Prevention and Control. (2021). *10 leading causes of non-fatal emergency department visits United States, 2021. All injuries, disposition: All cases, both sexes, all races, all age groups.* www.cdc.gov/injury

Centers for Disease Control and Prevention (CDC), National Center for Injury Prevention & Control. (2023a). *Teen drivers and passengers: Get the facts.* www.cdc.gov

Centers for Disease Control and Prevention (CDC), National Center for Injury Prevention and Control. (2023b). *Leading causes of death, all cases, both sexes, all races, all age groups, United States, 2021.* www.cdc.gov/injury

Centers for Disease Control and Prevention (CDC), Public Health Genomics & Precision Health Knowledge Base. (2023). *Genomics and precision health topics.* www. phgkb.cdc.gov

Chaves, E., Jeffrey, D., & Williams, D. (2023). Disordered eating and eating disorders in pediatric obesity. *International Journal of Environmental Research in Public Health, 20*(17), 6638. https://doi.org/10.3390/ijerph20176638

Chen, Y., Zhang, Z., & Zhu, B. (2023). The effect of an exercise intervention on adolescent idiopathic scoliosis: A network meta-analysis. *Journal of Orthopedic Surgery and Research, 18,* 655. https://doi.org/10.1186/s13018-023-04137-1

Cheung, A., Zucherbrot, R., Jensen, P., Laroque, D., & Stein, R. GLAD-PC Steering Group. (2018). Guidance for adolescent depression in primary care (GLAD-PC) Part II: Treatment and ongoing management. *Pediatrics, 141*(3), e2017–e4082.

Chew, K., & Temples, H. (2022). Adolescent eating disorders: Early identification and management in primary care. *Journal of Pediatric Health Care, 36*(6), 618–627. https://doi.org/10.1016/j.pedhc.2022.06.004

Cousins, J., Wong, K., & Chee, W. (2019). Multi-night sleep restriction impairs long-term retention of factual knowledge in adolescents. *Journal of Adolescent Health, 65,* 549–557.

Cucci, K., Thompson, J., & Derouin, A. (2022). Bridging the gap in adolescent depression: An action plan intervention. *Journal of Pediatric Health Care, 36*(3), 264–269. https://doi.org/10.1016/j.pedhc.2021.10.008

Curtin, S., & Garnett, M. (2023). Suicide and homicide death rates among youth and young adults ages 10 to 24: United States 2001 to 2021. In *National Center for Health Statistics Data Brief 471.* https://www.cdc.gov/nchs

DePaola, K., & Cuddihy, L. (2020). Pediatric spine disorders. *Pediatric Clinics of North America, 67*(1), 185–204.

Dow-Fleisner, S., Leong, A., & Lee, H. (2023). The interaction between peer bullying and school connectedness on youth health and wellbeing. *Children and Youth Services Review, 155,* 107147. https://doi.org/10.1016/j.childyouth.2023.107147

Erickson, C. C., Salerno, J. C., Berger, S., Campbell, R., Cannon, B., Christiansen, J., Moffatt, K., Pflaumer, A., Snyder, C. S., Srinivasan, C., Valdes, S. O., Vetter, V. L., Zimmerman, F., & Section on Cardiology and Cardiac Surgery, Pediatric and Congenital Electrophysiology Society (PACES), Task Force on Prevention of Sudden Death in the Young. (2021). Sudden death in the young: Information for the primary care provider. *Pediatrics, 148*(1), e2021052044.

Erikson, E. (1968). *Identity: Youth and crisis*. New York: Norton.

Fanous, Y., & Dorian, P. (2019). The prevention and management of sudden cardiac arrest in athletes. *Canadian Medical Association Journal, 191*(28), E787–E791. https://doi.org/10.1503/cmaj.190166

Flynn, J. T., Urbina, E. M., Brady, T. M., Baker-Smith, C., Daniels, S. R., Hayman, L. L., Mitsnefes, M., Tran, A., Zachariah, J. P., & Atherosclerosis, Hypertension, and Obesity in the Young Committee of the American Heart Association Council on Lifelong Congenital Heart Disease and Heart Health in the Young; Council on Cardiovascular Radiology and Intervention; Council on Epidemiology and Prevention; Council on Hypertension; and Council on Lifestyle and Cardiometabolic Health. (2022). Ambulatory blood pressure monitoring in children and adolescents: 2022 update: A scientific statement from the American Heart Association. *Hypertension, 79*(7), e114–e124, https://doi.org/10.1161/HYP.0000000000000215

Federal Interagency Forum on Child and Family Statistics. (2023). Youth victims of serious violent crimes. In *America's Children: Key National Indicators of Well-Being*. http://www.childstats.gov

Fredkove, W., Gower, A., & Sieving, R. (2019). Association among internal assets, bullying, and emotional distress in eighth grade students. *Journal of School Health, 89*(11), 883–889.

Gahagan, S. (2020). Overweight and obesity. In R. Kliegman, J. St. Geme, N. Blum, S. Shah, R. Tasker, K. Wilson, & R. Behrman (Eds.), *Nelson textbook of pediatrics* (21st ed., Chapter 60). St. Louis, MO: Elsevier.

Gangonil-Gagalang, E., Schultz, M., Badzek, L., & Calzone, K. (2023). Advancing nursing knowledge in precision health and genomics. *American Nurse Journal, 18*(9), 82.

Gaylor, E., Krause, K., Welder, L., Cooper, A., Ashley, C., & Mack, K. Crosby, A. E., Trinh, E., Ivey-Stephenson, A. Z., & Whittle, L. (2023). Suicidal thoughts and behaviors among high school students – Youth risk behavior survey, United States, 2021. *MMWR Supplements, 72*(1), 45–54. https://doi.org/10.15585/mmwr.su7201a6

Gerassi, L., Nichols, A., Cox, A., Goldberg, K., & Tang, C. (2021). Examining commonly reported sex trafficking indicators from practitioners' perspectives: Findings from a pilot study. *Journal of Interpersonal Violence, 36*(11–12), NP6281-NP6303.

Gilligan, C., Lyons, N., & Hanmer, T. (1990). Making connections: The relational worlds of adolescent girls at Emma Willard School. Cambridge, MA: Harvard University Press.

Greenbaum, J., Kaplan, D., Young, J., & AAP Council on Child Abuse and Neglect & Council on Immigrant and Family Health. (2023). Exploitation, labor, and sex trafficking of children and adolescents: Health care needs of patients. *Pediatrics, 151*(1), e2022060416.

Hahn, B., Blair Burnette, C., Hooper, L., Wall, M., Loth, K., & Neumark-Sztainer, D. (2023). Do weight perceptions in adolescents predict concurrent and long-term disordered behavior. *Journal of Adolescent Health, 72*, 803-810.

Halstead, M., Walter, K., & Moffatt, K., & Council on Sports Medicine and Fitness. (2018). Sport-related concussion in children and adolescents. *Pediatrics, 142*(6), e20183074.

Hampi, S., Hassink, S., Skinner, A. Armstrong S., Barlow S., Bolling, C. Avila Edwards, K. C., Eneli, I., Hamre, R., Joseph, M. M., Lunsford, D., Mendonca, E., Michalsky, M. P., Mirza, N., Ochoa, E. R., Sharifi, M., Staiano, A. E., Weedn, A. E., Flinn, S. K., Lindros, J., Okechukwu, K. (2023). Clinical practice guideline for the evaluation of children and adolescents with obesity. *Pediatrics, 151*, e2022060640.

Harrington, J., & Palmert, M. (2020). *Definition, etiology, and evaluation of precocious puberty*. www.uptodate.com

Hinckley, J. (2023). Fentanyl: Accelerant of the adolescent opioid crisis. *Child and Adolescent Psychiatry*.

Hockenberry, M. J., Duffy, E., & Gibbs, K. (2024). *Wong's nursing care of infants and children* (12th ed.). St. Louis, MO: Elsevier.

Hodder, R. K., Homer, S., Freund, M., Bowman, J. A., Lecathelinais, C., Colyvas, K., Campbell, E., Gillham, K., Dray, J., & Wiggers, J. H. (2018). The association between adolescent condom use and individual environmental resilience protective factors. *Australia and New Zealand Journal of Public Health, 42*(3), 230–235.

Hodges, A., & Ameringer, S. (2019). The symptom experience of adolescents with concussion. *Journal of Specialists in Pediatric Nursing, 24*, e12271.

Hornor, G. (2018). Bullying: What the PNP needs to know. *Journal of Pediatric Healthcare, 32*(4), 399–407.

House, H., Gaines, S., & Hawkins, L. (2019). Needs of our LGBTQ patients and their families. *Clinical Pediatric Emergency Medicine, 20*(1), 9–16.

Hudgins, J., Porter, J., Monuteaux, M., & Bourgeois, F. (2019). Trends in opioid prescribing for adolescents and young adults in ambulatory settings. *Pediatrics, 143*(6), e20181578.

Jiao, J., & Segrin, C. (2023). Moderating the association between overparenting and mental health: Open family communication and emerging adult children's trait autonomy. *Journal of Child and Family Studies, 32*, 652–662. https://doi.org/10.1007/s10826-022-02528-2

Juelich, J., Owens, R. Denny, D., Raatz, S., & Lindseth, G. (2023). Effects of sleep on adolescents' appetite, dietary intake, and weight. *Sage Open Nursing*, 1–10. https://doi.org/10.1177/23779608231206753

Kahn, L. (2019). Puberty: Onset and progression. *Pediatric Annals, 48*(4), e141–e145.

Khurana, A., Bleakley, F., Elliothorpe, M., Hennessey, M., Jamieson, P., & Weitz, I. (2019). Media violence exposure and aggression in adolescents: A risk and resilience perspective. *Aggressive Behavior, 45*, 70–81.

Kim, W. (2020). Acne. In R. Kliegman, J. St. Geme, N. Blum, S. Shah, R. Tasker, K. Wilson, & R. Behrman (Eds.), *Nelson textbook of pediatrics* (21st ed., Chapter 689). St. Louis, MO: Elsevier.

Kimball, H., Fernandez, F., Moskowitz, K., Kang, M., Alexander, L., & Conway, K. (2023). Parent perceived benefits and harms associated with Internet use by adolescent offspring. *JAMA Network Open, 6*(10), e2339851. https://doi.org/10.1001/jamanetworkopen.2023.39851

Kohlberg, L. (1981). *The philosophy of moral development*. San Francisco, CA: Harper & Row.

Kreipe, R., & Starr, T. (2020). Eating disorders. In R. Kliegman, J. St. Geme, N. Blum, S. Shah, R. Tasker, K. Wilson, & R. Behrman (Eds.), *Nelson textbook of pediatrics* (21st ed., Chapter 41). St. Louis, MO: Elsevier.

Laaksonen, M., Airikkala, E., Halkoaho, A., & Paavilainen, E. (2023). A scoping review: Do instruments measuring genomic competence in nursing incorporate ethics? *Nursing Open, 10*, 4932–4947. http://doi.org/10.1002/nop2.1805

Le, N., Belay, Y., Le, L., Pirkis, J., Mihalopoulous, C. (2023). Health related quality of life in children, adolescents, and young adults with self-harm or suicidality: A systematic review. *Australia and New Zealand Journal of Psychiatry, 57*(7), 952–965.

Lebet, R., Joseph, P., & Aroke, E. (2019). Knowledge of precision medicine and health care: An essential nursing competency. *American Journal of Nursing, 119*(10), 34–42.

Liu, Z., Zheng, C., Riggio, R., Day, D., & Dai, S. (2019). Leader development begins at home: Overparenting harms leader emergence. *Journal of Applied Psychology, 104*(10), 1226–1242.

López-Gil, J. F., García-Hermoso, A., Smith, L., Firth, J., Trott, M., Mesas, A. Jiménez-López, E., Gutiérrez-Espinoza, H., Tárraga-López, P. J., & Victoria-Montesinos, D. (2023). Global proportion of disordered eating in children and adolescents: A systematic review and meta-analysis. *JAMA Pediatrics, 177*(4), 363. https://doi.org/10.1001/jamapediatrics.2022.5848

Marzilli, E., Cerniglia, L., & Cimino, S. (2018). A narrative review of binge eating disorder in adolescence: Prevalence, impact, and psychological treatment strategies. *Adolescent Health Medicine and Therapeutics, 9*, 17–30.

Master, C., Bacal, D., Grady, M., Hertle, R., Shah, A., Strominger, M. Whitecross, S., Bradford, G. E., Lum, F., Donahue, S. P., & AAP Section on Ophthalmology, American Academy of Ophthalmology, American Association for Pediatric Ophthalmology and Strabismus, American Association of Certified Orthoptists. (2022). Evaluation of the visual system by the primary care provider following concussion. *Pediatrics, 150*(2), e2021056048.

Mendez, L., Modrowski, C., Mozeley, M., & Kerig, P. (2023). Trauma exposure and adolescent gang involvement: Distinguishing the roles of specific posttraumatic stress symptoms. *Psychological Trauma, Theory, Research, Practice, and Policy, 15*(S1), S92–S101. https://doi.org/10.1037/tra0001482

Menger, R., & Sin, A. (2023). *Adolescent idiopathic scoliosis*. www.ncbi.nlm.nih.gov

Mistovich, J., & Spiegel, D. (2020). Idiopathic scoliosis. In R. Kliegman, J. St. Geme, N. Blum, S. Shah, R. Tasker, K. Wilson, & R. Behrman (Eds.), *Nelson textbook of pediatrics* (21st ed., Chapter 699.1). Philadelphia, PA: Elsevier.

Montano, G. (2019). Homelessness among LGBT youth in the United States. *Pediatric News, 53*(2), 10.

Murray, B. (2019). Sexual health education for adolescents with developmental disabilities. *Health Education Journal, 78*(8), 1000–1011.

National Association of Anorexia Nervosa and Associated Disorders (ANAD). (2023). *Eating disorder statistics*. www.anad.org

National Association of Pediatric Nurse Practitioners, Evans, S., Derouin, A., Fuller, M., Heighway, S., & Shapiro, N. (2019). NAPNAP position statement on health risks and needs of lesbian, gay, bisexual, transgender, and questioning youth. *Journal of Pediatric Health Care, 33*, A12–A14.

National Institutes of Health Genetic Home Reference. (2019). *Adolescent idiopathic scoliosis*. https://ghr.nlm.nih.gov/condition/adolescent-idiopathic-scoliosis

National Institute on Drug Abuse. (2021). *What are the signs of having problems with drugs?* www.nida.nih.gov

National Institute of Mental Health. (2023). *Depression*. http://www.nimh.nih.gov

Norris, S., Frongillo, E., Black, M. Yanhui D., Fall, C., Lampl, M. Liese, A. D., Naguib, M., Prentice, A., Rochat, T., Stephensen, C. B., Tinago, C. B., Ward, K. A., Wrottesley, S. V., & Patton, G. C. (2022). Nutrition in adolescent growth and development. *Lancet (London, England), 399*, 172–184. http://doi.org/10.1016/S0140-6736(21)01590-7

Osinubi, A., Lewis-de-los Angeles, P., Poitevien, P., & Topor, L. (2022). Are Black girls exhibiting puberty earlier? Examining implications of race-based guidelines. *Pediatrics, 150*(2), e2021055595. https://doi.org/10.1542/peds.2021-055595

Osterman, M., Hamilton, B., Martin, J., Driscoll, A., & Valenzuela, C. (2023). Births: Final data for 2021. *National Vital Statistics Reports, 72*(1), 1–10.

Pediatric Endocrine Society. (2022). *Precocious puberty*. https://www.endocrine.org/patient-engagement/endocrine-library/precocious-puberty

Pender, N. J., Murdaugh, C., & Parsons, M. A. (2010). *Health promotion in nursing practice* (6th ed.). Upper Saddle River, NJ: Prentice-Hall.

Piaget, J. (1969). *The theory of stages in cognitive development*. New York, NY: McGraw-Hill.

Powers, M., Takagishi, J., & AAP Committee on Adolescence Council on Early Childhood. (2021). Care of adolescent parents and their children. *Pediatrics, 147*(5), e2021050919. https://doi.org/10.1542/peds.2021-050919

Quinn, H. (2023). How to care for inked skin. *Nursing Standard, 38*(2), 51–54.

Radhakrishnan, L., Leeb, R., & Bitsko, R. (2022). *Pediatric emergency department visits associated with mental health conditions before and during the COVID-19 pandemic – United States January, 2019-January 2022*. www.cdc.gov

Rafferty, J., AAP Committee on Psychosocial Aspects of Child and Family Health, & Committee on Adolescence Section on Lesbian, Gay, Bisexual and Transgender Health and Wellness. (Policy reaffirmed 2023). *Ensuring comprehensive care and support for transgender and gender diverse children and adolescents*. www.aap.org

Roberts, C. (2022). Persistence of transgender identity among children and adolescents. *Pediatrics, 150*(2), e202057693.

Schmitt, C., Koh, J., Borzutzky, C., & Wu, S. (2021). HEADSS up: Predictors for compliance of adolescent psychosocial screening by inpatient pediatric residents. *Pediatrics, 147*(3), 566.

Schulkind, L., & Sandler, S. (2019). The timing of teenage births: Estimating the effect on high school graduation and later life outcomes. *Demography, 56*, 345–365.

Seleckman, J., Monforto, K., & Seleckman, D. (2023). Violence toward and by youth: Part 1: Looking for the "whys." *NASN School Nurse, 38*(4), 187–193. https://doi.org/10.1177/1942602X231154549

Sieving, R., McRee, A., Mehus, C., O'Brien J., Wang S, Brar, P., Catallozzi, M., Gorzkowski, J., Grilo, S., Kaseeska, K., Santelli, J., Steiner, R. J., & Klein, J. D. (2021). Sexual and reproductive health discussions during preventive visits. *Pediatrics, 148*(2), e2020049411.

Splete, H. (2019). Vaping soars among American teens in 2018 survey. *Pediatric News, 53*(1), 2.

Stafford, A., Garbuz, T., Etter, D., Adams, Z., Hulvershorn, L., Downs, S., & Aalsma, M. (2020). The natural course of: Treatment in the primary care setting. *Journal of Pediatric Healthcare, 34*(1), 38–46.

Szucs, L., Pampati, S., Jingjing, L. Copen, C. Young, E., Leonard, S., DNP, & Carman-McClanahan, M. N. (2023). Role of the COVID-19 pandemic on sexual behaviors and receipt of sexual and reproductive health services among U.S. High School Students-Youth Risk Behavior Survey, United States, 2019-2021. *MMWR Supplements, 72*(1), 55–65.

Taba, M., Allen, T., Caldwell, P., Skinner, R., Kang, M., McCaffery, K., & Scott, K. (2022). Adolescents' self-efficacy and digital health literacy: A cross-sectional mixed methods study. *BMC Public Health, 22*, 1223. https://doi.org/10.1186/s12889-022-13599-7

Tang, C., & Damian, M. (2019). *Delayed puberty*. https://www.ncbi.nlm.nih.gov/books/NBK544322/#article-20323.s6

The Surgeon General. (2023). *My family health portrait*. https://cbiit.github.io/https://curehht.org/resource/family-health-portrait/

Thiboutot, D., Dreno, B., Sanders, V., Rudea, M., & Gollick, H. (2020). Changes in the management of acne, 2009-2019. *Journal of the American Academy of Dermatology, 82*(5), 1268–1269.

Townsend, M., Matthews, E., Miller, C., & Grenyer, B. (2023). Adolescent self-harm: Parents' experiences of supporting their child and help-seeking. *Journal of Child Health Care, 27*(4), 516–550.

Trent, M., Dooley, D., & Douge, J., & Section on Adolescent Health, Council on Community Pediatrics, & Committee on Adolescence. (2019). The impact of racism on child and adolescent health. *Pediatrics, 144*(2), e20191765.

US Department of Health and Human Services (USDHHS). (2018). *Physical activity guidelines for Americans* (2nd ed.), Washington, DC: USDHHS.

US Department of Health and Human Services (USDHHS). (2019). *What is the U.S. opioid epidemic?* http://www.hhs.gov

US Department of Agriculture (USDA) & US department of Health and Human Services (USDHHS). (2020). *Dietary guidelines for Americans 2020–2025* (9th ed.). www.DietaryGuidelines.gov https://www.dietaryguidelines.gov/sites/default/files/2020-12/Dietary_Guidelines_for_Americans_2020-2025.pdf

US Department of Health and Human Services, Office of Disease Prevention and Health Promotion. (2020). *Proposed objectives for Healthy People 2030*. Washington, DC: US Department of Health and Human Services, Office of Disease Prevention and Health Promotion.

US Preventive Services Task Force. (2018). *Adolescent idiopathic scoliosis screening*. https://www.uspreventiveservicestaskforce.org

Van Every, M. (2019). Male genital and reproductive functions. In J. Banasik & L. Copstead (Eds.), *Pathophysiology* (6th ed., Chapter 30). St. Louis, MO: Elsevier.

Vecchio, JM, & Carson, D. (2023). Understanding the role of violence and conflict in the stages of gang membership. *Youth Violence and Juvenile Justice, 21*(1), 27–43.

Wenhua, L., & Munoz-Laboy, M. (2023). Screening for depression and suicide risk in children and adolescents. *The Journal of Pediatrics, 261*, 113320. https://doi.org/10.1016/j.jpeds.2022.12.022

Williams, K., Monsman, H., & Chadwell, J. (2018). Why do adolescents engage in non-suicidal self-injury? *American Nurse Today, 13*(8), 37–40.

Wood, S., & Stevenson, E. (2023). Fertility planning is more critical now than ever. *Nursing for Women's Health, 27*(6), 403–406. https://doi.org/10.1016/j.nwh.2023.07.002

Xu, J., Murphy, S. L., Kochanek, D., & Arias, E. (2022). Mortality in the United States, 2021. In *National Center for Health Statistics Data Brief 456*. https://dx.doi.org/10.15620/cdc:122516

Yip, T., Wang, Y., Minguin, X., See, P. Fowle, J., & Buckhalt, J. (2022). School start times, sleep, and youth outcomes: A meta-analysis. *Pediatrics, 149*(6), e2021054068. https://doi.org/10.1542/peds.2021-054068

Zimlich, R. (2022). Teens, acne and mental health. *Dermatology Times, 43*(9), 21. www.dermatologytimes.com

Zucherbrot, R., Cheung, A., Jensen, P., Stein, R., & Laroque, D., & GLAD-PC Steering Group. (2018). Guidelines for adolescent depression in primary care Part I: Practice preparation identification, assessment, and initial management. *Pediatrics, 141*(3), e20174081.

22

Young Adult

Susan Natale

http://evolve.elsevier.com/Edelman/

OBJECTIVES

After completing this chapter, the reader will be able to:

- Identify the major developmental milestones of the young adult period.
- Summarize preventive health care recommendations for young adults.
- Analyze current trends in young adult health behaviors that may affect future health.
- Describe the nurse's role in reducing the rate of unintentional pregnancies in young adult females.
- Discuss the need for equitable access to sexual and reproductive health care for young adults.
- Evaluate strategies that the nurse can use to reduce risky behaviors in young adults.
- Critically analyze factors that contribute to health disparities in young adults.

KEY TERMS

Aerobic exercise
Assisted reproductive technology (ART)
Behavioral health integration
Binge drinking
Built environment
Cardiovascular assessment
Chronic traumatic encephalopathy (CTE)
Climate change
Clinician decision support tools
Deferred Action for Childhood Arrivals (DACA)
Direct-to-consumer genetic testing
Doxycycline Post-Exposure Prophylaxis Environmental justice
Expedited partner therapy (EPT)
Fetal neural tube defects
Food deserts
Genetic impairments
Gig economy
High-intensity interval training
Human immunodeficiency virus
Human papilloma virus
Infertility
Intimacy versus isolation
Maternal mortality rate
Metabolic syndrome
Noninvasive prenatal testing (NIPT)
Papanicolaou (Pap) smear
Patient-centered medical home
Point-of-decision prompts
Polycystic ovarian syndrome (PCOS)
Postconventional level of moral reasoning
Preexposure prophylaxis (PrEP)
Shared clinical decision-making
Sun protective factor
Syphilis
Unmet social needs

THINK ABOUT IT

Reproductive Health Disparities

Reproductive health disparities have existed for decades in the United States, primarily affecting females of color who experience higher maternal and infant death rates, higher rates of abortion, and an increased likelihood of contracting a sexually transmitted infection (STI) compared with White females (Hill et al., 2022). Recent events such as the COVID-19 pandemic and the overturning of Roe v. Wade have renewed focus on these disparities. States that have restricted abortion access have higher rates of maternal and infant deaths, fewer maternity care providers, and greater racial inequities compared with states without restricted abortion access (Declercq et al., 2022; Thompson et al., 2022).

- What can nurses do to decrease reproductive health disparities?
- What role does health policy play in reproductive health outcomes for young adults?
- Which geographic regions in the United States have the highest numbers of maternal and infant deaths? Which have the lowest?

The young adult period encompasses the ages from 18 to 35 years, a time that spans the end of adolescence to the beginning of middle adulthood. It includes the critical transition to adult roles and responsibilities, including navigating educational choices, attaining full-time employment, establishing an independent home, finding a partner, and possibly having children. This can be a challenging time, particularly for those from disadvantaged backgrounds or those who have experienced trauma or adverse childhood events (Berman et al., 2022). Although young adults are most often at their peak in terms of physical health, changing trends in the health of young adults make health-promotion efforts for this age group critical.

BIOLOGY AND GENOMICS

The young adult period is a time of many physical and emotional changes and is an opportunity for learning by experience and experimentation (Box 22.1: Quality and Safety Scenario). Young adulthood is characterized by greater complexity of thinking, appreciation for diverse views, further organization of emotional and cognitive development, and decision-making based on the effect on others and future consequences (Simpson, 2018). Today's young adults are better educated and more ethnically diverse than older generations. They are interested in health and wellness.

Developmental changes can vary by a number of factors, such as sex, education, race, sexual identity, temperament, substance use, and history of prior abuse or trauma (Simpson, 2018). Preventive health concerns for young adults can be separated into two categories: developing behaviors that promote a healthy lifestyle and decreasing the incidence of accidents, injuries, and acts of violence. The leading causes of death for young adults are largely preventable: unintentional injuries, suicides, and homicides. Deaths from unintentional injuries include injuries from traffic accidents, firearms, and poisoning, largely due to drug overdoses (Centers for Disease Control and Prevention [CDC], 2023a).

In 2022, approximately 20.5% of the US population was composed of adults aged 20 to 34 (US Census Bureau, 2023). Declining birth rates have led to projections that the young adult population will grow more slowly in future decades. The CDC (2023b) reports that the birth rate per 1000 for the population of all ages in 2021 was 11.0; this rate has been dropping since 1990, when it was more than 16.7 live births per 1000 people.

Physical maturation is mostly complete by the age of 20 years. The early 20s also sees peak physical development in healthy young adults, including muscle strength, reaction time, cardiac functioning, and sensory abilities (Taylor et al., 2022). Nursing goals for individuals of this age group are oriented toward prolonging this period of optimal physical energy; developing mental, emotional, spiritual, and social potential; encouraging proper health habits; anticipating and screening individuals for the onset of chronic disease and therefore being able to treat it at an early stage; and treating disease when appropriate. Health-promotion efforts are particularly important for young adults because health teaching for this age group has significant potential to directly influence future health for themselves and subsequent generations. *Healthy People 2030* (US Department of Health and Human Services [USDHHS], 2023) outlines a number of objectives designed to address health promotion and disease prevention that are pertinent to the young adult population (Box 22.2: *Healthy People 2030*).

BOX 22.1 QUALITY/SAFETY SCENARIO

Topic: Examining Problematic College Drinking Behaviors in Young Adults

Young adults between the ages of 18 and 25 report the highest drinking rates of any age group, and college students have been reported to drink at higher rates than non-college-age young adults. The 2021 National Survey on Drug Use and Health found that 49.3% of full-time college students aged 18 to 22 consumed alcohol in the past month, while 27.4% engaged in binge drinking. Binge drinking is defined as five or more drinks for males and four or more drinks for females. High-intensity drinking, or "extreme binge drinking" is defined as consuming 10+ drinks and is more common in males. Binge drinking and high-intensity drinking are associated with an increased risk of unintentional injuries and deaths, sexual assault, and sexually transmitted diseases. Binge drinking can also cause cognitive processing issues, such as blackouts (Patrick et al., 2022).

You are the clinic director and nurse at a small liberal arts college. Mary, a 19-year-old first-year student, has generally been a good student, easily making the adjustment to living away from home during her first 2 months in the dormitory. She comes to you to talk about an episode that occurred the previous weekend that frightened her. On Saturday night, she was at a party at a private residence in a rural, wooded setting away from the campus. She remembers consuming five or six alcoholic drinks; however, any memory after midnight is missing. She woke up in a fellow female student's dormitory room without any memory of leaving the party or returning to the dormitory. She was able to piece together information from her friends, who told her that she had consumed at least nine alcoholic drinks that night and that she had left the party with others who were returning to the dormitory, but they were not the friends with whom she had been seen all evening. She is concerned that she may have been drugged or that she may be having memory lapses. Assessment of her previous alcohol use reveals that she can recount at least four occasions during which she drank more than seven drinks at a party or family gathering. She describes her family as "social drinkers." On days that she anticipates drinking, she restricts her caloric intake. Last June, she was involved in a minor car accident that might have been related to her consumption of at least three drinks that afternoon. The road to this rural college has two roadside shrines dedicated to students who have died in automobile crashes near the college. To further analyze Mary's situation, you consider the following questions:

- Do you think that Mary has a problem with drinking? Would you classify her as a binge drinker? How do you clarify what she values?
- Is Mary engaging in risky behavior especially if she drives while drinking?
- What kind of physical assessment might assist you in making a determination that Mary has a drinking problem?
- What kinds of preventive educational programs could you advise?
- What kinds of monitoring and follow-up mechanisms might assist Mary in keeping her safe and in a treatment plan?

From Krieger, H., Young, C. M., Antheniem, A. M., & Neighbors, C. (2018). The epidemiology of binge drinking among college-age individuals in the United States. *Alcohol Research, 39*(1), 23–30.

BOX 22.2 ***HEALTHY PEOPLE 2030***

Selected National Health-Promotion and Disease-Prevention Objectives for the Young Adult

Symbol	Healthy People Objective
FP-10	Increase the proportion of females at risk for unintended pregnancies who use effective birth control
HIV-03	Reduce the number of new HIV diagnoses
IVP-03	Reduce unintentional injury deaths
MHMD-08	Increase the proportion of primary care visits where adolescents and adults are screened for depression
PA-06	Reduce the proportion of adults who do no physical activity in their free time
SDOH-02	Increase employment in working-age people
SDOH-06	Increase the proportion of high school graduates in college the October after graduating
SDOH-07	Increase the proportion of the voting-age citizens who vote
STI-03	Reduce the syphilis rate in females
TU-10	Eliminate cigarette smoking initiation in adolescents and young adults

From *Healthy People 2030*. US Department of Health and Human Services. https://health.gov/healthypeople

A classic public health indicator of a nation's health resources and services that involves young adults is the **maternal mortality rate**. The United States has one of the highest maternal mortality rates compared with other developed nations, and it has been steadily increasing. In 2021, the maternal mortality rate was 32.9 deaths per 100,000 births, a substantial increase from 23.8 in 2000 and 20.1 in 2019. In comparison, in 2020, Canada's maternal death rate was 8.4, and Japan's was 2.7 per 100,000 births (Commonwealth Fund, 2022). Significant disparities exist, particularly for Black females, who have 2.6 times the risk compared with non-Hispanic White females (Hoyert, 2023). Although the reasons for the increased rates are likely multifactorial, the COVID-19 pandemic is thought to have played a large role. *Healthy People 2030* has set an ambitious target of 15.7 deaths per 100,000 births. To reach this goal there is a need for robust national and statewide action to identify gaps in health disparities, access to health care, early prevention, treatment, and research (USDHHS, 2023).

Although young adulthood is generally assumed to be a period of relatively good health, there are several growing areas of concern (Box 22.3). In 2019, more than 53.8% of those aged 18 to 34 reported at least one chronic health condition, while 22.5% reported more than one. The most frequently reported conditions included obesity, depression, and hypertension. Those reporting chronic conditions were more likely to report physical inactivity, smoking, and binge drinking (Watson et al., 2022). Additionally, rates of obesity-related cancers, such as kidney, gallbladder, uterine, and colorectal, are increasing in young adult populations (Sung et al., 2019).

Economic and educational disparities, which may have been present in childhood and adolescence, can lead to health disparities in young adults. Higher education is closely linked to better employment opportunities and access to material resources such as housing. College-educated young adults report better health, and are less likely to report heart disease, diabetes, and mental health concerns, and are more likely to report healthy behaviors (USDHHS, 2023). Young adults (24–34 years) without college degrees have been found to have poorer cardiovascular health (body mass index [BMI], tobacco use, physical activity, diet, blood pressure, glucose, and cholesterol) compared with their more educated peers (Lawrence et al., 2018).

BOX 22.3 **Reductions in Life Expectancy**

Increases in life expectancy began to slow in the United States beginning in the 1980s and then began an actual decline starting in 2014. A 2019 report examining mortality rates for the period between 1999 and 2017 highlights the growing concerns about mortality data for young adults aged 25 to 34 years. The death rates for this group increased 29%, from 102.9 deaths/100,000 to 132.8 deaths/100,000 (Woolf & Schoomaker, 2019). Causes of the increased death rates include suicide, drug overdoses, and alcohol-related liver disease. Females have historically had an advantage over males in terms of life expectancy, and the data now show that gap is closing. It is critical to identify the root causes of these trends.

- What health system factors may be implicated in this decline?
- Suicide and drug- and alcohol-related deaths are sometimes referred to as "deaths of despair." What role does mental health play in these statistics?
- What are the implications for the nurse in terms of health-promotion counseling for the young adult?

GORDON'S FUNCTIONAL HEALTH PATTERNS

Health Perception–Health Management Pattern

Even though they may remain on their parents' health insurance until the age of 26, young adults become legally responsible for their own health care at the age of 18. Health care services for the young adult are important opportunities for disease prevention and health screenings. The majority of young adults consider their health to be very good to excellent (Grant et al., 2019). One goal for *Healthy People 2030* is to improve patient and provider communication. This goal focuses not only on in-person communication but also on the use of technology to improve online communication and increase patients' access to their own medical records (USDHHS, 2023).

At age 18 years (approximately the time of graduation from high school), a full health appraisal is recommended. The transition from pediatric care to an adult care provider is considered a developmental milestone and ideally has occurred at this point, although encouragement and support is sometimes required, and the process can be difficult to navigate (Simpson, 2018). The transition from pediatric to adult care can be particularly difficult for those with chronic disease and special health needs, resulting in fragmentation and lack of continuity in care (Box 22.4: Evidence-Based Practice). Despite initial increased insurance access under the Affordable Care Act (ACA), particularly for those 26 and under who can remain on their parents' plans, young adults have the highest uninsured rate of all age groups. In 2022, 14.0% of those aged 19 to 25 and 12.5% of those aged 26 to 34 were uninsured,

BOX 22.4 **EVIDENCED-BASED PRACTICE**

Transitioning to Adult Health Care

The transition from pediatric to adult health care can be difficult for young adults to navigate and may result in gaps in receiving needed or preventive health care services. This problem is magnified for young adults with intellectual disabilities, who often have complex medical and mental health comorbidities. A recent systematic review (Brown et al., 2019) examined the problems experienced by this group of young adults and their parents. The findings highlight the need for improved transition services. Majorities of young adults and their parents reported that transition planning was poorly executed or nonexistent. Parents experienced high levels of stress, frustration, and feelings of abandonment from the pediatric care team, and the need to advocate and "fight" for appropriate care for their child. Other challenges included difficulty finding adult providers willing to care for intellectually disabled and medically complex young adults, a lack of follow-up from adult providers, lost medical information, and a lack of support. The authors recommend early transition planning; greater collaboration between pediatric, adult care, and specialty providers; and identifying a lead agency to manage the transition. Additionally, knowledge is needed about the advanced care planning process, power of attorney, the guardianship process, and other legal issues that may arise with this population. It is suggested that nurses are uniquely suited for roles that facilitate this transition process, as transition management is a core nursing practice. These findings have implications for nursing practice, for nursing education, and at the policy level. More research is needed as to how nursing can best meet the needs of intellectually disabled young adults.

compared with a rate of 8.4% for all age groups (Keisler-Starkey et al., 2023). Access to health insurance makes it more likely that people seek out preventive care and receive recommended screening tests such as blood pressure checks, cholesterol screening, and others (USDHHS, 2023; Kaiser Family Foundation [KFF], 2019).

The health of young adults can vary considerably based on their health behaviors. For some, there is a focus on fitness and wellness. However, research has found that this age group is more likely to engage in unhealthy behaviors than past generations, have decreased physiologic status, and have increases in mental illness. More males than females engage in unhealthy behavior (Zheng & Echave, 2021). The rising prevalence of health-related misinformation can also alter health behavior, particularly misinformation concerning COVID-19, vaccinations, and reproductive health. Those without a college degree, racial minorities, and those living in rural areas have been found to be more susceptible to health misinformation (Lopes et al., 2023). Nurses play a critical role in educating young adults about healthy behaviors and correcting health-related misinformation.

Behavioral Health

Behavioral health encompasses mental health, including stress, substance misuse and health behaviors (Agency for Healthcare Research and Quality [AHRQ], 2023a). The United States Preventive Taskforce (USPTSF) recommends that all adults be screened for depression and anxiety at primary care visits (2023). A health history inclusive of behavior is particularly important for young adults. Risky behaviors are major causes of death and disability in this population. Both medical and behavioral health are important aspects of the overall health of young adults.

Preventive Care

The basic goals of preventive care are to maximize the period of optimal health status and detect risks for health problems. Studies indicate that young adults do not receive all the necessary preventive services they should (Alawode & Nicholson, 2023). The use of brief screening tools that are integrated into the electronic medical record (EMR), along with the use of **clinician decision support** (CDS) tools, improves the likelihood that young adults will receive timely screenings and required interventions while improving health outcomes (AHRQ, 2023b). These tools provide electronic reminders to the provider and health care team about which screening and preventive services are recommended at the time of the visit. The use of electronic patient registries allows the primary care practice to identify patients who have not received proper preventive services and aids efforts aimed toward population health. These approaches to preventive health care are cornerstones of the **patient-centered medical home** (PCMH), a team-based primary care delivery model. Nurses working in these settings have a unique role in population health management, while also providing opportunities for holistic nursing practice and care management (Ortiz, 2020).

Table 22.1 illustrates examples of preventive care that are important during the young adult period, along with the recommended frequency of screening. There has been an increased focus on identifying evidenced-based guidelines specifically designed for the young adult period, but current recommendations come from a number of different sources (National Adolescent and Young Adult Health Information Center, 2023). As a common expectation, the recommendation for most areas is a repeated health history and visit at approximately 2-year intervals, although assessment of individual risk factors should be taken into consideration. Under current ACA rules, compliant health insurance plans must cover an annual well physical exam and recommended preventive health services without cost or copays. Appropriate intervention at these visits is directed toward correcting health issues through history assessment and counseling about avoidance of adverse health behaviors. Subsequent counseling sessions focus on rechecking and updating information gathered in earlier meetings. Since **unmet social needs** (such as food insecurity, lack of transportation, or problems paying for utilities) contribute greatly to health status, screening for social determinants of health should also occur (Fraze et al., 2019; Onie et al., 2018) (Box 22.5: Best Practice). Table 22.2 is an example of a social needs screening tool.

A physical examination includes measurements of height, weight, BMI, and blood pressure, and blood tests. An emphasis should be placed on health behavior counseling, particularly the risk factors of tobacco use, poor nutrition, lack of physical activity, and excessive alcohol use. Screening for cervical cancer is strongly recommended in females who have been sexually active (**Papanicolaou [Pap] smear**). Current recommendations for cervical cancer screening include testing every 3 years for those aged ≥21 years. Beginning at the age of 30, the addition of high-risk human papillomavirus screening should occur every 5 years. Current guidelines recommend against cervical cancer screening

TABLE 22.1 Young Adult Preventive Health Monitoring (Examples)

	AGE 18–25 YEARS	
Health Issue	**Intervention**	**Frequency**
Tobacco screening and counseling	History and counseling	Each visit
Obesity/body mass index	History, weight, and counseling	Each visit
Alcohol screening and counseling	History and counseling	Each visit
Accidental injury, lap and shoulder belts, bicycle or motorcycle helmets, smoke detectors, safe firearm use	History and counseling	Each visit
Contraception	Counseling	Each visit
Depression	Counseling	Each visit
Illegal drug use screening	History and counseling	Each visit
Hypertension/blood pressure	Blood pressure measurement	Every 3–5 years with no other risks
Tetanus, diphtheria, pertussis	Tdap booster vaccine	Td booster every 10 years
Hepatitis B	Immunization	If not immunized
Diabetes, proteinuria, bacteriuria	Urinalysis	Once
Dyslipidemia	Cholesterol, triglyceride levels	Once between 17 and 21 years
Cervical dysplasia	Gynecological examination; Papanicolaou smear	Every 3 years, start at age 21 years
STI prevention	Counseling—offer HPV vaccine	Individually determined based on risk
Chlamydia (women)	Chlamydia screen	At gynecologic examination if sexually active
Gonorrhea	Vaginal culture	At gynecologic examination if sexually active
Influenza	Seasonal flu vaccine	Each year

Recommendations collated from National Adolescent and Young Adult Health Information Center, Bright Futures, American Congress of Obstetricians and Gynecologists (ACOG).
HPV, Human papilloma virus; STI, sexually transmitted infection.
Modified from National Adolescent and Young Adult Health Information Center (2023).

BOX 22.5 BEST PRACTICE

Screening for Social Needs

There is growing evidence that up to 60% or more of health outcomes are related to social and environmental factors. Social determinants, such as access to healthy food, safe and affordable housing, and transportation, have a great affect on a person's health. A shift in focus to population health, in addition to health reform efforts, has fueled a growing number of health care providers to screen their patients for social needs in addition to medical needs. Screening for these needs can help health care systems better plan services for their patients, meet individual patient needs, and facilitate referrals to outside community resources—all with the goal of improving health outcomes for those with unmet social needs (Onie et al., 2018; Woolf, 2019).

for females younger than 21 years (US Preventive Services Task Force [USPSTF], 2023). The USPSTF also currently recommends against teaching breast self-examination or testicular self-examination based on insufficient evidence of benefit, although some health care providers may continue to support the practice.

Chronic disease, such as cardiovascular disease and cancer, is the leading cause of mortality for adults. The young adult period offers opportunities to lower the risk of chronic disease in later years. **Cardiovascular assessment** of the young adult should begin at the age of 20 and occur at least every 4 to 6 years (Arnett et al., 2019). Risk factors for cardiovascular disease include obesity and unhealthy diets, hypertension, elevated cholesterol, diabetes, and physical inactivity. Other risk factors that should be assessed include family history of premature cardiovascular disease, the presence of metabolic syndrome, and chronic inflammatory conditions such as rheumatoid arthritis. Nurses can assist in gathering a comprehensive health history, including pertinent information about family history of cardiovascular disease. In females, a history of pregnancy-induced hypertension or preeclampsia is an important risk factor for cardiovascular disease (Carey & Whelton, 2018; Stone et al., 2022).

The prevalence of hypertension among young adults aged 18 to 39 during the period from 2017 to 2018 was 22.4%. Prevalence was higher for males than for females (31.2% compared with 13.0%) (Ostchega et al., 2020). Young adults diagnosed with hypertension have a significantly higher risk of adverse cardiovascular events in later life (Yano et al., 2018). Brain changes that may lead to cognitive decline in midlife have been linked to younger adults aged 20 to 40 with hypertension. This finding supports more aggressive management of hypertension in this age group (American Heart Association, 2022a).

Metabolic syndrome includes a cluster of cardiovascular risk factors associated with overweight and obesity, particularly abdominal obesity. It includes a constellation of disorders, including elevated blood pressure, hyperglycemia, hyper triglyceridemia, and reduced high-density lipoprotein cholesterol (HDL). Many studies have demonstrated that this cluster of symptoms is related to increased risk for type 2 diabetes and cardiovascular disease. A prominent sign of metabolic syndrome is central adiposity, or waist-centered obesity. The prevalence of metabolic syndrome has been increasing in the United States, and in 2021, 41.8% of the adult population had the disorder. The prevalence

TABLE 22.2 Social Needs Screening Tool

	Yes/No
In the past 12 months, did you ever eat less than you felt you should because there wasn't enough money for food?	
In the last 12 months, has the electric, gas, oil, or water company threatened to shut off your services in your home?	
Are you worried that in the next 2 months, you may not have stable housing?	
Do problems with childcare make it difficult for you to work or study? (Leave blank if you do not have children.)	
In the past 12 months, have you needed to see a doctor but could not because of cost?	
In the last 12 months, have you ever had to go without health care because you didn't have a way to get there?	
Do you ever need help reading hospital materials?	
Do you often feel that you lack companionship?	
Are any of your needs urgent? For example: I don't have food tonight, I don't have a place to sleep tonight	
If you responded YES to any boxes above, would you like to receive assistance with any of these needs?	

Adapted from the Health Leads Social Needs Screening Toolkit. Available at www.healthleadsusa.org.

of metabolic syndrome in young adults aged 20 to 39 years was 22.2% during the same period. First-step therapy includes lifestyle alterations, including weight management and increased physical activity (Liang et al., 2023).

Diabetes is the eighth-leading cause of death in the United States and significantly contributes to cardiovascular disease risk. In 2021, 38.4 million Americans had diabetes: 29.7 million who had been diagnosed and an estimated 8.7 million who had not been diagnosed. Minority populations (Black Americans, Native American/Alaska Natives, and Hispanics) have been disproportionately affected, with Native American populations experiencing twice the rate of new cases recorded in non-Hispanic White populations (CDC, 2023c). The incidence of diabetes, especially type 2 diabetes, and related complications (cardiovascular disease, blindness, lower limb amputations, and kidney disease) has been increasing in the United States. An estimated 18% of adolescents and 24% of young adults (19–34) are now living with prediabetes. The prevalence is higher in males and those who are obese. Prediabetes is a state characterized by elevated cholesterol, systolic blood pressure, central adiposity, and lower insulin resistance (Andes, Cheng, & Rolka, 2019). Prediabetes increases the risk of type 2 diabetes and cardiovascular disease. Because careful control can delay the beginning and progression of long-term complications, nursing efforts directed at early detection and monitoring of diabetes in young adults are important.

Decision-Making and Risk-Taking

The decision-making of a young adult directly affects health and well-being. Peak physical skills stimulate young adults to be venturesome, daring, enterprising, and aggressive. Young adults have less experience with the death of significant people in their lives, and they may take inordinate risks. The leading causes of death in individuals 15 to 24 years of age combined are unintentional injuries, homicide, and suicide (CDC, 2023a). The prevalence of adverse behaviors associated with sudden death illustrates a developmental lack of fear in young adults. Bullying, dating violence, and sexual violence are becoming more prevalent. Underuse of seat belts and helmets by motorcyclists and bicyclists are a cause of many accidental injuries and deaths. Some states still do not have laws that require the use of helmets.

Communicable Diseases and Adult Immunization

Communicable (infectious) diseases affect young adults with differing degrees of severity. Although increased availability of better drug treatments and/or vaccines, improved hygiene and food handling, and provision of cleaner water supplies have promoted prevention and control of infectious disease, new disease threats are continually emerging. The threat of emerging infectious disease is due to improvements in travel and changes in social, sexual, and other behaviors that expose broader populations of individuals to emerging pathogens. These threats must be understood in a global context because of increasing travel and migration, human encroachment into animal habitats, importation of foods, agriculture practices, and bioterrorism. New communicable disease threats may occur because of climate change, which is responsible for expanding the habitats of disease-carrying mosquitos. Other emerging threats are related to antibiotic resistance (Rector & Stanley, 2022).

COVID-19 is an example of a novel pathogen that emerged in 2019. Although older adults were more likely to be hospitalized and die from COVID-19 infection, young adults were also affected. In a study examining the clinical outcomes of young adults hospitalized with COVID during 2020, the presence of obesity, hypertension and diabetes increased the risks of adverse outcomes. Of those hospitalized, 36.8% suffered from obesity, 24.5% were morbidly obese, 18.2% were diabetic, and 16.1% had hypertension. A total of 21% required intensive care, and 2.7% of those died (Cunningham et al., 2021).

Seasonal influenza is a common threat for all ages. A goal of *Healthy People 2030* is to increase the percentage of persons who are vaccinated for seasonal influenza (USDHHS, 2023). During the 2021 to 2022 flu season, 37.1% of adults aged 18 to 49 were vaccinated. This age group typically has the lowest vaccination rate compared with others. Those that are very young or old have the greatest risk of adverse outcomes from the flu, however, young adults with chronic conditions, those who are pregnant, and those who work in health care are at higher risk (CDC, 2023d).

The incidence of tuberculosis (TB) is decreasing in the United States. In 2022, about 2.5 per 100,00 cases were reported, with most of those in non–US-born persons (CDC, 2023e).The nurse should be aware that many countries with high prevalence of TB use the BCG (Bacille Calmette-Guerin) vaccine in children, which may later result in false positive reactions with the tuberculin skin test (TST). Blood tests for TB are not affected (Okafor et al., 2023).

Injection drug users are at higher risk of developing hepatitis B (HBV), hepatitis C (HCV), and **human immunodeficiency virus** (HIV). Vaccination against HBV is available and is generally obtained during childhood. The vaccine should be offered to young adults who are not vaccinated. Currently, there is no vaccine for HCV. Injection drug users, hemodialysis patients, and those with HIV infection should therefore be screened. Curative advances in drug treatment for HCV have made better case findings more important (CDC, 2022a; CDC, 2023f).

Cases of meningococcal diseases have been declining since the 1990s, and most outbreaks are sporadic. However, the disease can be deadly in adults in as little as a few hours. Young adults up to the age of 23 are at particular risk. Brain damage, hearing loss, and learning challenges can result in permanent disability for survivors. Young adults living in college/university dormitories and military barracks have an increased risk compared with young adults not living in close settings (CDC, 2022b). Most colleges require proof of vaccination before entrance. Specific recommendations are also indicated to control sudden outbreaks of meningococcal disease.

Other viruses, such as **human papilloma virus** (HPV), commonly affect young adults. HPV is spread through sexual contact, and some strains of the virus are related to the later development of cervical dysplasia and cancer, in addition to vulvar, vaginal, anal, penile, and oropharyngeal cancers. The Advisory Committee on Immunization Practices recommends that all children and adults be vaccinated up to the age of 26. In 2018, the catch-up guidelines for vaccination were expanded to those aged 27 to 45 years based on **shared clinical decision-making** with a provider (CDC, 2022c). A *Healthy People 2030* goal seeks to reduce HPV infections that could have been prevented by vaccination. In 2021, 58.5% of 13- to 15-year-olds had received 2 or 3 doses of the HPV vaccine (USDHHS, 2023). More girls than boys have been vaccinated. Other STIs affecting young adults are discussed later in the chapter.

Nutritional-Metabolic Pattern

Young adults are body conscious—they value thinness, defined muscle tone, and athletic ability. However, over 74% of adults in the United States are overweight or obese, increasing cardiometabolic and other health risks (CDC, 2023g). During the young adult years, a number of life events increase the likelihood of weight gain: college, marriage, and beginning a family. Stress is also a contributing factor. Risk factors for obesity include consuming large amounts of energy-dense foods, unhealthy eating habits, increased screen time, and poor sleep quality (Lee et al., 2023).

Maintaining a healthy body weight is influenced by the amount of energy that is expended, closely linking body weight with physical activity. Regular physical activity increases muscle and bone strength, decreases body fat, aids in weight control, enhances well-being, and reduces depression. Females aged 19 to 30 typically require 1800 to 2400 calories per day, while males in the same age group require 2400 to 3000 calories per day. Caloric needs decrease somewhat after the age of 30, with females requiring 1600 to 2200 calories per day and males requiring 2200 to 3000 calories per day. Specific caloric needs are based on activity level, with less caloric need if sedentary and higher caloric need if active. Pregnant and lactating females require additional caloric intake. No additional caloric intake is recommended during the first trimester; an additional 340 calories daily is recommended during the second trimester; and 452 additional calories daily is recommended during the third trimester. Lactation during the first 6 months after birth requires an additional 330 calories daily, increasing to 400 calories daily beyond 6 months. Assuming a prepregnancy healthy weight, the typical females gains 25 to 35 pounds during pregnancy (US Department of Agriculture and USDHHS, 2020).

US dietary guidelines recommend eating foods that are nutrient dense and reflective of personal and cultural preferences, with consideration of budgetary factors (US Department of Agriculture and USDHHS, 2020). Increased caloric intake without a corresponding increase in energy expenditure can lead to obesity, which is a significant risk factor for hypertension, cardiovascular disease, and diabetes. Increasing rates of obesity-related cancers are becoming more prevalent in young adult populations (Sung et al., 2019).

The prevalence of obesity among US adults aged 20 to 39 years was 39.8% from 2017 to 2020 (CDC, 2023g). Hispanic and non-Hispanic Blacks had the highest levels of obesity. Nurses, with other health providers, can investigate weight problems by measuring waist circumference, blood pressure, cholesterol levels, and activity levels rather than weight alone. Assessments of weight and height are used to calculate BMI. Whereas BMI may be a good indicator for population screening, it may not be the best measurement for predicting health risks, as each individual's cardiovascular and obesity-related risks must be assessed (CDC, 2022d). A normal BMI is considered less than 25 kg/m^2. A BMI of between 25 and 29 kg/m^2 is considered overweight. Individuals with a BMI of 30 kg/m^2 should be offered or referred to intensive multicomponent behavioral interventions, which may include pharmacologic management. Those with a BMI greater than 35 kg/m^2 and with the presence of obesity-related comorbid conditions may be referred for bariatric surgery. Obesity comorbidities include diabetes, hypertension and other cardiovascular conditions, nonalcoholic fatty liver disease, obstructive sleep apnea, asthma, reproductive disorders, impaired renal function, impaired quality of life, and depression (Lim & Boster, 2023). Those with a BMI greater than 40 should be referred for surgical consideration regardless of comorbidities. However, the focus of nursing advice is conservative at first—recommending lifestyle management, careful diet appraisal, and increase in exercise patterns—and should be offered to all who are overweight or obese.

Pharmacologic interventions for obesity should be reserved for those with a BMI of 30 kg/m^2 or greater and for those with a BMI of between 27 and 29.9 kg/m^2 with weight-related comorbidities. Newer treatments include glucagon-like peptide

(GLP-1) receptor agonists, which are administered via subcutaneous injection. These drugs stimulate glucose-dependent insulin secretion, inhibit glucagon release, and delay gastric emptying, resulting in weight loss (Perreault, 2023).

For many Americans, food sources are abundant, portion sizes have increased, and lifestyles are becoming increasingly sedentary. Young adult diets should contain a variety of nutrient-dense foods, especially whole grains, fruits, vegetables, low-fat or fat-free milk, lean meats, and protein sources. Caloric intake and intake of saturated and trans fats, cholesterol, added sugars, sodium, and alcohol should be limited. Food label information on all processed and packaged foods should be read. Another challenge is the increasing consumption of food prepared and eaten away from home, which is generally higher in fat, cholesterol, and sodium and lower in fiber and calcium than food prepared in the home (CDC, 2023h). Many states have legislation that requires restaurants and fast food outlets to list food composition on menus. Low-income communities may be considered **food deserts**, areas that lack large supermarkets where fresher and healthier food can be purchased, and more often only provide neighborhood convenience stores or small markets that stock nutrient-poor snacks, sugar-sweetened drinks, and less-fresh fruits and vegetables. Food insecurity, or limited or uncertain access to adequate food, also increases the risk of obesity (USDHHS, 2023). A lack of transportation options in these communities contributes to the problem. Collective national action and community involvement are needed to promote healthful diets among all Americans across the life span.

Long-term weight management is a frustrating process. Weight loss approaches should be specifically tailored for the young adult population and can include technologic supports such as smartphone applications and social media. Interventions found promising include goal setting, self-monitoring tools, tailored feedback, social support, and behavioral prompts (Willmott et al., 2019). Applying principles of motivational interviewing and addressing the problems of obesity and overweight through use of a chronic care model offers potential for long-range weight management (Anderson et al., 2023). Addressing young adult obesity is a particularly challenging problem.

Proper nutrition is particularly necessary for the young adult female during the childbearing years. The factors contributing to iron deficiency in this age group are regular loss of blood (during menses) and pregnancy. Iron deficiency anemia can result from a blood loss of 2 to 4 mL/day (1–2 mg of iron). Young females who do not eat a healthy diet and have heavy periods or who use nonsteroidal antiinflammatory drugs are specifically at risk. Iron supplementation is recommended during pregnancy to promote growth of the fetus (Georgieff, Krebs, & Cusick, 2019). The USPSTF recommends that all females who are planning or capable of becoming pregnant take a daily folic acid supplement (400–800 mcg) to reduce the risk of **fetal neural tube defects**, including spina bifida (USPSTF, 2023). Since nearly half of all pregnancies are unplanned and neural tube defects occur in the first weeks of pregnancy, the recommendation for all females capable of becoming pregnant to take folic acid supplementation is especially important. Fortification of foods (cereals, bread) with folic acid has also aided in these efforts. Since these recommendations went into effect, neural tube defects have decreased (CDC, 2023i).

Most adolescent and adult females fail to meet their calcium requirements, placing them at risk of osteoporosis and bone fractures in later life. Low calcium intake is a direct result of low milk consumption related to soft drink ingestion. An increase in intake of calcium-containing foods is therefore recommended, particularly for teens and young females (see Chapter 11).

Elimination Pattern

Patterns of elimination are generally well established by young adulthood. Although eating disorders (anorexia and bulimia) typically begin at an earlier stage of development, they can persist during young adulthood. Gastrointestinal symptoms are common in the general population. In one study of college students, one-third of participants reported at least one gastrointestinal symptom of a severity beyond expected normal levels. Commonly reported symptoms included gas or bloating, nausea/vomiting, belly pain, constipation, and diarrhea (Vivier et al., 2020). The nurse plays a role in educating the young adult about common gastrointestinal complaints such as constipation, hemorrhoids, and occasional diarrhea, as well as in recognizing symptoms requiring further evaluation.

The overall incidence of colorectal cancer has been in decline for the general population; however, rates for young adults, aged 20 to 39, have been increasing. Risk factors for colorectal cancer include family history of the disease, excess body weight, high consumption of processed meats and alcohol, and low levels of physical activity and fiber consumption (You et al., 2020). Rising rates of obesity and poor diet are thought to be particular risk factors for young adults. Nurses should be aware of the increased risk for this population and provide timely follow-up for those with concerning symptoms. Common symptoms in those with early onset colorectal cancer include abdominal pain, rectal bleeding, diarrhea, and iron deficiency anemia (Wang, 2023).

Activity-Exercise Pattern

In addition to healthy eating, engaging in regular physical activity is one of the most important ways to promote health and prevent disease for people of all ages. A growing body of evidence highlights the benefits of regular physical activity: overall feeling better; decreased risks of anxiety, depression, and chronic disease; improved brain health; and reduction in some types of cancer. Sedentary behavior has been found to increase all cause and cardiovascular mortality in adults (USDHHS, 2023). Physical activity in young adults may be particularly important. A recent study found that those who engaged in physical activity as young adults had a decreased risk of diabetes and lower cholesterol levels, regardless of moderate to vigorous physical activity levels later in life (Nagata et al., 2022).

Current recommendations for physical activity for adults include at least 150 to 300 minutes of moderate-intensity aerobic activity weekly, with improved benefits for those engaged for longer periods. During pregnancy and the postpartum period, females should engage in at least 150 minutes of moderate-intensity activity.

Ideally, physical activity is spread out over the week, with muscle-strengthening exercise occurring on at least two of those days. **Aerobic exercise**, in which oxygen is metabolized to produce energy, develops an optimally functioning cardiorespiratory system.

The nurse should counsel young adults to engage in regular physical activity, sharing the many benefits and highlighting that any activity is better than sitting. Attaining adequate physical activity is a gradual process. Walking is one activity that is relatively easy to initiate for most young adults. The use of an activity tracker or smartphone application (app) can help young adults meet goals and provide support. Examples of moderate-intensity exercise include walking briskly, swimming, and some types of yoga, such as Vinyasa or power yoga. Engaging in yard work or home maintenance activities are other examples. Vigorous activities include jogging, hiking uphill, and engaging in **high-intensity interval training** (HIIT). This involves alternating short periods of high-intensity activity with less-intense recovery periods. Young adults with disabilities should also be encouraged to engage in physical activity on a regular basis. Those with disabilities are more likely to be obese and have higher rates of chronic disease. If able, those with disabilities should follow the same guidelines as previously outlined and should avoid inactivity as much as possible (CDC, 2022e). Walking is one activity that those with disabilities commonly engage in if able.

In addition to counseling young adults about the importance of engaging in regular physical activity, the nurse should advocate at the legislative level to promote policies that aim to improve the **built environment**, altering the physical environment to make it easier for people to be more active in their communities. These population-based interventions, such as the addition of bike lanes, sidewalks, and green space, offer an opportunity to help increase physical activity for all Americans. Other community-level interventions include **point-of-decision prompts**, such as signs that encourage people to make a more active choice, such as taking the stairs instead of the elevator, and bicycle share programs (The Community Guide, 2023; Omura et al., 2020) (Fig. 22.1). Workplace interventions such as health-education classes, discounted gym memberships, goal setting, and telephonic and digital interventions can also be helpful, particularly for those who work in sedentary jobs (The Community Guide, 2023).

In 2020, only 24.2% of adults over the age of 18 met physical activity guidelines for both aerobic and muscle strengthening (CDC, 2022e). People with higher incomes and college education have higher levels of physical activity. Young males (aged 18 to 24) with a college education are 27% more likely to engage in physical activity than young males with a high school diploma. Black and Hispanic females are less likely to report adequate physical activity than White females (Armstrong et al., 2018).

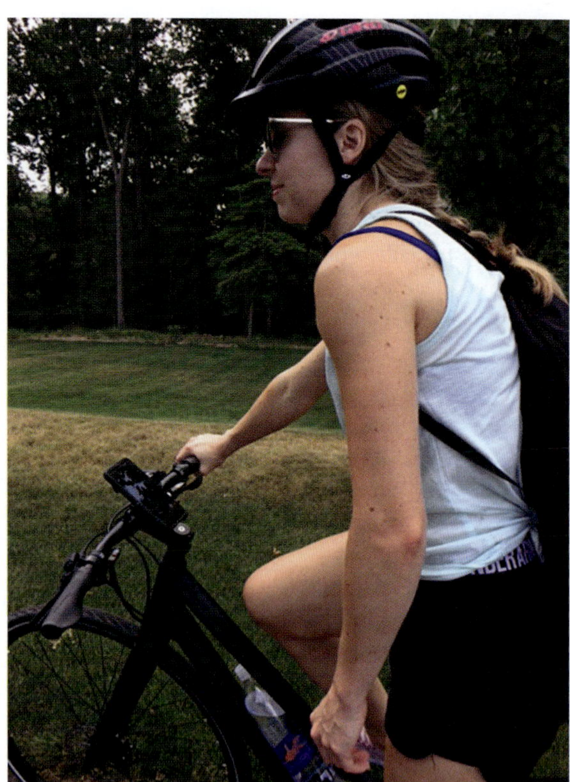

FIG. 22.1 Bike lanes are part of the built environment that encourages physical activity.

Radiation and Excessive Sun Exposure

Exposure to the sun, sun lamps, or tanning beds causes early aging of the skin and increases the risks of skin cancer. Those with fair skin tones are at highest risk, but all types of skin tones can develop cancer. Melanoma, a serious type of skin cancer, is one of the most common cancers in those under age 30, particularly for young females (American Cancer Society, 2023). Nurses need to educate young adults about the risks of sun exposure and tanning, the preventive use of sun-blocking agents and other protective factors, and skin symptoms that might indicate cancer.

Sun-blocking agents reduce sunburn or other skin damage with the goal of lowering the risk of skin cancer. **Sun protection factor** (SPF) index is a measure of the effectiveness of various preparations. For example, a rating of 30 means the sunscreen provides 30 times the protection of unprotected skin. The American Academy of Dermatology (2023) recommends that everyone use sun-blocking agents with an SPF of 30 or greater when outside. Other recommended sun-protecting behaviors include wearing long sleeves and pants, wide-brimmed hats, and sunglasses that block ultraviolet (UV) radiation. Some clothing contains an UV protection factor (UPF) that can be found on the label. Sunscreens should be broad spectrum—those that block both UV A and UV B light—and water resistant. Young adults should avoid sunbathing during the 2-hour period before and after noon, because two-thirds of the day's UV light comes through Earth's atmosphere during this time. The best protection is achieved by application of agents 15 to 30 minutes before exposure and then reapplying approximately every 2 hours and after sweating or swimming. Sun-protective measures such as use of sunscreen, use of sun-protective clothing, and avoidance of UV light are an essential part of young adult education. The nurse considers that the most effective skin cancer prevention activities for young adults include primary care counseling, sun protection, and avoidance of the use of tanning beds.

Sports and Fitness

Many young adults who are interested in improving their health attend fitness programs. After a decline during the COVID-19 pandemic, gym memberships and engagement in sports and fitness programs are returning to prepandemic levels. Young adults who are interested in alternative forms of transportation or who are concerned about the environmental affect of air pollution may bicycle. Growing numbers of bike-sharing programs in urban communities promote this activity. E-bike use is increasing and may be a good introduction to increased physical activity. Although less intense than typical cycling, it has been found to increase aerobic fitness and is associated with moderate to vigorous physical activity (Riiser et al., 2022). Young adults, typically males between the ages of 24 and 34 who are thrill seeking, may be involved with "extreme" sports. Extreme sports, sometimes called *action sports*, are those that involve a high degree of risk and are more likely to result in severe injury or death. Examples include BASE jumping, cliff diving, extreme skiing, and waterfall kayaking (Cohen, Baluch, & Duffy, 2018). Current fitness trends include wearable technology such as fitness trackers and smart watches, HIIT, virtual reality workouts, and holistic wellness programs (Thomas, 2023).

Regardless of the sport or activity, the risk of accident, injury, and death exists. The most commonly reported injuries are related to exercising, cycling, and basketball (National Safety Council [NSC], 2023a). The number of preventable deaths related to bicycles has been increasing, with 1260 deaths reported in 2020. The majority of bicycle deaths are caused by motor vehicles. Males account for 89% of all bicycle deaths (NSC, 2023b). Bicycle helmets are believed to be the single most effective preventive measure available to decrease the incidence of brain and head injuries. Helmets prevent 52% to 60% of bicycle-related head injury deaths (Consumer Product Safety Commission, 2021). Motorcycles are appealing to young adults, primarily because they have high performance and speed capabilities. Motorcycle helmets also prevent fatal injuries. The use of motorcycle helmets decreased from 69% in 2020 to 64.9% in 2021 (NSC, 2022).

Accidental deaths from drowning are a leading cause of death among those aged 29 and younger. Rates of drowning increased significantly in 2020 for those aged 20 to 29 (Moreland et al., 2022). Swimming, boating, and scuba diving are associated with the high number of water-related fatalities. Hang gliding, parachuting, and flying small aircraft are responsible for a large number of outdoor fatalities. Extreme sports, mountain climbing, hiking in poor weather conditions, downhill ski racing, and bobsledding are other hazardous activities. Many so-called accidents are not random, uncontrollable events, but are predictable and preventable if precautions and risks are analyzed (USDHHS, 2023).

Amateur and professional sports activities generally pose few hazards when rules and safety precautions are observed. Relatively few fatalities are associated with professionally organized contact sports, such as football, hockey, or boxing; however, there are concerns about neurodegenerative changes associated with repetitive head concussions. **Chronic traumatic encephalopathy (CTE)** is the term given to a cluster of symptoms with cognitive and psychiatric dimensions. Symptoms may include memory loss, confusion, impaired judgment, impulsivity and aggression, depression, and progressive dementia. CTE lacks established clinical criteria for diagnosis, and more research is needed to understand the full implications. It can only be diagnosed at autopsy after death (Filley et al., 2019). However, concerns have resulted in significant changes in professional football policies and sports concussion protocols. Although football remains Americans' favorite sport, participation in youth and high school football has been steadily decreasing because of parental concerns about repeated head trauma (Powell, 2019).

A comprehensive history of recreational activities alerts the nurse to specific needs about safety education. Young adults are encouraged to learn and abide by the rules of the sport in which they are engaged. Rules in many sports have evolved from health and safety concerns, enabling the individual to learn the sport well with appropriate instruction.

Sleep-Rest Pattern

Sufficient sleep is a critical component of health and well-being. Sleep plays a role in immunity and promotes growth and learning. Poor sleep habits in young adulthood may lead to longer-term sleep difficulties in later adulthood. Young adults are subject to poor sleep caused by work, stress, device use, and inactivity, leading to fatigue. Adults 18 and older should sleep 7 or more hours daily (CDC, 2022f). Sleep disorders in young adults are common and include obstructive sleep apnea, chronic insomnia, and restless leg syndrome. Addressing sleep disorders is critical for young adults, as lifetime health behaviors are set during this period (McArdle et al., 2020). Healthy sleep habits include maintaining a consistent sleep schedule, turning off electronic devices at least 30 minutes before bedtime, and avoiding alcohol and caffeine before bedtime. Moderate to vigorous physical activity is associated with improved quality of sleep, including taking less time to fall asleep and promoting a deeper sleep (USDHHS, 2023). A number of digital devices can record sleep as well as activity patterns.

Cognitive-Perceptual Pattern

Physical and Mental Patterns

Visual acuity is highest at approximately age 20 years and begins to decline at approximately age 40 years, when farsightedness frequently develops. Young adults under the age of 40 are recommended to have a comprehensive eye exam every 5 to 10 years. For young adults with diabetes, a yearly eye exam is recommended (Daiber & Gnugnoli, 2023). Hearing is also best at age 20 years; the ability to distinguish high-pitched tones decreases with age. The other senses—taste, smell, touch, and awareness of temperature and pain—remain stable until age 45 to 50 years (Weber & Kelly, 2022).

Further maturation requires young adults to learn skills and behaviors that increase the performance abilities they gained as adolescents. The factors that an individual young adult may perceive as essential to learn will depend on specific goals, values, attitudes, and practices as influenced by intrinsic (constitutional) and extrinsic (environmental or community) factors. Executive decision-making becomes better developed: calculation of risks versus rewards, prioritizing, self-evaluation, self-correction, and long-term planning become more sophisticated. The development of intellectual maturity influences the selection of behaviors and attitudes that affect health and well-being practices (Simpson, 2018).

Piaget's Theory

Several stage theorists have described the growth of young adult thought and moral development. It is important to note that these stages are fluid, and individual differences occur. Within Piaget's cognitive-developmental theory, formal operational thought evolves from concrete operational thought in adolescence and extends through the reasoning process of young adults (Piaget, 1972). Although more recent developmental theorists dispute Piaget's findings, this scheme of cognitive development assists the nurse in learning about and understanding young adult reasoning (Babakr et al., 2019). Achievement of formal operational thinking allows young adults to analyze all combinations of possibilities and construct hypotheses. Young adult thought becomes more perceptive and insightful; issues can therefore be evaluated realistically and objectively. Young adults are energetic and can therefore contribute substantially to social and occupational decision-making. Although they tend to take greater risks, young adults typically demonstrate the use of appropriate reasoning, anticipation, and analytical approaches.

Intellectual Growth

Organization of information influences memory. Evidence shows that recall performance diminishes with age: at its peak in the 20s, memory starts to diminish during the 30s. Improved strategies for organization of information, however, can enhance recall, and limitation of memory with increasing age is likely a result of retrieval rather than storage mechanisms. Recent evidence from brain development research indicates that during the early years of young adulthood, important frontal lobe brain development is still occurring; this is important for control of emotions and later for full adult rational decision-making (Simpson, 2018).

Erikson's Theory

Erikson (1993), another widely cited psychological theorist, reported that the most important goal for young adults is the development of an increased sense of competency and self-esteem. In developing self-esteem, the young adult learns to be truly open and capable of trust through the formation of intimate relationships that are characteristic of this period. This stage is described as a phase of psychosocial development termed **intimacy versus isolation** *and loneliness*.

Erikson's concept of genuine intimacy extends beyond sexual relations to a broader view of mutual psychosocial intimacy with a spouse or lover, parents, children, and friends. Characterized by the reciprocal expression of affection, intimacy requires mutual trust. These interchanges are spontaneous for the young adult; relationships should be free and allow self-disclosure. Young adults who are unsure of their identity may avoid intimate contact or engage in promiscuous behavior lacking in true intimacy, which can result in isolation and consequent self-absorption. Healthy adults search for continuity, regularity, or unity of meaningful relationships while avoiding situations of little commitment.

Moral Development

Young adults who have successfully mastered the previous cognitive, social, and moral stages are usually able to recognize or use principled reasoning. Kohlberg identifies this ability as the **postconventional level of moral reasoning** (Kohlberg & Lickons, 1986). During this phase the individual is able to differentiate the self from the rules and expectations of others and to define principles regarding rights in terms of self-chosen principles. The interests of individuals can be weighed against the needs of society and the state, and violations of law can be justified when individual interests are in accord with principles. Gilligan (1982, 2002, 2013), who studied the development of moral reasoning in adult and young females, asserts that their moral judgments reflect less of a "rights" perspective and more of an emphasis on responsibilities in relationships. Newer framing of this theory of women's emotions and relationships is now essential to understanding intelligence and self-awareness (Gilligan, 2013).

Although development of principled moral reasoning is possible during young adulthood, it may never occur if the cognitive and social factors that stimulate higher reasoning are not present. Acts of personal violence representative of lower moral reasoning should not be present; however, such acts do occur during this period, illustrating the need for moral developmental concerns to be addressed at earlier stages of education and socialization.

Self-Perception–Self-Concept Pattern

The young adult period is marked by a series of transitional events that help to shape adult identity. In non-Western cultures entrance to adulthood is generally defined and marked by social events such as marriage. In Western societies, maturation is defined through the individual's achievement of financial and residential independence, and is a more drawn-out, gradual process. The changing social and economic conditions of recent times have resulted in young adults attaining these traditional life milestones later than previous generations (Fry, 2023a).

Two emotional themes regarding the value of work and financial independence become evident during young adulthood. During their 20s, young adults yearn to explore and experiment, keeping structures temporary and reversible. These individuals may move from job to job and relationship to relationship, remaining in a transient state. At the opposite extreme is the urge to prepare for the future by making firm commitments. During this period, both males and females question their value to society, the merit of their accomplishments, their success as sexual beings, and the probability of attaining their unfulfilled goals (Arnett et al., 2020).

Transitioning to full-time employment is a major milestone of young adulthood and key to financial independence. It's also an important aspect of personal identity. Completion of a post-secondary degree is the strongest predictor of obtaining a high-quality job, in which wages, benefits, and hours are adequate, and results in a degree of job satisfaction (US Department of Labor, 2024). Young adults who grow up in low-income families have lower rates of high school graduation and college enrollment and completion, ultimately earning lower wages (Ross et al., 2018). The wage disparities between those who are college educated and those who are not are growing, and this is contributing to income inequality. Employment opportunities are rebounding after the COVID-19 pandemic, with 75% of females and 85% of males aged 25 to 34 reporting working in 2022 (National Center for Educational Statistics, 2023).

The nature of work is being transformed, with a continued trend toward longer hours, increased use of contracted and temporary workers, and increased telecommuting. The US workforce is changing dramatically as companies merge, restructure, downsize (right size), and shift employees around to account for changing market conditions, company mergers, and buyouts. There is increasing concern about "globalization," outsourcing, and moving jobs overseas, especially in industrial centers, the pharmaceutical industry, and the technology sector. The gig economy has provided workers with additional ways to make a living through technology-driven platforms such as remote work, ride-hailing apps, and other service-related work. Although offering flexibility to workers, these jobs lack the traditional benefits of a regular job, such as health insurance and paid time off, and contribute to stress caused by job insecurity. Job insecurity can not only cause economic stress but also affect the young adult's sense of personal identity and threaten their well-being (Anderson et al., 2021). Young workers are more likely to report lower job satisfaction than older generations. Among those aged 18 to 29, 32% report that they find their job stressful all or most of the time; however, a majority also say that their job shapes their self-identity. Personal connections with coworkers was one factor that ranked highest in job satisfaction (Leppert, 2023).

Females make up nearly half of the workforce in the United States. Despite gains, females still face challenges while at work compared with males. Wage gaps persist. In 2022 females earned 82% of what males earned. Other work-related issues for females include race and sex bias, exposure to sexual harassment, and lack of flexible work arrangements (Catalyst, 2023). Many young females postpone childbearing until they have established their careers. The majority of females with a young child work, and many experience high levels of stress and guilt as they attempt work-life balance. Compared with other Western countries, US employers provide limited support to working mothers.

Nurses working in occupational settings engage with workers to promote health and prevent illness and injury. When nurses advocate for healthy work sites, this increases the chance that young adults will have access to comprehensive health-promotion programs. Occupational health nurses can also advocate for policies that support the work environment for new mothers (American Association of Occupational Health Nurses, 2021).

Instead of transitioning to full-time employment, some young adults may consider serving their country by joining the military. Benefits include job security, good pay, educational and travel opportunities, and access to housing and health care. However, the armed forces requires that recruits be in top physical condition. The Department of Defense estimates that only 23% of 17 to 24-year-olds were eligible for military service in 2020, down from 29% in 2016. Reasons for ineligibility included obesity, poor nutrition, tobacco use, and excessive alcohol use (CDC, 2022e).

Attaining residential independence is another milestone in the transition to adulthood. Young adults today are living longer in the parental home. It is estimated that 20% to 50% of young adults who leave home ultimately return. There is some evidence that college debt is contributing to this "boomeranging." Approximately half of young adults live with their parents, particularly when they are younger than 30 (Fadeyi & Horowitz, 2022).

Roles-Relationships Pattern

Close friendships are a critical source of support for young adults. Young adult friendships are more complex and enduring than earlier relationships. The focus of the relationship is the sharing of feelings or confidences as well as common interests. True friendship is characterized by emotional closeness and reciprocity of support. Establishing interpersonal relationships involves agreeable and purposeful interactions with others. Interpersonal relationships can be created with people of the same or the opposite sex. Age is typically a less-important factor than it was during adolescence. The formation of intimate relationships develops within or outside a family context, the school setting, or work environment. A degree of trust is needed to develop relationships; otherwise, social and emotional isolation can occur (Fig. 22.2). The evidence supporting the importance of social connectedness is growing. Those who are isolated and lonely are at risk for premature mortality (Holt-Lunstad, 2022). Social connectedness is particularly important during times of stress. During the COVID-19 pandemic, young adults reported higher rates of loneliness, anxiety, and depression compared with older age groups. However, one study revealed that young adults with a greater number of friends and satisfying relationships reported fewer of these symptoms. Particularly important was the ability to connect with friends via digital platforms (Juvonen et al., 2022).

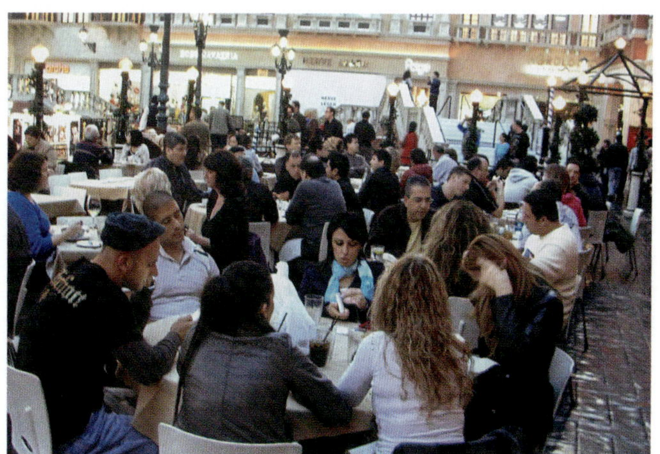

FIG. 22.2 Young adults enjoy gathering in a local café to socialize together.

The use of social networking websites, such as Facebook, Instagram, TikTok, and Snapchat, is prevalent in young adults. These sites allow the user to digitally communicate with "friends." Many young adults use these sites to maintain relationships. However, excessive social media use can lead to increased depression, anxiety, and stress (Shannon et al., 2022).

Developing romantic relationships is a key developmental milestone in young adults (Xia et al., 2018). In 2022, 63% of males aged 18 to 29 reported being single (not married or in a committed relationship) compared with 34% of females (Gelles-Watnick, 2023). As young adults age, more permanent, serious relationships develop. Young adults value marriage. However, like other developmental milestones, marriage is more delayed than in prior generations, with young adults often waiting until they are established in their careers and financially stable. The median age for marriage in 2021 was 30.2 years for males and 28.1 years for females (Tillman et al., 2019; US Census Bureau, 2023).

More young adults are reporting their sexuality as something other than heterosexual. Among those aged 18 to 34 years, 15.5% of non-Hispanic Whites, 12.1% of Blacks, and 15.5% of Hispanics report not being heterosexual (McCarthy, 2022). Same-sex marriage legislation has been upheld by the US Supreme Court and applies to all US states; this legislation legitimizes the legal rights of same-sex couples through marriage or civil union statutes. Support for same-sex marriage has increased in the United States. In 2022, 71% of Americans supported the legalization of same-sex marriage (McCarthy, 2022).

The concept of gender is complex and expanding and is core to self-identity for young adults. The LGBTQI+ (lesbian, gay, bisexual, transgender, queer, intersex, and other sexual orientation) population in the United States is diverse and experiences significant disparities across the life spectrum. Health disparities include worse-reported physical and mental health; unsafe sex practices resulting in an increased risk of STIs such as HPV and HIV; higher prevalence of substance abuse; and increased rates of suicide. This population is less likely to have a usual source of care and reports discriminatory practices by health care providers, creating distrust and fear. Other challenges for this group include a lack of consistent legal protection, higher rates of unemployment, exposure to stigma, harassment, and violence. Transgender young adults in particular face more discrimination and rising risks of violence (Medina & Mahowald, 2023; National Academies of Science, Engineering, & Medicine, 2022). Approximately 5.1% of young adults younger than 30 identify as transgender or nonbinary (Brown, 2022). A growing number of states have passed laws limiting the rights of transgender individuals. An estimated 42% of transgender women (born male) have HIV (CDC, 2023j). Strong social relationships are important for developing resilience in this group. It's important for the nurse to not make assumptions about gender, to treat everyone with equal respect, and appear nonjudgmental.

In addition to marriage, consideration must be given to decisions related to childbearing, such as finances, safety, family support, where to live, the relationship with extended family members, and the roles and responsibilities within the nuclear family unit. Young adults who are establishing a family must have open communication about self-development, which includes issues of dual careers, childrearing practices, and domestic duties. Although goals differ greatly among young adult couples, they are generally concerned with acquiring material comforts; the desire for housing, transportation, clothing, or recreation generally necessitates that both partners are employed to meet financial obligations. This desire necessitates the changing of roles and the sharing of responsibilities, and open communication becomes a crucial component.

In addition to achieving intimacy, the young adult must accomplish other developmental tasks to achieve true psychosocial maturation (Fig. 22.1). Decision-making about life and career direction is the developmental milestone that heralds the transition from adolescence to adulthood. In 2022, half of adults aged 18 to 29 lived with one or both parents (Fadeyi & Horowitz, 2022). Young adults frequently remain in their parents' home for economic reasons, particularly when life choices involve continued schooling, unemployment, or remaining unmarried (Fig. 22.3).

Fewer young adults are attending college, down by 1.2 million from the peak in 2011. This decline results more from fewer young males entering college than females. Males represent 44% of 18- to 24-year-old students at 4-year colleges. College enrollments have been slowly declining during the past several years. Rising college tuition, better work opportunities, and declining birth rates are believed to affect these numbers (Fry, 2023c). Although recent college enrollments have been declining, the overall number of 25- to 29-year-olds with an associate degree or higher has increased to 49% (National Center for Educational Statistics, 2023).

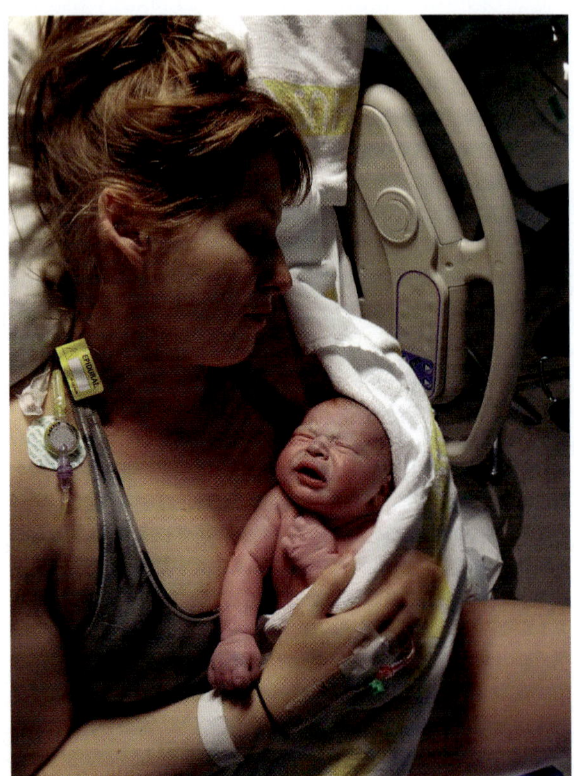

FIG. 22.3 A major developmental milestone for some young adults is parenthood.

Separation and Divorce

For many young adult couples, financial concerns, different careers, friends, and differing maturity levels place strains on their relationship. These circumstances can provide a basis for domestic difficulty. Excessive online social networking has also been found to affect romantic relationships, leading to less commitment and increased risk of divorce as a result of conflict and jealousy (Abbasi, 2018).

Divorce rates in the United States have been declining (US Census Bureau, 2023). Females are more likely to initiate divorce than males. Contemporary romantic relationships are less interdependent than in prior generations. Females now have higher incomes and are less likely to sacrifice their own happiness and well-being for a partner (Parker et al., 2022). Although dissatisfaction and unhappiness are frequent precursors to separation and divorce, the decision to dissolve a marriage is not necessarily easy. Considerable emotional strain exists for both partners, their children, their families, and their close friends. Divorce requires that young adults reevaluate their basic values, individual personality, spiritual beliefs, ego strength, job potential, and socioeconomic factors to ensure future security for themselves and their children. Some young adults are unable to adjust to role and status changes and to threats of self-concept. For these reasons, support systems in the form of groups, individual counseling, or special social activities are critical.

Increasing numbers of young adults do not marry but have children. One-third of children live in households with an unmarried parent: either with a solo parent, usually a mother, or with cohabitating parents (Livingston, 2018). The rate of living with an unmarried parent varies by race and ethnicity. Black children (58%) are most likely to live with an unmarried parent, followed by Hispanic children (36%) and White children (24%). Those living with a solo parent are more likely to experience financial difficulties (Livingston, 2018).

Nurses recognize the importance of relationships and social support for physical health and well-being. Nursing care and assessment can help to identify the feelings of guilt, grief, and loss that young adults experience during a separation or divorce. Nurses are also accepting of the varying family structures in those they care for. Referrals to a variety of resources can be made by the nurse to help young adults and their families cope with the dissolution of committed relationships and marriage.

Male and Female Risk of Violence

Violence is a global and national health problem. The recipients of violence may be older adults, children, and females and males (CDC, 2023k). Gun violence in particular has been increasing in the United States and is viewed as a public health problem. Violent deaths are intentional deaths that occur from physical force or power exerted against self, others, or a community (CDC, 2023k). The United States has some of the highest rates of violence compared with other developed countries. Homicide is a leading cause of death for young adults. Seventy-nine percent of all homicides in 2020 were from firearms. Males are the victims in 86% of firearm deaths and 87% of firearm injuries (CDC, 2023k; Gramlich, 2023). When compared with the general population, death rates are higher for males in poorer populations, in urban areas, and with less formal education. Homicide is closely associated with alcohol and drug abuse and is frequently related to other violent acts, such as assault and robbery. Other risk factors include a history of loss of employment, incarceration, access to firearms, abuse in the home, mental illness, social isolation, and homelessness. The presence of firearms in the home is associated with the increased risk of unintentional and intentional injury. A target of *Healthy People 2030* is to reduce firearm-related deaths. However, firearm death and injury rates have been increasing in recent years, The firearm-related death rate is highest for Black, American Indian, Alaska Native, and Hispanic males (USDHHS, 2023).

Intimate partner violence (IPV) is physical or psychological abuse that occurs in a close relationship. IPV can result in physical violence, sexual violence, stalking, or psychological aggression and can lead to long-term physical and mental health problems. Abuse crosses all socioeconomic, racial, ethnic, religious, gender, and age boundaries. Approximately 41% of females and 26% of males experience physical violence, sexual violence, and/or stalking during their lifetime (CDC, 2023k). Young adults who have had violent encounters with partners have an increased risk of cardiovascular events later in life (American Heart Association, 2022b). IPV can result in serious economic outcomes if the perpetrator prevents their partner from working or sabotages their employment, leading to job loss (Sullivan, 2018). The USPSTF (2023) recommends that all females of reproductive age be screened for IPV and be provided or referred to support and other resources. Preventive efforts for IPV include educating young adults about healthy relationships and improving safe environments. Services and support for survivors of IPV are often in short supply due to the pervasiveness of the problem and a lack of adequate funding. Supports and services needed include shelter programs, transitional housing, advocacy services, and support groups (Sullivan, 2018).

Sexuality-Reproductive Pattern

By young adulthood the menstrual cycle is generally well established in females, and it is an important consideration in evaluating reproductive health. Cyclical hormonal function is responsible for regularity of the cycle and normal functioning of the ovaries and uterus. The normal duration of menses is 2 to 7 days (with a flow of 5 to 79 mL). Blood loss greater than 80 mL per cycle is abnormal and may lead to anemia. Irregularities such as painful menstruation, premenstrual syndrome, and prolonged or heavy bleeding need further assessment. Although these problems are not always abnormal, the symptoms and the individual's reaction to them can signal functional disorders and the need for further investigation and treatment. A variety of newer menstrual products are available for those who are concerned about the cost and environmental effect of disposable products. Reusable items include menstrual cups (such as the Diva Cup) and reusable underwear (period underwear) and pads (Hatcher et al., 2018). Several brands of period underwear have been found to contain per- and polyfluoroalkyl substances (PFAS), "forever chemicals" associated with potential health risks such as cancer (Amenabar, 2023).

Reproductive Problems

Infertility is defined as the lack of conception in the presence of unprotected sexual intercourse for at least 12 months. Approximately 10% of females of reproductive age in the United States have difficulty conceiving or carrying a fetus to term, and the prevalence increases with age (USDHHS, 2023). Infertility can result from both male and female reproductive issues. For females, problems with ovulation and obstructed fallopian tubes may contribute. The most common cause of female infertility is **polycystic ovarian syndrome (PCOS)**, a condition with genetic, hormonal, metabolic, and reproductive factors that can cause obesity, cardiovascular disease, and diabetes. Male factors include abnormal production and quality of sperm, hormonal and genetic factors, and other medical conditions. Treatment varies based on the underlying cause and may include **assisted reproductive technologies (ART)** such as in vitro fertilization. Other options include surrogacy or the use of a gestational carrier, in which a woman's egg is fertilized by her partner's sperm and placed in a carrier's uterus. Success rates for ART are highest for females younger than 35 years (39%) (USDHHS, 2023). Infertility treatment can create great psychological and financial stress for couples, affecting the couple's relationship. Disparities in access to ART have been reported along racial/ethnic lines. Black and Hispanic females are twice as likely to report income and weight as a barrier to receiving ART as White and Asian females. Socioeconomic factors likely play a role given the high cost of ART treatments. Insurance coverage for infertility treatments is based on varying state laws (Galic et al., 2021).

Unintended Pregnancy

Family planning is one of the biggest public health achievements of the 20th century. Despite the advent of modern contraceptives, unintended pregnancy remains a persistent problem. Approximately half of all pregnancies are unintended, which may be either unwanted or mistimed (USDHHS, 2023). The highest rates of unintended pregnancies occur in females aged 18 to 24, females with incomes below the poverty level, and Black and Hispanic females Females with unintended pregnancies are more likely to delay prenatal care, and children resulting from an unintended pregnancy have a higher risk of physical and mental health issues (USDHHS, 2023). Although most young adults consider family planning services to be an essential basic health service, barriers to access are increasing and exist at the national, state, and local levels, particularly for pregnancy termination services. Significant disparities exist in reproductive care.

The overturning of Roe v. Wade in 2022 has resulted in increased abortion restrictions and outright abortion bans in many states, requiring females to travel out of state for the procedure. Limiting access to reproductive health care services results in reproductive health disparities (Center for Reproductive Rights, 2023a). States that limit abortion access are also more likely to have not expanded Medicaid under the ACA and have less funding for family social support services, increasing the burden for these females. Most states that have restricted or banned abortion access do have exceptions for the life and health of the mother, pregnancies resulting from rape or incest, and lethal fetal anomalies. However, many of these exceptions are vague and have caused confusion for health care providers and health care organizations. Reports of delayed care, as in the case of miscarriage management, have been reported (Felix et al., 2023).

More than half of abortions are medication abortions. The combined use of the drugs mifepristone and misoprostol is a safe and effective way to terminate an early pregnancy. However, these drugs are also restricted in states with abortion limits. There are concerns that access to mifepristone may be restricted in all 50 states, even in states where abortion is legal, with current legal challenges related to the initial approval of the drug. Mifepristone is also used for other reproductive health reasons, including ectopic pregnancies and miscarriages (Center for Reproductive Rights, 2023b).

Prevention of unintended pregnancy requires increased access and proper use of contraceptives. Approximately half of unintended pregnancies are the result of contraceptive failure. All young adults need information about contraceptives (Table 22.3) to decrease the number of unwanted pregnancies and the need for abortions. The nurse's role in contraceptive counseling includes discussion about reproductive goals and helping individuals choose the method most appropriate to their needs. New and improved contraceptive agents are continually becoming available (Hatcher et al., 2018), so the nurse must understand current techniques. Laws and policies in some settings restrict nurses and other health care providers from engaging in certain types of counseling, including providing abortion information. Title X is a federal grant program provided to improve access to reproductive services for low-income females. Recent changes to the program have reproductive advocates concerned that access to such services will be restricted, particularly in states that already had a small number of women's health clinics.

Emergency contraception can substantially reduce the number of unintended pregnancies. There are several forms of emergency contraception available that can be taken after episodes of unprotected sex or contraceptive failure. Several types of emergency contraceptive pills are also available and can be taken within 5 days of unprotected sex. In the United States, progestin-only emergency contraception is available over the counter without any age restriction (includes Plan B One-Step and generics). There is some evidence that this method may not be effective with females with weights greater than 80 kg. Another pill, ella, a single dose of ulipristal acetate, is more effective past the fifth day and with females with higher BMIs. This option does require a prescription for use. Placement of a copper intrauterine device (IUD) within 5 days of unprotected sex reduces the risk of pregnancy by 99% (Goldstuck & Cheung, 2019). Emergency contraception works by altering tubal transport of either sperm or ova or by inhibiting implantation. It will not terminate an existing pregnancy, and it does not provide protection against STIs. The choice to use emergency contraception is frequently made with the partner and may involve complex decision-making centering on responsibility, relationship power, and a woman's right to choose and autonomy over her body. Females who report repeated use of emergency contraception should be screened for contraceptive challenges, such as reproductive coercion by a partner (Hatcher et al., 2018).

TABLE 22.3 **Summary of Risks and Noncontraceptive Benefits of Selected Contraceptive Methods**

Contraceptive Method	Risks of Use	Noncontraceptive Health Benefits
Combined hormonal contraception (pill, patch, and vaginal ring)	Cardiovascular complications (CVA, MI, blood clots, HTN); Increased risk of breast, cervical, and liver cancer	Decreases dysmenorrhea, heavy menstrual bleeding, anemia, acne, risk of ectopic pregnancy, PID; protects against ovarian, endometrial, and colorectal cancer
Intrauterine devices	Infection, uterine perforation, expulsion, anemia (with copper IUD), ectopic pregnancy	Levonorgestrel IUD reduces menstrual blood loss and dysmenorrhea, can be used to treat endometriosis, reduces risk of endometrial cancer
Progestin implant (Nexplanon)	Rare migration, rare infection at implant site; problems with removal	Decreases dysmenorrhea, usually reduces menstrual bleeding, lactation not disturbed
Injectable (Depo-Provera)	Allergic reactions, pathologic weight gain, decreased bone mineral density	Lactation not disturbed, reduces risk of catamenial seizures, may protect against ovarian and endometrial cancers
Male condom	Anaphylactic reaction to latex	Reduced risk of STI and HIV transmission, delays premature ejaculation
Female condom	None known	Protects against STIs
Diaphragm, sponge	Vaginal and urinary tract infections, toxic shock syndrome, possible increase in susceptibility to HIV/AIDS if exposed to positive partner	None known
Spermicides	Vaginal and urinary tract infections, possible increase in susceptibility to HIV/AIDS if exposed to positive partner	Antiviral activity against HPV, decreased activity of other STIs, decreases risk of PID
Permanent contraception (male/female sterilization)	Anesthetic or surgical complications, if pregnancy occurs after tubal occlusion, high risk it will be ectopic	Tubal occlusion reduces risk of ovarian cancer and may protect against PIOD
Emergency contraception pills (ella, Plan B One-Step)	Generally safe	Not for routine use

CVA, Cerebrovascular accident; *HTN,* hypertension; *HPV,* human papilloma virus; *IUD,* intrauterine device; *MI,* myocardial infarction; *PID,* pelvic inflammatory disease; *STI,* sexually transmitted infection.
From Hatcher, R. A., Nelson, A. L., Trussel, J., Cwiak, C., Cason, P., Policar, M.S., Edelman, A. B., Aiken, A. R. A., Marrazzo, J. M., & Kowal, D. (2018). *Contraceptive technology* (21st ed.). New York: Ayer Company Publishers, LLC.

Prenatal Care

Access to prenatal care and financing of sufficient care are critical concerns. The well-being of mothers and their infants affects the next generation. Delayed prenatal care is associated with worse health outcomes for both females and babies. Lack of adequate prenatal care has been associated with females younger than 24 years of age, females with lower educational attainment, females who are not married, and females with lower incomes (Krukowski et al., 2022). *Healthy People 2030* has set goals directed toward increasing the proportion of mothers who receive both early (in the first trimester) and adequate prenatal care (USDHHS, 2023). The reasons females do not seek early prenatal care are varied but may include insensitivity and cultural biases of providers. Thirty percent of Black, Hispanic, and multiracial females report mistreatment during maternity care, such as poor communication, privacy violations, and verbal abuse (Vitalsigns, 2023).

Decreased access to prenatal and maternity care are the result of maternity care deserts, areas that lack hospitals with maternity services or birth centers and that lack obstetrical health care providers. This lack of services is often driven by financial challenges, with closure of maternity units or hospitals. The March of Dimes (2023) reports that 36% of counties in the US are considered maternity care deserts, and these are largely located in rural areas.

Sexually Transmitted Infections

STIs are common, and rates are increasing, especially for chlamydia, gonorrhea, and syphilis. STIs frequently occur without symptoms, particularly in females, and left untreated can result in infertility, ectopic pregnancy, and increased risk for HIV infection. Between 2017 and 2021, rates of syphilis increased by 74% and gonorrhea by 28% (CDC, 2023l). Chlamydia rates declined by 4%, however, which is thought to be a result of decreased screening during the COVID-19 pandemic rather than a decline in the number of cases, which had been on the rise. More concerning is a 203% increase in congenital syphilis. Syphilis transmitted to the fetus during pregnancy can cause miscarriage, stillbirth, and neonatal death (CDC, 2023l). Rates of STIs are highest for young adults younger than the age of 25, racial and ethnic minorities, and gay and bisexual males (CDC, 2023l). The list of other STIs includes HPV infection, genital herpes, HIV infection, genital mycoplasma infections, cytomegalovirus infection, HBV, and bacterial vaginitis (Table 22.4). There are 12 strains of HPV that are considered a high-risk type associated with the development of cancer (anal, cervical, oropharyngeal, penile, vaginal, and vulvar) (National Cancer Institute [NCI], 2023). A study of 14 countries found that HPV vaccination decreased the incidence of infections by 66% for those aged 20 to 24, a 54% decrease in anogenital warts, and 31% decline in precancerous lesions compared with the period before vaccination (National Cancer Institute, 2019). Screening for chlamydia should be done annually for all sexually active females aged 24 years and younger (Hatcher et al., 2018). The presence of multiple STIs increases the risk of HIV infection. STIs cost billions of dollars in screening, treatment, and

TABLE 22.4 Summary of Selected Sexually Transmitted Infections

Infections	Causative Agent	Diagnostic Methods	Treatment	Risks or Complications	Nursing Teaching
AIDS	HIV	Enzyme immune assay, Western blot, differentiation assay	Current recommendations include antiretrovirals; post-exposure prophylaxis; preexposure prophylaxis (daily antiretroviral) for those at high risk	Opportunistic infections, perinatal transmission	Monitor CD4 T lymphocyte analysis and HIV plasma viral load, monitor men who have sex with men, early pregnancy testing strongly recommended
Hepatitis B	Hepatitis B virus	Hepatitis B serology antibody test	Tenofovir, entecavir, lamivudine*Although not typical, hepatitis A and hepatitis C can be sexually transmitted	Perinatal transmission	Routine vaccination or vaccine before pregnancy
Genital herpes	Herpes simplex virus	Herpes simplex virus antibody test, culture, viral test	Acyclovir at first diagnosis or episode, famciclovir, valacyclovir	Urethral stricture, lymph node enlargement	Examine partners, abstain from sex while symptomatic
Genital warts	Human papilloma virus	Clinical inspection, colposcopy, biopsy	Podofilox, trichloroacetic acid, imiguimod, cryotherapy/laser, valacyclovir, famciclovir	Cervical dysplasia, cervical cancer	Offer vaccine and counseling, return for treatment as necessary, treat partner
Bacterial/Other STIs					
Gonorrhea	Neisseria gonorrhoeae	Culture	Ceftriaxone, cefixime, some strains becoming resistant	PID, infertility, ectopic pregnancy	Monitor antibiotic treatment, expedited partner therapy, repeat culture, check for chlamydia
Syphilis	Treponema pallidum	Fluorescent antibody tests of lesion or exudates, VDRL, RPR	Benzathine penicillin G	Secondary/late syphilis, congenital syphilis	Monitor treatment, test and monitor partner
Chlamydia	Chlamydia trachomatis	Culture, chlamydia monoclonal antibody test	Azithromycin, doxycycline	Infertility, ectopic pregnancy, urethral scarring, PID, endocervicitis, neonatal infection	Expedited partner therapy, condoms to prevent future infection
Bacterial vaginosis	Gardnerella vaginalis	Clinical criteria, wet mount (clue cells)	Metronidazole (Flagyl)	Asymptomatic infection	Sexual transmission not proven
Trichomoniasis	Trichomonas vaginalis	Trich rapid test, culture (protozoa)	Metronidazole (Flagyl)	Recurrence, excoriation of genital area	Use condoms to prevent new infection
Vulvovaginal candidiasis	Candida albicans, non–C. albicans	Wet mount/potassium hydroxide test (hyphae and spores)	Antifungal medication: butoconazole, miconazole, clotrimazole, fluconazole	Recurrence of disease	Reduce moisture/heat in genital area, recheck in 14 days

PID, Pelvic inflammatory disease; *RPR,* rapid plasma reagin test; *STI,* sexually transmitted infection; *VDRL,* Venereal Disease Research Laboratory test.
From Centers for Disease Control and Prevention (2023l); Hatcher et al. (2018)

reporting. In addition to creating a substantial problem for young adults, STIs impose tremendous demands on health care facilities (USDHHS, 2023). Health care providers are mandated to report cases of chlamydia, syphilis, gonorrhea, and HIV to state departments of public health. The CDC strongly recommends **expedited partner therapy (EPT)**, where health care professionals can provide prescriptions or medications to the partners of those treated with chlamydia and gonorrhea without their being seen in a health care setting. The vast majority of states allow EPT, although policies and regulations vary by state (CDC, 2023l). See Table 22.4 for commonly occurring STIs. One recent intervention for preventing STIs is **Doxycycline Post-Exposure Prophylaxis** (DoxyPEP), referred to a "morning-after pill" for STIs. A single dose of doxycycline is taken within 24 to 72 hours after sexual exposure and is effective against chlamydia, syphilis, and gonorrhea (CDC, 2023l).

Human Immunodeficiency Virus

More than 1.2 million people are estimated to have HIV infection in the United States, with approximately 31,800 new diagnoses in

2022 (HIV.gov, 2025). This is a 12% decrease since 2018. Screening and preventive measures have been attributed to declines in mother-to-child transmission during pregnancy and birth. Seventy percent of new diagnoses of HIV infection are the result of male-to-male sexual (MSM—men who have sex with men) contact (HIV.gov). An estimated 42% of transgender women (born male) have HIV (CDC, 2023j). Current HIV screening recommendations include adolescents and adults aged 15 to 65 and all pregnant females. Factors that increase risk include injection drug use, multiple sexual partners, other STIs, and exchange of sex for drugs or money. Those with increased risk should be screened more frequently. Early initiation of antiretroviral therapy reduces the risk of clinical progression to AIDS. Preexposure and postexposure prophylactic treatment with antiretroviral medications can also prevent HIV infection in those at risk. The USPSTF (2023) recommends that those at high risk for HIV (MSM, heterosexuals with HIV-infected partners, IV drug users who share equipment) be offered **preexposure prophylaxis (PrEP)**.

Prevention education is aimed at all high-risk groups, including heterosexuals and MSM. All sexually active individuals are counseled on the hazards of unprotected sexual activity and on the effective use and limitations of condoms, stressing that they must be used properly and can fail. Condom failures occur at an estimated rate of 13%; therefore, counseling should stress that condom use is not foolproof (Guttmacher Institute, 2020).

The nurse's role in intervening with regard to STIs includes providing treatment, early diagnosis, and education. When an individual is suspected of having an STI, the nurse obtains a complete history, including sexual history, sexual contacts, previous treatment and test results, signs or symptoms of a current infection, recent use of antibiotics, and allergic reactions to antibiotics. When treatment is required, the nurse ensures that the person understands the goals of treatment, including follow-up care with partners and adherence to the care plan. Appropriate health education for the individual with an STI includes the mode of transmission, incubation periods, signs and symptoms, methods of treatment, complications resulting from lack of treatment, and signs of recurrent infections. Nurses may also be responsible for reporting STIs to state departments of public health.

Coping–Stress Tolerance Pattern

Assessment of Stress Levels

Stress, the result of forces operating on the individual that disrupt physiologic or psychological equilibrium, is an integral part of young adulthood; therefore, a comprehensive health assessment should include questions to determine stress levels. Sources of stress include economic and social factors, including the rapid rate of change occurring in today's society. Technology makes it difficult to "shut down" and affects work-related stress. Anxiety, depression, or somatic complaints are indicators of stress. The role of the nurse is to listen, offer support, and demonstrate concern. The nurse may also screen for depression and anxiety and make referrals to appropriate health providers and support groups.

Job- and School-Related Stress

The nature of work is changing as a result of technologic advances. Sixty-five percent of US workers characterize their work as being a significant or somewhat significant source of stress, Fifty-four percent of workers report that work stress affects their home life (Occupational Safety and Health Administration [OSHA], 2023). Stress can affect work engagement, physical functioning, and job performance and productivity (CDC, 2023m). The digital economy has contributed to increased stress levels for workers due to longer work hours, compressed work weeks, and decreased job security. Being "hyper-connected" often means that workers are expected to work anywhere at any time. Overachievers in the workforce may develop symptoms of burnout, such as emotional exhaustion and depersonalization (Cheung et al., 2018). The **gig economy** has provided workers additional ways to make a living through technology-driven platforms such as ride-hailing apps and other service-related work. Although offering flexibility to workers, these jobs can increase stress levels (Hafeez et al., 2023).

Many young adults are high achievers and seek opportunities to be challenged. Employment problems are stressful and traumatic to an individual's self-esteem and self-worth, particularly in the current economic environment. The failure to obtain promotions or pay rises can accelerate the degree of stress. Employment is more than a source of income; it provides self-esteem and social interaction. Because the adjustment to the job market influences many other aspects of daily living, young adults frequently require assistance in developing coping mechanisms to manage stress. Properly managing the initial stress prevents further complications that can arise if the young adult uses unhealthy stress relievers such as alcohol or drugs.

Higher education can be an additional stressor to young adults. Stress experienced by college students can be related to academic performance, pressure to succeed, financial stressors, and postgraduation career options, and it is becoming increasingly prevalent (Jones et al., 2018). This stress can cause anxiety and depression and lead to future mental health conditions. Anxiety can cause insomnia, exacerbate existing medical problems, and affect academic performance (American Institute of Stress, 2019). The young adult should be informed about stress-reduction methods, including guided imagery, progressive muscle relaxation, mindfulness meditation, and activities such as yoga and tai chi (Weber & Kelley, 2022). Work site wellness programs and student counseling services should be encouraged and utilized by young adults in these settings.

Suicide and Depression

Suicide is a leading cause of death in the United States and was the second leading cause of death for those aged 20 to 34 in 2021. The suicide rate in young adults increased 39% from 2011 to 2021 (Saunders & Panchal, 2023). Rates of suicide in 2021 were 15.2 per 100,000 for those aged 15 to 24 and 19.5 per 100,000 for those aged 25 to 34. Males had four times the rate of suicide compared with females (CDC, 2023m). American Indian and Alaska Native young males, in particular, have higher rates of suicide compared with other ethnicities. Young adults may be thought of as "young invincibles"; however, they are in an age group exposed to multiple stressors, including the considerable stress caused by the transition to adulthood. Risk factors for suicide include alcohol use, a family member or friend having attempted suicide, exposure to violence, and symptoms of depression. Those with a higher risk include those who have experienced violence, including child abuse, bullying, and sexual violence. Young adults who identify as LBGTQI+ have a higher prevalence of suicidal thoughts and suicide attempts (CDC, 2023m). Having a firearm in the home increases the risk of suicide; more than 50% of suicides are committed with guns. For some people, pressure arises when they are dealing with interpersonal conflicts such as marital problems, family discord, or the loss of a close relationship; for others, the precipitating event is a lack of personal resources, unemployment, or dissatisfaction with work or school. Many young adults may try to solve their problems before the fatal incident but see no positive solutions; in many cases, a prior suicide attempt was a signal for help. In other instances, family and friends are completely unaware of the young adult's mental state.

Depression is a risk factor for suicide, although the majority of people who commit suicide have no known mental health conditions (CDC, 2023m). Depression often begins during the young adulthood period (Po et al., 2020). The USPSTF recommends depression screening for all adults aged 18 years or older, including pregnant and postpartum females, when adequate systems are available for diagnosis, treatment, and appropriate follow-up. A variety of depression screening tools are available. One tool used frequently in the primary care setting is the Patient Health Questionnaire-2 (PHQ-2). This tool uses two simple questions: Over the past 2 weeks, how often have you been bothered by any of the following problems? (1) Little interest in doing things; (2) Feeling down, depressed or hopeless? The PHQ-2 is scored based on frequency of the symptoms reported. Those screening positive require an in-depth assessment for depression (USPTSF, 2023). Social media usage has been associated with higher rates of depression and anxiety, so an assessment of social media use may be warranted in the young adult population (Karim et al., 2020). The USPTFS (2023) has concluded that there is insufficient evidence to universally screen for suicide risk, although it may be warranted in certain clinical settings and for those at higher risk.

Nursing interventions are directed toward identifying and supporting young adults at risk for depression and suicide, teaching coping and problem-solving skills, and promoting safe environments, including safe storage of firearms and medicines (CDC, 2023m). Access to mental health services is problematic, with demand far exceeding available services (National Council for Behavioral Health, 2018). Because physical and mental health are closely linked, experts advocate for **behavioral health integration** (Box 22.6) in the primary care setting to improve access and provide a more holistic approach to mental health care. In 2022, the federal government introduced a new crisis number, 988, for those who are suicidal or experiencing a mental health crisis. Here they can access crisis counseling, resources, and referrals to other mental health services (Saunders & Panchal, 2023).

BOX 22.6 Behavioral Health Integration

Physical health care needs are often closely linked to mental (behavioral) health needs. There are multiple barriers to access mental or behavioral health services in the United States, including a limited number of providers, long wait times for appointments, and insurance coverage issues. Young adults in particular may be affected—43% of those with a mental illness are in the 18 to 34 age range, and stigma and difficulty navigating the health care system can affect access to treatment. Additionally, only 40% of those aged 18 to 25 with a serious mental illness report receiving treatment. One innovative solution is behavioral health integration, a team-based care delivery model where behavioral health services are located within primary care practices. These types of models are often part of patient-centered medical homes. Clinicians are not just "colocated" in the same area but routinely interact to provide holistic health services to the individual. This includes a "warm handoff," where team members provide in-person introductions to behavioral health care providers. Behavioral health providers may work with primary care providers in chronic illness care, helping individuals cope with life stressors, and addressing barriers to wellness. Research has shown that the benefits of behavioral health integration include improved access to mental health and substance abuse services, improved outcomes, and reduced costs. More research is needed to fully assess the benefits of these models, particularly for the young adult population (Agency for Healthcare Research and Quality [AHRQ], 2023a; Blasi et al., 2018).

Ethnicity, Race, and Culture

Racism and discrimination are prevalent in the United States. The young adult whose ethnic background is different from that of the dominant culture may experience this discrimination, which can occur because of differences in race, creed, language, attitudes, values, preferences, or behaviors. The young adult may also face discrimination at work, at school, in health care delivery systems, and in the community (Box 22.7: Health and Social Determinants/Health Equity).

Race and ethnicity are closely connected to educational and work-related decisions, which subsequently affect income. Lower incomes limit the resources that young adults have, such as adequate housing, access to healthy food, and health insurance. Young adults with more resources are more likely to report good health (Wu et al., 2018). Minorities are more likely to live in poverty and experience health disparities. Research has shown that racial and ethnic minorities have higher morbidity and mortality compared with Whites. These disparities can result from difficulties in accessing quality health care. Discrimination can be overtly present in health care systems and can be encountered with providers who are biased, difficulties in communication because of language spoken, and lack of trust in the health care system, which may lead the young adult to not follow recommended care (Rector & Stanley, 2021).

Values-Beliefs Pattern

Young adults enter their 20s with habits, values, and beliefs acquired during childhood and adolescence. Many acquired habits foster continuance of practices that are hazardous to health and well-being in later life. Prevention is directed toward altering value and belief patterns that encourage poor health practices and reorienting them toward those that support

BOX 22.7 HEALTH AND SOCIAL DETERMINANTS/HEALTH EQUITY

The transition to adulthood can be especially challenging for some groups. Studies have shown that undocumented immigrants who were brought to the United States as children are one such group. Some authors have termed this period as the "transition to illegality," in which young adults experience increased restrictions related to immigration policies as they transition to adulthood. In 2012, President Barack Obama created the **Deferred Action for Childhood Arrivals (DACA)** program, which provided respite for a select group of immigrants brought to the United States as children. By the end of 2022, there were approximately 580,000 immigrants who participated in the program. The program allows access to many of the societal benefits young immigrants had been previously denied, facilitating their transition to adulthood. Studies show overwhelmingly that the DACA program has had positive effects, including improved high school graduation rates, increased employment opportunities, reductions in rates of poverty, and improvements to physical and mental health. However, political and legal challenges continue to plague the program, creating a sense of uncertainty for participants.

Immigration status is an important social determinant of health and is a major contributor to health inequities. Although the DACA program has improved many aspects of undocumented immigrants' lives, they remain ineligible for many federal programs. DACA recipients are unable to apply for financial aid, and studies have shown that they have lower rates of attendance at post-secondary schools. They also are ineligible for health coverage through Medicaid and the Affordable Care Act health insurance marketplaces, resulting in higher uninsured rates (Hamilton et al., 2021: Kaiser Family Foundation, 2023).

What do you think?

- How does the DACA program contribute to the well-being of young immigrants?
- What might be some of the physical and mental health effects related to undocumented immigration status?
- Discuss the role of the nurse caring for this population in terms of advocacy and social justice.

optimal health behaviors. Nursing care is more effective when the nurse can describe, compare, identify, and align value and belief patterns consistent with practices known to maximize health.

Values Involved in Parenting

Most young adults envision parenthood as an important developmental stage; therefore health-promotion and health-protection activities to ensure healthy offspring are crucial (see the case study at the end of this chapter). American young adults are now waiting longer to have children: the average age of first-time motherhood in 2021 was 27.3 years for females. Congenital malformations, which may be genetic in origin, are the leading cause of infant deaths, affecting approximately 3% of live births. **Genetic impairments**, caused by abnormal chromosomes or inborn errors of metabolism, are also responsible for perinatal deaths, although how much is uncertain because genetic disorders may not be considered, or an infant may die before diagnosis (Wojcik et al., 2018). Tests are now available for over 1000 genetic diseases, and more are being developed (National Institute of Health [NIH], 2023). Traditional genetic testing can be lengthy. New genetic testing modalities, such as rapid whole exome sequencing (WES) and whole genome sequencing (WGS), provide a more efficient way to diagnose many genetic disorders and are being increasingly used in clinical settings. **Noninvasive prenatal testing** (NIPT) is a newer method of testing for genetic disorders that requires a sample of a mother's blood and screens both the mother and fetus for certain genetic conditions (American College of Obstetricians and Gynecologists [ACOG], 2023). A positive screening indicates the need for more specific diagnostic testing. Genetic testing, in conjunction with genetic counseling, can help guide young adults make important decisions about their current and future pregnancies and can provide closure when a perinatal death occurs. Many young adults utilize direct-to-consumer genetic testing, gaining information about their own risk factors as well as information about ancestry (Box 22.8: Genomics).

BOX 22.8 GENOMICS

Direct-to-Consumer Genetic Testing

The use of direct-to-consumer genetic testing is growing, resulting in a $465 million market in 2020. This type of testing can be obtained without involvement of a health care provider, and it offers information about ancestry, genetic health risks such as cancer and Alzheimer disease, pharmacogenetics, and general wellness information. In a recent study of over 23,000 participants, nearly half reported engaging in testing because of general curiosity and seeking information about their family trees. Twenty-seven percent of consumers learned about previously unknown close relatives, such as siblings. Some found out that their parents, who they considered biologic, were not. Although most report that this information was received as either neutral or positively, such information can be disorienting to young adults as they develop their self-identity (Basch et al., 2023; Guerrini et al., 2022),

Values Regarding Prenatal Diagnosis and Genetic Impairment

Extensive prenatal diagnostic procedures have been available since the mid-1960s. This capability has enabled the identification of high-risk pregnancies and requires the cooperation and education of childbearing females and their partners, both of whom must provide accurate family health and obstetrical histories and comply with suggested screening and follow-up measures. Decisions about the advisability of reproduction are based on current information on genetics and known deleterious genetic factors. Genetic testing, while beneficial, also includes risks and limitations, complicating decision-making (ACOG, 2023).

The finding of a malformed or genetically impaired fetus may result in a parental decision to terminate the pregnancy. Theologic and political debates in addition to legislative mandates have greatly influenced family control over many of these decisions. Abortion restrictions are making these decisions even more complex (Felix et al., 2023). Genetic counseling is an important nursing intervention for young adults. A genetic specialist gives technical explanations of genetic disorders; however, nurses have a strong supportive role in helping young adults decide whether to have children or to carry through a pregnancy that is at risk.

ENVIRONMENTAL PROCESSES

Physical Agents

Accidents

Unintentional injuries are the leading cause of death in young adults and individuals younger than 44 years (CDC, 2023a). Motor vehicle accidents cause more fatalities than all other causes of death combined. Reducing speed limits contributes to lower fatality rates. The majority of states (49 out of 50) have seat belt laws, and all states have seat belt requirements for children. In 2022, 91.6% of motor vehicle drivers and front seat occupants used seat belts (US Department of Transportation, 2023). About 50% of those killed in motor vehicle crashes in 2021 were unrestrained. Distracted driving, texting while driving, and cell phone use are the cause of many motor vehicle crashes. Most states have enacted "hands-free" or Bluetooth wireless audio legislation that limits the use of hand-held cell phones. Texting while driving is banned in 49 states. A number of states have specific rules that limit cell phone use by novice drivers, and 16 states ban all drivers from hand-held device use (Federal Communications Commission, 2021; US Department of Transportation). Besides accidents caused by distracted driving, cell phones are increasingly involved in other injuries that are the result of tripping, falling, and walking into objects while using the device. These injuries are generally to the head and neck and are most common in 13- to 29-year-olds (Povolotskiy et al., 2020).

Accident-prevention education, long considered appropriate for young children, is an important part of young adult instruction. Most young, licensed drivers have participated in driver education courses, and a number of states have adopted progressive licensing programs. A number of states have "graduated driver licensing" programs (CDC, 2023k), which have been shown to reduce younger driver crash rates. The young adult must understand the potentially fatal consequences of distracted driving.

Biologic Agents

Noise Pollution

Environmental noise is a form of air pollution that can negatively affect health. Noise exposure is one the most preventable causes of hearing loss and can be found in many environments. Elevated noise levels may also contribute to acute and chronic stress, sleep disturbances, increased cardiovascular risks, and adverse reproductive outcomes (Sivakumaran, 2022).

Sources of environmental noise include road and airport traffic and occupational exposures. The National Institute for Occupational and Health (NIOSH) recommends taking hearing precautions with noise levels that are 85 A-weighed decibels (dBA) and above. Sounds at 85 dBA require you to raise your voice to be heard by someone who is 3 feet away (NIOSH, 2023).

Young adults are also at risk of hearing loss from recreational noise exposure, including using personal music devices, visiting nightclubs, attending concerts or festivals, or playing in a band (Degeest et al., 2022). Ear protection is necessary to prevent hearing disability. Recognition of hazards and corresponding appropriate preventive education are early nursing strategies for decreasing excessive noise exposure.

Air Pollution

There are multiple sources of air pollution, both natural and human made. Motor vehicles are the largest source of air pollution; vehicles release tons of particles and noxious gases each year, most of which is either carbon monoxide or hydrocarbon emissions. Industrial facilities, agriculture, and wildfires are other sources that contribute to poor air quality. In addition to respiratory diseases, air pollution has been found to be associated with a number of health-related concerns: higher serum lipid measures in young adults, increasing cardiometabolic risk (Kim et al., 2019), associations with diabetes, rheumatic diseases, neurodegenerative conditions, cognitive decline, and premature birth (Woychik, 2023). Fine particulate matter, one type of air pollution, has been linked to a higher risk of dementia, particularly from agriculture and wildfire sources (National Institutes of Health, 2023). A Swedish study implicated air pollution in an increased risk of long COVID in young adults (Yu et al., 2022).

Climate change is a global public health challenge. Climate change (global warming) is expected to affect human health in multiple ways, including by worsening air quality by decreasing the degradation of harmful substances and by resulting in changes to the ozone layer. Rising global temperatures are also implicated in the growing intensity and frequency of wildfires, droughts, extreme rainfall, rising sea levels, and more intense storms (National Aeronautics and Space Administration, 2023).

Environmental interventions aimed at reducing air pollution and carbon emissions at an individual level include better reliance on public transportation; use of vehicles with improved fuel economy, including electric and hybrid models; and greater use of ride-sharing services. Major policy shifts and global commitment to changing current carbon emissions will be necessary to combat this problem. Young adults have a vested interest in advocating for sound approaches to addressing climate change for their future health and the health of subsequent generations. Eco-anxiety is a term used to describe the mental health effects caused by the threats of climate change. Young adults aged 18 to 34 are more concerned with the effect of climate change and have higher anxiety scores compared with older generations (Coffey et al., 2021).

Occupational Hazards and Stressors

Occupational hazards pose a threat of illness, injury, or death in all age groups, and occupational safety standards have contributed greatly to the reduction of work-related accidents. The Occupational Safety and Health Act (1970) has resulted in the improvement of work conditions, along with the provision of health care facilities, in many companies.

Workers younger than 25 have the most work-related injuries. Young adults should not be allowed to work in certain industrial settings without vocational training to reduce hazards. Occupational training should include education about personal exposure risks, identification of work-related hazards, and identification of situations in which the severity of accidents is connected to personal behaviors or habits. For example, drivers of heavy construction machinery should be particularly observant, avoid reckless behaviors, and avoid fast driving. Working females who are pregnant can expose their fetuses to industrial chemicals. Proper evaluation and temporary reassignment may be necessary. The most common workplace safety violations cited by the Occupational Safety and Health Administration (OSHA, 2023) include fall protections, hazard communications, and respiratory, machinery, and eye and face protections. Racial and ethnic minorities, recent immigrants, younger and older workers, and those with disabilities are most at risk.

Occupational preventive intervention requires that known work hazards and risks be identified early. Health histories should include questions about the place of work, type of work, and young adults' understanding of the risks associated with their occupations. Occupational risk and health are closely related; stress associated with work, the use of alcohol or drugs, and negative work attitudes are predictive of occupational injuries. Job counseling aimed at changing the nature of employment can be an appropriate referral for some people with health conditions. Nurses in occupational settings can provide periodic health assessments, updates of the health history, promote wellness, and provide counseling.

Chemical Agents

Drug Use

Misuse and overuse of drugs, including prescription drugs and opioids, is widespread. Young adults are at particular risk. Young adults aged 18 to 25 have the highest rates of illicit drug use, with 23.2% reporting use (Substance Abuse and Mental Health Services Administration [SAMHSA], 2023). Although legal in a growing number of states, marijuana is the most commonly used drug, with one-third of 18- to 25-year-olds reporting use. Other drugs used by young adults include hallucinogens (LSD, MDMA, mescaline, psilocybin), cocaine, and opioids, among others. Drug use is associated with an increased risk of unintentional injury and death, disability, violence, homicide, suicide, and communicable disease. Stress, anxiety, and poor coping skills are closely linked to drug abuse. Sources of stress for the young adult include the challenges of adjusting to adult responsibilities, school- and work-related stress, and abuse, neglect, and trauma experienced during childhood (SAMHSA, 2023). Physical health problems associated with drug abuse may be short or long term and vary by which drugs are used, how much, and for how long they are used. Changes in appetite, sleep, heart rate, and blood pressure can be short-term effects. Heart and lung disease, cancer, mental illness, HIV, and hepatitis are longer-term health problems that can arise from drug abuse (SAMHSA, 2023). Mental illness and illicit drug use are common comorbidities. Over 13% of young adults aged 18 to 25 have both a substance use disorder and some mental illness.

Two-thirds of adults that are treated for opioid disorders report having first used opioids before the age of 25, and the majority of young adults (64%) have used illicit drugs by their late 20s (National Institute of Drug Abuse [NIDA], 2023). The current opioid crisis began in the 1990s with an increase in opioid prescribing. Many of those addicted turned to using heroin, which was cheaper and more accessible. Synthetic opioids, such as fentanyl, have greatly contributed to overdose deaths (CDC, 2023n). Death rates showed some stability between 2016 and 2017, but significant increases were seen in Blacks, American Indian/Alaska Natives, and those over the age of 65. Males aged 25 to 44 have the highest heroin death rate. Prevention efforts have been aimed at establishing prescribing guidelines and prescription drug monitoring programs, in addition to increasing the availability of naloxone. Naloxone can reverse opioid overdoses and save lives. The majority of states allow naloxone to be dispensed by pharmacists without a formal prescription to increase access by friends and family members of opioid users (SAMHSA, 2023). Other harm-reducing interventions include syringe services programs (SSPs), which provide sterile syringes and injection equipment, screening for infectious diseases, and referral to treatment programs. Medication-assisted treatment, in combination with counseling and other behavioral interventions, provides a holistic approach to opioid addiction. Buprenorphine (Suboxone) is a drug that can be prescribed in office settings and works to minimize withdrawal symptoms (SAMHSA, 2023).

In the United States, marijuana is the most abused drug. Recreational use of marijuana (cannabis) is now legal in a growing number of states. Although it may be legal, there are potential health risks associated with marijuana use, including memory, learning, and attention difficulties; anxiety and depression; sexually risky behaviors; and injuries and accidents. Marijuana that is smoked can increase the risk of lung and cardiovascular disease. Results of research on marijuana use in states where it is legal are mixed, but there is some evidence that marijuana use has increased.

Nurses employed in all settings encounter individuals who have drug abuse and addiction problems. Nursing activities involve prevention strategies that may include distribution of current drug literature, early treatment of complications, education about proper naloxone use, and information regarding drug treatment centers. Several tools are available that the nurse may use for screening, such as the Drug Abuse Screening Test (DAST) or the Screening, Brief Intervention, and Referral to Treatment (SBIRT) tool.

Alcohol Use

Alcohol-related accidents among individuals aged 15 to 24 years continue to be a leading cause of preventable morbidity, disability, and death. Heavy alcohol use, that is, consumption of five or more drinks on at least one occasion within a month, is more common in 18- to 24-year-olds than in younger or older adults (Krieger et al., 2018; USDHHS, 2023). All 50 states have now set a maximum blood alcohol concentration of 0.08% for driving while intoxicated enforcement and prosecution. In addition to motor vehicle accidents, excessive alcohol use contributes to other accidents such as falls, drownings, and burns, and it increases the risk of violence by homicide, suicide, interpersonal violence, and sexual assault. Alcohol abuse is directly related to health conditions such as cirrhosis, heart disease, and certain cancers. Modifying alcohol consumption in young adults can decrease the frequency of chronic and disabling conditions in later life.

In 2019, 26% of adults aged 18 years or older reported that they had engaged in **binge drinking** in the previous 30 days (USDHHS, 2023). Binge drinking is generally defined as five or more drinks for males, or four or more drinks for females, consumed in a 2-hour period (Krieger et al., 2018). Rates of binge drinking are higher in college student populations. In 2018, 28.3% of college students reported binge drinking in the previous 30 days. Although these rates have been declining, they remain a concern.

Sexual assault is common on college campuses, is estimated to affect 20% to 25% of students, and is frequently associated with alcohol use. Females and gender diverse students report the highest levels of sexual assault, although males also report sexual assault incidents. In the majority of incidences, alcohol is involved (John Hopkins Center for Injury, 2020). First-year college students are particularly vulnerable. To address sexual assault, colleges and universities have adopted educational interventions and stricter institutional policies.

Tobacco Use

Smoking is a leading cause of preventable death in the United States; therefore, smoking cessation is the single most important counseling topic for all people because of its potential to lower the risk of contracting many preventable diseases. The majority of smokers (90%) start before the age of 18; however, the age of smoking initiation has been rising. Cigarette smoking rates among people aged 18 years and older have been declining. In 2021, 11.5% of adults reported smoking cigarettes, including 5.3% aged 18 to 24 and 12.6% aged 24 to 44 (CDC, 2023o). However, there is continued concern about the use of electronic-cigarettes (e-cigarettes) and other vaping products in the young adult population. Young adults are more likely to vape than older people, and they are less likely to use cigarettes. Twenty percent of those aged 18 to 29 reported vaping either regularly or occasionally (Schaeffer, 2019). The use of flavoring is believed to be a contributor to the appeal for young users. These electronic devices can be used for other drugs also, most commonly marijuana (CDC, 2023n).

Individuals employed in high-risk occupations (e.g., mining, construction) are informed of the synergistic relationship between smoking and other environmental exposures, including exposure to asbestos, coal dust, and radiation. Fear tactics, nagging, preaching, and threats are generally ineffective at convincing people to stop smoking. A major barrier to smoking cessation is the presence of other smokers, particularly in situations where alcohol is also being consumed.

Decreasing the use of any tobacco products among adults is a *Healthy People 2030* goal. A number of interventions have been found to be effective in reducing tobacco use, including policies and programs that reduce the out-of-pocket costs for evidence-based treatment programs, smart phone apps that provide behavioral support, work-based incentives, smoke-free policies, increasing the cost of tobacco products, and restricting product access to minors (Community Guide, 2023). Nurses should be familiar with the antismoking resources in their state and community, enabling them to make the appropriate referrals. Motivational interviewing can be utilized to help individuals begin to consider tobacco cessation.

Carcinogens

Young adults are potentially exposed to multiple carcinogens. Environmental sources include food, personal care items, household cleaners, lawn care products, and work exposures. Exposure to a known carcinogen will not necessarily result in cancer but will depend on multiple factors, including the amount and duration of the exposure in addition to the genetic make-up of the individual (National Cancer Institute, 2023). Health behaviors that increase cancer risk include having multiple sexual partners, unhealthy diets, tobacco use, excessive sun exposure, and heavy alcohol use. In the work setting, environmental regulations have limited exposure to some hazardous chemicals, but the long-term effects on health of exposure to many industrial chemicals remains unknown, and cancers may develop many years after exposure (National Cancer Institute, 2023). In addition to individual counseling, nurses can join professional organizations and advocate at the policy level for healthy environments through the legislative process (Alliance of Nurses for Healthy Environments, 2023).

DETERMINANTS OF HEALTH

Social Factors and Environment

Community Resources

The environment of the community strongly influences the well-being of the young adult and sets the standard for the health of people and families living within a neighborhood. Healthy communities are those that provide safe neighborhoods, adequate availability of jobs, sources for healthy food, and access to transportation and health care services. Community resources for exercise and recreation can make important contributions to the young adult's physical and emotional health. The built environment, which refers to human-made structures and features, including sidewalks, bike lanes, and green spaces, encourages people to become more physically active. Public spaces and shady areas encourage social interaction. When these resources are available, the young adult has the opportunity to exercise and release stress in a positive fashion.

Environmental disparities exist and contribute to health disparities. Low-income communities have disproportionally higher rates of childhood asthma, elevated lead levels, cancers related to environmental exposures, and obesity. Minorities and those living in poverty are more likely to live in substandard housing, have poorer water quality, live on land that is contaminated, and have greater exposure to sources of pollution. **Environmental justice** addresses disparities that are based on higher exposure to environmental risks and hazards (Rector & Stanley, 2022).

Levels of Policymaking and Health

Civic engagement is another mark of the transition to adulthood and includes activities such as voting, volunteering, and activism. Young adults who participate in these activities have been found to have improved mental health, greater educational attainment, and higher incomes (Hope, 2022). A study involving 44 countries, including the United States, found that voters reported better health. Voting offers an opportunity to contribute to ideas and creates a sense of purpose and connection to communities. Encouraging young adults to be involved in their communities fosters a lifelong commitment to civic participation (USDHHS, 2023).

Half of young adults aged 18 to 29 years voted in the 2020 election, an increase of 11 points from 2016. Although turnout varied across the country, the young adult vote proved decisive in several states (Tufts Center for Information & Research on Civic Learning and Engagement, 2021). Participation in protests and demonstrations have also increased. Young adults report caring about issues including racial justice, abortion, climate change, gun violence, and student loan debt. Young adults also participate politically by making political donations and through consumer choices. Social media plays a critical role, with 59% of young adults reporting it is a way to engage with social and political issues (Hope, 2022).

Health Services/Delivery System

Access to health services is critical for supporting population health and eliminating health disparities. Improving health services generally means finding usual and continuing sources of primary/preventive care. Economic realities, however, influence the effectiveness of resources, particularly for the young adult who lives in economically depressed or rural areas (Box 22.9: Ethical Issues). In some communities, health services are lacking or, if available, are not culturally sensitive or adapted to the customs and beliefs of the people who are served. Rural areas can be particularly challenging for finding appropriate health services. Access to public transportation can be a critical problem, affecting the ability of the young adult to keep appointments. Young adults aged 18 to 24 years are the least likely of any age group to have a usual source of care (US Census Bureau, 2023); thus, a target of *Healthy People 2030* is to increase the proportion of adults with a usual primary care provider (USDHHS, 2023). Higher numbers of females report a usual place of care than males. Gaps in health care insurance coverage that occur between the end of schooling and the attainment of full employment can reduce the young adult's access to primary care. The ACA, passed in 2010, mandates coverage for young adults up to the age of 26 years within family health insurance coverage. This act has decreased the young adult uninsured rate and decreased the disparities between Hispanic and Black populations. However, in 2018, those aged 18 to 34 were the most likely to be uninsured (17%) compared with other age groups and more likely to report difficulty paying for care, particularly for prescriptions (Hensley, 2018). Racial minorities are more likely to be uninsured in addition to those who live in states that did not expand Medicaid access under the ACA (Kaiser Family Foundation [KFF], 2022). A number of other barriers of access to health care services exist, contributing to health disparities. Social determinants of health such as income, education level, and immigration status play a major role in health disparities. Those who are disabled, live in rural areas, and are sexual and gender minorities also experience disparities (KFF, 2023).

Health-delivery methods in the United States are based primarily on Western belief systems, which tend to be rigid in their applications. Young adults are interested in the convenience of health care and may utilize nontraditional sources of care more than older groups. These sources include increased emergency department use, urgent care centers, retail clinics, and online telemedicine visits. These sources of care are less likely to engage in preventive and health-promoting services. Greater transformation needs to occur in the health care system to improve patient engagement. A sustained relationship with a primary care provider can improve health outcomes. Nurses need to be able to identify health practices and health system gaps that are barriers to care and harmful to people.

Nursing accounts for the largest group of professionals within the US health care system. However, nurses may not be able to deliver care optimally within changing health care settings because of barriers to practice and ineffective workforce planning, data, and information infrastructure. A widely circulated report from the Institute of Medicine (2010) noted that the nursing profession cannot contribute optimally unless nurses fully participate in team planning and health care redesign with physicians and other health care professionals. In addition, business, government, health-delivery agencies, and the insurance industry must all participate in a newly designed health care system that provides accessible, affordable quality care, leading to increases in measurable health outcomes (see the case study at the end of this chapter).

BOX 22-9 Ethical Issues

Health care disparities are pervasive in the United States; however, there are growing geographic disparities, particularly between urban and rural communities. Rural populations have higher rates of poverty, fewer economic opportunities, increased mental health needs, higher mortality rates, aging populations, and fewer health care providers and community services than urban areas. These factors create unique challenges for young adults transitioning to adulthood. More research is needed to further contextualize the experiences of rural young adults and to identify resources and interventions that can improve health outcomes (Fenton et al., 2022; Rural Health Information Hub, 2023).

NURSING APPLICATION

Young adulthood is a critical period of transitions. Physical growth is complete by this stage. The physical abilities of the young adult are in peak condition, so the goals of the nurse are aimed at maintaining optimal physical condition, encouraging healthy habits, screening individuals for disease, and treating illnesses.

Preventive care is recommended to young adults in the form of screening and preventive care visits. Health examinations at recommended intervals are a crucial component of screening individuals for potential health concerns and providing education about measures to avoid disease and disability.

It is necessary to screen individuals for cardiovascular conditions after the age of 25 years as well as to provide education about risk factor modification. Intervention efforts should reflect diversity of age, sex, ethnicity, and socioeconomic status. As the nurse obtains an assessment of the individual and family history, the necessity of further screening, education, or monitoring is determined. Elements of education include smoking cessation and dietary modifications.

Young adults are encouraged to engage in physical activity and muscle-strengthening exercise. Lack of time or lack of access may be barriers to increased physical activity. The nurse working with the young adult population should consider implementing work site wellness programs. Group fitness or weight loss programs can be an effective means of promoting wellness at work while increasing employee satisfaction and productivity. Some workforce programs use incentive systems in which points are awarded for the achievement of particular milestones. Once a set level of points is reached, the employee is given a reward in the form of gift cards or movie tickets. These types of programs are often effective for smoking cessation, weight loss, and exercise. In addition, some companies encourage the formation of facility-sponsored sports teams for charities or sports, such as bowling leagues, softball teams, or a running club. This encourages camaraderie among colleagues and increases participation in people who respond well to group motivation. Nonworking young adults looking for a group fitness or sports program should be directed to resources within the community via Internet research.

CASE STUDY

Preparing for Childbearing: Kirsten

Kirsten is a healthy 22-year-old whose favorite sport is running. Most of the time she runs outside, but she also uses gym treadmills. Since this spring, Kirsten has believed that her breathing capacity is diminishing, and her levels of energy are decreasing. During her period these symptoms appear to worsen. Last week, while running up a rather steep course, Kirsten became much weaker, dizzier, and more fatigued than usual, and her best friend and running partner recommended that she make a physician's appointment for a physical examination. Kirsten's running partner also noted that she has appeared pale lately.

In the physician's office, Kirsten is noted to have a normal temperature, elevated heart and respiratory rates, and a blood pressure of 90/60 mm Hg. Kirsten's description of her period is that it tends to be heavy and has been this way for 5 years. For muscle aches and pains caused by running, she usually takes two aspirin tablets every 3 to 4 h for as long as 7 days. When her running increases during the summer, she takes aspirin or ibuprofen continually for 2 to 3 months. Diagnostic testing indicates that her hemoglobin level is 7 g/dL, and her red blood cells are pale and small. Kirsten has been in a long-term relationship for several years, her wedding is in several months, and there has been discussion of preconceptional health planning and future children.

Reflective Questions

- What common health alteration in young adult females is most likely for Kirsten?
- What contributing factors place Kirsten at risk?
- What lifestyle modifications can Kirsten implement to decrease her risk?

The nurse working with young adults provides education about skin cancer risk, the need for adequate sunscreen, and signs and symptoms of skin cancer. Safety education is provided about recreational and sports-related injuries and how to prevent them. Additional education is required for young adult females. The nurse may be in a position of providing counseling or referrals for contraception, prenatal care, unintended pregnancy, STIs, and HIV infection. It is imperative that females receive preconceptional and early prenatal care to maintain optimal health for themselves and the unborn child.

The nurse working with the young adult population often becomes a counselor. It is important to assess stressors, as prolonged stress, anxiety, or depression can negatively affect the health of the individual. Stressors may be related to relationships, divorce, employment, layoffs, or financial concerns. The nurse listens, offers support and concern, and provides the individual or family with resources or support groups specific to the stressor.

SUMMARY

- The young adult period is a critical developmental stage offering the nurse unique opportunities for health-promotion and disease-prevention efforts.
- Young adults transitioning to adulthood achieve major life milestones, including secondary education, full-time employment, independent living, romantic partnering, and parenthood.
- Changing trends in the health of young adults include higher incidences of unhealthy behaviors, increasing mental health challenges, and chronic health conditions.
- Unhealthy behaviors greatly contribute to an increased risk of cardiovascular disease, diabetes, and cancer in later life.
- Nurses can provide critical education to young adults in college and work settings and on social media platforms.
- Nurses are challenged to advocate for social justice, healthy environments, and the reduction of health disparities.

EVOLVE CHAPTER FEATURES

http://evolve.elsevier.com/Edelman/

- Study Questions

REFERENCES

Abbasi, I. S. (2018). Social media and committed relationships: What factors make our romantic relationship vulnerable? *Social Science Computer Review*, *37*(3), 425–434. https://doi.org/10.1177/0894439318770609

Agency for Healthcare Research and Quality. (2023a). *What is integrated behavioral health?* https://integrationacademy.ahrq.gov/?_gl=1*1uwq0fo*_ga*MTYwNDIzMzgxLjE2OTI5ODU5NDU.*_ga_1NPT56LE7J*MTcwNDIxNTA3NC4xNC4xLjE3MDQyMTUyNTYuMC4wLjA

Agency for Healthcare Research and Quality. (2023b). *Clinical decision support*. https://www.ahrq.gov/cpi/about/otherwebsites/clinical-decision-support/index.html

Alawode, O. A., & Nicholson, H. L. (2023). Health literacy and uptake of annual physical checkups among emerging adults in the United States: Findings from the behavioral risk factor surveillance system. *Sociology Compass*, *17*(4). https://doi.org/10.1111/soc4.13081

Alliance of Nurses for Healthy Environments. (2023). *About AHNE.* https://envirn.org/about/

Amenabar, T. (2023). 'Forever chemicals' found in period underwear, tampon wrappers. *The Washington Post.* https://www.washingtonpost.com/wellness/2023/08/10/forever-chemicals-pfas-period-underwear-tampons/

American Academy of Dermatology. (2023). *How to prevent skin cancer.* https://www.aad.org/skin-cancer-how-prevent

American Association of Occupational Health Nurses (AAOHN). (2021). *AAOHN position statement: Delivery of occupational and environmental health nursing services.* https://www.aaohn.org/Portals/0/docs/Delivery%20of%20Occupational%20and%20Environmental%20Health%20Nursing%20Services.pdf

American Cancer Society. (2023). *Key statistics in melanoma skin cancer.* https://www.cancer.org/cancer/types/melanoma-skin-cancer/about/key-statistics.html

American College of Obstetricians and Gynecologists (ACOG). (2023). *ACOG Explains: Prenatal genetic testing.* https://www.acog.org/womens-health/videos/prenatal-genetic-testing

American College of Sports Medicine. (2023). https://www.acsm.org/

American Institute of Stress. (2019). *Anxiety in college students: Causes, statistics, & how universities can help.* https://www.stress.org

American Heart Association. (2022a). *High blood pressure in younger adults linked to midlife brain changes.* https://newsroom.heart.org/news/high-blood-pressure-in-younger-adults-linked-to-midlife-brain-changes#:~:text=Younger%20adults%20who%20had%20higher,in%20mid%2D%20and%20late%20life

American Heart Association. (2022b). *Young adults who experienced intimate partner violence may face higher cardiac risks later.* https://newsroom.heart.org/news/young-adults-who-experienced-intimate-partner-violence-may-face-higher-cardiac-risks-later

Andes, L. J., Cheng, Y. J., & Rolka, D. B. (2019). Prevalence of prediabetes among adolescents and young adults in the United States, 2005-2016. *JAMA Pediatrics*, 174(2), e194498. https://doi.org/10.1001/jamapediatrics.2019.4498

Anderson, L. N., Alvarez, E., Incze, T., Tarride, J. E., Kwan, M., & Mbuagbau, L. (2023). Motivational interviewing to promote healthy behaviors for obesity prevention in young adults (MOTIVATE): a pilot randomized controlled trial protocol. *Pilot & Feasibility Studies*, *9*, 156. https://doi.org/10.1186/s40814-023-01385-0

Armstrong, S., Wong, C. A., Perrin, E., Page, S., Sibley, L., & Skinner, A. (2018). Association of physical activity with income, race/ethnicity, and sex among adolescents and young adults in the United States: Findings from the National Health and Nutrition Examination Survey, 2007-2016. *JAMA Pediatrics*, *172*(8), 732–740. https://doi.org/10.1001/jamapediatrics.2018.1273

Arnett, D. K., Blumenthal, R. S., Albert, M. A., Buroker, A. B., Goldberger, Z. D., Hahn, E. J., Himmelfarb, C. D., Khera, A., Llyod-Jones, D., McEvoy, W., Michos, E. D., Miedema, M. D., Munoz, D., Smith, S. C., Virani, S. S., Williams, K. A., Yeboah, J., & Ziaeian, B. (2019). 2019 ACC/AHA guideline on the primary prevention of cardiovascular disease: A report of the American College of Cardiology/American Heart Association task force on clinical practice guidelines. *Circulation*, *140*, e596–e646. https://doi.org/10.1161/CIR.0000000000000678

Arnett, J. J., Lachman, M. E., & Robinson, O. (2020). Rethinking adult development: Introduction to the special issue. *American Psychologist*, *75*(4), 425–430. https://doi.org/10.1037/amp0000633

Babakr, Z. H., Mohamedamin, P., & Kakamad, K. (2019). Piaget's cognitive developmental theory: Critical review. *Education Quarterly Review*, *2*(3), 517–524. https://doi.org/10.31014/aior.1993.02.03.84

Basch, C. H., Hillyer, G. C., Samuel, L., Datuowei, E., & Cohn, B. (2023). Direct-to-consumer genetic testing in the news: A descriptive study. *Journal of Community Genetics*, *14*, 63–69. https://doi.org/10.1007/s12687-022-00613-z

Berman, I. S., McLaughlin, K. A., Tottenham, N., Godfrey, K., Seeman, T., Loucks, E., Suomi, S., Danese, A., & Sheridan, M. A. (2022). Measuring early life adversity: A dimensional approach. *Development and Psychopathology*, *34*, 499–511. https://doi.org/10.1017/s0954579421001826

Blasi, P. R., Cromp, D., McDonald, S., Hsu, C., Coleman, K., Flinter, M., & Wagner, E. H. (2018). Approaches to behavioral health integration at high performing primary care practices. *Journal of the American Board of Family Medicine*, *31*, 691–701. https://www.jabfm.org/content/31/5/691

Brown, A. (2022). *About 5% of young adults in the U.S. say their gender is different from their sex assigned at birth.* Pew Research. https://www.pewresearch.org/short-reads/2022/06/07/about-5-of-young-adults-in-the-u-s-say-their-gender-is-different-from-their-sex-assigned-at-birth/

Brown, M., Macarthur, J., Higgins, A., & Chouliara, Z. (2019). Transitions from child to adult health care for young people with intellectual disabilities: A systematic review. *Journal of Advanced Nursing*, *75*, 2418–2434. https://doi.org/10.1111/jan.13985

Carey, R. M., & Whelton, P. K. (2018). Prevention, detection, evaluation, and management of high blood pressure in adults: Synopsis of the 2017 American College of Cardiology/American Heart Association hypertension guideline. *Annals in Internal Medicine*, *168*(5), 351–358.

Catalyst. (2023). *Workplaces that work for women.* https://www.catalyst.org/

Centers for Disease Control and Prevention. (2022a). *Hepatitis B Information.* https://www.cdc.gov

Centers for Disease Control and Prevention. (2022b). *Meningococcal disease.* https://www.cdc.gov/meningococcal/index.html

Centers for Disease Control and Prevention. (2022c). *HPV vaccination for adults aged 27-45 years.* https://www.cdc.gov/vaccines/hcp/admin/downloads/isd-job-aid-scdm-hpv-shared-clinical-decision-making-hpv.pdf

Centers for Disease Control and Prevention. (2022d). *Body mass index (BMI).* https://www.cdc.gov

Centers for Disease Control and Prevention. (2022e). *Physical activity.* https://www.cdc.gov

Centers for Disease Control and Prevention. (2022f). *Sleep and sleep disorders.* https://www.cdc.gov/sleep/index.html

Centers for Disease Control and Prevention (CDC). (2023a). *Leading causes of death and injury.* https://www.cdc.gov/injury/wisqars/leadingcauses.html

Centers for Disease Control and Prevention (CDC). (2023b). *Births and Natality.* National Center for Health Statistics. https://www.cdc.gov/nchs/fastats/births.htm

Centers for Disease Control and Prevention (CDC). (2023c). *National diabetes status report: Estimates of diabetes and its burden in the United States.* https://www.cdc.gov

Centers for Disease Control and Prevention (CDC). (2023d). *About flu.* https://www.cdc.gov/flu/about/index.html

Centers for Disease Control and Prevention (CDC). (2023e) *Tuberculosis.* https://www.cdc.gov

Centers for Disease Control and Prevention (CDC). (2023f). *Hepatitis C.* https://www.cdc.gov/hepatitis/hcv/index.html

Centers for Disease Control and Prevention (CDC). (2023g). *Obesity and overweight*. National Center for Health Statistics. https://www.cdc.gov/nchs/fastats/obesity-overweight.htm

Centers for Disease Control and Prevention (CDC). (2023h). *Nutrition*. https://www.cdc.gov/nutrition/index.html

Centers for Disease Control and Prevention (CDC). (2023i). *Facts about neural tube defects*. https://www.cdc.gov

Centers for Disease Control and Prevention (CDC). (2023j). *HIV*. https://www.cdc.gov/hiv/default.html

Centers for Disease Control and Prevention (CDC). (2023k). *Injury prevention and control*. https://www.cdc.gov/injury/index.html

Centers for Disease Control and Prevention (CDC). (2023l). *Sexual transmitted diseases*. https://www.cdc.gov

Centers for Disease Control and Prevention (CDC). (2023m). *Mental health*. https://www.cdc.gov

Centers for Disease Control and Prevention (CDC). (2023n). *Drug basics*. https://www.cdc.gov

Centers for Disease Control and Prevention (CDC). (2023o). *Smoking and tobacco use*. https://www.cdc.gov

Center for Reproductive Rights. (2023a). *Abortion*. https://reproductiverights.org/our-issues/abortion/

Center for Reproductive Rights. (2023b). *Nationwide threat to medication abortion*. https://reproductiverights.org/fda-lawsuit-threatens-medication-abortion-nationwide/

Cheung, F., Tang, C. S. K., Lim, M. S. M., & Koh, J. M. (2018). Workaholism on job burnout: A comparison between American and Chinese employees. *Frontiers in Psychology*, *9*, 1–11. https://doi.org/10.3389/fpsyg.2018.02546

Coffey, Y., Bhullar, N., Durkin, J., Islam, A. S., & Usher, K. (2021). Understanding eco-anxiety: A systematic scoping review of current literature and identified knowledge gaps. *Journal of Climate Change and Health*, *3*, 100047. https://doi.org/10.1016/j.joclim.2021.100047

Cohen, R., Baluch, B., & Duffy, L. J. (2018). Defining extreme sport: Conceptions and misconceptions. *Frontiers in Psychology*, *9*, 1974. https://doi.org/10.3389/fpsyg.2018.01974

Commonwealth Fund. (2022). *The U.S. maternal mortality crises continues to worsen: An international comparison*. https://www.commonwealthfund.org/blog/2022/us-maternal-mortality-crisis-continues-worsen-international-comparison#:~:text=New%20international%20data%20show%20the,most%20other%20high%2Dincome%20countries

The Community Guide. (2023). https://www.thecommunityguide.org/index.html

Cunningham, J. W., Vaduganathan, M., Claggett, B. L., Jering, K. S., Bhatt, A. S., Rosenthal, N., & Solomon, S. D. (2021). Clinical outcomes in young US adults hospitalized with COVID-19. *JAMA Internal Medicine*, *181*(3), 379–381. https://doi.org/10.1001/jamainternmed.2020.5313

Daiber, J. F., & Gnugnoli, D. M. (2023). Visual acuity. In *StatPearls*. StatPearls Publishing. https://www.ncbi.nlm.nih.gov/books/NBK563298/

Declercq, E., Barnard-Mayers, R., Zephyrin, L. C., & Johnson, K. (2022). *The U.S. maternal health divide: The limited maternal health services and worse outcomes of states proposing new abortion restrictions* [Issue Brief]. Commonwealth Fund. https://doi.org/10.26099/z7dz-8211

Degeest, S., Corthals, P., & Keppler, H. (2022). Evolution of hearing in young adults: Effects of leisure noise exposure, attitudes, and beliefs toward noise, hearing loss, and hearing protection devices. *Noise & Health*, *24*(113), 61–74. https://doi.org/10.4103/nah.nah_7_21

Erikson, E. H. (1993). *Childhood and society*. New York: W.W. Norton.

Fadeyi, D., & Horowitz, J. M. (2022). Americans more likely to say it's a bad thing than a good thing that more young adults live with their parents. Pew Research Center. https://www.pewresearch.org/short-reads/2022/08/24/americans-more-likely-to-say-its-a-bad-thing-than-a-good-thing-that-more-young-adults-live-with-their-parents/

Federal Communications Commission. (2021). *The dangers of distracted driving*. https://www.fcc.gov/consumers/guides/dangers-texting-while-driving

Felix, M., Sobel, L., & Salganicoff, A. (2023). *A review of exceptions in state abortion bans: Implications for the provision of abortion services*. Kaiser Family Foundation. https://www.kff.org/womens-health-policy/issue-brief/a-review-of-exceptions-in-state-abortions-bans-implications-for-the-provision-of-abortion-services/

Fenton, M. P., Forthun, L. F., Aristild, S., & Vasquez, K. B. (2022). The role of the rural context in the transition to adulthood: A scoping review. *Adolescent Research Review*, *7*(1), 101–126. https://doi.org/10.1007/s40894-021-00161-6

Filley, C. M., Arciniegas, D. B., Brenner, L. A., Anderson, A., & Kelly, J. P. (2019). Chronic traumatic encephalopathy: A clinical perspective. *Journal of Neuropsychiatry and Clinical Neuroscience*, *31*(2), 170–172. https://doi.org/10.1176/appi.neuropsych.18100223

Fraze, T. K., Brewster, A. L., Lewis, V. A., Beidler, L. B., Murray, G. F., & Colla, C. H. (2019). Prevalence of screening for food insecurity, housing instability, utility needs, transportation needs, and interpersonal violence by US physician practices and hospitals. *JAMA Network Open*, *2*(9), 1–14. https://doi.org/10.1001/jamanetworkopen.2019.11514

Fry, R. (2023a). *Young adults in the U.S. are reaching key life milestones later than in the past*. Pew Research. https://www.pewresearch.org/short-reads/2023/05/23/young-adults-in-the-u-s-are-reaching-key-life-milestones-later-than-in-the-past/#:~:text=Adults%20who%20are%2021%20are,married%20and%20having%20a%20child

Fry, R. (2023c). *Fewer young men are in college, especially at 4-year schools*. Pew Research Center. https://www.pewresearch.org/short-reads/2023/12/18/fewer-young-men-are-in-college-especially-at-4-year-schools/#:~:text=College%20enrollment%20among%20young%20Americans,fewer%20young%20men%20pursuing%20college

Galic, I., Negris, O., Warren, C., Brown, D., Bozen, A., & Jain, T. (2021). Disparities in access to fertility care: Who's in and who's out. *F&S Reports*, *2*(1), 109–117. https://doi.org/10.1016/j.xfre.2020.11.001

Gelles-Watnick, R. (2023). *For Valentine's Day, 5 facts about single Americans*. Pew Research Center. https://www.pewresearch.org/short-reads/2023/02/08/for-valentines-day-5-facts-about-single-americans/

Georgieff, M., Krebs, N. F., & Cusick, S. E. (2019). *The benefits and risks of iron supplementation in pregnancy and childhood. Annual Review of Nutrition*, *39*, 121–146. https://doi.org/10.1146/annurev-nutr-082018-124213

Gilligan, C. (1982). *In a different voice*. Cambridge, MA: Harvard University Press.

Gilligan, C. (2002). *The birth of pleasure*. New York: Alfred A. Knopf.

Gilligan, C. (2013). *Joining the resistance*. Malden, MA: Polity Press.

Goldstuck, N. D., & Cheung, T. S. (2019). The efficacy of intrauterine devices for emergency contraception and beyond: A systematic review update. *International Journal of Women's Health*, *11*, 471–479. https://doi.org/10.2147/IJWH.S213815

Grant, R., Becnel, J. N., Giano, Z. D., Williams, A. L., & Matinez, D. (2019). A latent profile analysis of young adult lifestyle behaviors. *American Journal of Health Behaviors, 43*(6), 1148–1161. https://pubmed.ncbi.nlm.nih.gov/31662173/

Gramlich, J. (2023). *What the data says about gun deaths in the U.S.* Pew Research. https://www.pewresearch.org/short-reads/2023/04/26/what-the-data-says-about-gun-deaths-in-the-u-s/

Guerrini, C. J., Robinson, J. O., Bloss, C. C., Brooks, W. B., Fullerton, S. M., Kirkpatrick, B., Soo-Jin Lee, S., Majumder, M., Pereira, S., Schuman, O., & McGuire, A. L. (2022). Family secrets: Experiences and outcomes of participating in direct-to-consumer genetic relative-finder services. *American Journal of Human Genetics, 109*, 486–497. https://doi.org/10.1016/j.ajhg.2022.01.013

Guttmacher Institute. (2020). *Contraceptive effectiveness in the United States.* https://www.guttmacher.org/fact-sheet/contraceptive-effectiveness-united-states

Hafeez, S., Gupta, C., & Sprajcer, M. (2023). *Stress and the gig economy: It's not all shifts and giggles. Industrial Health, 61*(2), 140–150. https://doi.org/10.2486/indhealth.2021-0217

Hamilton, E. R., Patler, C., & Langer, P. D. (2021). The life-course timing of legalization: Evidence from the DACA program. *Socius: Sociological Research for a Dynamic World, 7*, 1–14. http:/doi.org/10.1177/23780231211058958

Hatcher, R. A., Nelson, A. L., Trussel, J., Cwiak, C., Cason, P., Policar, M. S., Edelman, A. B., Aiken, A. R. A., Marrazzo, J. M., & Kowal, D. (2018). *Contraceptive technology* (21st ed.). New York: Ayer Company Publishers, LLC.

Hensley, S. (2018). *Poll: Young people more likely to defer health care because of cost.* National Public Radio. https://www.npr.org/sections/health-shots/2018/12/07/674567886/poll-young-people-most-likely-to-defer-health-care-because-of-cost

Hill, L., Artiga, S., & Ranji, U. (2022). *Racial disparities in maternal and infant health: Current status and efforts to address them.* Kaiser Family Foundation. https://www.kff.org/racial-equity-and-health-policy/issue-brief/racial-disparities-in-maternal-and-infant-health-current-status-and-efforts-to-address-them/

HIV.gov. (2025). *U.S. statistics.* https://www.hiv.gov/hiv-basics/overview/data-and-trends/statistics/

Holt-Lunstad, J. (2022). Social connection as a public health issue: The evidence and a systemic framework for prioritizing the "social" in social determinants of health. *Annual Review of Public Health, 43*, 193–213. https://doi.org/10.1146/annurev-publhealth-052020-110732

Hope, E. C. (2022). *Rethinking civic engagement.* Brennan Center For Justice. https://www.brennancenter.org/our-work/research-reports/rethinking-civic-engagement

Hoyert, D. L. (2023). *Maternal mortality rates in the United States, 2021.* National Center for Health Statistics. https://www.cdc.gov/nchs/data/hestat/maternal-mortality/2021/maternal-mortality-rates-2021.htm

Institute of Medicine (IOM). (2010). *The future of nursing: Leading change, advancing health.* National Academies Press. https://www.ncbi.nlm.nih.gov/books/NBK209880/pdf/Bookshelf_NBK209880.pdf

Johns Hopkins Center for Injury Research and Policy. (2020). *Reducing alcohol-related sexual assault on college campuses: A public health approach.* Johns Hopkins Bloomberg School of Public Health, Baltimore, MD, 21205. https://publichealth.jhu.edu/sites/default/files/2023-03/jhsph-cirp-reducing-alcohol-related-sexual-assult.pdf

Jones, P. J., Park, S. Y., & Lefevor, G. T. (2018). Contemporary college student anxiety: The role of academic distress, financial stress, and support. *Journal of College Counseling, 21*(3), 252–264. https://doi.org/10.1002/jocc.12107

Juvonen, J., Lessard, L. M., Kline, N. G., & Graham, S. (2022). Young adult adaptability to the social challenges of the COVID-19 pandemic: The protective role of friendships. *Journal of Youth and Adolescence, 51*, 585–597. https://doi.org/10.1007/s10964-022-01573-w

Kaiser Family Foundation. (2019). *The uninsured and the ACA: A primer - Key facts about health insurance and the uninsured amidst changes to the Affordable Care Act.* https://www.kff.org/report-section/the-uninsured-and-the-aca-a-primer-key-facts-about-health-insurance-and-the-uninsured-amidst-changes-to-the-affordable-care-act-how-does-lack-of-insurance-affect-access-to-care/

Kaiser Family Foundation. (2023). *Key facts on deferred action for childhood arrivals (DACA).* https://www.kff.org/racial-equity-and-health-policy/fact-sheet/key-facts-on-deferred-action-for-childhood-arrivals-daca/#:~:text=To%20be%20eligible%2C%20individuals%20must,as%20of%20June%2015%2C%202012

Karim, F., Oyewandes, A. A., Abdalla, L. F., Ehsanullah, R. C., & Khan, S. (2020). Social media use and its connection to mental health: A systematic review. *Cureus, 12*(6), e8627. https://doi.org/10.7759/cureus.8627

Keisler-Starkey, K., Bunch, L. N., & Lindstrom, R. A. (2023). *Health insurance coverage in the United States: 2022.* US Census Bureau. https://www.census.gov/content/dam/Census/library/publications/2023/demo/p60-281.pdf

Kim, J. S., Chen, Z., Alderete, T. L., Toledo-Corral, C., Lurmann, K. B., Berhane, K., & Gulliland, F. D. (2019). Associations of air pollution, obesity and cardiometabolic health in young adults: The Meta-AIR study. *Environment International, 133*, 1–10. http://doi.org/10.1016/j.envint.2019.105180

Kohlberg, L., & Lickons, T. (1986). *The stages of ethical development: From childhood through old age.* San Francisco, CA: Harper.

Krieger, H., Young, C. M., Antheniem, A. M., & Neighbors, C. (2018). The epidemiology of binge drinking among college-age individuals in the United States. *Alcohol Research, 39*(1), 23–30.

Krukowski, R. A., Jacobson, L. T., John, J., Kinser, P., Campbell, K., Ledoux, T., Gavin, K. L., Chiu, C. Y., Wang, T., & Kruper, A. (2022). Correlates of early prenatal care access among U.S. women: Data from the pregnancy risk assessment monitoring system (PRAMS). *Maternal and Child Health Journal, 26*, 328–341. https://link.springer.com/article/10.1007/s10995-021-03232-1

Lawrence, E. M., Hummer, R. A., & Domingue, B. W. (2018). Wide educational disparities in young adult cardiovascular health. *SSM Population Health, 5*, 249–256. https://pubmed.ncbi.nlm.nih.gov/30094320/

Lee, M. K, Lee, J. K., Sohn, S. Y., Ahn, J., Hong, O. K., Kim, M. K., Baek, K. H., Song, K.H., Han, K., & Kwon, H. S. (2023). Cumulative exposure to metabolic syndrome in a national population-based cohort of young adults and sex-specific risk for type 2 diabetes. *Diabetology & Metabolic Syndrome, 15*, 78. https://doi.org/10.1186/s13098-023-01030-z

Leppert, R. (2023). *Young workers express lower levels of job satisfaction than older ones, but most are content with their job.* Pew Research Center. https://www.pewresearch.org/short-reads/2023/05/25/young-workers-express-lower-levels-of-job-satisfaction-than-older-ones-but-most-are-content-with-their-job/

Liang, X., Or, B., Tsoi, M. F., Cheung, C. L., & Cheung, B. M. Y. (2023). Prevalence of metabolic syndrome in the United States Nutritional Health and Nutrition Examination Survey 2011-18. *Journal of Postgraduate Medicine, 99*(1175), 985–992. https://doi.org/10.1093/postmj/qgad008

Lim, Y., & Boster, J. (2023). Obesity and comorbid conditions. In *StatPearls*. StatPearls Publishing. https://www.ncbi.nlm.nih.gov/books/NBK574535/

Livingston, G. (2018). *About one-third of U.S. children are living with a single parent*. Pew Research. https://www.pewresearch.org/short-reads/2018/04/27/about-one-third-of-u-s-children-are-living-with-an-unmarried-parent/

Lopes, L., Kearney, A. Washington, I., Valdes, I., Yilma, H., & Hamel, R. (2023). *KFF health misinformation tracking poll pilot*. Kaiser Family Foundation. https://www.kff.org/coronavirus-covid-19/poll-finding/kff-health-misinformation-tracking-poll-pilot/

McArdle, N., Ward, S. V., Bucks, R. S., Maddison, K., Smith, A., Huang, R. C., Pennell, C. E., Hillman, D. R., & Eastwood, P. R. (2020). The prevalence of common sleep disorders in young adults: A descriptive population-based study. *Sleep*, *43*(10), zsaa072. https;//doi.org/10.1093/sleep/zsaa072

McCarthy, J. (2022) *Same sex marriage support inches up to new high of 71%*. Gallup. https://news.gallup.com/poll/393197/same-sex-marriage-support-inches-new-high.aspx

Medina, C., & Mahowald, L. (2023). *Discrimination and barriers to well-being: The state of the LGBTQI+* community in 2022. Center for American Progress. https://www.americanprogress.org/article/discrimination-and-barriers-to-well-being-the-state-of-the-lgbtqi-community-in-2022/

Moreland, B., Ortmann, N., & Clemens, T. (2022). Increased unintentional drowning deaths in 2020 by age, race/ethnicity, sex, and location, United States. *Journal of Safety Research*, *82*, 463–468. https://doi.org/10.1016/j.jsr.2022.06.012

Nagata, J. M., Vittinghoff, E., Gabriel, K. P., Garber, A. K, Moran, A. E., Rana, J. S., Reis, J. P., Sidne, S., & Bibbins-Domingo, K. (2022). Moderate-to-vigorous intensity physical activity from young adulthood to middle age and metabolic disease: A 30-year population-based cohort study. *British Journal of Sports Medicine*, *56*(15), 847–853. https://doi.org/10.1136/bjsports-2021-104231

National Academies of Science, Engineering, & Medicine. (2022). *Measuring sex, gender identity, and sexual orientation*. National Academies Press. https://doi.org/10.17226/26424

National Aeronautics and Space Administration. (2023). *Understanding our planet to benefit humankind*. https://climate.nasa.gov/

The National Institute for Occupational Safety and Health (NIOSH). (2023). https://www.usa.gov/agencies/national-institute-of-occupational-safety-and-health

National Adolescent and Young Adult Health Information Center. (2023). *Summary of clinical preventive services guidelines for young adults ages 18–25*. San Francisco: University of California. https://nahic.ucsf.edu/wp-content/uploads/2023/08/CPSG-YA.August.2023.pdf

National Cancer Institute. (2023). *Risk factors for cancer*. https://www.cancer.gov/about-cancer/causes-prevention/risk

National Center for Education Statistics. (2023). *Employment and unemployment rates by educational attainment*. https://nces.ed.gov/programs/coe/indicator/cbc

National Institute on Alcohol Abuse and Alcoholism. (2023). *Harmful and underage college drinking*. https://www.niaaa.nih.gov/publications/brochures-and-fact-sheets/college-drinking

National Institute of Drug Abuse. (2023). *Trends & statistics*. https://www.drugabuse.gov/drug-topics/trends-statistics

National Institute of Health. (2023). *Genetics and genomics*. https://irp.nih.gov/our-research/scientific-focus-areas/genetics-and-genomics

National Safety Council. (2023a). *Sports and recreational injuries*. https://injuryfacts.nsc.org/home-and-community/safety-topics/sports-and-recreational-injuries/

National Safety Council. (2023b). *Bicycle deaths*. https://injuryfacts.nsc.org/home-and-community/safety-topics/bicycle-deaths/

Occupational Safety and Health Administration. (2023). *Workplace stress*. https://www.osha.gov/workplace-stress

Omura, J. D., Carlson, S. A., Brown, D. R., Hopkins, D. P., Kraus, W. E., Staffileno, B. A., Thomas, R. J., Lobelo, F, Fulton, J. E., & American Heart Association Physical Activity Committee of the Council on Lifestyle and Cardiometabolic Health; Council on Cardiovascular and Stroke Nursing; and Council on Clinical Cardiology. (2020). Built environment approaches to increase physical activity: A science advisory from the American Heart Association. *Circulation*, *142*, e160–e166. https://doi.org/10.1161/CIR.0000000000000884

Onie, R. D., Lavizzo-Mourey, R., Lee, T. H., Marks, J. S., & Perla, R. J. (2018). Integrating social needs into health care: A twenty-year case study of adaptation and diffusion. *Health Affairs*, *37*(2), 240–247. https://doi.org/10.1377/hlthaff.2017.1113

Ortiz, M. R. (2020). Patient-centered medical (health) home: Nursing theory-guided policy perspectives. *Nursing Science Quarterly*, *33*(1), 91–96. https://doi.org/10.1177/0894318419881795

Ostchega, Y., Fryer, C. D., Nwankwo, T., & Nguyen, D. T. (2020). *Hypertension prevalence among adults aged 18 and over: United States, 2017-2018 (Data Brief No. 364)*. National Center for Health Statistics. https://www.cdc.gov/nchs/data/databriefs/db364-h.pdf

Parker, G., Durante, K. M., Hill, S. E., & Haselton, N. G. (2022). Why women choose divorce: An evolutionary perspective. *Current Opinion in Psychology*, *43*, 300–306. https://doi.org/10.1016/j.copsyc.2021.07.020

Patrick, M. E., Terry-McElrath, Y. M., & Bonar, E. E. (2022). Patterns and predictors of high-intensity drinking and implications for intervention. *Psychology of Addictive Behaviors*, *36*(6), 581–594. https://doi.org/10.1037/adb0000758

Perreault, L. (2023). *Obesity in adults: Drug therapy*. UptoDate. https://www.uptodate.com/contents/obesity-in-adults-drug-therapy?search=drugs%20for%20obesity&source=search_result&selectedTitle=1~150&usage_type=default&display_rank=1

Piaget, J. (1972). Intellectual evolution from adolescence to adulthood. *Human Development*, *15*, 1–12.

Po, J., Brindis C. D., Adams, S., Teipel, K., Park, M. J., & Sieving, R. (2020). *Improving young adult health: State & local strategies for success*. San Francisco: National Adolescent and Young Adult Health Information Center, University of California. https://nahic.ucsf.edu/resource_center/ya-strategies/

Povolotskiy, R., Gupta, N., Leverant, A. B., Kandinov, A., & Paskhover, B. (2020). Head and neck injuries associated with cell phone use. *JAMA Otolaryngology - Head and Neck Surgery*, *146*(2), 122–127. https://doi.org/10.1001/jamaoto.2019.3678

Powell, M. (2019). This helmet will save football. Actually, probably not. *The New York Times*. https://www.nytimes.com/2019/12/12/sports/concussions-football-helmet.html Rector, C, & Stanley, M. J. (Eds.). (2022). *Community and public health nursing* (10th ed.). Wolters Kluwer.

Riiser, A., Bere, E., Anderson, L. B., & Nordengen, S. (2022). E-cycling and health benefits: A systematic literature review with meta-analyses. *Frontiers in Sports and Active Living*, *4*, 1031004. https://doi.org/10.3389/fspor.2022.1031004

Rural Health Information Hub. (2023). *Healthcare access in rural communities*. https://www.ruralhealthinfo.org/topics/healthcare-access

Schaeffer, K. (2019). *Before recent outbreak, vaping was on the rise in U.S., especially among young people*. Pew Research. https://www.pewresearch.org/fact-tank/2019/09/26/vaping-survey-data-roundup/

Shannon, H., Bush, K., Villeneuve, P. J., Hellemans, K. G. C., & Guimond, S. (2022). Problematic social media use in adolescents and young adults: Systematic review and meta-analysis. *JMIR Mental Health*, *9*(4), e33450. https://doi.org/10.2196/33450

Saunders, H., & Panchal, N. (2023). *A look at the latest suicide data and change over the last decade*. Kaiser Family Foundation. https://www.kff.org/mental-health/issue-brief/a-look-at-the-latest-suicide-data-and-change-over-the-last-decade/

Simpson, R. (2018). *MIT: Young adult development project*. https://hr.mit.edu/static/worklife/youngadult/

Sivakumaran, K., Ritonja, J. A., Waseem, H., AlShenaiber, L., Morgan, E., Ahmadi, S. A., Denning, A., Michaud, D., & Morgan, R. L. (2022). Impact of noise exposure on risk of developing stress-related obstetric health effects: A systematic review and meta-analysis. *Noise & Health*, *24*(114), 137–144. https://doi.org/10.4103/nah.nah_22_22

Stone, N.J., Smith, S. C., Orringer, C. E., Rigotti, N. A., Navar, A. M., Khan, S. S., Jones, D. W., Goldberg, R., Mora, S., Blaha, M., Pencina, M. J., & Grundy, S. M. (2022). Managing atherosclerotic cardiovascular risk in young adults: *JACC* state-of-the-art review. *Journal of the American College of Cardiology*, *79*(8), 819–836. https://doi.org/10.1016/j.jacc.2021.12.016

Substance Abuse and Mental Health Services Administration (SAMHSA). (2023). *Mental illness and substance use in young adults*. https://www.samhsa.gov/young-adults

Sullivan, C. M. (2018). Understanding how domestic violence support services promote survivor well-being: A conceptual model. *Journal of Family Violence*, *33*, 123–131. https://doi.org/10.1007/s10896-017-9931-6

Sung, H., Siegel, R. L., Rosenberg, P. S., & Jemal, A. (2019). Emerging cancer trends among young adults in the USA: Analysis of a population-based cancer registry. *Lancet Public Health*, *4*, e137–e147. http://doi.org/10.1016/s2468-2667(18)30267-6

Taylor, C. R., Lynn, P. B., & Bartlett, J. L. (Eds.). (2022). *Fundamentals of nursing: The art and science of person-centered care*. Wolters Kluwer.

Tillman, K. H., Brewster, K. L., & Valle Holway, G. (2019). Sexual and romantic relationships in young adulthood. *Annual Review of Sociology*, *45*, 133–153. https://doi.org/10.1146/annurev-soc-073018-022625

Thomas, W. (2023). Worldwide survey of fitness trends for 2023. *American College of Sports Medicine (ACSM) Health & Fitness Journal*, *27*(1), 9-18. doi:10.1249/FIT.0000000000000834

Thompson, T. M., Young, Y. Y., Bass, T. M., Baker, S., Njoku, O., Norwood, J., & Simpson, M. (2022). Racism runs through it: Examining the sexual and reproductive health experience of black women in the South. *Health Affairs (Project Hope)*, *41*(2), 195–202. https://doi.org/10.1377/hlthaff.2021.01422

Tufts Center for Information and Research on Civic Learning and Engagement. (2021). *Half of Youth Voted in 2020, an 11-point increase from 2016*. https://circle.tufts.edu/latest-research/half-youth-voted-2020-11-point-increase-2016

US Department of Agriculture, & US Department of Health and Human Services. (2020). *Dietary guidelines for Americans, 2020-2025* (9th ed.). https://www.dietaryguidelines.gov/sites/default/files/2020-12/Dietary_Guidelines_for_Americans_2020-2025.pdf

US Census Bureau. (2023). *Age & Sex Composition in the United States: 2022*. https://www.census.gove/data/tables/2022/demo/age-and-sex/2022-age-sex-composition.html

US Department of Health and Human Services. (2023). *Healthy People 2030 objectives*. Office of Disease Prevention and Health Promotion. https://health.gov/healthypeople

US Department of Labor. (2024). *Career Outlook: Education pays, 2023*. https://www.bls.gov/careeroutlook/2024/data-on-display/education-pays.htm#:~:text=Workers%20with%20graduate%20degrees%20had%20the%20lowest%20unemployment%20rates%20and%20highest%20earnings.&text=Note%3A%20Data%20are%20for%20persons,Labor%20Statistics%2C%20Current%20Population%20Survey.

US Department of Transportation. (2023). *Traffic safety facts: Seat belt use in 2022-overall results*. https://crashstats.nhtsa.dot.gov/Api/Public/ViewPublication/813407.pdf

US Preventive Services Task Force (USPSTF). (2023). *Published recommendations*. Rockville, MD: Agency for Healthcare Research and Quality. https://www.uspreventiveservicestaskforce.org/uspstf/

Vitalsigns. (2023). *Many women report mistreatment during pregnancy and delivery*. Centers for Disease Prevention and Control. https://www.cdc.gov/vitalsigns/respectful-maternity-care/index.html

Vivier, H., Ross, E. J., & Cassisi, J. (2020). *Classification of gastrointestinal symptom patterns in young adults. BMC Gastroenterology*, *20*(1), 326. https://doi.org/10.1186/s12876-020-01478-7

Watson, K. B., Carlson, S. A., Loustalot, F., Town, M., Eke, P. I., Thomas, C. W., & Greenlund, K. J. (2022). Chronic conditions among adults aged 18–34 years — United States, 2019. *MMWR. Morbidity and Mortality Weekly Report*, *7*(30), 964–970. https://www.cdc.gov/mmwr/volumes/71/wr/pdfs/mm7130a3-H.pdf

Weber, J. R., & Kelley, J. H. (2022). *Health assessment in nursing* (7th ed.). Wolters Kluwer.

Willmott, T. J., Pang, B., Rundle-Thiele, S., & Badejo, A. (2019). Weight management in young adults: Systematic review of electronic health intervention components and outcomes. *Journal of Medical Internet Research*, *21*(2), e10265. https://doi.org/10.2196/10265

Wojcik, M. H., Schwartz, T. S., Yamin, I., Edward, H. L., Genetti, C. A., Towne, M. C., & Agrawal, P. B. (2018). Genetic disorders and mortality in infancy and early childhood: Delayed diagnoses and missed opportunities. *Genetic Medicine*, *20*(11), 1396–1404. https://doi.org/10.1038/gim.2018.17

Woolf, S. H. (2019). Necessary but not sufficient: Why health care alone cannot improve population health and reduce health inequities. *Annals of Family Medicine*, *17*(3), 196–199. https://doi.org/10.1370/afm.2395

Woolf, S. H., & Schoomaker, H. (2019). Life expectancy and mortality rates in the United States, 1959–2017. *JAMA*, *322*(20), 1996–2016. http://doi.org/10.1001/jama.2019.16932

Woychik, R. (2023). *Wildfire smoke, other air pollution can harm brain health, expert says*. National Institute of Environmental Health Sciences. https://factor.niehs.nih.gov/2023/8/feature/4-air-pollution-and-brain-development

Wu, S., Wang, X., Wu, Q., & Harris, K. M. (2018). *Household financial assets inequity and health disparities among young adults: Evidence from the national longitudinal study of adolescent to adult health. Journal of Health Disparities Research and Practice*, *11*(1), 122–135.

Xia, M., Fosco, G. M., Lippold, M. A., & Feinberg, M. E. (2018). A developmental perspective on young adult romantic relationships: Examining family and individual factors in adolescence. *Journal of Youth and Adolescence*, *47*, 1499–1516. https://doi.org/10.1007/s10964-018-0815-8

Yano, Y., Colangelo, L. A., Shimbo, D., Viera, A. J., Allen, N. B., Gidding, S. S., Bress, A. P., Greenland, P., Munter, P., & Lloyd-Jones, D. M. (2018). Association of blood pressure classification in young adults using the 2017 American College of Cardiology/American Heart Association blood pressure guideline with cardiovascular events later in life. *Journal of the American Medical Association*, *320*(17), 1774–1782. https://doi.org/10.1001/jama.2018.13551

You, Y. N., Lee, L. D., Deschner, B. W., & Shibata, D. (2020). Colorectal cancer in the adolescent and young adult population. *JCO Oncology Practice*, *16*(1), 19–27. https://doi.org/10.1200/JOP.19.00153

Yu Z, Bellander, T., Bergström, A., DIllner, J., Eneroth, K., Engardt, M. Georgelis, A., Kull, I., Ljungman, P. L., Pershagen, G., Stafoggia, M. Melén, E., & Gruzieva, O. (2022). Association of short-term air pollution exposure with SARS-CoV-2 infection among young adults in Sweden. *JAMA Network Open*, *5*(4), e22810. https://doi.org/10.1001/jamanetworkopen.2022.8109

Zheng, H., & Echave, P. (2021). Are recent cohorts getting worse? Trends in US adult physiological status, mental health, and health behaviors across a century of birth cohorts. *American Journal of Epidemiology*, *190*(11), 2242–2255. https://doi.org/10.1093/aje/kwab076

23

Middle-Aged Adult

Miriam Ford and Susan Moscou

http://evolve.elsevier.com/Edelman/

OBJECTIVES

After completing this chapter, the reader will be able to:

- Describe three psychosocial changes that frequently occur during middle age.
- Explain the usual biologic changes that occur because of the aging process.
- Identify the major causes of death in the middle-aged adult.
- Describe frequently occurring health patterns of middle-aged adults.
- Discuss the health problems commonly experienced by adults aged 35 to 65 years.
- Analyze the influence of psychosocial stressors on the middle-aged adult.

KEY TERMS

Advance directive
Body mass index
Calcium
Cardiac output
Cataract
Constipation
Degenerative joint disease
Durable power of attorney
Empty nest syndrome
Functional aerobic capacity
Generativity versus stagnation
Gingivitis
Glaucoma
Health care agent
High blood pressure
Kyphosis
Living will; Macular degeneration
Menopause
Obesity
Osteoarthritis
Osteopenia
Osteoporosis
Overweight
Perimenopause
Periodontitis
Presbycusis
Presbyopia
Sandwich generation
Sleep disorders
Vitamin D

THINK ABOUT IT

The "Sandwich Generation"

The sandwich generation refers to middle-aged adults who support both aging parents and growing children. Charles Shelton is 48 years old and has been in excellent health. Mr. Shelton operates heavy machinery for a construction team that clears environmentally polluted sites. These sites are known to be contaminated with lead, mercury, and other chemicals, so he visits the occupational health nurse regularly for intermittent blood testing and physical examinations. Mr. Shelton has two children who are 15 and 18 years old. Sarah Jones, his partner, worked as a licensed practical nurse in a skilled nursing facility until she injured her back, and she now receives disability insurance payments. Ms. Jones is also the sole caretaker of her 80-year-old mother, who needs increasing assistance. Their oldest child plans to enter college next fall. Although Mr. Shelton and Ms. Jones have saved money, they are worried about college costs, funding their eventual retirement, and the cost of care for Ms. Jones's mother. Ms. Jones's injury has made them more conscious of workplace hazards and exposures. Based on this scenario, consider the following:

- What type(s) of health care providers do Mr. Shelton and Ms. Jones (the couple) need to address their health concerns and psychosocial issues?
- How can health care providers guide and support this couple through their stressors?
- Describe health-promotion and wellness strategies this couple can implement.
- What community organizations are available to this couple to assist with an aging parent?
- What are the responsibilities of health care providers and policymakers to encourage health promotion to middle-aged adults?

The CDC Workplace Health Promotion website is an excellent resource to answer the previously mentioned questions: https://www.cdc.gov/workplace-healthpromotion/index.html.

Middle adulthood spans a 30-year interval between 35 and 65 years of age. During their midlife years, many adults experience expanded responsibilities and increased productivity. In most cases, there is a concomitant increased sense of accomplishment. Within this age interval, significant biologic, physiologic, social, and psychological changes occur. Some individuals experience spiritual changes. Vital statistics reports published by the Centers for Disease Control and Prevention (CDC) divide middle-aged adulthood into three categories for ease of describing mortality and morbidity data. These are 35 to 44 years, 45 to 54 years, and 55 to 65 years. This age group (30-year span) accounts for nearly 40% of the population of the United States.

Many changes related to aging and health that occur during this time frame will be discussed in this chapter. Health promotion addresses individual practices and community opportunities that optimize health and well-being for adults in midlife. This concept is the central focus of the presentation of materials and related figures and study aids.

An examination of the gains achieved for *Healthy People 2020* will be compared with the national goals and objectives for *Healthy People 2030*. Along with an analysis of these findings, information related to the role of nurses will appear throughout the text. Nurses are integral to the health of the American people; their role includes fostering health promotion and health maintenance.

BIOLOGY AND GENETICS

Although the time of onset differs, biologic changes occur during the middle years, affecting most body systems. The hair of the adult begins to thin and turn gray. The skin's moisture and turgor decrease, and with the loss of subcutaneous fat, wrinkling occurs. Excessive sun exposure through the years makes some changes more pronounced, especially increased coarseness of facial features.

Fat deposition increases during these years, often with concomitant increases in weight. Body height decreases as a result of decreased bone density and mass. This combination of changes results in increased **body mass index**. The body contour changes as fat deposits on the hips, commonly called love handles and outer thighs (saddlebags) appear. Sedentary lifestyles and unchanged dietary habits contribute considerably to these changes.

The inactive lifestyle is further compromised by a decrease in energy; "I'm not as young as I used to be" is a common remark. This proclamation is legitimate because the capacity for physical work decreases. As **functional aerobic capacity** decreases, there is a resulting decrease in **cardiac output**. For individuals who maintain regular exercise programs that provide stretching and strengthening of skeletal muscle, cardiac output remains essentially undiminished for many years.

In the musculoskeletal system, bone density and mass progressively decrease. When 55-year-old adults say that they were 1 inch taller when they were 18 years of age, the observation is likely to be true. A 1- to 4-inch (2.5- to 10-cm) loss in height occurs as a person ages; thinning of the intervertebral disks accounts for approximately 1 inch. However, dramatic losses in height (more than 4 inches) can occur with thoracic **kyphosis**, an angulation of the posterior spine (commonly known as hunchback). The wear and tear on joints predispose the adult to **degenerative joint disease**, deterioration of the joint(s), with more frequent painful backaches. The general decrease in muscle tone, categorized by many as flab, reduces physical agility.

Degenerative joint disease, specifically **osteoarthritis**, has its peak onset in middle age and can greatly influence activity and endurance, which affects employment. Most frequently the knees and hands, followed by the hips, spine, shoulders, and ankles, are involved. *Healthy People 2020* and *Healthy People 2030* identify targets for arthritis, osteoporosis, and chronic back pain. The goal continues to be to prevent illness and disability related to arthritis and other rheumatic conditions, osteoporosis, and chronic back conditions.

Osteopenia is a condition of sub-normal mineralized bone, usually as a result of a rate of bone lysis that exceeds the rate of bone matrix synthesis. **Osteoporosis** is a disorder characterized by abnormal loss of bone density and deterioration of bone tissue, with an increased fracture risk. It occurs most frequently in small, sedentary postmenopausal females and in people using corticosteroids on a long-term basis. Furthermore, frequency of osteoporosis increases with age (Leboff et al., 2022).

The functional capacity of all organ systems generally decreases. For example, in the gastrointestinal tract, the following chain of events occurs: decreased metabolism leads to less enzyme production, resulting in lower hydrochloric acid levels, which decreases tone in the large intestine. As a result, middle-aged adults may experience acid indigestion with increased belching. When an adult leads a sedentary lifestyle, the effects of the diminished motility through the gastrointestinal tract can be more pronounced. It is well known that Americans eat more refined foods (foods that are low in bulk) than residents of developing nations. A low-bulk diet can contribute to the problem of **constipation**, a change in bowel habits characterized by decreased frequency or passage of hard, drier stools and difficult defecation, and is believed to be a primary contributor to the increased incidence of colon cancer in the United States. Kidney function also decreases. Between age 25 and age 85, a 35% loss of nephron units occurs. The remaining nephrons increase in size and undergo degenerative changes. The entire weight of the kidneys decreases. Because blood supply is also diminished, the glomerular filtration rate is decreased by nearly half.

Significant changes occur in the cardiovascular system as the blood vessels lose elasticity and become thicker. This process predisposes middle-aged adults to coronary artery disease, hypertension, myocardial infarctions, and strokes. Heart disease remains the leading cause of death in middle-aged adults (CDC, 2023b).

Menopause is the cessation of menses. It is an expected physiologic change related to aging, and it marks the end of a woman's reproductive function. Menopause is determined retrospectively after cessation of menses for 12 consecutive months. In North America the median age for menopause is 50.5 to 51.4 years (North American Menopause Society, 2023). Females now expect to live one-third of their lives after menopause. The National Institutes of Health's study on females' health over the past 25 years includes findings on menopause. Menopause enables many females to engage in personal creativity while gradually adapting to the many expected biologic, psychological, social, and spiritual changes of menopause. Others, however, enter a period of depression, particularly as work life changes (Jones et al., 2020). During menopause, production of ovarian estrogen and progesterone ceases; the remaining estrogen is produced by the adrenal glands. As a result of the diminished estrogen level, secondary sex characteristics regress. These include loss of pubic hair and decrease in breast size. Female reproductive organs shrink, and vaginal secretions decrease, which may require additional lubrication during intercourse.

As males approach the end of the middle years, they experience changes in their sexual response cycle as testosterone levels plateau and then decrease. The testes undergo degenerative changes, the number of viable spermatozoa diminishes, and the volume and viscosity of semen decreases. In men, sexual energy gradually declines; achieving an erection takes longer, but it is sustained longer. Stress, however, can significantly diminish function (National Institute on Aging [NIA], 2020).

Life Expectancy and Mortality Rates

Americans are expected to see gains in life expectancies in the coming decades. By 2060, life expectancy projections for the total population will increase by 6 years, from an average of 77 in 2020 to 85.6 in 2060. Males will see larger increases in life expectancy than females, but females will still outlive males, on average, in 2060. In the coming decades, all racial and ethnic groups will see longer life expectancies, but the greatest gains will be native-born males who are Black non-Hispanic and non-Hispanic American Indian or Alaska Native alone. In 2060, foreign-born males and females are projected to sustain longer life expectancies than their native-born peers, regardless of race or Hispanic/Latinx origin (Medina et al., 2020).

The leading causes of death during middle adulthood are heart disease, cancer, and accidents (CDC, 2020). Box 23.1 shows a breakdown for each 10-year interval for middle-aged adults. Reducing disabilities and deaths from these chronic conditions are national health-promotion and disease-prevention objectives.

The CDC uses a multifaceted approach to mitigate the chronic disease burden: epidemiology and surveillance to monitor trends, environmental strategies to promote healthy behaviors, health-system interventions to advance clinical and preventive services, and community resources to improve clinical management of chronic conditions. Box 23.2 outlines selected objectives and target goals for *Healthy People 2030*. These leading health indicators provide some perspective of the many tasks and opportunities that lie ahead for Americans.

BOX 23.1 Leading Causes of Death in Middle-Aged Adults

Age 35 to 44 Years
- Unintentional injuries (34,589)
- Heart disease (12,177)
- Malignant neoplasms (10,730)

Age 45 to 54 Years
- Malignant neoplasms (34,589)
- Heart disease (34,169)
- Unintentional injury (36,119)

Age 55 to 64 Years
- Malignant neoplasms (110,243)
- Heart disease (88,551)
- COVID-19 (42,090)

From CDC 10 Leading Causes of Death by Age Group, United States—2020 https://wisqars.cdc.gov/lcd/?o=LCD&y1=2022&y2=2022&ct=10&cc=ALL&g=00&s=0&r=0&ry=2&e=0&ar=lcd1age&at=groups&ag=lcd1age&a1=0&a2=199

BOX 23.2 *HEALTHY PEOPLE 2030*

National Health-Promotion and Disease-Prevention Objectives for the Middle-Aged Adult

Objectives

Arthritis, Osteoporosis, and Chronic Back Conditions (AOBC)

AOCBC-01: Reduce the proportion of adults with provider-diagnosed arthritis who experience a limitation in activity due to arthritis or joint symptoms

AOCBC-07: Reduce the prevalence of adults having high-effect chronic pain

Diabetes (D)

D-01: Reduce the annual number of new cases of diagnosed diabetes in the population

D-02: Reduce the rate of all-cause mortality among adults with diagnosed diabetes

Occupational Safety and Health (OSH)

OSH-2030-04: Reduce work-related assaults

OSH-2030-05: Reduce the rate of elevated blood lead levels in adults with work-related lead exposure

Heart Disease and Stroke (HDS)

HDS-2030-01: Increase overall cardiovascular health in US adults

HDS-2030-02: Reduce coronary heart disease deaths

US Department of Health and Human Services (USDHHS). [Internet]. *Healthy People 2030*. Office of Disease Prevention and Health Promotion. https://www.health.gov/healthypeople/objectives-and-data/browse-objectives.

Healthy People initiatives were established in 1980 to provide structure for health-promotion and disease-prevention programs. Every 10 years, revised objectives and target goals are established for each leading indicator.

Most of the leading indicators identified in *Healthy People 2020* and *Healthy People 2030* are preventable, or at least modifiable. Knowledge of the direction of the program offers professional nurses an incentive to modify their practice and their health-promotion education efforts to best help Americans achieve the target goals specified in the *Healthy People* initiative. Health education, often conducted by professional nurses, has been effective with adults who want to or must change their lifestyle behaviors. Nursing professionals have contributed extensively to helping the nation to meet the target goals for heart disease, stroke, and many types of cancer.

Hypertension and obesity are conditions that significantly affect middle-aged adults. These chronic illnesses often lead to heart disease, stroke, and the development of diabetes. There was a significantly increased trend in obesity between 1999 to 2000 and 2015 to 2016. Obesity, a growing problem, is associated with health risks. Obesity increases the risk of complications in coronary heart disease (CHD) and end-stage renal disease. Among males, the prevalence of obesity is 40.3% among those aged 20 to 39, 46.4% among those aged 40 to 59, and 42.2% among those aged 60 and over. Among females, the prevalence of obesity is 39.7% among those aged 20 to 39, 43.3% among those aged 40 to 59, and 43.3% among those aged 60 and over (Hales et al., 2020).

In summary, there has been evidence of progress in meeting approximately 670 of 955 leading health indicator target goals. Projecting ahead for 2030, efforts must be directed toward the following: increasing awareness of the *Healthy People 2030* initiative as a tool to improve the overall health of Americans; expanding knowledge of the initiative in schools, tribal communities, and local health agencies through the use of public service announcements carried on radio, television, and Internet-based programs; and linking the objectives and goals to preventive health provisions associated with work sites (occupational health programs) and health insurance policies. The good news is the *Healthy People 2030* target goals are more achievable (less ambitious than projected for 2010), and the objectives focus on individuals more than on "big" programs. There are goals that involve health counseling and behavior-modification strategies provided by nurses, advanced practice nurses, and mental health nursing specialists in addition to physicians. In the larger picture, Americans will benefit when nurses, in all roles, incorporate the *Healthy People 2030* objectives into their practice.

In 2019 the death rate from heart disease for men was 161.5 per 100,000 deaths compared to 126.2 per 100,000 for women (CDC, 2024a). Although cardiovascular disease death rates are declining for both sexes, heart disease remains one of the primary causes of death. The risk factors for heart disease include obesity, lack of physical activity, smoking, high total cholesterol level, hypertension, and genetics. Obesity is common, serious, and costly. (See Chapter 11 for a discussion of overweight, obesity, and *Healthy People* target goals.)

Gender and Relationship Status

Studies show that almost 38% of adults aged 25 to 54 are living without a partner (Fry & Parker, 2021). Partnered adults report better health than unpartnered adults. In addition, partnered adults also have better economic outcomes than unpartnered adults. According to Fry and Parker (2021) the growth in the single population is driven by a decline in marriage among young and middle-aged adults.

Social Determinants of Health

The economic and social conditions in communities where people live, learn, work, and play affect a wide range of health risks and outcomes known as social determinants of health (SDOH). SDOH is one of the three key areas of focus of *Healthy People 2030*, along with health literacy and health equity (CDC, 2022). SDOH also refers to societal conditions that affect health, such as poverty, environmental hazards, education, racism, sexism, ageism, and income. An SDOH goal of *Healthy People 2030* is to create social and physical environments that promote equity in health for all. Understanding the effects of SDOH can improve population health and advance health equity.

Income Inequality

Income inequality refers to the disparity in the distribution of income between individuals, groups, populations, and social classes (Carter & Howard, 2019). Income inequality contributes to an individual's health status. The overall median household income grew relative to the 2018 overall median household income, but income growth remains uneven by race and ethnicity. Real median income increased 4.6% among Asian households (from $83,376 to $87,194), 1.8% among African American households (from $40,963 to $41,692), 1.1% among non-Hispanic White households (from $69,851 to $70,642), and only 0.1% among Hispanic households (from $51,390 to $51,450) (Wilson & Williams, 2019).

Wealth, a measure of an individual's or family's financial net worth, is a better indicator than income. In 2023, the top 10% of US households held 69% of the wealth and the bottom half of households held less than 3% of the wealth (USAFacts.org, 2024).

BOX 23.3 GENOMICS

Lung cancer is the second most common cancer in both males and females in the United States, not including skin cancer; however, it is the leading cause of cancer-related death. Prostate cancer is more common in males and breast cancer is more common in females. The American Cancer Society estimates that in 2024 there will be approximately 234,580 new cases of lung cancer (116,310 in males and 118,270 in females, resulting in 125,070 deaths from lung cancer—65,790 in males and 59,280 in females) (American Cancer Society, 2023). Both the number of new cases of lung cancer and lung cancer deaths are on the decline, attributed to decreases in smoking and increases in detection (American Cancer Society, 2023).

Several types of cancer treatment are available—surgery, radiation therapy, chemotherapy, immunotherapy, hormone therapy, and stem cell transplant. Molecular and genomic profiling of lung tumors has revolutionized the treatment of metastatic non–small cell lung cancer (NSCLC).

The Adjuvant Lung Cancer Enrichment Marker Identification and Sequencing Trials (ALCHEMIST) involve genetic screening of resected NSCLC specimens (Cardarella & Johnson, 2013). Patients whose tumors test positive for either epidermal growth factor receptor gene or anaplastic lymphoma kinase gene mutations will be referred to the ALCHEMIST for genotype-directed targeted therapies. Adjuvant targeted therapy, based on tumor mutation genotyping, will likely improve outcomes for all NSCLC patients.

American Cancer Society, 2023. https://www.cancer.org/cancer/types/lung-cancer/detection-diagnosis-staging/how-diagnosed.html
Centers for Disease Control and Prevention. Lung cancer statistics (http://www.cdc.gov)

Genetics

The middle-aged adult is at greater risk than the young adult for diseases associated with genetics (i.e., familial characteristics). These conditions include diabetes, hypertension, Huntington chorea, arteriosclerosis, gout, obesity, heart disease, and alcoholism. Some malignancies are related to genetics; for example, females with a personal or family history of breast cancer are at a higher risk of developing this type of malignancy. In addition, individuals with a family history of colorectal cancer, rectal or colon polyps, or ulcerative colitis have an increased risk of developing this type of cancer (Box 23.3: Genomics).

GORDON'S FUNCTIONAL HEALTH PATTERNS

Health Perception–Health Management Pattern

To promote health in middle-aged adults, the nurse performs a health assessment that includes the person's values and beliefs, lifestyle patterns, general perceptions of health, and health practices (Murdaugh et al., 2019).

Habits used for coping that have been practiced for years (cigarette smoking, excessive alcohol use, and overeating) begin to have visible consequences in middle age. As pressures increase, adults may be tempted to turn to substances such as these as a crutch for coping with stress. Prevention is extremely important, primarily because withdrawal from any of these substances is a difficult process. Motivational interviewing and harm-reduction measures have been found to work for many people (Miller & Rollnick, 2023; Lopez, et al., 2022).

Health Indicators

The leading cause of morbidity and mortality in middle-aged and older adults include cancer, chronic obstructive pulmonary disease, congestive heart failure, diabetes, back pain, hypertension, a fractured hip, myocardial infarction, rheumatism or arthritis, and stroke.

Nutritional-Metabolic Pattern

Dietary factors are correlated with many of the leading causes of death in the United States: CHD, some cancers, stroke, non–insulin-dependent diabetes mellitus, and atherosclerosis (CDC, 2022b). The lack of healthy diet may be closely related to social determinants of health, including the inability to afford healthy food and a lack of access to food stores (food deserts).

High Saturated Fat Diet

Lipid levels and ratios have a significant influence on cardiovascular and cerebrovascular morbidity and mortality rates. The National Heart, Lung, and Blood Institute considers 1) total blood cholesterol level less than 200 mg/dL, 2) low-density lipoprotein (LDL) cholesterol level less than 100 mg/dL, 3) high-density lipoprotein (HDL) cholesterol level greater or equal to 60 mg/dL, and 4) triglycerides level less than 150 mg/dL as desirable (CDC, 2020b). Much of the success in lowering cholesterol levels and increasing HDL levels (considered the good cholesterol) is attributed to the use of statin drugs. Statin medications lower the level of LDLs (considered bad cholesterol) in the blood.

The incidence of elevated cholesterol in middle-aged adults is greater than the incidence in adults younger than 40 and older than 60 (MacDonald, 2022). Over 50% of American adults have elevated LDL levels, with more than a third of those having untreated elevated levels (Hill & Bordoni, 2023). Interprofessional care, including care from nutritionists, is essential to helping people lower their cholesterol. Diet and exercise along with medication can provide primary and secondary prevention of heart disease.

Calcium and Vitamin D

Adequate **calcium** intake is essential for developing and maintaining bone mass. Additionally, calcium is needed for other physiologic processes, including muscle contraction and blood pressure regulation. Males and females need a minimal daily intake of 1000 mg of calcium. Pregnant and nursing females need 1200 mg, and postmenopausal females need either 1000 mg (when taking estrogen) or 1500 mg (when not taking estrogen). When daily intake of calcium is less than adequate, the serum calcium level will be maintained by leaching calcium from bone, resulting in osteoporosis. Weight-bearing exercise contributes to bone mass by increasing mechanical stress on the bones, whereas **vitamin D** promotes calcium absorption and regulates serum calcium and phosphate concentrations to maintain bone health (LeBoff et al., 2020). Calcium and vitamin D taken together help protect older adults from osteoporosis.

Vitamin D also plays an important role in overall health and the prevention of chronic diseases. Emerging studies suggest an association between inadequate levels of vitamin D and an increased risk of chronic diseases such as osteoporosis, diabetes, heart disease, hypertension, cancers, obesity, depression, cognitive decline, fractures, and falls, and autoimmunity. Possible causes of vitamin D deficiency include an insufficient consumption of vitamin D–fortified foods, lack of dietary supplements, and limited exposure to sunlight. It is difficult to achieve sufficient vitamin D levels through dietary sources alone, as few foods naturally contain vitamin D. The food sources that provide vitamin D include fatty fish, dairy products, liver, and fortified cereals and beverages. The best way to ensure adequate vitamin D serum levels is through supplementation (National Institutes of Health [NIH], Office of Dietary Supplements, 2020).

Vitamin D is unique because it can be synthesized endogenously when the skin is exposed to ultraviolet B radiation. Many factors can interfere with ultraviolet B exposure and the body's ability to synthesize vitamin D from sunlight: seasons, time of day, length of day, location, cloud cover, smog, skin melanin content, and use of sunscreen (NIH, Office of Dietary Supplements, 2020). Aging may also impede cutaneous synthesis of vitamin D. As people age, the skin cannot synthesize vitamin D as efficiently as when they are younger. Older adults are also more likely to spend more time indoors (homebound or in occupations that limit sun exposure). Prolonged sun exposure to prevent vitamin D deficiency is not generally recommended because exposure to ultraviolet radiation increases the risk of skin cancer. The exact definition of a low vitamin D level is not well established. Daily vitamin D intake of 600 IU in adults aged 18 to 70 years and 800 IU in adults older than 70 years will meet the needs of most adults.

Caffeine

Caffeine is a popular stimulant found in coffee, tea, and some soft drinks, such as colas. Caffeine prolongs the amount of time that physical work can be performed and appears to decrease boredom and increase attention span. On the negative side, coffee has recently been the subject of significant scrutiny from the media, with reports of a link between cancer of the pancreas and coffee consumption. There is controversy regarding whether daily moderate intake of caffeine has any detrimental effects.

Like alcohol and nicotine, caffeine is readily available and has become an accepted part of daily living. Because caffeine is a strong stimulant with effects that are typically taken for granted, its importance as an addictive substance must be emphasized. Ingestion of 0.5 g of caffeine (three to four cups of coffee) can increase the basal metabolic rate by an average of 10% and possibly as much as 25% for some people.

Long-term stimulation of the central nervous system results in restlessness, sleep disturbances, cardiac stimulation, and withdrawal effects. Nurses' assessments should screen individuals for stimulating and addictive substances that may be producing these symptoms.

High-Sodium Diet

High-sodium diets play a significant role in hypertension, especially when consumed over many years. The result may be an increase in the amount of total body fluids, which increases peripheral vascular resistance. Salt contains approximately 40% sodium and is a contributing factor for hypertension in the 10% to 20% of Americans who are at risk. On average, Americans consume 4 to 5 g of sodium per day. A major contributor to dietary sodium is the salt found in processed foods.

In the past 3 decades, many clinical studies have demonstrated the effectiveness of lowering blood pressure by lowering dietary sodium intake. Other studies have described the relationships between urinary and sodium excretion and the change of blood pressure with age and the relationship between increased salt intake and blood pressure (Grillo, et al., 2019).

Alcohol

The Dietary Guidelines for Americans, issued jointly by the US Department of Agriculture and the US Department of Health and Human Services (USDHHS) https://www.nutrition.gov/ defines *moderate drinking* as no more than one drink per day for females and no more than two drinks per day for males. Females are more vulnerable than males to the effects of alcohol because, pound for pound, females have less water in their bodies, and they tend to weigh less than males. This means that identical doses of alcohol per kilogram of body weight will result in significantly higher blood alcohol levels in females. A female's brain and other organs are exposed to more alcohol and its toxic by-products as it is metabolized. A female is more likely to drink excessively if her parents, siblings, or other blood relatives have problems with alcohol; if she was abused physically or sexually as a child; if her partner drinks heavily; if she is experiencing difficulties with intimate and close relationships; or if she has a history of depression (CDC, 2019).

Alcohol use disorders are associated with motor vehicle accidents, violence, homicides, suicides, drownings, heart disease, strokes, liver disease, pancreatitis, and fetal alcohol syndrome. Fetal alcohol syndrome is the most known preventable cause of mental impairment. The brain damage that occurs with fetal alcohol syndrome can result in lifelong problems with learning, memory, attention, and problem-solving (NIH, National Institutes of Alcohol Abuse and Alcoholism, 2024).

Initially, alcohol appears to be a stimulant, but it is a central nervous system depressant and anesthetic. Long-term alcohol use produces tolerance, thereby necessitating a gradual increase in dose to achieve the same effect. Alcohol contributes to problems with safety because of decreased reaction time and depression of the central nervous system. Those experiencing alcohol use disorders may report symptoms such as heartburn and gas, stomach distention, poor eating habits, nausea and vomiting, gastric pain, right upper quadrant pain, and irritation of the mouth, throat, and esophagus. Two additional subtle findings are spider angiomata and palmar erythema. Researchers believe that even moderate alcohol use may result in accumulated harm to the brain by middle age (Immonen, 2020).

Primary prevention for substance and alcohol abuse is complex, especially because adults consume these agents for many reasons, including peer pressure, loneliness, alienation, frustration, anxiety, and low self-esteem. Heavy drinkers may also be following the example established by influential people in their lives. Merely telling people about the potential physical, emotional, and legal hazards appears to have little effect as a preventive measure. Promotion of more realistic portrayals of substance abuse through the media is difficult to implement. Although techniques such as assertiveness training and teaching adults to resist persuasion are helpful, more useful approaches might include helping them learn to manage anxiety and increase their self-esteem.

Early detection and intervention can decrease ongoing and future physical and psychosocial problems resulting from alcohol abuse. Nurses use a variety of screening strategies to identify individuals' perceptions and consequences of drinking. The CAGE questionnaire is one of the most popular screening tools used in primary care. The Michigan Alcohol Screening Test https://www.oregon.gov/oha/HSD/AMH/docs/MAST.pdf and the Alcohol Use Disorders Identification Test https://auditscreen.org/ are examples of other screening instruments.

Abnormal laboratory test results, including elevations in aspartate aminotransferase level, erythrocyte mean corpuscular volume, and serum glutamyl transferase level, are not adequately sensitive and specific enough to detect alcohol use disorders, as these may be a result of other causes, including trauma, disease, and medications.

A variety of treatments are known to be effective, but no single "best" intervention has been identified. Effective treatments may be to address other problems with use of interventions such as pharmacologic agents, stress management, acupuncture, individual and family therapy, and supportive environments.

Oral Health

Gingivitis

Gingivitis is found commonly among adults who fail to brush their teeth and use dental floss regularly. Redness and swelling develop around the teeth. Bleeding of the gums, while the teeth are being brushed, is an early sign of gingivitis. The gums may or may not be tender. When inflammation is not adequately treated and controlled, **periodontitis**, involving bone destruction, can develop in addition to tooth loss.

Dental Hygiene and Decay

Dental health is essential to overall health. Brushing the teeth and flossing after eating, receiving routine dental checkups, and consuming fewer carbohydrates (especially simple sugars) are important interventions to prevent dental caries. Adults in their middle years have responsibility not only for their own regular dental care but also for the care of their children and parents. Fluoridation of water (versus bottled or tap water) and use of applied sealants are additional health choices that support prevention of dental caries and, possibly, tooth loss.

Dental health is one of the leading indicators identified in *Healthy People 2030*. There is increasing evidence to show that periodontal, or gum disease, is closely linked to diabetes, heart disease, and stroke. For the middle-aged woman, poor oral health can cause premature births and low-birth-weight infants (Brailer et al., 2019).

There are many conditions that begin with changes in the oropharyngeal mucosa, such as cancer of the mouth and esophageal cancer. Consequently, twice yearly dental visits are important because dental professionals (dentists or dental hygienists) may be the first to detect a symptom or irregularity that points to a potentially dangerous condition (American Dental Association, 2022).

The findings described on the *Healthy People 2020* oral health webpage indicate that approximately 41.2% of Americans, regardless of race and ethnicity, receive annual health care by a dentist. The target goals for oral health services use (OH-7 outlined in the objectives for *Healthy People 2030*) indicate an expectation of a 10% increase in the proportion of adults and children aged 2 or older who receive dental care annually. The goal of reducing the percentage of the population unable to get dental care when needed has been met. Only 18% of the population is unable to get dental care when needed; the goal was to decrease it below the 20.2% reported in 2019 (CDC, 2023a).

People who are in vulnerable populations (individuals whose annual income is below the poverty line, others who are chronically ill or disabled, or still others whose medical or psychiatric treatment plans are very complicated) may not receive adequate or proper oral health care. The Surgeon General commented that, whereas there is evidence of progress being made to increase access to oral health services for a greater proportion of the population, those who are vulnerable because of illness, such as people with HIV/AIDS, still find difficulty in obtaining proper and adequate oral health care (Feng et al., 2020). The Oral Health Care Initiative will help address the multilayered complexities that people with HIV/AIDS face. The factors that frequently deter oral health care in this population include lack of dental insurance, lack of transportation, limitations of disability, increasing costs of treatment, inability to afford the cost of oral health care, and discrimination on the part of dental health care providers. Nurses are an essential part of the interprofessional team incorporating oral health in the care of people living with HIV and AIDS (Damian, 2023).

National data also indicate that the cost of dental care is a major deterrent to sustained oral health. About 16% of adults aged 18 to 64 years reported an unmet dental need because of cost in the previous 12 months. Among adults aged 18 to 64 years, the main reason to forgo a dental visit in the previous 6 months was cost; 42% could not afford treatment or did not have insurance. About one-half (50.2%) of dentate adults aged 18 to 64 in the United States had private health coverage with dental coverage during 2014 to 2017. Among those with private health insurance and dental coverage, less than one-fourth (22.1%) had not seen a dentist in the past 12 months, and 4.4% had unmet dental needs due to cost in the past 12 months (CDC, 2023a; Blackwell, Villaroel, & Norris, 2019).

Tobacco use in any form (cigarettes, pipes, and smokeless [spit] tobacco) raises the risk of gum disease. Dental health is often poorer among smokers (currently smoking) compared with former smokers and with those who have never smoked. Smokers who were interviewed said that they had three or more dental problems. In addition, current smokers reported infrequent visits to their dentist (in some cases, more than 5 years) or never seeing a dentist. Research findings indicate that the prevalence of gum disease is two times greater in individuals who smoke cigarettes than in individuals who have never smoked (CDC, 2020a, 2020c).

In summary, oral disease is preventable. Regularly scheduled dental care with a dentist and dental hygienist is highly recommended for good dental hygiene and early treatment of dental decay and periodontal diseases such as gingivitis. In addition, dentists can provide screening for oropharyngeal cancer. Oral health is essential to the overall digestive and elimination processes.

Elimination Pattern

Aging brings a gradual decrease of tone in the large intestine. This change, accompanied by a sedentary lifestyle, lack of fiber in the diet, and inadequate fluid intake, can predispose the adult to constipation. Advertising on television and other forms of media presents strong arguments that encourage individuals to rely on external controls rather than on exercise and dietary means to solve this problem. Consequently, many adults are dependent on taking fiber products, as well as laxatives, for regular bowel movements.

In the kidneys, degenerative changes in the nephron units gradually increase during the middle years. In most cases, adults do not have any appreciable alteration in kidney function unless the person has experienced repeated infections, trauma, or the long-term effects of diabetes mellitus or hypertension.

Alteration in bladder control (incontinence) can occur in both females and males because of weakening of the muscles of the pelvic floor or damage to pelvic nerves. Urinary incontinence is problematic in females who have experienced multiple births. Inmales, urinary incontinence frequently occurs as a complication of surgery for prostate cancer. Incontinence can be socially embarrassing, but the condition can be relieved with Kegel (pelvic floor) exercises (Radzimińska et al., 2018).

Activity-Exercise Pattern

Regular physical activity increases life expectancy and the quality of life. Exercise helps prevent CHD, hypertension, diabetes, osteoporosis, and depression. Research findings show a strong correlation between physical exercise and lower rates of osteoporosis (Beck & Winters-Stone, 2020), back injury, stroke, and colon cancer. Weight-loss programs that incorporate physical activities also make significant contributions to health promotion as evidenced by increased life expectancy and quality of life.

One of the objectives of *Healthy People 2030* is to continue to decrease deaths related to heart disease. Evidence suggests that a significant percentage of Americans in the middle-aged adult bracket do not engage in regular moderate physical activity for at least 30 minutes on 5 or more days per week. Physical Activity objective 2, which measures the percentage of people who meet the recommendation for exercise, has shown little movement (47.9% in 2020 and 48.1% in 2022). Sedentary behavior increases with aging. This finding may be due to the onset of conditions that affect mobility and strength.

Continuous, rhythmic exercise maintained for a period sufficient to stress the cardiac system (increase heart rate and blood pressure) is desirable. Suggested activities include brisk walking, jogging, swimming, bicycling, and skipping rope, as well as walking or biking to work or getting off public transportation before the desired stop. Activities that focus on strength training, skill, and coordination should be attempted by adults older than 40 years rather than activities necessitating speed and strength. Moderation is key for all groups of individuals. Caution is recommended for adults nearing 65 years of age to prevent muscle strains and/or falls. Overexertion, as evidenced by dizziness, chest pressure or chest pain, and unresolved shortness of breath, should be avoided. Additionally, in hot weather, strenuous exercise should be balanced with rest periods and increased intake of fluids to prevent heat stroke.

Nurses play significant roles in assessing, teaching, and evaluating individuals relative to activity-exercise programs. Advanced practice nurses are often instrumental in creating and guiding weight loss programs; nurses working in the community may see local residents at health fairs or health-promotion events, and other nurses or therapists may visit individuals at home for care following hospitalization for surgery or acute illness as home health professionals. Activity programs are initiated to restore health (following heart attack) or to improve cardiac function (such as cardiac and pulmonary rehabilitation), and in some cases to control blood glucose levels. A thorough assessment, including a cardiac stress test, is necessary when an individual has not exercised regularly in the past. Parameters for heart rate, blood pressure, and length and frequency of exercise sessions are set in advance by a cardiologist. Nurses support and guide individuals by helping them determine program goals, monitoring their progress, and teaching them how to modify lifestyle behaviors to obtain particular objectives.

To achieve maximal effectiveness, physical exercise should involve as many muscles as possible and be performed on a regular basis. Adults should spend 30 minutes or more in brisk physical activity every day for a total of 3 to 4 hours per week. The optimal performance level differs for each individual and should be based on parameters set by the individual's physician in advance of the individual starting a fitness program. Even very modest amounts of exercise may increase cardiac muscle tone.

To summarize, routine exercise is essential to the health of the heart and overall muscle strength. The type of activity and style is an individual choice. Program goals are achieved more readily when exercise is incorporated into leisure activities or is part of a group activity.

Sleep-Rest Pattern

Middle-aged Americans may not get as much sleep as young adults because of increased demands in their lives. Caring for immediate family, including children and sometimes parents, and fulfilling employment responsibilities consume most of a 24-hour period.

Insomnia is a common finding in this age category. It may be the result of overstimulation resulting from drinking too many caffeinated beverages, strenuous exercise within 2 hours of bedtime, or failure to have a regular sleep-wake schedule in a 24-hour period (National Sleep Foundation, 2020). Insomnia that occurs frequently can lead to distractibility, irritability, and fatigue during the daytime hours.

Sleep apnea is a common disorder during which normal breathing is disrupted by breathing pauses or shallow breaths. Breathing pauses may occur 30 times or more each hour and can last from a few seconds to minutes. Because of collapsed or blocked airways, a loud snorting or snoring sound is produced when normal breathing resumes. This pattern of pauses and shallow breathing is typical for the most common type of sleep apnea: obstructive sleep apnea. Although obstructive sleep apnea may be experienced by anyone, this type of sleep apnea commonly affects obese adults. Central sleep apnea is the least common type of sleep apnea. It occurs because of a disruption of central nerve signals to the diaphragm, resulting in brief periods of not breathing while asleep.

Sleep apnea is a chronic condition and may increase the risk of myocardial infarction, stroke, arrhythmias, and heart failure. Treatments include lifestyle changes, such as weight loss, continuous positive airway pressure therapy, and the use of mouthpieces, or surgical intervention. Femalesare often not diagnosed with sleep apnea because many health care providers consider this a disease only evident inmales. Studies show that sleep apnea in females is likely underestimated and undertreated because premenopausal females exhibit different signs and symptoms compared withmales. For example, some females do not snore or experience undue daytime sleepiness. Further, sleep apnea in postmenopausal females is as common as in males of the same age (National Heart, Lung, and Blood Institute, 2020).

Rest is essential to allow restorative functions of the body to occur. The effects of insomnia can be counteracted by regularly scheduled, high-quality sleep and occasional napping when fatigued. If insomnia becomes a chronic problem, cognitive-behavioral therapy has also been demonstrated to be an effective treatment option (Rossman, 2019). The National Sleep Foundation offers detailed information about treating sleep disorders at https://www.cdc.gov/oralhealth/about/healthy-people.html.

Cognitive-Perceptual Pattern

Learning is a phenomenon that occurs across the life span. The need to increase knowledge or information and the need to acquire new skills are constants as adults develop through a variety of experiences. Employment demands or new roles in life, such as becoming a parent or needing to care for an elderly family member, thrust the middle-aged adult into numerous different learning situations. The ability to learn a range of skills or to acquire knowledge through observing, performing, or participating in play activities begins in childhood as described by Gardner (1983, 1993) and extends into the middle years and beyond. The capacity to perform intellectually (i.e., to reason through critical thinking, to use/increase vocabulary, and to apply spatial perception skills) stays constant through the 35- to 65-year-old age range. However, some decreases in reaction time and cognitive flexibility become more apparent as age increases.

Skill Acquisition

The ability to acquire new knowledge or skills accumulates through formal education and life experiences and continues to increase throughout life. The evidence of this phenomenon is demonstrated by the many scholars and artists who become more productive in their middle years than when they were young adults. Some individuals discover "new talents" later in life because they have more leisure time or motivation to explore new areas or interests.

The theories of Havighurst and Orr (1956), Piaget (1970), and Bloom (1984) are relevant to the middle-aged adult. These theorists conclude that the prime time to be in the learner role is when the developmental task for that role is to be accomplished. The adult in the middle years as the learner-performer is a case in point. For example, to balance the responsibilities of caring for children and parents and being employed outside the home, the adult may explore new career options or creative endeavors.

Havighurst and Orr (1956) defined developmental tasks as the basic tasks of living that must be achieved for the adult to live successfully. These tasks are dictated by the expectations of society, the physiologic changes of the body throughout life, and the individual's own value system and goals. Although initially described in 1956, Havighurst and Orr's developmental tasks of middle age remain relevant (Box 23.4: Developmental Tasks of Middle Age).

If career goals have been previously identified, then attaining them can be highly rewarding, both psychologically and financially. In addition to career activities, the mature adult has an increased social awareness and often assumes more civic responsibility.

In Piaget's theory of cognitive development, formal operations are the highest or most complex level. This stage begins at approximately age 12 and continues throughout life. Piaget describes the thoughts of adults as being both flexible and effective. The adult can deal efficiently with complex problems of reasoning, including hypothesis testing (Piaget, 1970).

Bloom (1984) developed a hierarchy of cognitive levels in the adult learner. Knowledge is the simplest or most basic cognitive level. Knowledge is the acquisition of information. The adult learner defines "high blood pressure" in lay terms.

Comprehension is the second level, as indicated by the learner grasping the meaning of the communicated message and relating the term(s) to other material. For example, the individual can state one way in which obesity influences high blood pressure.

The third level is application of knowledge. At this level, the learner demonstrates an understanding of ideas and concepts by extending them to describe or relate them to real-life situations. For example, the individual with hypertension becomes involved in an exercise program.

The fourth level is analysis. At this level, all aspects of learning are united in thought, and the individual is cognizant of the relationships and interactions of all the parts. For example, the individual considers their values and life goals when making decisions about taking action in regard to understanding health care needs. The highest order of learning involves synthesis and evaluation. The person is able to combine various elements to form a plan and then is able to judge the extent to which the actions and results satisfy the original objectives. For example, people may develop plans to improve their health status and increase their disease self-management responsibilities.

BOX 23.4 Developmental Tasks of Middle Age

- Helping children become responsible and contented adults
- Rediscovering or developing satisfaction in the relationship with one's spouse (for the single adult, this can occur in a relationship with a sibling or significant other)
- Developing an affectionate, but independent, relationship with aging parents
- Reaching the peak in one's career
- Achieving mature social and civic responsibility
- Accepting and adapting to biologic changes
- Maintaining or developing friendships
- Developing leisure-time activities

The next step is to validate the results of ongoing health care programs in relation to their projected expectations. Genetic and personality factors, in combination with environmental conditions and lifestyle practices, account for the large difference in the ways in which individuals maintain mental abilities. Factors that may help to maintain cognitive function in later life are as follows:

- Absence of chronic diseases
- Healthy blood pressure
- Involvement in complex social activities
- Flexible personality style
- Relationship with partner or friends with high cognitive function
- High levels of performance speed
- Personal satisfaction with accomplishments in midlife and early old age (see Box 23.4)

Perceptual Changes

Presbyopia (farsightedness) is common in middle-aged adults, even in individuals who have had no previous problems with their vision. This condition occurs because of the loss of elasticity in the lens of the eye so that the adult cannot focus on objects that are in close range, such as reading without using prescription lenses. Presbyopia is corrected with prescription lenses, which may be needed only for reading or for close work.

Other visual conditions that may not be as easily corrected include decreased peripheral vision and decreased visual sensitivity in the dark. Both conditions are slow and insidious in their development and occur as the cornea becomes less transparent. Because all these conditions are not readily detected by the individual, middle-aged adults should undergo a routine professional eye examination every year.

Glaucoma occurs as a result of increased intraocular pressure, which can damage the optic nerve, resulting in vision loss and blindness (National Eye Institute, 2023). Loss of peripheral vision, or tunnel vision, is a common condition associated with glaucoma. Damage to the optic nerve is irreversible, but visual loss can be prevented if damage is identified early and treatment is initiated. Information at www.aao.org/eyecare-america shows that glaucoma is the leading cause of blindness among Black Americans in the United States. A current estimate is that three times the number of Black Americans compared with White

Americans have glaucoma; in addition, the rate of blindness attributable to glaucoma is four times greater in Black Americans relative to White Americans. The importance of regular eye examinations by an ophthalmologist cannot be overstated.

A **cataract**, opacity of the lens, can develop and cloud the vision in the later years of middle age. Often cataracts develop in people who have diabetes. Another disorder, diabetic retinopathy, gradually causes rupture of vessels in the retina, which leak into the eye, causing a lack of color differentiation and central vision changes.

Macular degeneration is often referred to as age-related macular degeneration (AMD). This age-related disorder is a progressive deterioration of the maculae of the retina and choroid structures of the eye and results in damaged sharp and central vision. Approximately 1.8 million Americans aged 40 years or older are affected by AMD, and the number of people with AMD was estimated to reach 2.95 million by 2020 (CDC, 2022a). This condition is very serious because it represents the effects of several disorders. Once a diagnosis of macular degeneration has been made, retinal ophthalmologists should be involved in the care of the individual.

Another common perceptual change in middle age is **presbycusis** (impaired auditory acuity). The first sounds to be lost are higher frequencies, such as a woman's voice. This is important in the work environment and situations that require social interaction. Because this process is subtle, middle age is a time for auditory evaluations as a part of routine examinations.

Beginning in the middle years, the sense of taste diminishes in a progressive and predictable manner. The taste buds located toward the anterior of the tongue are the first to be affected, causing an inability to detect sweet and salty flavors. When the effectiveness of the posterior taste buds declines, detection of bitter and sour flavors is lost. Consequently, this change can alter a person's food preferences and present problems for people who insist on adding salt to compensate for the deficit. Nurses involved in the care of the middle-aged adult, perhaps in the community or in home health care, can show the individual how the use of various herbs and spices can enhance flavor.

Self-Perception–Self-Concept Pattern and Transitions

Levinson's Theory

In Levinson's (1986a, 1986b) research on males and females (Levinson, 1996), a theory on "individual life structures" is posed. Levinson describes age-associated seasons or eras. The midlife transition, beginning at age 38 to 40 years, appears to include reappraising one's life, integrating the polarities, and modifying one's life structure toward being who one wants to be. Middle-aged adults struggle with meaning, value, and direction of their lives.

Erikson's Theory

In Erikson's eight stages of the life cycle (Erikson & Erikson, 1998), the last three stages are related to adulthood. Stage 7, **generativity versus stagnation** or self-absorption, is most frequently associated with the middle years. Erikson identifies generativity as the primary task to achieve during adulthood. Generativity includes a sense of productivity and creativity as evidenced by reaching previously established goals versus stagnation, the failure to achieve lifelong goals (Hornstein, 1986; Reifman et al., 1991; Thomas, 1995). Generativity also encompasses a desire to care for others versus self-absorption, the tendency to direct most of one's interest and attention to oneself, thereby excluding others.

Middle age is a time of critical self-review. For some, this review may prompt sadness, disappointment, self-doubt, and regret if the desired and expected life goals have not been met. For others, this may be a time of renewal, freedom to explore new ways of living, and a new sense of confidence.

Meleis's Theory

The nursing theory of transition was developed and expanded upon by Meleis (2010). Describing transition as the passage from one stage to another, it has been used to understand developmental, situational, health-illness and organizational changes (Schumacher & Meleis, 1994; Lindmark et al., 2019). Middle age is a time of significant transition in terms of health, work, and inward and outward perspectives. Application of Meleis's theory can assist individuals in framing and reframing the changes that occur as they get older.

Physiologic Changes

The effect of physiologic changes on mental health is nearly as critical during the middle years as it is during adolescence. Some of the most obvious changes that influence self-esteem are graying hair, an increasing number of wrinkles, decreasing visual and auditory acuity, and changes in body shape. The extent to which these changes are tolerated depends largely on the person's level of self-satisfaction and acceptance. People address these changes in varied ways.

Before 2002, hormone therapy (estrogen alone or estrogen and progesterone) was given to millions of postmenopausal females. Estrogen is still the only therapy approved by the Food and Drug Administration for the treatment of hot flashes associated with menopause. Millions of females took hormone therapy not only to relieve hot flashes but also because they were told hormone replacement may prevent heart disease, the number one cause of death in postmenopausal females. All of this changed in 2002 when data from the Women's Health Initiative (WHI) showed that postmenopausal females who took estrogen and progesterone increased their risk of cardiac events and other health problems, including stroke, blood clots, and breast cancer.

Follow-up analysis of the WHI data showed that the effects of hormone therapy depended on a woman's age and the length of time since menopause. In younger postmenopausal females, between 50 and 59 years of age, hormone use did not increase the risk of cardiac events as it did in older females. There is new evidence that hormone therapy may be beneficial for younger postmenopausal females, but timing and evaluation of risk and benefit is essential (Maas, 2021).

It is difficult to separate menopause from the physical and psychological changes that females experience as they age. The stressors common to females in their 40s and 50s include raising a family, helping parents as they age, coping with divorce or death of a spouse, retirement, and financial insecurity. Menopause happens in the midst of all this. All the events in a woman's life influence her experience of menopause and perimenopause, a period that precedes menopause and lasts approximately 4 years. Symptoms such as mood swings, nervousness, agitation, fatigue, and depression are often ascribed to the decline in estrogen levels that occurs during this time. The physiologic changes are important, but a woman's experience in menopause is profoundly affected by all the events in her life (Lowdermilk et al., 2019).

Males also experience physical and psychological reactions to middle age. The hormonal changes in males are gradual, typically beginning between 40 and 55 years of age. The symptoms are similar to those experienced by females, with emotional effects related to other life events, past coping patterns, and general feelings of self-esteem.

Roles-Relationships Pattern

Middle age is frequently a time of reassessment and change. This may be a turning point that occurs for several reasons. Over time, middle-aged adults become aware of subtle and compromising changes in physical, cognitive, and emotional agility. Furthermore, the inevitability of one's own death is recognized, perhaps for the first time. Middle-aged adults must accept that lifestyle choices have been made, unintended consequences may have lasting repercussions, and the opportunity to amend prior decisions may no longer be possible. Alternatively, middle-aged adults may be quite satisfied with prior life choices and the resultant personal satisfaction and contentment (Box 23.5: Evidence-Based Practice).

Family

Duvall and Miller (1985) delineate eight stages of the family life cycle, with stages 5, 6, and 7 in the middle years (see Chapter 7):

- Stage 5: Families with children, with the oldest child aged 13 to 20 years; lasts approximately 7 years
- Stage 6: Families launching young adults, from the first leaving until the last; lasts approximately 8 years
- Stage 7: Families from empty nest to retirement; lasts approximately 15 years

Family arrangements may consist of children residing with individuals identified as parents, a single-parent household, or children living with individuals other than parents, such as grandparents. The developmental tasks identified for families in stages 6 and 7 are similar to those described by Havighurst and Orr (1956); they focus on changes from a nuclear family to a marital couple with other responsibilities. For example, in stage 6, parents who are helping their children to become independent may also be caring for their aging parents. Additionally, middle-aged adults fulfill multiple complex responsibilities within a variety of career, social, and civic positions.

In 2022, 65% of children up to age 17 lived in a household with two married parents, and another 5% lived with two cohabitating parents. Regarding households with two married parents, there was significant racial disparity as follows: White alone 75%; Hispanic 60%; Black alone 38% (Childstats, 2024).

Families with young adolescent or young adult children have been described in research studies as both postparental and launching families. In contrast, criticism of this emphasis on the separation of children (regardless of age) from their families is increasing. Gilligan (1982) criticizes the work of many human development theorists who identify human development in terms of separation from the family. Middle-aged parents are encouraged to continue to care for and nurture their adolescent and adult children while recognizing the increasing interdependence of their relationships.

By supporting their children's efforts, parents can increase the self-esteem of their children while being effective role models. The parent assumes less of a parent-child relationship while interacting more on an adult-to-adult level. As the children are "launched," the parents may have uninterrupted time alone and time to share activities. The "launching" may be prolonged as young adult children return home to live after a period away. The challenges of the economy and cost of living make it difficult for many young people to live away from home and may force them to return home. This may create difficulty in family life, particularly given that young adult children may want the privacy and independence of living away from home while parents may expect adherence to rules and behaviors established when the children were younger. This may vary from having to give up a newly created hobby room to frustration over a lack of participation in home maintenance or learning how to balance substance use. Family life may also be threatened by opposition to a child's partner or the inability to establish satisfactory relationships with potential or actual partners or sons- and daughters-in-law. For many parents, the idea of their children leaving home is anticipated with either relief that the heavy care responsibilities of parenting are over or with dread over having to fill the void of time and inactivity. Empty nest syndrome may be exacerbated if parents never learned to communicate with each other effectively or to enjoy each other's company without the children.

At the other end of the family spectrum, aging parents can place demands on adult children primarily because older adults

BOX 23.5 EVIDENCE-BASED PRACTICE

"Regrets are the natural property of grey hairs"—Charles Dickens

Disappointment and regret are common emotions experienced across all ages. The dominant narrative about midlife is that it is full of regrets; the disconnection between goals and outcomes may have both a positive and negative yield. Midlife is a time of challenges and is a time period that has been studied less than time periods such as childhood and aging adulthood. The Midlife in the United States Study examines individuals in midlife across psychosocial, cognitive, and health developments; dynamics of daily life; and physiologic and neurologic correlates (Infurna et al., 2020). Midlife brings new opportunities, particularly in terms of connections to family and community. This is affected by individual health, both physical and mental, as well as societal expectations of people based on race, ethnicity, and gender. Areas where nurses have an effect on helping to improve well-being at midlife include encouraging physical activity, working to make neighborhoods greener and more accessible, and encouraging social support and engagement. Nurses can advocate at local and national levels for policies that support midlife well-being and work toward promoting an equity model of health.

are frequently beset with health problems. A caring relationship is in order, in which the aging parent's need for independence is recognized. Because of society's emphasis on youth, the middle-aged adult must associate feelings of self-worth with personal integrity rather than with body appearance or physical prowess.

Friends can provide invaluable support systems. When children have left home, middle-aged adults may have more free time to share favorite activities and learn new ones. Middle-aged adults without financial constraints have greater opportunities to pursue activities that contribute to better health outcomes and a sense of well-being.

Work

Perhaps the most common role that middle-aged adults share is that of a worker. Much of their pride and sense of satisfaction is derived from their work. Work is equated with being "grown up." One can easily recall the "What do you want to be when you grow up?" questioning of youth. Success and achievement are evaluated in terms of careers and family life. Research has shown that middle-aged adults are more satisfied with their jobs than younger adults (Goedereis, et al., 2023).

Middle-aged adults constitute most of the US workforce. For many, vocations play a major role in defining personal levels of wellness. There were 5486 fatal work injuries recorded in the United States in 2022, a 5.7% increase from 5190 in 2021 (US Bureau of Labor Statistics, 2023). The largest percentage of these fatalities related to transportation incidents. Exposure to harmful substances and contact with objects and equipment accounted for the bulk of the remainder of fatalities. The highest rates of nonfatal injuries occur in construction, manufacturing, and health services. Thirty percent of nonfatal injuries and illnesses requiring days away from work continue to be due to overexertion and repetitive motion.

Poor housekeeping and poor design predispose workers to falls and other accidents; exposure to noise and toxic chemicals also make employees susceptible to injury and illness. Many injuries that contribute significantly to the morbidity and mortality of adults can be prevented. Fixing faulty steps, repairing faulty electrical wires, and securing carpets are only a few of the many preventive measures.

Accidents are twice as common among smokers as among nonsmokers (National Institute for Occupational Safety and Health, 2023; CDC 2023c). Possible explanations include the loss of attention, the use of one hand for smoking, and irritation of the eyes. Other work-related problems include exposure to harmful substances resulting in lung diseases, cancers, and workplace violence.

The effect of life events on mental health depends on the personal strength of the individual, the availability of support, and the nature and number of events and their significance for the person. Three common examples of life events with potential disruptive effects are partner separation or divorce, having two or more jobs, and caring for aging parents. Their negative effects may be alleviated if assistance is provided early in the process of a change. In some organizations, resources for managing problems of addiction, life transitions, emotional issues, financial problems, stress reduction, and grief counseling are available off-site to all employees. These resources are offered without cost to the individual and, in some cases, to their family members or support persons.

Two-or-More-Job Family: Family and Work Responsibilities

Historically, females have always participated in the labor force. However, this participation rests onfemales' family roles, discrimination, changes in the economy, changes in technology, and personal choice (Jacobs & Bahn, 2019). During the second half of the 20th century, there was a rapid growth in the number of females in the labor force. There was a dramatic increase from 1960 to 1980s, which reached a peak in 1999. There was decline from 2007 to 2009, when there was a recession. In 2015, females represented 56.7% of the labor force, and in 2017, they represented 57% of the workforce. Participation in the labor force varies by marital status and gender. Females who never married have higher participation rates (64.3% in 2017) compared with divorced females (61.5%), separated females (61.7%), and married females (58.2%). Widows and widowers were the least likely to participate in the labor force (US Bureau of Labor Statistics, 2018).

Females' participation in the labor market has changed since the 1940s because of socioeconomic factors and educational attainment. The number of females aged 25 to 64 who held a college degree nearly quadrupled from 1970 to 2017, whereas the number of males in the same age range only about doubled during the same period. Additionally, females were more likely to work full-time and year-round. However, females' earnings as a proportion of males' earnings remain lower (US Bureau of Labor Statistics, 2018).

Job-related travel has also increased during the last few years for both males and females. Travel by either partner means additional responsibilities for the one who remains at home. Additionally, if one partner travels more than the other travels, feelings of resentment may develop, or the common ground for discussion of work events may be altered. The one who stays at home may feel "put upon" when their spouse is perceived as having fun. In contrast, travel is tiring and is not usually as exciting as it appears to observers. The traveling partner may come home tired, irritable, and desiring peace and quiet, which may conflict with the expectations of other family members.

Traveling for work may become much less frequent as more people work from home and more meetings are set up online. The number of people working from home increased during the COVID-19 pandemic. People in occupations that were conducive to working remotely were sent home, and many of them continue to work from home. This may both create and alleviate stress in families. Balancing childcare expectations and interruptions, the lack of space for separate and private work areas, and the lack of socialization may increase stress on families. However, decreases in transportation costs, as well as the possibility of interrupting the workday with household tasks or restorative breaks, may help families create new patterns of interaction that are not as stressful. Opportunities to discuss changing family roles can be helpful and may be offered to family members who experience these changes as stressful. Family members should be referred to support groups with volunteers or professionals who provide services to various agencies and community resources.

The effect of work on families can be emotionally draining, particularly when it is filled with conflict, and poses threats to family stability. When adults come home tired, angry, or frustrated from their work experiences, they likely have limited emotional support to share with other family members. When people gain self-esteem from their jobs and generally enjoy going to work, they tend to experience less frustration and dissatisfaction with themselves and their positions, enabling them to give more of themselves to other members of the family.

Middle age is important when one is looking at the career clock. Issues that need to be considered include midcareer changes and preretirement planning. Retirement is a major turning point; to many people, it is the transition from middle age to old age and from the period of work to the period of leisure or different work.

Many adults are working up to and beyond the age of retirement. Many are entering new careers later in life because they are living longer and need more financial resources to successfully enter the older adult years. As adults progress through the middle years, they become increasingly aware of the time remaining. Some may choose to try new types of work or avocation; others may be working in areas where physical stamina is vital, including unit-based nursing. Some nurses who have worked in hospitals at the bedside may choose to enter nursing education.

Comprehensive health-promotion programs at the work site contain these elements: 1) health education focusing on developing skills, 2) lifestyle changes, 3) information dissemination and awareness building tailored to employee interests and needs, 4) supportive social and physical work environments, 5) policies promoting healthy behaviors at work (e.g., safer work site policies, smoking policies, healthy nutritional alternatives in the cafeteria and vending machines, opportunities to obtain regular physical activity), and 6) integration of the work site programs with administrative structures (e.g., employee assistance programs, screening programs, linking the delivery of health care services to ensure follow-up, appropriate treatment, and adherence). These efforts should be part of a comprehensive occupational health and safety program (Box 23.6: Quality and Safety) (CDC, 2020a).

Caring for Aging Parents

The needs of aging parents and of the middle-aged adult's own children can create additional demands during the middle years (Fig. 23.1). The middle-aged adult can feel caught between the children and the parents. Both children and older parents can present unrealistic, excessive demands and be difficult to please. However, it can also be a time of great joy as children and grandparents interact and learn from each other.

Middle-aged adults may be faced with having frail and ill parents living within their own family unit or placing them in a nursing home. These dilemmas are complicated by the reality that their parents are growing older and may not have long to live. The recognition of the parents' impending death heightens middle-aged adults' awareness of their own aging and mortality.

BOX 23.6 QUALITY AND SAFETY SCENARIO

Lifetime Prevention of Cardiovascular Disease in Females

Heart disease is a leading cause of death in females. Healthy diet; exercise; maintaining blood pressure and cholesterol control; limiting salt, sugar, and alcohol; and eliminating tobacco use all contribute positively to heart health. Lack of access to places to exercise, living in food deserts, and the absence of health insurance or economic resources all contribute negatively to heart health. As nurses encourage females to achieve heart health, they need to be aware of the nonmodifiable factors that affect females' health.

- Eat a healthy diet with fruits, vegetables, whole grains, and fat-free or low-fat milk and milk products. Choose foods low in saturated fats, cholesterol, salt (sodium), and added sugars.
- Exercise regularly. Adults need 2 hours and 30 minutes (or 150 minutes total) of exercise each week. Activity can be spread out during the week and broken up into smaller chunks of time during the day.
- Be tobacco free. The US Department of Health and Human Services has a website providing information about quitting smoking (https://betobaccofree.hhs.gov/).
- Smoke Free has information about quitting smoking for different groups (e.g., veterans, elders, females, teens). Information is also available in Spanish (https://smokefree.gov/).
- Limit alcohol use, which can lead to long-term health problems, including heart disease and cancer. If choosing to drink, do so in moderation, which is no more than one drink per day for females. Do not drink at all if pregnant.
- Know your family history. Certain factors may increase your risk for heart disease and stroke.
- Manage any medical condition you might have. Learn the ABCs of heart health and keep them in mind every day, especially when speaking to your health provider:
- Appropriate aspirin therapy for those who need it
  - Blood pressure control
  - Cholesterol management
  - Smoking cessation

From the Centers for Disease Control and Prevention (CDC, 2017). *Lower your risk for the number 1 killer of women.* https://www.cdc.gov.

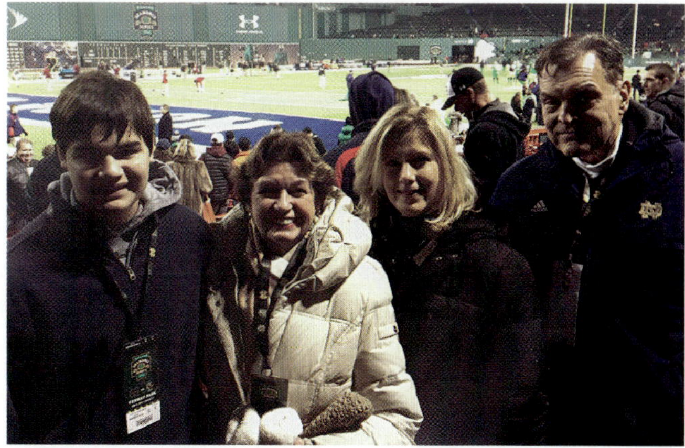

FIG. 23.1 Middle-aged adults, young adults, and older adults can enjoy meaningful relationships with one another.

Difficulties in caring for older parents can be somewhat lessened when potential situations are discussed before a crisis arises. This is particularly true when all members of the middle-aged adult family are working, space in their home is limited, and the community has few resources for well or ill older adults. Although institutionalization is undesirable to many families, the care of ill, older parents may eventually require it. By anticipating these needs and preparing for them, middle-aged adults and their parents can develop more meaningful relationships with one another.

Divorce and Separation

Divorce or separation may be considered a major disruption to a marriage, committed relationships, and family. This event may result in short-term and long-term health consequences. Although the divorce rate has decreased in recent years, the need for individuals and families to address and find solutions to new and multiple problems may affect their health (US Census, 2023). When a divorce occurs, each family member must confront the necessity of examining and, in many cases, modifying an accustomed style of living and adapting. Some states now mandate that divorcing parents participate in programs to support their children (Divorcewriter, 2023). This mandate comes in part due to the recognition of the effect separation or divorce may have on children's mental health (D'Onofrio & Emery, 2019).

Parents may interact with the health care system often as a result of their children's sickness and well visits. The American Academy of Child and Adolescent Psychiatry has developed a source to assist nurses and other health providers in discussing divorce with parents: https://www.aacap.org/AACAP/Families_and_Youth/Facts_for_Families/FFF-Guide/Children-and-Divorce-001.aspx.

Death

Death of a partner or close friends can result in grieving for the loss of companionship and the loss of an anticipated future free from the responsibilities of work and children. The surviving spouse may be unprepared to be single again, to be the only parent, or to live alone. The loneliness may be exacerbated by ill or dying peers or parents. Middle-aged adults become increasingly aware of the finite nature of life, thinking not only of the number of years since birth but also of the number of years left to live. The midlife review is a common outcome of this recognition.

Sexuality-Reproductive Pattern

Research suggests that a high proportion of people remain sexually active well into later life. People can continue to have a satisfactory pattern of sexual functioning throughout the middle and older adult years (NIA, 2020). As they would in any other developmental phase, middle-aged adults may need counseling to make health-promoting decisions about their sexual and reproductive behaviors and health.

Unintended pregnancies are high across all ages of American females but are highest (77% of all pregnancies) in middle-aged females. Fertility begins to decline for females between 35 and 40 years of age; however, perimenopausal females are still at risk of an unintended pregnancy. Unintended pregnancy rates decrease with age (Guttmacher Institute, 2019).

The pregnancy-related mortality rate for all females in the United States continues to rise. In 2021, 1205 females died of maternal causes in the United States compared with 861 in 2020 and 754 in 2019 (CDC, 2021). Research indicates that an increasing number of pregnant females in the United States have chronic health conditions such as hypertension, diabetes, and chronic heart disease that increase the risk of complications. Considerable disparities in pregnancy-related mortality exist based on the individual's race, ethnicity, age, education, and state of delivery. Data show significantly higher pregnancy-related mortality ratios among Black and American Indian/Alaska Native females (Njoku et al., 2023).

Achieving the *Healthy People 2030* target goals of reducing maternal deaths will require that national, state, and local policies address females' needs before and during pregnancy and that gaps in research and prevention programs be identified through improved monitoring. A focus on health equity and reproductive justice is vital at the local and national levels (Njoku et al., 2023).

Changes in the reproductive systems of males and females result in changes in sexual function throughout adulthood. During middle adulthood, sexual arousal is slower, orgasms are less intense, and a return to prearousal levels is more rapid, with males having longer refractory periods between ejaculation and their next erection. When a person continues to be sexually active, these functional changes occur over decades and are minimally noticeable until later in adulthood unless external factors, such as the negative effects of some antihypertensive and antidepressant agents, are present.

Middle-aged females may confront their own aging for the first time and may be perplexed as to symptomatic factors and changing roles. Females can experience vaginal dryness, difficulty finding a partner, less interest in initiating sex, and longer times to reach orgasm. However, perceived emotional closeness during sex was found to be associated with more frequent arousal, lubrication, and orgasm (David et al., 2018).

Although males and females frequently enjoy satisfactory sexual relationships throughout the middle adult years, males in their middle age are more vulnerable to sexual dysfunction than are females. Erectile dysfunction, the inability to attain or maintain an erection sufficient for sexual activity, is a common disorder among older males. The gradual decline of age-related physiologic function combined with chronic comorbidities may impair erectile function (Pelligrino et al., 2023). Common disorders related to erectile dysfunction include cardiovascular disease, diabetes, lower urinary tract symptoms, and depression—all of which should be considered by health care providers when assessing middle-aged males experiencing erectile dysfunction. Several readily available, nonsurgical treatments for erectile dysfunction exist, including medications, supplements, hormonal therapy, penile injection, and external vacuum devices. The successful treatment of erectile dysfunction has the potential to increase sexual performance satisfaction, intimacy between partners, and overall quality of and satisfaction with life. Health care providers should not hesitate to initiate a sexual wellness assessment with middle-aged adults. Discussions should include specific sexual wellness strategies designed to prevent sexually transmitted infections (STIs).

Abnormal genital bleeding and secondary amenorrhea are common gynecologic conditions that indicate serious physical problems. Abnormal genital bleeding is the most common reason for gynecologic office visits by adult females. Although pregnancy and menopause are the most common causes of secondary amenorrhea, other conditions related to abnormal pregnancy, functional disorders, physiologic changes, and pathologic factors must be considered.

STIs continue to be a major public health problem for middle-aged adults. Consequences of untreated STIs are sterility, ectopic pregnancy, fetal and infant deaths, birth defects, and fetal cognitive deficits. Virtually all cases of cervical cancer are caused by human papilloma virus (HPV), and two HPV types (16 and 18) are responsible for approximately 70% of all cases (NCI, 2023). As with many other health behaviors and diseases, the full effect on the life of an individual and the family may not be realized until middle age.

According to the CDC (2023e), about 1.2 million people in the United States had HIV at the end of 2021, and approximately 87% knew they had HIV. The annual number of new diagnoses of HIV decreased 7% from 2017 to 2021 (CDC, 2023e). Knowledge of HIV status increases with age. Middle-aged Americans are more likely to receive a diagnosis of HIV infection later in the course of their disease, which can lead to a poorer prognosis and shorter survival after an HIV infection diagnosis (CDC, 2023e).

The US Preventive Services Task Force now recommends HIV screening for adolescents and adults between 15 and 64 years, those who engage in risky behaviors, and all pregnant females, including those who present in labor whose HIV status is unknown (CDC, 2023e).

Coping–Stress Tolerance Pattern

Kobasa (1979) was the first to investigate the concept of stress hardiness. Kobasa identified hardiness as an aspect of personality that included control, commitment, and challenge. Her theory is clinically relevant because it suggests that hardiness acts as a mediator between perceived stress and self-efficacy across many dimensions: physical, psychological, mental, and emotional. According to Kobasa, across the health continuum, individuals who demonstrate hardiness appear to be more resistant to the effects of stress (Iwanowicz-Palus et al., 2022).

Stress is an unavoidable human life experience that triggers a reactive physiologic response often derived from perceived psychological stressors. The many negative effects of perceived stress on physical health are well documented. Physiologically, stress causes the hormones cortisol, epinephrine, and norepinephrine to activate or exacerbate medical conditions, including chronic physical, mental, and comorbid health conditions (Palus et al., 2022). Stress tolerance is a learned behavior. Almost 50 years ago, Benson first described the "relaxation response" as a reproducible state of deep rest (Benson & Klipper, 1975; Benson-Henry Mind Body, 2020). The immediate and long-lasting effects of stress can be mitigated with effective coping skills, including holistic mind-body interventions such as meditation, yoga, tai chi, and deep breathing (Toussaint et al., 2021). Evidence-based research demonstrates how the mind-body connection helps individuals cope with a wide range of illnesses and stressful life events (Box 23.7: Best Practice).

BOX 23.7 BEST PRACTICE

Benson-Henry Mind Body Institute of Massachusetts General Hospital, Harvard Medical School Stress Management and Resiliency Training (SMART)

Research demonstrates that many health care visits are for symptoms such as headaches, insomnia, weakness or fatigue, and gastrointestinal symptoms, all of which are frequently stress related. Stress Management and Resiliency Training is designed to help individuals who have chronic illnesses (including life-threatening illnesses) or stress-related symptoms to better manage their health problems and optimize their quality of life. The interventions combine conventional medical care with knowledge of the effects of behaviors and attitudes on health. The following are included in the biopsychosocial-spiritual approach of the assessment and treatment plans:

- Eliciting the relaxation response, a state of deep rest that changes responses to stress (decreases vital signs and muscle tenseness, increased mindfulness)
- Enhancing coping skills through cognitive-behavioral strategies
- Encouraging exercise or physical activity
- Providing nutritional counseling
- Monitoring and adjusting medication, when necessary, in consultation with the physician

Because health insurance policies differ, coverage and reimbursement differ, insurance claims for these outpatient visits are submitted directly to each person's insurance carrier. A patient advocate works with patients to understand their insurance coverage for these services and submitting claims for reimbursement from their carrier. Evidence supports the effectiveness of these interventions:

- Persons with pain reduced their number of clinician visits.
- Visits to a health maintenance organization were reduced after a relaxation response–based intervention, resulting in significant cost savings.
- Blood pressure was lowered, and use of medications decreased in hypertensive persons.
- Sleep patterns were improved for 100% of persons with insomnia; 90% reduced or eliminated the use of sleep medication.
- Infertile females reported decreased levels of depression, anxiety, and anger.
- Females with severe premenstrual syndrome experienced a reduction in physical and psychological symptoms.
- Health-promoting behaviors such as nutrition, social support, self-esteem, health responsibility, and exercise increased after the program and were maintained by the follow-up visit.
- Six months after the program, a majority of participants continued to experience reduction of their physical symptoms.
- Anxiety and depression normalized for most participants and were maintained.
- Females with menopause reported fewer hot flashes, lower blood pressure, improved sleep, and decreased depression, anxiety, and anger.

From the Benson-Henry Institute website (https://www.bensonhenry-institute.org/).

Stress and Heart Disease

As reiterated throughout this chapter, heart disease is a leading cause of death in middle-aged adults. In landmark studies, Haynes and colleagues (1978, 1980) described the relationship of psychosocial factors to CHD using the Framingham study. In the study, 24 measures of psychosocial stress were used. Inmales, aging worries correlated significantly with systolic and diastolic blood pressure. Partner stress and personal worries correlated significantly with diastolic blood pressure. Both diastolic and systolic pressure correlated significantly with work changes and anxiety in employed females between 45 and 64 years of age. Anger suppressed, anger discussed, tension, and anger symptoms correlated significantly with diastolic blood pressure in this age group.

The death of a parent enhances awareness of one's vulnerability to illness and death. The more opportunities and time people have to prepare for these stressful events, the more likely they will be to feel in control and the less likely they will be to feel anxious and helpless. When individuals assume more responsibility for their life, decisions lead to concrete behaviors, such as drafting a will, developing an advance directive (which includes **living will, health care agent**, and granting a durable power of attorney), and making funeral prearrangements. An **advance directive** is a legal document prepared when an individual is alive, competent, and able to make decisions to provide guidelines for health care providers in the future, when the individual is not able to make decisions because of physical disability (being unconscious) or mental incompetence. By granting a **durable power of attorney**, the individual designates another person (spouse, son, daughter, or friend) to make health care decisions (especially decisions about aggressive treatment to forestall death) when an individual becomes unable to make such decisions. The nurse helps middle-aged adults anticipate stressors so that they are better prepared to cope with and prevent additional physical, psychosocial, and spiritual stressors, thereby optimizing their health.

Values-Beliefs Pattern

When adults make decisions affecting their lives, this is usually the result of a personal, complex pattern of values and beliefs. Much of what people value or believe to be true is formed early in life and can be difficult to alter. Usually, people do not spend a great deal of conscious thought on abstract explanations of the meaning of life and why certain things are valued. However, during times of illness or crisis, most people will take time to review their value systems and seek meaning about what is important.

A crisis at any age can be a turning point during which both increased vulnerability and increased potential are present. When the crisis is managed successfully, a virtue or strength will evolve. Erikson and Erikson (1998) identified caring as a middle-aged adult virtue that is often developed during times of crisis.

Committed responsibilities for the care and welfare of others promote moral development. When middle age is lived with generativity, many opportunities are afforded to live life by one's higher principles. The middle-aged adult can differentiate among personal wants and needs, duties demanded by society, and principles by which to live. Kohlberg's work on moral development delineated these phases as conventional and postconventional. His studies of males described stage 3 as an interpersonal definition of morality, whereas stage 4 is a societal definition based on law and order. Kohlberg concludes that most American adults are in these phases of moral development. In contrast, stage 5 is the concern and willingness to sacrifice oneself for the well-being of others (Kohlberg & Lickona, 1986). Subsequent studies by Gilligan (1982) on moral development in females and males demonstrate sex differences when describing high morality. Females discussed issues of selfishness versus responsibility, of exercising care with decision-making, and avoiding hurting others. Males described terms of justice, fairness, and rights of individuals. Gilligan (1982, 1990) and Gilligan and Snider (2018) conclude that females possess a process of moral development different from that ofmales.

Valuing others, having relationships, and being responsible to others enable middle-aged adults to make the transitions of moral development. This process is accomplished through raising children, developing more junior employees, and serving the community. As people fulfill these commitments, they increasingly treat others as equals and gradually develop a sensitivity and desire to change barriers to human worth and equality, such as racial prejudice, homelessness, inadequate access to health care, and the availability of stockpiles of weapons.

ENVIRONMENTAL PROCESSES

Environmental factors are significant variables in health promotion. Public health initiatives have played an important role in reducing and controlling the spread of infectious diseases such as influenza. Our continued efforts at improving sanitation and controlling pollution (air, water, noise) have resulted in a reduction of health problems such as lung disease, transmission of bacterial and viral infections, and hearing loss. On the individual level, the effect of handwashing in controlling illness cannot be overstated.

Because there are approximately 100 million workers in the United States, occupational hazards are a serious threat to national health. Exposure to toxic chemicals, asbestos, coal dust, cotton fiber, ionizing radiation, physical hazards, excessive noise, and stress can precipitate numerous health problems (Nguyen et al., 2018). For the middle-aged worker, these problems include cancers, lung and heart diseases, decreased hearing, physical injuries, and mental health problems (Friis, 2018).

Physical Agents

Ionizing radiation is a physical agent that can cause cancer. One example of this is cancer caused by medical procedures that include the use of diagnostic radiography and therapeutic radiation.

Water pollution has become another major concern. Many industrial and agricultural wastes, such as benzene and chlordane, have been recovered in rivers and lakes from which drinking water is obtained. These substances can potentially lead to carcinomas and other health problems.

Air pollution from automobile emissions, burning fuels, and industrial incineration has warranted smog alerts and air pollution indices. This issue is especially important to the individual with chronic respiratory or cardiovascular disease. Noise pollution in industry is a potential problem for the middle-aged adult worker. Hearing loss is the most common occupational disease, but it can be prevented if federal guidelines regarding noise exposure levels and hearing conservation programs are followed, especially prevention activities aimed at miners and construction workers, for whom hearing loss is a major problem. Exposure to excessive noise, radon, radiation, sunlight, and vibration can produce problems such as chronic obstructive lung disease, cancer, and degenerative diseases (EPA, 2024).

Biologic Agents

As noted throughout this text, health and disease are influenced by the interactions among the agent, host, and environment. Agent factors can be biological, physical, chemical, or psychological. The biologic causes of diseases include bacteria, viruses, fungi, parasites, and food poisoning. Because these causes are often limited to identifiable occupations, they can be readily diagnosed, treated, and prevented. Many of these agents are transmitted through the air or by contact with certain media, such as water, food, blood, or feces.

Hepatitis A is caused by viral infection, with transmission occurring primarily through the fecal-oral route. This host-agent interaction typically occurs in the middle-aged adult living in an environment with poor sanitation and having close contact with an infected person. The person may also be exposed to contaminated food and water. The hepatitis B viral agent is transmitted primarily in the blood or plasma of the infected individuals, which is particularly significant for the adult who is employed in a health care setting. Among medical and dental personnel (with surgeons, oral surgeons, and pathologists at the highest risk), the risk of contracting hepatitis B is six times higher than that of the general population.

There are two other infections of concern for middle-aged adults: pneumonia and varicella/herpes zoster (shingles). Both can be prevented through vaccinations, which adults aged 60 years and older are advised to receive (CDC, 2024b).

Chemical Agents

Chemicals include a wide variety of substances that increase the risk of morbidity and death in the middle-aged adult. When a home is located near an industry, there is the risk of exposure to toxic chemicals that pollute the air. Contaminants can also be carried home from the workplace on clothing.

Workers at increased risk include coal miners, wood handlers, and those who work with asbestos and coal. Pneumoconiosis is caused by breathing in certain types of dust particles; when the dust is from coal, it is commonly called black lung disease and is found in approximately 15% of coal miners. Wood handlers have increased risk of certain cancers. The asbestos worker has an increased risk of mesothelioma and asbestosis. Approximately two million workers each year are exposed to benzene and vinyl chloride, which may be carcinogens. Among American industrial workers, 9 in 10 may be inadequately protected from exposure to at least 10 of the 163 most common hazardous chemicals. More than 2000 of the 50,000 chemicals found in the workplace are suspected human carcinogens (CDC, 2023f).

Tobacco

While cigarette smoking and tobacco continue to be the leading causes of preventable death, disease, and disability in the United States, the percentage of smokers has dropped and remained steady since 2015. Data on smoking patterns by age, gender, race, and ethnicity can be found at https://www.statista.com/statistics/184418/percentage-of-cigarette-smoking-in-the-us/.

Goals that have been met toward *2030 Healthy People* objectives include the reduction of cigarette smoking by adolescents, the reduction of use of smokeless tobacco by adolescents, and the increase in the number of states requiring 21 as the minimum age to purchase tobacco products (CDC.gov, 2024). The proportion of US adults who smoke cigarettes declined from 20.9% in 2005 to 14.2% in 2019. However, disparities in cigarette smoking remain. In 2015, the rate of cigarette smoking was higher among male adults aged 25 to 44 years, those who had a General Education Development certificate (GED), those who lived below the federal poverty level, and those who lived in the Midwest, those who were insured by Medicaid or uninsured, those who had a disability/limitation and were experiencing psychological distress (Statistica.com, 2023).

Among Americans, cigarette smoking and exposure to secondhand smoke results in more than 480,000 deaths every year, including 41,000 deaths from secondhand smoke. Smoke recipients are at increased risk of heart disease as well as colds, chronic bronchitis, emphysema, and cancers of the mouth, lungs, esophagus, pancreas, and bladder. More than 16 million Americans are living with smoking-related illnesses (CDC, 2022d). Quitting smoking not only reduces premature death but may add as many as 10 years to life expectancy (CDC, 2023d, 2023f).

Few smokers realize that cigarettes contain 2000 known chemicals, including tar, nicotine, hydrogen cyanide, formaldehyde, and ammonia. Cigarette smoking is, for most smokers, an addiction to nicotine, which is absorbed into the bloodstream. Nicotine acts on the two divisions of the nervous system: central (brain and the spinal cord) and peripheral (autonomic nervous system and motor and sensory fibers to the arms and legs). The effects of nicotine stimulation can be observed both in electroencephalographic changes and in hand tremors. Nicotine also stimulates the heart, leading to an increased pulse rate and elevated blood pressure. Although smokers frequently believe that cigarettes have a calming effect, this notion is misleading. Nicotine stimulates the body, whereas carbon monoxide causes lethargy. Smokers may feel calm, although they are having their sensations dulled by carbon monoxide. Additive effects such as those from chlorine, cotton dust, and γ-radiation can lower midexpiratory flow values. Profound effects can also be observed with asbestos interaction.

DETERMINANTS OF HEALTH

Social Factors and Environment

An individual's set of beliefs, practices, norms, customs, rituals, and assumptions about life are learned during the early years of socialization (Spector, 2016). Nurses need to explore the potential influences of health beliefs with the patient and not presume these beliefs represent a specific culture. Culture is mediated by an individual's education, assimilation status, income, and occupation. Additionally, employing cultural awareness reduces nurses' biases about a patient's culture. Cultural awareness is the "self-examination of and in-depth exploration of one's own cultural and professional background" (Campinha-Bacote, 2002). Practicing cultural awareness enables the nurse to listen to the middle-aged adult's interpretation of their symptoms and how they relate those symptoms to a clinical diagnosis.

The health of middle-aged adults is varied and affected by a variety of factors (Box 23.8: Health and Social Determinants). Health problems are a result of long-term environmental and social exposures. Structural racism, social determinants, and implicit bias each affect how individuals and communities can access health care. These exist as people interact with providers and health care systems (Egede et al., 2021). Implicit bias is a negative attitude one is not aware they have toward certain groups of people based on factors such as ethnicity, race, gender, size, or sexual orientation. Nursing education is now underscoring the importance of nurses being aware of implicit bias, how to address it, and how to minimize its effect; many health professions require training as part of professional licensure and recertification (Feeney, 2023). Resources include implicit bias training developed by the American Academy of Family Practice (https://www.aafp.org/family-physician/patient-care/the-everyone-project/toolkit/implicit-bias.html).

Poverty rates are important indicators of community well-being and the health status of community members. Economic adversity results in disproportionate access to health services, which may contribute to lower life expectancy and a disproportionate disease burden.

Life expectancy in the United States in 2023, on average, was 79 years for females and 74 years for males. Life expectancy decreased in the United States by 1.3 years from 2019 to 2022, during the COVID-19 pandemic. In peer countries, life expectancy fell by 0.5 years during the same period. Peer countries of the United States, according to the Peterson-Kaiser Family Foundation (KFF) Health System Tracker, include Australia, Austria, Belgium, Canada, France, Germany, Japan, the Netherlands, Sweden, Switzerland, and the United Kingdom (https://www.healthsystemtracker.org/chart-collection/u-s-life-expectancy-compare-countries) (Peterson-KFF, 2024). Life expectancy is influenced by societal factors such as the quality of health care and access to preventive health services. Other factors that rest with both the individual and society are lifestyle, diet, violence, and accidents.

Because most people begin to interact with the health care system as they get older, measuring life expectancy at older ages may provide a better sense of how well the health care system performs. Disparities in access between the United States and comparable countries remains but is less pronounced at older ages, when older Americans have access to Medicare.

Aging confers many benefits to middle-aged adults as well as declines in health. Nurses who engage in cultural awareness can ensure that appropriate health promotion is provided, especially for vulnerable populations and those individuals, families, and communities who have special health care needs.

Levels of Policymaking and Health

Adults in the middle years are frequently at the peak of their careers. Although their net income may be greater than it was during early adulthood, they frequently have significant additional financial obligations. For many individuals in their late 50s or early 60s, retirement may be in the planning stages (Fig. 23.2). However, leaving full-time employment for retirement may not be possible for many middle-aged adults. Reasons that many middle-aged adults give are as follows:

- Technologic advances in health care may extend the limits for life expectancy for those individuals who can afford and are able to access those advances. Individuals are living longer than previous generations; therefore, they cannot "afford" to retire in their mid-60s because they have a financial need to "fund" another 25 to 30 years of life.

BOX 23.8 HEALTH AND SOCIAL DETERMINANTS

Patients should expect the highest standard of care regardless of their gender, race, ethnicity, income, age, or education. However, clinicians may have unconscious or conscious biases about a patient's perceived gender, race, age, income, and education level. These biases contribute to negative associations about the patient and may lead to less-than-optimal care (Fitzgerald & Hurst, 2017). Clinicians' implicit attitudes about race, ethnicity, gender, or class may facilitate differential treatment in patients, which in turn contribute to health disparities in care.

Nurses need to be aware of potential stereotypes they may have about patients and examine whether they do have biases. We encourage nurses (as well as clinicians) to take The Implicit Association Test (IAT), which measures implicit attitudes and stereotypes about groups (race, age, disability, sexuality, religion, and weight to name a few). The following is a link to the IAT items that will be contained in the online survey: https://www.implicit.harvard.edu (Fitzgerald & Hurst, 2017).

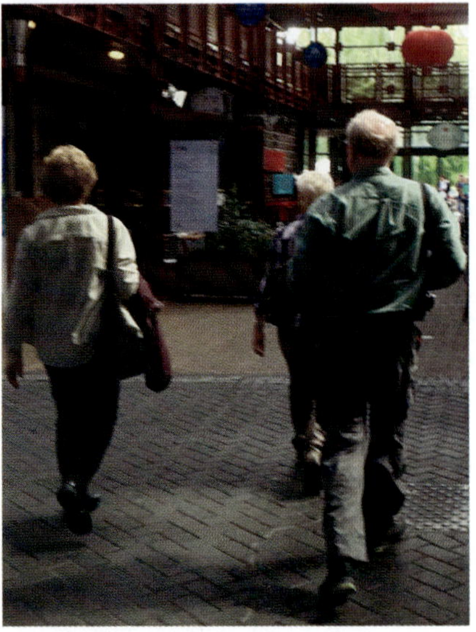

FIG. 23.2 Middle-aged adults may enjoy travel after retirement.

- Quality health care is expensive. Because the United States is a predominately employer-based health care system, many middle-aged adults remain at their employment until they are eligible for Medicare. Because the health care system spends less on prevention, chronic illnesses require more care and interventions, which in turn influences the financial burden borne by almost all Americans.
- Changes in the US economy in the past 10 years have necessitated significant changes in family patterns. Increasingly, more than one generation may live in the same home to afford the rising costs of commodities that have been taken for granted. For example, the costs of a college education funded by middle-aged adults are not necessarily balanced by a full-time position at the end of the 4 or 5 years needed to obtain a college degree. Young adults may not leave home at 22 or 23 years of age. Consequently, their parents, if still employed, may need to continue to work to support adult children and pay the debt of the college educational experience.
- Individuals may have accrued increasing debt to pay for health insurance that is becoming more costly. As people develop health conditions that are related to accumulated stress and the aging process, they require more use of their benefits from their health insurance companies.
- In addition, they may be supporting elderly parents or children with chronic health issues. They may have consumed their savings and home investment to pay for medications, hospitalizations, and/or nursing home expenses. When the adult or family members have ongoing health problems, the economic status of the family can be compromised further.
- Unemployment is cyclical, may be industry-specific, and may be related to a variety of factors, such as the COVID-19 pandemic. When people lose their jobs, they often lose their health insurance. If they develop illness or a medical condition associated with the middle years, they often exhaust their savings. Such changes may precipitate mental health strain, which may result in ongoing mental health problems. The individual's economic status plays a role in their ability to seek care. Unemployment can result in a higher incidence of mental illness, with higher rates of anxiety, depression, and phobias.
- Technologic changes have opened opportunities for individuals to work at home and/or at remote sites. These extensions of the workplace often require individuals to change their routines and to take educational courses to either keep up with current job requirements or increase competency to take on more responsibilities. Training to increase skills or knowledge can be expensive and often must be funded by the individual.

Health Services/Delivery System

Numerous agencies are geared toward providing information and other resources for the middle-aged adult. These can be categorized as official, voluntary, and service agencies. Councils of community services frequently publish a directory. Official agencies include those that are state and federally funded, such as public health departments and drug treatment centers. Voluntary agencies include the American Heart Association, the American Cancer Society, the American Lung Association, and Alcoholics Anonymous. Many educational and self-help programs are sponsored by these organizations. The American Lung Association sponsors a smoking cessation program, which can be conducted on a group basis in a work or community setting. Service agencies include professional organizations such as state nurses' associations, the American Medical Association (sponsor of the Tel-Med program), bar associations, the YMCA, hospice programs, and the Women's Occupational Health Resource Center.

NURSING APPLICATION

Interventions focused on health promotion vary and depend on work location (e.g., community, hospital, outpatient work site). Consequently, nurses interact with middle-aged adults in many ways.

Individuals in this middle age range will likely need the services of a professional nurse several times before they reach their 60s. They may meet a nurse when seeking care for themselves in a clinician's office or primary care center. If they parent, they are likely to accompany their school-age child to the emergency room for a sports-related injury or their elder parent who has fallen. In the employment realm, some individuals will have their initial experience with a nurse through a preemployment evaluation visit. As a company employee, the same person may receive first aid for a minor injury or have their blood pressure monitored periodically by a nurse working in the occupational health department.

If the individual needs surgery or hospitalization, they may meet a home health nurse after discharge. Nurses are also available in rehabilitation settings to instruct and coach people regarding lifestyle changes following a heart attack or other acute events. Community health nurses provide health-promotion activities, which consist of health fairs that include "flu clinics" where adults are vaccinated against influenza. Life events such as the death of a partner, sudden unemployment, or disability may cause anxiety, depression, or other stress-related symptoms. Nurses who specialize in mental health can provide counseling and other forms of treatment for grief support or mental health issues resulting from trauma or sudden losses.

In a variety of settings, nurses are health educators. For example, the nurse who works in the community or in occupational health initiates events that raise awareness to identify health risks among middle-aged adults. Nurses teach strategies for controlling symptoms and working toward lifestyle changes that reduce morbidity or mortality. These interventions can be provided on a one-to-one basis, in groups, or as a lecture presented in a health seminar.

The target groups identified by occupational health nurses frequently have common needs for information, interventions, and periodic monitoring. The following are common concerns in the workplace: ergonomics, exposure to chemical or toxic substances, tobacco, alcohol, substance use and addiction, and ongoing problems with fatigue attributable to frequent changes in scheduled shifts.

The occupational health nurse has a wide range of responsibilities. For example, they may evaluate patterns of absenteeism to identify a source of infection that is affecting a group of employees.

The nurse participates in policy development focused on preventing or reducing the incidence of work site injuries or incidents. In another instance, the nurse provides clarification of Occupational Safety and Health Administration (OSHA) regulations when new machinery is brought into operation. The nurse invites a diverse group of employees to participate in or join the company safety committee because the primary purpose is keeping the work site safe for employees. Strategies to achieve optimal workplace safety include determining health hazards that exist in each department of the company and developing or refining procedures that promote safety, creating policies that address infection control, and enacting procedures such as fire drills. If the nurse has certification from the American Heart Association, they can offer classes in cardiopulmonary resuscitation and use of the automated external defibrillator.

The scope of practice for community health nurses (CHNs) differs from state to state. CHNs may derive their authority through the city or state health department. The role of the CHN focuses on health promotion and disease prevention for a population living in a specific area. The CHN interfaces with nurses working in the municipality and surrounding areas such as medical offices, state health department offices, hospitals, urgent care clinics, schools, emergency services, YMCA/ YWCA, and local businesses. Frequently, lectures or demonstrations are sponsored by the CHN at the request of community service organizations such as the Lions or Kiwanis clubs. The CHN may combine efforts with nurses who volunteer with faith-based or other organizations. Together they may present an annual health fair or senior health fair to serve the broad scope of health-information needs of the local community.

The features of the fair could include 15 to 20 displays that offer some of the following, all on a single occasion: demonstrations of the use of car seats and seat belts; short presentations on fall prevention; screening measures to identify risk factors for heart disease, cancer, and diabetes; town planning guides for emergency preparedness; massage therapy for stress reduction; informational guides for the regional poison control center; and recommended immunizations for middle-aged adults (e.g., flu shot). Health fairs allow the CHN to generate interest and enthusiasm among middle-aged adults about improving their health and well-being as well as to educate the residents living in the local community.

Health-promotion strategies will become more widely recognized as the objectives and target goals of *Healthy People 2030* are incorporated into health plans supported by health insurance policies, employers, wellness programs, and health care providers. With the passage of the Affordable Care Act in 2010, accessibility and utilization of health care services, especially for uninsured adults, are expected to increase. Nurses in leadership roles will organize and implement early detection and screening programs. They will survey communities, identify the needs of specific populations, and evaluate the effectiveness of public health measures already in place. They will be called on to develop educational programs and create online information sites that disseminate current medical research findings to the public, showing how changes in lifestyle behaviors can positively influence health outcomes. Information about the target goals of *Healthy People 2030* can be made available on these websites or blogs for individuals to see and incorporate into their lifestyles to improve the overall population health statistics in the United States.

Health promotion and well-being must be stressed for those midlife adults who are themselves working in health care. Stress is one of the factors that affect people in health care, particularly nurses. Learning coping mechanisms as well as changing health care systems decreases stress and promotes well-being (Iwanowicz-Palus et al., 2022). In summary, better health and enhanced well-being of the American people are expected outcomes of health promotion. The *Healthy People 2030* objectives and target goals provide the framework and direction for improving health awareness and practices among US residents.

In this chapter, health needs and potential diseases and conditions relevant to middle-aged adults have been addressed along with strategies to mitigate symptoms, prevent complications, and foster well-being. Normal changes expected with the aging process have also been presented. In addition, the effect of social processes such as relationships, family, work, belief systems, disability, death, and finances completed the discussion.

Nurses provide important strategies for fostering health promotion. Nurses are employed in most settings where middle-aged adults live, work, play, and raise their families. Because of their integral position in society, nurses are highly influential in identifying health concerns, organizing interventions, and evaluating the effectiveness of program outcomes. *Healthy People 2030* is presented as one approach for health professionals to use in their mission to improve the health and well-being of the American people.

OSHA mandates that employees work in a healthy and safe environment. The Occupational Safety and Health Act (1970) is applicable to every employer engaged in a business that affects commerce. The employer must ascertain that the workplace is free from recognized hazards and must comply with the act. OSHA has offices in most major cities and can provide recommended standards for occupational agents. Because of OSHA, the role of the nurse in supporting employee health is to obtain a complete health history, which should contain medical and social histories. The nurse should ask about current chronic medical illnesses such as hypertension, asthma, arthritis, cancer, heart disease, or hernia; past medical illnesses; and the individual's family medical history. The nurse should ask about current and past medication use. Social history would include questions about smoking—whether the person smokes, when they started, and the number of cigarettes they smoke per day. If the person is an ex-smoker, questions should include when they stopped and the number of cigarettes they smoked per day. The nurse should address medical limitations; for example, decreased visual acuity may mean no driving, and dermatitis may mean no skin exposure to oils, chemicals, or solvents. Removing a worker from a particular job may be indicated if the worker might endanger coworkers, if the worker has a disease condition that might be aggravated by the job, or if the worker is taking prescribed medications with potentially harmful side effects.

The nurse in the community and in industry should reiterate key safety directives (e.g., wearing seat belts, observing speed limits, using hands-free telephone communication, and not texting while driving) to the middle-aged adult.

With an increase in leisure time, the middle-aged adult is at greater risk of recreational accidents. As noted, moderation should be stressed. Alcohol is a depressant and should be avoided in activities that require attentiveness. Protection from burns is essential; 56% of fatal residential fires are directly related to cigarette smoking while in bed. Falls can occur at any age; safety measures should be considered for the entire family, including specific preparatory planning for the very young and for aging parents. A few suggestions to the middle-aged adult might be to avoid highly waxed floors, correct poor environmental lighting, avoid high beds, and avoid bathtubs lacking nonslip bottoms.

Handgun availability is controversial at best; however, approximately 20% of US households have handguns. When the individual believes strongly that it is necessary to have a firearm, safety measures to avoid accidental injury, such as security locks and proper storage, should be discussed.

The Occupational Safety and Health Act (1970) works to ensure that workers are employed under safe and healthy working conditions.

Nurses can participate actively in the safety committee of the industry in which they are employed. When no such committee exists, many protection measures will fall within the nurse's domain. The following suggestions can facilitate safer and healthier working conditions:

- Tour work facilities on a regular basis. Become familiar with resource books, laws, and codes.
- Develop a toxicology chart with symptoms of overexposure and recommended treatments. Update this chart frequently.
- Become a role model for safety issues by wearing safety glasses, protective footwear, and gloves. Do not smoke.
- Discuss the preemployment physical examination with the employee with an emphasis on risk factors and strategies to modify risks. Monitor health problems and exposure levels in the work setting.

The worker must be aware of OSHA and their role in maintaining a safe work environment. Workers should wear protective clothing if applicable, practice sanitation measures for the work environment, practice general hygiene measures, and obtain recommended immunizations. The food handler, for instance, should have an annual tuberculosis test, wear clean clothing and appropriate hair protection, and use proper handwashing techniques. The nurse should not assume that workers know how to protect themselves and others.

Since 1996, the National Occupational Research Agenda has become the research framework for the National Institute for Occupational Safety and Health and the nation. Partners work together to identify and address the critical issues in workplace safety (https://www.cdc.gov/niosh/about.htm).

A major challenge for the nurse is to encourage workers to participate in workplace safety measures to protect their health. Increasingly, organizations are interested in promoting the health of their employees because minimizing lateness, absenteeism, and turnover and reducing physical disabilities and emotional issues reduce disability costs, insurance costs, and life insurance costs. Health-promotion programs are increasingly recognized for their vital contributions to the financial viability of organizations.

Health-promotion programs within an organizational setting can be categorized into one of three levels: awareness, lifestyle change, and supportive environment. The goal of a health program, at the level of awareness, is to increase the individual's knowledge of or interest in a health issue such as smoking cessation. Examples of

CASE STUDY

Reducing Caregiver Role Strain

A caregiver is an individual who is responsible for the physical care or emotional support of a family member, relative, or close friend. Caring activities can range from minor involvement, such as assisting with grocery shopping, to major involvement in activities of daily living. Caregiver role strain occurs when caregivers feel overwhelmed by the responsibility and find it difficult to perform their role. To reduce the effects of caregiver strain, the nurse assists with health-promoting behaviors such as scheduling respite care, providing exercise activities, and supporting optimal nutrition.

Sandra Graham, a 52-year-old woman, lives in a three-floor walk-up with her 62-year-old sister, Susan Jones, a professor of nursing at a local community college. Six months ago, Ms. Graham was diagnosed with early onset dementia after multiple visits to the emergency room and the neurologist. Ms. Jones has been trying to balance her teaching with caring for Ms. Graham. Coming home between classes, preparing meals that could be reheated in the microwave, and asking the neighbor to check in worked for the first few months. Recently, Ms. Graham's dementia has progressed, and she is not able to remain alone during the day, as she is unable to use the toilet by herself and becomes agitated when she wants to go to the store. Ms. Jones plans to work until age 65 and is not financially or emotionally ready to leave her job. She finds herself torn between guilt and resentment and has begun to neglect her health. Climbing the three flights to the apartment has become more difficult, and Ms. Jones has begun to dread leaving the apartment or returning home. A colleague with experience in dementia and strong ties to local service agencies has insisted on meeting with Ms. Jones. She expresses sympathy for the situation, lets Ms. Jones talk about her feelings, and helps her set out a plan for her own care and that of her sister.

The main issues involved are Ms. Jones's need to seek knowledge about her sister's illness, treatment modalities, side effects of medication, physical and mental symptoms of the disease, and strategies to reduce caregiver role strain. A focused plan of care with community support could address knowledge deficits, impaired comfort, and anticipatory grieving when working with an uncertain future.

Reflective Questions

- What are the main stressors for Ms. Jones?
- What are the potential problems Ms. Graham, Ms. Jones, and their families might experience?
- What resources are available to support Ms. Graham and reduce caregiver stressors for Ms. Jones?
- Describe Ms. Graham's feelings about dependency and potential loss of autonomy.
- Describe the processes, for Ms. Jones, of learning to balance caring for her sister while maintaining her own health.

awareness programs include special events, flyers, lunch seminars, meetings, and newsletters. Changing health behaviors or status is not the goal of awareness programs, but it is the goal of lifestyle change programs. Lifestyle change programs last at least 8 to 12 weeks and include assessment, education, and evaluation components to help individuals implement long-term modifications in health behaviors and experience the results of the instituted changes. To maintain long-term changes and to develop a healthy lifestyle, individuals need a supportive organizational environment. This type of environment may include health-promoting physical settings, corporate policies and culture, ongoing programs, and employee ownership of programs. Nurses need to be at the forefront of the health of the country, ensuring that justice and equity are the centerpiece of care (Dillard-Wright & Shields-Haas, 2021).

SUMMARY

- Nurses help middle-aged adults improve their quality of life, both for the present and for the future, through identification of risk factors, health promotion, and other nursing interventions.
- Nurses work in a variety of health care settings utilized by middle-aged adults: outpatient clinics, occupational health clinics, and private practice.
- Health-promotion and disease-prevention strategies are aimed at modifying existing habits and lifestyles to improve health outcomes in the middle-aged adult.
- These strategies aid in the achievement of optimal levels of health because they are informed by modifying identified risk factors (social and physical), providing self-help information, and describing available resources relevant to the middle-aged adult.
- Using these strategies, the nurse can motivate middle-aged adults to prioritize their own health and quality of life while maintaining their multiple roles as parents, partners, siblings, and offspring.
- By maintaining a healthy lifestyle begun as a young adult or making lifestyle changes, the middle-aged adult reduces their risk of disability from chronic disease and promotes a better quality of life.

EVOLVE CHAPTER FEATURES

http://evolve.elsevier.com/Edelman/

- Study Questions

REFERENCES

American Cancer Society. (2023). *Key statistics for lung cancer*. https://www.cancer.org/cancer/types/lung-cancer/about/key-statistics.html

American Dental Association. (2022). *Home oral care*. https://www.ada.org

Beck, B. R., & Winters-Stone, K. M. (2020). Exercise in the prevention of osteoporosis-related fractures. In B. Leder, & M. Wein (Eds.), *Osteoporosis. Contemporary endocrinology*. Humana: Cham. https://doi.org/10.1007/978-3-319-69287-6_11

Benson, H., & Klipper, M. Z. (1975). *The relaxation response*. New York, NY: Hapertorch.

Benson-Henry Mind Body. (2020). *Benson-Henry Institute for Mind Body Medicine*. https://bensonhenryinstitute.org/

Blackwell, D. L., Villarroel, M. A., & Norris, T. (2019). Regional variation in private dental coverage and care among dentate adults aged 18–64 in the United States, 2014–2017.

Bloom, B. S. (1984). *Taxonomy of educational objectives: Handbook 1, cognitive domain*. New York, NY: Longman.

Brailer, C., Robison, V., & Barone, L. (2019). Protect tiny teeth toolkit: an oral health communications resource for providers of pregnant women and new mothers. *Journal of Women's Health*, 28(5), 568–572. https://doi.org/10.1089/jwh.2019.7657

Campinha-Bacote, J. (2002). The process of cultural competence in the delivery of healthcare services: A model of care. *Journal of Transcultural Nursing*, *13*(3), 181–184. https://doi.org/10.1177/10459602013003003

Carter, V. J., & Howard, M. W. (2019). *Income inequality*. In Encyclopedia Britannica. https://www.britannica.com/topic/income-inequality

Centers for Disease Control and Prevention (CDC). (2019). Excessive alcohol use and risks to women's health. https://www.cdc.gov

Centers for Disease Control and Prevention (CDC). (2020a). *Public safety program*. https://www.cdc.gov/niosh/programs/pubsaf/default.html

Centers for Disease Control and Prevention (CDC). (2020b). *Expected new cancer cases and deaths in 2020*. https://www.healthypeople.gov

Centers for Disease Control and Prevention (CDC). (2020c). *Getting your cholesterol checked*. https://www.cdc.gov/cholesterol/cholesterol_screening.htm

Centers for Disease Control and Prevention (CDC). (2020d). *Smoking, gum disease, and tooth loss*. www.cdc.gov/tobacco/campaign/tips/diseases/periodontal-gum-disease.html

Centers for Disease Control and Prevention (CDC). (2021). *Maternal mortality rates in the United States, 2021*. https://www.cdc.gov/nchs/data/hestat/maternal-mortality/2021/maternal-mortality-rates-2021.htm

Centers for Disease Control and Prevention (CDC). (2022a). *Social determinants of health at CDC*. https://www.cdc.gov

Centers for Disease Control and Prevention (CDC). (2022b). Prevalence of age-related macular degeneration. https://www.cdc.gov/visionhealth/vehss/estimates/amd-prevalence.html

Centers for Disease Control and Prevention (CDC). (2022c). *Poor nutrition*. https://www.cdc.gov

Centers for Disease Control and Prevention (CDC). (2023a). *Healthy people 2030: Oral health objectives*. https://www.cdc.gov/oralhealth/about/healthy-people.html

Centers for Disease Control and Prevention (CDC). (2023b). *Heart disease deaths*. https://www.cdc.gov/nchs/hus/topics/heart-disease-deaths.htm

Centers for Disease Control and Prevention (CDC). (2023c). *Chronic disease: Tobacco*. https://www.cdc.gov/chronicdisease/programs-impact/pop/tobacco.htm

Centers for Disease Control and Prevention (CDC). (2023d). *Smoking and tobacco use: Benefits of quitting*. https://www.cdc.gov/tobacco/quit_smoking/how_to_quit/benefits/index.htm

Centers for Disease Control and Prevention (CDC). (2023e). *HIV: Basic statistics*. https://www.cdc.gov

Centers for Disease Control and Prevention (CDC). (2023f). Adverse health effects of smoking and the occupational environment. https://www.cdc.gov/niosh/docs/79-122/default.html

Centers for Disease Control and Prevention (CDC). (2024a). *Age-adjusted death rates for selected causes of death*. https://www.cdc.gov/nchs/

Centers for Disease Control and Prevention (CDC). (2024b). *Recommended adult immunization schedules for adults ages 19 years or older.* https://www.cdc.gov/vaccines/schedules/downloads/adult/adult-combined-schedule.pdf

Centers for Disease Control and Prevention (CDC). (2024c). *Smoking and tobacco use.* https://www.cdc.gov/tobacco/index.html

Childstats. (2024). https://www.childstats.gov/

David, P. S., Kling, J. M., Vegunta, S., Faubion, S. S., Kapoor, E., Mara, K. C., Schroeder, D. R., Hilsaca, K. F., & Kuhle, C. L. (2018). Vasomotor symptoms in women over 60: Results from the data registry on experiences of aging, menopause, and sexuality (DREAMS). *Menopause (New York, N.Y.), 25*(10), 1105–1109. https://doi.org/10.1097/GME.0000000000001126

Damian, T. (2023). Patient and patient advocates' reflections on oral health care challenges for patients living with HIV/AIDS. *Academy Health.* https://academyhealth.org

Dillard-Wright, J., & Shield-Haas, V. (2021). Nursing with the people: Reimagining futures for nursing. *Advances in Nursing Science, 44*(3), 195–209. https://pubmed.ncbi.nlm.nih.gov/33624989

Divorcewriter. (2023). *Divorce parenting classes: State requirements.* https://www.divorcewriter.com/parent-education-class-divorce

D'Onofrio, B., & Emery, R. (2019). Parental divorce or separation and children's mental health. *World Psychiatry, 18*(1), 100–101. https://www.ncbi.nlm.nih.gov/pmc/articles/PMC6313686/

Duvall, E. M., & Miller, B. (1985). *Marriage and family development* (6th ed.). New York, NY: Harper Collins.

Egede, L. E., Walker, R. J., & Williams, J. S. (2021). Intersection of structural racism, social determinants of health, and implicit bias with emergency physician admission tendencies. *JAMA Netw Open, 4*(9), e2126375. https://jamanetwork.com/journals/jamanetworkopen/fullarticle/2784402

Environmental Protection Agency (EPA). (2024). *Health risk of radon.* https://www.epa.gov/radon/health-risk-radon

Erikson, E. H., & Erikson, G. M. (1998). *Life cycle completed.* New York, NY: W.W. Norton.

Feng, I., Brondani, M., Bedos, C., & Donnelly, L. (2020). Access to oral health care for people living with HIV/AIDS attending a community-based program. *Canadian Journal of Dental Hygiene, 54*(1).

Feeney, A. (2023). Combating implicit bias in nursing. *Nurse Journal.* https://nursejournal.org/articles/combating-implicit-bias-in-nursing

Fitzgerald, C., & Hurst, S. (2017). Implicit bias in healthcare professionals: A systematic review. *BMC Medical Ethics, 18*, 19.

Friis, R. H. (2018). *Essentials of environmental health* (3rd ed.). Burlington, MA: Jones and Bartlett.

Fry, R., & Parker, K. (2021). *Rising share of U.S. adults are living without a spouse or partner.* Pew Research Center. https://www.pewresearch.org/social-trends/2021/10/05/rising-share-of-u-s-adults-are-living-without-a-spouse-or-partner

Gardner, H. (1983). *Frames of mind: The theory of multiple intelligences.* New York, NY: Basic Books.

Gardner, H. (1993). *Multiple intelligences: The theory in practice.* New York, NY: Basic Books.

Gilligan, C. (1982). *In a different voice: Psychological theory and women's development.* Cambridge, MA: Harvard University Press.

Gilligan, C. (1990). *Mapping the moral domain.* Cambridge, MA: Harvard University Press.

Gilligan, C., & Snider, N. (2018). *Why does patrimony persist?* Cambridge: Polity Press.

Goedereis, E., Mehta, C., Jones, J., & Ayotte, B. (2023). "I want to focus on something that I feel really good about every day": Career development in established adulthood. *Acta Psychologica.* https://doi.org/10.1016/j.actpsy.2023.103863

Grillo, A., Salvi, L., Coruzzi, P., Salvi, P., & Parati, G. (2019). Sodium intake and hypertension. *Nutrients*, 11(9):1970. https://pubmed.ncbi.nlm.nih.gov/31438636/

Guttmacher Institute. (2019). *Fact sheet: Unintended pregnancy in the United States.* https://www.guttmacher.org/fact-sheet/unintended-pregnancy-united-states

Hales, C. M., Carroll, M. D., Fryar, C. D., & Ogden, C. L. (2020). Prevalence of obesity and severe obesity among adults: United States, 2017–2018. https://www.cdc.gov/nchs/data/databriefs/db360-h.pdf

Havighurst, R. I., & Orr, B. (1956). *Adult education and adult needs.* Chicago, IL: Center for Study of Liberal Education for Adults.

Haynes, S. G., Levine, S., Scotch, N., Feinleib, M., & Kannel, W. B. (1978). The relationship of psychosocial factors to coronary heart disease in the Framingham Study. I. Methods and risk factors. *American Journal of Epidemiology*, 107(5), 362–383.

Haynes, S. G., Feinleib, M., & Kannel, W. B. (1980). The relationship of psychosocial factors to coronary heart disease in the Framingham Study. III. Eight-year incidence of coronary heart disease. *American Journal of Epidemiology, 111*(1), 37–58. https://pubmed.ncbi.nlm.nih.gov/7352459/

Hill, M. F., & Bordoni, B. (2023). *Hyperlipidemia.* In *StatPearls* [Internet]. Treasure Island (FL): StatPearls. https://www.ncbi.nlm.nih.gov/books/NBK559182/

Hornstein, G. (1986). The structuring of identity among midlife women as a function of their degree of involvement in employment. *Journal of Personality, 54*, 551–575. https://doi.org/10.1111/j.1467-6494.1986.tb00412.x

Immonen, S., Launes, J., Järvinen, I. Maarit, V., Vanninen, R., Schiavone, N., Lehto, E., Tuulio-Henriksson, A., Lipsanen, J., Michelsson, K., & Hokkanen, L. (2020). Moderate alcohol use is associated with decreased brain volume in early middle age in both sexes. *Nature: Scientific Reports, 10*, 13998. https://doi.org/10.1038/s41598-020-70910-5

Infurna, F. J., Gerstorf, D., & Lachman, M. E. (2020). Midlife in the 2020s: Opportunities and challenges. *American Psychologist, 75*(4), 470–485. https://www.ncbi.nlm.nih.gov/pmc/articles/PMC7347230

Iwanowicz-Palus, G., Mróz, M., Kowalczuk, K., Szlendak, B., Bień, A., & Cybulski, M. (2022). Nurses coping with stressful situations: A cross-sectional study. *International Journal of Environmental Research in Public Health, 19*(17), 10924.

Jacobs, E., & Bahn, K. (2019). *Women's history month: U.S. women's labor force participation.* Washington Center for Equitable Growth. https://www.equitablegrowth.org/womens-history-month-u-s-womens-labor-force-participation

Jones, H. J., Gillis, C., & Lees, K. (2020). Depressive symptoms associated with physical health problems in midlife women: A longitudinal study. *Journal of Affective Disorders, 263*, 301–309. https://doi.org/10.1016/j.jad.2019.11.166

Kobasa, S. (1979). Stressful life events, personality and health: An inquiry into hardiness. *Journal of Personality and Social Psychology, 37*, 1–11. https://doi.org/10.1037/0022-3514.37.1.1

Kohlberg, L., & Lickona, T. (1986). *The stages of ethical development: From childhood through old age.* New York, NY: Harper Collins.

LeBoff, M. S., Greenspan, S. L, Insogna, K., Lewiecki, E., Saag, K., Singe, A., & Siris, E. S. (2022). The clinician's guide to prevention and treatment of osteoporosis. *Osteoporosis International, 33*, 2049–2102. https://doi.org/10.1007/s00198-021-05900-y

LeBoff, M. S., Chou, S. H., Murata, E. M., Donlon, C. M., Cook, N. R., Mora, S., Lee, I. M., Kotler, G., Bubes, V., Buring, J.E., & Manson, J. E. (2020). Effects of supplemental vitamin d on bone health outcomes in women and men in the Vitamin D and OmegA-3

Trial (VITAL). *Journal of Bone and Mineral Research, 35*(5), 883–893. https://doi.org/10.1002/jbmr.3958

Levinson, D. (1986a). A conception of adult development. *American Psychologist, 41*, 3–13.

Levinson, D. (1986b). *The seasons of a man's life*. New York, NY: Ballantine.

Levinson, D. (1996). *The seasons of a woman's life*. New York, NY: Knopf.

Lindmark, U., Bulow, U., & Martensson, J. (2019). The use of the concept of transition in different disciplines within health and social welfare: An integrative literature review. *Nursing Open*, 6(3), 664–675. https://doi.org/10.1002/nop2.249

Lopez, A., Thomann, M., Dhatt, Z., Ferrera, J., Al-Nassir, M., Ambrose, M., & Sullivan, S. (2022). Understanding racial inequities in the implementation of harm reduction initiatives. *American Journal of Public Health, 112*(S2), S173–S181. https://doi.org/10.2105/AJPH.2022.306767

Lowdermilk, D., Perry, S., Cashion, M., Alden, K., & Olshansky, E. (2019). *Reproductive system concerns. Maternity and women's health care* (12th ed.). St. Louis, MO: Mosby.

MacDonald, T. (2022). Prevalence of high cholesterol among the adult U.S. population: NHANES 2013–2018. *Current Developments in Nutrition, 6*(Suppl 1), 925. https://www.ncbi.nlm.nih.gov/pmc/articles/PMC9194142/

Maas, A. (2021). Hormone therapy and cardiovascular disease: Benefits and harms. *Best Practice & Research Clinical Endocrinology & Metabolism, 35*(6), 101576. https://doi.org/10.1016/j.beem.2021.101576

Medina, L., Sabo, S., & Vespa, J. (2020). *Living longer: Historical and projected life expectancy in the United States, 1960 to 2060*. US Department of Commerce, US Census Bureau.

Meleis, A. (Ed.). (2010). *Transitions theory: Middle-range and situation-specific theories in nursing research*. New York: Springer Publishing Company.

Miller, W., & Rollnick, S. (2023). *Motivational interviewing: Helping people change*. Guilford, CT: Guilford Press.

Murdaugh, C. L., Pender, N., & Parsons, M. A. (2019). *Health promotion in nursing practice* (8th ed.). New York, NY: Pearson.

National Cancer Institute. (2023). *HPV and cancer*. https://www.cancer.gov/about-cancer/causes-prevention/risk/infectious-agents/hpv-and-cancer

National Eye Institute. (2023). *Glaucoma*. https://www.nei.nih.gov/learn-about-eye-health/eye-conditions-and-diseases/glaucoma

National Institue on Aging (NIA), 2020. https://www.nia.nih.gov/

National Institutes of Alcohol Abuse and Alcoholism. (2024). *Alcohol and the human body*. https://www.niaaa.nih.gov/alcohols-effects-health/alcohol-topics/alcohol-facts-and-statistics/alcohol-and-human-body

National Institute for Occupational Safety and Health. (2023). www.cdc.gov/niosh/topics/cwhsp

National Institutes of Health (NIH), National Heart, Lung, and Blood Institute. (2020). *What is sleep apnea?* http://www.nhlbi.nih.gov/health/health-topics/topics/sleepapnea

National Institutes of Health. (2020). *Vitamin D*. https://www.ods.od.nih.gov

National Institutes of Health (NIH), Office of Dietary Supplements. (2020). *Vitamin D fact sheet for health professionals*. https://ods.od.nih.gov/factsheets/VitaminD-HealthProfessional

National Sleep Foundation. (2020). *What to do when you can't sleep? 8 techniques you can do*. https://www.sleepfoundation.org/insomnia/treatment/what-do-when-you-cant-sleep

Nguyen, H. T. T., Kitaoka, K., Sukigara, M., & Thai, A. L. (2018). Burnout study of clinical nurses in Vietnam: Development of job burnout model based on Leiter and Maslach's theory. *Asian nursing research, 12*(1), 42-49.

Njoku, A., Evans, M., Nimo-Sefah, L., & Bailey, J. (2023). Listen to the whispers before they become screams: Addressing Black maternal morbidity and mortality in the United States. *Healthcare (Basel, Switzerland), 11*(3), 438. https://pubmed.ncbi.nlm.nih.gov/36767014/

North American Menopause Society. (2023). The 2023 nonhormone therapy position statement of The North American Menopause Society. *Menopause (New York, N.Y.)*, 6(30), 573–590. https://doi.org/10.1097/GME.0000000000002200

Pellegrino, D., Sjoberg, D. D., Tin, A. L., Benfante, N. E., Briganti, A., Montorsi, F., Eastham, J. A., Mulhall, J. P., Vickers, A. J. (2023) Relationship between age, comorbidity, and the prevalence of erectile dysfunction. *European Urology Focus, 9*(1), 162–167. https://doi.org/10.1016/j.euf.2022.08.006

Peterson-KFF. (n.d.) Health System Tracker. https://www.healthsystemtracker.org/

Piaget, J. (1970). *Structuralism*. New York, NY: Basic Books.

Radzimińska, A., Strączyńska, A., Weber-Rajek, M., Styczyńska, H., Strojek, K., & Piekorz, Z. (2018). The impact of pelvic floor muscle training on the quality of life of women with urinary incontinence: a systematic literature review. *Clinical Interventions in Aging, 13*, 957. https://doi.org/10.2147/CIA.S160057

Reifman, A., Biernat, M., & Lang, E. (1991). Stress, social support, and health in married professional women with small children. *Psychology of Women Quarterly, 15*, 431–445. https://doi.org/10.1111/j.1471-6402.1991.tb00419.x

Rossman, J. (2019). Cognitive-behavioral therapy for insomnia: An effective and underutilized treatment for insomnia. *American Journal of Lifestyle Medicine, 13*(6), 544–547. https://www.ncbi.nlm.nih.gov/pmc/articles/PMC6796223/

Schumacher, K. L., & Meleis, A. I. (1994). Transitions: A central concept in nursing. *Image Journal of Nursing Scholarship, 26*(2), 119–127. https://pubmed.ncbi.nlm.nih.gov/8063317/

Spector, R. E. (2016). *Cultural diversity in health and illness* (9th ed.). Upper Saddle River, NJ: Prentice Hall.

Statistica.com. (2023). *Cigarette smoking in the US between 1965 and 2019*. https://www.statista.com/statistics/184418/percentage-of-cigarette-smoking-in-the-us

Thomas, S. P. (1995). Psychosocial correlates of women's health in middle adulthood. *Issues in Mental Health Nursing, 16*, 285–314. https://doi.org/10.3109/01612849509072526

Toussaint, L., Nguyen, Q. A., Roettger, C., Dixon, K., Offenbächer, M., Kohls, N., Hirsch, J., & Sirois, F. (2021). Effectiveness of progressive muscle relaxation, deep breathing, and guided imagery in promoting psychological and physiological states of relaxation. *Evidence Based Complementary Alternate Medicine*. https://www.ncbi.nlm.nih.gov/pmc/articles/PMC8272667/

USAFacts (2024). *Wealth and savings*. https://usafacts.org/topics/wealth-savings/

US Bureau of Labor Statistics. (2023). *National census of fatal occupational injuries in 2022*. https://www.bls.gov/news.release/pdf/cfoi.pdf

US Bureau of Labor Statistics. (2018). *Women in the labor force: A databook (Report 1077)*. https://www.bls.gov/opub/reports/womens-databook/2018/home.htm

US Census Bureau. (2023). *U.S. marriage and divorce rates declined in last 10 years*. census.gov

Wilson, V., & Williams, J. (2019). *Racial and ethnic income gaps persist amid uneven growth in household incomes*. Economic Policy Institute. https://www.epi.org/blog/racial-and-ethnic-income-gaps-persist-amid-uneven-growth-in-household-incomes/

24

Older Adult

Susan Moscou, Miriam Ford and Renu Varughese

http://evolve.elsevier.com/Edelman/

OBJECTIVES

After completing this chapter, the reader will be able to:

- Describe health-promotion activities specifically targeted to older adults.
- Discuss *Healthy People 2030* objectives as they relate to health promotion for older adults.
- Describe how expected aging changes in the older adult relate to health-promotion strategies and coincide with aging theories.
- Discuss preventive strategies related to risk factors that could lead to health problems in older adults.
- Discuss how social determinants of health affect environmental, physical, biologic, and chemical agents that contribute to disability, morbidity, and mortality in older adults.
- Discuss international trends in aging.

KEY TERMS

Activities of daily living
Alzheimer disease
Atrophy
Cognition
Decubitus ulcer
Delirium
Dementia
Depression
Euthanasia
Glaucoma
Health literacy
Impotence
Influenza
Instrumental activities of daily living
International Aging
Life review
Mild cognitive impairment
Mini-Mental State Examination
Nutritional screening
Osteoporosis
Physician-assisted suicide
Polypharmacy
Postoperative cognitive dysfunction
Presbycusis
Presbyopia
Reminiscence
Restless legs syndrome
Sclerosis
Social portfolio
Stress incontinence
Theories of aging
Urge incontinence

THINK ABOUT IT

Sexually Transmitted Infections in Older Adults

You are a community health nursing student whose clinical rotation is at a senior center. You just attended several lectures about the increase in sexually transmitted infections (STIs) in older adults.

STIs in adults aged 65 and older have doubled in the last 10 years. Rates of primary and secondary syphilis cases per 100,000 increased from 91 in 2007 to 349 in 2017; chlamydia cases were 809 in 2007 and 2178 in 2017; gonorrhea rates increased from 707 in 2007 to 2178 in 2017 (Smith et al., 2020).

Given these statistics, you ask your instructor if you can develop a project related to education about STIs and safer sexual practices. The director acknowledges that an educational program about STIs for elders would be useful for this population.

- What additional information do you need to determine the potential efficacy of developing an educational activity about STIs and safer sexual practices in your center?
- What types of resources are available to help you obtain the necessary assistance for this type of program?
- What provisions are available under Medicare and the Affordable Care Act of 2010 to assist a person with this educational activity?
- What policy changes might be instituted at the senior center to ensure that elders are adequately educated about STIs and safer sex practices?

Older adults, those aged 65 and older, are living longer and healthier lives because of technologic advances, better health care services, public health interventions (e.g., sanitation and immunizations), and utilizing health services research to promote optimal health outcomes (Fulmer et al., 2021).

There has been a consistent increase of aging of Americans since the 1900s. In 2020, older adults represented 17% of the population (55.7 million). By 2040, there will be about 80.8 million US residents aged 65 and older. This number is more than double the 65 and over population in 2000. Adults aged 85 and older will nearly quadruple between 2000 and 2040 (Searing, 2023).

Because Americans are living longer, we will see a growth in the number of older adults developing cognitive disorders. As people age, the number diagnosed with Alzheimer dementia increases. Five percent of elders aged 65 to 74, 13% of elders aged 75 to 84, and 33% of elders aged 85 and older are expected to be diagnosed with Alzheimer dementia. About one in nine people aged 65 and older (10.7%) have been diagnosed with Alzheimer dementia (Alzheimer's Association, 2023).

Rogers et al. (2019) found that aging adults are at higher risk for chronic diseases (e.g., hypertension, diabetes, and Alzheimer disease). More than 80% of adults aged 65 and older have at least one chronic condition, and 60% have at least two chronic illnesses. Chronic illnesses may result in higher rates of disability affecting activities of daily living (Fong, 2019). Older adults with chronic conditions may have a lower quality of life.

As older adults are living longer, it is important that society meet their needs by providing health insurance, supportive environments, healthy communities, and social safety nets so all older adults can age well and live as independently as possible. In addition, changes in policies are necessary to address disparities in education, employment, and income (Fulmer et al., 2021).

Who is the older adult today? The World Health Organization (WHO) notes that most developed countries accept the chronologic age of 65 years as a definition of an older adult. Aging baby boomers (born between 1946 and 1964) fueled this rapid growth as they began turning 65 in 2011. By 2030, all baby boomers will be 65 and over, and the growth of older Americans is projected to start slowing. The 75-to-84 age group is expected to grow in the next decade as baby boomers age into this group. The 85-to-94 age group experienced slower growth (12.6%) than other older age groups, increasing from 5.1 million in 2010 to 5.7 million in 2020. The 95-and-older population experienced a large growth rate (48.6%), increasing from about 425,000 in 2010 to 631,000 in 2020 (US Census, 2023).

SOCIAL AND ECONOMIC STATISTICS OF OLDER ADULTS

Demographic Shifts for Elders

The Population Reference Bureau's (2024) *Fact Sheet: Aging in America* details the demographic shifts affecting elders aged 65 and older:

- Americans ages 65 and older are projected to increase from 58 million in 2022 to 82 million by 2050 (a 47% increase), and the 65-and-older age group's share of the total population is projected to rise from 17% to 23%.
- Elder Americans are becoming more racially and ethnically diverse. Between 2022 and 2050, the share of the older population that identifies as non-Hispanic White is projected to drop from 75% to 60%.
- Education levels increased among people 65 and older. In 1965, only 5% had completed 4 years of college or more. By 2023, this had risen to 33%.
- Older adults are working longer. By 2022, 24% of males and about 15% of females ages 65 and older were in the labor force. These levels are projected to rise further by 2032, to 25% for males and 17% for females.
- More older adults can meet their daily care needs because they are functioning better on their own. Home modifications and assistive devices such as walkers have helped older Americans maintain their independence.
- More older adults are divorced compared with previous generations. The share of divorced females aged 65 and older increased from 3% in 1980 to 15% in 2023, and the share of divorcedmales aged 65 and older increased from 4% to 12% during the same period.
- More older females are living alone. About 27% of females aged 65 to 74 lived alone in 2023. This increased to 39% among females aged 75 to 84 and 50% among females aged 85 and older.
- There is a caregiving gap for older Americans, especially those with lower incomes and diagnosed with dementia. The number of elders requiring elder care is expected to increase because more Americans are living with Alzheimer disease, and this number could more than double from 6 million to 13 million by 2050.
- Social Security and Medicare expenditures will increase from a combined 9.1% of gross domestic product (GDP) in 2023 to 11.5% by 2035 because of the large share of older adults.

Aging in Place

More older adults are "aging in place" in the community, with new living options that include retirement communities and independent living facilities or assisted living facilities (ALFs), as well as skilled care institutions. These changes in longevity and living arrangements have implications for health-promotion planning and interventions.

Health care expenditure grew 4.17% to reach $4.5 trillion, or $13,493 per person, in 2022, which represented 17.3% of GDP. Adults aged 65 and older accounted for 17% of the population but approximately 37% of all spending in 2020.

The slower growth in 2021 was driven by a 3.5% decline in federal government expenditures for health care, which followed strong growth in 2020 that occurred largely in response to the COVID-19 pandemic as well as the effect of greater use of health care goods and services and increased insurance coverage in 2021.

GDP increased 10.7% in 2021, contributing to a drop in the share of the economy devoted to health care from 19.7% in 2020 to 18.3% in 2021, but up from 17.6% in 2019. In 2021, uninsured individuals declined for the second consecutive year as Medicaid and Marketplace enrollment increased.

In 2021, Medicare spending grew 5.9% to $944.3 billion, or 21% of total national health expenditure. Private health care spending on older adults was $1.2 trillion ($22,356 per person) in 2020. Health care spending for females 65 and over accounted for 55% of all health care spending for older adults in 2020 ($683 billion), while health care spending for males 65 and over accounted for the remaining 45% ($560 billion). These expenditure shares are equal to the female and male shares of the population aged 65 and over. Per capita spending for males was 2% more than females.

The Inflation Reduction Act will lower the out-of-pocket expenses for older adults because the government began negotiating prescription medication costs with pharmaceutical companies. Per capita spending for older adults (65+) grew at an average rate of 4.5% between 2018 and 2020. Both males and females aged 65 to 84 experienced the fastest spending growth from 2018 to 2020 (9.7%), is partially because of an increase in the population of this age group relative to other age groups as well as an increase in Medicare and Medicaid spending from 2018 to 2020 that was greater in this age group compared with others (CMS, 2023).

There may be misconceptions surrounding health promotion for older adults; thus, it is essential that nurses and other health providers offer care that enhances healthy aging. Overcoming these misconceptions or biases about older adults will enable nurses and clinicians to discuss health-promotion interventions that maintain an active and healthy lifestyle for older adults.

Health promotion is as important in later adulthood as it is in childhood. Older adults derive the same benefits from health-promotion activities as do their younger counterparts. You are never too old to stop smoking, start exercising, change your diet, or participate in a healthier lifestyle. Specific health-promotion strategies may differ for adults aged 65 to 74 years (considered young-old), adults aged 75 to 84 years (considered middle-old), and adults aged 85 and older (considered oldest-old). For example, strength training may be very appropriate for the young- and middle-old groups but may not be feasible for the oldest-old group. Balance exercises are essential for adults in older age groups. The potential for health improvements is great in all groups; therefore, nurses have a key role in educating older adults about health-promotion strategies as well as in advancing our understanding of health promotion for older adults.

The diverse representation of populations in the United States (e.g., socioeconomic status, race and ethnicity, first- or second-generation immigrants) may influence life transitions associated with aging.

Social Isolation

The US Surgeon General's advisory on loneliness and isolation was issued to call attention to a phenomenon of social isolation. Loneliness and isolation can be viewed as a public health crisis at the epidemic level. Elders who find themselves alone because of the death of a spouse or partner, retirement, separation from friends or family, loss of mobility, and lack of transportation are at particular risk. Loneliness and social isolation in older adults are serious public health risks affecting a significant number of people in the United States and putting them at higher risk for dementia and other serious medical conditions. Nurses should understand the connection between health and isolation and receive training about the relevance of social connections and health, the importance of routinely screening elders for their level of social connection, and the importance of educating patients about the benefits of social connection and the risk factors for social disconnection (Murthy, 2023).

Race and Ethnic Demographic Shifts

By 2060, people of color will account for about half of the US population aged 65 and older. In 2020, 24% of persons aged 65 and older were members of racial or ethnic minority populations: 9% were African American (not Hispanic), 5% were Asian American (not Hispanic), 0.6% were American Indian and Alaska Native (not Hispanic), 0.1% were Native Hawaiian/Pacific Islander (not Hispanic), and 0.8% identified as being of two or more races (Administration for Community Living [ACL], 2022).

Given the change in demographics, nurses need to develop an awareness about population health and identify the social determinants of health that influence health outcomes.

Life Expectancy

Life expectancy in the United States decreased by a half-year between 2020 and 2021, from 77 years to 76.4 years, according to final 2021 mortality data from the National Center for Health Statistics. Life expectancy in 2021 was at its lowest level since 1996 (Kuehn, 2023). Reasons for the drop were increased deaths from COVID-19 and drug overdoses. In 2019, individuals reaching age 65 had an average life expectancy of an added 19.6 years (20.8 years for females and 18.2 years formales). A child born in 2019 could expect to live 78.8 years, more than 30 years longer than a child born in 1900 (47.3 years) (Kochanek et al., 2020). Life expectancy in the United States remains lower than in other comparable countries. In addition, racial and ethnic disparities in life expectancy persist: Life expectancy for Black adults at age 65 is 18 years, life expectancy for White adults 19.4 years, and life expectancy for Latino/Hispanic adults is 21.4 years. Life expectancy among adults in all three groups at age 65 is higher for females than males (Ochieng et al., 2021).

Median Income

In 2022, there were 57.6 million Americans aged 65 and older. The yearly income for half of all individual adults was less than $29,740, and half of older households received less than $50,290 in yearly income from all sources (Social Security, pensions, private pensions, and government employee pensions). One out of five older adults has income from earnings. In 2022, the median income of adults aged 65 and older and fully retired was $24,190. The amounts were similar among all older age groups (Pension Rights Center, 2023).

In 2020, the median income of older persons was $26,668. The median income was $35,808 for males and $21,245 for females. From 2019 to 2020, the real median income, which is the inflation-adjusted amount of money a median household earns annually, decreased by 3.3%.

In 2020, households headed by persons aged 65 and older reported a median income of $68,067 ($72,855 for non Hispanic White, $46,183 for Hispanic/Latino, $54,909 for African American, and $67,378 for Asian American). About 5% of family households with an older adult householder had incomes less than $15,000, and 79% had incomes of $35,000 or more (ACL, 2022).

Poverty

Poverty rates are important indicators of community well-being and the health status of older adults. In 2022, the poverty rate was

11.5%, with 37.9 million people in poverty. The poverty rate by race was 10.5% for Whites, 17.1% for Blacks, 8.6% for non-Hispanic Whites, 8.6% for Asians, 25% for American Indians and Alaska Natives, 12.2% for individuals who identified as two or more races, and 16.9% for Hispanic/Latino any race. The poverty rate for Black individuals decreased between 2021 and 2022, with the 2022 rate being the lowest on record (Shrider & Creamer, 2023).

The poverty rate for Americans 65 and older has dropped nearly 30% during the past 50 years because of Social Security. Social Security continues to be the most important antipoverty program. In 2022, Social Security income moved 28.9 million people out of poverty.

Older adults who are isolated, have lower levels of education, or reside in economically depressed areas and medically underserved communities are at higher risk of poverty.

Healthy People 2030

Healthy People 2030 is the fifth edition of the US national effort to improve the health and well-being of people in the United States. *Healthy People* national objectives are multiyear processes that reflect input from a diverse group of individuals and organizations (Ochiai, 2021).

Healthy People 2030 developed 23 leading health indicators (LHIs). LHIs are a subset of high-priority *Healthy People 2030* objectives selected to improve health and well-being. LHIs cover the life span and include objectives across topic areas. LHIs address factors that affect major causes of death and disease in the United States and help organizations, communities, and states focus their resources and efforts on improving the health and well-being of all people.

Healthy People 2030 has an increased focus on social determinants of health. Social determinants of health examine the environments where people reside and how their environment affects their health.

Selected national health-promotion and disease-prevention objectives for older adults are listed in Box 24.1. The objectives focus on increasing health-promotion programs, which decrease morbidity and mortality in chronic and acute diseases.

As the population of older adults increases, diversity within this population also increases. Patients' cultural background, race, and ethnicity may influence the treatment they receive in the health care system. How populations access health care and the treatments they receive contribute to the prevalence of disease in the United States. However, inequities persist among medically underserved and under-resourced communities. The disparities that occur are access, care coordination, affordability, person-centered care, and effective treatments. Language barriers are also associated with decreased quality of care and decreased safety. The goal is to increase quality and access to health care to achieve equitable health care for all.

BOX 24.1 *HEALTHY PEOPLE 2030* OBJECTIVES

Symbol	*Healthy People 2030* Objectives
OA 01	Increase the proportion of older adults with reduced physical or cognitive function who engage in light, moderate, or vigorous leisure-time physical activities
OA 04	Reduce the rate of pressure ulcers in hospitalized older adults
OA 05	Reduce the rate of hospital admissions for diabetes
DIA 01	Increase the proportion of older adults with diagnosed Alzheimer disease and other dementias, or of their caregivers, who are aware of the diagnosis
DIA 02	Reduce the proportion of preventable hospitalizations in older adults with dementia
DIA 03	Increase the proportion of adults experiencing cognitive decline who discuss their symptoms with a provider
OA 07	Reduce the rate of hospital admissions for urinary tract infections among older adults
IVP 08	Reduce fall-related deaths among older adults
OA 02	Reduce the proportion of older adults who use inappropriate medications
OA 03	Reduce the rate of emergency department visits because of falls among older adults
OH 04	Reduce the proportion of older adults with untreated root surface decay
OH 05	Reduce the proportion of adults aged 45 years and over who have lost all of their natural teeth
OH 06	Reduce the proportion of adults aged 45 years and over with moderate and severe periodontitis
O-02	Reduce hip fractures among older adults
O-D01	Increase the proportion of older adults (aged 65 and over) screened for osteoporosis
O-D02	Increase the proportion of older adults (aged 65 and over) treated for osteoporosis following a fragility fracture
OA 06	Reduce the rate of hospital admissions for pneumonia among older adults
RD-D03	Reduce hospitalizations for asthma among older adults (aged 65 years and over)
V 07	Reduce visual impairment cause by age-related macular degeneration

From US Department of Health and Human Services. [Internet]. *Healthy People 2030.* Office of Disease Prevention and Health Promotion. https://health.gov/healthypeople/objectives-and-data/browse-objectives/older-adults

BIOLOGY AND GENETICS

Age-Related Changes

Although there is a serious need to promote the health of the older population, there are numerous challenges in meeting this need. One of the great challenges to health promotion for older adults lies in the misconceptions about the benefits of disease prevention and health promotion. Another challenge relates to the difficulty in separating normal changes of aging from pathologic processes and illness. Age-related changes are frequently regarded as inevitable and irreversible. However, there is a large amount of variability in age-related changes within each individual. Environmental, economic, physiologic, genetic, psychological, and social factors may influence the aging process. A recent interest in consumer genetic testing has resulted in some older adults learning about their genetic makeup and whether it may influence their aging process and

BOX 24.2 PERSONAL GENOMIC TESTING

Older adults are increasingly interested in learning about their own DNA to find clues about their heritage and about factors that may affect their future health. With technological developments in recent years, it is now possible to purchase low-cost genetic kits for as little as $100. The question arises as to whether the results of these tests prompt older adults to change their habits to more healthy lifestyles.

In the United States, three companies have dominated the market for do-it-yourself, direct-to-consumer (DTC) genetic kits that allow consumers to bypass medical intermediaries: 23andMe, Navigenics, and DeCODEme. These genetic tests offer a wide array of information about ancestry, physical traits, and health information. (Ancestry.com does not provide health information.) Health-related genetic tests include predictive tests for alterations in genes known to be strongly associated with disease onset (e.g., Alzheimer disease and several cancer syndromes), along with susceptibility tests that give feedback of much lower increased risk of developing common health conditions (e.g., type 2 diabetes).

Bioethicists and health researchers have raised concerns about the health-risk genre of these tests, and the US Food and Drug Administration asked 23andMe to stop marketing the health tests until it could provide evidence that the results are reliable. Those who favor DTC health-related testing argue that direct access to personal genetic information is a fundamental right and helps to preserve autonomy and privacy by eliminating health care intermediaries. Others argue that providing genetic information directly to consumers without health professional support to explain the information could result in numerous harms, in that consumers may not have adequate information to make determinations about the meaning of the results. There is concern that individuals who are told they carry genetic risk variants may have harmful psychological responses, such as feeling fatalistic about their potential to reduce their risk of health problems. However, early users of the DTC kits have not reported strong emotional response to test results, regardless of whether the findings show increased risk.

Consumers state that genetic susceptibility tests for conditions such as obesity would motivate them to adopt a healthier lifestyle and could also provide information that would help their primary care provider monitor their health.

Very few studies have evaluated whether individuals change their lifestyle after receiving genetic risk results. However, early evidence suggests that, thus far, genetic test results have not had a demoralizing effect on consumers' efforts or desire to change health habits. There is mixed evidence on how susceptibility testing may influence use of health services. The bottom line is that when consumers receive the results of their testing, they often find that their personalized risk results are matched with the same health recommendations they already know. Most experts believe that potential breakthroughs that could enable genomic risk information to be used routinely to prevent disease and foster healthy aging are still in the future (McBride, 2015).

development of disease. Box 24.2 provides information about personal genomic testing.

Most researchers agree that biologic changes show that growth and development peak during early adulthood, with subsequent linear decline until death. These normal changes must be distinguished from pathologic changes to focus health-promotion interventions on behaviors that can be changed. For example, it is normal for older adults to experience a decline in their respiratory vital capacity; therefore, when nurses recommend exercise programs, older adults should start gradually, which will allow them to experience exercise free from respiratory distress. Selected changes will be discussed in the Gordon's Functional Health Patterns section.

Another challenge in promoting the health of older adults relates to the prevalence of chronic illness and multiple health problems. Although chronic illness is not a normal part of aging, years of environmental assault, less-than-optimal health behaviors, and stress have placed older adults at a higher risk to develop chronic illnesses. Table 24.1 lists the percentage of older adults with chronic conditions. Illness influences the older adult's capacity and motivation to undertake health-promoting activities to fit functional abilities. Chronic conditions may contribute to greater functional limitation and disability. Almost 50% of people with chronic conditions have some type of activity limitation, which is associated with decreased ability to perform activities of daily living (Fong, 2019).

Most of these limitations are associated with the physical changes of aging and chronic diseases such as arthritis, heart disease, stroke, and respiratory disease. The prevalence of preventable illness and the concomitant physical limitations associated with chronic disease indicate a greater need for health-promotion and disease- and injury-prevention activities for older adults. It is important to note that health-promotion practices among older adults may vary because of the individual's self-perception of health status and the individual's economic resources, access to health providers, and resources, consistent with the individual's expressed cultural background (Box 24.3: Health and Social Determinants/Health Equity).

Theories of Aging

The study of how and why people age has continued over many years and has been the source of ongoing debates. For many years, the cause of death on many older adults' death certificates was listed as old age. At the 55th Gerontological Society of America annual meeting, Butler and Olshansky (2002) explored this mindset in a presentation entitled "Has Anyone Ever Died of Old Age?" As the study of aging (gerontology) has progressed, researchers have clarified the physiologic, social, and psychological reasons for death.

There is no formula to predict how a person will age or how long that individual will live. Many **theories of aging** continue to be examined, including those regarding metabolism, the role of free radicals, stress, the immune system, genetics, epigenetics (the blending of nature/genetics and nurture/environment), and diet. Genetic markers may predict the development of disease and play a role in how a person ages and their longevity. In addition, researchers report that calorie-restricted diets have resulted in an increase in longevity in animals; however, the role of calorie intake and longevity is still being debated. The role of antioxidants in binding free radicals as an important influence on increasing longevity is also under consideration, but there is no consensus about the entire aging process. The theory of epigenetic age is that an individual's rate of aging is based on myriad factors, which include diet, lifestyle, genetics, and disease (Li et al., 2022). However, exciting theories continue to be advanced. Some of the theories used to explain aging are briefly described in Box 24.4.

TABLE 24.1 Average Percentage of People Aged 65 Years or Older Who Have Chronic Health Conditions

Chronic Condition	Total Population	Less Than 65 Years	65 Years and Older	Males	Females
Depression	17.9%	31%	15%	13%	22%
Diabetes	27.2%	27%	27%	29%	26%
Drug abuse/Substance abuse	3.4%	12%	2%	4%	3%
Heart failure	13.9%	10%	15%	14%	13%
Hyperlipidemia	40.7%	28%	43%	41%	41%
Hypertension	57.1%	43%	60%	56%	58%
Ischemic heart disease	26.9%	17%	29%	32%	22%
Osteoporosis	6.4%	2%	7%	1%	10%
Schizophrenia/Other psychotic disorders	3.1%	10%	2%	3%	3%
Stroke	3.8%	3%	4%	4%	4%

From Centers for Medicare and Medicaid Chartbooks. (2017). https://www.cms.gov

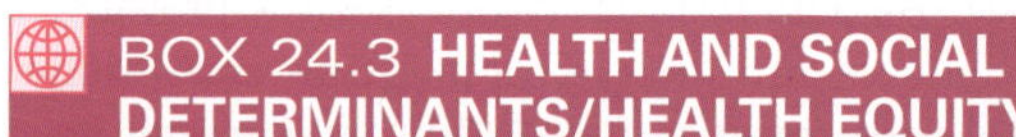

BOX 24.3 HEALTH AND SOCIAL DETERMINANTS/HEALTH EQUITY

Reported Importance and Access to Health Care Providers Who Understand or Share Cultural Characteristics with Their Adult Patients by Race and Ethnicity

The Centers for Disease Control and Prevention National Health Interview Survey (2017) examined whether patients thought it was important to be seen by providers who looked like them and shared their culture. Studies have shown that disparities in health care delivery and quality are profound and related to inadequate health care, which results in higher mortality in minority populations. Research has also found that adults receive better care in health care settings where providers share similar cultural characteristics, language, or ethnicity. Health care providers who are fully cognizant of cultural awareness and social determinants of health have a more comprehensive understanding of health equity issues.

Non-Hispanic White adults believed it was less important to see a health care provider who looked like them or shared similar cultural traditions, whereas Latinx or Hispanic adults thought it was slightly important. However, Latinx/Hispanic adults also reported that being seen by a provider that looks like them or shares their culture was unlikely (Terlizzi et al., 2019).

GORDON'S FUNCTIONAL HEALTH PATTERNS

Health Perception–Health Management Pattern

Motivation is an important factor in maintaining health. Nurses who care for older adults know that the best nursing care cannot make an individual do something they believe is unnecessary. A primary factor in the older adult's motivation to promote personal health is the perception of health and its subsequent management. For older adults who have always been healthy and receive a diagnosis of a serious disease, it is important to find ways to promote health while living with the disease. For example, new research shows that many of the debilitating aspects of Parkinson disease can be minimized through active exercise, including bicycling (Bouça-Machado et al., 2020). Older adults with a diagnosis of spinal stenosis or back pain that prevents walking long distances may think they can no longer travel. Mobility devices such as scooters allow individuals to ride through the airport and make travel possible. These devices also provide independence for older adults to participate in activities outside of their homes (Fig. 24.1).

Nurses can be very helpful in working with older adults to achieve their health and social goals. If a person dislikes group activity, it may not be effective to encourage them to take exercise or nutrition classes. Suggesting exercising at home or reading about nutrition may be more helpful. It is also important not to underestimate the abilities of older adults, as many continue to participate in competitive sports such as tennis, pickleball, bowling, bicycle riding, and marathon running. Even chronic illnesses do not need to prevent health-promotion activities. Older adults should be encouraged to continue with their self-care activities. Because some memory impairment may be present in cognitively healthy older adults, memory aids and familiar environments should be encouraged because the goal is to keep one's mind active, continue learning, and maintain self-confidence.

A variety of activities promote health and prevent frailty. These include maintaining healthy weight and diet, staying active, practicing fall prevention, maintaining relationships, and keeping regular medical appointments. Clinical preventive screening recommended for older adults include the following immunizations: Tdap every 10 years, COVID-19, respiratory syncytial virus, pneumococcal disease, and shingles (Murthy et al., 2023). It also includes screenings for early detection of breast cancer, colorectal cancer, diabetes, lipid disorders, and osteoporosis (Jin, 2022). Adults who smoke should be offered smoking-cessation counseling. Under the Affordable Care Act of 2010, many preventive services are provided at no cost to Medicare-eligible beneficiaries. SilverSneakers is a popular exercise program that is available at no cost to many older adults through their Medicare or private insurance plan (Flores et al., 2022). Older adults can access many different online and mobile applications to aid in monitoring exercise. Assisting older adults in maintaining or initiating healthier lifestyles is an essential nursing role.

Health-maintenance behaviors include exercise, good nutrition, sexual safety, and appropriate sleep-rest patterns.

BOX 24.4 Theories of Aging

Biologic Theories of Aging

- Programmed theories of aging: Aging is the result of predictable cellular death.
- Immunity theory: Aging is a programmed accumulation of damage and decline in the function of the immune system resulting from oxidative stress.
- Neuroendocrine control/pacemaker theory: Aging is a programmed decline in the functioning of the nervous, endocrine, and immune systems. The cells lose their ability to reproduce.
- Gene theory: Longevity may be associated with a genetic trait or a "longevity gene"; "juvenescent" genes mediate youthful vigor and mature adult well-being; "senescent" genes promote functional decline and structural deterioration.
- Error theories of aging: Aging is the result of an accumulation of random errors in the synthesis of cellular DNA and RNA.
- Oxidative stress theory (free radical theory): Errors are a result of random damage from free radicals.
- Cross-linkage theory: Aging is a product of accumulated damage from errors associated with cross-linked proteins where cross-linked proteins become stiff and thick.
- Wear-and-tear theory: Cellular errors are the result of deterioration over time because of continued use.
- Calorie restriction theory: In animal models, calorie restriction increased the life span and the health of the animals.

Sociological Theories of Aging

- Activity theory: Continued activity is an indicator of successful aging.
- Disengagement theory: During aging, the individual slowly withdraws from former roles and activities.
- Role theory: The ability of an individual to adapt to changing roles throughout life is predictive of adjustment to the changing roles associated with aging.
- Continuity theory: In normal aging, personality remains consistent. Personality influences role activity and life satisfaction.
- Age stratification theory: Focus is placed on the relationship between age as an element of social structure and aging people as a cohort.
- Subculture theory: Older people have their own norms, habits, and beliefs and interact better among age peers than with other age groups.

Developmental Theories of Aging

- Erikson's developmental theory: There is a predetermined order of development, and specific tasks are associated with specific periods in a person's life. For older adults, the developmental stage is integrity versus despair. Peck's developmental theory: This theory expands on Erikson's theory with identification of discrete tasks of late life that, when accomplished together, result in ego integrity.
- Havighurst's developmental theory: There are specific tasks associated with aging, including adjusting to the losses of aging (e.g., health, income, death of spouse and age peers), adapting to change and new roles, and accepting life's experiences.
- Tornstam's theory of gerotranscendence: Aging is viewed as the movement from birth to death and maturation toward wisdom. Gerotranscendence involves achieving wisdom through personal transformation.

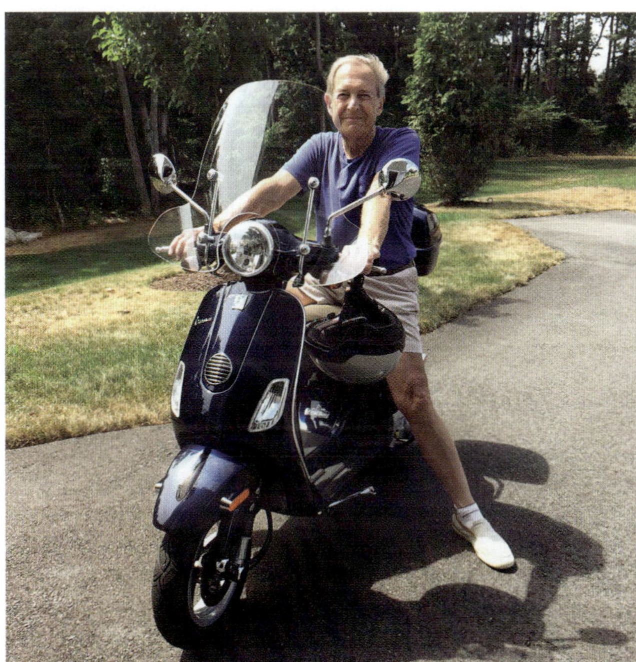
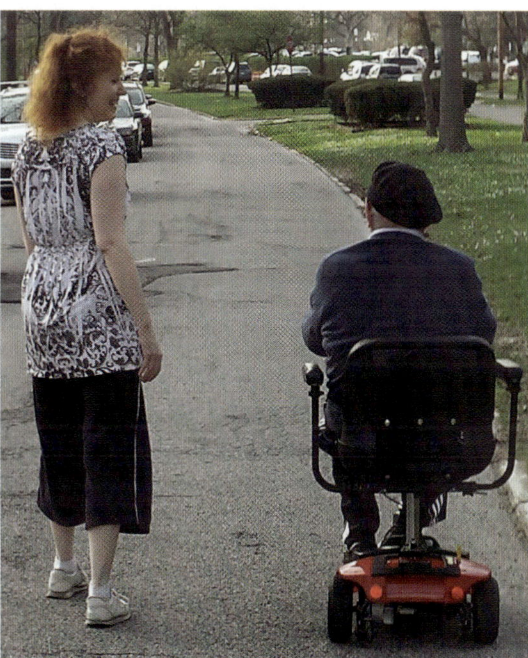

FIG. 24.1 Mobile devices provide independence for older adults with limited mobility.

Health-maintenance practices also include regular health care checkups to detect disease and management of chronic illness. The perception of the benefit of health-promoting activities determines the level of engagement. Practicing health-promoting activities varies by the economic and social resources of individuals and their neighborhoods. It is essential that nurses recognize the social determinants of health that contribute to older adults' access to health-promoting activities. In addition, understanding the individual's access to health-promotion activities will enable the nurse to be most effective in helping them make the changes necessary to improve their health (Box 24.5: Best Practice).

BOX 24.5 BEST PRACTICE/INNOVATIVE PRACTICE

Geriatric Assessment

The health care system, with its emphasis on acute care, busy office schedules, and fragmented delivery systems, often frustrates older people and their families. The very old or frail person's health problems are often overlooked, ignored, or only partially treated. Many communities have a health care service that uses a team approach to meet the special needs of older adults. This service is known as geriatric assessment.

Goals of Geriatric Assessment and Care

- Maintain health and health-maintenance practices.
- Promote disease prevention through routine immunizations and health screenings.
- Implement fall-prevention strategies to decrease the incidence of falls and fall-related injuries.
- Minimize hospitalizations.
- Establish complete diagnoses that are often missed or overlooked, including hearing impairment, vision deficits, early dementia, depression, and poor nutrition.
- Decrease misuse of medications, including prescription medications, over-the-counter medications, vitamins/minerals/supplements, and herbal remedies.

Geriatric care uses an interdisciplinary team consisting of a geriatric nurse practitioner, a physical therapist, and a social worker. Each member of the team evaluates the person from a health care, functional, cognitive, or psychosocial perspective. Additional members of the team might include a geriatric psychiatrist, geriatrician, nutritionist, pharmacist, dentist, or podiatrist. The program team evaluates the home environment, risk of falls, incontinence, vision and hearing impairments, memory loss, depression and anxiety, functional decline, physical deconditioning, caregiver stress, economic resources, advance directives, and quality-of-life issues. The team is coordinated by the geriatric nurse practitioner.

A baseline geriatric assessment should be completed during a primary care visit to evaluate medical, psychosocial, and functional limitations of the older adult. Additional geriatric assessments should be based on problems identified by the primary care provider, family members, caregivers, or the older adult. The people who benefit are those who are often frail. An example of an older person who might benefit from geriatric assessment is as follows:

- Is older than 80 years
- Has a history of frequent falls
- Is losing weight
- Is depressed; has mild memory loss
- Has been hospitalized three times in 2 months
- Takes more than five medications regularly and frequently gets them confused
- Has no close family or other support persons in the community
- Needs health teaching

Geriatric assessment usually identifies the strengths and weaknesses of the older adult and evaluates that person's situation, including family and other social support. Following the assessment, the geriatric nurse practitioner begins developing a care plan to incorporate usable strengths and assist with weaknesses.

The primary care physician, family physician, internist, geriatrician, family nurse practitioner, adult nurse practitioner, or geriatric nurse practitioner is a key link between the geriatric assessment team and the individual, primarily because this provider carries out the team's recommendation and monitors the person's progress. In most cases the nurse practitioner coordinates between the team and the person's primary care provider and family.

Geriatric assessment clinics are available in many larger cities. As the US health care system changes from costly methods of treating acute health problems with frequent office and hospital visits to a more cost-controlled, coordinated, comprehensive health-management system, geriatric assessment will play a key role in identifying individual strengths, correcting problems, and maintaining the health and quality of life of older citizens.

Nutritional-Metabolic Pattern

Nutrition plays an important role in preventing cancer, obesity, and gastrointestinal disorders. In addition, adequate nutritional intake provides older adults with the energy required to function in all **activities of daily living**. One measure of adequate nutritional intake is whether the individual is meeting the recommended daily allowance (RDA) for caloric intake.

The US Department of Health and Human Services (USDHHS) and US Department of Agriculture (USDA, 2020) provide dietary guidelines for Americans. Currently, the RDAs are 2000 (sedentary), 2200 (moderately active), and 2600 (active) calories formales aged 66 to 75 years. The RDAs for males aged 76 and older are 2000 (sedentary), 2200 (moderately active), and 2400 (active) calories. The RDAs are 1600 (sedentary), 1800 (moderately active), and up to 2200 (active) calories for females aged 66 and older (USDHHS & USDA, 2020).

Poor nutrition in older adults affects overall health and contributes to increased health care costs. Specific nutritional risk factors for US older adults include solitary living, lower socioeconomic status, social isolation, and lack of social support. Many older adults experience food insecurity, which is limited access to adequate nutritious food. Food insecurity affects 40 million people in the United States, including 5.5 million people aged 60 and older. This represents approximately 11.3% of older adults in that age range. Residents at long-term nursing facilities are at higher risk of being malnourished. These data underscore the problems of maintaining good nutrition. For independent elders, the barriers that may interfere with the ability to obtain adequate and nutritional food include limited transportation, income, and social support resources (Jung et al., 2019; Gundersen & Ziliak, 2015).

Problems with access to food are compounded by the effect of normal changes of aging. Declines in gastrointestinal organ function can lead to changes in digestive metabolism and the absorption and elimination of nutrients. A deterioration of the smell, vision, and taste senses and the high frequency of dental and swallowing problems make maintaining adequate daily nutrition even more difficult. In addition, side effects of required medications may affect appetite. Cultural food preferences and lifelong eating habits, such as diets high in fat and cholesterol, are other obstacles to maintaining optimal nutrition.

Because of physiologic and metabolic changes associated with aging, nutritional problems are more difficult to quantify and evaluate in older adults. A nutritional assessment for an older adult entails a comprehensive approach that includes health history, physical examination, laboratory data, dietary data, and measurement of functional status. However, initial **nutritional screening** is more straightforward. Nutritional screening evaluates the risk of malnutrition and may identify the need for a more formal nutrition assessment. A variety of tools, such as the Mini Nutritional Assessment (MNA), can be used for nutritional screening in older adults. The MNA contains an initial set of questions that, if scored less than 11, indicates risk of malnutrition and requires the completion of additional questions to confirm the likelihood of malnutrition (Mastronuzzi & Grattagliano, 2019). The MNA and other screening tools can identify the risk of malnutrition, but a formal nutritional assessment is needed to establish a diagnosis of malnutrition and appropriate interventions.

The living environment further affects nutritional status. Community-dwelling seniors are at higher risk of nutritional disorders because access to food may be limited (Whitelock & Ensaff, 2018). Older adults in long-term care facilities do not have a problem with availability of food, but the meals may contain excessive fat, cholesterol, or salt and may lack enough fiber. In addition, fresh fruit and vegetables are less available. Institutional food may be unappealing, and institutions may not be able to adapt their meals to the cultural and religious preferences of their residents. Encouraging family members to bring in special foods that the resident enjoys is helpful. Nurses who work in institutional settings can make an important difference for older adults by assessing the person's food preferences and difficulties in eating. The nurse can then plan an appropriate menu to encourage healthy eating.

A pleasant setting with social interaction enhances the desire to eat. In one study, an expert panel of nutrition practitioners concluded that the two most important enablers of healthy eating among older adults are accessibility and social support. Many older adults want to age in their own home without having to relocate to a long-term care facility. Nutritional support plays a critical role in older adults' ability to remain in their homes. Food assistance from friends and family in the form of cooking or food sharing is also an important facilitator of nutritional health and being able to age in place.

Anorexia, or lack of appetite, can accompany disease. Medications, poor dentition, difficulty swallowing, or a lack of dentures can also cause older people to eat less than is optimal. Those in acute care hospitals or long-term care facilities may experience a lack of appetite because of illness. The hospital stay is a time during which good nutrition is most important to heal wounds and to restore energy; however, a lack of interest in or energy for eating during hospitalization places the older adult at a higher risk of developing nutritional disorders.

Obesity is also a problem for older adults. The rate of obesity in adults aged 60 years and older is 41.5% (CDC, 2023a). Obesity is associated with several chronic health conditions, including hypertension, diabetes, and heart disease. However, it is important to recognize that scientists have described a phenomenon called "the obesity paradox," in which obesity in older adults, unlike in younger individuals, does not appear to be clearly associated with a shorter life span. Some studies have suggested that the "ideal" protective weight might be higher in the older population (Tutor et al., 2023). However, there is still much debate about this, and because obesity is clearly linked to a lesser quality of life, it is important to discuss options for weight reduction. During weight loss, muscle is lost as well as fat. This is an important consideration when one is planning a weight-loss program for older adults. Because of normal aging and often deconditioning, older adults are likely to have less muscle mass and more fat than when they were younger. However, studies have found that a moderate weight loss of 5% to 10% in older adults results in significant health benefits and that even a weight loss of 3% significantly reduces inflammation, blood pressure, cholesterol levels, and blood glucose levels (Tahrani & Morton, 2022). For nurses working with older adults trying to lose weight, it is important to recognize that these individuals may have struggled with weight issues for years and may be very frustrated with their unsuccessful efforts to achieve an ideal weight. Factors such as living alone, cooking for one person, the ability to access fresh fruits and vegetables, medications, fast food accessibility, lack of green space, and difficulty exercising make weight loss more difficult. Nurses can assist older adults in identifying strategies to attain and maintain a healthy weight.

Nurses assist older adults in maintaining the highest possible nutritional level by educating them about the food needed to maintain optimal nutritional status as well as providing information about resources to purchase food. An important social resource is the supplemental nutrition assistance program (SNAP), a federal program. SNAP is available to older adults who meet the economic criteria; SNAP assistance allows older adults to obtain nutritious food at participating markets without depleting their limited budgets. Approximately 5.2 million seniors take advantage of this benefit. However, many older adults eligible for SNAP benefits do not apply because of embarrassment, difficulty in applying for the program, and lack of awareness about the program. The American Association of Retired Persons (AARP) assists older adults in determining SNAP eligibility as well as with the application process (Dean et al., 2022).

In addition to SNAP, there are other federally supported food assistance programs available to older adults. These programs include the Commodity Supplemental Food Program, the Emergency Food Assistance Program, and the Senior Farmers' Market Nutrition Program (SFMNP).

The Nutrition Services Program was authorized under Title III of the Older Americans Act (OAA). This program gives grants to states and US territories to support nutrition services programs for seniors. The OAA Nutrition Programs include the Congregate Nutrition Program, which serves healthy meals and provides opportunities for adults to engage in social, health, and wellness activities. The Home-Delivered Nutrition Program delivers healthy meals to the home, as well as providing an informal safety check for those homebound elders. The Title III grants authorize programs for State and Community Programs on Aging; and the Title VI grants authorize programs for American Indians, Alaska Natives, and Native Hawaiians. The objectives are to (1) reduce hunger and food insecurity, (2) promote socialization, (3) promote health and well-being, and (4) delay adverse health conditions. The purpose is to develop community-based nutrition services available to older adults who are at risk of losing their independence and their ability to remain in the community (Administration for Community Living, 2024). Meals on Wheels provides nutritional services specifically to older adults. Detailed information about this program, as well as other important nutritional information related to older adults, is described in Chapter 11.

Elimination Pattern

Bowel and bladder functions in the older adult are altered by normal changes of aging. The bladder retains its tone, but its capacity decreases. Gastrointestinal motility decreases as people age. In addition to some of the normal changes of aging, diet plays a significant role in problems with intestinal motility and constipation. Decreased intake of fluids and fiber contributes in large part to constipation. Many medications taken by older adults also cause elimination concerns. Lack of physical activity and changes in the environment that decrease privacy contribute to elimination problems. Many older adults may believe elimination problems are a necessary part of aging and may be embarrassed to mention their concerns to health care providers. It is important to reassure them that, through diet and exercise, they can gain control of most elimination problems.

Constipation is often a major problem for older adults and has far-reaching effects on their quality of life. There are several bowel elimination problems described by older adults as constipation: hard stools, infrequent stools, the need for excessive straining, and a feeling of incomplete bowel evacuation often associated with abdominal cramping or feeling bloated. Although inadequate diet and inactivity are common causes of constipation, it is important to consider whether constipation is related to metabolic disease such as hypothyroidism, neurologic disease such as Parkinson disease, psychological illness such as depression, or medications. Nurses can assess the cause of constipation and develop an appropriate plan of care. Encouraging older adults to exercise and increase their fluid intake helps reduce the incidence of constipation. Integrating more fiber into the diet and eating prunes each day can also be very effective for preventing constipation.

Urinary incontinence, often underreported and underdiagnosed, increases with age. Sources provide estimates that vary from approximately 10.4% of adults 60 and older (Shaw & Wagg, 2017) to approximately 23% for females 60 and older (Russo et al., 2021). The rate of incontinence for adults residing in long-term facilities is 65% to 70% (Stefanacci et al., 2022). Incontinence is classified as either acute (transient) or chronic (established). Acute incontinence has a sudden onset, has been present for less than 6 months, and is usually secondary to a treatable condition. Chronic incontinence has either a sudden or a gradual onset and is categorized into four major types: **stress incontinence**, which is the most common and occurs during exercise, laughing, coughing, or sneezing; **urge incontinence**, or the inability to delay voiding after the bladder is full; urge, mixed, or stress incontinence with high post void residual incontinence; and functional incontinence, which is associated with environmental barriers, physical limitations, or cognitive impairment where the person is unable to reach the toilet. High post void residual incontinence occurs when the bladder does not empty completely and becomes overdistended, which may be caused by an obstruction in the urinary elimination tract, such as an enlarged prostate gland.

Incontinence may affect psychological and physical health, including depression, urinary tract infections, skin breakdown, and falls. Nurses can help older adults to understand incontinence as a manageable problem. Implementing appropriate management is important for the older adult's continued good health and self-esteem. Pelvic floor or Kegel exercises can be taught to strengthen the musculature of the urinary system. Modified Pilates exercises have also been shown to be effective in treating incontinence (Lausen et al., 2018). Management programs may include scheduling regular times to void, improving access to toileting facilities, managing diet and fluids, and using disposable absorbent undergarments. Voiding schedules are most effective when the person selects specific times during the day for urination. Eliminating dietary caffeine helps some people with urge incontinence, and increasing fiber in the diet helps those whose incontinence is related to pressure caused by constipation.

Activity-Exercise Pattern

Approximately 80% of adults do not meet the key guidelines for both aerobic and muscle-strengthening activity (Piercy et al., 2018). Males are more likely to meet the guidelines than females, and older adults living in lower-income communities may exercise less. Reasons for disparities in exercise are related to neighborhood characteristics such as lack of green spaces and facilities, safety considerations, free time, and economic resources. The benefits of regular exercise in promoting health and preventing disease are widely accepted. The overwhelming evidence of the positive effects of exercise has led the USDHHS to develop within its *Healthy People 2030* program national objectives for increasing the percentage of adults who exercise regularly. Regular physical activity helps and may even prevent many chronic health problems associated with aging, including hypertension, obesity, diabetes, and depression. Regular physical activity can increase both the years of life and the quality of those years. Strength training can improve balance and reduce the risk of falls, strengthen bones, and reduce blood glucose levels. Normal changes of aging, pathologic conditions, and environmental deterrents do not need to prevent the older adult from exercising (Fig. 24.2).

The CDC recommends a combination of aerobic exercise and muscle-strengthening activities every week. Aerobic exercise may range from moderate intensity to vigorous intensity depending on the older person's level of fitness, and muscle-strengthening activities can include exercises that work all major muscle groups (Abildso et al., 2023). Teaching the many benefits of exercise is the first lesson in motivating older adults to engage. Understanding barriers that prevent exercise needs to be explored with the older adult. Individual counseling is needed to identify exercises that can be enjoyed and continued (Fig. 24.3). The nurse or physical therapist can assist in designing an appropriate exercise program that helps maintain strength, flexibility, and balance. Walking can be done in community settings and health care facilities and is a popular form of exercise among older adults.

Other popular activities for older adults include swimming, weight-bearing exercises, and aquatic exercises. Weight-bearing

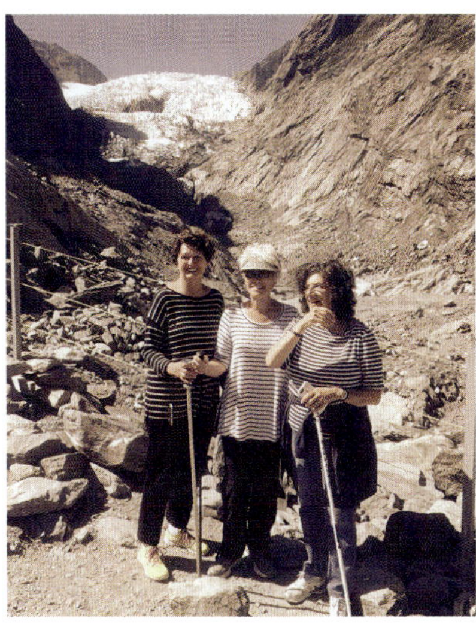

FIG. 24.2 Normal changes of aging and environmental deterrents do not prevent older adults from exercising.

and muscle-building exercises help maintain functional mobility, promote independence, and prevent falls. Weight-bearing exercises are highly effective in reducing bone wasting associated with osteoporosis. Regular exercise promotes maintenance of bone mineral density in older adults. People with conditions such as spinal stenosis and arthritis often find that they can exercise in a swimming pool without pain, so this is an important way for them to maintain an exercise plan and increase their functional ability. Box 24.6 lists many benefits that can be derived from participation in an exercise program.

Before beginning any exercise program, an older person who has not been exercising should consult a physician or nurse practitioner. After the program begins, activity levels can be increased gradually. Maintaining adherence to exercise programs is a major problem for all populations. The best strategies to encourage continued exercise among older adults are to communicate the importance of exercise in maintaining quality of life and to help them choose an exercise they enjoy

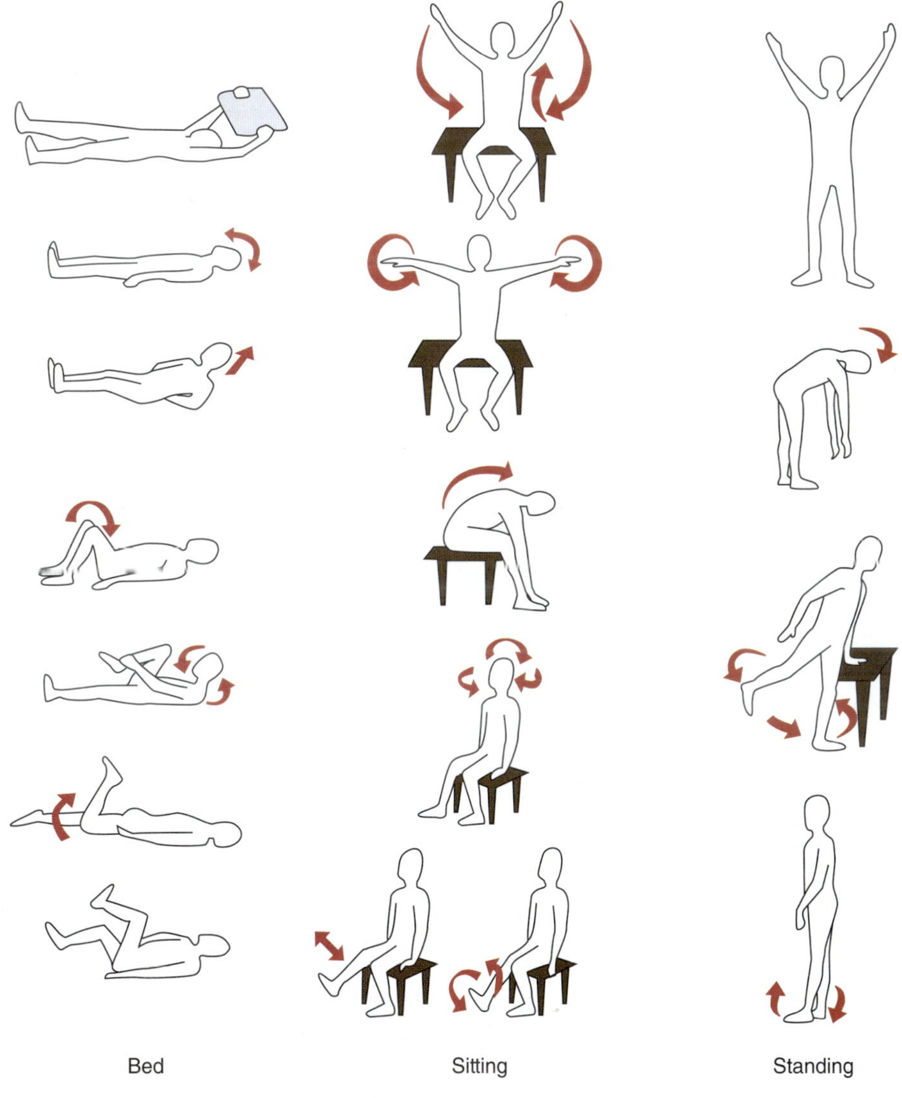

FIG. 24.3 Bed-lying, sitting, and standing exercises. (Redrawn from Ebersole, P., & Hess, P. [1998]. Toward healthy aging: Human need and nursing response [3rd ed.]. St. Louis: Mosby.)

BOX 24.6 Benefits of Exercise in the Older Adult

- Better sleep
- Reduced constipation
- Lower cholesterol level
- Lower blood pressure
- Better digestion
- Weight loss
- Socializing opportunities
- Greater sense of well-being

From Langhammer, B., Bergland, A., & Rydwik, E. (2018). *The importance of physical activity exercise among older people.* BioMed Research International. https://doi.org/10.1155/2018/7856823

that is easily accessible. Exercising with a family member or friend is also helpful in motivating older adults to exercise.

Sleep-Rest Pattern

Inability to sleep is a frequent concern of older adults. Sleep difficulties may include sleep apnea, the inability to fall asleep, the inability to stay asleep, the inability to fall back to sleep when awakening in the night, or the feeling of not being refreshed when awakening in the morning (Yaremchuk, 2018). Sleep-disordered breathing, or sleep apnea, is associated with an increased risk of stroke and death (McDermott et al., 2018). **Restless legs syndrome**, characterized by unpleasant throbbing, pulling, or creeping sensations in the legs and an almost uncontrollable urge to move the legs, is a neurologic disorder that affects many older adults (National Institute of Neurological Disorders and Stroke, 2019). Because the sensations are worse when the person is lying down and trying to sleep, the disorder can seriously limit sleep quality. Older adults (20%–30%) are more likely to report excessive daytime sleepiness, which means they find it difficult to remain awake or alert at appropriate times during the day (Petrovsky et al., 2020). The high prevalence of sleep disorders in older adults indicates that it is an important area for health care providers to address.

The benefits of a good night's sleep are numerous. Quality sleep results in overall increases in energy, motivation to continue a high quality of life, and improved immune function. Because of overall problems with sleep, the *Healthy People 2030* sleep health goal is to increase public knowledge about the need for adequate sleep. Nurses assist older adults in achieving a good night's sleep through assessment that might reveal possible causes of sleep disturbances. The Pittsburgh Sleep Quality Index is a subjective tool that is helpful in assessing the quality and patterns of sleep in older adults (Sancho-Domingo et al., 2021). The tool measures seven areas: subjective sleep quality, sleep latency, sleep duration, habitual sleep efficiency, sleep disturbances, use of sleeping medication, and daytime dysfunction. Educating older adults about normal changes may provide reassurance that sleep patterns change but are not necessarily harmful. This information may decrease anxiety. Identifying helpful bedtime rituals, such as drinking a glass of milk, taking a relaxing bath, reading, or meditating, can assure the older adult that these practices may help to establish normal sleep routines.

Increasing physical activity during the day also helps with falling asleep more readily at night. In addition, pain medication or using alternative pain-relief methods before going to bed can help those who suffer from painful conditions to obtain better rest at night.

Residents of nursing facilities or acute care facilities may have difficulty adjusting to the environment at night. Adjustments in noise and lighting help these individuals sleep better. Emotional disorders that interfere with sleep should be identified so that therapy and medication can be administered during the day to assist in restful sleep at night. Although a nap may be beneficial, it is important to ensure that daytime napping does not interfere with nighttime sleep (Box 24.7: Best Practice).

Sleep medications may be helpful for short-term use; however, the American Geriatric Society (2023) Beers Criteria recommend avoidance of long-term use of benzodiazepines, barbiturates, and chloral hydrate for treatment of insomnia in older adults because of older adults' increased sensitivity

BOX 24.7 BEST PRACTICE/INNOVATIVE PRACTICE

Measures to Promote Sleep

Sleep problems can be caused by many things, including stress; medications; medical conditions such as angina, asthma, anxiety, or depression; poor sleeping habits; and sleep disorders. The following are some suggestions to improve sleep in older adults.

Do

- Plan a regular bedtime and wake-up schedule.
- Participate in exercise, hobbies, and other activities during the day.
- Develop specific bedtime rituals, such as reading, meditating, drinking a glass of milk, or taking a warm bath. These tell the body it is almost time for sleep.
- Ensure a comfortable and quiet sleep environment, which is dark except for night safety lights.
- Sleep on a comfortably firm mattress with comfortable pillows and bedclothes.
- Use the bed only for sleep and sexual activities.
- Check with a physician about prescription and over-the-counter medications that may interfere with sleep.

Avoid

- Long daytime naps that may interfere with nighttime sleep
- Exercise or vigorous activity immediately before bedtime
- Caffeine after midmorning
- Drinking alcohol before going to bed
- Sleep medications
- Tobacco products
- Driving when tired or sleepy

When Sleep Problems Persist

- Keep a sleep log, recording times and duration of sleep throughout 24-hour periods for at least 1 week.
- Ask sleep companion about sleep habits, such as snoring or restlessness.
- See health care provider.

From Sleep Foundation: https://www.sleepfoundation.org/articles/sleep-hygiene

to these drugs and increased risk of dependency, along with their decreased metabolism of long-term agents, resulting in an increased risk of cognitive impairment, falls, and overdose.

Cognitive-Perceptual Pattern

Cognition

Thinking processes (**cognition**) in old age have been the subject of intensive study in the past few decades. Brain weight decreases with aging, and a shift occurs in the proportion of gray matter to white matter. The ways in which these changes manifest in individuals differ based on lifestyle, environmental exposures, and social factors. There is a growing body of research that shows obesity may affect cognitive aging, which includes the processing of information, memory, comprehension, problem-solving, and decisions (Boidin et al., 2020). It is important to consider how even subtle changes in cognition may affect older adults in their day-to-day activities. For example, older adults are more at risk for targeted scams asking them to send money or personally identifiable information to callers who appeal to their sense of fear or the promise of a reward.

There is a common belief that older adults will eventually develop dementia; however, cognitive problems are not a normal change of aging, and many individuals live well into old age without ever experiencing dementia. It is important to be cautious in assessing older adults who present with confusion. Confusion is not always indicative of dementia and can be the result of many treatable health problems, including electrolyte imbalances, diabetic ketoacidosis, and hypoxia. **Mild cognitive impairment** is a pathologic collection of symptoms that results in memory loss, language difficulties, and impairments in judgment and reasoning. A review of **instrumental activities of daily living** will help identify changes in higher executive functions, such as paying bills, taking medications as ordered, using the phone, and driving safely.

A condition that is receiving increased attention in older adults is **postoperative cognitive dysfunction** (POCD), a temporary deterioration in cognition that is associated with surgery and anesthesia (Brodier & Cibelli, 2021). As the population of older adults has increased dramatically in recent years, surgery is more common at advanced ages. Individuals with POCD experience postoperative cognitive changes that may include anxiety, blurred vision, inability to sleep, hallucinations, and depression. POCD is not the same as **delirium**, which is a short-term change in cognition that may develop in the immediate postoperative period. Cognitive changes in POCD are more subtle and extend over a longer period—sometimes for months after discharge from the hospital. These changes can be very distressing to the older adult and the older adult's family. POCD is thought to be related to the type or amount of anesthesia administered during surgery, but more research needs to be done to establish the cause of POCD and how to prevent it. It is important for nurses in all health care contexts to be aware of the possibility of POCD in older adults and to identify ways in which they can intervene. Because there is no specific treatment for POCD, nurses need to anticipate the needs of both older adults and their families. Educating older adults and their families about POCD and emphasizing that it is usually temporary can help decrease anxiety.

Dementia is not accepted as a normal change of aging. Dementia is an umbrella term for a group of cognitive disorders that affect memory and lead to difficulty in areas of language, motor activity, object recognition, and ability to plan and organize. The high incidence of dementia and Alzheimer disease in older adults prompted the USDHHS to add dementia, including Alzheimer disease, as a separate topic in *Healthy People 2030* with a goal to decrease morbidity and costs associated with dementia and maintain or enhance the quality of life for people with these cognitive disorders.

Dementias include **Alzheimer disease**, the most common dementia, as well as Parkinson-related dementia, Huntington disease, Creutzfeldt-Jakob disease, Pick disease, and Lewy body dementia. The Alzheimer's Association estimates that approximately 5.1 million Americans older than 65 years have Alzheimer disease and that approximately 81% of individuals with Alzheimer disease are 75 years or older (Alzheimer's Association, 2023).

The symptoms of dementia include forgetfulness, inattentiveness, disorganized thinking, altered levels of consciousness, perceptual disturbances, sleep-wake disorders, psychomotor disturbances, and disorientation. Assessment for dementia should be part of the routine assessment of older adults, especially if symptoms arise. An instrument that is used to screen older adults for cognitive impairments is the **Mini-Mental State Examination** (MMSE) (Gallegos et al., 2022; Folstein et al., 1975) (Fig. 24.4).

The MMSE assesses the baseline mental status of older adults and evaluates change or decline in mental functioning. The instrument is a 30-point scale that measures the level of awareness and orientation, appearance and behavior, speech and communication, mood and affect, disturbances in thinking, problems with perception, and abstract thinking and judgment. The higher the examination score, the more intact the mental status. Examination scores of 23 or lower indicate a problem with cognition. It is important to note that this instrument is problematic because of its limited sensitivity for early stages of cognitive impairment (Creavin et al., 2016). In addition, this instrument is difficult to use for individuals who speak languages other than English, those who are visually impaired, and older adults with low literacy levels.

The MMSE is relatively easy to perform after a little practice and is used for initial and subsequent evaluations of older adults in a variety of settings. The most effective way to perform the assessment is to make the older adult comfortable and establish a rapport. Eliminating extraneous noise and promoting attention and concentration will allow individuals to answer questions to the best of their ability. After the examination, the computed score can be used as a basis for care planning and further evaluation.

There is no cure for Alzheimer disease (Alzheimer's Association, 2023). Treatment of Alzheimer disease includes the use of medications for memory loss, including cholinesterase inhibitors and memantine; treatments for behavioral changes associated with Alzheimer disease; and treatment for sleep changes. There are three cholinesterase inhibitors commonly prescribed to treat

Mini Mental Status Examination Sample Items

Orientation to Time

"What is the date?"

Registration

"Listen carefully,

I am going to say three words.

You say them back after I stop.

Ready? Here they are...

HOUSE (pause), CAR (pause), LAKE (pause).

Now repeat those words back to me."

[Repeat up to 5 times, but score only the first trial.]

Naming

"What is this?"

[Point to a pencil or pen.]

Reading

"Please read this and do what it says."

[Show examinee the words on the stimulus form.]

CLOSE YOUR EYES

FIG. 24.4 Mini-Mental State Examination sample items. (Reproduced by permission of Psychological Assessment Resources, Inc., Lutz, FL, from the Mini-Mental State Examination, by Marshal Folstein and Susan Folstein, Copyright 1975, 1998 by Mini Mental LLC, Inc. Published 2001 by Psychological Assessment Resources, Inc. Further reproduction is prohibited without permission of Psychological Assessment Resources, Inc. The Mini-Mental State Examination can be purchased from Psychological Assessment Resources, Inc., by calling 800-331-8378.)

Alzheimer disease at all stages. These medications are donepezil (brand name Aricept), galantamine (brand name Razadyne), and rivastigmine (brand name Exelon). Razadyne has also been approved to treat mild to moderate dementia associated with Parkinson disease. The cholinesterase inhibitors are most effective during the early stages of the disease, as they prevent the breakdown of acetylcholine (which is needed to support communication among the nerve cells) in the brain. These medications treat symptoms related to memory, thinking, language, judgment, and other thought processes. Memantine (brand name Namenda) is an NMDA (short for N-methyl-D-aspartate) receptor antagonist also used to treat Alzheimer disease. Memantine regulates the activity of glutamate, a chemical involved in information processing, storage, and retrieval.

Nonpharmacologic techniques for managing the problems associated with dementia include developing and keeping routines; working in a calm, gentle, and unhurried manner; encouraging self-care activity; and reducing sensory overload. Interventions to keep the older adult safe include curtailing wandering behavior and preventing falls and other injury.

Sensory Factors

Older adults experience age-related changes in vision, hearing, taste, smell, and touch sensation. Because of the normal changes and potential pathologic changes associated with the senses, older adults benefit from routine assessment and appropriate nursing interventions. Safety, particularly while driving, is a concern for older adults and society. Sensory changes affect a person's ability to drive safely. As technology advances, self-driving cars may become an option for older adults. Until then, nurses can encourage older adults to take senior driving classes to learn how to become safer drivers as these changes occur.

A variety of structural changes cause visual acuity to decrease, color discrimination to become less acute, pupil size and constriction ability to decrease, and peripheral vision to diminish. **Presbyopia** is a loss of accommodation that occurs as people age and results in the inability to maintain focus on objects close to the eye. The lens of the eye thickens and becomes yellow and predisposes the older adult to cataracts. The older adult is also at increased risk of **glaucoma**, a group of eye disorders characterized by increased intraocular pressure. Because of the normal changes in the aging eye and the high risk of disease, a baseline eye assessment should be done to identify age-related changes and any disease processes. Follow-up eye appointments should be scheduled annually.

The nurse routinely assesses the older adult for the accumulation of cerumen (earwax), to ensure optimal hearing (see the case study at the end of this chapter). Hearing deficits are common in old age, resulting from inner ear **atrophy** or **sclerosis** of the tympanic membrane. The inner ear also undergoes several changes, including those that are cell degenerative and nerve related. **Presbycusis** is a progressive sensorineural hearing loss associated with aging that results in difficulty filtering background noise and understanding higher-pitched voices. Sound threshold changes, with an associated difficulty in understanding what others are saying. Like changes of the eye, changes in hearing and the increased risk of pathologic conditions indicate that older adults should have ear and hearing screening. Hearing loss occurs in approximately one in three persons between 65 and 74 years and in almost half of those older than 74 years (National Institute on Deafness and Other Communication Disorders, 2023). Loss of hearing can result in decreased quality of life because it may lead to miscommunication, loss of self-esteem, depression, falls, safety risks, and cognitive decline. Hearing aids assist those with hearing loss to communicate more effectively.

Taste changes with aging because of a loss of taste buds. The flavors of sweet, sour, salty, and bitter become less distinguishable with this loss. The sensations brought about by touch may also diminish with the decrease in sensory nerve endings, especially in the presence of debilitating diseases such as diabetes, stroke, or Parkinson disease. The ability to smell and the acuity of the olfactory nerve also decrease with age. Because of the loss of smell and taste sensations, older adults may increase the amounts of salt and sugar in their food, which may negatively affect chronic health conditions. Educating older adults about safe cooking and the use of alternative seasonings in food may help them adjust to sensory changes. In addition, when the sense of smell is impaired, the inability to sense warning signals such as smoke or rotten food may occur. It is helpful to educate older adults to check expiration dates on food packages and to be attentive when cooking and preparing meals to ensure safety.

The decline in taste and smell sensations, combined with problems of obtaining adequate nutrition, makes dental care of vital importance to this population. Lack of fluoridated water and preventive dentistry during the developmental years may have led to tooth and periodontal problems in older populations. Periodontitis, or gum disease leading to tooth loss, is a common contributor to decreased taste sensation and poor nutrition. The inability to chew and swallow food in a comfortable manner works synergistically with decreased smell and taste sensations and other problems that inhibit proper nutrition. The American Dental Association recommends that adults be seen for oral hygiene checks and counseling at least twice a year. During the initial evaluation, follow-up visits are scheduled to ensure that teeth and gums remain in good condition and that appropriate dental care devices are being used.

The skin of the older adult changes, becoming thinner, less elastic, wrinkled, and more fragile. Although sweating decreases and injuries take longer to heal, the skin remains capable of sensing and performing its protective role. Chronic disease, however, can place an individual at risk of decreased sensation throughout the body. Cerebrovascular accidents (strokes) and neuropathies resulting from diabetes are two examples of diseases that disrupt the ability to feel pain and pressure through the skin. This lack of sensation can threaten safety. Older adults benefit from information about safety when cooking on a hot stove and about the appropriate temperature for bathing and showering to prevent burns.

Nurses should perform frequent skin assessments to detect alterations in skin integrity at an early stage and implement appropriate interventions. The potential for skin impairment is common for those who have sensory impairment from physical disease or dementia. A pressure sore (**decubitus ulcer**) is a localized area of tissue necrosis that develops when soft tissue is compressed between two bony prominences or between a bony prominence and an external surface for a prolonged period. In addition to prolonged pressure on the skin, friction, moisture, shearing, and inadequate nutrition place the older adult at risk of developing a decubitus ulcer, which is difficult to treat. Preventing ulcers is the best method for maintaining intact skin. People at risk of decubitus ulcers should change their position at least every 2 hours to redistribute pressure appropriately throughout all areas of the skin. Elevating the lower extremities and maintaining proper body alignment are imperative to prevent decubitus ulcers. Specialty beds are readily available in most care settings to decrease pressure and assist in positioning individuals who are at risk. Positioning pillows and other orthopedic devices provide ways to help maintain the proper support of body parts and body alignment. Proper nutrition, including adequate amounts of zinc and vitamins C and E, will help to prevent this skin problem.

Self-Perception–Self-Concept Pattern

The variability of self-concept in the older adult is similar to the variability seen in the general population. As in all aspects of health, culture, environment, family, lifestyle factors, and heredity are integral to forming self-concept. Self-concept includes an individual's attitudes, perception of abilities (cognitive, affective, or physical), body image, identity, general sense of worth, and general emotional pattern.

Developmental Theories of Aging

Many believe that adults no longer grow emotionally or physically in their later years. In truth, although the rate of physical decline exceeds the rate of physical growth, no evidence was found that emotional growth declines in any way. The film *The Best Exotic Marigold Hotel* illustrates that older adults go through many developmental changes in the 30 to 40 years that often make up older adulthood. Erikson's (1998) theory of development asserts that older adults must pass through developmental stages as do infants, children, and younger adults. As in all stages of psychosocial development, unsuccessful passage through a stage can result in psychological illness, and successful passage through the stage promotes health.

Ego integrity versus despair is the developmental stage of older adults. The quality associated with successful passage of this stage is to achieve a balance between integrity and despair. "The process of bringing into balance feelings of integrity and despair involves a review of and a coming to terms with the life one has lived thus far" (Erikson et al., 1986, p. 70). Based on the increasing life span, this stage of development is expanded into three additional stages: ego differentiation versus work role preoccupation, which involves achieving identity apart from work; body transcendence versus body preoccupation, which focuses on adjusting to normal aging changes; and ego transcendence versus ego preoccupation, which involves accepting death (Erikson, 1998).

Other developmental theorists have built upon Erikson's work. Some of their theories are included in Box 24.4: Theories of Aging. Levinson moved away from Erikson's focus on the role of tensions that emerge during successive stages and instead emphasized that major life transitions are influenced by evolving physiologic, psychological, and role-oriented life changes. Vaillant also moved from an emphasis on "stages" to focus on developmental tasks of life. Vaillant theorized that generativity grows out of one's career. His studies suggested that successful generativity tripled the chances for a person to experience more joy than despair in their 70s. Gilligan criticized Erikson, Levinson, and Vaillant for proposing theories that addressed only male development and focused her work primarily on the unique role of interpersonal connections in female development (Agronin, 2013).

Dr. Gene Cohen is considered the founding father of geriatric psychiatry. Dr. Cohen brought forth the modern concept of old age and focused on the continued potential for growth that occurs in old age. Dr. Cohen's work demonstrates how the brain continually resculpts in response to experience and learning and that creativity increases in old age. Dr. Cohen proposes that older adults develop a **social portfolio** to facilitate moving through various phases of aging. The social portfolio consists of individualized lists of vital activities that individuals can engage in. The activities are a result of an active review of lifelong personal assets. The social portfolio should include vital activities that a person can engage in even when faced with serious disability or loss (Agronin, 2013).

Nurses working in all settings are charged with helping older adults accomplish the task of balancing ego integrity and despair. Two successful methods of support for older adults at all cognitive levels are **reminiscence** and **life review**. An increasing number of researchers have found that reminiscence programs provide older adults with substantial psychosocial health benefits. The beneficial outcomes are enhanced moods, increased socialization, improved cognitive functioning, and enhanced well-being (Tam et al., 2021). There are a variety of reminiscence programs designed to engage participants in discussing their memories, sometimes with reflection prompts such as food or objects from the person's past. Reminiscence therapy helps individuals with dementia remember events, people, and places from their past lives. As part of the therapy, care partners use objects in various activities to help individuals with recall of memories. Reminiscence programs have also been used to treat older adults with mild to moderate depression and older adults residing in nursing homes (Liu et al., 2021). Life review is a more formal therapy technique that takes the person through their life in a structured and chronologic order. Both therapeutic approaches can be done individually or in groups, orally or through writing.

Roles-Relationships Pattern

Although the general framework of self-perception remains constant throughout the life span, the source of an individual's self-perception often changes with older adulthood. The formation of self that focuses on a person's role in a family changes when children become independent or a spouse dies. Roles such as daughter, son, sister, brother, wife, husband, or committed partner may be lost because of death or illness. The loss of these roles can result in grieving, sadness, and potentially depression in some older adults. However, new roles evolve, such as becoming grandparents, great aunts, and uncles (Fig. 24.5).

Approximately 2.55 million children reside in a household with their grandparent(s). In 2022, 486,000 children younger than age 3 lived in a household where a grandparent was present (US Census Bureau Statista, 2023). The role of grandparent frequently brings the older adult great joy and happiness at a time when they feel loss; however, grandparents who rear grandchildren encounter both emotional and physical stress. Their new role as grandparent-caregiver may lead to role confusion and increased health-related problems. However, researchers have also found that these grandparents may show positive levels of physical activity and self-care, especially if they do not perceive caretaking responsibility as highly stressful (Stephan, 2023). Thus it is important for nurses to explore with these individuals what activities may help to reduce stress. Coping strategies or techniques can assist older adults in managing stress. Adults in the caretaking role can manage stress via acceptance of responsibility, self-control, positive reappraisal, planned problem-solving, and distancing. Support groups, counseling, and education to help them manage stress more effectively are other resources that should be explored. Encouraging and supporting older adults in their caregiving role is important to help them ease the stress

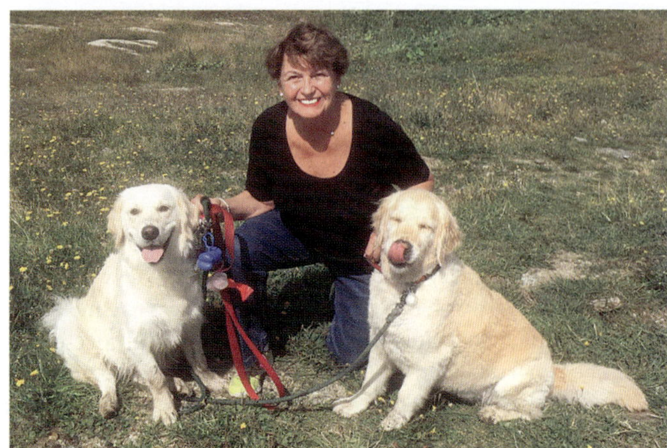

FIG. 24.5 Loss of some roles can provide an opportunity for new roles. As family members grow up and move away, the older adult may decide to devote time to training dogs to be pet therapy dogs.

and strain of changes that come with the caregiving experience. In addition, nurses can work with older adults to identify their approaches to coping strategies. Recognizing whether coping strategies are problem focused versus emotion focused, active versus passive, cognitive versus behavioral, or approach versus avoidant can reduce stressors (Stephan, 2023).

With the average life span increasing, older adults can spend many more years in retirement than previous generations. There were approximately 70.6 million Social Security beneficiaries as of December 2022 (Social Security Administration [SSA], 2022). A variety of factors are predictors of satisfaction with retirement. These factors include good health and functional ability, adequate income, a suitable living environment, a strong social support system, and a positive outlook. An important factor is the autonomy of the retiree in choosing retirement and the preparation for retirement while still working. Retirees in committed relationships and who share similar interests are more satisfied with retirement. Participating in retirement activities that provide an opportunity to feel useful, to learn and grow, and to enjoy oneself is important. Many retirees enjoy sports and hobbies they developed during their working years, and many become more active in volunteerism, community, civic, and political activities (La Rue et al., 2022).

Volunteering can be an effective method for older adults to continue to feel engaged in the community as a productive, contributing member of society. Older adults who volunteer have an external incentive for getting dressed and going out of the house in the morning; they take a great amount of pride in their work. Filling a volunteer position provides a feeling of self-worth and helps to change negative feelings about retirement and other role changes. It also makes important contributions to society.

Federal and state funding has created several subsidized work programs for older adults. With the assistance of this funding through private agencies and local area agencies on aging, older adults are given the opportunity to work for pay. Although the pay may not be comparable with that earned before retirement, the earnings can be a necessary supplement to Social Security benefits. These programs allow older adults to work in programs such as those involving children in day care centers or disabled and ill older adults at home and in administrative positions. Nurses can provide interested individuals with information about these programs.

Downsizing from the family home to a smaller residence, widowhood, retirement, and relocation may elicit profound feelings of loss. Older adults who remain engaged in a variety of activities and relationships are happier and healthier. Personality and its expression over time are considered major determinants of how engaged or active a person will be late in life. Other variables such as culture, health, bereavement, and habit affect activity as well.

Health-promotion activities center on an understanding of the individual's usual behavior and any unexpected or unexplained deviation from that behavior. Nurses can help older adults identify the meaning of their lost roles, the results of those losses, and how to work through reactions to the losses. In more traumatic cases, support groups, such as bereavement groups, can be helpful. The nurse supports older adults going through role changes by eliciting reactions and facilitating communication about these reactions. Significant others, such as children, neighbors, and friends, can provide important support. The nurse is integral in helping older adults to develop and explore their new roles in their older years.

Family Caregiving

Family has always played a role in caring for elders. In the United States, there has been a rise in elder spouses and partners providing this care. Approximately 53 million people help a family member support their health, maintain quality of life, and maintain independence, with the family member requiring assistance because of age, a disability, or a chronic health condition. Grandparent caregivers and relatives account for 2.7 million people. Many older adults and people with disabilities would not be able to live at home and in their communities without this essential support. The cost of unpaid caregiving is estimated at $470 billion each year (USDHHS, 2022).

Nearly 8 out of 10 caregivers report paying for expenses out of pocket. The typical annual total is $7,242, which is a significant amount. Family caregivers, on average, spend 26% of their income on caregiving activities (Skufca & Rainville, 2021).

Caregivers experience physical and emotional strains (Table 24.2). The strains of caregiving not only jeopardize the health of the caregiver but place the individual receiving support at risk for increased medical problems and the potential of losing their caregiver.

Given the burdens of caregiving, the USDHHS, through its Administration for Community Living, released the 2022 National Strategy to Support Family Caregivers. Under this initiative the federal government will support family caregivers of all ages (youth to grandparents) regardless of where they live and whether they are related. Caregivers will be compensated for their role in providing long-term care. These actions recognize that many caregivers often lack resources to maintain their health, well-being, and financial security while providing the necessary support for their family (USDHHS, 2021). Nurses can play an important role in providing families with information about this program and referring families to agencies that determine eligibility and assist in the application process.

Sexuality-Reproductive Pattern

The WHO defines sexual health as "a state of physical, emotional, mental and social well-being in relation to sexuality" (2020). In older adults, as in all adults, sexual health is characterized by an approach to sexual relationships that is positive and respectful. There has been much debate regarding the presence or absence of sexual desire among older adults, and many assume that older adults do not participate in sexual relationships. There are numerous myths about sexual activity among older adults. These include (1) most older males have erectile dysfunction (**impotence**) and are therefore unable to have sexual intercourse; (2) after menopause, older females no longer have sexual desire; (3) physical and psychological impediments in older adults make them unable to have sexual intercourse; (4) an aging body is not sexy; and (5) older people should not

TABLE 24.2 Safety Risk Areas and Related Interventions

Area of Attention	Intervention
Stairways	Secure handrails. Illuminate stairways with light switches at both top and bottom. Eliminate clutter on all steps and stair landings. Use nonskid treads on steps.
Bedroom	Use nightlights. Tack down carpet. Discourage use of throw rugs. Arrange furniture so that it will not obstruct clear pathways. Secure extension cords and telephone wires and remove them from walking areas. For smokers, never smoke in bed.
Bathroom	Use handrails near tub and toilet. Use nonskid mats in tub area and on floor. Use a bath thermometer to measure hot water in tub. Use nightlights.
Kitchen	Wear nonflammable, lightweight clothing when cooking. Place dishes and cooking utensils at reasonable heights. Use stepstools with a handrail according to specifications and only when not alone. Keep off wet floor and refrain from using slippery wax. Never climb on chairs. Keep emergency numbers near the telephone. Ensure locks can be easily opened in times of emergency. Cook on the front burners of the stove rather than on the back ones Do not use electrical appliances with frayed cords.
Living room	Use furniture that is easy to get in and out of. Eliminate clutter on all floor areas. Install fire detectors at appropriate places.
Outdoors	Make sure stairs are free of breaks and cracks and clear of snow and ice. Use safe handrails. Provide good lighting for stairs and walkways.

have sex. It is important to realize that sex does not belong solely to the young and that sexual contact correlates with enhanced health, positive relationships, and improved stress management.

Older adults who do not identify as heterosexual experience health disparities because of their gender orientation. Based on population estimates, 2.7% of adults aged 50 to 64 and 1.8% of adults aged 65 and older identify as lesbian, gay, bisexual, transgender, or queer or questioning (LGBTQ) (Flores & Conron, 2023).

Healthy People 2030 includes goals to achieve health equity and improve the health, safety, and well-being of LGBTQ individuals; however, research suggests that these individuals continue to face health disparities linked to social stigma, discrimination, and denial of their civil and human rights (Valdiserri et al., 2019). The LBGTQ older adult population is more likely to delay seeking treatment for health problems and thus have higher incidences of disease transmission and progression, mental health problems, and physical ailments, resulting in increased health care costs and decreased longevity. Nurses who use compassionate and nonjudgmental approaches and use open-ended questions about relationship status and sexual orientation provide a supportive environment in which LGBTQ older adults can openly express their concerns about their health and well-being (Brown et al., 2019).

The most accurate predictor of sexual interest in older adulthood is the enjoyment and frequency of sex at a younger age. There is no evidence that males or females lose interest in sexual activity as they age. Older adults also need to fulfill the human needs for intimacy and love and to touch and be touched. Touch is an overt expression of closeness and an integral part of sexuality. Although the need to express sexuality continues, older adults are susceptible to many chronic medical conditions, such as cardiac problems, arthritis, and normal aging changes that can make sexual intercourse difficult. The reduced availability of sex hormones results in less rapid and less extreme vascular responses to sexual arousal. The lack of circulating hormones in males and females results in changes in four areas of the sexual system: arousal, orgasm, post orgasm, and extragenital changes. In females the vagina becomes narrower, shorter, and thinner, and there is less natural lubrication. Males experience less intense and slower erections, increased difficulty regaining an erection, decreased force of ejaculation, and an extended refractory time. Medications and other measures to manage medical conditions can also hinder sexual response.

Nurses are in an ideal position to help older adults find ways to fulfill their sexual desires by compensating for normal aging changes and chronic medical conditions and medications. Knowledge is essential to the successful fulfillment of sexual needs. After conducting a sexual assessment, nurses can intervene to prevent or correct problems, but nurses often choose not to consider sexuality when planning care. Reasons for not assessing older adults sexually may be that nurses believe the societal myths about sexuality of older adults. With proper education and experience, they may be sufficiently confident to venture into this delicate area.

One way in which nurses can gain knowledge of the sexual needs of older adults is through a staff development program using role-play to discuss and process feelings associated with an older person's limitations in fulfilling intimate and sexual relationships. The expression of intimacy and sexuality among older adults results in a higher quality of life achieved through fulfilling a natural desire. In long-term care facilities, the need to address sexual needs of residents is great because of difficulties related to their chronic illnesses and because of a lack of resident privacy to engage in intimate and sexual relationships. Long-term care facilities can develop policies to assist residents in effectively fulfilling the need for intimacy and sexuality.

Many nurses believe that acquired immunodeficiency syndrome (AIDS) and other sexually transmitted diseases (STDs) are not problems for older adults. However, the number of cases of human immunodeficiency virus (HIV) infection and AIDS in older adults continues to increase because greater numbers of older adults are becoming newly infected with HIV, and an increasing proportion of those who have HIV are reaching their older years (CDC, 2023b). Two areas that are so important for successful aging—cognition and social engagement—are of concern for those aging with HIV because declines in both areas have been observed in this population. Approximately 50% of individuals with HIV experience cognitive problems, and as people age, they may be at increased risk of developing cognitive changes. Social support and engagement often decline for many older adults and may be exacerbated by stigma and depression in older adults with HIV (Brown & Adeagbo, 2021). It is important for nurses to suggest ways to promote social engagement, as this may help improve both mood and cognitive functioning.

Older adults are just as susceptible to STIs as younger adults. STIs have doubled among adults aged 55 and older from an average rate of 11.8 per 100,000 people in 2014 to a population-adjusted rate for chlamydia, gonorrhea, and primary and secondary syphilis of 24.5 per 100,000 people (Shaw, 2020).

A survey conducted by the American Sexual Health Association showed that only 5.1% of males older than 61 years had used a condom in recent sex (Esposito, 2016). Older adults may not perceive they are at risk for a STI even though there has been a dramatic increase among those who are widowed and divorced (Smith et al., 2020). Because STIs are noted in younger individuals, elders do not see themselves reflected in brochures. Brochures do not provide images of individuals with gray hair and wrinkles (Esposito, 2016). Given the invisibility of older adults and their sexuality, it is important that older adults are educated about the disease risks in their sexual relationships and follow the recommended guidelines for safer sex.

Coping–Stress Tolerance Pattern

An individual's ability to cope with the common stresses of older adulthood is a key factor in maintaining self-concept. As people age, they tend to encounter many losses, such as the loss of a home, spouses, friends, siblings, and even children. They also experience declines in income, health, and physical functioning. The nurse who cares for the older adult can provide support related to these losses during the coping process. Trying to find the positive and developmental benefits of losses is preferable to continually thinking about a loss or bad event. Negative associations have been found between depressive symptoms and rumination, catastrophizing, and self-blame. After assessing the most appropriate way in which the individual desires to cope with a situation, the nurse may help create a suitable environment for coping.

Spirituality is also an important consideration in helping some older adults cope with stressful situations. The concept of spirituality is broad and is framed by the individual. Spirituality may be exercised privately or through a religious framework. However, the effect of spirituality on quality of life has been well documented among older adults and often has a strong relationship with their ability to cope with the changes and losses of aging.

Depression

Among older adults, **depression** may mainly affect those with chronic illnesses and cognitive impairment and result in suffering, family disruption, and disability. Depression can worsen the outcomes of many illnesses and increase mortality. Aging-related and disease-related processes, including arteriosclerosis and endocrine and immune system changes, compromise the integrity of front striatal pathways, the amygdala, and the hippocampus and increase vulnerability to depression. Heredity factors may also play a part. Psychosocial adversity—economic impoverishment, disability, isolation, relocation, caregiving, and bereavement—contributes to physiologic changes, further increasing susceptibility to depression or triggering depression in already vulnerable older individuals.

It is important to know that most older adults are not depressed; however, the stigma associated with mental health may deter older adults from seeking treatment. Estimates of major depression in community-dwelling older adults range from less than 1% to 5%, but these percentages rise to 13.5% in those who need home health care (CDC, 2022a). The National Institute of Mental Health (2023) notes that the risk of depression increases in older adults as they experience chronic illnesses and their ability to function becomes impaired. The numerous losses experienced by older people may also play a role. Depression is also caused by physiologic changes in the aging body. Although depression appears to affect older adults in much the same way that it affects younger individuals, certain patterns of symptoms and older adults' overall susceptibility are different from those of younger counterparts.

Nurses are integral in helping to diagnose and manage depression in older adults. Depression can be found in all care environments. Some common signs are lack of appetite and weight loss, sleep disorders, fatigue, decreased ability to think or concentrate, psychomotor agitation, decreased participation in daily living and social activities, social withdrawal, and suicidal ideation. There are instruments available to assist nurses in assessing depression in older adults. The Geriatric Depression Scale (Yesavage et al., 1982) is available in several formats (30, 15, 5, or 1 question) and is easily administered. Positive results on the screening examinations require a referral to social services for further evaluation. After depression has been diagnosed, successful management may include implementation of antidepressant medications and psychosocial therapy.

Suicide

The suicide rate for older Americans is disproportionally high in the American population and is a major public health problem. Suicide rates are particularly higher among older males, with males ages 85 and older having the highest rate of any group in the country. Suicide attempts by older adults are much more likely to result in death than among younger persons because (1) older adults plan more carefully and use more deadly methods, (2) older adults are less likely to be discovered and rescued, and (3) the physical frailty of older adults means they are less likely to recover from an attempt. In 2021, the suicide rate for males aged 55 and older was 29.6 deaths per 100,000, and for females it was 6.2 deaths per 100,000. This number rises for adults aged 75 to 84 (38.2 per 100,000) and is even higher for adults aged 85 and older (55.7 per 100,000). Common suicide methods used by older adults are firearms, poison, overdose of pills, gas, and suffocation (Garnett et al., 2023).

The reason for the high number of suicides in the older adult population continues to be explored. The elevated rates of depression in older adults may assist the medical community with motives for suicide. Many older adults have serious medical illnesses, which can play a large part in suicidal ideations. Risk factors for suicidal ideation and suicide attempts include social isolation, alcohol and substance use, psychosis, bereavement, and ongoing medical illnesses.

The importance of different aspects of life also differs by the older adult's self-reported culture. However, it is important for nurses and clinicians to recognize that culture is mediated by an individual's education, assimilation status, income, and occupation. Using cultural awareness reduces biases about a patient's culture. Some older adults may visit a health care provider with a somatic problem before the suicide attempt. This action may be a call for help; therefore, nurses working with older adults must be aware of the high rate of suicide in this age group and be alert for the risk factors. Older adults exhibiting signs of depression must be asked about possible suicidal thoughts, and suicide threats must be taken seriously, with interventions implemented to keep the older adult safe.

The incidence of chronic illness that frequently accompanies old age raises a concern for ethical care. Many members of society believe that with the increased life span, individuals may be subjected to more suffering. A solution to ending the suffering of those with chronic illness has been **euthanasia**, or **physician-assisted suicide**. Physician-assisted suicide is legal in nine US states and the District of Columbia. Individuals have an option by law in the District of Columbia, Hawai'i, Maine, New Jersey, Oregon, Vermont, and Washington and by court decision in Montana and California.

Nurses can educate patients, families, politicians, and clinicians about the benefits of being an older adult and the ways in which extended life spans bring about positive and negative issues. Nurses caring for chronically ill older adults have the added responsibility of assessing pain and ensuring that chronically ill older adults are comfortable and pain free using pharmacologic and nonpharmacologic interventions. Nurses are instrumental in making sure that the older person experiences a pain-free death by advocating for an appropriate pain-management program and working with other health care professionals toward this goal. Nurses should also not dismiss chronically ill adults who want to discuss physician-assisted suicide in those states in which this option is legal.

Values-Beliefs Pattern

Every person nurses care for will have a different sense of spirituality. For many older adults, spirituality may have an influence on the way they choose to live and their decisions about health care. Many older adults describe themselves as both spiritual and religious. A spiritual life may help some older adults overcome the pain and distress of chronic health and psychosocial problems that arise in their later years (Forlenza & Vellada, 2018).

Nurses should understand that for some older adults, spirituality plays a significant role in meaning-making in relation to attitudes and beliefs about the world, self, and others. Because of the highly personal quality of spirituality, nurses should be unobtrusive and sensitive toward the older adult's need to achieve spiritual health. Spiritual assessment tools are available as a guide for nurses to ask questions to better understand the person's spirituality. Open-ended questions such as "What is your perception of a higher being and spirituality?" encourage discussions about the person's innermost spirituality. The nurse can provide an environment that is supportive to the practice of the person's spirituality. Helping older persons actualize their spirituality can provide them with great comfort and lead nurses to a deeper understanding of their own spirituality.

ENVIRONMENTAL PROCESSES

Physical Agents

Accidents

Healthy People 2030 identifies goals of preventing unintentional injuries and violence, as well as reducing the consequences of these problems (USDHHS, n.d.). One important focus for injury prevention in older adults is falls. Falls are a leading cause of morbidity and death among older adults. One in three older adults falls each year, and one in five falls results in a serious injury, such as a fracture or head injury (National Institute of Aging [NIA], 2022). Each year 2.5 million older adults are treated for fall injuries in emergency departments. More than 95% of hip fractures are caused by falls, and each year 250,000 older adults are hospitalized for a hip fracture. It is essential that nurses are knowledgeable about interventions for prevention (Box 24.8: Quality and Safety Scenario).

Some of the causes of falls in older adults are neuromuscular dysfunction, osteoporosis, stroke, and sensory impairment. Falls can result in decreased mobility, decreased ability to live independently, and increased risk of an early death. Although a fall in a younger individual may not be problematic, a fall in an older adult can have devastating consequences. Falls account for 40% of admissions to nursing homes each year. Even if older adults are not injured in a fall, they may develop a fear of falling and limit activities that increase their risk of future falls.

Because of the higher risk of osteoporosis in the older population, a fall can result in a fracture. **Osteoporosis** is a disease of bone loss common to females aged 70 years or older and males aged 80 years or older. The disease develops six times more frequently in women than it does in males. The rapid decline in estrogen secretion at the onset of menopause signals the calcium in the bones to move into the bloodstream, which causes the bones to become weak and brittle. Because of this weakness, falls in older adults with osteoporosis frequently result in fractures, which place these individuals in a spiral of iatrogenic risk, beginning with weeks of decreased mobility and possibly resulting in decubitus ulcers, psychological trauma, pneumonia, and even death.

BOX 24.8 QUALITY AND SAFETY SCENARIO

Fall Prevention for Older Adults in the Community

Falls in community-dwelling older adults are a critical problem for nurses to address, as falls are the leading cause of injury in older adults. Between 30% and 40% of community-dwelling adults aged 65 years and older fall at least once per year. The US Preventive Services Task Force (USPSTF) makes and periodically updates recommendations about the effectiveness of specific clinical preventive services for older adults. The recommendations are based on evidence of both the benefits and harms of the service. These recommendations are intended to provide helpful information for clinicians, but the USPSTF emphasizes that clinical decisions involve more considerations than evidence alone and that clinicians need to individualize decision-making for a specific client.

The USPSTF notes that various approaches to identify people at increased risk are helpful. There is no single evidence-based instrument that accurately identifies older adults at increased risk of falling. Clinicians need to assess risk based on a variety of factors, such as a history of falls and impaired mobility and balance. Early intervention is important for people assessed to be at risk, as these interventions can prevent serious injury.

The USPSTF states that more research is needed for clinical validation of tools to identify older adults at risk of falling. It also recommends efficacy trials for interventions related to vision correction, medication withdrawal, protein supplementation, education or counseling, and home hazard modification.

Summary of Recommendations

- The USPSTF recommends exercise interventions to prevent falls in community-dwelling adults 65 years and older who are at increased risk for falls.
- The USPSTF recommends against vitamin D supplementation to prevent falls in community-dwelling adults 65 years and older.
- The USPSTF recommends that clinicians selectively offer multifactorial interventions to prevent falls in community-dwelling adults 65 years and older who are at increased risk for falls.

From US Preventive Services Task Force. (2024). *Falls prevention in community-dwelling older adults: Interventions.* https://www.uspreventiveservicestaskforce.org/uspstf/search_results?searchterm=Falls%20prevention%20in%20community-dwelling%20older%20adults%3A%20Interventions.%20

The risk factors for osteoporosis include a small, thin frame; family history of osteoporosis; excessive thyroid medication or high doses of cortisone-like drugs for treatment of asthma, arthritis, or cancer; a diet low in dairy products and other sources of calcium; physical inactivity; smoking cigarettes; and drinking alcohol. Osteoporosis is typically diagnosed after an older adult sustains a fracture. However, bone density testing is available to determine the risk of a bone fracture. This test helps to estimate the density of one's bones and the chance of breaking a bone. Calcium intake remains vitally important and will continue to reduce the normal bone loss of aging. Health care providers frequently monitor calcium and vitamin D levels as a part of wellness care in older adults. Most females need 1000 mg daily before menopause and 1500 mg daily after menopause. Consuming this amount of calcium from the current average diet is difficult; therefore, a calcium supplement is essential. Vitamin D is also essential for bone health. Although one can obtain adequate vitamin D by daily exposure to the sun, because of concerns about the amount of sun exposure necessary, 400 to 800 IU of vitamin D via supplements is usually recommended in conjunction with calcium. For the prevention of osteoporosis and the optimal maintenance of both psychological and physical well-being in the older adult, regular physical activity is necessary.

Governmental concern about falls among older adults has resulted in a *Healthy People 2030* objective to prevent emergency room visits and decrease the rate of fall-related deaths (Moncada & Mire, 2017). Less than half of older adults tell their health care provider about a fall, so it is important for nurses to inquire about falls. Because many factors contribute to falls, risk assessment is essential. If a fall has been sustained, the older adult is at increased risk of falling again, and fall-prevention strategies must be implemented. Several fall risk assessment tools have been developed, but more research is needed to validate their use in different settings. By identifying the risks of falls and assessing an older adult's vision, hearing, medication use, blood pressure, mobility, and other factors, nurses can predict and prevent many falls (CDC, 2023c).

Table 24.2 lists frequent causes of accidents that occur in the home and nursing interventions to prevent them. Home care nurses are in an ideal position to prevent injuries. During the initial and subsequent assessments, the nurse can evaluate individuals' homes for common factors leading to fires, poisoning, and falls, such as frayed wires on electrical appliances that can produce sparks and start fires, improperly labeled cleaning products that can be accidentally ingested, loose rugs on the floor, absence of handrails on stairs or in bathrooms, and poor lighting that can cause falls. Appropriate health teaching incorporates the concept of accident prevention for all older adults living not only in the community but also in acute care facilities and long-term care facilities.

The older adult's ability to feel changes in heat and cold may be impaired because of normal and pathologic changes of aging. This process can cause older adults to die of the effects of excessive heat or cold. During periods of high temperature and humidity, older people should increase fluid and salt intake, stay in a cool and shaded environment, remain calm, have more rest periods, and refrain from going outdoors when the temperature is higher than 90°F. Sweating, which is reduced in older adults, can be accommodated by the wearing of light-colored, lightweight cotton clothing. If sweating ceases or is inadequate, the older person is at risk of heat stroke. Heat stroke can contribute to sepsis, myocardial infarction, and cerebrovascular accidents, particularly in people with diabetes. Reduced body heat can also present problems in older adults. Symptoms of and interventions for hypothermia are listed in Box 24.9.

Preventing Injury

Falls and fires are leading causes of unintentional injury and death in people 65 years and older. Other unintentional injuries and deaths in older adults are caused by motor vehicle accidents, suffocation, and poisoning. Because of normal age-related changes and the increased incidence of chronic illness, older adults can experience decreased muscle strength and delayed reaction time and subsequently become more vulnerable to environmental hazards. Decreased sensory acuity and

BOX 24.9 Nursing Interventions for Hypothermia

Symptoms

- Cold to touch
- Slow respiration
- Bradycardia
- Low blood pressure
- Slurred speech
- Drowsiness
- Temperature 95°F rectally

Interventions

- Warm hands and feet
- Cover with blanket
- Set room temperature to 70°F
- Wear cap to bed at night
- Wear socks to bed at night
- Wear several layers of clothing
- Increase activity
- Decrease alcohol intake
- Use extreme caution with space heaters, heating pads, and electric blankets

BOX 24.10 When to Stop Driving

Poor driving skills that are warning signs of unsafe driving include the following:

- Delayed response to unexpected situations
- Becoming easily distracted while driving
- Decrease in confidence while driving
- Having difficulty moving into or maintaining the correct lane of traffic
- Hitting curbs when making right turns or backing up
- Getting scrapes or dents on car, garage, or mailbox
- Having frequent close calls
- Driving too fast or too slow for road conditions

From the American Association of Retired Persons (AARP). (2016). *We need to talk: The difficult driving conversation.* https://www.aarp.org/auto/driver-safety/info-2016/when-to-stop-driving-in-older-age.html

impaired balance further diminish their ability to interpret the environment.

As the percentage of older adults living in the United States increases, the number of older drivers also increases. In 2022 there were 52 million licensed drivers 65 years of age or older. Each day an average of 740 older adults experience an injury from a car crash (CDC, 2024). Age-related changes in vision, joint mobility, and cognitive changes may affect the older person's ability to drive. Because of these changes, older adults often avoid driving at night, in bad weather, in heavy traffic, on long trips, or on highways or high-speed roads (CDC, 2022b).

Because of changes in neuromuscular and sensory abilities, which slow response time in emergency situations, older adults are at increased risk of severe injury resulting in hospitalization, disability, or death from motor vehicle injuries.

In 2020, 7500 older adults were killed in motor vehicle crashes, and more than 200,000 were treated in emergency departments for motor vehicle crash injuries (CDC, 2022b). Most traffic fatalities involving older adults occur during the daytime and involve other vehicles. In two-vehicle fatal crashes involving both older and younger drivers, the older driver's vehicle was more than twice as likely to be struck than the younger person's, indicating a decline in defensive driving as opposed to an increase in aggressive driving among older adults. However, older drivers involved in fatal automobile accidents had the lowest blood alcohol level.

Older adults are encouraged to take senior driving safety courses to understand how aging can affect their driving and learn strategies for safer driving. Nurses working in the community may encourage older drivers to contact the AARP or the American Automobile Association (AAA) for driving classes designed to meet their needs. In addition, attending these classes often provides savings on vehicle insurance. At some point, it may be better for older adults to stop driving. Box 24.10 offers warning signs that suggest when an older adult should limit or stop driving. Older adults are often resistant to stopping driving because driving is an important sign of independence. When an older adult has a motor vehicle accident, it may be time for families to talk about not driving. In the case of an older adult with dementia, health care providers may need to talk with family members about preventing the person from driving. If an older adult has been found to be an unsafe driver and refuses to stop driving, a family member may take away the car keys or mechanically disable the car so that it cannot be driven. However, it is important to find ways for the older adult to continue to participate in pleasurable activities and not to become isolated. For example, a loss of spiritual connections may occur when older adults can no longer drive to their place of worship. In rural areas, many older adults manage farms and depend on their ability to drive to obtain needed supplies and services. Family members or friends may be able to set up a schedule to alternate driving the person to the supermarket, church, entertainment activities, and other places. Driving older adults to their activities also provides important social interactions.

Elder Mistreatment

Elder abuse (elder mistreatment) refers to intentional or neglectful acts by a caregiver or trusted person that results in, or may lead to, harm of a vulnerable elder. Elder abuse is defined as mistreatment, physical abuse, neglect, emotional or psychological abuse, verbal abuse and threats, financial abuse and exploitation, sexual abuse, and abandonment. In many states, self-neglect is also considered mistreatment (Storey, 2020).

Approximately 1 in 10 Americans aged 60 and older has experienced some form of elder abuse. Some estimates range as high as five million elders abused each year. One study estimated that only 1 in 14 cases of abuse are reported to authorities. Warning signs of elder abuse are physical abuse, neglect, or mistreatment (bruises, pressure marks, broken bones, abrasions, burns); emotional abuse (unexplained withdrawal from normal activities, sudden changes in alertness, unusual depression, strained or tense relationships, frequent arguments between the caregiver and older adult); financial abuse (sudden changes in financial situations); neglect (bedsores, unattended medical needs, poor hygiene, unusual weight loss); and verbal or emotional abuse (belittling, threats, other uses of power and control by individuals) (CDC, 2021a).

Victims of elder abuse are more likely to be single females older than 75 years who are dependent on the caregiver for food and shelter. They are more likely to be frail, to be incontinent, or to have mental disability. The abuser is usually the adult son or daughter of the victim, who has poor impulse control and low self-esteem (Nies & McEwan, 2019). Nurses have a responsibility to identify abuse, provide appropriate care for injuries, and report suspected abuse to appropriate state agencies or law enforcement personnel. The nurse may consult social services to find a more suitable living arrangement for the victim. The most important consideration is to provide a safe environment for the older adult who is in immediate danger.

Biologic Agents

Because of decreased immune system responses, older adults are susceptible to bacterial and viral disease. In many cases, older adults have not received primary immunization against diphtheria and tetanus. A large emphasis is placed on immunizing young children against communicable disease; however, older adults can also be protected by commonly available vaccines that have been shown to lower both morbidity and mortality. Influenza and pneumonia are two disease processes that are associated with higher mortality and morbidity.

Influenza remains a significant cause of morbidity and death in older adults. Flu vaccinations play an important role in reducing morbidity and mortality of influenza. The influenza vaccine, composed of inactivated whole virus or viral subunits grown in chick embryo cells, is given annually to older adults. Vaccinating high-risk adults with chronic conditions such as pulmonary or cardiac problems and those in long-term care facilities is especially important. Vaccination is contraindicated in individuals who had a previous reaction to the vaccine and are allergic to eggs. However, in 2019, two vaccines licensed for use were manufactured without using eggs and are considered egg free. The vaccine Flublok quadrivalent is licensed for use in adults 18 years and older, and Flucelvax quadrivalent is licensed for use in age groups 4 years and older. Both egg-free vaccines can be given to those who were previously allergic to the egg-based vaccine (CDC, 2019).

COVID-19 was first detected in December 2019. Approximately 1.3 million cases have been reported worldwide, of which approximately 330,000 cases were in the United States. COVID-19 hospitalization rates increase with age. As of April 2020, the hospitalization rate for adults aged 65 to 74 was 2258 per 100,000, and the rate for adults aged 75 to 84 was 3913 per 100,000 (Garg et al., 2020).

Pneumococcal Infections

Deaths from pneumococcal infections have declined in recent years, indicating the value of public health initiatives to spread information about the importance of immunization against pneumonia and influenza. Implementation of immunization programs in public places such as supermarkets and pharmacies, in addition to medical offices and clinics, has enhanced access to this preventive measure. Nevertheless, many older adults remain unvaccinated. The Centers for Disease Control and Prevention (CDC) recommends that adults aged 65 years and older receive the pneumococcal vaccination. It is important that nurses inform the public about the importance of immunizations and counteract the myth that receiving the vaccination will result in the disease, which often prevents older adults from receiving immunization (CDC, 2023a).

Cancer

Cancer rates for older adults are disproportionately high in the United States. Although only 12% of the population is considered to be older adults, more than 50% of all diagnosed cancers are found in this population, and the death rate for cancer is highest among adults aged 65 years and older. The reason for the large proportion of cancer in the United States is unknown. Theories include longer exposure to carcinogens, increased susceptibility to cancer in the older body, decreased cellular healing ability, loss of tumor-suppressing genes, and decreased immune function. Although the exact cause cannot be determined, cancer is a significant problem for older adults in the United States.

The types of cancer common to older adults are listed by sex in Table 24.3. Prostate cancer is the second leading cause of cancer deaths in males in the United States. It is estimated that 8% of all males in the United States will receive a diagnosis of prostate cancer during their lifetime. Early detection of prostate cancer allows treatment while it is still localized in the prostate gland and highly curable. Evidence suggests that by using a combination of screening techniques, such as prostatic specific antigen and digital rectal exam, and asking about symptoms may detect prostate cancer earlier. The four major treatment options for prostate cancer are surgery, radiation therapy, watchful waiting, and hormone therapy.

Breast cancer is the most common cancer in females. Only lung cancer surpasses breast cancer death rates. About one in nine females will develop breast cancer in her lifetime. Breast cancer typically occurs in middle-aged and older females. The median age for breast cancer diagnosis is 62. The risk of breast cancer increases in females whose close female relatives (mothers or sisters) have had the disease. Females who have never had children or who had their first child after age 30 years appear to have an increased risk. The causes of breast cancer remain unclear. The best protection is early detection and prompt treatment.

Breast cancer screening in older women should continue until age 74 or 75. However, the decision to screen beyond 75 should be a shared decision process (Schrager et al., 2020). Screening should continue if a female is in good health and is expected to live at least 10 more years. Nurses can provide education about mammogram screening.

Nurses can help older adults change the habits that place them at high risk of developing cancer. Following nutritional guidelines (as suggested earlier in this chapter), reducing stress, adopting a program of regular exercise, and stopping smoking and other use of tobacco products are a few of the approaches nurses can advise to promote individual wellness. Periodic monitoring and screening in the form of regular visits to a primary health care provider or community screening can alert older adults to early signs and symptoms of cancers that occur during the later years.

TABLE 24.3 **Long-Term Care Housing and Assessment Continuum**

	Independent Living	Retirement Community	Assisted Living	Nursing Facility
Description	Covers a broad range of housing options (residential houses, apartments, condominiums, townhouses, subsidized senior housing) for older people who are functionally and socially independent	Provides a living arrangement that integrates shelter and services for older people who do not need 24-hour protective oversight	Provides a living arrangement that integrates shelter and services for frail older people who are functionally and/or socially impaired and require 24-hour protective oversight	Provides a living arrangement that integrates shelter with medical, nursing, psychosocial, and rehabilitation services for older people who require 24-hour nursing supervision
Primary services	**A** Environmental security Possible coordination of resident services (transportation, activities, housekeeping) Or no services are available	**B** A plus: Meals (one to three per day) Transportation Activities Housekeeping assistance Assistance with coordination of community-based services	**C** A and B plus: Assistance with activities of daily living Medication monitoring, with 24-hour protective oversight	**D** A, B, and C plus: Medication administration, with 24-hour nursing supervision
Mobility	Capable of moving about independently or ambulatory with cane or walker Independent with wheelchair, but needs help in an emergency	Capable of moving about independently Able to seek and follow directions Able to evacuate independently in emergency or ambulatory with cane or walker Independent with wheelchair, but needs help in an emergency	Mobile, but may require escort or assistance resulting from confusion, poor vision, weakness, or poor motivation, or requires occasional assistance to move about but is usually independent	May require assistance with transfers from bed, chair, and toilet, or requires transfer and transport assistance Requires turning and positioning in bed and wheelchair
Nutrition	Able to prepare own meals; eats without assistance	Able to prepare own meals; eats without assistance Generally, a minimum of one meal a day is available	All meals and snacks are provided May require assistance getting to dining room, or requires minimal assistance (opening cartons or other packages, cutting food, or preparing trays)	May be unable or unwilling to go to dining room May be dependent on staff for eating or feeding needs, or may be fully dependent on staff for nourishment (includes reminders to eat)
Hygiene	Independent in all care, including bathing and personal laundry	Independent in all care, including bathing and personal laundry	May require assistance with bathing or hygiene, or may require assistance, initiation, structure, or reminders May be able to complete tasks	May be dependent on staff for all personal hygiene
Housekeeping	Independent in performing housekeeping functions (includes making bed, vacuuming, cleaning, and laundry)	Independent in performing housekeeping functions (includes making bed, vacuuming, cleaning, and laundry), or may need assistance with heavy housekeeping, vacuuming, laundry, and linens	Housekeeping and laundry services provided	Housekeeping and laundry services provided
Dressing	Independent and dresses appropriately	Independent and dresses appropriately	May require occasional assistance with shoelaces, zippers, or medical appliances or garments, or may require reminders, initiation, or motivation	May be dependent on staff for dressing
Toileting	Independent and continent	Independent and completely continent, or may have incontinence, colostomy, or catheter, but independent in caring for self through proper use of supplies	Same as for retirement community, or may have occasional problem with incontinence, colostomy, or catheter, and may require assistance in caring for self through proper use of supplies	May have problem with incontinence, colostomy, or catheter and require assistance, or may be dependent and unable to communicate needs

TABLE 24.3 Long-Term Care Housing and Assessment Continuum—cont'd

	Independent Living	Retirement Community	Assisted Living	Nursing Facility
Medications	Responsible for self-administration of all medications	Responsible for self-administration of all medications, or may arrange for family or home health agency to establish a medication administration system	Able to self-administer medications, or facility staff may remind the person about or monitor the process, or facility staffed by registered nurses or licensed practical nurses who administer medications	Medications administered by staff personnel or self if assessed as capable
Mental status	Oriented to person, place, and time Memory intact, but may have occasional forgetfulness Able to reason, plan, and organize daily events Mentally capable of identifying needs and meeting them	Oriented to person, place, and time Memory intact, but may have occasional forgetfulness without consistent pattern of memory loss Able to reason, plan, and organize daily events Mentally capable of identifying environmental needs and meeting them	May require occasional direction or guidance in getting from place to place, or may have difficulty with occasional confusion that results in anxiety, social withdrawal, or depression Orientation to time, place, or person may be impaired	Judgment can be poor, and may attempt tasks that are not within capabilities, or may require strong orientation and reminder program May need guidance in getting from place to place May be disoriented to time, place, and person, or memory is severely impaired
Behavioral status	Deals appropriately with emotions and uses available resources to cope with inner stress	Deals appropriately with emotions, and uses available resources to cope with inner stress Deals appropriately with other residents and staff, or may require periodic intervention from staff to resolve conflicts with others to cope with situational stress	May require periodic intervention from staff to facilitate expression of feelings to cope with inner stress, or may require periodic intervention from staff to resolve conflicts with others to cope with situational stress	May require regular intervention from staff to facilitate expression of feelings and to deal with periodic outbursts of anxiety or agitation Maximal staff intervention may be required to manage behavior

Chemical Agents

Chemical agents can be both therapeutic and harmful depending on their use. The increased use of prescription and over-the-counter medications can result in increased adverse drug events. The use of alcohol and tobacco products can be especially harmful for older adults.

Drug Use

Normal changes of aging have a significant effect on the pharmacodynamics of drugs in older adults. The ways in which medications are absorbed, distributed, metabolized, and excreted from the body are affected by normal physiologic changes and by illness. Even when medications are taken as prescribed, age-related changes and disease increase the risk of undesirable side effects. Older adults are more likely to take multiple medications, resulting in increased risk of serious drug interactions. In addition to potential adverse effects caused by prescription drugs, older adults may take over-the-counter nonprescription substances such as vitamins, minerals, supplements, herbal remedies, and other remedies used to resolve common ailments. **Polypharmacy**, or the use of multiple medications for the same or for different health problems, is a major concern for older adults. Approximately one-third of older adults in the United States take five or more prescription drugs. The higher rate of polypharmacy in older adults compared with younger groups is related to increased health problems in older adults and new medications that effectively treat these conditions. The Beers Criteria provides guidelines for potentially inappropriate medications for the elderly. The guidelines list medications known to place older adults at risk of adverse reactions (American Geriatric Society, 2023).

Many older adults who reside at home take their medications independently. Although self-medication with prescription and nonprescription substances is an effective method of disease management, little is known about how older adults take their medications after leaving the health care practice or facility. Although it is generally assumed that medications are taken as prescribed, sensory disturbances; lack of knowledge; and alternative drug, alcohol, and nutrition practices may present challenges to medication self-administration, as well as interfere with medical management of health problems. Nurses should take a thorough medication history to assess the older adult for past drug reactions and identify currently prescribed and nonprescription substances. Typically, new medications are prescribed at their lowest effective dose and increased slowly as necessary. Nurses should be aware of this medical practice, review dosage information, and contact the prescriber if this does not seem to be the case.

One of the major barriers to drug adherence in the older adult is affordability. Medicare provides prescription drug coverage to everyone eligible for Medicare under Medicare Part D. One can get Medicare drug coverage in one of two ways: a Medicare Prescription Drug Plan (PDP) or a Medicare Advantage Plan (preferred provider organization [PPO] or health maintenance organization [HMO]). Lower-income older adults who are not eligible for Medicaid (dual coverage) may need assistance in purchasing their medications. Affordable prescription drugs are available via several methods: switching coverage to a less-costly drug plan or applying to pharmaceutical company assistance programs, state pharmaceutical assistance programs, national- and community-based charitable programs, and the Extra Help program through Medicare and Social Security.

Alcohol and Drug Abuse

Substance abuse among Americans aged 60 years and older, including misuse of prescription drugs, is estimated to affect approximately 17% of older adults (Yarnell et al., 2020). Alcohol is widely used among older adults. Sixty-five percent of adults aged 65 and older report high-risk drinking. High-risk drinking is defined as exceeding daily guidelines at least weekly in the past year (National Institute of Drug Abuse [NIDA], 2020). Alcohol and drug abuse problems among older adults have been underestimated. In 2020, alcohol-related deaths in adults aged 65 and older were recorded at 11,616 adults. Although these deaths account for less than 1% of all deaths in this age group, age-adjusted death rates for alcohol-induced causes have been increasing since 2011 and rose by 18.2% from 2019 (17.0 deaths per 100,000 standard population) to 2020 (20.1 deaths per 100,000 standard population) (CDC, 2021c). Alcohol-Related Disease Impact application estimates that each year there are more than 140,000 deaths (approximately 97,000 male deaths and 43,000 female deaths) attributable to excessive alcohol use, making alcohol one of the leading preventable causes of death in the United States, behind tobacco. Alcohol and drug abuse in older adults are often unreported and unnoticed because the presenting symptoms may be similar to those of other common problems of aging. In addition, health care providers often do not ask elders about alcohol or nonprescription drug use. The longer the problem remains undetected, the greater it becomes, and the more potential harm it can cause related to other chronic health problems (CDC, 2021c).

Older adults are more vulnerable to the effects of alcohol and illicit drugs because their detoxification and excretion systems are not as efficient as those of younger people. Alcoholism and drug abuse predispose older adults to accidents and injury, cognitive decline, physical debility, nutritional deficiencies, disease, and decreased function. In addition, alcohol use while taking medications can interfere with the desired effect of the medication.

Tobacco Use

Tobacco use includes cigarette smoking, cigar smoking, pipe smoking, and chewing tobacco. Use of tobacco products is associated with cardiovascular disease, several types of cancer, and chronic lung disease (CDC, 2021b). Some older males and females may be the first generation to have smoked throughout their lives, starting in their teens or 20s when smoking seemed fashionable. Although smoking-related health problems occur slowly over time, smoking is an important predictor of longevity. Smoking also poses problems for older adults because it can increase or decrease the effectiveness of medications.

Older adults can experience the benefits of smoking cessation even after the age of 65 years. These people may be more motivated to quit smoking than when they were younger, as they are likely to see some of the damage that smoking has caused and anticipate that smoking cessation will restore or improve their health. Nurses can assist older adults in making the commitment to quit smoking through education and referral to smoking-cessation programs.

SOCIAL DETERMINANTS OF HEALTH

Social Factors and Environment

The incidence of chronic and acute illnesses and the subsequent decline in functional status, changes in economic status, and changes in family structure frequently place older adults in situations in which they are admitted to acute care facilities or must make a temporary or permanent move into a residential or long-term care facility. When providing health-promotion services to older adults, nurses must consider the type of setting in which the person lives. Box 24.11: Evidence-Based Practice provides helpful information about transitional care for older adults with chronic illness as well as their caregivers.

When older adults leave their homes, they may enter a continuum of care extending from an independent living center and ALFs to skilled care facilities or nursing homes, with possible short-term stays in acute care settings. Nurses who work in each of the settings on the continuum can promote health to this population in many ways. From the acute care setting through each stage of the continuum, opportunities are available for nurses to introduce older adults and their families to community resources (Table 24.4). The acute care nurse has the opportunity to offer health-promotion strategies to older adults who would benefit from lifestyle changes that will improve their health status. In most cases, an acute care admission is an opportunity to introduce health-promotion teaching, and the acute care nurse should consider developing a care plan that includes health-promotion strategies. Many older adults are open to information that will prevent future hospital admissions and restore their health. Home health nursing is an important service because assisting the older adult with appointments, transportation services, housekeeping services, adult day care, and assistance with grocery shopping or home-delivered meals allows older adults to return to their home environment, which is a better place to recover from an illness. Helping older adults and their families locate adult day care programs, smoking-cessation programs, stress-management workshops, or weight-loss and exercise programs before leaving the hospital will encourage older adults to enter these programs immediately after discharge, while they are motivated.

Long-term care nurses can locate and plan community resources during the resident's stay. Some community services

BOX 24.11 EVIDENCE-BASED PRACTICE

Evidence-Based Transitional Care for Chronically Ill Older Adults and Their Caregivers

A transitional care model (TCM) is a multidisciplinary approach used to address the needs of very-high-risk chronically ill older adults who are transitioning from the hospital to the home following an acute illness. TCM is led by an advanced practice nurse (APN) using a holistic person-centered and family care–centered approach. The APN acts as the "point person" throughout the episode of care, facilitating timely exchange of information across all settings. The criteria identified to determine high-risk persons include those who are 80 years or older, those who have moderate to severe functional deficits, and those who are unable to complete self-care or manage daily tasks.

The tools used to assess potentially affected persons include the Hospital Admission Risk Profile, the Katz Index of Independence in Activities of Daily Living or the Lawton Instrumental Activities of Daily Living Scale, and the Mental Status Assessment of Older Adults (Mini-Cog). Potentially affected persons are also screened with use of the Geriatric Depression Scale—Short Form to assess symptoms of depression. The following risks associated with readmission have been identified: having four or more active coexisting health problems, being treated with six or more prescribed standing medications, having two or more hospitalizations within the previous 6 months, being hospitalized within the previous 30 days, having been hospitalized with baseline dementia, being treated for delirium, lacking formal or informal family caregiver support, and having low health literacy.

With APN services under the TCM, mutual goals are developed, there is improved communication and collaboration among health care providers; there is improved medication and dietary adherence; there are decreased numbers of rehospitalizations during the 52 weeks of follow-up; and there is high person, caregiver, and physician satisfaction. The barriers to widespread adoption of the TCM identified include the organization of current systems of care, barriers of regulation, lack of quality and financial incentives, and culture of care issues.

From Berthelsen, C., Møller, N., & Bunkenborg, G. (2024). Transitional care model for older adults with multiple chronic conditions: An evaluation of benefits utilising an umbrella review. *Journal of Clinical Nursing, 33*(2), 481–496. https://doi.org/10.1111/jocn.16913
From Leithaus, M., Beaulen, A., de Vries, E., Goderis, G., Flamaing, J., Verbeek, H., & Deschodt, M. (2022). Integrated care components in transitional care models from hospital to home for frail older adults: A systematic review. *International Journal of Integrated Care, 22*(2), 28. https://doi.org/10.5334/ijic.6447
From Hirschman, K., Shaid, E. McCauley, K., Pauly, M., & Naylor, M. (2015). Continuity of care: The transitional care model. *The Online Journal of Issues of Nursing, 20*(3). https://doi.org/10.3912/OJIN.Vol2No03Man01

will enable an older person to return home to an environment in which active health promotion continues. Community resources that may help older adults who are discharged from long-term care facilities include adult day care programs, support groups and medical resources, telephone and Internet information, and referral services. In addition to their role in individual care planning, long-term care nurses can be more involved in institutional policy changes. Recommendations about smoking policies, healthy diets, and exercise programs may prompt interdisciplinary changes that will result in improved health for the entire institution.

The geriatric care manager who visits older adults in their homes or in other residential facilities may be charged with individual health-promotion planning. Home care nurses provide health care information and services to individuals and their families. The resources available to community health nurses are frequently rich and enable the nurses to draw on a variety of sources to assist in promoting the health of community-dwelling older adults. Transportation options, home-delivered meals, assistance with housekeeping, socialization activities, exercise programs, and self-help groups are only a few of the health-promotion resources available within the community. Nurses in all settings can consult a social worker or contact the community older adult services office for information on available resources.

It is important for the nurse to consider the health literacy level of the older adult and their family when providing information and health teaching. **Health literacy** is defined as "the degree to which individuals have the capacity to obtain, process, and understand basic health information needed to make appropriate health decisions and services needed to prevent or treat illness" (Rudd et al., 2023, p. 175). Health literacy also includes the ability to work with and understand numbers. For example, calculating cholesterol and blood sugar levels, measuring medications, and understanding nutrition labels all require math skills. Choosing between health plans or comparing prescription drug coverage requires calculating premiums, copays, and deductibles.

Inadequate health literacy skills are associated with poorer physical and mental health outcomes. Older adults at risk for lower health literacy skills are non-English speakers, have lower

TABLE 24.4 Common Caregiving Problems

Mental Health	Physical Health	Functional or Cognitive Impairments	Secondary Strains	Care Decisions	Resources	Family Challenges	Advocacy
• Depression • Anxiety • Subclinical stress • Anticipatory grief • Negative affect	• Fatigue • Sleep problems • Weakened immune system • Increased risk for injury, illness, mortality	• Memory difficulty • Concentration	• Employment • Financial • Relationship stress • Loss of self-care • Reduced quality of life	• When is it time? • Residential placement • End of life care	• Housing • Health care • Respite • Community services	• Conflict • Behavioral issues • Caregiver lack of support • Balancing needs of healthy and ill family members	• Service systems liaison • Care coordination

American Psychological Association. (2020). *Common caregiving problems.* https://www.apa.org/pi/about/publications/caregivers/practice-settings/common-problems

educational levels, are from lower socioeconomic strata, and reside in medically and economically underserved communities. Older adults with low health literacy may have difficulty finding appropriate health care providers, seeking preventive health care, filling out health forms, managing chronic illness, following directions, understanding the relationship between risk behaviors and health problems, and following medication and treatment plans (Nutbeam & Lloyd, 2021). It is important for nurses to identify older adults who have low health literacy skills and develop instructional materials that use simple language and short sentences, avoiding or defining technical terms. Nurses can assist older adults who have difficulty completing forms. For older adults who have limited English skills, written and oral instruction can be provided in their native language.

In recent years, there has been a substantial increase in the use of palliative and hospice care by older adults. Palliative care is provided for people with a serious illness who will continue to receive curative treatment and symptom relief. Palliative care is available to anyone with a serious illness, whereas hospice care requires a terminal prognosis with an expected death within 6 months. Once the person is placed in hospice care, treatment to relieve pain and other symptoms is continued, but curative treatment ends. In 2018, approximately 1.55 million Medicare recipients received hospice care. This was a 4% increase from 2017.

Hospice services consist of direct clinical care for individuals and bereavement services for the person and the family (National Hospice and Palliative Care Organization [NHPCO], 2020). Older adults in a hospice are empowered to live with dignity, alert and free of pain. The goal of hospice care is to facilitate a "good death" for individuals. Families and loved ones are consistently engaged in caregiving for the dying and helping them maintain the highest possible quality of life. The hospice environment promotes quality of life within the context of differing cultural and spiritual values and beliefs. Nurses in all settings may identify and refer individuals for palliative or hospice care and facilitate the use of these services to promote wellness during serious or terminal illness.

Older adults can be overwhelmed by the amount of advertising that is directed at them about such "necessities" as nutritional supplements, drugs, hearing aids, alarms to use if they fall, phones, Internet sites, and digital devices. Nurses can help them sort out the confusion related to this advertising and direct them to reliable sources of information. The AARP provides many services to people older than 50 years, including excellent educational materials and community program packages. The topics reflect a broad range of concerns and are generally presented in a self-help manner. Among the topics covered are smoking, exercise, nutrition, and wellness. Each program serves as a guide to negotiate a system or learn more about a health problem. These topics are written in easily understood language and are printed in large print to accommodate vision changes. This self-help method is especially important for those who feel uncomfortable addressing questions on finances or sexuality with nurses and physicians.

The National Institute for Aging conducts research to examine many aspects of aging to improve the quantity and quality of life in older years. It provides free educational publications called Age Pages that can be given to older adults to help them adapt safely and successfully to the many changes and concerns encountered as a person ages. Age Pages are easily accessed on the Internet and are written in large font and language easily understandable to the lay public.

Two additional environments of care emerged in the United States in the second half of the 20th century: continuing care retirement communities (CCRCs) and ALFs. CCRCs are full-service communities offering long-term contracts that provide older adults with a continuum of care, extending from retirement services through assisted living to skilled nursing, all in one location. The mission behind CCRCs is "aging in place." CCRCs are expensive and require an entrance fee and a monthly payment. Residence in a CCRC requires commitment to a long-term contract that specifies the housing, services, and nursing care provided. ALFs are defined as homelike settings that promote resident autonomy, privacy, independence, dignity, and respect while providing necessary support. The lower cost of ALFs in comparison with skilled nursing facilities and the greater emphasis on functional autonomy make these facilities appealing to older consumers and their families. Although residents of ALFs have many long-term health care needs, it is important to understand that the role and availability of nurses in these facilities differ greatly by state guidelines.

One additional social factor that should be considered is age discrimination. Even now when many older adults are active contributors to society, they experience discrimination because of their age. Ageism refers to attitudes, ideas, beliefs, and practices that result in biases about groups based on their age. Ageism is a barrier to older adults seeking employment even though the Age Discrimination in Employment Act (ADEA) does not permit age discrimination against people aged 40 and older.

Older adults have described situations in which health care providers do not address them but direct their inquiries to a family member. Many of these older adults are highly educated, cognitively aware, and capable of adhering to advice from health care providers. Older age should not be stigmatized, because older adults are able to enrich the lives of others via the knowledge and experience they have accumulated through the years.

Diversity Awareness

The percentage of older adults who are White is expected to decrease from 1990 to 2030, whereas the percentages of Black, Asian, and Hispanic older adults are expected to increase. These changes in diversity require the US health care delivery system to meet the health care needs of all populations. Challenges will continue to present themselves as the United States experiences more diverse populations. Meeting the health care needs of diverse populations requires that health care providers look like their patients, speak the language of their patients, and recognize their implicit biases about diverse communities.

Nurses must be aware of the cultural diversity of older adults for whom they care and communicate about health care decisions. Nurses need to explore the potential influences of health beliefs with the patient and not presume these beliefs represent a specific culture. Culture is mediated by an individual's education, assimilation status, income, and occupation. In addition, using cultural awareness reduces nurses' biases about a patient's culture. Cultural awareness has been classically described as the self-reflection of an individual's self-reported cultural experiences and professional identity that may contribute to biases about the patient's health beliefs (Campinha-Bacote, 2002).

Nurses may best accomplish cultural awareness by conducting a bias assessment about their understanding of a specific culture. After identifying personal cultural biases that influence care, nurses must bracket these beliefs to make sure they do not affect delivery of care. After this step has been accomplished, it is important to increase understanding about population-specific health-related values, beliefs, and behaviors. It is important to remember that, although an older person may be part of a cultural group, the individual may have become acculturated while living in the United States. When conducting cultural assessments, the nurse must remember that some of the standardized assessment tools, such as the Geriatric Depression Scale and the MMSE, are available in languages other than English. Caution must be taken in interpreting a tool that has not been formally translated, because the meanings of many words and phrases may not have an appropriate translation. The final stage in attaining cultural awareness is to develop skills for working with diverse populations, which includes using interpreters and translation services (if applicable), engaging in self-awareness about structural inequity, and actively working toward improving health care. Nurses can also practice cultural competence and cultural humility in caring for elders of diverse backgrounds (Stubbe, 2020).

Levels of Policymaking and Health

This chapter has attempted to emphasize the need for health-promotion services for older adults. Federal, state, and local agencies have programs in place to improve health promotion and illness/injury prevention. The Affordable Care Act of 2010 strengthens Medicare by providing new and additional benefits, including free or low-cost preventive services, free annual wellness visits, and discounts on prescription drugs in Medicare Part D or in Medicare Part C, which is Medicare Advantage. Preventive services include immunizations for influenza, pneumonia, and hepatitis B. Preventive examinations include screening for diabetes, cholesterol, cardiovascular diseases, colorectal cancer, breast cancer, cervical cancer, and prostate cancer. Counseling services for smoking cessation and medical nutrition therapy for those with diabetes or kidney disease are also provided.

Medicare, Medicaid, and Social Security for older adults (direct or indirect) constitute a large portion of the federal budget. Medicare represented 15% of the 2018 federal budget and is projected to rise to 18% of the budget by 2029; Medicaid represented 11%, and Social Security represented 24% (Cubanski & Neuman, 2019).

Medicare Part A covers hospitalizations, Medicare Part B covers medical services, and Medicare Part C covers Medicare Advantage Plans (health maintenance organizations [HMOs], preferred provider organizations [PPOs], medical savings accounts, and other expenses covered in Parts A and B). Medicaid provides health coverage to approximately 7.2 million low-income elders who are also enrolled in Medicare. Approximately 12 million people are "dually eligible" and enrolled in both Medicaid and Medicare, accounting for approximately 15% of all Medicaid enrollees. Older adults who are enrolled in both Medicaid and Medicare, by federal statute, can be covered for both optional and mandatory categories (Medicare.gov, n.d.).

Social Security plays an important role in reducing poverty levels of older adults. Without this benefit, approximately 22.1 million Americans would be below the poverty level. The poverty level of older adults (aged 65 and older) would be 39.2% without Social Security, but with Social Security, the poverty rate is 9.2%. Approximately 15,333,000 older adults have been lifted above the poverty line because of Social Security (Romig, 2019).

Medigap policies are purchased from private insurance companies to pay health care costs not covered by Medicare (e.g., copayments and deductibles). Medigap policies vary and provide different levels of coverage. Older adults purchasing Medigap policies should be clear about the level of coverage needed and their medical needs (e.g., durable health care supplies, prescription medications, and other medical charges) before selecting a policy. Nongovernmental organizations also influence policy decisions, which may affect older adults and health. Professional health care provider organizations such as the American Nurses Association, the National Gerontological Nurses Association, and the American Medical Association conduct research to determine best practices in elder care and to provide information to policymakers. AARP and the Gray Panthers are examples of two consumer organizations that gather information, fund research related to issues of older adults, and act as advocates for older adults in policymaking organizations.

Because the US health system is fragmented, medical expenditures are higher than in other developed countries. Controlling medical expenditures continues to be debated at the federal and state levels. However, nurses can play a key role in promoting health, implementing prevention strategies, and preventing older adults from becoming impoverished.

Health Services/Delivery Systems

In the United States, many people are not financially prepared for older adulthood. Although some older adults receive supplemental income from pensions or individual retirement accounts, many do not, and the amount of income from these sources is often very limited. Many older adults live on a limited income. There are several federal programs available to help older adults with limited finances. These programs help lower-income older adults improve their quality of life. Medicaid, authorized by Title 19 of the Social Security Act, was created to assist older adults receiving public assistance to pay for medical expenses. Both federal and state governments fund the Medicaid program. To qualify for Medicaid, an individual must have a limited income and assets. Medicaid coverage is more extensive than that of Medicare in that Medicaid covers stays in long-term care facilities, transportation for health care visits, and prescription drug services. Medicare covers these services only in medically acute situations and for a limited time. Older adults who require long-term care may be forced to "spend down" their assets to be eligible for Medicaid.

Careful financial planning before the onset of illness is optimal because it will avoid the need to spend down assets as well as provide the older adult with a desirable income level. Financial planning, if possible, can be accomplished through meetings with lawyers and financial planners early in life. Adults should consider financial planning at or around 30 years of age. Other essential planning activities are completing advance directives and naming a conservator in advance of illness. Advance directives and naming a conservator assist caregivers and family in making difficult decisions at the end of life for a person who is no longer able to make decisions about their medical care. The better prepared the older adult is, the easier it is to receive appropriate care and treatment during times of illness.

Reverse mortgages are becoming more popular with older adults who have equity in their homes and want to supplement their income. A reverse annuity mortgage is obtained when a bank or private business purchases the residence of an older adult. The bank pays a set amount of money each month until the house, cooperative, or condominium is paid in its entirety. This approach enables older adults to remain in their home while providing an income. Reverse mortgages often negate the need for older adults to move or sell their home if an illness arises. When the older adult (mortgagee) is deceased, the bank or mortgager then owns the property.

Long-term care insurance is an option for those planning for the possibility of long-term care. As with other insurance programs, younger adults can purchase a policy, which is now widely available from insurance agents. A premium is paid each month that entitles the beneficiary to receive long-term care benefits at home, in an ALF, in a day care facility, or in a long-term care facility. Older adults should explore all of the options available for this type of insurance. The benefits and coverage differ, and exclusions are frequently written into the contract to prevent care in certain situations. An important feature of these policies is the option to hire a personal caregiver if the need arises.

Because population shifts have resulted in many older adults in the United States, political movements protecting the rights of older adults are abundant and strong. Older adults are actively engaged in political activity and play a large role in shaping social and health policies for this age group. Interestingly, it was the development of Social Security that facilitated political activism in seniors. Social Security benefits have made it possible for older adults to have a regular income, better health, and free time to engage in politics. By receiving Social Security benefits, seniors now have an interest in making sure the program remains viable. Social Security also provides the basis for political parties and interest groups such as the AARP to gain traction.

The nurse who specializes in the care of older adults can facilitate and promote health and well-being through education, research, and practice. Educational curricula require ongoing evaluation to ensure that content is appropriate and accurate for older adults. The quality of care depends on the clinician's knowledge base; thus, providing education to older adults is equally important and begins with an assessment of the individual's level of understanding of health-promotion activities.

Health-promotion and illness and injury-prevention research for this population is only beginning. More research needs to be done to explore the concepts of health promotion and to relate these concepts to developing research studies. Research is needed to change incorrect beliefs, myths, and stereotypes about aging. Defining concepts of health promotion, such as quality of life and functional ability, will yield data that can be studied and tested. Health promotion facilitated by qualified nurses can lead to improving the quality of older adults' lives.

International Aging Trends

Aging populations are not unique to the United States. Life-expectancy increases and reductions in family sizes have resulted in dramatic increases in the percentage of the population of adults aged 60 and older. In 2022, Monaco had the oldest population of the world with 36% of adults aged 60 and older, followed by Japan at 29% (Dyvik, 2023).

The world's population is expected to increase by two billion people in the coming years, from 7.7 billion at present to 9.7 billion in 2050. Older adults, aged 65 and above, are considered the largest-growing age group. Globally, for the first time in 2018, older adults outnumber children under the age of five, and by 2050, older adults will outnumber adolescents and youth (ages 15 to 24). (See Table 24.5.) Europe and Eastern Asia already face challenges in supporting and caring for their older populations. As life expectancy continues to increase and fertility rates decline, older adults will play more significant roles in societies and economies (United Nations, n.d.).

Population aging is occurring along with broader social and economic changes that are taking place around the world. Globally, there were 727 million people aged 65 years or over in the world in 2020. Over the next 3 decades, the global number of older persons is projected to more than double, reaching over 1.5 billion in 2050.

All regions will see an increase in the size of their older population between 2020 and 2050. The share of the global population aged 65 years and older is expected to increase from 9.3% in 2020 to 16.0% by 2050 (United Nations, 2019a). From 2021 to 2050, the population aged 65 and older in Eastern and South East Asia and in Central and South Asia is projected to grow by more than 540 million, accounting for more than 60% of the global increase (United Nations Department of Economic and Social Affairs, Population Division, n.d.).

Today, Europe and North America combined have the highest share of older persons. North Africa, West Asia, and sub-Saharan Africa are expected to experience the fastest growth in the number of older people over the next 3 decades. Globally, the number of people aged 80 years and older is rising even faster than the number aged 65 or above. By 2050, the world will have an estimated 459 million persons aged 80 or older, almost triple the number in 2021 at around 155 million (United Nations, n.d.).

Nursing education must adapt to aging population shifts to ensure that we meet the health care needs for this growing age group.

TABLE 24.5 International Aging Trends

Age	Number	Percent	Male	Percent	Female	Percent
62–64 years	68,662	20.9	31,629	19.5	37,033	22.2
65–74 years	56,193	17.1	25,647	15.8	30,546	18.3
75 years and over	22,489	6.8	9817	6.1	12,672	7.6

Source: US Census Bureau. (2022). *Current population survey, annual social and economic supplement, 2022.*

NURSING ACTIONS AND APPLICATION

Nurses can provide optimal care to older adults by focusing on health promotion, population health, maintaining self-care, preventing disease and its complications, and understanding social determinants of health. Nursing activities with older adults often focus on the management of chronic conditions instead of engaging older adults in health-promotion activities. When nurses deliver care within a holistic framework, they address the functional and psychosocial needs of the older adult.

Health-promotion activities consist of healthy weight and diets, exercise activities, fall prevention, home safety strategies, and keeping medical appointments for screening and medical management. Immunizations for COVID-19, pneumococcal disease, and influenza are important for the older adult. In addition, educating the older adult about screenings to detect cancer, diabetes, late-onset heart disease, osteoporosis, and hypertension is necessary. An effective method of engaging older adults to participate in screenings is coordinating health fairs in senior centers. When the nurse can provide an accessible location for older adults to obtain vaccinations, health education, blood pressure checks, and glucose monitoring, the nurse is ensuring that older adults participate in their health needs. The nurse should always offer counseling as needed and refer the older adult to their primary care provider for follow-up.

CASE STUDY

Unsafe Driving: Larry Johnson

Larry Johnson is a healthy 75-year-old. Mr. Johnson resides alone in an apartment and is completely independent in activities and instrumental activities of daily living. Last Friday morning, Mr. Johnson left his apartment complex at 8:00 a.m. to go shopping. While backing out of the driveway, he did not see an approaching school bus even though his car had a rear camera and was beeping a warning, and his car struck the bus. Although no one was injured, this incident indicated the need for a sensory and neurologic assessment. The assessment revealed both hearing and visual deficits.

Reflective Questions

- How does the nurse assist in the assessment and interpreting the results?
- Should Mr. Johnson undergo further neuropsychological tests?
- How would the nurse approach Mr. Johnson about not being able to drive?
- How can Mr. Johnson's family be helpful in this situation?

SUMMARY

- Life expectancy is now beyond 75 years for both males and females, with the fastest-growing age group being those older than 85 years.
- The aging process brings about physiologic changes in many body functions, and older adults have a higher frequency of illness than the younger population.
- The physical, emotional, and role changes of older adults are part of aging, and the nurse has a role in assisting older adults in understanding this process.
- It is essential that nurses engage in cultural awareness when working with older adults who speak different languages, may be immigrants, or are first generation.
- The more the nurse engages with the older adult, the more they can provide appropriate health-promotion strategies, which can lead to a fuller, healthier life.

EVOLVE CHAPTER FEATURES

http://evolve.elsevier.com/Edelman/

- Study Questions

REFERENCES

Abildso, C. G., Daily, S. M., Umstattd Meyer, M. R., Perry, C. K., & Eyler, A. (2023). Prevalence of meeting aerobic, muscle-strengthening, and combined physical activity guidelines during leisure time among adults, by rural-urban classification and region — United States, 2020. *Morbidity and Mortality Weekly Reports*, *72*, 85–89. http://dx.doi.org/10.15585/mmwr.mm7204a1

Administration for Community Living (ACL). (2022). *2021 profile of older Americans.* https://acl.gov/programs/health-wellness/nutrition-services

Administration for Community Living (ACL). (2024). *Nutrition services.* https://acl.gov/programs/health-wellness/nutrition-services#:~:text=The%20Home-Delivered%20Nutrition%20Services%20of%20the%20OAA%20authorizes%20meals%20and

Agronin, M. E. (2013). From Cicero to Cohen: Developmental theories of aging, from antiquity to the present. *The Gerontologist*, *54*(1), 30–39. https://doi.org/10.1093/geront/gnt032

Alzheimer's Association. (2023). Alzheimer's disease facts and figures. *Alzheimers & Dementia*, *19*(4), 1598–1695. https://doi.org/10.1002/alz.13016

American Geriatrics Society Beers Criteria® Update Expert Panel. (2023). American Geriatrics Society 2023 updated AGS Beers Criteria® for potentially inappropriate medication use in older adults. *Journal of the American Geriatrics Society*, *71*(7), 2052–2081. https://doi.org/10.1111/jgs.18372

Boidin, M., Handfield, N., Ribeiro, P. A., Desjardins-Crépeau, L., Gagnon, C., Lapierre, G., Gremeaux, V., Lalongé, J., Nigam, A., Juneau, M., Gayda, M., Bherer, L., Gayda, M. (2020). Obese but fit: The benefits of fitness on cognition in obese older adults.

Canadian Journal of Cardiology, 36(11), 1747–1753. https://doi.org/10.1016/j.cjca.2020.01.005

Bouça-Machado, R., Rosário, A., Caldeira, D., Castro Caldas, A., Guerreiro, D., Venturelli, M., Tinazzi, M., Schena, F., Ferreira, J. (2020). Physical activity, exercise, and physiotherapy in Parkinson's disease: Defining the concepts. *Movement Disorders Clinical Practice*, *7*(1), 7–15. https://doi.org/10.1002/mdc3.12849

Brodier, E. A., & Cibelli, M. (2021). Postoperative cognitive dysfunction in clinical practice. *BJA Education*, *21*(2), 75–82. https://doi.org/10.1016/j.bjae.2020.10.004

Brown, L., Huffman, J. C., & Bryant, C. (2019). Self-compassionate aging: A systematic review. *The Gerontologist*, *59*(4), e311–e324. https://doi.org/10.1093/geront/gny108

Brown, M. J., & Adeagbo, O. (2021). HIV and aging: double stigma. *Current epidemiology reports, 8*, 72–78.

Butler, R., & Olshansky, S. J. (2002). Has anybody ever died of old age? *The Gerontologist*, *42*(Special Issue 1), 285–286.

Campinha-Bacote, J. (2002). The process of cultural competence in the delivery of healthcare services: A model of care. *Journal of Transcultural Nursing*, *13*(3), 181–184.

Centers for Disease Control and Prevention (CDC). (2019). *Flu vaccination coverage, United States, 2018–19 influenza season*. https://www.cdc.gov/

Centers for Disease Control and Prevention (CDC). (2021a). *Preventing elder abuse*. https://www.cdc.gov/violenceprevention/elderabuse/fastfact.html#:~:text=Elder%20abuse%20is%20an%20intentional,a%20person%20the%20elder%20trusts

Centers for Disease Control and Prevention (CDC). (2021b). *Smoking and tobacco use*. https://www.cdc.gov/tobacco/index.html

Centers for Disease Control and Prevention (CDC). (2021c). *About underlying cause of death, 2018–2022, single race*. CDC Wonder. https://wonder.cdc.gov/ucd-icd10-expanded.html

Centers for Disease Control and Prevention (CDC). (2022). *Depression is not a normal part of growing older*. https://www.cdc.gov

Centers for Disease Control and Prevention (CDC). (2023a). *Pneumococcal disease*. https://www.cdc.gov/pneumococcal/index.html#:~:text=Pneumococcal%20%5Bnoo%2Dmuh%2DKOK,to%20help%20prevent%20pneumococcal%20disease

Centers for Disease Control and Prevention (CDC). (2023b). *Adult obesity facts*. https://www.cdc.gov/obesity/data/adult.html

Centers for Disease Control and Prevention (CDC). (2023c). Estimated HIV incidence and prevalence in the United States, 2017–2021. *HIV Surveillance Supplemental Report, 28*(3). https://www.cdc.gov

Centers for Disease Control and Prevention (CDC). (2023d). *WISQARS™ — Web-based Injury Statistics Query and Reporting System.*

Centers for Disease Control and Prevention (CDC). (2024). Older adult drivers. https://www.cdc.gov/older-adult-drivers/about/index.html

Centers for Medicare & Medicaid Services. (2023). *National health expenditure data*. https://www.cms.gov/data-research/statistics-trends-and-reports/national-health-expenditure-data

Creavin, S. T., Wisniewski, S., Noel-Storr, A. H., Trevelyan, C. M., Hampton, T., Rayment, D., Thom, V. M., Nash, K. J., Elhamoui, H., Milligan, R., & Patel, A. S. (2016). Mini-Mental State Examination (MMSE) for the detection of dementia in clinically unevaluated people aged 65 and over in community and primary care populations. *Cochrane Database of Systematic Reviews, 1*, CD011145. https://doi.org/10.1002/14651858.CD011145.pub2

Cubanski, J., & Neuman, T. (2019). *The facts on Medicare spending and financing*. https://digirepo.nlm.nih.gov/master/borndig/101740287/Issue-Brief-Facts-on-Medicaid-Spending-and-Financing.pdf

Dean, O., Gothro, A., Bleiweiss-Sande, R., Navarro, S., & Reynolds, M. (2022). *Boosting SNAP participation among older adults to reduce food insecurity*. Washington: AARP Public Policy Institute.

Dyvik, E.H. (2023). The countries with the largest percentage of total population over 65 years 2023. In *Statista*. https://www.statista.com/statistics/264729/countries-with-the-largest-percentage-of-total-population-over-65-years/

Erikson, E. H. (1998). *The life cycle completed (extended version)*. W.W. Norton and Company.

Erikson, E. H., Erikson, J. H., & Kivnick, H. Q. (1986). *Vital involvement in old age: The experience of old age in our time*. W.W. Norton and Company.

Esposito, L. (2016). *Seniors and sexual health: What older adults should know*. U.S. News and World Report. https://health.usnews.com/health-news/patient-advice/articles/2016-03-16/seniors-and-sexual-health-what-older-adults-should-know

Flores, E., Nakagawa, S., Moyer, R., & Bluethmann, S. M. (2022). Assessment of a community-based exercise program for older adults in a mixed rural/urban catchment area: Silver Sneakers in Central Pennsylvania. *Preventing Chronic Disease*, *19*, 210–283. http://dx.doi.org/10.5888/pcd19.210283

Folstein, M. E., Folstein, S. E., & McHugh, P. (1975). Mini-mental state: A practical method for grading the cognitive state of patients for the clinician. *Journal of Psychiatric Research*, *12*, 189–198.

Fong, J. H. (2019). Disability incidence and functional decline among older adults with major chronic diseases. *BMC Geriatrics*, *19*(1), 323. https://doi.org/10.1186/s12877-019-1348-z

Forlenza, O. V., & Vallada, H. (2018). Spirituality, health and well-being in the elderly. *International Psychogeriatrics*, *30*(12), 1741–1742. https://doi.org/10.1017/S1041610218001874

Fulmer, T., Reuben, D. B., Auerbach, J., Fick, D. M., Galambos, C., & Johnson, K. S. (2021). Actualizing better health and health care for older adults. *Health Affairs*, *40*(2), 219–225. https://doi.org/10.1377/hlthaff.2020.01470

Gallegos, M., Morgan, M. L., Cervigni, M., Martino, P., Murray, J., Calandra, M., Razumovskiy, A., Caycho-Rodríguez, T., & Gallegos, W. L. A. (2022). 45 Years of the Mini-Mental State Examination (MMSE): A perspective from Ibero-America. *Dementia & Neuropsychologia*, *16*(4), 384–387. https://doi.org/10.1590/1980-5764-DN-2021-0097

Garg, S., Kim, L., Whitaker, M., O'Halloran, A., Cummings, C., Holstein, R., Prill, M., Chai, S. J., Kirley, P. D., Alden, N. B., Kawasaki, B., Yousey-Hindes, K., Niccolai, L., Anderson, E. J., Openo, K. P., Weigel, A., Monroe, M. L., Ryan, P., Henderson, J., ... Fry, A. (2020). Hospitalization rates and characteristics of patients hospitalized with laboratory-confirmed Coronavirus Disease 2019—COVID-NET, 14 States, March 1–30, 2020. *MMWR. Morbidity and Mortality Weekly Report*, *69*(15), 458–464. http://doi.org/10.15585/mmwr.mm6915e3

Garnett, M. F., Spencer, M. R., & Weeks, J. D. (2023). *Suicide among adults age 55 and older, 2021*. (Data Brief No. 483). National Center for Health Statistics. https://www.cdc.gov/nchs/data/databriefs/db483.pdf

Gundersen, C., & Ziliak, J. P. (2015). Food insecurity and health outcomes. *Health Affairs*, *34*(11), 1830–1839. https://doi.org/10.1377/hlthaff.2015.0645

Jin, J. (2022). Routine checkups for adults. *Journal of the American Medical Association*, *327*(14), 1410. https://doi.org/10.1001/jama.2022.1775

Jung, S. E., Kim, S., Bishop, A., & Hermann, J. (2019). Poor nutritional status among low-income older adults: Examining the interconnection between self-care capacity, food insecurity, and depression. *Journal of the Academy of Nutrition and Dietetics, 119*(10), 1687–1694. https://doi.org/10.1016/j.jand.2018.04.009

Kochanek, K. D., Xu, J. Q., & Arias, E. (2020). *Mortality in the United States, 2019: NCHS data brief, no 395*. Hyattsville, MD: National Center for Health Statistics.

Kuehn, B. M. (2023). US life expectancy in 2021 lowest since 1996. *Journal of the American Medical Association, 329*(4), 280. https://doi.org/10.1001/jama.2022.23562

La Rue, C. J., Haslam, C., & Steffens, N. K. (2022). A meta-analysis of retirement adjustment predictors. *Journal of Vocational Behavior, 136*, 103723. https://doi.org/10.1016/j.jvb.2022.103723

Lausen, A., Marsland, L., Head, S., Jackson, J., & Lausen, B. (2018). Modified Pilates as an adjunct to standard physiotherapy care for urinary incontinence: A mixed methods pilot for a randomised controlled trial. *BMC Women's Health, 18*(1), 16. https://doi.org/10.1186/s12905-017-0503-y

Li, A., Koch, Z., & Ideker, T. (2022). Epigenetic aging: Biological age prediction and informing a mechanistic theory of aging. *Journal of Internal Medicine, 292*(5), 733–744. https://doi.org/10.1111/joim.13533

Liu, Z., Yang, F., Lou, Y., Zhou, W., & Tong, F. (2021). The effectiveness of reminiscence therapy on alleviating depressive symptoms in older adults: A systematic review. *Frontiers in Psychology, 12*, 709–853. https://doi.org/10.1016/j.ijnurstu.2020.103847

Mastronuzzi, T., & Grattagliano, I. (2019). Nutrition as a health determinant in elderly patients. *Current Medicinal Chemistry, 26*(19), 3652–3661. https://doi.org/10.2174/0929867324666170523125806

McBride, C. (2015). Personal genomic tests for healthy aging: Neither feast nor foul. Generations. *Journal of the American Society on Aging*. https://api.semanticscholar.org/CorpusID:68580240

McDermott, M., Brown, D. L., & Chervin, R. D. (2018). Sleep disorders and the risk of stroke. *Expert Review of Neurotherapeutics, 18*(7), 523–531. https://doi.org/10.1080/14737175.2018.1489239

Moncada, L. V. V., & Mire, L. G. (2017). Preventing falls in older persons. *American Family Physician, 96*(4), 240–247. https://www.aafp.org/afp/2017/0815/p240.pdf

Murthy, N., Wodi, P. A., McNally, V., Cineas, S., & Ault, K. (2023). Advisory committee on immunization practices recommended immunization schedule for adults aged 19 years or older — United States. *Morbidity and Mortality Weekly Report, 72*(6), 141–144. http://dx.doi.org/10.15585/mmwr.mm7206a2

Murthy, V. (2023). *Our epidemic of loneliness and isolation: The U.S. surgeon general's advisory on the healing effects of social connection and community*. https://www.hhs.gov/sites/default/files/surgeon-general-social-connection-advisory.pdf

National Hospice and Palliative Care Organization. (2020). *NHPCO facts and figures: 2020 edition*. https://www.nhpco.org/wp-content/uploads/NHPCO-Facts-Figures-2020-edition.pdf

National Institute of Aging. (2022). *Falls and fractures in older adults: Causes and prevention*. https://www.nia.nih.gov/health/falls-and-falls-prevention/falls-and-fractures-older-adults-causes-and-prevention

National Institute of Mental Health. (2023). *Depression*. https://www.nimh.nih.gov/health/topics/depression

National Institute of Neurological Disorders and Stroke. (2019). *Restless legs syndrome*. https://www.ninds.nih.gov/disorders/all-disorders/restless-legs-syndrome-information-page

National Institute on Deafness and Other Communication Disorders. (2023). *Age-related hearing loss (Presbycusis)*. https://www.nidcd.nih.gov/health/age-related-hearing-loss

Nies, M. A., & McEwan, M. (2019). *Community/public health nursing: Promoting the health of populations* (7th ed.). Philadelphia, PA: Saunders.

Nutbeam, D., & Lloyd, J. E. (2021). Understanding and responding to health literacy as a social determinant of health. *Annual Review of Public Health, 42*(1), 159–173. https://doi.org/10.1146/annurev-publhealth-090419-102529

Ochiai, E., Kigenyi, T., Sondik, E., Pronk, N., Kleinman, D. V., Blakey, C., Heffernan, M., & Brewer, K. H. (2021). *Healthy People 2030* leading health indicators and overall health and well-being measures: Opportunities to assess and improve the health and well-being of the nation. *Journal of Public Health Management and Practice, 27*(1), S235–S241. https://doi.org/10.1097/PHH.0000000000001424

Ochieng, N., Cubanski, J., Neuman, T., Artiga, S., & Damico, A. (2021). *Racial and ethnic health inequities and Medicare*. https://www.kff.org/medicare/report/racial-and-ethnic-health-inequities-and-medicare/

Pension Rights Center. (2023). *Income of today's older adults*. https://pensionrights.org/resource/income-of-todays-older-adults/

Petrovsky, D. V., Hirschman, K. B., Varrasse McPhillips, M., Sefcik, J. S., Hanlon, A. L., Huang, L., Brewster, G. S., Hodgson, N. A., & Naylor, M. D. (2020). Predictors of change over time in subjective daytime sleepiness among older adult recipients of long-term services and supports. *International Psychogeriatrics, 32*(7), 849–861. https://doi.org/10.1017/S1041610220000782

Piercy, K. L., Troiano, R. P., Ballard, R. M., Carlson, S. A., Fulton, J. E., Galuska, D. A., George, S. M., Olson, R. D. (2018). The physical activity guidelines for Americans. *Journal of the American Medical Association, 320*(19), 2020–2028. https://doi.org/10.1001/jama.2018.14854

Population Reference Bureau. (2024), *Fact sheet: Aging in the United States*. https://www.prb.org/resources/fact-sheet-aging-in-the-united-states/

Romig, K. (2019). *Social Security lifts more people above the poverty line than any other program*. https://www.cbpp.org/research/social-security/social-security-lifts-more-americans-above-poverty-than-any-other-program

Rudd, R. E., Anderson, J. E., Oppenheimer, S., & Nath, C. (2023). Health literacy: an update of medical and public health literature. *Review of Adult Learning and Literacy, 7*, 175–204.

Russo, E., Caretto, M., Giannini, A., Bitzer, J., Cano, A., Ceausu, I., Chedraui, P., Durmusoglu, F., Erkkola, R., Goulis, D. G., Kiesel, L., Lambrinoudaki, I., Hirschberg, A. L., Lopes, P., Pines, A., Rees, M., van Trotsenburg, M., & Simoncini, T. (2021). Management of urinary incontinence in postmenopausal women: An EMAS clinical guide. *Maturitas, 143*, 223–230. https://doi.org/10.1016/j.maturitas.2020.09.005

Sancho-Domingo, C., Carballo, J. L., Coloma-Carmona, A., & Buysse, D. J. (2021). Brief version of the Pittsburgh Sleep Quality Index (B-PSQI) and measurement invariance across gender and age in a population-based sample. *Psychological Assessment, 33*(2), 111–121. https://doi.org/10.1037/pas0000959

Schrager, S., Ovsepyan, V., & Burnside, E. (2020). Breast cancer screening in older women: The importance of shared decision making. *Journal of the American Board of Family Medicine, 33*(3), 473–480. https://doi.org/10.3122/jabfm.2020.03.190380

Searing, L. (2023). More than 1 in 6 Americans now 65 or older as U.S. continues graying. *Washington Post*. https://www.

washingtonpost.com/wellness/2023/02/14/aging-boomers-more-older-americans/

Shaw, C., & Wagg, A. (2017). Urinary incontinence in older adults. *Medicine, 45*(1), 23–27. https://doi.org/10.1016/j.mpmed.2016.10.001

Shrider, E.A., & Creamer, J. (2023). *Poverty in the United States: 2022. Current population reports, P60-280*. Washington, DC: US Government Publishing Office. https://www.census.gov/content/dam/Census/library/publications/2023/demo/p60-280.pdf

Skufca, L., & Rainville, C. (2021). Caregiving can be costly—even financially. *AARP Research*. https://doi.org/10.26419/res.00473.001

Social Security Administration. (2022). *Fast facts & figures about social security, 2022*. https://www.ssa.gov/policy/docs/chartbooks/fast_facts/2022/fast_facts22.pdf

Stefanacci, R. G., Yeaw, J., Shah, D., Newman, D. K., Kincaid, A., & Mudd Jr, P. N. (2022). Impact of urinary incontinence related to overactive bladder on long-term care residents and facilities: A perspective from directors of nursing. *Journal of Gerontological Nursing, 48*(7), 38–46. https://doi.org/10.3928/00989134-20220606-06

Stephan, A. T. (2023). Grandparent caregiver wellbeing: A strengths-based approach utilizing the positive emotions, engagement, relationships, meaning, and accomplishment (PERMA) framework. *Journal of Family Issues, 44*(5), 1400–1418. https://doi.org/10.1177/0192513X211058818

Storey, J. E. (2020). Risk factors for elder abuse and neglect: A review of the literature. *Aggression and Violent Behavior, 50*, 101339. https://doi.org/10.1016/j.avb.2019.101339

Stubbe, D. E. (2020). Practicing cultural competence and cultural humility in the care of diverse patients. *Focus, 18*(1), 49–51. https://doi.org/10.1176/appi.focus.20190041

Tahrani, A. A., & Morton, J. (2022). Benefits of weight loss of 10% or more in patients with overweight or obesity: A review. *Obesity, 30*(4), 802–840. https://doi.org/10.1002/oby.23371

Tam, W., Poon, S. N., Mahendran, R., Kua, E. H., & Wu, X. V. (2021). The effectiveness of reminiscence-based intervention on improving psychological well-being in cognitively intact older adults: A systematic review and meta-analysis. *International Journal of Nursing Studies, 114*, 103847. https://doi.org/10.1016/j.ijnurstu.2020.103847

Terlizzi, E. P., Connor, E., Zelaya, C., Ji, A. M., & Bakos, A. (2019). Reported importance and access to health care providers who understand or share cultural characteristics with their patients among adults, by race and ethnicity. *National Health Statistics Reports, 130*, 1–11. https://www.cdc.gov/nchs/data/nhsr/nhsr130-508.pdf

Tutor, A.W., Lavie, C. J., Sergey, K., Milani, R. V, & Ventura, H. O. (2023). Updates on obesity and the obesity paradox in cardiovascular diseases. *Progress in Cardiovascular Diseases, 78*, 2–10. https://doi.org/10.1016/j.pcad.2022.11.013

US Census Bureau. (2023). *U.S. older population grew from 2010 to 2020 at fastest rate since 1880 to 1890*. https://www.census.gov/library/stories/2023/05/2020-census-united-states-older-population-grew.html

US Census Bureau. (2023). *Historical poverty tables: People and families - 1959 to 2023*. https://www.census.gov/data/tables/time-series/demo/income-poverty/historical-poverty-people.html

US Census Bureau Statista. (2023). *Number of children living with grandparents in the United States in 2023, by age of child (in 1,000s)*. https://www.statista.com/statistics/769741/us-children-living-with-grandparents-by-age-of-child/

US Department of Agriculture and US Department of Health and Human Services. (2020). *Dietary Guidelines for Americans, 2020-2025*. https://health.gov/our-work/nutrition-physical-activity/dietary-guidelines/current-dietary-guidelines

US Department of Health and Human Services (USDHHS). (n.d.). *Injury and violence prevention*. https://health.gov/healthypeople/objectives-and-data/browse-objectives/older-adults

United Nations. (n.d.). *Shifting demographics*. https://www.un.org/en/un75/shifting-demographics#:~:text=Globally%2C%20for%20the%20first%20time,caring%20for%20their%20older%20populations

Valdiserri, R. O., Holtgrave, D. R., Poteat, T. C., & Beyrer, C. (2019). Unraveling health disparities among sexual and gender minorities: A commentary on the persistent impact of stigma. *Journal of Homosexuality, 66*(5), 571–589. https://doi.org/10.1080/00918369.2017.1422944

Whitelock, E., & Ensaff, H. (2018). On your own: Older adults' food choice and dietary habits. *Nutrients, 10*(4), 413. https://doi.org/10.3390/nu10040413

World Health Organization. (2020). *Defining sexual health*. https://www.who.int/reproductivehealth/topics/sexual_health/sh_definitions/en/

Yaremchuk, K. (2018). Sleep disorders in the elderly. *Clinics in Geriatric Medicine, 34*(2), 205–216. https://doi.org/10.1016/j.cger.2018.01.008

Yarnell, S., Li, L., MacGrory, B., Trevisan, L., & Kirwin, P. (2020). Substance use disorders in later life: A review and synthesis of the literature of an emerging public health concern. *The American Journal of Geriatric Psychiatry, 28*(2), 226–236. https://doi.org/10.1016/j.jagp.2019.06.005

Yesavage, J. A., Brink, T. L., Rose, T. L., Lum, O., Huang, V., Adey, M., & Leirer, V. O. (1982). Development and validation of a geriatric depression screening scale: A preliminary report. *Journal of Psychiatric Research, 17*(1), 37–49. https://doi.org/10.1016/0022-3956(82)90033-4

25

Health Promotion for the 21st Century: Throughout the Life Span and Throughout the World

Lynnette Leeseberg Stamler, Louise LaFramboise and Jessica Semin

http://evolve.elsevier.com/Edelman/

OBJECTIVES

- Compare the relationships among the social determinants of health, the United Nations (UN) Sustainable Development Goals, and the 2019 UN 10 threats to humans (updated 2023).
- Analyze problems and implications of various communicable diseases, including viruses, COVID -19, and drug-resistant bacterial diseases.
- Discuss noncommunicable disease threats to human health and compare with communicable disease threats.
- Describe the linkages between climate change, pollution, and human health.
- Discuss and synthesize the importance of strong primary health care at the global level.

KEY TERMS

Air pollution
Antimicrobial resistance
Communicable diseases
COVID-19
Dengue fever
Ebola virus
Fragile states
Fragility
Global warming
Herd immunity
HIV/AIDS
Influenza pandemic
Life course approach
Life expectancy
Noncommunicable diseases
One Health
Pandemic
Primary health care
Primary health care progression model
Social determinants of health
Telemedicine network
Vaccine hesitancy
Zika virus

THINK ABOUT IT

One of the social determinants of health is the physical environment. Two very important aspects of that are the presence of dependable electricity and wireless internet capability. These two aspects influence much of our current daily lives, whether it be running a hospital or clinic, taking online classes, completing everyday banking, or ensuring communication and support locally or globally with friends and family members. Whether one is in a rural and remote area or in the middle of a concrete jungle, and wherever one is throughout the world, the absence of either of these aspects could strongly impinge on the individual or family being able to manage their health needs and daily lives.

- What efforts are being made where you live to ensure dependable electricity and wireless internet? Are any of your classmates and/or faculty experiencing difficulties with these factors?
- Select another country of your choice and find out information on the state of these two factors in that country. How could that affect health promotion and health care?
- What effect does local, national, and international politics have on access to these factors?

INTRODUCTION

The potential for and challenges to health promotion on a global scale are well illustrated by the intersection of the social determinants of health from the World Health Organization (WHO), the Public Health Agency of Canada (PHAC), the United Nations (UN) 10 Threats to Global Health, and the UN Sustainable Development Goals (SDGs). Social determinants identify factors that affect health, the 10 threats delineate current threats to health, and the SDGs outline where humans, as a global community, can focus their actions for improvement of global health. Each of these documents has been highlighted in a text box at the end of this chapter, and students are encouraged to note the similarities and differences among them. In the previous sections of this book, health promotion has been examined from a variety of perspectives, from assessment to interventions, and from pregnancy to death. In each of these chapters, a wealth of information related to the US health care system and society has been presented. In this chapter, the focus will be on global health issues that may be similar to or different from those that are seen in the United States. The guiding framework for this chapter is the 10 Threats to Global Health in 2019 as identified by the WHO (2019a). The top 10 threats are part of the WHO's 5-year strategic plan known as the "Thirteenth General Programme of Work." An updated strategic plan and list of threats is slated to be approved at the World Health Assembly in 2024 (WHO, 2024). Current emerging trends include: the aging population, mental health conditions, communicable disease, malnutrition, climate change, and health system structures. Students are encouraged to read each document in light of the other two documents.

WHO Social Determinants of Health

The WHO has defined **social determinants of health** as "the conditions in which people are born, grow, live, work and age" (WHO, n.d.). The WHO brought together member states in 2011 to consider the social determinants of health. The resulting declaration signed by member states indicates a "global political commitment for the implementation of a social determinants of health approach to reduce health inequities" (WHO, 2011). The determinants as outlined by the WHO and the government of Canada through the PHAC are found in Box 25.1 (Government of Canada, 2023). The PHAC added race/racism to the determinants of health. This is in recognition that "experiences of discrimination, racism and historical trauma are important social determinants of health for certain groups" (PHAC, 2023). In examining these determinants, it is clear that they touch on almost every facet of everyday life across the life span. Health inequities arise when some members, groups, or populations experience significantly higher or lower levels of specific determinants (e.g., physical environment). Although not every determinant can be controlled by the individual (e.g., genetics), many of the determinants can be influenced by deliberate action. Health promotion, on an individual or global scale, can be deliberate interventions to improve one or more of the determinants. In 2021, the World Health Assembly requested the WHO develop a new operational framework for how social determinants of health and health inequities will be measured, assessed, and addressed (WHO, 2023a,b). Throughout 2023, the draft of the operational framework was reviewed by member states, with many being supportive of the draft. A final report is expected to be released in 2024 with the hope that it will provide policymakers information and resources to make informed decisions in relation to collection of data related to the social determinants of health and health equity (WHO, 2023c; see Box 25.1).

BOX 25.1 HEALTH AND SOCIAL DETERMINANTS OF HEALTH/HEALTH EQUITY

- Income and social status: Higher income and social status are linked to better health. The greater the gap between the richest and poorest people, the greater the differences in health.
- Employment and working conditions: People in employment are healthier, particularly those who have more control over their working conditions.
- Education and literacy: Low education levels are linked with poor health, more stress, and lower self-confidence.
- Childhood experiences: Living safely, with shelter and plentiful food, and being loved are linked to better health.
- Physical environment: Safe water and clean air, healthy workplaces, safe houses, communities, and roads all contribute to good health.
- Social support networks and coping skills: Greater support from families, friends, and communities is linked to better health. The development of positive coping skills contributes to better health.
- Culture: Customs, traditions, and the beliefs of the family and community all affect health.
- Genetics: Inheritance plays a part in determining life span, healthiness, and the likelihood of developing certain illnesses.
- Personal behavior: Balanced eating, keeping active, smoking, drinking, and how we deal with life's stresses and challenges all affect health.
- Health services: Access to and use of services that prevent and treat disease can influence health.
- Sex: Males and females suffer from different types of diseases at different ages.
- Race/racism: Status in society can depend on one's race combined with where one lives.

Source: Government of Canada (2023)

Health on a global scale is frequently talked about using a variety of comparable statistics. One of the most common is **life expectancy**. Although conventional wisdom posits that underdeveloped countries experience shorter life expectancy, there are other factors to consider. The United States has enjoyed significant increases in life expectancy over the past few decades; however, in a ranking of just over 200 countries in terms of life expectancy, the United States ranked 40th (World Population Review, 2023), with a total life expectancy of 79.74 years versus the highest level of 87.01 years. The average life expectancy figure fluctuates depending on the data source and timing of calculations. However, researchers agree that the United States is lagging behind peer countries in life expectancy over the past several years (Venkataramani et al., 2021). The Centers for Disease Control and Prevention (CDC) reported that data from 2021 indicated the life expectancy at birth fell to its lowest level since 1996 (CDC, 2022a). There are multiple factors contributing to these data. In recent years, the declines in life expectancy were largely related to the pandemic. However, a factor in the

BOX 25.2 Ten Threats to Global Health

1. Air pollution and climate change
2. Noncommunicable diseases
3. Global influenza pandemic
4. Fragile and vulnerable settings
5. Antimicrobial resistance
6. Ebola and other high-threat pathogens
7. Weak primary health care
8. Vaccine hesitancy
9. Dengue
10. Human immunodeficiency virus (HIV)

From WHO (2019a)

United States has been the opioid crisis/drug overdose as well as increasing suicide and unintentional injuries. The WHO, as part of its emergency response, has created lists of the greatest threats to human life and therefore human life expectancy. The most recent list was created for the year 2019 and is being used as a framework for this chapter; the list of threats can be found in Box 25.2. It is noteworthy that many of the 10 threats are disease-based, but the number one threat is **air pollution** and climate change. The most effective health promotion strategy for the disease threats is prevention, which is frequently through vaccines or other health behaviors. Health promotion strategies for both disease-based and nondisease threats may be strongly linked to the social determinants of health, which in themselves provide healthy behaviors and protection. In November 2023, the WHO identified an additional global issue, social isolation and loneliness, based on estimates that one in four older adults and between 5% and 15% of adolescents experience loneliness (WHO, 2023d). Social isolation and loneliness are risk factors for anxiety, depression, suicide, dementia, stroke, and cardiovascular disease, resulting in early deaths. A commission has been formed to gather more evidence and develop promising solutions to reduce the incidence and prevalence of social isolation and loneliness.

UN Millennial Goals and Healthy People 2030

At the start of the new millennium, in 2000, the UN developed millennial goals for global development. In 2015, they announced a new agenda for global sustainable development for 2015 to 2030. They called the agenda "Transforming Our World" and identified that world poverty was an area that affected every other facet of life. Five broad areas were presented that would guide the world and populations on a more sustainable pathway. These areas were people, planet, prosperity, peace, and partnership (UN Sustainable Development, n.d.). As part of this new agenda, 17 SDGs and 169 actions were announced. Although the actions are not reprinted in this chapter, the SDGs are listed in Box 25.3. The heads of state of the 193 member states who signed the declaration agreed to commit to enacting actions to meet the goals by 2030. Periodic reports are produced by the UN to outline global progress in meeting the SDGs. For example, an SDG Report 2023 is available via the internet (https://unstats.un.org/sdgs/report/2023/). The most recent report indicates that progress towards the goals has been hindered worldwide due to the lingering effects of the COVID-19 pandemic, climate crisis, the war in Ukraine, and a weak global economy. The authors report that the lack of progress is worldwide. Partnerships and collaborative goals are imperative to moving the SDG forward despite worldly challenges. In and among some countries, partnerships have been identified. For example, Sigma Theta Tau International Honor Society of Nursing was granted consultative status to the UN Economic and Social Council in 2012 because of the global expertise of Sigma's members. This brings a very formal link between nursing and the UN that enhances health and health promotion work throughout the world.

BOX 25.3 United Nations Sustainable Development Goals

Goal 1: End poverty in all its forms everywhere
Goal 2: End hunger, achieve food security and improved nutrition, and promote sustainable agriculture
Goal 3: Ensure healthy lives and promote well-being for all at all ages
Goal 4: Ensure inclusive and quality education for all and promote lifelong learning
Goal 5: Achieve gender equality and empower all adult and young females
Goal 6: Ensure availability and sustainable management of water and sanitation for all
Goal 7: Ensure access to affordable, reliable, sustainable, and modern energy for all
Goal 8: Promote sustained, inclusive, and sustainable economic growth, full and productive employment, and decent work for all
Goal 9: Build resilient infrastructure, promote inclusive and sustainable industrialization, and foster innovation
Goal 10: Reduce inequality within and among countries
Goal 11: Make cities and human settlements inclusive, safe, resilient, and sustainable
Goal 12: Ensure sustainable consumption and production patterns
Goal 13: Take urgent action to combat climate change and its effects
Goal 14: Conserve and sustainably use the oceans, seas, and marine resources for sustainable development
Goal 15: Protect, restore, and promote sustainable use of terrestrial ecosystems, sustainably manage forests, combat desertification, halt and reverse land degradation, and halt biodiversity loss
Goal 16: Promote peaceful and inclusive societies for sustainable development, provide access to justice for all, and build effective, accountable, and inclusive institutions at all levels
Goal 17: Strengthen the means of implementation and revitalize the Global Partnership for Sustainable Development

From United Nations Sustainable Development (n.d.)

As each individual ponders the topics listed in these three complementary documents, patterns become clear. Although absence of poverty is listed as an overall goal, attention to climate change must also be accomplished or other efforts will be in vain. The documents are unique but complementary; however, the actions and goals are indivisible. Focusing on only one to the exclusion of others will not assist the world to achieve health or health equity.

The United States also has health goals, called *Healthy People 2030.* Although these have been developed for the US health care system and society, selected goals that have global applicability can be found in Box 25.4. There are 359 core objectives,

BOX 25.4 *HEALTHY PEOPLE 2030* OBJECTIVES

AHS-04	Reduce the proportion of people who can't get medical care when they need it
AHS-07	Increase the proportion of people with a usual primary care provider
ECBP-01 -	Increase the proportion of adolescents who participate in daily school physical education
EH-D02	Reduce diseases and deaths related to heat
GH-D01	Increase the number of individuals grained globally to prevent, detect, or respond to public health threats
HAI-02-	Reduce MRSA bloodstream infections that people get in the hospital
HC/HIT-01	Increase the proportion of adults whose health care provider checked their understanding
IID04-	Maintain the vaccination coverage level of two doses of the MMR vaccine for children in kindergarten
PHI-04	Increase the proportion of state and territorial jurisdictions that have a health improvement plan
PREP-01	Increase the rate of bystander CPR for nontraumatic cardiac arrests
SDOH-01	Reduce the proportion of people living in poverty

CPR, Cardiopulmonary resuscitation; *MMR,* measles, mumps, rubella; *MRSA,* methicillin-resistant *Staphylococcus aureus.*
From Healthy People 2030 (n.d.)

which tend to be more specific than SDGs. These objectives are associated with evidence-based interventions. The plan also includes over 100 developmental and research objectives. Developmental objectives highlight issues with evidence-based interventions but lack current, reliable data. Research objectives highlight emerging issues that do not yet have evidence-based interventions. Both developmental and research objectives may become core objectives in the future. For the first time in the initiative's history, the concept of health literacy was added at both personal and organizational levels (US Department of Health and Human Services, 2023). This highlights the growing complexity of social determinants on health and health equity.

Many of the major health issues and threats throughout the world are interdependent and closely linked. The concept of One Health can help to illustrate the connectedness.

"**One Health** recognizes that the health of humans, animals, and ecosystems are interconnected. It involves applying a coordinated, collaborative, multidisciplinary and cross-sectoral approach to address potential or existing risks that originate at the animal-human-ecosystems interface" (Mackenzie & Jeggo, 2019). As communicable diseases, such as COVID-19, continue to emerge and mutate, it is clear that humans, animals, and the environment are interlinked. In 2021, the WHO formed the One Health High-Level Expert Panel (OHHLEP) to bring experts from a variety of disciplines linked to human, animal, and ecosystem health together to collaboratively assess and provide guidance on a long-term strategic approach to reduce the risk of zoonotic-related pandemics (WHO, 2023e). These experts continue to examine how world leaders and organizations can further understand and address the interdependent cause and effect relationships humans, animals, and the environment have on each other.

In the next section of the chapter, the authors have used the WHO's 10 Threats to examine the dangers that these threats present and to look at current evidence and health promotion activities for each of the threats. Some of the named threats have been combined for ease of understanding. Many of the threats have links to humans, animals, and the environment as described by the One Health approach. Global health challenges can quickly change as we saw during the COVID-19 pandemic. Lucero-Prisno et al. (2023) suggest emerging global health trends include "health systems, the mental health crisis, substance abuse, infectious diseases, malnutrition and food insecurity, sexual and reproductive health challenges, environmental pollution, the climate crisis, cancer, and diabetes." The chapter will focus on the most recent WHO strategic plan released in 2019, but as previously discussed, many new and returning issues are on the horizon that all health professionals will need to be aware of to best care for patients, families, and populations.

AIR POLLUTION AND CLIMATE CHANGE

For many years, concerns about air pollution and climate change have been brought forth by scientists. For the general population of citizens, there are believers and nonbelievers of the data cited by scientists. But for the nonbelievers, just looking at the environment around them should offer some concrete evidence of the data put forth by environmental scientists. Already, climate change threatens clean air, safe drinking water, nutritious food supply, safe shelter, and disease incidence and prevalence.

Air Pollution

Depending on the source referenced, up to 99% of the Earth's population breathes air that is polluted beyond acceptable standards, which contributes to about 6.7 million premature deaths globally each year, with about 89% of those deaths occurring in low- and middle-income countries (WHO, 2022, 2023f). **Air pollution** is a result of fine particles in the air as a result of pollutants released into the air. These fine particles penetrate deep into the lungs and are transported into the circulatory system and brain. As a result of these particles' deposition in the lungs and distribution to the rest of the body, the population living in areas of greater pollution is at increased risk for stroke, heart disease, lung cancer, chronic obstructive pulmonary disease (COPD), and infections such as pneumonia. In fact, air pollution was the cause of premature death in 37% of stroke and heart disease, 18% of COPD, 23% of lower respiratory tract infection, and 11% of lung cancer mortalities (WHO, 2022a). But no one on

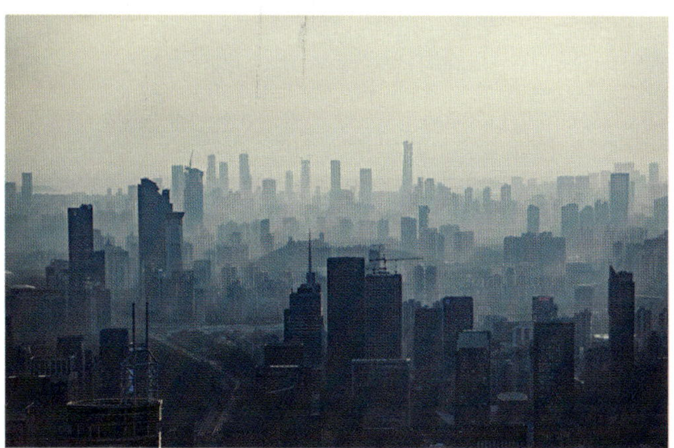

FIG. 25.1 Air pollution can affect safety and health in all facets of human life. (From iStock.com/real444.)

the Earth is immune to the effects of air pollution. Air pollution is a global problem and, while worse in some areas of the globe, is prevalent across the globe (Fig. 25.1). A systematic review of the literature indicates air pollution may also be associated with impaired neurocognitive development in infancy and childhood and dementia in older adults (Chandra et al., 2022).

Almost 70 years ago, the United States recognized the importance of decreasing air pollution and on July 14, 1955, passed the Air Pollution Control Act (Environmental Protection Agency [EPA], 2022). This act was intended to provide research and technical assistance in the management of air pollution, but left states in charge of managing pollution at the source. This resulted in a variety of different standards and limited effectiveness in the actual control of pollution. In 1963, the Clean Air Act was passed to better define air quality criteria. The EPA was established in 1970 and additional legislation to diminish air pollution was passed in 1990. The nation's air quality has improved significantly since 1990, but people are traveling farther and driving more so challenges remain (EPA, 2023a).

The challenges in achieving clean air are varied. There is the cost-benefit ratio of pollution control measures and their affect on overall health. There is also the influence of the politicians involved. If the cost of environmental protection measures will affect the bottom line of a politician's constituents, how likely is that politician to vote for statutes and regulations that support managing air pollution?

China, the world's largest emitter of climate-warming greenhouse gases, is more recently responding to local and global pressure to reduce air pollution. China's economy is heavily industry-based and making changes in polluting emissions will take time and considerable effort. China is followed by the United States and India as the second and third top emitters, respectively. Together, these three countries account for 42.6% of the world's total greenhouse gas emissions (Friedrich et al., 2023). All three will need to implement ambitious measures to change the effect on global warming.

Global Warming

Global warming (the continual increase in temperature of the Earth's surface, oceans, and atmosphere) is contributing to climate change (Oka, 2023) and increased incidence of extreme weather events (National Aeronautics and Space Administration [NASA], 2023). With global warming, the environmental determinants of health, that is, clean air, safe drinking water, food supply, and safe shelter, are affected.

With global warming, there is an increase in ice melt, leading to release of long-buried microbes, a rise in sea levels (8–9 inches since 1870 with an accelerated rise in levels expected in coming years; National Oceanic and Atmospheric Administration [NOAA], 2022), and increased acidity of sea water (due to absorption and dissolution into carbonic acid of atmospheric CO_2).

Global warming is affecting almost every stage of the water cycle, including evaporation, precipitation, surface runoff and stream flow, oceans, snowpack, and clouds. Warmer air holds more moisture and will pull more water from lakes, oceans, soil, and plants, affecting drinking water supply and agriculture. The warmer, wetter air, when combined with a cold front, will cause heavier rains and snowfall, contributing to more flooding from rain and potentially more flooding with heavier snow melt. Global warming will also affect where the precipitation falls, leading to more precipitation in the Northeast and less in the Southwest. With drier vegetation, wildfires in the West will likely be more frequent and cause greater areas of devastation (Federation of American Scientists, 2023). As precipitation patterns change, the food supply is also likely to be affected. Heavier rainstorms have the potential to deplete agricultural land of nutrients important to the crops grown and to pollute rivers and streams with a variety of substances not currently present in the water supply. In addition to contaminating our drinking water, it may also be harmful to fish, causing a decrease in that food supply (EPA, 2023b).

Temperature changes are changing ocean currents, which will change atmospheric weather patterns globally. Increasing temperatures in the oceans are also causing the fish to migrate to cooler waters, which may affect ocean life and viability. Increased heat is contributing to decreased cloud cover. This will lead to an increased need to irrigate crops or hydrate livestock. As the water supply diminishes due to increased evaporation, the ability to support food sources will decrease (EPA, 2023b; Crimmins et al., 2023).

Some current animal sources of food are likely to become extinct if they cannot migrate and/or cannot survive in the new climate. Some plants will not thrive in a warmer environment. Additionally, as warmer temperature expands the range of disease-causing pathogens, plant species will succumb. The loss of both plant and animal food sources will leave the Earth's population with fewer options for and a diminished supply of food. Plant sources of food, particularly protein-based, tend to be the most reproduceable and inexpensive to obtain. Due, in part, to climate change, plant-based food sources are not consistently adequately available to sustain protein needs (Nithiyanantham et al., 2019).

Global attention has been given to managing climate change in an effort to stop the negative effects on global health. The Paris Agreement, a formal effort to combat climate change, was developed in 2015. The major aim of this agreement is to strengthen the global response to maintaining a near-steady temperature for the Earth, with the agreement limiting the increase in temperature during the 21st century to 2°C. A more ambitious goal was also discussed that would keep the rise in temperature to 1.5°C. In all, the Paris Agreement does the following: holds participating countries legally accountable for limiting global temperature increase and decreasing greenhouse gas emissions; has participating countries take stock every 5 years of their progress toward the goals; encourages conserving and enhancing efforts through activities such as replanting forests that have been cut down; encourages countries to set even higher ambitions for stopping the negative effects than those that are identified in the agreement; encourages adaptation and resilience to diminish vulnerability to climate change; stresses the importance of averting, minimizing, and managing damage due to climate change; stresses the responsibility of developed countries to assist developing countries relative to these efforts; and provides climate change education to the public (United Nations, 2023a; see Box 25.5: Quality and Safety Scenario).

Although global efforts are critical to combating climate change, the effect by individuals will also be imperative. It is the efficiencies in lifestyle created over time with our "advances" in technology and conveniences available to us that contribute to the development of greenhouse emissions. As individuals, it will be important to make lifestyle changes as well. Suggestions include: (1) eating less meat as it requires more energy to produce than plant-based food; (2) consider modes of transportation and choose those that require less fuel; (3) plant trees to help remove carbon dioxide from the atmosphere; (4) use renewable energy to power your home; (5) use energy-efficient appliances; (6) use less water; (7) don't buy more food than you will use to avoid having to throw food out; (8) use energy-efficient light bulbs; and (9) unplug electronic devices rarely used (UN, 2023b; see Box 25.6: Ethical Issues for critical thinking questions).

DISEASES

Noncommunicable Diseases

Noncommunicable diseases (NCDs), which account for 74% of all deaths globally, are those that cannot be transmitted directly from one person to another, are chronic, and have a slow progression. With NCDs, there are often strategies individuals can employ to prevent the disease and/or to slow its progression.

The four main types of NCDs are cardiovascular diseases (e.g., heart attacks and stroke), cancer, chronic respiratory diseases (e.g., COPD and asthma), and diabetes. These four types of NCDs account for over 80% of all premature NCD deaths. And 77% of those premature deaths occur in low- and middle-income populations (WHO, 2023g). Contributing factors to the development of NCDs include unhealthy diets, physical inactivity, exposure to tobacco smoke, and the harmful use of alcohol. Recent information suggests global climate change also has an effect.

There are a variety of risk factors that lead to development of NCDs, with some being more easily modified than others. Tobacco use, physical inactivity, unhealthy diet, and harmful use of alcohol are all risk factors that would be relatively easy

BOX 25.5 QUALITY AND SAFETY SCENARIO

A recent article in *The Journal for Nurse Practitioners* highlighted the effect of climate change on older adults (Kriebel-Gasparro, 2022). The author noted that the population of older adults aged 65 and older is growing. In the United States, the population is projected to double in size over the next 40 years. Changes in weather patterns have brought extreme weather to all parts of the world. Natural disasters, such as heat waves, forest fires, droughts, hurricanes, and cold spells, have caused much destruction and devastation to humans, animals, and the environment in recent years. Older adults are more vulnerable to extreme weather. Researchers have found that older adults are more likely to experience respiratory, cardiovascular, and psychological harm in weather events, especially heat waves. The author states that health care professionals, especially nurses and nurse practitioners, need to understand the effects of extreme weather events on older adults.

You are a practicing nurse and trusted community member in a rural town with a population of approximately 3500 people. The mayor has recently heard the upcoming summer season is slated to be one of the hottest on record with little rain. He comes to you concerned and asks your opinion on what can be done to prepare for the hot weather and to prevent people from getting sick from the heat. The mayor is especially worried about older adults as they make up 40% of the town's population. He is also worried about the local farming community as the possibility of drought is high and the hot temperatures can be dangerous for livestock. You have been asked to help your local community build a public health plan for the upcoming summer season to reduce the risk of heat-related illness.

- Why are older adults more vulnerable to extreme heat?
- What actions can older adults take to minimize their risk of heat-related illness? How can friends and family of older adults help them to minimize their risk? What can the local town do to help reduce the incidence of heat-related illnesses?
- What role does the health care system have in the prevention of heat-related illness?
- In your town, there is a primary care clinic and a critical access hospital. You have identified nurse champions at both the clinic and hospital. What role can these nurses play in reducing the incidence of heat-related illnesses?
- The extreme temperatures are predicted to have effects on human, animal, and environmental health in your local community. You have decided to introduce the concept of One Health to the mayor. How would you describe this framework? What can your local community do to address One Health?

BOX 25.6 Ethical Issues

Global Ethical Dilemmas

- Is it ethical for the current inhabitants of the Earth to ignore the factors that contribute to global warming, considering the potentially catastrophic affect of climate change on the survival of future generations?
- Considering the resources available in developed countries, ethically what is the role of policy makers within the country and the role of international delegates?
- Should individuals be allowed to make choices of convenience that contribute to additional release of global-warming greenhouse gases or should emissions be regulated with consequences for exceeding limits?

to modify. Metabolic risk factors, such as raised blood pressure, overweight/obesity, hyperglycemia, and hyperlipidemia would require more effort, but again could be modified. Socioeconomic risk factors, such as poverty, are much more difficult to modify. Being poor also affects an individual's ability to choose more healthy foods, which tend to be more expensive. Getting adequate physical activity if you can't afford a gym membership or if you live in an area where personal safety would be a concern if you were to walk or run outdoors is also more difficult to modify (see Box 25.7: Best Practice).

Strategies that have been somewhat effective in reducing use of tobacco and alcohol include regulation of availability and taxation because increased cost often leads to decreased use. Transformed marketing practices have also led to consumers making healthier food choices. Education in the form of one-to-one work with health care professionals and the public as well as group efforts have been offered to teach the lay public about strategies to manage modifiable risk factors, and for some individuals this is very effective. But regulation, marketing, and education are clearly not enough. Even among health care professionals, who are well educated in the strategies important to prevent and manage NCDs, there is smoking, physical inactivity, unhealthy diets, excess alcohol use, hypertension, obesity, hyperglycemia, and hyperlipidemia.

BOX 25.7 BEST PRACTICE

Changing lifestyles and behaviors may be factors in the rising prevalence of cardiovascular- related diseases (hypertension, hyperlipidemia, stroke, etc.) and diabetes across the globe. Researchers estimate 15 million people die per year globally due to these diseases, with a greater proportion of deaths occurring in low- and middle-income countries. Researchers from the United States and South Africa recently came together to test and adapt an evidence-based intervention aimed at reducing hypertension, hyperlipidemia, and diabetes (Catley et al., 2022). The study took place in a Xhosa-speaking urban township in Cape Town, South Africa, with high rates of poverty. Participants were adults who were overweight or obese (i.e., BMI >25 kg/m^2). The randomized controlled trial compared participants who participated in the Lifestyle Africa program to those receiving usual care. The Lifestyle Africa program used local community health workers to deliver 17 video-based group sessions at community clubs. The curriculum encouraged physical activity and dietary changes using behavior change theories. Additionally, participants received twice daily text tips. A health assessment consisting of blood pressure, weight, cholesterol, and HbA1c was conducted before the intervention and within 7 to 9 months after the trial. A total of 240 participants received the Lifestyle Africa program and 254 participants received usual care. Researchers found that the intervention had no effect on weight loss, blood pressure, or cholesterol. However, the intervention resulted in a statistically significant reduction in HbA1c compared to those in usual care. This study highlighted several key points. Evidence-based interventions in high-income countries can be feasibility modified and adapted to fit the needs of populations at risk in low- and middle-income countries. The use of community health workers along with the statistically significant effect on HbA1c were positive outcomes of the study that need to be further explored for future studies. This study is foundational in helping researchers and NGOs better understand how to build and deliver noncommunicable disease community-based prevention programs in a variety of global settings.

BMI, Body mass index; *HbA1c*, hemoglobin A1c; *NGO*, nongovernmental organizations.

Research has demonstrated that a mother's behavior during pregnancy can influence health and behavior of the child for a lifetime (Bekkhus et al., 2022). It would be reasonable then to begin education and intervention for human beings in utero during prenatal care. Not only would this support the health and well-being of the mother but provide a strong beginning for the infant. During childhood when much of the time is spent in school, it's critical that children have ample time for physical activity and are provided healthy meals to teach them about good nutrition and appropriate physical activity. Some of the challenges are that many schools do not offer much physical activity except for the 10 to 15 minutes that remain after lunch is eaten, and the meals offered at schools of all levels typically are not examples of good nutritional choices. What families offer for meals at home is equally important. Considering the rising obesity rate in the United States alone, especially in children, the conclusion may be drawn that good examples of physical activity and healthy nutrition are not consistently occurring in the home either. Data that quantify the obesity epidemic indicate that in female children, the United States ranks 15th in the world for highest obesity rate at 20%, preceded by 14 underdeveloped countries; in male children, the United States is the 12th highest country at 23%, preceded by 11 underdeveloped countries (Global Obesity Observatory, 2017; NCD Risk Factor Collaborative, 2020). As a leading developed country with one of the most advanced health care systems in the world, the United States should be able to achieve better outcomes.

The good examples that should be provided in schools and at home during childhood should continue into adolescence. Typically, as individuals move from going to school to having a full-time job, they trade sitting in school all day to sitting at work. They may also start their own family, and finding time to be active may be a bit challenging. This is one point in life when shortcuts will be more common because of time constraints, and finding time for physical activity and healthy eating will be more challenging. And the final transition, from working to retirement, will present additional opportunities to consider how individuals will work to maintain health.

Mikkelsen and colleagues (2019) suggest a life course approach. Unlike the disease-oriented approaches commonly used to manage one condition, a **life course approach** considers the critical stages, transitions, and settings individuals will experience in their life and through which they will work to maintain health. This approach would also take into consideration the social determinants of health, sex, equity, and human rights and would involve a close partnership with health care providers or health coaches who can offer guidance at various points of transition. This approach would also require improved health literacy through work with individuals, institutions, communities, and countries to achieve success in preventing and/or managing NCDs.

Heat-related illnesses are also NCDs, including heat stroke (body has lost temperature control ability), heat exhaustion (excessive sweating resulting in excessive loss of fluids and electrolytes), rhabdomyolysis (rapid breakdown, rupture, and death of muscle due to prolonged physical activity during heat stress), heat syncope (fainting due to prolonged heat exposure),

BOX 25.8 EVIDENCE-BASED PRACTICE

Cooling interventions among agricultural workers: A pilot study

Objective: Worldwide temperatures are on the rise. With higher temperatures, a greater incidence of heat-related illness occurs. Agricultural workers are 35 times more likely than the general workforce to die of a heat-related illness (Gubernot et al., 2015). The nature of their work requires them to be outside for long periods of time and is physically demanding. The environmental and exertional heat can elevate one's core body temperature. When the core body temperature rises to 38°C or higher, heat exhaustion can occur. Symptoms include headache, excessive sweating, nausea and vomiting, muscle cramps, and so forth. If symptoms are not managed, death can occur. This study aimed to better understand the effectiveness of selected cooling devices to prevent a rise in core body temperature to 38°C or higher (Chicas et al., 2021).

Methods: Agricultural workers (n = 84) in Florida were randomized to one of four groups: (1) no intervention; (2) cooling bandana; (3) cooling vest; or (4) both a cooling bandana and a cooling vest during a typical workday. Participants wore biomonitoring equipment to capture their core body temperature along with an accelerometer to capture their level of physical activity. At the end of the day, workers were asked to fill out a survey asking about the occurrence of any heat- related symptoms.

Results: Seventy-eight agricultural workers completed at least one intervention during a typical workday. Those wearing the bandana had lower odds of exceeding 38°C core body temperature (odds ratio [OR] = 0.7, 90% confidence interval [CI] = 0.2, 3.2). Those wearing vests had higher odds of exceeding a body temperature of 38°C (OR = 1.8, 90% CI = 0.3, 5.6). Using both the bandana and cooling vest had little effect from the control (OR = 1.3, 90% CI = 0.3, 5.6).

Conclusions: The use of a cooling bandana was found to lower the chances of agricultural workers' core body temperatures from rising to 38°C or higher, which is associated with a higher chance of heat-related illnesses.

Nursing implications: Cooling bandanas are inexpensive, easy to obtain, light weight, and reusable. They can help to reduce the incidence of heat-related illnesses among agricultural workers and other vulnerable occupational groups exposed to high environmental and exertional heat. Nurses are uniquely poised to suggest feasible health-related suggestions, such as the use of a cooling bandana, in a variety of settings, including primary care and occupational health clinics.

heat cramps (due to heat induced sweating and electrolyte loss), and heat rash (due to excessive seating) (CDC NIOSH, 2022). Box 25.8 offers a recent study to examine interventions to assist migrant workers struggling with excess heat.

Vector-borne (e.g., ticks, mosquitoes) diseases are also NCDs and are on the rise. There is a two-fold increase in tick-borne diseases and an alarming increase in mosquito-borne illnesses. Warmer global temperatures have elongated the tick and mosquito seasons, leading to a prolonged opportunity for transmitting disease (Advisory Board, 2023). Global warming has also had a negative affect on the natural predators (e.g., bats) of these vectors, resulting in a larger population able to spread diseases (Festa et al., 2023). Of major concern is that only one of the 16 vector-borne diseases, yellow fever, has a Food and Drug Administration–approved vaccine available (Advisory Board, 2023).

Communicable Diseases

Communicable diseases are those that are passed from one human to another, or from an animal to a human, with or without an intervening vector (e.g., mosquito). They may be relatively harmless or life-threatening. Unlike most NCDs, if the individual survives the disease, it is more likely that there are few sequelae or life-lasting complications. In this section, communicable diseases that have been in the public discourse over the last few years will be addressed.

COVID-19 Pandemic

A **pandemic** is an "outbreak of infectious disease that occurs over a wide geographical area and that is of high prevalence, generally affecting a significant proportion of the world's population, usually over the course of several months" (Rogers, 2024). Since early 2020, the world has been engaged in a global pandemic of a novel coronavirus that leads to the disease known as **COVID-19**. Originating in China, it spread to almost every corner of the world. With a very strong presence over 2020 and 2021, the world continues to experience outbreaks and new variants of this disease.

Over time, the world has faced different pandemic situations. Each time, governments and organizations believe they are learning from the challenges that could not be met in the previous situation. However, each time it is also clear that those same governments and organizations were not adequately prepared to manage the challenges of the current pandemic, that some global agency failed to sound the alarm early enough, or that countries and populations failed to take warnings seriously. The response to the pandemic has differed from country to country, as has the incidence and mortality rate, with those countries heeding the warnings and responding more quickly demonstrating better outcomes.

Historically, pandemics have occurred approximately every 10 years or so. More recently, pandemics are occurring with greater frequency. Examples of recent pandemics include severe acute respiratory syndrome (SARS) (2003), influenza A H1N5 (bird flu) (2007), H1N1 (swine flu) (2009), Middle East respiratory syndrome (MERS) (2012), Ebola (2014), Zika (2016), and COVID-19 (Council on Foreign Relations, 2023).

The main questions are, why is the frequency of pandemics increasing and what can be done to reverse the course? First, why is the frequency increasing? This chapter has discussed the effect of climate change and global warming on the overall health of the world. Scientists have been warning that global warming would lead to an increased incidence and prevalence of communicable diseases. Now the legitimacy of those warnings is becoming evident. One of the major contributing factors is deforestation of the Earth. Only approximately 15% of the Earth's forests remain intact. As animals lose their natural environment, they relocate. Often, animal relocation and human movement into the area cleared of the forest contribute to humans and animals living in closer proximity. This increases the potential for animal-to-human transmission of diseases previously occurring only in the animal population. Currently, approximately 60% of new human illnesses come from an animal source (Lustgarten, 2020). Even today, after much discussion and debate, there are two major hypotheses for the origins of COVID-19, one being a zoonotic disease moving to humans through exposure in a market and the other a leak of matter from the Institute of Virology in Wuhan, China (Gostin & Gronvall, 2023). Regardless of the origin of

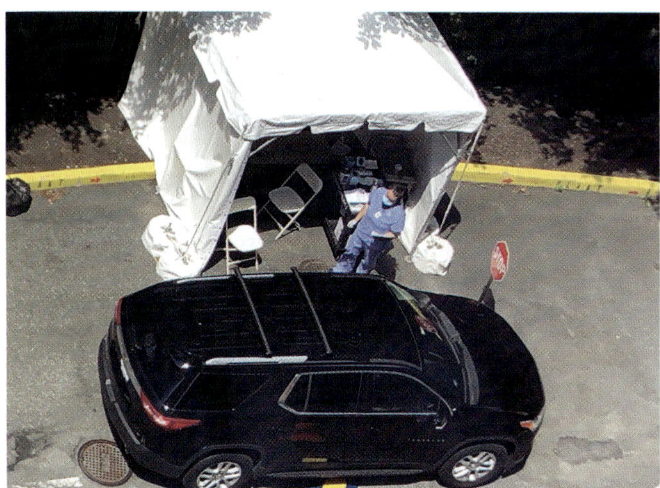

FIG. 25.2 Testing sites are in place to identify if an individual is positive for COVID-19.

a pandemic, the ease and amount of human travel, which has increased markedly over the last few decades, has contributed significantly to the spread of a pandemic disease.

Fragile and vulnerable settings are also at higher risk for the development and transmission of and death from emerging infections. COVID-19 is particularly problematic because it can be spread by an individual for up to 14 days even when the individual has no symptoms and never exhibits the disease. Fragile states lack the resources and infrastructure for clean water, safe food handling, protective housing, and adequate health care. In the situation with COVID-19, we know that millions of people became ill, and thousands died even in places where there was a safe, stable environment and a well-developed health care system readily available. Fragile states or autocratic governments can carry greater risk for disease development of, transmission of, and death from COVID-19 because of the lack of resources in the environment or lack of political will to follow the science (Fig. 25.2).

So, what is the solution to the current threats from global pandemics? Many of the changes needed to prevent pandemic outbreaks have been addressed in other sections in this chapter, but a primary approach would be to work effectively to achieve the UN SDGs outlined in Box 25.3. The health of the world is dependent on it, and survival of the planet is questionable unless those goals are everyone's priority.

Influenza Pandemic

Influenza is highly contagious. Individuals are most likely to infect others 3 to 4 days after symptoms begin, but for some the range of contagion can vary from 1 day before symptoms to 5 to 7 days after demonstrating illness. Symptoms include fever/chills, cough, sore throat, nasal stuffiness, muscular aches, and fatigue (WHO, 2023h). Influenza can strike at any age, although the very young, elderly, and persons with other chronic diseases are more susceptible to complications and severe cases. Influenza is often mild and frequently resolves on its own. However, the attack can be severe and lead to death. There are multiple strains of influenza virus, and frequent mutations within the viruses ensure that there are always new strains arising. The best prevention for influenza is an annual vaccine. Every 6 months, the WHO Global Influenza Surveillance and Response System updates the current influenza viruses present in the world (WHO, 2023i). From these data, an annual vaccine is recommended that addresses the identified strains. However, even with this strong monitoring, it is difficult to ensure they have the right "mix," because these decisions must be made long before an influenza season begins, to ensure that sufficient amounts of that year's vaccine are developed, produced, and disseminated across the globe for use in clinics and other health care facilities.

As noted with COVID-19, given the current amount of global travel in the modern world, a virus that begins anywhere can rapidly move across the globe, attached to travelers who spread it wherever they go. A pandemic can happen at any point in time. The WHO has prepared a global influenza strategy for dealing with a future pandemic (WHO, 2019b). Elements within that strategy include two high-level outcomes, which include "better tools to prevent, detect, control and treat influenza" and "strong national capacities for preparedness and response against influenza" (WHO, 2019b, p. 3). Four strategic objectives are also included in that plan (Box 25.9).

BOX 25.9 Strategic Objectives for Global Influenza Strategy 2019–2030

1. Promote research and innovation to address unmet public health needs
2. Strengthen global influenza surveillance, monitoring, and data utilization
3. Expand seasonal influenza prevention and control policies and programs to protect the vulnerable
4. Strengthen pandemic preparedness and response for influenza to make the world safer

From WHO (2019b, p. 6)

Dengue Fever

Dengue fever is a virus that is spread to humans through being bitten by an infected mosquito of the Aedes species. The same mosquitos can spread other diseases such as Zika. Close to half of the world's population lives in areas where this mosquito can spread disease, which are generally tropical and subtropical areas, including parts of the United States. Mosquitos tend to be more prevalent in urban and suburban areas, where humans are more plentiful. There are four variations of **dengue fever**, and mosquitos in a given area can carry all four. An individual can get each kind in his or her lifetime. One in 20 persons who are symptomatic progress to severe dengue and about 40,000 die annually (CDC, 2023a). The CDC is now tracking dengue fever within the United States, where cases may be travel-related or locally acquired (CDC, 2023b). Health promotion and prevention activities for dengue primarily focus on avoidance of mosquito bites, although there is a dengue vaccine. The recommendation for the vaccine is that it be given only to persons (including children) who have already experienced one of the versions of dengue fever (CDC, 2024).

Avoidance of mosquito bites takes many forms. Insect repellent that has been recognized by the EPA can be used on most individuals, including pregnant and breastfeeding women. The other huge protection is the use of mosquito netting. This can take the form of screens in buildings or netting around baby carriages/strollers or beds. Other prevention efforts include wearing clothing that covers arms and legs and monitoring and cleaning places where standing water can accumulate (e.g., bird baths, planters, trash containers; CDC, 2020). These are prime receptacles for the laying of mosquito eggs.

For those persons who are exposed through mosquito bites, approximately 25% will actually become ill. Fever is the primary symptom, with variations of pain behind the eyes and in muscles, joints, and bones; nausea/vomiting; and rash. Treatment is symptom-related, as well as supporting the individual. Most cases will not require hospitalization, and recovery is common in approximately 1 week (CDC, 2020).

Zika Virus

Zika is another disease spread through the bite of the Aedes species mosquito. There is currently documented evidence of transmission from sexual contact and from mother to fetus during pregnancy; there have been no confirmed cases of transmission of Zika through blood transfusion (CDC, 2025). Although discovered in humans in 1952, this disease has been documented primarily since 2007. The actual disease is generally mild, and many persons may experience it without symptoms or, indeed, without realizing that they have it. The larger concern with Zika is the influence on other diseases and conditions. This is particularly true for the pregnant female who experiences Zika virus. This infection may result in preterm birth, miscarriage, microcephaly, and other congenital concerns (CDC, 2025). Furthermore, it has been linked to neurologic complications, which can include Guillain-Barré syndrome (CDC, 2025).

Health promotion and prevention strategies for Zika virus are similar to those of dengue fever, highlighting the avoidance of mosquito bites. Females who are pregnant and wanting to become pregnant should take extra precautions, including planning or avoiding travel to affected global areas where possible.

Human Immunodeficiency Virus

Human immunodeficiency virus (HIV) is a type of virus known as a "retrovirus." It is spread through body fluids. The effect of the virus is that the individual's immune system is slowly destroyed, sometimes to the point that the person cannot fight off other diseases or infections. This virus originated in animals and was probably present in humans by the late 1800s. However, it was not until the mid-1970s that it became recognized as a strong threat to human life. When the medical community realized the scope of the issue, one of the responses was the creation and implementation of universal precautions, which currently remain in use (CDC, 2022b). On a global scale, the UN Program on HIV/Acquired Immunodeficiency Syndrome (AIDS) (UNAIDS) reports that 39.0 million persons lived with HIV in 2022, with only 76% of adults receiving treatment. In 2022, 1.3 million were newly diagnosed, which is 40% of the number diagnosed in 1995. Approximately 86% of those with HIV were aware of their diagnosis (UNAIDS, 2023).

AIDS is the final state of HIV infection. During the 1970s and 1980s, a diagnosis of HIV signaled certain death, with often just a few years between HIV diagnosis, AIDS, and death from complications of AIDs. Significant misinformation was present in the early years, with fears of infection from shaking a diagnosed person's hand and from using the same toilet as an infected person. Further research resulted in the knowledge that HIV was transmitted though specific body fluids, including semen, blood, rectal and vaginal fluids, and breast milk. However, excellent precautions and the discovery of antiretroviral drugs have changed the outlook globally for persons with HIV. Better treatment also includes the early diagnosis of infections that arise in persons with altered immune systems (called "opportunistic infections"). With all the treatments available nowadays, individuals with HIV can enjoy almost the same length of life as those who do not have HIV (CDC, 2022b).

There are several health promotion and prevention activities that can be used with HIV/AIDS. The first is knowledge. Because individuals with HIV can now enjoy near-normal lives, it is important that everyone understand how to protect themselves, and others, and how to seek treatment. This includes safe sex activities, no sharing of drug utensils such as needles, accessing testing if engaging in potentially harmful behaviors, and ensuring the affected person continues treatment as prescribed (CDC, 2022b). One of the global health issues has been the presence, dissemination, and cost of the drugs involved. Countries with fewer resources may not be able to make the drugs available to their populations. The UN estimates that only 65% to 89% of diagnosed adults have access to retroviral drugs, depending on the population (UNAIDS, 2023). A second is the stigma that comes with HIV—in some cultures it was completely denied, and in others, lack of knowledge ensured that the spread continued. Because the disease was first present in populations of males having sex with males, a homophobic moral response sometimes hindered diagnosis and treatment of these patients. Global health was and can still be compromised when there is a lack of knowledge, diagnosis, or treatment. With the advent of strong opportunities for HIV control in the infected individual, another issue has come forward. Now infected persons must learn to live their lives with HIV, which means, for example, planning for sexual encounters, birth of a baby, and parenting (CDC, 2022b).

Ebola virus

Ebola virus is a deadly virus that can be transmitted from animals to humans or from humans to humans. Although this virus is primarily present in sub-Saharan Africa, the nature of global travel can ensure that the potential for spread is clearly worldwide. There are several Ebola virus strains that have been identified; however, only certain ones affect humans (CDC, 2023c). Human-to-human transmission is through blood or body fluids from an infected person with signs and symptoms, the corpse of a person who died with Ebola, or contaminated bedding or clothing of an infected person. It is noted that Ebola can be found in semen of recovered persons (CDC, 2023c). Although few people in North America have been affected, there were some highly publicized cases during the 2014 outbreak. During that outbreak, more than 28,000 persons were infected and more than 11,000 died (CDC, 2023a).

Following an incubation period of 2 to 21 days, symptoms generally appear. The first symptoms are known as "dry" symptoms—fatigue, fever, aches, and pains. The disease then progresses to "wet" symptoms—diarrhea and vomiting, bruising, and hemorrhaging. Part of the difficulty in diagnosing is the similarity of dry symptoms to other diseases. If precautions are not observed, the period of incubation or dry symptoms can provide an excellent path to spreading the virus to other persons (CDC, 2023c). Scientists around the world have been working on a vaccine for Ebola. One such vaccine, which was trialed for use in 2018 to 2019, was approved by the European Commission in November 2019, and it was approved by the USFDA in December 2019 (CDC, 2023c). Vaccination is encouraged for persons who are at occupational risk for the disease (CDC, 2023c). A significant thrust of health promotion is for all health care workers to ask questions of every patient—about travel to affected areas and possibility of exposure. A second health promotion strategy is the consistent use of universal precautions, especially handwashing. At the community level, prevention and protection go hand in hand and include "case management, infection prevention and control practices, surveillance and contact tracing, a good laboratory service, safe and dignified burials and social mobilization" (WHO, 2023j).

FRAGILE AND VULNERABLE SETTINGS

Definitions and Components of Fragile States

Countries that don't have the capacity to manage the political, social, economic, environmental, and security risks they face are referred to as **fragile states** (Klassen, 2019; World Bank, 2023). The risks may be internal, external, or both, but in the end they significantly affect the economic stability of a country. Extreme poverty, premature mortality, and ill health are highly concentrated in areas characterized by **fragility** and conflict (Christianson et al., 2023). In fact, over half of preventable maternal deaths and deaths of children under 5 years of age occur in settings of conflict, displacement, and natural disasters (Primo Braga et al., 2020). Many assume these effects are confined to countries that experience internal and/or external conflict and those whose economic stability is uncertain. However, that is not the case. In countries experiencing conflict and economic and political challenges, citizens who are able relocate to other countries. Those individuals seek a geographic location in which they feel safe and are able to meet basic human needs. As a result, developed countries that are generally considered to be economically and politically stable have pockets of fragility as immigrants who lack health care and, typically, the economic means to support personal basic needs, arrive.

When considering the hierarchy of needs, food, water, and shelter come first (Maslow, 1970). If an individual cannot feed and shelter themselves or their family, health promotion and prevention strategies will not be a priority. Research has shown that individuals who have reached a level of self-actualization are considerably more likely to engage in health-related behaviors than those who have not. In fact, obvious indicators of a health problem will be ignored until the basic needs of all those for whom an individual is responsible are met (Thompson et al., 2016).

The United States has known for more than 20 years the effect of fragile states on US soil. If there was no recognition before, the incidents on September 11, 2001, were a significant wake-up call. Terrorist training bases, transnational crime networks, and poverty, disease, and humanitarian emergencies create crises in developing countries that influence the current foreign policy and security challenges. In some developing countries, the government has failed or is too weak to protect its citizens from internal and external threats, provide basic health care and education, and respond to the overall needs of its citizens (Organization for Economic Cooperation and Development, 2020).

Conflict, disease, and economic collapse in developing countries globally will have spillover effects in developed countries. This will not be resolved by developing more weapons and creating larger armed forces to better protect the citizens of any country. To address the global chaos created when a country cannot meet the needs of its population, the global community must work together to ensure the needs of every human being are met. This global chaos extends to surveillance, prevention, and management of disease outbreaks. A number of epidemics have been experienced over the years. The slow response of international organizations to identify them as epidemics and mobilize resources has led to wider disease spread and increased number of deaths. The question to consider is how might that epidemic course have been different if the disease started in a developed country rather than a fragile state? And what if the international organizations became involved at an early point in the process? Could outcomes have been different? Consider the West African Ebola epidemic that came to the world's attention in 2014. It took international agencies 6 months to proclaim the outbreak an epidemic and mobilize resources. In those 6 months, there were more than 28,000 diagnosed cases of Ebola and 11,000 deaths (CDC, 2019). In that time, international travel continued, with the potential to make Ebola a global epidemic. But we're learning. With the more recent outbreak of COVID, international agencies moved more quickly to alert the world. But did they move quickly enough? On December 12, 2019, a cluster of patients in Wuhan, China, were diagnosed with an atypical pneumonia-like illness that did not respond well to standard treatment. It wasn't until January 17, 2020, that the CDC began screening passengers arriving from China. By this time, COVID had been identified in four countries, including China, Thailand, Japan, and Korea. On January 20, 2020, the first case was identified in the United States. It took international agencies more than a month to start screening and restricting travel. In that time, COVID was allowed to spread worldwide (CDC, 2023d). So, while the global response to COVID was considerably more timely, it wasn't fast enough to prevent a global pandemic.

Challenges in Fragile States

The challenges in fragile states include:

- Capacity for local health governance to recognize, report, and respond to infectious outbreaks
- Lack of sustainable communication and trust between global health governance agencies and local health governance
- A rapidly growing private market for health care that weakens public health efforts

- Lack of community engagement and mobilization as part of the risk mitigation framework
- Weak health systems fail to identify microbial threats, epidemics further weaken such systems, and the momentum to break that cycle is lacking (Adrian et al., 2023; International Monetary Fund, 2023).

As discussed, drivers that lead to fragility include weak political systems, poor economic resources, availability of natural resources, violence and conflict, external stressors, geography, climate and disease, and international political and economic relationships. There have been lengthy discussions for many years about the contributing factors of fragility and strategies to address the issues that result. And a variety of strategies have been tried, but with limited success.

The complex nature of the drivers contributing to fragility creates challenges that require multifaceted strategies to significantly affect fragile states. However, in this chapter we discuss strategies that support health promotion and disease prevention.

Globally, developed countries have traditionally responded to epidemics, natural disasters, and other unexpected crises. In addition to the rising risks associated with fragility and the effects of climate change, crisis response will soon not be sustainable. Rather, global efforts need to shift to sustainable solutions. A place to begin efforts is in working to decrease the incidence of NCDs and the persistence of communicable diseases (Primo Braga et al., 2020).

This situation also presents opportunities for widespread collaboration. The United States has a well-developed **telemedicine network.** In this country, small rural hospitals collaborate with larger urban medical centers to provide expert care to rural residents. Telemedicine strategies include nurses who monitor and teach as well as providers who diagnose and treat. The urban health care professionals partner with those in rural settings to provide state-of-the-art strategies for health promotion, disease prevention, and acute care. There are about 16 billion mobile devices worldwide (Larrichia, 2023), suggesting that telemedicine might be an opportunity to reach populations in serious need of care to monitor, teach, diagnose, and treat. A Healthy People 2030 objective currently in research status (i.e., it doesn't currently have evidence-based research interventions developed to address it) is to "increase the use of telehealth to improve access to health services (Healthy People 2030, n.d.). When considering the number of mobile devices worldwide, it would seem this objective would be within reach in the very near future if the number of providers is sufficient.

The UN recognizes the global threat created by fragility. Fragility drives conflict and reverse development. But fragility is not just the result of conflict. The five dimensions that drive fragility are economic, environmental, political, security, and societal. And climate change exacerbates fragility (Roberts & Pompei, 2018). But the countries who have signed the SDG (see Box 25.3) have pledged to work with fragile countries, beginning with those that are furthest behind, so that globally, no one is left behind in a state of crisis (UN, 2023c). A global effort has the greatest potential to support a future that eliminates conflict, poverty, and crisis response and instead provides stable, well-supported management of health and well-being regardless of location (Box 25.10: Genomics, on using genomics to benefit global health).

BOX 25.10 GENOMICS

The five dimensions that drive fragility are continuing to rapidly change. Research and public health organizations continue to work together to identify best methods to prevent, mitigate, and reduce the drivers of fragility. Part of this work also involves building strong foundational knowledge on the various factors and how they interact. One way to do this is to better understand each of the factors' genomics, which includes its basic structure, function, and evolution. The study of genomics is vast and can encompass many different domains. The study of microbial genomes has helped to control infectious disease. Researchers are better able to prevent, diagnose, manage, and treat genetic conditions through a better understanding of human genomics. Agricultural experts are able to better understand genetic traits of plants, animals, and insects that can enhance food production. Forensic scientists are able to accurately identify deceased individuals. In 2022, the WHO's Science Council published a report along with 15 actions for member states to consider with the goal of accelerating access to genomics to benefit global health (WHO, 2022d). The recommendations are grouped into four themes: (1) promotion of genomics through advocacy; (2) implementation of genomic methodologies; (3) collaboration among entities engaged in genomics; and (4) attention to the ELSIs raised by genomics. They suggest that access and use of genomics can significantly benefit the health of both individuals and populations.

ELSI, Ethical, legal, and social issues; *WHO*, World Health Organization.

CHALLENGES TO MAINTAINING GLOBAL HEALTH

Antimicrobial Resistance

Antimicrobial resistance (or drug resistance) is the situation in which the treatment (e.g., antibiotics) of an infection is no longer effective because the microorganism has mutated to the point that the bacteria, parasite, virus, or fungus no longer is susceptible to the treatment. It is best known in the areas of drug-resistant tuberculosis (TB). When this happens, the microorganism can be spread to other persons at a greater speed and effectiveness—leading to greater numbers of infected persons in the population. In addition to increasing the spread of the disease, the individual is much less protected and can more easily die from a disease that was treatable a short time ago. When combined with vaccine hesitancy (see next section), the result is a global population at greater risk for disease and greater illness, disability, and death. Although TB is a widely recognized bacterium that is becoming more and more drug-resistant, HIV, malaria, and infections due to *Escherichia coli* and *Staphylococcus aureus* also present higher risks to humans (WHO, 2023k). This situation also increases the risk for anyone having surgery, including caesarean section, or chemotherapy, which in themselves increase the risk of an infection. Although there is no specific cause for antimicrobial resistance, it is thought that overuse of antibiotics in humans and animals has contributed to the genetic changes in microorganisms that have resulted in resistance. The CDC has identified antimicrobial resistance as "an urgent global public health threat," noting that "at least

BOX 25.11 Health Protection and Promotion

1. Know your risk, ask questions, and take care
2. Clean your hands
3. Get vaccinated
4. Use antibiotics and antifungals appropriately
5. Be aware of changes in your health
6. Practice healthy habits with animals
7. Prepare food safely
8. Stay healthy when traveling abroad
9. Prevent sexually transmitted diseases

From CDC (2023e)

2.8 million people get an antibiotic-resistant infection" each year in the United States and "more than 35,000 people die" (CDC, 2022c). The CDC has also linked antibiotic resistance to social determinants of health, noting that it is a health equity issue (CDC, 2022d)

The CDC has identified multiple health promotion and protection strategies for antimicrobial resistance. These can be read in Box 25.11. The authors have listed them in this section, but the items can be applied to a myriad of health issues.

Vaccine Hesitancy

Vaccine hesitancy refers to the failure of individuals or families to participate in vaccination programs even when the vaccines are available. Larson et al. (2022) describe it as "a state of indecision and uncertainty that precedes a decision to become (or not become) vaccinated." Headlines from around the world have highlighted not only groups that are refusing vaccinations on religious and other grounds but that faith in the efficacy and necessity of vaccinations is waning even in global areas where uptake was previously excellent (Dube et al., 2015; Larson et al., 2022). Larson et al. (2022) note that social media has increased this indecision and uncertainty, which may result in hesitancy to a specific vaccine or to vaccines in general.

When segments of the population engage in vaccine hesitancy or refusal, the outcome can be a decrease in herd immunity. **Herd immunity**, also known as community immunity, is "a situation in which sufficient proportion of a population is immune to an infectious disease (through vaccinations and/or prior illness) to make its spread from person to person unlikely. Even individuals not vaccinated (such as newborns and those with chronic illnesses) are offered some protection because the disease has little opportunity to spread within the community" (CDC, 2022e).

The vaccination process for COVID-19 may have precipitated increased concerns about vaccines in general, leading to greater hesitancy. In addition, the pandemic itself resulted in missed vaccines for several other conditions. For example, the WHO estimated that almost 40 million children missed a measles vaccine dose in 2021 (WHO, 2022c). They and other international partners are prioritizing raising global immunization levels for several diseases to prepandemic levels–known as The Big Catch-up (WHO, 2023l). The good news is that global immunization levels are recently showing signs of increasing (WHO, 2023m;

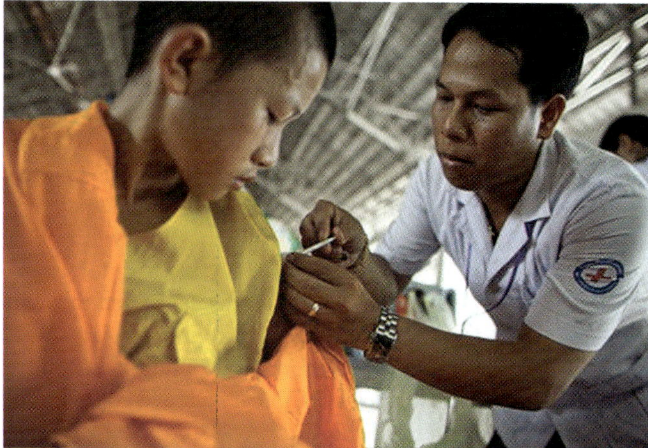

FIG. 25.3 Vaccinations can mitigate the effects of many communicable diseases.

Fig. 25.3) What is important to remember is that vaccine hesitancy is as individual as the person or the group. Nurses and other health professionals, as trusted advisors for health care, "need to offer support and encouragement and listen to what matters from the patient's perspective" (Larson et al., 2022) and be aware of the information and misinformation readily available to community members (see the Case Study at the end of the chapter).

Weak Primary Care and Poor Access

Primary health care is usually the first point of contact people have with their health care system, and ideally it should provide comprehensive, affordable, community-based care throughout life and be "rooted in a commitment to social justice, equity, solidarity, and participation" (WHO, 2023n). Several authors posit that primary health care is the backbone of universal health care systems. Regardless of one's stance or beliefs on universal health care, the fact remains that many of the actions and strategies already mentioned in this chapter and throughout this book rely on the presence of and reasonable access to primary health care. Even in the United States, where there is significant debate on whether health care is a right or a privilege to be purchased, the increasing preparation of and emphasis on primary care nurse practitioners and telehealth delivery systems testifies to the importance of a strong and accessible primary health care system. Global emphasis on primary health care is not new. The first primary health care declaration was signed at Alma-Ata in 1978 and remains the touchstone for all future efforts (WHO, 2023o). More recently, in 2018, the WHO hosted a conference in Astana, Kazakhstan. At this conference, there was a renewed global commitment to primary care (WHO, 2023p).

Over time, a myriad of strategies has been proposed and implemented to strengthen primary care. An example of a global partnership is the Primary Health Care Performance Initiative (PHCPI). This group began in 2015 through the Melinda and Bill Gates Foundation, the WHO, and the World Bank Group, in collaboration with other global partners. Their overall stance is that "strong primary health care saves lives" and their three primary goals are measure, improve, and engage (PHCPI, 2022).

One example of an activity that contributes to all goals of PHCPI is the **primary health care progression model** for measuring primary health care system capacity, performance, and effect. Although primarily targeting middle- and low-income countries, this model can be used anywhere. The goal of this tool is to use common metrics to measure capacity, performance, and effect within a given country. These data can then not only point the way for strategies for improvement within that country, but they can also provide comparable data for global progress. The original 32-measure tool was developed through participatory methods and piloted in five countries (Argentina, Ghana, Rwanda, Senegal, and the United Republic of Tanzania) in 2018. Each country formed a team that included government officials as well as other stakeholders, in collaboration with one of the founding partners of PHCPI. Although data collection methods varied across countries, the results, presented in the Vital Signs Profile, were compiled and presented at the aforementioned Astana Conference. Analysis and refinement of the measurement tool has been on-going, with a new beta version released for use and evaluation in 2021 (Feil et al., 2021).

In addition to such global cooperation, smaller, more constrained studies also have the ability to enhance primary health care in terms of specific health care issues or more widely.

CASE STUDY

Mr. and Mrs. Singh are parents of a 6-month-old baby male in New Delhi, India. During antenatal care, both expressed a strong desire to have their child vaccinated because they had been vaccinated as children. Now, however, they are expressing concerns. These concerns include that government should not dictate what happens to their child, that pharmacologic companies are using vaccination encouragement to profit from parents, and finally, that Western countries sell only substandard vaccines to developing countries and their young child will be harmed by all the vaccines. Although they accepted the hepatitis B and polio vaccines at birth, they have refused the recommended 6-week vaccinations (e.g., polio; diphtheria, pertussis, tetanus [DPT]). They are now trying to decide about the doses scheduled for 6 months (e.g., influenza).

Reflective Questions

1. Why might these parents have changed their minds about vaccination?
2. How might the nurse approach the topic with the parents when they come in for the next well child check?
3. Are there actions the health care provider can suggest that meet the parents' needs?
4. What community-based interventions could the local clinic in conjunction with community leaders consider implementing to ensure parents are equipped with accurate vaccination information to guide their decision-making?

SUMMARY

- The interconnectedness of social determinants of health, UN sustainable development goals, and US Healthy People 2030 was demonstrated.
- One Health, which incorporates human-animal interface as part of the big picture, was introduced.
- The UN top 10 public health threats were utilized as chapter framework, explaining the threat as well as health promoting activities employed to mitigate the threat.

EVOLVE CHAPTER FEATURES

http://evolve.elsevier.com/Edelman/

- Study Questions

REFERENCES

Adrian, T., Bousquet, F., Desruelle, D., Gaspar, V., & Kroese, B. (2023). *Fragile states need customized support to strengthen institutions*. https://www.imf.org/en/Blogs/Articles/2023/09/21/fragile-states-need-customized-support-to-strengthen-institutions#:~:text=In%20addition%20to%20limited%20room,are%20also%20taking%20a%20toll

Advisory Board. (2023). *The dramatic rise of tick- and mosquito-borne diseases, charted*. https://www.advisory.com/daily-briefing/2018/05/04/vector-ticks-mosquitos

Bekkhus, M., Lee, Y., Samuelsen, S. O., Tsotsi, S., & Magnus, P. (2022). Maternal and paternal anxiety during pregnancy: comparing the effects on behavioral problems in offspring. *PLoS One*, *17*(10), e0275085. https://doi.org/10.1371/journal.pone.0275085

Catley, D., Puoane, T., Tsolekile, L., Resnicow, K., Fleming, K. K., Hurley, E. A., et al. (2022). Evaluation of an adapted version of the Diabetes Prevention Program for low-and middle-income countries: a cluster randomized trial to evaluate "Lifestyle Africa" in South Africa. *PLoS Medicine*, *19*(4), e1003964. https://doi.org/10.1371/journal.pmed.1003964

Centers for Disease Control and Prevention (CDC). (2019). *Ebola outbreak in West Africa*. https://www.cdc.gov/

Centers for Disease Control and Prevention (CDC). (2020). *Dengue: prevent mosquito bites*. https://www.cdc.gov/

Centers for Disease Control and Prevention (CDC). (2022a). *Life expectancy in the U.S, dropped for the second year in a row in 2021*. https://www.cdc.gov/nchs/pressroom/nchs_press_releases/2022/20220831.htm

Centers for Disease Control and Prevention (CDC). (2022b). *HIV basics*. https://www.cdc.gov/

Centers for Disease Control and Prevention (CDC). (2022c). *Antibiotic/antimicrobial resistance*. https://www.cdc.gov/drugresistance/about.html

Centers for Disease Control and Prevention (CDC). (2022d). *CDC's priority to address health equity issues across antimicrobial-resistant threats*. https://www.cdc.gov/

Centers for Disease Control and Prevention (CDC). (2022e). *Glossary (vaccines and immunizations)*. https://www.cdc.gov/

Centers for Disease Control and Prevention (CDC). (2023a). *About Dengue: what you need to know*. https://www.cdc.gov/dengue/about/index.html

Centers for Disease Control and Prevention (CDC). (2023b). *Dengue, current year data*. https://www.cdc.gov/

Centers for Disease Control and Prevention (CDC). (2023c). *Ebola*. https://www.cdc.gov/vhf/ebola/index.html

Centers for Disease Control and Prevention (CDC). (2023d). *CDC Museum COVID-19 timeline*. https://www.cdc.gov/museum/timeline/covid19.html

Centers for Disease Control and Prevention (CDC). (2023e). *Protect yourself and your family*. https://www.cdc.gov/drugresistance/protect-yourself-family.html

Centers for Disease Control and Prevention (CDC). (2024). *About a Dengue vaccine*. https://www.cdc.gov/dengue/vaccine/index.html

Centers for Disease Control and Prevention (CDC). (2025) *Zika Virus*. https://www.cdc.gov/zika/index.html

Centers for Disease Control and Prevention (CDC) & National Institute for Occupational Safety and Health (NIOSH). (2022). *Heat stress-heat related illness.* https://www.cdc.gov/niosh/topics/heatstress/heatrelillness.html

Chandra, M., Rai, C. B., Kumari, N., Sandhu, V. K., Krishna, M., Kota, S. H., et al. (2022). Air pollution and cognitive impairment across the life course in humans: a systematic review with specific focus on income level of study area. *International Journal of Environmental Research and Public Health, 19*(1405), 1–39.

Cherian, V., Saini, N. K., Sharma, A. K., & Philip, J. (2022). Prevalence and predictors of vaccine hesitancy in an urbanized agglomeration of New Delhi, India. *Journal of Public Health, 44*(1), 70–76. https://doi:10.1093/pubmed/fdab007

Chicas, R., Xiuhtecutli, N., Elon, L., Scammell, M. K., Steenland, K., Hertzberg, V., et al. (2021). Cooling interventions among agricultural workers: a pilot study. *Workplace Health & Safety, 69*(7), 315–322. https://doi.org/10.1177/2165079920976524

Christianson, J., Stiles Herdt, C. S., & Nadolny, G. (2023). *The global fragility act: unlocking the full potential of interagency cooperation.* https://www.csis.org/analysis/global-fragility-act-unlocking-full-potential-interagency-cooperation#:~:text=Promoting%20stability%20is%20imperative%20to,both%20U.S.%20national-%20interests%20and

Council on Foreign Relations. (2023). *Major epidemics of the modern era 1899-2023.* https://www.cfr.org/timeline/major-epidemics-modern-era

Crimmins, A. R., Avery, C. W., Easterling, D. R., Kunkel, K. E., Stewart, B. C., & Maycock, T. K. (2023). *USGCRP 2023: fifth national climate assessment. U. S. Global Change Research Program.* https://doi.org/10.7930/NCA5.2023

Dube, E., Gagnon, G., MacDonald, N., & The SAGE Working Group on Vaccine Hesitancy. (2015). Strategies intended to address vaccine hesitancy: review of published reviews. *Vaccine, 33*(34), 4191–4203. https://doi.org/10.1016/j.vaccine.2015.04.041

Environmental Protection Agency (EPA). (2022). *Evolution of the clean air act.* https://www.epa.gov/clean-air-act-overview/evolution-clean-air-act

Environmental Protection Agency (EPA). (2023a). *Air pollution: current and future challenges.* https://www.epa.gov/clean-air-act-overview/air-pollution-current-and-future-challenges

Environmental Protection Agency (EPA). (2023b). *Climate change impacts on agriculture and food supply.* https://www.epa.gov/climateimpacts/climate-change-impacts-agriculture-and-food-supply

Federation of American Scientists (FAS). (2023). *Wildfire statistics.* https://sgp.fas.org/crs/misc/IF10244.pdf

Feil, C., Wahnschafftt, S., Okara, L., Villar-Uribe, M., Vincencio, J., Ramadan, M., et al. (2021). *Primary health care performance measurement in World Bank health, nutrition and population projects.* https://documents1.worldbank.org/curated/en/099816005262234609/pdf/IDU0e1bb0d1401b61042de0878f0c51d2166a397.pdf

Festa, F., Ancillotto, L., Santini, L., Pacifici, M., Rocha, R., Toshkova, N., et al. (2023). Bat responses to climate change: a systematic review. *Biological Reviews, 98,* 19–33.

Friedrich, J., Ge, M., Pickens, A., & Vigna, L. (2023). This interactive chart shows changes in the world's top 10 emitters. https://www.wri.org/insights/interactive-chart-shows-changes-worlds-top-10-emitters#:~:text=The%20top%20three%20GHG%20emitters,only%20account%20for%20only%202.9%25

Global Obesity Observatory. (2017). *Ranking: % obesity by country.* https://data.worldobesity.org/rankings/?age=a&sex=m

Gostin, L. O., & Gronvall, G. K. (2023). The origins of Covid-19 – Why it matters (and why it doesn't). *New England Journal of Medicine, 388,* 2305–2308.

Government of Canada. (2023). *Social determinants of health and health inequalities.* https://www.canada.ca/en/public-health/services/health-promotion/population-health/what-determines-health.html

Gubernot, D. M., Anderson, G. B., & Hunting, K. L. (2015). Characterizing occupational heat-related mortality in the United States, 2000–2010: an analysis using the census of fatal occupational injuries database. *American Journal of Industrial Medicine, 58*(2), 203–211. https://doi.org/10.1002/ajim.22381

Healthy People 2030. (n.d.). *Increase the use of telehealth to increase access to health services.* https://health.gov/healthypeople/objectives-and-data/browse-objectives/health-it/increase-use-telehealth-improve-access-health-services-ahs-r02

International Monetary Fund. (2023). *Fragile and conflict affected states.* https://www.imf.org/en/Topics/fragile-and-conflict-affected-states#:~:text=Research%20and%20Publications-,Overview,forced%20displacement%2C%20and%20cven%20war

Klassen, J. (2019). *Resilience, refugees, and fragile states.* https://globalwa.org/issue-brief/resilience-refugees-and-fragile-states/

Kriebel-Gasparro, A. (2022). Climate change: effects on the older adult. *The Journal for Nurse Practitioners, 18*(4), 372–376.

Larrichia, F. (2023). *Forecast number of mobile devices worldwide from 2020 to 2025 (in billions).* https://www.statista.com/statistics/245501/multiple-mobile-device-ownership-worldwide/#:~:text=In%202021%2C%20the%20number%20of,devices%20compared%20to%202020%20levels

Larson, H. J., Gakidou, E., & Murray, C. J. L. (2022). The vaccine -hesitant moment. *New England Journal of Medicine, 387,* 58–65.

Lucero-Prisno, D. E., Shomuyiwa, D. O., Kouwenhoven, M. B. N., et al. (2023). Top 10 public health challenges to track in 2023: shifting focus beyond a global pandemic. *Public Health Challenges, 2,* e86. https://doi.org/10.1002/puh2.86

Lustgarten, A. (2020). *How climate change is contributing to skyrocketing rates of infectious disease.* https://www.propublica.org/article/climate-infectious-diseases

Mackenzie, J. S., & Jeggo, M. (2019). The One Health approach—Why is it so important? *Tropical Medicine and Infectious Disease, 4*(2), 88. https://doi.org/10.3390/tropicalmed4020088

Maslow, A. (1970). *Motivation and personality* (2nd ed.). New York, NY: Harper & Row.

Mikkelsen, B., Williams, J., Rakovac, I., Wickramasinghe, K., Hennis, A., Shin, H., et al. (2019). Life course approach to prevention and control of non-communicable diseases. *British Medical Journal, 364,* 1257. https://www.researchgate.net/publication/330693775_Life_course_approach_to_prevention_and_control_of_non-communicable_diseases

National Aeronautics and Space Administration (NASA). (2023). *Extreme weather and climate change.* https://climate.nasa.gov/extreme-weather/

National Oceanic and Atmospheric Administration (NOAA). (2022). *Climate change: global sea level.* https://www.climate.gov/news-features/understanding-climate/climate-change-global-sea-level

NCD Risk Factor Collaborative. (2020). Height and body-mass index trajectories of school-aged children and adolescents from 1985 to 2019 in 200 countries and territories: a pooled analysis of 2181 population-based studies with 65 million participants. *The Lancet, 396,* 1511–1524.

Nithiyanantham, S., Kalaiselvi, P., Mahomoodally, M. F., Zengin, G., Abirami, A., & Srinivasan, G. (2019). Nutritional and functional roles of millets – A review. *Journal of Food Biochemistry, 43*(7), e12859. https://doi.org/10.1111/jfbc.12859

Oka, K., Honda, Y., Phung, V. L. H., & Hijioka, Y. (2023). Prediction of climate change impacts on heat stroke cases in Japan's 47 prefectures with the effect of long-term heat adaptation. *Environmental Research, 232*, 1–9.

Organization for Economic Cooperation and Development. (2020). *Developing countries and development co-operation: what is at stake?* https://read.oecd-ilibrary.org/

Pediatric Academy of India. (2014). *IAP guidebook on immunization 2018–2019. IAP recommended immunization schedule 2018.* https://iapindia.org/pdf/124587-IAP-GUIDE-BOOK-ON-IMMUNIZATION-18-19.pdf

Primary Health Care Performance Initiative (PHCPI). (2022). *Measuring progress on PHC.* https://www.improvingphc.org/measuring-progress-phc

Primo Braga, C. A., Henderson, J. E., Yu, H. H., Fischer, W. A., Avagyan, K., & Stehli, S. (2020). *Health and fragile environments.* https://www.imd.org/research-knowledge/strategy/articles/health-in-fragile-environments/

Public Health Agency of Canada (PHAC). (2023). *Social determinants of health and health inequities.* https://www.canada.ca/en/public-health/services/health-promotion/population-health/what-determines-health.html

Roberts, M., & Pompei, A. (2018). *Unpacking fragility: insights from the OECS's new state of fragility report.* https://unfoundation.org/blog/post/unpacking-fragility-insights-from-the-oecds-new-states-of-fragility-report/

Rogers, K. (2024). *Pandemic.* https://www.britannica.com/science/pandemic

Rozbroj, T., Lyons, A., & Lucke, J. (2020). Vaccine-hesitant and vaccine-refusing parents: reflections on the way parenthood changed their attitudes to vaccination. *Journal of Community Health, 45*, 63–72. https://doi:10.1007/s10900-019-00723-9

Thompson, T., Kreuter, M., & Boyum, S. (2016). Promoting health by addressing basic needs: effect of problem resolution on contacting health referrals. *Health Education Behavior, 43*(2), 201–207. https://doi:10.1177/1090198115599396

United Nations (UNAIDS). (2023). *Global HIV statistics –2022 fact sheet.* www.unaids.org/sites/default/files/media_asset/UNAIDS_FactSheet_en.pdf

United Nations. (2023a). *Framework convention on climate change.* https://unfccc.int/process-and-meetings/what-is-the-united-nations-framework-convention-on-climate-change

United Nations. (2023b). *Actions for a healthy planet.* https://www.un.org/en/actnow/ten-actions

United Nations. (2023c). *High-level political forum on sustainable development.* https://hlpf.un.org/

United Nations Sustainable Development (UN). (n.d.). *Transforming our world: the 2030 agenda for sustainable development.* https://sustainabledevelopment.un.org/content/documents/21252030%20Agenda%20for%20Sustainable%20Development%20web.pdf

U.S. Department of Health and Human Services. (2023). *Healthy people 2030.* https://health.gov/our-work/national-health-initiatives/healthy-people/healthy-people-2030

Venkataramani, A. S., O'Brien, R., & Tsai, A. C. (2021). Declining life expectancy in the United States: the need for social policy as health policy. *Journal of American Medical Association, 325*(7), 621–622. https://doi:10.1001/jama.2020.26339

World Bank. (2023). *Classification of fragility and conflict situations.* https://thedocs.worldbank.org/en/doc/fb0f93e8e3375803bce211ab1218ef2a-0090082023/original/Classification-of-Fragility-and-Conflict-Situations-FY24.pdf

World Health Organization (WHO). (n.d.). *Social determinants of health.* https://www.who.int/health-topics/social-determinants-of-health#tab=tab_1

World Health Organization (WHO). (2011). *World conference on social determinants of health.* https://www.who.int/publications/m/item/rio-political-declaration-on-social-determinants-of-health#:~:text=The%20declaration%20expresses%20global%20political,national%20action%20plans%20and%20strategies

World Health Organization (WHO). (2019a). *Ten threats to global health in 2019.* https://www.who.int/news-room/spotlight/ten-threats-to-global-health-in-2019

World Health Organization (WHO). (2019b). *Global influenza strategy 2019-2030.* https://apps.who.int/iris/bitstream/handle/10665/311184/9789241515320-eng.pdf

World Health Organization (WHO). (2022a). *Ambient (outdoor) air pollution.* https://www.who.int/news-room/fact-sheets/detail/ambient-(outdoor)-air-quality-and-health

World Health Organization (WHO). (2022b). *Zika virus.* https://www.who.int/news-room/fact-sheets/detail/zika-virus

World Health Organization (WHO). (2022c). *Nearly 40 million children are dangerously susceptible to growing measles threat.* https://www.who.int/news/item/23-11-2022-nearly-40-million-children-are-dangerously-susceptible-to-growing-measles-threat

World Health Organization (WHO). (2022d). *Accelerating access to genomics for global health: promotion, implementation, collaboration, and ethical, legal, and social issues: a report of the WHO Science Council.* https://www.who.int/publications/i/item/9789240052857

World Health Organization (WHO). (2023a). *Social determinants of health report.* https://apps.who.int/gb/ebwha/pdf_files/WHA76/A76_7Rev1Add1-en.pdf

World Health Organization (WHO). (2023b). *Operational framework.* https://www.who.int/initiatives/action-on-the-social-determinants-of-health-for-advancing-equity/operational-framework

World Health Organization (WHO). (2023c). *Operational framework draft report.* https://cdn.who.int/media/docs/default-source/documents/social-determinants-of-health/who_operational-framework-for-monitoring-social-determinants-of-health-equity_16052023.pdf?sfvrsn=1dd8a53b_3

World Health Organization (WHO). (2023d). *WHO commission on social connection.* https://www.who.int/groups/commission-on-social-connection

World Health Organization (WHO). (2023e). *One health high-level expert panel.* https://www.who.int/groups/one-health-high-level-expert-panel

World Health Organization (WHO). (2023f). *Air pollution.* https://www.who.int/health-topics/air-pollution#tab=tab_1

World Health Organization (WHO). (2023g). *Non communicable diseases.* https://www.who.int/news-room/fact-sheets/detail/noncommunicable-diseases

World Health Organization (WHO). (2023h). *Influenza (seasonal).* https://www.who.int/news-room/fact-sheets/detail/influenza-(seasonal)

World Health Organization (WHO). (2023i). *Global influenza surveillance and response system (GISRS).* https://www.who.int/initiatives/global-influenza-surveillance-and-response-system

World Health Organization (WHO). (2023j). *Ebola virus disease.* https://www.who.int/news-room/fact-sheets/detail/ebola-virus-disease

World Health Organization (WHO). (2023k). *Antimicrobial resistance.* https://www.who.int/en/news-room/fact-sheets/detail/antimicrobial-resistance

World Health Organization (WHO). (2023l). *Global partners announce a new effort – "The Big Catch-up" – to vaccinate millions of children and restore immunization progress lost during the pandemic.* https://www.who.int/news/item/24-04-2023-global-partners-announce-a-new-effort-the-big-catch-up-to-vaccinate-millions-of-children-and-restore-immunization-progress-lost-during-the-pandemic

World Health Organization (WHO). (2023m). *Immunization coverage.* https://www.who.int/news-room/fact-sheets/detail/immunization-coverage

World Health Organization (WHO). (2023n). *Primary health care.* https://www.who.int/news-room/fact-sheets/detail/primary-health-care#:~:text=Primary%20health%20care%20ensures%20people,feasible%20to%20people's%20everyday%20environment

World Health Organization (WHO). (2023o). *Declaration of Alma-Ata.* https://www.who.int/teams/social-determinants-of-health/declaration-of-alma-ata

World Health Organization (WHO). (2023p). *Global conference on primary health care.* https://www.who.int/teams/primary-health-care/conference

World Health Organization (WHO). (2024). *Fourteenth general programme of work, 2025-2028.* https://www.who.int/

World Population Review. (2023). *Life expectancy by country, 2023.* https://worldpopulationreview.com/country-rankings/life-expectancy-by-country

INDEX

A

Note: Page numbers followed by "f" indicate figures, "t" indicate tables, and "b" indicate boxes.

B

E

F

H

O

T

U

V